# HAVENER'S
# OCULAR PHARMACOLOGY

*Disclaimer*

We have made every effort to ensure that the dosage of drugs and the indications for their use are in accordance with current recommendations. We recommend referring to the package insert or *Physician's Desk Reference* before using a drug for the first time. Some of the drugs described in this book have not been approved by the Food and Drug Administration for that particular indication. Caution should be exercised in their use, and the prescriber should have full knowledge of their supporting literature.

Havener's

# Ocular Pharmacology

*Edited by*

THOMAS F. MAUGER, O.D., M.D.

Assistant Professor of Ophthalmology
The Ohio State University
William M. Havener Eye Center
Columbus, Ohio

ELSON L. CRAIG, M.D.

Associate Professor of Ophthalmology
Associate Professor of Pathology
The Ohio State University
William M. Havener Eye Center
Columbus, Ohio

**SIXTH EDITION**

*with* 152 *illustrations*

Mosby

St. Louis Baltimore Berlin Boston Carlsbad Chicago London Madrid
Naples New York Philadelphia Sydney Tokyo Toronto

Mosby
Dedicated to Publishing Excellence

Editor: Laurel Craven
Associate Developmental Editor: Wendy Buckwalter
Project Managers: Nancy Baker, Patricia Tannian
Cover Designer: Teresa Breckwoldt
Manufacturing Supervisor: Betty Richmond

SIXTH EDITION



Printed in the United States of America
Composition by Graphic World, Inc.
Printing/binding by Maple-Vail Book Mfg. Group

Mosby–Year Book, Inc.
11830 Westline Industrial Drive
St. Louis, Missouri 63146

**Library of Congress Cataloging in Publication Data**

Havener's ocular pharmacology—6th ed./edited by Thomas F. Mauger, Elson L. Craig.
p. cm.
Rev. ed. of: Ocular pharmacology/William H. Havener. 5th ed. 1983.
Includes bibliographical references and index.
ISBN 0-8016-6767-4
1. Ocular pharmacology. I. Mauger, Thomas F. II. Craig, Elson L. III. Havener, William H. (William Henry), 1924- . Ocular pharmacology. IV. Title: Ocular pharmacology.
[DNLM: 1. Eye Diseases—drug therapy. WW 166 H3864 1993]
RE994.H35 1993
617.7′061—dc20
DNLM/DLC
for Library of Congress 93-47912
CIP

94 95 96 97 98 / 9 8 7 6 5 4 3 2 1

# Contributors

KENNETH V. CAHILL, M.D.
Clinical Assistant Professor of Ophthalmology, Ohio State University College of Medicine, Columbus, Ohio

ROBERT B. CHAMBERS, D.O.
Associate Professor of Ophthalmology, Ohio State University College of Medicine, Columbus, Ohio

ELSON L. CRAIG, M.D.
Associate Professor of Ophthalmology and Pathology, Ohio State University College of Medicine, Columbus, Ohio

ROBERT J. DERICK, M.D.
Assistant Professor of Ophthalmology, Ohio State University College of Medicine, Columbus, Ohio

LOUIS DESANTIS, Jr., Ph.D.
Senior Director and Research Ocular Pharmacologist, Glaucoma Research, Alcon Laboratories, Fort Worth, Texas

THOMAS F. MAUGER, O.D., M.D.
Assistant Professor of Ophthalmology, Ohio State University College of Medicine, Columbus, Ohio

MARY LOU KACHMER McGREGOR, M.D.
Clinical Assistant Professor of Ophthalmology, Ohio State University College of Medicine, Columbus, Ohio

E. MITCHEL OPREMCAK, M.D.
Assistant Professor of Ophthalmology and Director, Ocular Immunology and Uveitis Service, Ohio State University College of Medicine, Columbus, Ohio

KARL S. PAPPA, M.D., PHARM. D.
Clinical Assistant Professor of Ophthalmology, University of Ohio College of Medicine, Columbus, Ohio

POPAT N. PATIL, Ph.D.
Professor, Division of Pharmacology, Ohio State University College of Pharmacy, Columbus, Ohio

DAVID K. SCALES, M.D.
Department of Pathology
Wilford Hall USAF MC, Lackland Air Force Base, San Antonio, Texas

PAUL A. WEBER, M.D.
Professor and Chairman of Ophthalmology, Ohio State University College of Medicine, Columbus, Ohio

*This book is dedicated to the memory of*

**William H. Havener, M.D.**
(1924 to 1991)

Professor and Chairman of the
Department of Ophthalmology at
The Ohio State University College of Medicine.
Dr. Havener was an innovative and skilled surgeon,
considerate and thoughtful physician, dedicated teacher,
creative thinker, and prolific writer, but most important he was
mentor to most of the contributors to this sixth edition of his
*Ocular Pharmacology*.

# Preface to the Fifth Edition

The old anecdote about the professor who always used the same examination questions but changed the answers is certainly applicable to ocular pharmacology. Our understanding of drug actions is constantly changing. Epinephrine, for example, had changed from a medication too unstable for use to the best drug for initial treatment of glaucoma. However, since the last edition of this text was published, this drug-of-choice status has been lost to timolol. It was formerly thought that epinephrine acted to reduce intraocular pressure by reducing aqueous production; now it is known that it increases both aqueous production and outflow via unconventional pathways. Next, it may be recognized that epinephrine does not affect aqueous production in any way but only acts to reduce vanadate to inactive vanadyl. (Vanadate inhibits aqueous production; vanadate reduction by epinephrine releases this inhibition.)

The moral is Nietzsche's: "Truth is an error that is temporarily irrefutable." Do keep an open mind as to the ways in which our treatments work and also to whether their apparent working is nothing but coincidence interpreted hopefully.

**William H. Havener, M.D.**

# Preface to the Sixth Edition

Doctor Havener originally asked us to help with a "minor" revision of his ocular pharmacology text. After he died and the task became our full responsibility, we discovered the enormous amount of work that would be required to accomplish a "minor" revision. Furthermore, it soon became clear that because a decade has passed since the last edition was published, a minor revision would not suffice. As we proceeded, we realized that, unlike Dr. Havener, we did not have a sufficient breadth and depth of knowledge in many of the areas to be included. We therefore recruited a number of our colleagues to write sections of the revision. We are very appreciative of the tireless efforts of the contributing authors. The book could not have been completed without them. Any deficiencies in the text are, of course, the responsibility of the editors.

Thomas F. Mauger
Elson L. Craig

# Contents

# HAVENER'S
# OCULAR PHARMACOLOGY

CHAPTER 1

# Evaluation of Therapeutic Response

William H. Havener

Thomas F. Mauger

Somewhere long ago I read of an early American physician who prescribed cabbage for the relief of certain symptoms suffered by a blacksmith. The blacksmith recovered. In due time a preacher became ill with similar symptoms. Cabbages were prescribed, but, alas, the preacher died. The physician thereupon concluded that for these symptoms cabbages would cure blacksmiths but would kill preachers. I hope that this book will help somewhat to put ophthalmic medications on a more rational basis than cabbages for symptoms.

Post hoc, ergo propter hoc (after this, because of this). Do clinical coincidences unjustifiably influence our treatment of patients today? Of course, they will always do so. The emotional impact of a single dramatic clinical occurrence often creates lasting but unwarranted impressions as to the effect of a given medication or procedure. As an example of this fallacy, the following actual case is cited.

An 84-year-old woman underwent an uncomplicated cataract extraction. The surgeon had planned to use α-chymotrypsin for zonulysis but decided against it at the last minute because he had never previously used it. Although there had been no bleeding and the eye looked perfect at the close of surgery, at the first dressing on the following day the anterior chamber was almost filled with fresh red blood. No history of trauma could be obtained. The hemorrhage grew progressively worse, filling the anterior chamber. On the seventh postoperative day, bright red blood still completely filled the anterior chamber, and no trace of iris detail was visible. Miraculously, on the eighth day the blood had entirely disappeared, and the eye was in perfect condition without even the tiniest hyphema. No medication was responsible for this amazing improvement.

Clearly evident is the unpredictability of an individual case. Had that surgeon used α-chymotrypsin, he would have been sure that it caused the hemorrhage. Any medication (carbonic anhydrase inhibitor, trypsin, blood transfusion, miotic, and the like) used on the seventh day would have received credit for the cure. Similarly, surgical evacuation of the blood would have been interpreted as the cause of improvement. This case also illustrates the importance of watchful nontreatment in our therapeutic armamentarium. This should not be confused with neglect but instead is a rational alternative to premature therapeutic interventions that may distort the clinical picture and complicate future therapeutic decisions.

## CONTROLLED OBSERVATION

Clinical trials of therapy vs. control are required to determine best management. The basic question is, "With what patient should the treated patients be compared?" Ideally the control group should be virtually identical to the treated patients in all respects. Control cannot be an equal number of patients accumulated 5 years ago. Because of observer bias, controlled does not mean strictly alternated groups of patients. Rather, a random selection (designed in an orderly fashion to invoke the laws of chance and not synonymous with haphazard) is important to eliminate the observer and patient factors that are not related to the treatment response being evaluated.[1, 2]

Guidance by a statistical expert is almost always necessary if a physician is to design a truly valid clinical trial. Surprisingly, often we are so naive as to believe that we know the natural course of the disease well enough to conclude that the observed rate of improvement after therapy will confirm the efficacy of treatment. This is simply not true.[3]

For example, 95% diethyl ether is known to destroy herpes simplex virus. A 10-minute topical application of ether to less than 1-day-old recurrent herpetic ulcers of the lip caused the vesicle to disappear within 2 days and complete healing of the crusted scar within 10 days. Pain disappeared within 5½ days. Subjectively, 75% of the ether-treated patients believed that the treatment had effectively accelerated healing. Ether diluted to 5% does not inactivate herpes virus but smells the same, so it was used as the control, resulting in vesicle disappearance in 1.6 days, less pain in 2.7 days, healing in 9 days, and subjective satisfaction in 77% of patients. The virus titer from the lesions was measured daily and decreased rapidly and spontaneously at the same rate for 5 days in both treated and untreated patients. Conclusion: A "cure" of 75% of cases was simply the normal course of the disease.[4]

## DOUBLE-BLIND CONTROLLED OBSERVATION

The ultimate in scientific objectivity and indisputable accuracy is supposedly represented by the double-blind tests. Obviously (supposedly) such a format will eliminate errors of judgment, control, and prejudice. To quote Spaeth[5]:

> Since the design of this study was of the double-blind, placebo-controlled type, the coded medication and placebo were identical in appearance and their identity was not known to the investigator, the nursing staff, or the patient until the termination of the study, at which time the code was broken and the findings recorded.

The author reports that when the code was broken, of the total 111 patients, 52 had received placebo medication and 59 active medication. All 52 placebo patients were male and all 59 active medication patients were female! The possibility that this distribution occurred by chance is about one in 10, not very likely. This means that despite all the care and work lavished on this experiment, someone misunderstood the instructions and introduced a methodical error by giving the medications on the basis of sex. This methodical error apparently was undetected by the author until he broke the code and discovered the impossible male-female distribution. A reasonable inference from this accident would be that one is justified in regarding with caution even the most careful scientific study if its results conflict with other sources of information or if it is not subsequently confirmed by other studies.

In this study there were two large wards segregated for men and women. The placebo box was placed in the male ward and the active medication box in the female ward. As Murphy's law states, if anything can go wrong, it will do so. O'Toole's law adds that "Murphy was an optimist."

## EVALUATION OF VITAMIN A TREATMENT OF RETINITIS PIGMENTOSA

The difficulty of making a true evaluation of therapeutic response is well illustrated by the history of a 10-year research project concerning the effect of 11-*cis* vitamin A in the treatment of retinitis pigmentosa.[6] As background for this project, recall that we ordinarily ingest vitamin A in the all-*trans* form, which is then isomerized in the eye to the 11-*cis* form. Only the 11-*cis* form can be used to manufacture retinene, the visual pigment. One theory of the causation of retinitis pigmentosa has postulated an inherited biochemical defect of the isomerization of vitamin A, with consequent degeneration of the retinal rods.

Animal experimentation demonstrated that retinal degeneration in vitamin A–deficient rats could be prevented by extremely small doses of 11-*cis* vitamin A but not by comparable doses of all-*trans* vitamin A.

An exploratory clinical experiment was performed by treating seven patients with retinitis pigmentosa with oral 11-*cis* vitamin A, 100,000 units daily for 1 month and then 50,000 units daily for 2 months. Of these seven patients, three showed significant improvement in visual field, and one showed significant improvement in the dark adaptation curve.

Another group of eight patients with retinitis pigmentosa received intramuscular injections of 100,000 units of 11-*cis* vitamin A twice daily for 1 year. Two of these patients showed significant improvement in visual fields, and two showed significant improvement in dark adaptation.

Understandably encouraged by these results, the authors undertook a 2-year study of 20 patients, administering 100,000 units of 11-*cis* vitamin A intramuscularly twice weekly. Vision improved significantly in six patients, visual fields improved in eight patients, and dark adaptation improved in two patients. Three patients interrupted treatment, suffered relapses, and improved when treatment was resumed.

From these data is it safe to conclude that 11-*cis* vitamin A treatment will at least arrest the progress of retinitis pigmentosa over a 2-year period, if not actually improve the condition, in approximately one third of patients? Certainly this would seem to be a conservative conclusion and would apparently justify such treatment of this previously hopeless disease.

Fortunately, these authors were critical scientists and formulated a rigidly controlled study of 88 retinitis pigmentosa patients matched in pairs according to history, progress, and status of the disease. The treatment group received 11-*cis* vitamin A, 100,000 units intramuscularly twice weekly for 3 years. The control group received an identical dosage of all-*trans* vitamin A. The final results, shown in Table

**TABLE 1–1.**

Final Results of 11-*cis* Vitamin A Treatment of Patients With Retinitis Pigmentosa

| | 3 yr | | 2½ yr or Less | |
|---|---|---|---|---|
| | 11-*cis* | All-*trans* | 11-*cis* | All-*trans* |
| Improved | [illegible] | 1 | 2 | 1 |
| Same | 4 | 9 | 0 | 1 |
| Regressed | 2[illegible] | 17 | 7 | 3 |
| Not qualified | [illegible] | 3 | 0 | 0 |
| TOTAL | 2[illegible] | 30 | 9 | 5 |

1–1, indicate absolutely no benefit from treatment with 11-*cis* vitamin A.

This 10-year study illustrates an all too common sequence of events. An attractive basic hypothesis receives initial confirmation from animal experimentation. Preliminary clinical studies show encouraging results. Additional clinical studies, still uncontrolled, independently verify the encouraging results. At this stage, unfortunately, the given therapy usually is released from the laboratory and becomes generally used in medical practice. Established in the medical literature and in drug handbooks, the treatment acquires the respectability of usage and inevitably receives credit for an encouraging number of satisfied patients. But, alas, as years go by some skeptical clinician finally arranges a controlled clinical study. (Can you imagine the effort required to evaluate 88 patients with retinitis pigmentosa, match them in severity, and inject them twice weekly for 3 years!) Of such experience is skepticism of new treatments born.

You may think that this example of 11-*cis*-vitamin A treatment of retinitis pigmentosa is not representative; after all, it has not been recommended. Preliminary reports from a committee (personal experience, Food and Drug Committee) on therapeutic evaluation suggest that two thirds of the older drugs available today are of unproved value and probably worthless. These useless drugs entered our armamentarium via the path outlined in the 11-*cis*-vitamin A example. Perhaps we are not as far from the bad old days of purging and bloodletting as we would like to imagine.

## STATISTICAL SIGNIFICANCE

Statistical significance is another misunderstood term. Often it is accepted as a sort of a seal of approval that verifies the conclusion of the author. Actually, all that is established by a "statistically significant difference" is that the control and experimental groups do indeed differ in some respect. This difference is not necessarily the use or nonuse of the given treatment but often will be another factor in selection of the two groups. These factors may be obvious to the reader or may be quite subtle, perhaps even concealed completely by inadequate reporting of selection methods. To cite a well-known example, there is a statistically significant correlation between the number of marriages performed by the Church of England and the new cases of venereal disease that occur during the same year. However, this does not mean that the marriage ceremony causes disease; rather, both marriage and disease rates are related to the number of individuals existing in the marriageable age group in a given year.

A statistical dilemma particularly relevant to ophthalmology disputes whether we should count eyes or subjects. The answer depends on the experiment. Because the eyes of an individual usually react very similarly, any analysis of the sum or average of measurements should be based on the number of subjects. Calculating this type of study on the basis of two eyes rather than one individual does not result in twice as much information. On the other hand, comparison of differences in response to a given treatment is ideally carried out by observing the differences in response of the paired eyes of a series of individuals.[7]

Both statistical significance and gambling are governed by the laws of chance. Just as the most enthusiastic gambler would hesitate to take on odds of 20 to 1, so the statistician says a finding is "significant" if it occurs by chance less than once in 20 times (values $<0.05$). For practical purposes we may rely on statistical significance if the experiment is properly designed and deals with a single predetermined contrast between two groups. However, the problem of multiple contrasts refers to a "fishing expedition" in which a computer makes multiple comparisons between the two groups (experimental and control). If six comparisons are made between two groups, the random chance of finding a spurious 0.05 association is 1 in 3 ($6 \times 0.05 = 0.3$). To call significant a finding from a six-contrast study would require demonstration of a frequency of 0.008 (0.05 divided by 6).[8] In fact, when an unsuspected positive result is encountered in a multiple-contrast fishing expedition, it probably has no validity whatsoever until the work is reproduced in another investigation designed to establish this specific relationship.

A classic example of such a flawed conclusion was the discovery that drinking coffee was positively associated with pancreatic cancer. Detailed analysis of this finding established it to be a statistical quirk, of no value unless subsequently independently verified.[8] The multiple-contrast problem is the reason we learn from the daily newspaper that almost everything causes cancer.

Case and control selection and retention pose almost insuperable problems in anything but a randomized, controlled prospective study. For example, Berkson's selective hospitalization bias may elevate relative-risk ratios in a hospital population to as much as 17 times their true value in the general population.[8] Migration bias refers to loss of follow-up, which may conceal important late changes in the control group. Exclusion bias arbitrarily discards cases or controls and easily results in selective changing of the sample. Protopathic bias refers to early disease, the presence of which may alter exposure to a suspected etiologic agent. For example, women with benign breast disease may be advised to avoid estrogen therapy. Subsequent study of the female population will then falsely disclose that estrogen therapy reduces the prevalence of benign breast disease.

Our choice of a control group against which we compare the experiment group is the key in performing a meaningful study. Various factors such as age, sex, race, and presence of possibly compounding disease need to be controlled in most prospective clinical studies. The question arises, "Where do we recruit these controls?" The practical answer is to select the controls from our office practices.[9] The advantages of this population include the relative ease of recruitment and follow-up compared with controls selected from the general population. Controls selected from an ophthalmology practice tend to be slightly older and have an increased risk of other eye diseases developing during the study. We must be aware of potential biasing as a result of selecting from specific subgroups rather than from the population as a whole.

When we propose a therapeutic intervention to a patient, a discussion of risk/benefit ratio should ensue. We may quote retrospective, prospective, or antidotal evidence (or combination thereof) during this discussion. It is usually helpful to the patient if the physician can interpret these studies into a percentage chance of an unfavorable event. How are we to interpret a nonevent found in a clinical study?[10, 11] Suppose a new topical corticosteroid medication is prepared that is intended to have a lower incidence of significant intraocular pressure elevation than older agents. We test it in 50 patients and find no instances of elevated intraocular pressure. Intuitively we know that there is still a chance that this event may occur when large numbers of patients are given the drug. The maximum risk may be estimated by $3/N$ at the 95% confidence level.[10] In our hypothetical case the maximum risk would be $3/50$, or 6%. If 1,000 subjects were in the study, the maximum risk would fall to 0.3%. We must therefore also pay attention to the N, or denominators, in a clinical study when interpreting risk/benefit ratios.

The well-known computer maxim, "Garbage in, garbage out," applies equally well to statistical evaluations. In retrospective case-controlled studies, the primary data are seldom verifiable. Discrepancies of major magnitude easily creep in and lead to entirely irrelevant conclusions being blessed with "statistical significance." Because all the details of basic data acquisition cannot be included in a paper of publishable length, data flaws are almost undetectable.

This brief recital of sources of error reveals why the prospective random-controlled trial is the only type of experiment that provides data good enough to permit valid statistical study.

## ACCURACY OF OBSERVATION

Even when the known distortions of prejudice and bias are excluded, our own ability to perceive details is far more limited and less reliable than we think it is. One needs only to discuss a series of previously observed patients with a group of competent ophthalmologists to realize the amazing differences of opinion as to the physical findings in a given eye. Our own record when compared with objective documentation such as a photograph is little better. I am quite certain that at least a 50% change, for better or for worse, must occur before I can reliably say the eye has improved or worsened since yesterday's observations. Repeatedly we have been convinced that a fundus lesion was substantially better or worse; yet when the photograph was returned, the lesion was found to be entirely unchanged. Many studies have documented these considerable variations in clinical and laboratory observations.

The accuracy of competent clinical work is high, and these comments should not be construed as adverse criticism of medical skills. Indeed, recognition of the possibility of faulty determination and observations is part of the skill of an astute physician.

It is instructive and sobering to specify the magnitude of potential clinical error. The interpretation of x-ray films lends itself well to such critical evaluation, because the same films remain available for repeated study.[12] In a study of the effectiveness of x-ray methods for mass survey detection of chest disease, experienced physicians missed 25% of the cases of x-ray-visible pulmonary disease. Reading the same films 3 months later, individual physicians missed 20% of the positive findings they had themselves previously diagnosed.

Still more thought provoking were the results of comparison of full-sized serial chest x-ray films to determine whether pulmonary disease had improved, worsened, or was unchanged. In such comparisons, experienced radiologists disagreed with each other in 30% of the cases, and a single physician disagreed with his own previous interpretation 20% of the time.[12]

Similar study of the histopathologic diagnosis of cancer suggests that an expert pathologist is about 85% reliable in his or her diagnosis. Clinical diagnoses suffer equal variability. Five pediatricians classified 221 children as to nutritional status. Malnutrition was diagnosed in 90 children by one or another physician, but all five agreed on the diagnosis of malnutrition in only seven children.[12]

Many other examples of variations in clinical and laboratory observations were cited in the same article. Although no reference was made to ophthalmology, the significance of these facts to ophthalmic therapy is clear. In our search for the scientific truths on which our medical or surgical treatments should be based, we must distinguish between the truly reliable and well-written paper and the potboiler that purports to reach a conclusion through "clinical impression." We must admit, at least to ourselves, the possibility that our case of unilateral chronic simple glaucoma might turn out to be a carotid-cavernous fistula, that pyrimethamine may do more harm than good in a given case of uveitis, or that convergence exercises in a particular case of exophoria may simply be of psychologic value. It is uncomfortable but stimulating to have residents perpetually ask, "Why do you do this?" In short, this is a plea for continuing self-evaluation of our diagnostic and therapeutic habits.

## LABORATORY VALIDITY

Modern automated laboratory technology is highly accurate, but machines cannot prevent human error in misidentification of specimens and faulty recording. An electrocardiogram or a chemical profile can easily be placed on the wrong chart by a hurried ward clerk. During the 18-month period from January 1979 through June 1980, in the Division of Chemistry of The Ohio State University, 284 improperly identified specimens (of a total of 493,000) were recognized because of the incompatible information on the request.[13] The number of unrecognized laboratory errors is, of course, unknown but is estimated to approximate 1%.[14] Of the 500,000,000 laboratory determinations performed annually at The Ohio State University Hospital, 1% would be 50,000 errors!

## ACCURACY AND PRECISION

Accuracy refers to closeness to the true value. Precision refers to the closeness of replicate measurements to each other. If a given blood urea nitrogen value is 25 mg/dl, and if 10 measurements on the same sample are all within 1 mg/dl, the measurement is highly precise but may be very inaccurate. The need for accuracy and precision in laboratory tests is obvious. Less appreciated is the importance of the concepts that follow.

## SENSITIVITY AND SPECIFICITY

The diagnostic sensitivity of a laboratory test means the percent positive in patients having the disease. The diagnostic specificity means the percent negative in those that do not have the disease.

Tests that are highly sensitive will give more false-positive results. Those that are highly specific will give more false-negative results. Experienced physicians understand that a false-positive test result for syphilis may occur for a considerable number of reasons and that this results in the problem of suspecting a disease that is not actually present. Conversely, a false-negative test result will miss the disease. However, not many of us know about Bayes' theorem.

## BAYES' THEOREM

Bayes' theorem is a statistical assessment of the probability of disease when the results of a test or examination are known. The important message is that the meaning of a test is not absolute but depends on circumstances such as the prevalence of disease in the population being tested. (Prevalence is the number of cases existing at a given time in a given population. Incidence is the number of new cases occurring during a given time period.) The diagnostic meaning of a given positive test result may vary from 2% to 95%, depending on the prevalence of the disease, as shown in Table 1–2.[15]

Table 1–2 is formulated to show the meaning of an unusually good test, one with a 95% sensitivity and a 95% specificity (most tests are not nearly that good), in relation to relevance of the disease. Note how greatly the predictive value of the test rises as prevalence increases.

Improvement of the sensitivity and specificity of a given test is difficult. Therefore, the key to making laboratory tests work for you is to increase the prevalence of the disease. This is accomplished by making a presumed diagnosis of the disease by means of careful history and physical examination or by previous less sensitive (and less expensive) laboratory tests. In this way we can limit the population in question to a group with a high probability of having disease.

An example in ophthalmology is the finding of a positive aqueous humor culture for *Staphylococcus epidermidis.* This organism may be a harmless culture contaminant or a cause of a sight-threatening, low-grade endophthalmitis. This test result may be ignored if the culture became positive 2 days after being aspirated from the anterior chamber of a lacerated globe and the eye is showing no clinical signs of endophthalmitis. Conversely, a positive *S. epidermidis* culture from an aspirate of a chronically inflamed, pseudophakic eye will have a much higher predictive power in showing the cause of the disease.

**TABLE 1–2.**

Influence of Prevalence of a Disease on the Likelihood of a Positive Test Result (Indicating the Presence of the Disease) in a Given Individual

| Prevalence (%)* | Predictive Value of a Positive Test Result (%) |
|---|---|
| 0.1 | 1.9 |
| 1.0 | 16.1 |
| 2.0 | 27.9 |
| 5.0 | 50.0 |
| 50.0 | 95.0 |

*Effect of prevalence: sensitivity, 95%; specificity, 95%.

Bayes' theorem is important to clinicians because it places on a scientific basis our intuitive knowledge that clinical and laboratory findings (the raw material from which we practice medicine) must be judged with wisdom before any given finding results in a course of action.

## THE COST OF DIAGNOSTIC CERTAINTY

We spend billions of dollars each year[16] on diagnostic laboratory tests that are being increasingly scrutinized by the government, insurers, and our peers. Before we order a test we must ask ourselves if the result will alter the management of the patient. When a disease is a near certainty, additional confirmatory tests add little useful information.[17] A patient seen in your office with a red eye might have a 1% or 2% chance of having herpes simplex keratitis (depending on the nature of your practice). Your clinical examination reveals the presence of a dendritic corneal ulcer with terminal bulbs. The possibility that the patient has herpes simplex keratitis has now risen to 99%. A viral culture to confirm the herpes infection will render little of importance to the management of this patient. A negative result will be ignored. The value of the viral culture is negligible compared with the clinical examination. The same viral culture may be enormously valuable in the patient with an atypical corneal lesion suspected of being an active herpes simplex keratitis by clinical examination. In the latter case, the possibility of a herpes infection may be only 50% after clinical examination but may rise to 98% with a positive culture or lower to 25% with a negative culture.

Tests with equal sensitivity and specificity performed consecutively will become less valuable as the probability of the disease increases. Simultaneous performance of tests (examination, laboratory, radiologic) will often result in needless overconfirmation.

One may come to the false conclusion from Bayes' theorem that because a test is more predictive when the probability of disease is high, it is also a more useful test. Fig. 1–1 demonstrates that quite the inverse is true. A test performed when the diagnosis is nearly certain will be very predictive if the results are positive, but its real usefulness in making the diagnosis is negligible.

Unnecessary laboratory testing is not only expensive but can lead to false diagnostic directions.[18] The reflex ordering of an admission battery of 20 or 30 laboratory tests on every patient is an example of inefficient simultaneous information gathering. Changes in physician ordering patterns are difficult to effect despite intensive education. Protocols and routines imprinted during our training are difficult to shed even when contradictory information is presented. A study performed in 1984 tested the effectiveness of education on the ordering habits of resident physicians.[19] Both lectures and chart audits were performed with regularity without any significant changes in the overall hospital charges as a result of physician orders. Better results were achieved in other studies,[19–21] indicating that we are capable of some (limited) change in our ordering patterns. It is useful to utilize a mental flowchart during diagnosis to visualize the value of a particular diagnostic test. If a test will not alter our future diagnostic and therapeutic interventions, the test is valueless and should not be performed.

## COST-EFFECTIVE THERAPY

Appropriate cost-effective therapy should be the goal in each of our patient encounters. The key concept is appropriateness. Until recently physicians had almost complete control of therapeutic decisions. We are now being asked to justify our choices in terms of costs/benefit ratio. I can easily justify the use of an aminoglycoside drop to treat a potentially blinding, gram-negative bacterial keratitis. However, I would have difficulty proving the cost-effectiveness of the chronic use of cyclosporin A eye drops ($200–$300/bottle) in the treatment of keratoconjunctivitis sicca.

This concept is difficult to execute in the large scale because of our inability to meaningfully measure the value of treatments. How does the ability to see compare with the use of our legs or two additional years with our family? One state is currently considering using cost-benefit analysis to determine a priority list from which to allow medical care of its citizens.[22] Advocates of this system argue that health care is currently being rationed according to income level. A more rational approach, they contend, is to ration

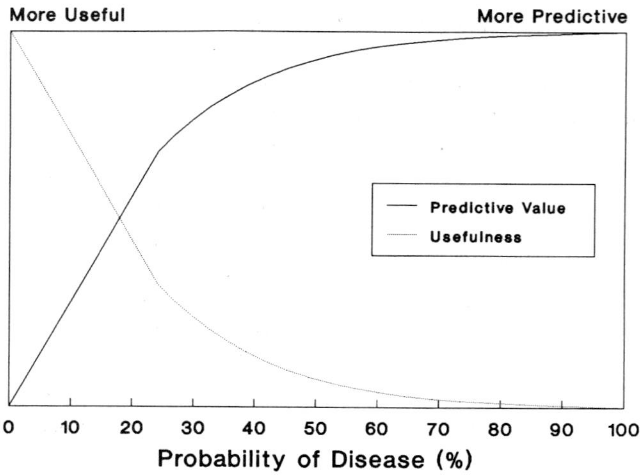


**FIG 1–1.**
The predictive value of a positive test result increases with greater probability of the disease. The usefulness of a positive test result reaches zero when diagnostic certainty is achieved.

expensive and ineffective therapy to allow everyone to have access to more cost-effective therapies. Opponents allege that the concept of assigning priorities using cost-effectiveness is inherently unworkable. The value of a therapeutic intervention is too complicated to quantitate and rank. The underlying dilemma is the difference between our limited resources and unlimited health care demands.

## VALIDITY OF DIAGNOSIS AND PROGNOSIS

Is it senile macular degeneration, macular histoplasmosis, chloroquine intoxication, tuberculosis, myopic degeneration, the result of old trauma, thermal injury from prolonged welding, or an early melanoma? If we combine the correct diagnosis with the correct treatment, perhaps we will achieve cure, or at least improved prognosis. You will recognize that evaluation of therapy, the subject of this chapter, is impossible without an accurate diagnosis.

Bayes' theorem applies to clinical methods of medical diagnosis, as well as to laboratory tests.[23] (This precise definition of the interrelationships of sensitivity, specificity, and prevalence was developed by Rev. Thomas Bayes and published posthumously in 1763.[24]) Unfortunately, information as to the specificity or sensitivity of a finding of a given small fundus hemorrhage or of diplopia is not at all accurate. Also, prevalence is not helpful when you are dealing with a single undiagnosed individual. The problem is that the extreme complexity of the clinical situation renders quantitative statistical models too cumbersome to be helpful. (See Harris[25] for the Bayes' formula.) When the problems of clinical diagnosis are evaluated by statistical models, it becomes apparent that many medical diagnoses must be uncertain and tentative—and so they are.

Even if an etiologic diagnosis is accurate, sample selection invalidates statistical predictions of prognosis.[26, 27] Samples of hyphema from a hospital group of patients, for instance, will always have a much worse outcome than will samples from the physician who first sees the patient. This is the reason that an individual ophthalmologist comparing the results of a favorite hyphema management with the results previously published by a large university hospital will always find the new method to be better. Results of therapy cannot be extrapolated from one population to another.

## PHARMACOGENETICS

Even if we are certain the proper medication has been administered as directed, constitutionally determined individual variations in response occur. Allergy, idiosyncrasy, and hypersensitivity are common examples of pharmacogenetic differences.[28]

The hypersensitivity of a person with Down syndrome (mongolism) to atropine is an example of a pharmacogenetic response of ophthalmologic interest. Topical atropine will produce abnormally great mydriasis in a patient with Down syndrome. This finding has been attributed to a structural anomaly of the iris. However, the cardioacceleratory effects of atropine are twice the normal magnitude in these patients, indicating that a difference in drug response is present throughout the body and not just within the iris.[29] Such pharmacogenetic differences are an often unappreciated cause of response variation

Succinylcholine, the muscle relaxant routinely used before intubation of patients' airways during general anesthesia, is inactivated within minutes by cholinesterase. However, individuals who have a genetic deficiency of cholinesterase may be paralyzed and apneic for many hours after succinylcholine administration.

## VALIDITY OF ANIMAL DATA

Although we are indebted to animal research for a great deal of our basic and clinical knowledge, therapeutic conclusions cannot be extrapolated directly to use with humans. For example, because the rabbit does not have a Bowman membrane, comparative studies of corneal surface injury give different results in monkeys and rabbits.[30]

Another well-known species difference is that many strains of rabbits possess an atropine esterase, which inactivates the effect of belladonna derivatives far more rapidly than that which occurs in humans.

## TOXIC EFFECTS

The evaluation of therapeutic response must also take into account the possibility of adverse side effects. Recognize that pilocarpine toxicity may cause nausea and vomiting wrongly attributed to acute glaucoma. Glaucoma secondary to corticosteroid therapy is well publicized but not always recognized. The somewhat confused mental state of the unreliable old woman with glaucoma could be caused by acetazolamide toxicity. Continuing superficial punctate keratitis may be caused by irritation from the medication long after the primary disease etiology has vanished. Glaucoma patients with iatrogenic cholinesterase deficiency should not undergo abdominal surgery in an attempt to find the cause of stomach pains.

A compact review of toxic drug effects is presented in the apocryphal story of a physician who treated himself*:

> About ten years ago this busy physician developed acute pharyngitis and, seeking quick relief, self-medicated himself with penicillin. The pharyngitis improved rapidly, but to his great distress, 48 hours later he developed a severe urticarial reaction to the penicillin and was confined to his bed for one week. After several days of misery, hydrocortisone was administered and in due course the urticaria subsided. Not long thereafter he experienced abdominal pain and gastrointestinal bleeding, and radiographic studies demonstrated a duodenal ulcer, a well-known complication of steroid therapy. Because of headaches resulting from the loss of blood, he was given acetophenetidin and to his utter chagrin, developed a fixed drug eruption on the genitalia, which consisted of a painful ulceration persisting for several weeks. But the worst was yet to come. The duodenal ulcer was treated with Sippy powders containing calcium carbonate and calcium phosphate to control gastric acidity; shortly thereafter he experienced painful urethral calculi, which fortunately subsided when these powders were discontinued. In addition, pro-Banthine was administered to control gastric secretion. The patient then noted some visual disturbances; after several months, it was discovered that he had glaucoma. The intraocular pressure was controlled with physostigmine salicylate solution; however, the use of these drops created a severe conjunctival congestion, resulting in great embarrassment and damage to the psyche.

One wonders if he might not have been better off had the original pharyngitis been treated with simple aspirin gargles and rest.

## MEDICATION ERRORS

Despite mimeographed reference sheets, repeated instructions, and personal attention to the proper bedside medications to be continued in home use, I find errors of frequency of use. Even errors regarding the medication to be used are not uncommon. Confusion is especially likely in the case of multiple medications.

Unlabeled drugs are a particularly dangerous source of error. As a consultant, I often see a patient who brings a purseful of bottles, some old, some new, labeled only with the frequency for use. Invariably such patients do not know which medications they should use. Accurate identification of something so important as a medical prescription should be legally required in every state.

Tribute to the accuracy and conscientiousness of our nurses and pharmacists is certainly appropriate. Nevertheless, allowance must be made for occasional human errors. Do not exclude the possibility of error in medication if the response of a given eye is greatly different from that expected.

The frequency of medication errors in hospitals has been estimated to be as high as 12%.[31] Most of these errors are insignificant, such as delays in timing. Near the top of the list as a cause of serious errors is illegible physician's handwriting. Verbal instructions

*From Dunphy EB: *Trans Am Acad Ophthalmol Otolaryngol* 70:9, 1966. Used by permission.

are even worse, because many drug names sound alike. Look-alike names are also a problem. For example, acetazolamide is similar to acetohexamide (a hypoglycemic drug) and has caused serious hypoglycemic problems with coma when given by mistake to patients with glaucoma.[32]

The problem of counterfeit drugs is of unknown magnitude, but it is known to exist in our nation. Penalties for drug counterfeiting are only token, and potential profits are great. Detection of a spurious antibiotic or corticosteroid preparation would be beyond my capability, except insofar as the expected therapeutic response is absent.

## DRUG INSTABILITY

Inactivation or alteration of medications occurs with time and adverse conditions (heat, light, oxidation). The deterioration of epinephrine is well known to all of us and can easily be recognized by obvious discoloration of the solution. But how many ophthalmologists alert the patient to this easily observed sign of loss of potency?

Tetracycline deterioration to a nephrotoxic product is a far more serious situation than mere loss of therapeutic effect.

Even well-known incompatibilities are commonly disregarded. Preoperative surgical cleaning may include consecutive scrubbing with hexachlorophene (pHisoHex) and benzalkonium (Zephiran) chloride. These are, of course, anionic and cationic detergents, respectively. Their combined effect is to neutralize each other.

## GENERIC INEQUIVALENCE

Discrepancies between reports of the effects of a given drug occur in both experimental situations and clinical therapy. Such discrepancies may sometimes be explained by differences in preparation of the drug by different manufacturers. Many factors may influence the therapeutic usefulness of a drug even though the preparation contains the stated amount of the active ingredient. Such factors include solubility of the dosage form, effect of other ingredients, pH, particle size, stability, age, compression of the tablet, binders, thickness and type of enteric coating, taste, comfort of use (for eye drops), appearance, uniformity of suspension, and type of liquid vehicle.

As an example of the great effect of differences in formulation, two lots of tolbutamide (Orinase) tablets were prepared, each containing 0.5 g of the drug and both meeting United States Pharmacopeia (USP) specifications. All composition and manufacturing details of these two preparations were identical except that one lot contained only half the amount of disintegrant gum. This single and seemingly minor pharmacy change more than tripled the tablet disintegration time from 2 to 7.6 minutes. An even more important but less conspicuous change occurred in dissolution time—from 3.8 to 103 minutes.[33]

As would be expected, this solubility difference was reflected in greatly reduced serum levels after administration of the less soluble drug. During the 8-hour period after tablet administration, the cumulative drug content in the serum was three and one-half times greater for the commercial preparation than for the experimental preparation with half the amount of disintegrant gum. Serum glucose levels were measured in these normal subjects. The cumulative 8-hour glucose drop was more than twice as great for the commercial preparation as for the experimental preparation.

The generic inequivalence of different brands of chloramphenicol has been the subject of much comment in the medical literature and presumably is well known to all physicians. Another significant generic inequivalence exists in penicillin preparations. The USP requires penicillin G preparations to contain at least 85% penicillin G. In fact, commercially available penicillin G from reputable manufacturers contains 98% or more of penicillin G. The less pure generic equivalent preparations offered inexpensively from other sources may contain many contaminating allergens. These contaminants are believed to be responsible for some of the allergic reactions attributed to penicillin, inasmuch as the pure drug may not cause a comparable allergic response.[34]

In a study of tetracycline inequivalence, the Achromycin brand resulted in an average plasma level of 5.29 μg/ml (dosage 250 mg four times daily). The use of Tetrachel brand produced a level of 3.74 μg/ml. In this study, therefore, the bioavailability of Tetrachel tablets was only 70% that of Achromycin capsules.[35]

Similarly, levothyroxine products are inequivalent. Synthroid produced a lesser response than Levothroid in every one of 34 patients.[36]

## PSYCHOLOGIC FACTORS IN THERAPEUTIC RESPONSE

Emotional and attitudinal factors substantially affect the therapeutic response of a patient. By far the most important of these are noncompliance and the placebo effect. Ability to deal with factors such as this is the skill that is known as the art of medicine. Such a term may be misinterpreted to mean that noncompliance and the placebo effect cannot be understood, characterized, or managed in a scientific manner. This is not true.

## PATIENT (UN)RELIABILITY

A delightful and ostensibly true anecdote describes an elderly woman, somewhat of a hypochondriac, who regularly and frequently with multiple complaints, visited her favorite physician. On her death, her will specified that a very large, securely locked trunk in her attic was to be given to the faithful physician. With great anticipation and considerable difficulty, he forced open the heavy lid. Within the trunk he found, unused, every single bottle of medication he had dispensed to her over the years.

This woman is representative of 30% to 40% of our patients. Multiple independent investigations document the astonishing fact that one third of our patients fail to use the medications we prescribe. Failure to cooperate cannot reliably be correlated with environment, education, socioeconomic status, or patient characteristics such as age or sex. Reliability of clinic attendance and of obtaining drugs does not correlate with cooperation in actually taking the medication. About the only consistent factor is duration of therapy. Patients become progressively less cooperative in using medication during a long course of treatment. (Glaucoma is a classic example of a long-term treatment disease.) Also, multiple medications are less likely to be taken properly.

Dropper and pill bottles may be fitted with microprocessors to record the date and time of medication dispensing. This type of system has been proved to be one of the only reliable ways to monitor compliance in clinical studies. Patients being treated for epilepsy would seemingly be among those most likely to use prescribed medications to prevent seizures. Only 39% of patients using four times daily oral dosing took the medication as instructed, and only 76% of the total doses were taken as prescribed. Two thirds of the seizures occurring during the study were associated with missed doses. We must be cognizant of the possibility of poor compliance in patients with unresponsive or relapsing conditions. The patients in this study were informed of the recording device in the pill bottle and would therefore be expected to demonstrate increased compliance. Patient characteristics that are associated with noncompliance include memory impairment and anxiety.[37]

Compliance with ophthalmic medications may be grossly overestimated by patient interview and the physician's perception of the patient's reliability. A study of four times daily pilocarpine use demonstrated that although patients reported taking more than 97% of doses prescribed, the medication monitor proved that only 76% of the intended doses were used.[38]

Noncompliance may not be reflected in poor intraocular pressure control because the medication will be used as prescribed immediately before an office visit. This may result in a glaucoma patient with progressive optic nerve damage and visual field loss despite seemingly adequate intraocular pressure measurements. Pupil size and reactivity have also been found to be unreliable indicators of compliance with pilocarpine use. Patient education with particular emphasis on incorporating the patient's schedule and life-style with his or her medication requirements may improve compliance.[39]

Repeated verbal and written instructions are helpful in improving compliance, but no education program will be successful if the medication protocol is too complex for the patient to use appropriately. Remember, "suboptimal" therapy that the patient uses is actually more effective than "optimal" therapy that is not used.

Some patients give their medications a low priority because the importance of the drug has not been emphasized to them. Ignorance of the disease and its natural course may be recommended by education. Disbelief may involve a lack of confidence in their physician, which may be dispelled with a well-selected second opinion confirming the diagnosis and proposed therapeutic regimen.

## NONCOMPLIANCE

Your instructions do the patient no good if they are not followed. The preceding section has established that failure to cooperate with instructions is common, if not characteristic, in the treatment of chronic illness. For practical purposes, glaucoma is the only major eye disease in which noncompliance is likely to cause serious consequences. The facts in this section, therefore, apply importantly to your patients with glaucoma. Patients who miss appointments are particularly likely to neglect their medication and should be scrutinized carefully for evidence of optic nerve deterioration.[40] The more frequent the dosage, the more likely a dose will be missed, especially the noon dose. (Apparently morning and evening doses are easier to remember.) Shorter intervals between office visits improve compliance.[41] Noncompliers are more likely to be men and to have had annoying side effects from treatment.[42] Evidently during noncompliance the patient does not have side effects and will not complain of them.

A "usefulness product" has been calculated by multiplying the percent of effectiveness by the percent of tolerance or compliance.[43, 44] For example, pilocarpine may be effective in lowering pressure in 80% of patients but tolerated in only 70%. This equals a usefulness product of 56%. Epinephrine is effective in 70% and tolerated over a long term in 30%, for a usefulness of 21%. Carbonic anhydrase inhibitors are 60% effective and 60% tolerated, for a usefulness of 36%. Timolol does better, with 75% effect and 95% (!) compliance, for a 71% usefulness. Sustained-release 500-mg acetazolamide capsules were found to have a particularly high incidence of annoying side effects.[45]

Any number of factors have been cited for noncompliance, including faulty instructions,[46] forgetfulness,[47] cost, poor commitment to health in general,[48] complexity and duration of the regimen, long wait in physician's office, and unfavorable impression of the physician.

I am personally convinced that the "negative placebo effect" is a major cause of noncompliance. This is the opposite of a placebo effect and refers to physician actions that displease or discomfort the patient. Such physician ineptness causes (1) patient non-well-being (the patient is worried and scared and does not feel good), (2) physician misdiagnosis (the physician thinks something is wrong because the patient does not feel good), (3) noncompliance (patient will not cooperate with an untrusted physician), and (4) medicolegal litigation (suing is a form of revenge).[49]

A practical suggestion: Check your own appointment schedule at the end of each day to see how many broken or canceled appointments have occurred. One form of patient noncompliance is disappearance. In one group of 89 patients with ocular hypertension and glaucoma, 37% failed to return within 12 to 21 months after diagnosis.[50] Loss to follow-up of more than one third of patients with such a potentially serious eye problem cannot be dismissed lightly. I personally have been reluctant to send missed appointments notices, thinking that it was the patient's privilege not to return to me. However, the implications of neglected glaucoma are so great that perhaps the matter should be reconsidered. Should we institute selective reminder and recall systems in our own office practice, as many dentists do? It might not be a bad idea, especially for glaucoma patients.

## THE PLACEBO EFFECT

Lest we forget the importance of our interpersonal relationships with patients and assume that medical care is accomplished only with drugs or surgery, I quote Dr. Charles Dunlap[51]:

> Among the tools used by a doctor, words both heard and spoken are as necessary and as powerful as drugs or instruments. Used carelessly, they can produce deep wounds that fester and never heal. But when skillfully and gently used, they can ease pain, inspire hope, bring joy, allay despair, and even put a fretful child to sleep.

The words, as well as the attitudes and the actions of a physician, cause a measurable patient response that may be termed the placebo effect. The placebo may be defined as a medication given to please the patient. The physician knows the mechanism of action of the placebo is psychologic. Actually, of course, the placebo effect will also account for part of the response of a patient of a potent drug. Even if the potent drug is ineffectual against the given disease, measurable subjective improvement can be expected in a significant number of cases. Here exists a trap for the unwary physician, who may readily confuse the placebo response with specific therapeutic benefit. This explains many of the enthusiastic but subsequently unconfirmed reports in the literature. In general, the greater a physician's interest in a treatment, particularly if the physician was the one to discover it or has recently been converted to its use, the more effective that treatment will appear to be.[52]

About 35% of patients will show a significant response to placebo therapy.[53] Stated in another way, almost any drug (provided that it is not harmful) will cause subjective improvement in one of every three patients suffering from almost anything. Objective improvements will also occur in the parameters ordinarily recognized as psychosomatic (e.g., pulse, respiration, gastric acid secretion, and fatigue). Interestingly, toxic side effects such as drowsiness, dry mouth, and nausea can be elicited in substantial numbers (10%–50%) of patients receiving a placebo, depending on the amount of suggestion present. Even skin rashes (dermatitis medicamentosa and angioneurotic edema) may be precipitated by placebo therapy of predisposed individuals. The placebo effect is greatest in situations where the stress and psychologic reaction of the patient are greatest. It does not matter in the least of what the placebo is made or how large the dose as long as it is not detected as a placebo by the patient.

Some 7,000 years ago a chronically ill Asian warrior recovered miraculously from his primary disease after an arrow wound. Fortunately the arrow struck him at the acupuncture site specific for the cure of his disease. Subsequent empirical clinical trials led to the discovery of the multiple acupuncture sites that are recorded on the charts of the traditional practitioners of Chinese medicine. The almost unbelievable capability of acupuncture to counteract virtually any type of disease or disorder is attested to by veteran reporters and by experienced physicians, including ex-President Nixon's own physician.[54–56]

But why does acupuncture work? Is it a mysterious technique, the details of which are unknown to science? Or is it but a variant of well-established principles of medical management? Does stimulation of the xiang-yang point with a needle alter a malfunctioning sympathetic system resulting in resolution of central serous retinopathy?[57] This study of 600 Chinese patients treated with acupuncture (no controls) showed improvement in 98% over 1 year. A truly remarkable success rate until we compare this with the natural course of the disease in the United States, which is quite similar.[58]

The absence of controls limits the value of this study. We might suspect that the acupuncture had no effect on the course of the disease, but we cannot rule out the possibility that there is an aggressive variant that was effectively improved with treatment. A placebo control of acupuncture is difficult to design and will always limit these studies. Pills, drops, and even laser allow the construction of believable controls in a way that procedures such as acupuncture cannot.[58] Without further ado, let us define acupuncture as simply the Chinese version of placebo therapy. The Chinese have skillfully perfected a format within which the placebo effect is maximized.

A placebo effect may be defined as the result of a therapy (or a component of a therapy) that has a demonstrable effect but that objectively is without specific activity for the condition being treated.

Do not minimize the value of the placebo effect. For centuries physicians have held an honored place in society despite the worthlessness of their remedies. No treatment of any specific value is found in the writings of Hippocrates. Witness the bloodletting and the purges that were advocated in comparatively modern times. As recently as 1952 as many as one third of 17,000 prescriptions in England were considered to have only placebo value.[59] The skill of the physician was (and still is) to treat illness by encouragement and ineffective medications. Many therapeutic successes can be attributed to the enthusiasm and support of the physician and the faith of the patient.

Lest we fail to comprehend the potency of emotional attitudes and believe that only psychosomatic illnesses respond to placebo therapy, let us refer to the control of pain from severe wounds. At the Anzio beachhead during World War II only 25% of the severely injured battle casualties required morphine.[60] In contrast, of the civilians studied, 80% required analgesic medication postoperatively. The difference was attributed to the fact that pain caused civilians to become apprehensive about their operations, whereas wounded soldiers knew injuries represented a ticket to the shelter of a hospital and then to home.

The therapeutic effect of the placebo is by no means limited to the management of disorders commonly accepted as being psychosomatic. A significant placebo therapeutic effect was demonstrated in 35% of 1,082 patients suffering from such diverse afflictions as wound pain, angina pectoris, headache, nausea, cough, seasickness, the common cold, and anxiety.[53] This placebo effect was demonstrable in 26% to 58% of the patients suffering from these various conditions. Please note that this percentage variability was not related to the responsiveness of the given medical condition. Placebo responsiveness is a property of the patient and the environment and not a characteristic of the disease (except insofar as the cure of a self-limited condition may be attributed to an unrelated factor, such as a placebo).

Angina pectoris responds nicely to placebo therapy; 38% of 90 patients experienced pain relief. In view of the emotional aspects of the disorder, such a placebo response is not surprising. The technique of selective coronary arteriography is now available and permits separation of patients with the anginal syndrome into two distinct groups, one with coronary atherosclerosis and the other with no detectable coronary abnormalities. Placebo therapy in 95 patients with angina and coronary vessel disease helped only 4%, whereas 25% of 27 patients with the anginal syndrome and normal coronary arteries responded to placebo therapy.[61] Perhaps the relatively low rate of placebo response resulted from the fact that the amount of psychic suggestion was deliberately minimized. However, the primary reason for commenting on this study is to emphasize that diagnostic inaccuracies may greatly alter the therapeutic (and placebo) response obtained in a given report.

In four separate studies of psychiatric outpatients, placebo response rates were 24%, 35%, 74%, and 76%.[62] The difference in response in these various studies was a result of the management of the patients. The lowest rate of placebo reactivity, 24%, was obtained in a study that included no testing of the patients. The highest rate of placebo reactivity, 76%, was achieved in a study that included detailed psychologic testing (eight separate tests, including some impressive examinations as the Minnesota Multiphasic Personality Inventory and Wechsler Adult Intelligence Scale) at the time of each clinic visit. These multiple tests and contacts with the research personnel caused the emotional impact that resulted in relief of the symptoms.

Not only the placebo response but also the effect of an active tranquilizer medication is affected by the circumstances of patient care. Specifically, the effectiveness of tranquilizing medications varied from 30% to 87%, depending on the amount of attention given to the patient. A very large proportion of the measured drug response in these patients was a placebo response entirely unrelated to specific drug activity. As an example, in one series of patients the placebo response was 76% and the chlordiazepoxide (Librium) response was 87%. This means that the true chlordiazepoxide response was only 11%, because 76% of the responses were attributable to the placebo effect. (This difference is statistically significant, providing it is reproducible.)

Clearly the clinical setting in which a new drug is evaluated is of great importance. Comparison of drug evaluations performed under different circumstances may be quite misleading.

Sir William Osler[63] advised that new remedies be used quickly while they are still efficacious. This astute, tongue-in-cheek statement illustrates this great clinician's understanding of the placebo effect, which is related to the enthusiasm and confidence of the physician.

So much for documentation of the placebo principle; now, what good is this knowledge to the ophthalmologist?

Wise physicians realize that they themselves cause the placebo effect. They do not really need to prescribe sugar pills or to twirl acupuncture needles. All they must do is present themselves to the patient as trustworthy, knowledgeable, genuinely interested persons who are offering specific recommendations for the patient. Reasonably detailed, rational explanations and discussions of the patient's problem are appropriate but probably benefit the patient via a placebo mechanism and not because of their intellectual value. Acquiring identical knowledge by reading a book from the library is not an adequate substitute for the physician placebo.

The placebo does not have to be the physician or a pill. The physician can invest patients or their relatives and attendants with the placebo mantle. One does this via specific instructions such as the application of warm compresses for 15 minutes four times daily, daily walks, and so on. What patients do is irrelevant as long as they believe it will help them. If you advise sensible, moderate physical exercise and intellectual contact with friends, so much the better, because this actually is beneficial.

A particularly excellent and comprehensive review of the placebo effect[64] presents an overwhelmingly convincing outline of the power of the placebo, which deserves conscious use in the therapy of conditions that do not respond to specific treatment. A remarkable list of severe toxic side effects associated with placebo use is also presented. The physician should be aware that such side effects will be encountered. There is even the apocryphal tale of the psychologist who committed suicide by taking an overdose of placebo.

In summary, intelligent and understanding use of the placebo effect can greatly benefit and comfort even those patients with genuine and serious eye problems. To avoid misunderstanding, I am not suggesting that psychologic hocus-pocus is any substitute for accurate diagnosis and specific therapy for eye disease. As we have already established, specific therapy automatically has placebo value, but by definition placebo therapy has no specific pharmacologic value.

One final comment about the placebo for those who think it is an unrecognized subject of no importance in medicine: A Medline literature search on the subject of placebos for the years 1976, 1977, and 1978 disclosed the existence of 1,500 published articles.[65] I have devoted so much time to the placebo because it is indeed a vital part of our therapy and of our evaluation of therapy.

## REASSURANCE THERAPY

The term placebo therapy conveys the impression of cheating the patient by giving the patient a worthless sugar pill. I much prefer to name this important aspect of medical practice reassurance therapy.[66]

With such a name, reassurance is readily recognized as being an important part of every patient-physician relationship. Reassurance sufficient to the patient's needs should be provided to every patient as a routine component of what we consciously plan as the patient's management. To be effective, reassurance therapy requires the following six steps. Omission of any of these steps detracts from or nullifies the value of the reassurance.

1. Obtain a sufficiently detailed history of the symptoms. Never try to reassure the patient during the initial history. Premature attempts at reassurance inhibit the patient from continuing with the history, usually reflect anxiety or impatience on the part of the physician, and are not effectively reassuring to the patient.

2. Determine the affective meaning of the symptoms. Although this step can be done almost simultaneously with step one, it is commonly overlooked or poorly performed. One reason for this is that the physician is concentrating on the verbal description and not on the affect. A second reason is that affect is communicated nonverbally, by tone of voice and mannerisms (body language). You must be aware that no patients come to you unless they are concerned or frightened by something. Therefore, it is necessary to evaluate consciously the amount of patient concern in every history. The amount of patient concern will, of course, determine the amount of reassurance therapy required.

A useful suggestion: Whenever you detect that a given patient makes you feel anxious[67] or that you actively dislike[68] a patient, you should recognize that the patient has successfully conveyed to you via body language that he or she is in need of reassurance therapy.

3. Examine the symptomatic portion of the body. Appropriate steps in physical diagnosis are necessary to establish the presence or absence of disease. Furthermore, touching the patient is in itself therapeutic and will dramatically enhance the effectiveness of the subsequent verbal reassurance.

4. Make a diagnosis. You should identify the presence or absence of disease in the traditional medical manner. You are unable to give reassurance or explanation until you are reasonably sure of the nature of the problem.

5. Explain the pathophysiology of the symptom to the patient. Paradoxically, patients do not really need to understand all details, but they must be able to recognize three attitudes in the physician. First, they must believe that the physician understands the symptoms. Second, they must believe that the physician is concerned about them as individuals but is not anxious, frightened, or uncertain as to the management of the symptoms. Third, patients must believe that the physician is sympathetic about the symptom. We tend to be annoyed by patients whose symptoms persist; they frustrate us and we convey an attitude of displeasure. Physicians must accept the fact that they cannot eradicate all physical and emotional symptoms and must not be affronted by the audacity of the persistent symptom.

6. Only after this preamble of history, examination, diagnosis, and explanation is reassurance appropriate. Reassurance may be defined as a credible and acceptable prognosis. Essentially, reassurance is a prediction of the future, an outline of the reasonable expectations of the patient. For benign conditions, reassurance may be categorical and absolute. For proposed surgery, reassurance must be qualified, perhaps with regard to the percentage of successful outcome or some comparable condition prediction. In some conditions the prognosis is hopeless; the eye is irreparably damaged. Even (and especially) under such circumstances, reassurance is appropriate and consists of a reasonable outline of the anticipated care and convalescence and of the type of lifetime activity subsequently possible. Reassurance cannot deny the facts of life, and no attempt should be made to evade genuine problems. Reassurance does stress the positive aspects of the situation and banishes the fears that are without foundation.

Do not neglect reassurance, because it is one of the most important contributions you make to the welfare of every patient. Indeed, for a very large proportion of your patients, you have absolutely nothing to offer them but reassurance. Do not overlook the component of reassurance in the evaluation of therapy, or otherwise you will grossly overestimate the value of your medications.

## PATIENT-PHYSICIAN NEGOTIATION[69]

Almost all physicians on occasion will speak deprecatingly of the noncompliance of patients who seem to be obnoxious and stupid little beggars, determined to thwart our attempts to cure them. Psychiatrists know better. They speak of "alliance" rather than compliance. Their concept of a patient-physician relationship goes through the stages of alliance, contract, undertaking, and termination. We, too, should do this, because noncompliance is the natural consequence of failure to reach a mutual understanding of what is the best management of a problem.

These words are essentially self-explanatory. Alliance is the attitude of having a common goal to achieve. Contract is the verbalizing and agreeing on what is to be done. Undertaking is the actual work involved in the management of the problem. Termination is the parting, with the patient aware of how to conduct himself or herself and under what circumstances he or she should return. Actually, this is nothing more than any other purposeful interpersonal relationship. Do not treat patients as if they were subhuman primates. Treat them as you would like to be treated, and they will respond with willingness to form an alliance for their own benefit.

## THE RANDOMIZED CONTROLLED CLINICAL TRIAL

Knowing about all these pitfalls that affect the outcome of therapy, how do we avoid them? Anyone planning a clinical study really should prepare for the ordeal by reading a symposium devoted to the subject, such as one published by the National Eye Institute.[70] It is sobering to realize that we do not really know whether coronary artery surgery is beneficial in all cases or whether emergency surgery is good for bleeding peptic ulcers. In our own field, we do not even know whether we should use photocoagulation for retinal holes (I do not think that asymptomatic holes discovered on routine examination should be treated, unless the other eye is already detached, and even then I am not sure), let alone whether we should photocoagulate venous occlusions, chorioretinitis, or senile macular degeneration.

Paradoxically, for 20 years I have tried to teach rational ophthalmic therapy and yet am daily unable to define what is rational. I know that osmotherapy will reduce intraocular pressure, but I am not convinced that intravenous mannitol is desirable before cataract extraction. So how should this be dealt with? The only answer that I can offer is that a medical or surgical treatment should not be used unless the physician is reasonably sure that it will be of benefit. That the treatment "might not hurt" is not enough indication for its use. Unfortunately, it is very difficult to prove that antibiotics do or do not favorably alter the normal surface bacterial flora preoperatively, that corticosteroids are or are not good for toxoplasmosis, and that pilocarpine is or is not good for hyphema.

Ultimately I must admit that I will never know whether a given retinal hole should be treated, even though I have personally operated on more than 10,000 retinal detachments. There are so many clinical variations, limitations of follow-up and technique, problems of informed consent, and malpractice hazards that there is just no way to answer the question except with vague generalization. I do not mean to condemn scientific attempts to seek knowledge but to place them in a proper perspective. Do not worship randomized controlled trials but recognize that they are far better than clinical impressions, which are truly misleading.

Two quotes: "Scientific truth is that which you believe at that moment."[71] "Truth is an error that is temporarily irrefutable" (Nietzsche).

## SUMMARY

We have an unfortunate tendency to permit our diagnostic and therapeutic responses to become stereotyped to such a degree that these intellectual exercises degenerate into controlled reflexes. When vitreous hemorrhage automatically means placebo pills and a waiting period of 2 weeks, our patients are in trouble. The scientific method is applicable to each patient. Gather all available facts (history and physical examination). Formulate a tentative hypothesis. Seek additional corroborative or conflicting facts (look at the patient again to confirm the findings pertinent to the diagnosis). From this information, assemble a theory (presume the diagnosis is correct). Finally, check the theory against other known facts (prescribe the appropriate medication and observe whether the expected therapeutic response occurs).

Most faults in patient management originate from insufficient fact gathering. The step most overlooked is the second check of the patient, intended to elicit subtle corroborative or conflicting facts. These inconspicuous details usually determine whether a macular lesion is a melanoma or a disciform degeneration. Such details require intellectually guided seeking (e.g., are sinusoids present?) rather than hopeful looking. This intellectually guided seeking is mandatory in evaluation of therapeutic response. Otherwise, if the patient finally recovers at the end of the self-limited disease, the unwary physician will attribute the "cure" to the final medication prescribed, but it will not work the next time (just as the cabbages at the beginning of this chapter failed to cure the preacher).

## REFERENCES

1. Hayden GF, Kramer MS, Horwitz RI: The case-control study; a practical review for the clinician, *JAMA* 247:326, 1982.
2. Horwitz RI, Feinstein AR: Improved observational method for studying therapeutic efficacy, *JAMA* 246:2455, 1981.
3. Schwartz D, Flamant R, Lellouch J: Clinical trials, New York, 1980, Academic Press.
4. Guinan ME, MacCalman J, Kern ER, and others: Topical ether and herpes simplex labialis, *JAMA* 243:1059, 1980.
5. Spaeth GL: The effects of bromelains on the inflammatory response caused by cataract extraction: a double-blind study, *Eye Ear Nose Throat J* 47:634, 1968.
6. Chatzinoff A, Nelson E, Stahl N, and others: Eleven-CIS vitamin A in the treatment of retinitis pigmentosa, *Arch Ophthalmol* 80:417, 1968.
7. Ederer F: Shall we count numbers of eyes or numbers of subjects? *Arch Ophthalmol* 89:1, 1973.
8. Feinstein AR, Horwitz RI, Spitzer WO, and others: Coffee and pancreatic cancer: the problems of etiologic science and epidemiologic case-control research, *JAMA* 246:957, 1981
9. Hawkins BS: Selection of controls for clinical research studies in ophthalmology, *Arch Ophthalmol* 106:835, 1988.
10. Manley JA, Lippmin-Hand A: If nothing goes wrong, is everything all right? *JAMA* 249:1743, 1983.
11. Hulka BS: When is the evidence for "No Association" sufficient? 252:81, 1984 (editorial).
12. Garland LH: Clinical and laboratory observer variations, *J New Drugs* 1:65, 1961.
13. Clinical laboratory update, Department of Pathology, The Ohio State University, Columbus, Ohio, vol 3, No 11, November 1981.
14. Senhauser D: Personal communication, 1981.
15. Clinical laboratory update, Department of Pathology, The Ohio State University, Columbus, Ohio, vol 2, No 3, March 1980.
16. Kreig AF, Gambino R, Galen RS: Why are clinical laboratory tests performed? When are they valid? *JAMA* 223:76, 1975.
17. Johnson MA: Diminishing returns on the road to diagnostic certainty, *JAMA* 265:2229, 1991.
18. Wong ET, Lincoln TL: Ready! Fire! Aim! An inquiry into laboratory test ordering, *JAMA* 250:2510, 1983.
19. Schroeder SA, Myers LP, Stephen JM, and others: The failure of physician education as a cost containment strategy, *JAMA* 252:225, 1984
20. Martin AR, Wolf MA, Thibodeau LA, and others: A trial of two strategies to modify the test ordering behavior of medical residents, *N Engl J Med* 303:1330, 1980.
21. Griner PF: Use of laboratory tests in a teaching hospital: long term trends, *Ann Intern Med* 90:243, 1979.

22. Eddy DM: Oregon's methods: Did cost-effectiveness analysis fail? *JAMA* 266:2135, 1991.
23. Jones RJ: Bayes' theorem, the exercise ECG, and coronary artery disease, *JAMA* 242:1067, 1979.
24. Bayes T: An essay toward solving a problem in the doctrine of chance, *Philos Trans R Soc Lond (Biol)* 53:370, 1763.
25. Harris Jr JM: The hazards of bedside Bayes, *JAMA* 246:2602, 1981.
26. Ellenberg JH, Nelson KB: Sample selection and the natural history of disease, *JAMA* 23:1337, 1980.
27. Gerber LM, Wolf AM, Braham RL, and others: Effects of sample selection on the coincidence of hypertension and diabetes, *JAMA* 27:43, 1982.
28. Wessler S, Avioli LV: Pharmacogenetics, *JAMA* 205:679, 1968.
29. Harris WS, Goodman RM: Hyperreactivity to atropine in Down's syndrome, *N Engl J Med* 279:407, 1968.
30. Hirst LW, Kenyon KR, Fogle JA, and others: Comparative studies of corneal surface injury in the monkey and the rabbit, *Arch Ophthalmol* 99:1066, 1981.
31. Shaw J: Medication errors a "great hidden problem," *Am Med News,* Jan 1–8, 1982, p 18.
32. Raab EL: Substitution of acetohexamide for acetazolamide, *Am J Ophthalmol* 87:848, 1979.
33. Varley AB: The generic inequivalence of drugs, *JAMA* 206:1745, 1968.
34. Friend DG: Generic drug and therapeutic equivalence, *JAMA* 206:1785, 1968.
35. Wood JH, Flora KP, Dunma RJ: Tetracycline: another example of generic bioinequivalence, *JAMA* 239:1874, 1978.
36. Ramos-Gabatin A, Jacobson JM, Young RL: In vivo comparison of levothyroxine preparations, *JAMA* 247:203, 1982.
37. Cramer JA, Mattson RM, Prevey ML, and others: How often is medication taken as prescribed? A novel assessment technique, *JAMA* 261:3273, 1989.
38. Kass MA, Meltzer DW, Gordon M, and others: Compliance with topical pilocarpine treatment, *Am J Ophthalmol* 101:515, 1986.
39. Kass MA, Gordon M, Meltzer DW: Can ophthalmologists correctly identify patients defaulting from pilocarpine therapy? *Am J Ophthalmol* 101:524, 1986.
40. Ashburn Jr FS, Goldberg I, Kass MA: Compliance with ocular therapy, *Surv Ophthalmol* 24:237, 1980.
41. Norell SE: Monitoring compliance with pilocarpine therapy, *Am J Ophthalmol* 92:727, 1981.
42. Bloch S, Rosenthal AR, Friedman L, and others: Patient compliance with glaucoma, *Br J Ophthalmol* 61:531, 1977.
43. Worthen DM: The "usefulness" product: concern for cupping, control, and compliance, *Ann Ophthalmol* 10:1393, 1978.
44. Worthen DM: Patient compliance and the "usefulness product" of timolol, *Surv Ophthalmol* 23:403, 1979.
45. Alward PD, Wilensky JT: Determination of acetazolamide compliance in patients with glaucoma, *Arch Ophthalmol* 99:1973, 1981.
46. Van Camerik SB: Why don't patients do what you tell them? *Leg Aspects Med Pract* 6:18, 1978.
47. Gillette RD: An aid to patient compliance, *JAMA* 244:659, 1988.
48. Barclay WR: Staying is harder than getting there, *JAMA* 239:53, 1978.
49. Miller LJ: Informed consent: IV, *JAMA* 244:2661, 1980.
50. Bigger JF: A comparison of patient compliance in treated vs. untreated ocular hypertension, *Trans Am Acad Ophthalmol Otolaryngol* 81:277-285, 1976.
51. Dunlap C: *Med World News,* July 3, 1964.
52. Shapiro AK: Etiologic factors in placebo effect, *JAMA* 187:712, 1964.
53. Beecher HK: The powerful placebo, *JAMA* 159:1602, 1955.
54. Thach W: I have seen acupuncture work, *Today's Health* 50:50, 1972.
55. Dimond EG: Medical education and care in People's Republic of China, *JAMA* 218:1551, 1971.
56. Dimond EG: Acupuncture anesthesia, *JAMA* 218:1558, 1971.
57. Lu J, Friberg TR: Idiopathic central serous retinopathy in China: a report of 600 cases (624 eyes) treated by acupuncture, *Ophthalmic Surg* 18:608, 1987.
58. Robertson D, Ilstrup D: Direct, indirect, and sham laser photocoagulation in the management of central serous retinopathy, *Am J Ophthalmol* 95:457, 1983.
59. Dunlop D: Survey of 17,301 prescriptions, *BMJ* 1:292, 1952.
60. Beecher H: Control of suffering in severe trauma, *JAMA* 173:534, 1960.
61. Amsterdam E: New aspects of the placebo response in the angina pectoris, *Am J Cardiol* 24:305, 1969.
62. Lowinger P, Dobie S: What makes a placebo work? *Arch Gen Psychiatry* 20:84, 1969.

63. Osler W: Editorial, *BMJ* 2:437, 1970.
64. Honigfeld G: Nonspecific factors in treatment, *Dis Nerv Syst* 24:145, 1964.
65. Silber TJ: Placebo therapy, the ethical dimension, *JAMA* 242:245, 1979.
66. Sapira JD: Reassurance therapy, *Ann Intern Med* 77:603, 1972.
67. Sutton R: Anxiety and the doctor-patient relationship, OSMA, *Ohio Med* 77:689, 1981.
68. Goodwin JM, Goodwin JS, Kellner R: Psychiatric symptoms in disliked medical patients. *JAMA* 241:1117, 1979.
69. Benarde MA, Mayerson EW: Patient-physician negotiation, *JAMA* 239:1413, 1978.
70. National Eye Institute: The randomized controlled clinic trial, *Am J Ophthalmol* 79:752, 1975.
71. Henkind P: Interactions with the public, *Ophthalmology* 88:21A, 1981.

CHAPTER 2

# Pharmacokinetics

Louis M. DeSantis, Jr.

Popat N. Patil

## PHARMACOKINETICS

Pharmacokinetics involves the study of the time course of changes in the concentration of drugs and their metabolites in tissues and involves the determination of the rates of the four processes or phases of drug disposition: absorption, distribution, metabolism, and excretion.[1–3] Pharmacokinetic analyses elaborate on the factors that cause changes in drug concentration and response. A knowledge of pharmacokinetics is useful to understand (1) whether the drug itself or a metabolite is responsible for the effect, (2) the optimum route of administration and dosage regimen, (3) the relationship between drug concentration in tissue and pharmacologic or toxicologic response, and (4) the consequence of a change in the kinetics of the processes just stated. However, in contrast to the abundance of pharmacokinetic data for systemic drugs, few data in humans are available for ophthalmic drugs.[4–7]

## BIOPHARMACEUTICS

Biopharmaceutics pertains to the study of the influence of drug formulation on pharmacologic and therapeutic activity.[8, 9] The subject deals with the relationship between the physicochemical properties of a drug, its dosage form, and the biologic response. The study of biopharmaceutics gives insight into the relationship between the drug response and the drug's physical state, salt form, particle size, crystalline structure, surface area, and dosage form, along with the pharmaceutical process by which it is made and the influence of any adjuvants or excipients present in the formulation. Biopharmaceutic and pharmacokinetic data allow better informed judgments on drugs and comparisons among drugs and their formulations and may permit selection of an appropriate drug, dosage regimen, and method of drug delivery to achieve the desired therapeutic outcome.

Drug-receptor interactions are governed by the laws of mass action. The concentration of a drug in the biophase at its receptor site primarily determines the intensity of the pharmacologic response.[10] The greater the free drug concentration at the vicinity of the receptor, the higher the statistical probability of a greater pharmacologic effect. The kinetics of the decline of drug concentration in the biophase determines the time course of the response. Dose, dosage regimen, and route of administration influence the concentration of drug in the target tissue and are variables over which the clinician usually has some control. Outside the clinician's control are the physicochemical characteristics of the drug molecule and the formulation or dosage form of the drug. Therefore, these factors should be taken into account when the drug is being designed, selected, and formulated, and pharmacokinetic and biopharmaceutic data for the drug in its dosage form should be obtained. Present knowledge about ocular pharmacokinetics is the result of intensive study of relatively few drugs, usually investigated in rabbits.[11] The study of fluorescein, which is readily detected by fluorophotometry, has contributed greatly to formulation of the basic principles of ocular pharmacokinetics.

This chapter reviews the processes of drug disposition as they relate to the eye and examines various approaches that have been taken to modify the rates of these processes for improving ophthalmic therapy.

## COMPARTMENTAL ANALYSIS AND MODELING

Compartmental analysis is a technique used to develop descriptive and predictive mathematical models to fit a drug's pharmacokinetic data.[6] *Compartment* is a pharmacokinetic term that refers to the physiologic or anatomic spaces within an organ separated by some barrier to drug transfer (Fig. 2–1). Within a compartment the drug is assumed to be homogeneously distributed, and exchange of drug between adjacent compartments occurs at some rate subject to prevailing biochemical and physiologic conditions. This transfer rate is the coefficient taken from the equation describing the change in drug concentration with respect to time in reference to a particular compartment. Data of this type are usually obtained from experiments in rabbits by sampling tissues at various times after drug administration. A sensitive analytical assay is required to obtain accurate drug concentration data. Typically, different groups of animals are used to obtain individual data points. The consecutive time intervals must be selected to adequately describe the kinetics of the process under study.

Compartmental modeling is used to analyze the changes in drug concentration over time.[12, 13] Components of systemic compartments are the blood, plasma, erythrocytes, urine, cerebrospinal fluid, brain, stomach, and intestines. From the standpoint of the body as a whole, the eye is a component of the systemic compartment, which, in turn, comprises multiple subcompartments, such as tears, cornea, aqueous

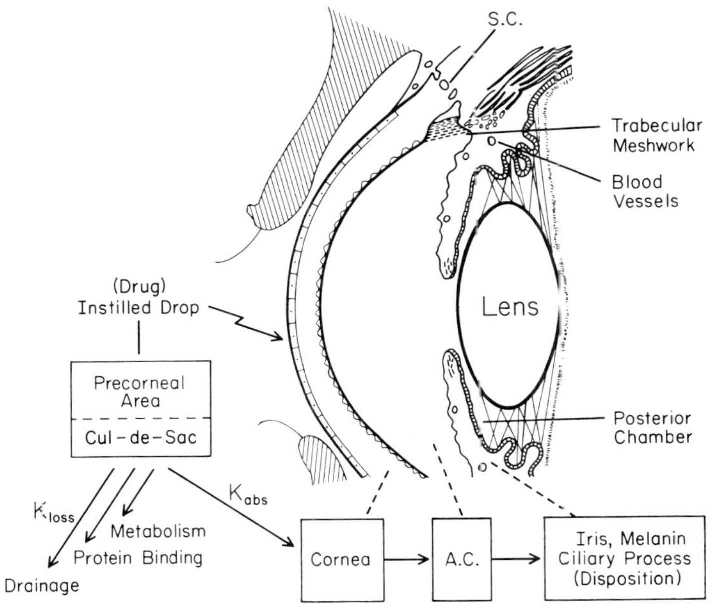


**FIG 2–1.**
Modeling of ocular compartments for the absorption ($K_{abs}$) and the disposition ($K_{loss}$) of a drug.[6] *A.C.* = anterior chamber; *S.C.* = Schlemm's canal. (From Mishima S, Masuda K, Tamura T: Drugs influencing aqueous humor formation and drainage. In Dickstein S, editor: *Drugs and ocular tissues,* New York, 1977, S Karger, pp 128–287; and Maurice DM, Mishima S: Ocular pharmacokinetics. In Sears ML, editor: *Pharmacology of the eye: handbook of experimental pharmacology,* vol 69, New York, 1984, Springer-Verlag New York, p 21. Used by permission.)

humor, iris, ciliary body, vitreous, sclera, retina, and lens. Although it is widely practiced among pharmacokineticists, compartmental analysis has more conceptual utility than practical value for the clinician. It is, however, a useful aid to visualize how drugs distribute in the eye and to evaluate whether a therapeutically active concentration of drug is reached in the ocular target tissue in question.

## TOPICAL OCULAR PHARMACOKINETICS AND BIOPHARMACEUTICS

### Corneal Permeability

Often the first pharmacokinetic data obtained for a drug are the corneal permeability coefficient (CPC).[7, 9] The CPC, in units of centimeters per second, is the corneal flux divided by the product of the initial drug concentration *times* the corneal surface area *times* 360 (to convert hours to seconds). Kinetic data for the flux of drug across the isolated cornea, using excised rabbit or human corneas mounted in Ussing-type chambers, permit the calculation of corneal permeability coefficients. In a typical experiment the drug solution is added to the bathing medium on the epithelial side of the cornea, and the drug concentration as a function of time is measured in the fluid on the endothelial side. The values obtained for a large number of compounds of ophthalmic interest ranged from $0.44 \times 10^{-6}$ to $78.8 \times 10^{-6}$ cm/sec. Values smaller than $10 \times 10^{-6}$ cm/sec indicate poor penetration.[9] Low corneal permeation may be compensated to some degree by high pharmacologic potency.

A parabolic relationship between log permeability coefficient (LPC) and log octanol/water partition coefficient has been shown for a group of corticosteroids (Fig. 2–2). The optimum range for log partition coefficient was between 2.5 and 3.0.[9] For ionizable drugs, a similar relationship is obtained for the log distribution coefficient (LDC) and LPC. Thus, the introduction of functional groups into the chemical structure to alter the LPC or LDC value of a drug is a means of modifying the permeability coefficient.

Under the steady-state conditions that prevail in the isolated cornea experiments, the factors that normally influence corneal absorption in vivo, such as blinking, dilution by tear flow, nasolacrimal drainage, and conjunctival absorption, are absent.[9] Thus, the isolated cornea approach has both advantages and limitations for predicting the ocular absorption of a drug in the living organism. Nonetheless, it is useful to assess

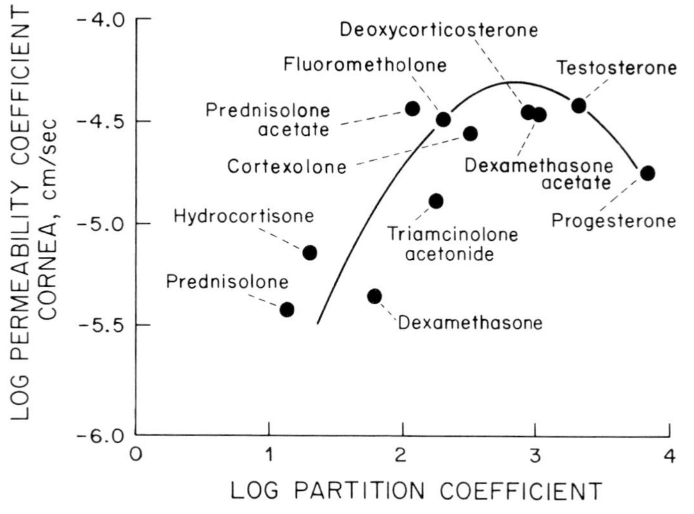


**FIG 2–2.**
Curvilinear relationship between the log permeability coefficient of corticosteroids and the respective log octanol/water partition coefficient. (From Schoenwald RD, Ward RL: *J Pharm Sci* 67:786, 1978. Used by permission.)

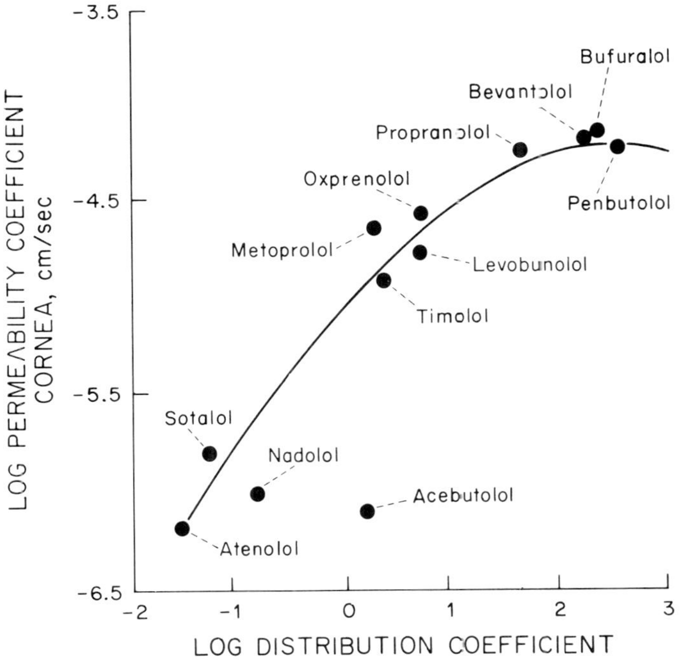


**FIG 2–3.**
The plot similar to that in Figure 2-2, except that data are for β-adrenoceptor-blocking drugs. The meaning of distribution coefficient is similar to partition coefficient except that it is preferred for ionizable drugs. (From Schoenwald RD, Huang HS: *J Pharm Sci* 72:1266, 1983. Used by permission.)

different drugs according to their relative permeability rates. This approach can assist in the selection of the drug in a series that exhibits the highest relative CPC and in the evaluation of substances that modify drug corneal penetration rates. The plot of log CPC vs. LDC measured in octanol/buffer for a series of β-adrenoceptor blockers exhibited an increase in permeability with an increase in distribution coefficient that reached a plateau at log values between 1.5 and 2.5 (Fig. 2–3).[9, 14]

## Ocular Bioavailability

Ocular bioavailability studies, which relate the amount of drug absorbed to the amount administered, are usually done in rabbits for reasons of economy and suitability. However, some significant dissimilarities in rabbit and human ocular anatomy and physiology such as a lower blink rate, a slower tear turnover rate, and the presence of the nictitating membrane make rabbits less than the ideal choice for ocular pharmacokinetic studies.[9] Furthermore, until recently, most studies have used albino rather than nonalbino rabbits, thereby ignoring such factors as drug binding to melanin pigment and drug metabolism within ocular tissues. Limited data have been obtained for human eyes by sampling the aqueous humor in patients undergoing anterior segment surgery, but considerable interindividual variability is seen, and only a single time point after administration is sampled in each individual. Noninvasive approaches using γ-scintigraphy and fluorophotometry have been used to study the kinetics of technetium-99m and fluorescein, respectively, in the precorneal area.[15, 16] Notwithstanding these efforts to obtain human data, the bulk of the information about ocular pharmacokinetics has come from rabbits.

## Transfer of Drug by Diffusion and Active Transport

Drug molecules pass between compartments by diffusion and active transport processes. Diffusion of a drug follows its concentration gradient and is related inversely to molecular size and directly to the temperature. Drug transport, active and passive, depends on the chemical structure and steric configuration of the molecule and is affected by competition of other substances for the transport system. Permeability coefficients for drugs are determined by measuring the drug concentration in compartments at various times.[4,6] It is common to determine the coefficients for the transfer of drug between cornea and aqueous humor, the removal of drug from the anterior chamber to the blood, the loss of drug with the tears, and the entry of drug from the plasma to the anterior chamber. The cornea and anterior chamber have dominant roles in the distribution of drugs within the eye. The symbols A and B are commonly used to denote the apparent elimination and absorption coefficients, respectively, between the cornea and the anterior chamber.[3] Thus, transfer coefficients can be used as a basis for drug comparisons and to gain a better understanding of the relative importance of each transfer process in the overall pharmacokinetic behavior of a drug.[4,6] Refer to the disposition of fluorescein in Fig. 2–4.

### Rates of Pharmacokinetic Processes

The order of kinetics of a pharmacokinetic process is a quantity obtained from the equation derived from experimental measurement of the process rate as a function of concentration. Many drug transfer processes follow first-order kinetics, in which the rate constant of transfer is proportional

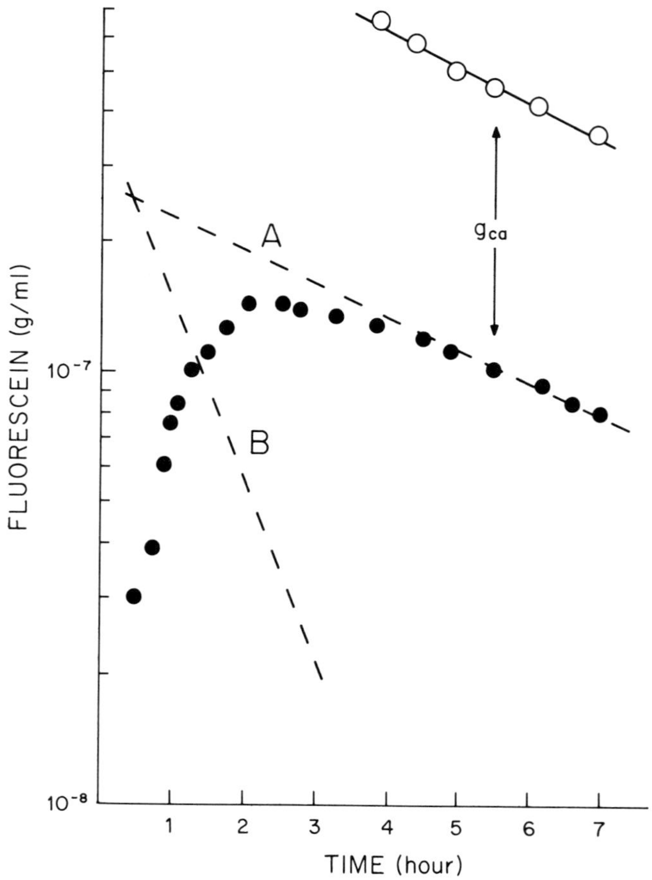


**FIG 2–4.**
Kinetics of fluorescein concentration in human eyes after instillation of 10% solution. The corneal concentration is in the upper curve and the aqueous humor concentration in the lower curve. The latter permits calculation of *A* and *B*, the *apparent* elimination and absorption rate constants. Cornea/aqueous concentration ratio ($g_{ca}$) in the parallel decrease phase. (From Mishima S: *Invest Ophthalmol* 21:504, 1981. Used by permission.)

to the drug concentration, and the drug half-life ($t\frac{1}{2}$) is a constant time regardless of the amount of drug administered. This is apparent from the equation for first-order half-life, $t\frac{1}{2} = 0.693/k$, where 0.693 is the natural logarithm of 2 and k is the proportionality constant from the differential equation relating the rate of change of concentration with time.[17] In a first-order process, concentration decreases exponentially with time, and on the curvilinear plot of concentration vs. time the concentration asymptotically approaches some final value as time advances toward infinity. The plot of log drug concentration (C) vs. time (t) is linear, and the value of C decreases by one half over each time interval corresponding to the half-life. For example, if the $t\frac{1}{2}$ is 1 hour and the initial drug concentration is 100 units, 50 units will remain after the first hour, 25 units after the second hour, 12.5 units after the third hour, and so forth. It is apparent that less than 1 unit will remain after the passage of seven half lives of the process. It is sometimes more convenient to think in terms of the time constant rather than the half-life. The time constant is the reciprocal of the first-order rate constant, that is, 1/k, or 1.443 times the half-life. It is the time interval required to reduce the initial concentration by 1/e of its initial value where e is the base of natural logarithms.[17] Commonly used ophthalmic drug formulations, such as solutions, gels, suspensions, and ointments, deliver drugs at rates that follow first-order kinetics unless the release characteristics of the formulation are altered to produce zero-order delivery.

A zero-order rate constant is not proportional to the drug concentration but is related to some functional capacity involved in the transfer of drug. Active transport systems change drug kinetics from first to zero order. When the transfer capacity is fully utilized, a higher concentration of the drug will not increase the transfer rate. Normally, it is free drug that diffuses between compartments. Drugs bound to tissue proteins or melanin must be free from their binding sites before the molecules diffuse. Pharmacologic response correlates best with the concentration of free drug at the site of action.[10]

Zero-order delivery of a drug to the eye would result if a constant concentration of the drug were maintained in the precorneal tear film to create a steady-state concentration in the tissues. The pilocarpine Ocusert is an example of a diffusion-controlled ophthalmic drug delivery system that delivers pilocarpine at a zero-order rate. Thus, the Ocusert releases pilocarpine at a constant rate to the tears over a finite time (Fig. 2–5).[1, 18 19]

## OCULAR ABSORPTION

Absorption of an ocular medication in the cul-de-sac begins with mixing of the drug with the tears to give some unknown dilution. The efficiency of ocular absorption depends on the adequate mixing of drug with the precorneal tear film and the residence time of the drug in the precorneal area.[6] The relatively stagnant precorneal tear film layer has a thickness of about 7 to 9 μm and forms a coacervate with mucin as it spreads over the corneal surface. A superficial oily layer secreted by the meibomian gland stabilizes the tear film.[20] Eyelid movements during blinking facilitate mixing of the drug with the precorneal tear film. There is incomplete saturation of the tear film with drug of about 46%. Data obtained for fluorescein show an increase in saturation with increasing instilled volume from 5 to 20 μL.[6]

A gradient of drug concentration between the precorneal tear film and the corneal and bulbar conjunctival epithelia acts as a driving force for passive drug diffusion into those tissues.[9] The time between the instillation of drug and its appearance in the aqueous humor is known as the lag time and it reflects the rate of diffusion of drug across the cornea. The amount of drug penetrating the eye is linearly related to its concentration in tears unless the drug interacts with other molecules present in the cornea or the cornea becomes saturated because of limited drug solubility.

The rate of decline of the drug concentration in the tears is proportional to the amount of drug remaining in the tears at the time; thus, it approximates first-order kinet-

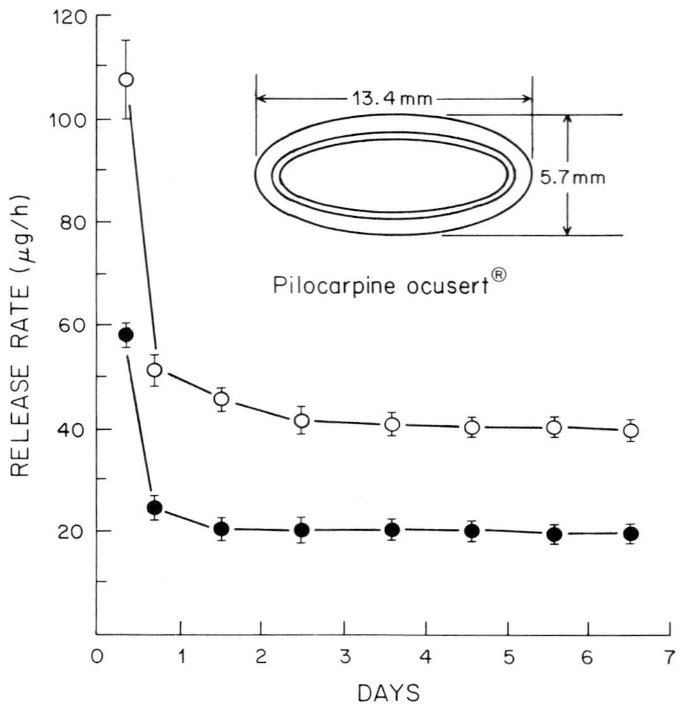


**FIG 2–5.**
In vitro, the zero-order rate of release of pilocarpine from the Ocusert. Pilo-20 and Pilo-40 ocular therapeutic system. (Courtesy of ALZA Corporation, Palo Alto, Calif.)

ics. It depends on the degree and rate of dilution by fresh tears and the drainage rate of tears from the cul-de-sac.[21, 22] The basal rate of tear flow in normal humans is approximately 1 μl/min and the physiologic turnover rate is 10% to 15%/min, which decreases with age. Basal tear flow is lower in patients with keratoconjunctivitis sicca and slightly higher in contact lens wearers.[21, 23] In rabbits, the average tear flow rate is 0.66 to 0.78 μl/min.[6] The half-life of the exponential decline of fluorescein in the precorneal tear film in normal humans measured by fluorophotometry varied from 2 to 20 minutes. Such variability applies to other substances as well. The loss rate constant for fluorescein varies depending on the amount of tearing. Reflex tearing caused by stinging on instillation of an irritating drug produces a higher loss rate. Eyelid closure, local anesthesia, and general anesthesia can decrease the tear flow rate. Physical, psychic, and emotional factors can increase tearing. Blinking movements force part of the instilled volume out through the puncta into the nasolacrimal duct. Each blink eliminates about 2 μL of fluid from the cul-de-sac.[6]

Aside from elimination by drainage through the nasolacrimal route and evaporation of tears and deposition of drug on the lid margins, drug may be bound to proteins in the tears and metabolized by enzymes in tears and tissue.[24] Such nonproductive processes tend to limit the amount of drug entering the eye. As a result of the limitation on residence time in the precorneal area imposed by these factors, but primarily because of rapid drainage, only a small fraction of the instilled dose (about 1%–10%) reaches the internal structures of the eye.[4] This fraction may be increased by prolonging the residence time of the drug at the ocular absorptive surfaces and enhancing the penetration rate of the drug through the corneal epithelium, generally by making the molecule more lipophilic. An example of the latter approach is the conversion of epinephrine to its dipivalyl ester derivative, which is more lipophilic but serves as a prodrug.[24] Transcorneal movement of a drug can be altered also by changes in the barrier properties of the corneal epithelium, for example, by applying a corneal anesthetic agent or after the damage of the epithelium.[9]

## DISTRIBUTION

### Blood to Aqueous Humor Transfer of Drug

The eye is relatively sequestered from the systemic circulation by the blood-retinal, blood-vitreal, and blood-aqueous barriers.[25] These barriers comprise the tight junctions between the capillary endothelial cells in the retina and iris, between the cells of the ciliary epithelium, and between the retinal pigment epithelium.[6] They exclude large molecules, such as plasma proteins, from entering the eye through the circulation but allow many small molecules (molecular weight ≤ 500 daltons) and drugs to pass. This barrier selectivity is evidenced by the low concentration of protein in the aqueous humor and the failure of fluorescein to appear in the aqueous humor after its intravenous injection unless the eye is inflamed. Organic acids are transported out of the eye by carrier-mediated transport systems, thus limiting the accumulation of a variety of these and related substances in ocular fluids.[26, 27] Because of the blood-ocular barriers, many drugs in the circulation find difficulty in reaching the ocular tissues.

### Aqueous Humor to Blood Transfer of Drug

The fraction of a drug that is absorbed into the eye can enter the systemic circulation along with the bulk flow of aqueous humor by way of the trabecular meshwork, Schlemm's canal, aqueous collecting channels, and intrascleral plexus into the circulation or by being absorbed into the blood vessels of the uvea, choroid, and retina. A drug that leaves with aqueous humor through the uveoscleral outflow pathway may be reabsorbed into the choroidal vessels from the suprachoroidal space.

### Drug Movement Within and Between Tissues and Fluids

Drug loss from the precorneal area limits the time available for absorption into the eye. The time to peak drug level in the eye is determined by the residence time.[28] Most drugs delivered topically to the eye exhibit similar apparent times to peak concentration in aqueous humor as the material drains out of the cul-de-sac within the first 5 minutes. For this reason, the time it takes for most drugs to reach their peak concentration in the aqueous humor falls within a rather narrow range of 20 to 60 minutes.[3, 4] Within the cornea, drugs may diffuse laterally to the limbus and enter the eye at the iris root. Drug also may be absorbed from the cul-de-sac across the conjunctiva and enter the eye through the sclera. The sclera poses less of a barrier to hydrophilic drugs than does the cornea, but both are comparable toward lipophilic drugs.[4] However, the main route of drug entry to the anterior chamber is through the cornea. A drug partitions between the vehicle and the tears thence into the cornea and conjunctiva. Drugs in the aqueous humor equilibrate with drugs in the tissues in contact with that fluid. Drugs are not distributed uniformly within the eye. Molecules may selectively concentrate in certain parts, for example; phenothiazine concentrates in pigmented cells and silver in Descemet's membrane. Drugs are eliminated from the anterior chamber by bulk flow of aqueous humor for the most part. Normally the turnover of aqueous humor in human eyes is rapid, with a half-life of approximately 52 minutes. The aqueous humor turnover of rabbit eyes has a half-life of about 46 minutes.[7] In the case of drugs that act to decrease the flow of aqueous humor, their effect on the turnover of aqueous humor may alter the rate of disappearance of drug to favor a longer duration of action. Half-lives of topically applied drugs in aqueous humor of rabbits are presented in Table 2–1. This is a possibility for the interaction between a β-blocker and a carbonic anhydrase inhibitor, both of which decrease aqueous secretion. The duration of action of either drug may be prolonged by the other

**TABLE 2–1.**
Half-Lives (t½) of Drugs Applied Topically to the Rabbit Eye

| t½h* | Drug |
|---|---|
| 5.8 | Dapiprazole |
| 4.5 | 6-Mercaptopurine |
| 2.8 | Fusidic acid |
| 2.6 | Suprofen |
| 2.2 | Histamine |
| 2.2 | Cimetidine |
| 1.9 | Gentamicin |
| 1.7 | Diclofenac |
| 1.7 | Flurbiprofen |
| 1.5 | Fluorometholone acetate |
| 1.5 | Cefamandole |
| 1.2 | Timolol |
| 1.2 | Lincomycin |
| 1.0 | Cefsulodin |
| 1.0 | Fluorouracil |
| 1.0 | Aztreonam |
| 0.75 | Fluorometholone |
| 0.75 | Tobramycin |
| 0.72 | Pilocarpine |
| 0.61 | Pyrilamine |
| 0.34 | 1,3-*Bis*(2-chloroethyl)-1-nitrosourea (BCNU) |

Data from Schoenwald R: *Clin Pharmacokinet* 18:255, 1990.
*In aqueous humor.

through decreased turnover of aqueous humor. The aqueous humor half-lives reported for a number of drugs representing multiple pharmacologic classes, administered either topically, intracamerally, or subconjunctivally to rabbit eyes, vary from 0.23 hour for ethoxzolamide to 5.8 hours for dapiprazole.[4]

Pulsed delivery exhibits peaks and valleys in drug concentration, the effect may wax and wane, and the dosing frequency must be chosen to obtain a steady effect level.[5] For example, pilocarpine solution must be given three or four times daily because of its relatively short duration of action. This repeated administration results in the recurrence of the side effects, miosis and induced myopia, each time a drop is instilled, which is troublesome to the patient. As a result, patient compliance is adversely affected, and some glaucoma patients may be undertreated. To overcome the disadvantages of pulsed drug delivery and achieve sustained delivery are the objectives of developing controlled delivery systems.[24]

The distribution of drugs from the anterior chamber to the tissues of the posterior segment by anteroposterior diffusion is hindered by the presence of barriers such as the iris, ciliary body and lens, as well as by the bulk flow of aqueous humor forward through the pupil. Thus, the action of most topical ophthalmic drugs is largely expressed in the anterior segment tissues, because insufficient drug concentration is achieved in the posterior tissues. The occurrence of epinephrine-induced maculopathy in the aphakic eye is probably caused by lack of the lens. There are significant challenges to the delivery of drugs to the retina that must be met to obtain the benefits of local administration of ophthalmic medicaments for diseases of the retina.

After topical instillation, the highest concentrations of most drugs in descending order are found in the cornea, iris, ciliary body, aqueous humor, sclera, and conjunctiva. Much lower concentrations of drug occur in the lens, vitreous, and retina. When a drug is absorbed through the conjunctival route, the distribution pattern changes to conjunctiva, cornea, ciliary body, and aqueous humor.[4]

After the drug has transferred from precorneal area to the cornea, it can diffuse laterally within the corneal epithelium, stroma, and endothelium into the contiguous cells of adjoining tissues, but primarily it enters the aqueous humor.[4] From the aqueous humor, the drug can be taken up by the iris, ciliary body, and lens. Within the iris and ciliary body the drug may be absorbed into the blood vessels or transported into the circulation. Ultimately the drug enters various cells and acts on enzymes or receptors present in those cells. Drug molecules may be bound to proteins or pigment and are unavailable to act until freed from these binding sites.

### Drug-Melanin Interactions

As early as 1929 the curious relationship between the iris color and ocular drug effects was quantified.[29] After topical application the mydriatic effects of drugs were slower in onset in heavily pigmented irides compared with that of the lightly pigmented

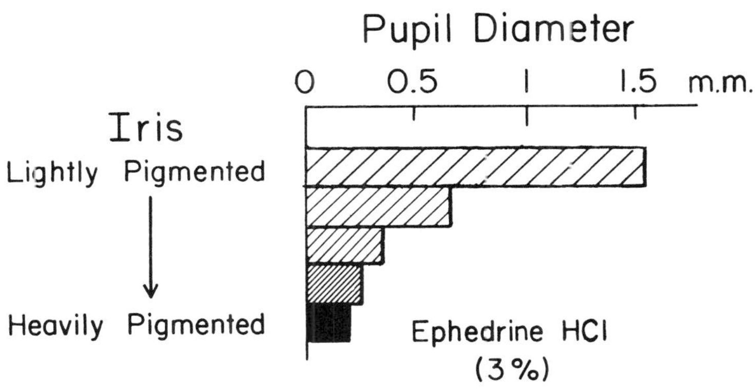


**FIG 2–6.**
Pupillary response to 3% ephedrine HCl applied topically to human eyes of various intensities of melanin pigmentation of iris. (From Obianwu HO, Rand MJ: *Br J Ophthalmol* 49:264, 1965. Used by permission.)

irides of human volunteers.[30] The maximum pupillary dilatation was also limited in the dark iris (Fig. 2–6). It has been demonstrated that large amounts of labeled atropine are bound by the melanin-containing iris of nonalbino rabbits compared with that of albino rabbits. Onset, as well as duration of drug action after topical application, correlated well with the retention of the drug in the melanin-containing iris. Duration of action of atropine was short in albino irises where very little drug was bound to the tissue.[31] Binding of drugs by melanin appears to be a very important factor in the control of drug action in ocular compartments. Many liposoluble drugs such as chloroquine, chlorpromazine, pilocarpine, timolol, propranolol, and antibiotics are bound by melanin from which the drugs can be slowly disposed (Figs. 2–7 and 2–8).[32] Accumulation of a high concentration of chloroquine in the retinal pigment epithelium can lead to local toxicity. The capacity of melanin to bind many liposoluble drugs is extensive. The binding of charged quaternary molecules is less extensive. In the case of atropine, the drug bound by mela-

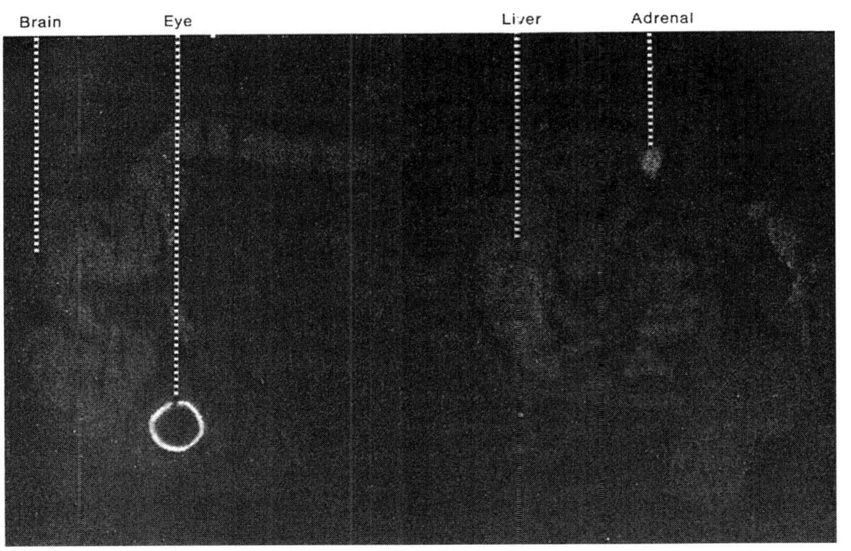


**FIG 2–7.**
Autoradiogram of a nonalbino mouse fetus 1 hour after an intravenous injection of chlorpromazine labeled with sulfur-35 to the pregnant mouse. (From Lindquist NG: *Acta Radiol* 325[suppl]:1, 1973. Used by permission.)

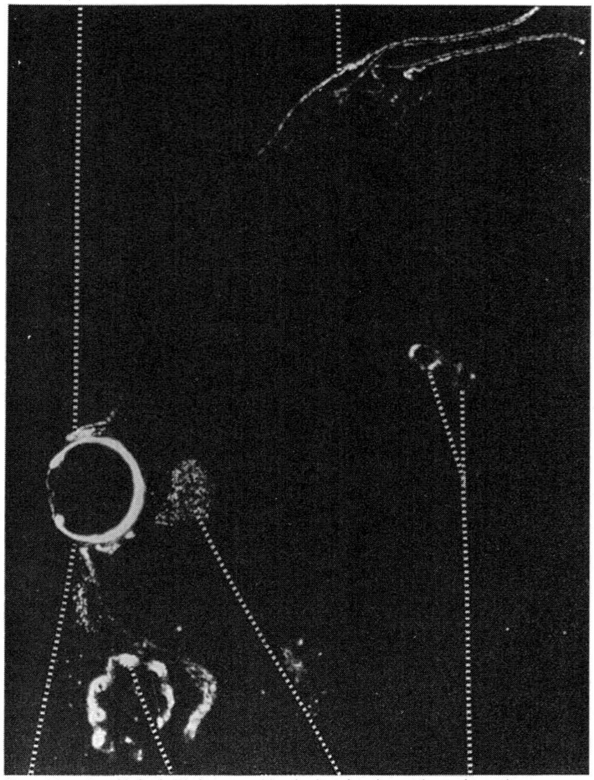


**FIG 2–8.**
Autoradiogram depicts the accumulation after 30 days of intravenous (±)-chloroquine labeled with carbon-14 in the melanin-containing ocular tissues, eyelids, Harder's gland, and superficial lymph nodes. (From Lindquist NG: *Acta Radiol* 325[suppl]:1, 1973. Used by permission.)

nin can be slowly released onto muscarinic receptors. In vitro, the miotic response of albino or nonalbino rabbit irises to the charged molecule carbachol is equal.[32] Thus, ocular drug response parameters may vary from individual to individual, depending on the degree of melanin pigmentation of the iris.

## OCULAR DRUG METABOLISM

Instilled drug can be metabolized by enzymes in the tears, adnexa, and ocular tissues.[33, 34] A broad range of active enzymes are reported in eye tissues. These include esterases (Table 2–2), oxidoreductases, lysosomal enzymes, peptidases, glucuro-

**TABLE 2–2.**
Esterase Activity in the Corneal Epithelium, Corneal Stroma, and Iris–Ciliary Body of Ocular Tissues

| | $10^2$ μmoles/min/mg Protein | | |
|---|---|---|---|
| Ocular Tissue | Albino Rabbit | Nonalbino Rabbit | Human |
| Corneal epithelium | 5.43 | 9.43 | 23.05 |
| Corneal stroma | 3.13 | 2.91 | 6.95 |
| Iris–ciliary body | 5.17 | 5.88 | 8.07 |

From Lee VHL, Robinson JR: *J Ocul Pharmacol* 2:67, 1986. Used by permission.

nide and sulfate transferases, glutathione-conjugating enzymes, catechol-O-methyltransferase, monoamine oxidase, and corticosteroid β-hydroxylase. Butyrylcholinesterase, acetylcholinesterase, and carboxylesterase were found in the anterior tissues of rabbit eyes. The esterases in some rabbits can easily limit the duration of mydriatic action of atropine (Fig. 2–9). Butyrylcholinesterase comprises the largest fraction of cholinesterase activity in rabbit ocular tissues, except for the albino rabbit corneal epithelium. Esterase activity in the cornea is involved in the conversion of ester prodrugs, for example, dipivalylepinephrine, to their parent compounds. Cholinesterase inhibitors may interfere with prodrug ester hydrolysis in the eye, thereby modifying the drug effect.[35] Moreover, butyrylcholinesterase is more susceptible to substrate than to product inhibition, and physiologic substrates such as peptides and amino acids may affect prodrug hydrolysis. The metabolite of levobunolol, dihydrobunolol, was present in aqueous humor of albino rabbits after topical administration of a racemic mixture of that β-adrenoceptor blocker.[36] This is in contrast to the lack of pilocarpine metabolism in albino rabbit eyes after topical administration. Significant metabolism of pilocarpine to pilocarpic acid was found in rabbit eyes containing melanin.

### Stereochemical Factors

Chiral molecules possess an asymmetric carbon atom in the structure and exist in two enantiomeric forms, dextro (*d*) and levo (*l*), which rotate polarized light in opposite directions.[37] Well-known chiral molecules are amino acids and the catecholamines epinephrine and norepinephrine. The equal mixture of the two enantiomers is called a racemate. Drug transfer across biologic membranes, drug metabolism, and drug-receptor interaction can be stereoselective. One of the stereoisomers is generally preferred by the enzyme, the transporter, or the receptor. Naturally occurring *l*-epinephrine or *l*-norepinephrine is physiologically

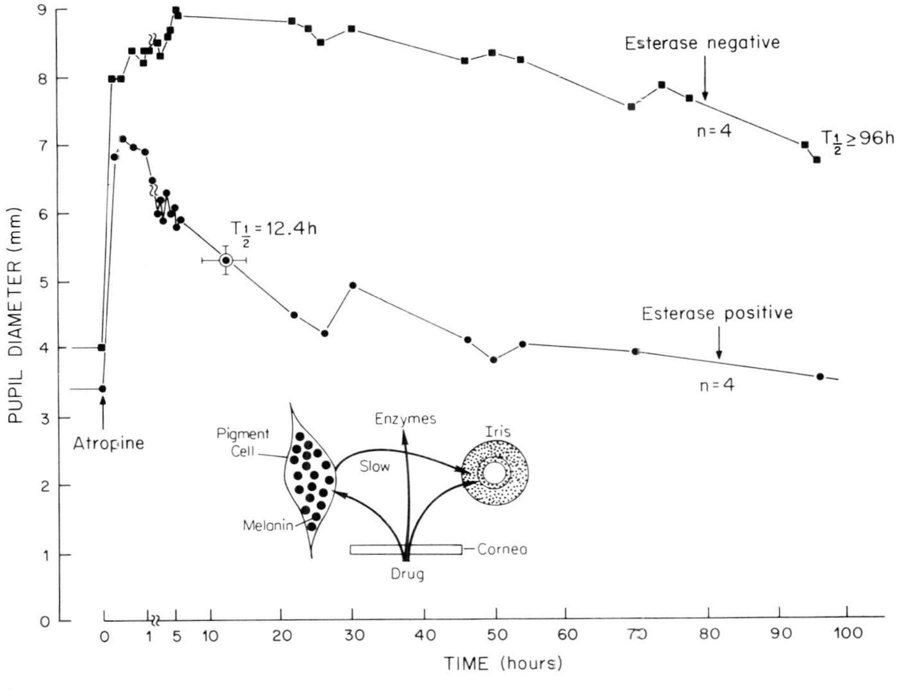


**FIG 2–9.**
Duration of mydriatic response to 0.05 ml of topical 2% atropine sulfate in rabbits with heavily pigmented irides. Note the contribution of aqueous esterases and the drug binding to melanin in limiting the intensity and the duration of the response. Schematic illustration depicts the routes of drug disposition. (From Patil PN: *Trends Pharmacol Sci* 5:201, 1984. Used by permission.)

more active than the unnatural *d*-isomer.[38] When infused, more *l*-norepinephrine is readily taken up by the transport system in noradrenergic neurons than the *d*-form. The *l*-propranolol is 100 times more potent as a β-adrenoceptor blocker than is *d*-propranolol. The local anesthetic effects of both propranolol isomers, however, are equal. The antimuscarinic action of (−)-tropicamide is at least 30 times greater than that of the (+)-isomer (*l* and *d* isomers may be designated as [−] and [+], respectively). Occasionally drugs containing chiral centers are available as racemates even though the therapeutic benefit may be derived primarily from one isomer. The less active isomer may compete with the more active one for an enzyme, a transport system, or the receptor. The metabolic disposition of the racemic drug may appear highly complex because the ratio of the molecular species; *d/l* can change in an unpredictable way. In body fluids, one isomer may be converted into the other, leading to racemization of the drug. Occasionally the "inactive" isomer may exhibit toxicity. Generally where there is an advantage to the use of a single isomer over a racemate, it will become the preferred form of the drug made available. The possible differences in behavior between isomers and racemate should be kept in mind when new medications are investigated clinically.[39]

## PHYSICOCHEMICAL FACTORS

For most topically applied ophthalmic drugs, the transcorneal route of absorption is the dominant one. Drugs may move across the corneal epithelium transcellularly and intercellularly or paracellularly. Nevertheless, the transconjunctival and transscleral routes serve as alternate pathways, particularly for hydrophilic drugs and to the iris and ciliary body.[3, 6] Administration of drugs intended to affect different parts of the eye must be guided by knowledge of the permeability of the various ocular structures.

The penetration of medications through the intact cornea is not a matter of simple diffusion but is best explained by a differential solubility concept. The cornea may be thought of as a fat-water-fat multilayered sandwich. Within the cornea, the epithelial cell layer poses the major barrier to absorption and more so for hydrophilic (water-loving) than for lipophilic (fat-loving) drugs or fat-soluble substances. Chemical analysis shows the lipid content of the epithelium and endothelium to be 100 times greater than that of the corneal stroma. The corneal stroma is more of a barrier to lipophilic than to hydrophilic drugs. The corneal epithelium is more tortuous but less porous than the stroma. However, the stroma and the monolayer of corneal endothelial cells act as a single barrier or compartment. Therefore, a drug with an optimum ratio of hydrophilicity and lipophilicity is best suited for transfer through the cornea. Very hydrophilic drugs will not diffuse well through the corneal epithelium, whereas high accumulation of lipophilic drugs will hinder the transport system (Table 2–3). The water solubility should not be confused with the partitioning behavior of a molecule, which is its preference to reside in either the lipid or aqueous phase at equilibrium. A highly water-soluble drug may be more or less lipophilic. Certainly it is only a drug in solution that can passively diffuse to be absorbed.

The differential solubility theory of penetration of the cornea by an alkaloidal weak base, for example, atropine, or other amino substituted compound such as epinephrine, is illustrated in Figure 2–10, in which $R_3N$ represents the nonionized, more lipophilic, less hydrophilic form of the drug. This exists in equilibrium with the ionized, more hydrophilic, less lipophilic form, $R_3NH^+$. The ratio of ionized to nonionized substance is determined by the pH and the dissociation constant (the negative log of which is denoted as $pK_a$ for weak acids and $pK_b$ for weak bases) according to the Henderson-Hasselbalch equation: $pH = pK_a + \log[\text{salt}]/[\text{acid}]$ for weak acids or $pH = (14 - pK_b) + \log[\text{base}]/[\text{salt}]$ for weak bases.[40] The salt and the acid or base forms represent the ionized and the nonionized forms, respectively. The sum of $pK_a$ and $pK_b$ equals 14, which is the range of the pH scale. Rearranging the equation for weak bases gives $\log[\text{base}]/[\text{salt}] = pH + pK_b - 14$. When the pH is numerically the same as the $pK_a$, a weak acid exists as a 50:50 mixture of its

**TABLE 2–3.**

Percentage Contribution of Each Corneal Barrier to Drug Permeability*

| Drug | Percentage Resistance of Corneal Barrier: Epithelium | Stroma | Endothelium | Log DC† |
|---|---|---|---|---|
| Lipophilic | | | | |
| Bevantolol | 7 | 44 | 49 | 2.19 |
| Bufuralol | 18 | 50 | 32 | 2.31 |
| Penbutolol | 1 | 46 | 53 | 2.53 |
| Propranolol | 7 | 45 | 48 | 1.62 |
| Slightly lipophilic | | | | |
| Cyclophosphamide | 72 | 10 | 13 | 0.38 |
| Levobunolol | 58 | 15 | 27 | 0.72 |
| Metoprolol | 48 | 18 | 34 | 0.28 |
| Oxprenolol | 45 | 21 | 34 | 0.69 |
| Timolol | 68 | 9 | 23 | 0.34 |
| Hydrophilic | | | | |
| Acebutolol | 91 | 1 | 8 | 0.20 |
| Atenolol | 97 | 1 | 2 | −1.52 |
| Nadolol | 95 | 1 | 4 | −0.82 |
| Phenylephrine | 95 | 1 | 4 | −1.00 |
| Sotalol | 95 | 1 | 4 | −1.25 |
| Tobramycin | 95 | 1 | 4 | < −2.00 |

Data from Schoenwald R: The control of drug bioavailability from ophthalmic dosage forms. In Smolen VF, Ball LA, editors: *Controlled drug bioavailability*, vol 3, New York, 1985, John Wiley & Sons, p. 257.
*Values determined from various excised rabbit corneal preparations in which epithelium and endothelial layers were removed to interpret individual barrier resistances to drug permeability
†Octanol/buffer (pH 7.65) distribution coefficient.

ionized and nonionized forms. For each unit of pH change, the ratio of acid or base to salt in the mixture changes tenfold, and the two forms occur in equilibrium in solution. Thus, the pH of the tears or the physiologic compartment in which the drug resides and the dissociation constant of the drug determine its degree of ionization, which influences its absorption characteristics. For example, atropine is a weak base with a $pK_b$ of 4.35. At the physiologic pH of tears, 7.4, the ratio of atropine in base form to salt form is 1:5,620. Thus, at pH 7.4 there will be 5,620 times more molecules of the atropine present in the ionized form than in the nonionized form. Although both ionized and nonionized alkaloid exists in the tears, the nonionized form penetrates more readily into the corneal epithelium but subsequently less readily into the stroma. In the stroma, it is the ionized form that traverses more readily than the nonionized form. The endothelium may or may not pose a significant barrier to the passage of the ionized form, and frequently the stroma and endothelium behave as a single barrier to drug distribution. An ionized and/or unionized form of a drug may interact with the receptor.

Positively charged quaternary amines, such as carbachol, exist in their ionized form and pass through the corneal epithelium with great difficulty. Likewise, fluorescein, a carboxylic acid, in its negatively charged form penetrates the epithelium quite poorly and is delivered more effectively to the aqueous humor by use of iontophoresis. Biomicroscopy shows no staining of the cornea or aqueous after fluorescein instillation on the normal intact cornea. However, if the epithelium is damaged, fluorescein enters the stroma. Disruption of epithelial integrity modifies its barrier property and allows poorly penetrating drugs to be absorbed more freely.

The structural and physiologic similarity of the conjunctival epithelium to that of the cornea is well known. That this similarity

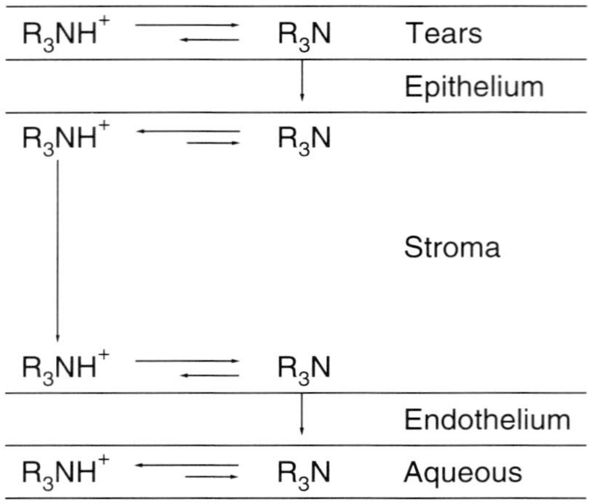


**FIG 2–10.**
Transcorneal movement of ionized and nonionized form of a drug into aqueous humor.

includes permeability characteristics is demonstrated clinically with the application of fluorescein.[6] The normal intact conjunctiva and the underlying subconjunctival, episcleral, and sclera tissues do not stain with fluorescein; thus, the surface must be resistant to the penetration of this and other electrolytes. The intact conjunctiva is resistant to the passage of molecules. This has been demonstrated by the appearance of 5.5% of the total dose of radiolabeled hydrocortisone in the tears after its subconjunctival injection because of leakage of the drug out of the opening created by the needle. When the injection of hydrocortisone was given through the eyelid, no hydrocortisone entered the tears across the intact conjunctiva.[41]

The transconjunctival-scleral route serves as a possible alternative to the transcorneal one for penetration of drugs into intraocular tissues, although current examples of delivery systems (aside from injections) that employ that route are not available.[42] The sclera is a relatively porous structure, far less of a barrier than the corneal epithelium, and permits the passage of large molecules such as dextran (molecular weight 40,000 daltons). However, the pressure gradient produced by the intraocular pressure results in a strong unidirectional outward flow, and even from the suprachoroidal location, labeled molecules do not penetrate readily inward. Clearly, the intraocular penetration of substances injected into Tenon's space will be minimal because of this rapid transscleral outflow.

There is some evidence that the transconjunctival route is a more common one for substances that are more hydrophilic. Inulin, a linear polymer of D-glucose and D-fructose (molecular weight approximately 5,000 daltons), is absorbed into the eye via the noncorneal route, which is responsible for nearly 40% of its entry into ocular tissues. Perhaps this route will be used more to permit delivery of drugs to more posterior tissues within the eye once it is better understood.

### Cul-de-sac Compartment

The cul-de-sac compartment is the space into which topical eye medications are instilled. The human cul-de-sac has a volume of about 7 μl, which can expand momentarily and variably to 30 μl. That fraction of an instilled drop that is in excess of the cul-de-sac volume drains into the nasolacrimal duct within 15 seconds after instillation or is lost by overflow to the cheek with forceful blinking. A normal blink eliminates about 2 μl of excess fluid from the cul-de-sac.[6]

### Eye Drop Volume

The volume of eye drops delivered from commercial product containers is typically in the 25- to 35-μl range but can be as high as 75 μl. Currently the practical lower limit of drop volume deliverable from commercial containers is about 20 to 25 μl without further modification of the container's tip. Studies with specially constructed drop delivery tips using phenylephrine have shown that similar pupillary dilatation is achieved when the drop size is reduced from 30 to 8 μl. Furthermore, the systemic absorption of the drug decreases substantially when the drop volume is reduced. For optimum ocular bioavailability, the drop size should be 20 μl or less.[43–46]

Instillation of multiple drops at one time, in the belief that it will increase ocular bioavailability, achieves little more than to increase the possibility for delivering a larger systemic dose, which could result in a higher incidence of side effects or toxicity. If a drop of one medication is followed closely by a drop of another medication or of saline solution, a substantial washout occurs with a concomitant lessening of the effect.[47–50] A 30-second interval between drops results in a 45% washout loss of drug effect, whereas a 2-minute interval results in only 17% loss of effect. After a 5-minute interval, a second drop will cause almost no washout effect on the first drop. When instillation of 1% prednisolone phosphate solution was followed by an antibiotic drop at 30 seconds, the corneal concentration of prednisolone was reduced from 8.96 to 3.89 μg/g. If the second drop was given at 60 seconds, the corticosteroid concentration was reduced only to 5.09 μg/g. After 120 seconds, the washout reduced the concentration by a still lesser degree to 6.85 μg/g.[51]

In the normal, nonirritated eye, the tear turnover rate averages 16%/min. Instillation of the average drop stimulates lacrimation to increase the turnover rate to 30%/min. The washout effect of this spontaneous tear flow results in almost complete disappearance of an instilled drug from the cul-de-sac within 5 minutes. At least 80% of the eye drop–applied drug leaves via lacrimal drainage and not by entering the eye. In general, drugs are readily absorbed across the highly vascularized nasopharyngeal mucosa into the systemic circulation.

### Nasolacrimal Occlusion

Much study has been given to punctal occlusion as a means of decreasing systemic absorption and increasing ocular absorption of topical ophthalmic drugs, thereby improving the therapeutic index.[48, 49] Nasolacrimal occlusion for 3 minutes during and immediately after drug instillation did not alter the intraocular pressure response to 0.5% and 2% epinephrine or 0.1% dipivefrin in normal healthy individuals or to all except 0.5% epinephrine in glaucoma patients.[50] However, it has been claimed that nasolacrimal occlusion allows a reduction in the dosage and frequency of administration of the antiglaucoma drugs, carbachol, timolol, and pilocarpine but results in similar efficacy as that obtained by the usual dosage regimens for these drugs.[51] The benefit of nasolacrimal occlusion should be determined individually for patients, and assurance as to the patient's compliance and proper performance of the procedure should be obtained before relying on it. The patient must be trained to perform punctal occlusion properly or its benefit is not realized. Improper performance of nasolacrimal occlusion can have a massaging effect and may promote the passage of drug into the nasolacrimal duct. Simple eyelid closure, so that the lacrimal pump system is not activated, also can reduce nasolacrimal drainage of topical medication. Care should be taken that it is done gently and not forcefully or repetitively. When this was done in conjunction with forming a pouch of the lower cul-de-sac by holding the lower eyelid everted while the patient looked upward, 53% of the instilled drug remained after 5 minutes in contrast to only 16% when the patient was allowed normal blinking and eye movement.[52]

## PERMEABILITY OF OCULAR STRUCTURES

### Absorption from the Systemic Compartment

#### *Blood-Ocular Barriers*

The blood-ocular barriers comprise the tight junctions between the vascular endothelial cells of the capillaries in the retina and iris, between the retinal epithelial cells, and between the nonpigmented ciliary epithelial cells.[25] The permeability or leakiness of the iris blood vessels increases during inflammation. The ciliary epithelium blocks the entry of most molecules from the circulation (e.g., proteins and antibiotics) into the aqueous humor. Damage to the blood-ocular barriers, resulting from injury or inflammation and manifested clinically by aqueous flare from protein leakage into the aqueous humor, may result in greatly increased entry into the eye of molecules otherwise excluded. Otherwise, drug access to the eye from the circulation is governed by the same factors that influence absorption through the corneal and conjunctival barriers. Transport systems, such as the anion transport within the ciliary body, can remove acceptable substrates such as prostaglandins from the eye and prevent their accumulation.

The bioavailability of drugs into the eye from the circulation is not well studied. Certainly drugs taken systemically do exert effects in the eye. Small molecules of less than 500-dalton molecular weight may pass readily through the blood-ocular barrier. Oral carbonic anhydrase inhibitors are useful to lower intraocular pressure. The intraocular pressure–lowering effect of β-adrenoceptor blockers was first described from their oral administration. Ocular tissues are no doubt the target site for circulating endogenous hormones. The oral route for the delivery of drugs to the eye is considered as inefficient because higher doses must be given. Substantial blood levels are required to achieve active concentrations in the eye, and systemic side effects may be a problem. Nevertheless, it is common practice to use systemic antibiotics in the therapy of ocular infection. More study is needed regarding the ocular bioavailability of systemic medication.

### *Topical Application*

Placing a drop of medication directly on the eye incorrectly implies that the drug is indeed delivered solely to the eye and remains there to carry out its function.[53, 54] This misconception is reflected in the multiple reports of adverse systemic reactions to ocularly instilled drugs. Such reports have increased with alarming frequency because ophthalmic drugs have become increasingly potent and possess the potential to cause significant effects in other parts of the body. The use of β-adrenergic blockers in treating glaucoma is an important example. Ocular instillation of some β-blockers poses a significant health hazard to patients with cardiopulmonary disease, particularly to patients who have previously undiagnosed asthma or chronic obstructive pulmonary disease.[54] Plasma levels of some topically applied medications are listed in Table 2–4. The use of cyclopentolate and other anticholinergics in children has been associated with psychotic reactions and behavioral disturbances, as well as other toxic manifestations.[55] A commonly heard admonition to parents is to press over the tear sac of the child after atropine instillation. Indeed, when properly executed, nasolacrimal occlusion can be an effective means of decreasing the systemic absorption of an instilled drug.[48, 49]

It must be borne in mind that drugs entering the circulation via nasolacrimal absorption are carried first to the heart and lungs, bypassing the liver, and thereby avoid the first-pass metabolism that normally can occur when drugs are absorbed from the gastrointestinal tract. In fact, in some instances, ocular instillation can be tantamount to intravenous injection. Thus, the metabolism and pharmacokinetic behavior of drugs absorbed after ocular instillation are likely to be different from those with other routes of administration. Indeed, ocular instillation is being considered as a route of administration for metabolically labile substances, for example, peptide hormones such as insulin and growth hormone.

Although modern ocular drug delivery methods under investigation are aimed at increasing or prolonging the ocular absorption of instilled drugs, some seek to minimize the systemic absorption to avoid side effects. So-called soft metabolizable drugs are known that are rapidly metabolized and inactivated when absorbed into the circulation but not so in the eye.[24] If ocular tissues that are targets for drug action were found

**TABLE 2–4.**
Peak Plasma Concentration and 1-Hour Concentration After Topical Application of Drug Eye Drops* to Healthy Adult Volunteers or Patients

| Drug | Dose (μg) | 1-hr Plasma (ng/ml) | Peak Plasma (ng/time) |
|---|---|---|---|
| Timolol | 150* | 1 4 | ND‡ |
| Timolol | 100 | 0 5 | 0.7/30 min |
| Levobunolol | 250† | 0.2–0.3 | ND |
| | 500† | 0.4–0.6 | ND |
| Atropine | 400 | 0 4 | 0.9/8 min |
| Cyclopentolate | 300 + 300 | 3 3 | 8.3/5–15 min |
| Scopolamine | 100 | 0 2 | 0.5/8 min |
| Phenylephrine | 1,250† | 0 2 | 3.0/10 min |
| | 5,000 | 1 7 | 10.2/10 min |
| Betamethasone | 25† | 0 2 | 0.2/3 hr |
| | 50† | 0 5 | 0.5/30 min |

From Salminen L: *J Ocul Pharmacol* 6:243, 1990. Used by permission
*Eye drop volume 40 μl.
†No eye drop volume, estimation 30 μl.
‡ND, Not determined.

to possess unique receptors different from those found in other organs, perhaps systemic side effects could be avoided altogether. It is possible that site-directed drug delivery can be achieved, for example, drugs that are preferentially absorbed through the cornea instead of the conjunctival or nasolacrimal mucosae. Should the cornea possess different esterases than these tissues, it might be possible to use a prodrug ester that is preferentially cleaved in the cornea to obtain site-directed delivery of inactive drug moiety. Alternatively, a substance that enhances corneal penetration over conjunctival or nasolacrimal penetration might make this possible. An ion pairing approach between drugs that are large organic anions or cations and counterions, for example, benzalkonium chloride, to mask the charge has been proposed. The modification of the pharmacokinetic properties of a drug by combining it with an entity to promote corneal absorption offers a practical approach to site-directed delivery of ophthalmic drugs.

It is possible to limit the access of drug to the brain across the blood-brain barrier, thereby reducing the chance for an action on the central nervous system (CNS). This may be achieved by modifying the drug's physicochemical properties to increase its degree of ionization at physiologic pH or to increase its hydrophilicity. Apraclonidine is an example of a drug that employs this approach.[56] It is both hydrophilic and highly ionized at physiologic pH so that very little enters the CNS where it may cause sedation and lower blood pressure. However, making a drug less permeable to the blood-brain barrier may also render it less permeable to the cornea, which could result in reduced ocular bioavailability. To some degree, this can be overcome by including a corneal penetration enhancer in the drug vehicle to promote the drug's absorption into the eye. Because the vehicle comes in contact with the cornea to exert its effect on it but does not with the blood-brain barrier, some degree of selective ocular over systemic absorption can be achieved.

### Influences of Vehicle on Drug Ocular Bioavailability

The vehicle in which a drug is applied affects the kinetics of its corneal and conjunctival penetration. The residence time of the drug in contact with the cornea and conjunctiva determines the extent of absorption. More viscous vehicles prolong ocular contact and thereby may increase the fraction of drug absorbed into the eye. However, there is a limited range of viscosities at the low end over which residence time is prolonged and its full benefit is achieved. Furthermore, in the case of highly viscous gels, the effectiveness depends on such factors as the shearing of the gel by blinking movements to provide a fresh surface for release of drug to the cornea, the hydrophilicity of the gelling polymer, and the diffusion constant of the drug within the gel vehicle.

The rate at which a drug is absorbed depends on its partitioning behavior, that is, its ability to move between the aqueous and lipid phases of the vehicle, tears, cornea, and conjunctiva. Oily vehicles, such as ointments, compete with the corneal epithelium for lipophilic substances and may retard their absorption somewhat. However, this has limited clinical significance because the concentration of drug in the formulation has usually been chosen to compensate for this and to give the desired pharmacologic effect.

Many other factors, such as pH, tonicity, electrolyte composition, wetting effects, and stability, enter into the design of the vehicle. Preservatives, buffers, and antioxidants may be added. Drug incompatibilities must be avoided, particularly when a combination of drugs is involved. Optimal drug concentrations and useful drug combinations are selected on the basis of preclinical and clinical test results. Accuracy is vital. Sterility in the original container is required by law. Stringent regulatory criteria are applied to the efficacy of the preservative system in the formulation to assure that it can safely and adequately handle the contamination that is inevitable during repeated use of the product. Because of these many requirements, drug compounding for ophthalmic use has become the responsibility of highly specialized pharmaceutical manufacturers; however, the local pharmacist will occasionally formulate ophthalmic solutions, such as fortified antibiotics, and must be aware of the principles involved that are unique to the eye.

#### *Hydrogen Ion Concentration (pH)*

The pH of an ophthalmic formulation is based on many factors and may influence the comfort of the ophthalmic formulation. The pH-stability profile of the drug is studied, and the pH needed to achieve the optimum conditions of chemical and physical stability for the formulation is selected. Hopefully that is a suitable pH to ensure the solubility of the active ingredient, as well as of the adjuvant ingredients, such as the preservative and any viscosity-imparting polymers. A buffer system may be included to overcome the drift in pH that might occur as carbon dioxide enters the container or is driven off in a high ambient temperature. In some instances, if the drug is a weak acid or weak base, it may itself provide the necessary buffering action should its $pK_a$ be in the appropriate range. The preservative effectiveness may be influenced by the pH, and this must be taken into account. Depending on the volume of the eye drop, the pH of the tears, which have their own buffer system, may be temporarily altered after instillation because of the overwhelming effect of the product's buffer. The buffering strength is kept to a minimum whenever possible to avoid this, so that the tears are able to resist a prolonged change in their pH. On the other hand, changing the pH of the tears momentarily to increase the amount of unionized drug present may be useful to increase the bioavailability of a drug with a $pK_a$ that is too high or too low. Although the eye tolerates a rather broad range in pH without tissue changes, very low pH may cause discomfort and elicit reflex tearing. This can cause excessive washout of the drug to interfere with absorption. Gels and other highly viscous formulations that contain buffers can change the pH of the cul-de-sac environment for more prolonged periods of time. The pH of the tears may modify the drug effectiveness.[57, 58]

#### *Osmolality and Tonicity*

Tear osmolality arises from the dissolved electrolytes, proteins, and crystalloids.[59] It varies between 302 and 318 mOsm/kg with the eyelids open, increasing by 1.43 mOsm/kg/hr during the day and 288 and 293 mOsm/kg after prolonged eyelid closure. Ophthalmic solutions that provoke discomfort or irritation have been found to have osmolalities less than 266 and greater than 445.[58] The osmolality of the tears can be altered in certain disease states, such as keratoconjunctivitis sicca.[20, 21] The tonicity of ophthalmic products is generally adjusted to a physiologically compatible value by using sodium chloride. In cases where a "salting out" effect of sodium chloride may reduce the solubility of the drug or other ingredients, the nonionizing substance mannitol may be used. The eye probably tolerates hypotonic solutions better than it does hypertonic ones. Excessive ranges of tonicity can elicit reflex tearing.

### *Viscosity*

Viscosity is an important formulation parameter because it can influence the residence time of a drug vehicle in the cul-de-sac.[7, 9, 15, 60] By prolonging the residence time, the flux (amount per unit of time) of drug through the cornea is increased, thereby increasing its ocular bioavailability. Prolonging contact time is presently achieved by increasing the viscosity of the drug vehicle using, for example, such cellulosic hydrophilic polymers as hydroxypropylmethylcellulose (HPMC) and hydroxyethylcellulose (HEC),[61] polyvinylpyrrolidone, carbopol, hyaluronan,[62] and polyvinylalcohol (PVA).[63] An example of this approach is the pilocarpine delivery system employing carbopol gel.[64, 65] In some cases, the surface tension of the formulation is reduced by the polymers that may facilitate mixing with the tears. The viscosities of solutions containing 0.5% HPMC and 1.4% PVA, which are the concentrations usually used in ophthalmic products, are about 20 and 10 cp or less, respectively. The addition of drug and adjuvants to the solutions may add to the viscosity. For a pilocarpine solution, when HPMC was added, the drainage rate from rabbit eyes was decreased by threefold as viscosity increased from 1 to 12.5 cp, and the aqueous humor levels increased by 60%. Another threefold decrease in drainage rate occurred over the viscosity range from 12.5 to 100 cp. Apparently the bulk of the benefit of viscosity is obtained within the range of 12 to 15 cp. Furthermore, at viscosities of 30 cp and higher, the polymers can impart a sticky feel to the formulation, making it uncomfortable to use.[61, 63]

Maintaining a drug in contact with the cornea and conjunctiva longer permits a greater fraction of it to enter the eye, with correspondingly less available to enter the systemic circulation. However, even if the amount entering the eye were to double, for example, from 5% to 10%, there remains 90% of the drug that is available for systemic absorption. Solid drug, representative of a zero volume dosage form, dissolves in the normal tear volume present and is least likely to result in excessive dilution and washout. This too reduces the chance for systemic absorption and increases the fraction of drug absorbed through the cornea and conjunctiva.

In lieu of increasing residence time, the bioavailability can be increased by increasing the rate constant for penetration so that more drug enters per unit time. An example of this approach is to make the dipivalyl ester of epinephrine, which is more lipophilic and acts as a prodrug.

### *Chemical Degradation of Drugs*

Depending on their chemical nature, drugs can undergo various chemical reactions that could result in their inactivation or the formation of an unacceptable compound.[66] In the case of an ester, hydrolysis is the reaction requiring control in formulating the drug. Hydrolysis may be acid or base catalyzed, so adjustment of the pH with appropriate buffering may be all that is needed to maintain a useful shelf life, desirably 2 years, for the formulation. When spontaneous hydrolysis occurs at an unacceptable rate, it may be necessary to formulate the drug in its freeze-dried (lyophilized) form for reconstitution by the pharmacist. In this case, the drug solution is made when the vehicle and the drug are mixed together by the pharmacist at the time of dispensing. Even then, the stability of the reconstituted product may be so limited as to require special storage conditions (e.g., refrigeration) and its discarding after a stated amount of time. Oxidation, for example, as occurs with epinephrine, may be catalyzed by light and affected by pH and temperature. The use of opaque containers, the use of antioxidants, and buffering of the pH serve to inhibit this degradative process.

The presence of adjuvants in a formulation to control pH, instability, and viscosity adds to its complexity and can be a source of discomfort or irritation, which may reduce the acceptability of the product to the patient. The achievement of a pharmaceutically elegant, comfortable, stable, safe, and effective ophthalmic product is dependent on skill and multiple factors. Some otherwise worthwhile drugs may never be made available because of the infeasibility of meeting all the necessary requirements of an acceptable formulation. The combination of two drugs, each with its own formulation requirements, can be exceedingly difficult to achieve.

## Ophthalmic Drug Delivery Systems

### *Solutions*

The clear, colorless aqueous solution of drug has become the most commonplace and possibly preferred ophthalmic dosage form.[7, 9] Drugs in solution are immediately available for absorption. However, solutions with a low viscosity drain rapidly from the cul-de-sac. The aqueous solution dosage form can be considered only for drugs with sufficient aqueous solubility to prevent them from precipitating under adverse storage conditions. In some cases, one or more cosolvents, such as polysorbate 80 (Tween 80) may be added to the formulation to facilitate dissolution or maintain the drug in solution.

### *Suspensions*

Suspensions are dispersions of drugs with low water solubility in finely divided forms. Although the drug solubility generally is insufficient to completely dissolve it, the aqueous phase becomes saturated with the drug.[24, 67] Some drugs that are soluble in water as salts may become less soluble or insoluble in their free-acid or free-base form. Different salts of the same drug can vary in water solubility, so a salt may be obtained that renders an otherwise soluble drug insoluble in water. Thus, it may be possible to reduce the stinging or discomfort of a drug by using a suspension of its poorly soluble salt instead of a solution. Because solubility is usually a function of temperature, a marginally soluble drug may cycle in and out of solution (temperature cycling) with extremes of temperature during transit or storage. Crystals of the drug may grow with varying temperature too.

Drug surface area is a function of particle size and can influence the rate of dissolution of drug.[9] Drug particles remaining in the cul-de-sac after instillation of a suspension can prolong the availability of drug. Here again, particle size may be important for determining the particle retention time. The presence of particulate matter in the cul-de-sac may cause a foreign body sensation. Suspensions are typically necessary to formulate corticosteroids with low solubility. Particle size also influences the rate of settling of suspended material and the ease with which the drug particles are resuspended on shaking the container. Micronization or reduction of particle size may or may not improve the performance of a drug suspension. A suspension of very small particles can drain from the cul-de-sac similarly to a plain solution, and few particles may stay in the precorneal area. Larger particles tend to remain longer in the cul-de-sac. Note the aqueous humor levels of a drug applied topically in different dosage forms (Fig. 2–11).

### *Gels*

Polymer-based aqueous gels are used for ophthalmic drug delivery as an alternative to ointments.[24, 68, 69] Gels prolong the residence time of the drug in the cul-de-sac and effectively increase ocular bioavailability. The polymers used in ophthalmic gels include the cellulosic ethers (hydroxypropyl cellulose, methyl cellulose, hydroxypropylmethylcellulose), polyvinyl alcohol, carbopol, polyacrylamide, polymethylvinyl ether–maleic anhydride, poloxamer 407, and pluronic acid. Mucoadhesiveness of the polymer has a role in its retention in the cul-de-sac.

Soluble polymers having thermosetting, pH-setting, or electrolyte-setting properties have been studied to serve as novel prolonged drug delivery systems.[70] Because of the reversible thermal gelation phenomenon the poloxamers exhibit, these polymers have been studied. Their micellar size has a marked temperature dependence, and their hydrophobic : hydrophilic ratio can be varied by modifying the molecular weight of

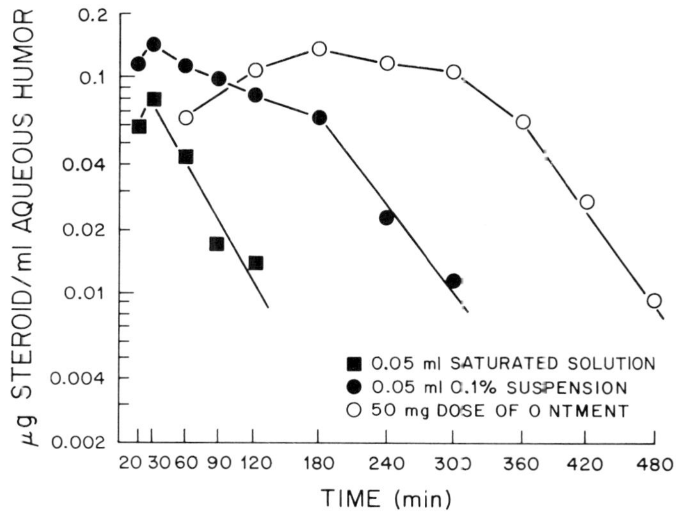


**FIG 2–11.**
Comparison of rabbit aqueous humor levels of tritiated fluorometholone after different topical dosage forms. (From Sieg JW, Roninson JR: *J Pharm Sci* 64:931, 1975. Used by permission.)

the poloxamer. Thus, the viscosity can be varied over a broad range. Electrolyte-setting and pH-setting polymers can be used to formulate gellable systems that form in situ when placed into the cul-de-sac. The electrolytes in tears and tear pH contribute to gel formation.

Drug release from gels occurs by diffusion and by erosion of the gel surface. Release is rapid for water-soluble drugs because the tears are able to enter the gel to dissolve the hydrophilic polymer and cause leaching out of the drug. Reducing the drug's water solubility could be used to control the leaching process. This mode of delivery, like eye drops, provides pulsed drug delivery, but it allows up to five times more of the drug to enter the cornea. Thus, the cornea may become saturated with the drug and serve as a reservoir for the drug, thereby prolonging the effect. However, zero-order delivery from a highly viscous vehicle has not yet been achieved. Gels may help to maintain the desired effect level of a drug with a short biologic half-life and may reduce the frequency and dose required. The carbopol gel containing 4% pilocarpine effectively reduces the number of instillations to once daily as required to provide up to 24-hour control of intraocular pressure.[64, 65] By applying the gel at bedtime, one can largely avoid the troublesome nature of the visual side effects of pilocarpine.

#### *Ointments*

Ophthalmic ointments usually contain anhydrous lanolin in a mineral oil and petrolatum base. Lanolin is considered to be a sensitizing agent and can cause a local allergic reaction. It is used in emulsion-like ointments to facilitate the dispersion of an aqueous solution component containing the drug into the solid and liquid hydrocarbon ointment bases In other cases, the drug is dispersed, usually in its micronized form, homogenously throughout the petrolatum. Peanut oil is also used as a liquid oily vehicle. Ointments are preserved using methylparaben and propylparaben. Ointments provide for an increased degree of absorption of drugs into the eye compared with viscous aqueous solutions because of their increased retention time in the cul-de-sac.[71, 72] Ointments can become entrapped within the fornices and act as a drug reservoir. The shearing action of the eyelid during blinking exposes a fresh surface from which more drug is available for absorption. The turnover rate for a drug in an ointment within the cul-de-sac is very low compared with that of tears, being on the order of 0.5%/min. Ophthalmic ointments are toxic to the intraocular tissues, causing endothelial damage, corneal edema, vascularization, and scarring.[73] For this reason, ophthalmic medications in ointment or oily liquid vehicles should not be instilled into the interior of the eye or used in such a way during surgery that they may accidentally enter the eye.[74, 75] Severe reaction with secondary glaucoma and eventual loss of the eye was observed in rabbits when 0.1 ml of these substances was introduced. Smaller amounts were less destructive.

Because of the messiness associated with their greasy nature and the temporary blurring of vision they produce, ointments are not readily accepted by patients. Accurate dosage with an ointment, or a gel for that matter, is difficult because the patient cannot easily measure the ribbon as it is being placed in the eye. Lipophilic drugs dissolve readily in ointment base and, in some cases, are not easily released from the formulation. On the other hand, hydrophilic drugs such as pilocarpine are released rapidly from oleaginous ointments. Ointments can prolong the delivery of drugs to the eye because they are less rapidly cleared from the cul-de-sac. Ointments containing antibiotics are convenient to use after surgery when patching the eye makes it cumbersome to repeatedly administer drops. They also serve to soften and eliminate crusts of bloody discharge that may form.

Concern has been expressed in the past for an adverse effect of ointment base on corneal wound healing or the inclusion of ointment particle beneath the healing epithelium or under conjunctival wounds. Experimentally, ointment entrapment could not be produced as a consequence of epithelial abrasions or corneal incisions. Actual injection of ointment was required before it would be retained within the corneal stroma or beneath the conjunctiva. Even here, the only consequence was transient neovascularization.[73]

### *Solid Inserts*

Ideally, if the effective concentration of a drug could be maintained by matching its rate of delivery to its rate of elimination from the site of action, the desired therapeutic action could be maintained until the drug reservoir becomes exhausted. This happens with a zero-order rate of delivery, such as has been achieved with solid insert dosage forms. However, solid inserts have limited acceptance by patients, particularly the elderly, because of their difficulty of placement and some problems associated with their retention in the cul-de-sac. Should these objections be overcome, zero-order delivery devices could be ideal ophthalmic dosage forms.

The release of the drug from a solid insert may be controlled by either the diffusion rate of the drug through the polymer or the erosion rate of the polymer itself.[76] Diffusion-controlled systems are either the reservoir type or the matrix type. A reservoir insert consists of a core of the drug in powder or liquid form that is encapsulated within a polymer layer that does not biodegrade and serves as a rate controlling barrier to diffusion. The drug diffuses through the polymer at a rate determined by the characteristics of the drug and of the polymer. Release of drug is determined by the surface area and thickness of the polymer layer, and uniformity can be achieved as long as the thickness of the polymer does not change. Should a hole develop in the polymer layer, instantaneous release of the drug will occur. The Ocusert Pilo-20 and Pilo-40 (ALZA Corporation, Palo Alto, California) are diffusion-controlled inserts using ethylene/vinyl acetate polymeric membranes and release pilocarpine at steady-state rates of 20 and 40 μg/hr, respectively.[77–80]

In the matrix type of solid insert, the drug is dispersed throughout the polymer matrix and must diffuse through the matrix structure to be released. Erodible solid inserts are biodegradable or bioerodible and release the drug, which is uniformly dispersed throughout the polymer matrix, as the polymer disintegrates. Unlike the nonbioerodible inserts, the erodible type does not require removal from the cul-de-sac and can be used to formulate water-insoluble drugs. Biocompatibility, biodegradability, permeability to water, and tensile strength are desirable attributes of the polymer used in a biodegradable insert. Ideally the solid insert should not elicit a foreign body sensation in the eye. Mucoadhesiveness is a useful property of a polymer to be used in an ocular drug delivery system.

Solid inserts avoid pulse delivery of drugs and provide delivery of the drug at a controlled rate. They require fewer doses because they last a long time; therefore, they improve compliance. However, inserts may be lost from the eye during sleep without the patient noticing it, and the patient then does not have the benefit of the drug.

#### *Soft Contact Lenses*

Soft contact lenses made of hydrophilic polymers such as hydroxyethyl methacrylate may be used as a drug delivery system when they are presoaked in the drug solution.[81, 82] Hard lenses may not be used in this manner. Highly soluble drugs such as pilocarpine are released rapidly from such lenses, with more than 90% being released within the first 20 to 30 minutes after being applied. Because the concentration of drug in the cornea rises more rapidly than the drug can diffuse into the aqueous humor, the cornea acts as a reservoir for the drug and maintains its delivery to the aqueous humor longer. Hydrophilic soft contact lenses do not provide constant drug release. The drug at the surface is released first, and the path of diffusion for the drug from the inner layers of the lens lengthens as the outer layers become depleted of drug; thus, the release rate decreases with time. The degree of hydration of the lens influences the release rate of the drug. Care must be taken to avoid an accumulation of the preservative benzalkonium chloride (which is widely used in ophthalmic solutions) in the lens during soaking because it may reach levels toxic for the cornea. Apparently it is not necessary to remove a soft contact lens from the eye before drops of most medications are instilled.

#### *Collagen Shields*

Collagen shields are biodegradable contact lens–shaped devices that have been used to deliver drugs to the eye, provide protection to the cornea, and promote corneal epithelial healing.[83, 84] They require rehydration before using, so shields may be saturated with drug by soaking them in drug solution. The drug may become entrapped within the collagen matrix or bind to the collagen. Current shields are made of collagen from porcine sclera or bovine corium and vary in degree of hydration between 65% and 83%. The amount of collagen cross-linking can be varied using ultraviolet irradiation to produce shields lasting 12, 24, or 72 hours on the eye. Collagen shields may provide prolonged drug delivery compared with simple drug solutions.

## COLLOIDAL PREPARATIONS FOR OPHTHALMIC USE

### Liposomes

In aqueous suspension, phospholipids can be made to form multilamellar or unilamellar vesicles ranging from 0.01 to 10 μm. The name liposome (fat body) is given to these tiny vesicles that consist of alternating bilayers of phospholipids and aqueous spaces. Drugs in solution may be entrapped within this lipoidal microsphere, either within the phospholipid or the aqueous phases. Typical phospholipids used to form liposomes are phosphatidylcholine, phosphatidylethanolamine, phosphatidylserine, phosphatidic acid, sphingomyelins, cardiolipins, plasmalogens, and cerebrosides. The physical, biologic, and chemical properties of liposomes may be modified by incorporation of other substances such as glycolipids, polymers, and sterols such that the drug delivery properties can be varied. Liposomes are prepared by a variety of methods, including, sonication, calcium-induced fusion, reverse phase evaporation, and detergent removal.

Because liposomes are colloidal systems and are unable to cross vascular membranes, their intravenous use as a drug delivery system is limited. To serve as an ocular drug delivery system, liposomes must remain in the cul-de-sac long enough to release their contents. It is likely that liposomes adsorb to the surface of cells, possibly fusing with the cell membranes. Alternatively, endocytosis appears to be a mechanism for liposomes to release their drug charge into the cell. Liposomes have yet to be demonstrated as effective for prolonging the release of drugs instilled in the cul-de-sac. Their advantage may be to bring the drug they carry into close contact with the corneal and conjunctival surfaces. The potential role of liposomes for ophthalmic drug delivery has been reviewed recently.[85–88]

## Nanoparticles

Nanoparticles are ultrafine solid particles of polymeric materials, ranging from 10 to 1,000 nm, that can have drug incorporated within them or adsorbed onto their surface.[88] Typical polymers used to make nanoparticles are the poly(alkylcyanoacrylates), for example, polybutylcyanoacrylate, polymethylmethacrylate, and polyhexylcyanoacrylate.[89] Such carriers may be made biodegradable and may exhibit bioadhesive properties. The release of drug may be controlled either by the rates of desorption from the particles or of degradation of the particle matrix and is determined by the method of manufacture. Retention characteristics of nanoparticles in the eye can be influenced by size, density, composition, charge density, and hydrophobicity.

The ocular disposition of poly(butyl-2-cyanoacrylate) nanoparticles labeled with indium-111 was studied in the rabbit using γ-scintigraphy.[90] The corneal and inner canthus clearance half-lives were found to be 2.15 minutes and 9.27 minutes, respectively, for nanoparticles compared with 1.3 and 5 minutes, respectively, for a solution containing $^{111}$In oxime. In that study, a comparison was made to small unilamellar liposomes and reverse-phase vesicles carrying positive, negative, or no surface charges, and the authors concluded that nanoparticles do not offer advantages over liposomes in the size range of 100 nm to 4 μm in ocular drug delivery. Using poly-hexyl-2-cyano[3-$^{14}$C]acrylate nanoparticles, Wood et al.[91] found approximately 19% degradation of the nanoparticles in tears within the first hour, and their rapid removal from the precorneal area occurred from drainage. However, retention was better for nanoparticles compared with simple solutions, and an estimated 1% of the initial dose remained for the 360-minute duration of the experiment.

In rabbit studies using biodegradable 310-nm poly-*n*-butyl-2-cyanoacrylate nanoparticles to which 2% pilocarpine nitrate had been adsorbed, the aqueous humor level of drug was elevated above that for an aqueous solution of pilocarpine formulation at 30 minutes. Furthermore, there was a prolonged duration of miosis and intraocular pressure lowering in the betamethasone-induced ocular hypertensive rabbit model from the nanoparticle formulation.[92]

The drug load of betaxolol hydrochloride, a β-adrenergic blocker, adsorbed to isobutylcyanoacrylate nanoparticles could be varied from 22% to 65% by modification of the particle surface charge. When the intraocular pressure effect of these particles was evaluated in rabbits with ocular hypertension (induced by intracameral injection of α-chymotrypsin), those carrying the highest percentage of drug unexpectedly produced much less intraocular pressure decrease than the lower concentrations and the solution drug formulation. It was suggested that the surface charge of the particles and the type of binding between the drug and the particles are important parameters for determining the rate of desorption of drug.[93]

Thus, drug release rates and retention in the precorneal area of the eye for nanoparticles must be worked out if they are to provide novel ophthalmic drug delivery systems in the future.[16, 94, 95]

## Subconjunctival, Sub-Tenon's, and Retrobulbar Injection

It is difficult to extrapolate to humans and to accurately assess the bioavailability of drugs injected subconjunctivally based on data reported from animal experiments.[6, 96] The main difficulty lies in the uncertainty of knowing whether corneal access was avoided or that the drug did not actually leak out the entry hole of the injection and enter the eye through the cornea from the tears. To what degree this leakage phenomenon contributes to bioavailability from subconjunctival injections made clinically is not clearly known. However, this phenomenon can be used to deliver drugs to the corneal surface over a longer period, for example, to treat bacterial corneal ulcers.[96, 97]

Certainly, subconjunctival injection should be considered to deliver drugs, such as antibiotics, which penetrate the cornea poorly.[98–101] This route is common for antiproliferative agents such as 5-fluorouracil, which are used to prevent scarring of filtering blebs associated with glaucoma surgery. Drugs with low water solubility, such as corticosteroids, may provide a repository of drug lasting over days to weeks after subconjunctival injection. However, repeated topical instillations may deliver adequate amounts of most drugs to achieve the desired response. The injection of drugs under the conjunctiva results in rapid (within 30 minutes) and nearly complete entry of drug into the systemic circulation. Vasoconstriction caused by epinephrine added to the injected material slows the rate of systemic absorption of the drug from the subconjunctival depot and can increase the amount penetrating the eye.

Besides entering the eye through the cornea from the tears, drugs injected subconjunctivally can enter the eye through the sclera and, ultimately, through the corneal stroma, the trabecular meshwork at the iridocorneal angle, the uveoscleral pathway, the vitreous body, the iris stroma, and the stroma of the ciliary body.[6, 102] As mentioned elsewhere, the diffusion of drug from Tenon's space into the eye is opposed by the outward pressure gradient and flow of fluid. Drug distribution within the ocular tissues from subconjunctival injection is not uniform.

Because the bleb of material spreads posteriorly after subconjunctival and anteriorly after retrobulbar injections, there are small differences in the distribution of drug between the two approaches. Less drug appears in the cornea and aqueous humor from retrobulbar injection than after subconjunctival.[100]

The disadvantages of periocular injection (patient apprehension, subsequent inflammation and pain, inconvenience, expense, and possible intraocular perforation) are great enough to nullify almost all advantages that might be expected from this route of administration. Probably its greatest clinical value is realized in the emergency management of acute infection of the anterior segment. When subconjunctival antibiotics are used, the preliminary use of topical or subconjunctival anesthetic to reduce pain is advised. The addition of lidocaine to most antibiotics does not reduce their in vitro antibacterial activity. Topical proparacaine and subconjunctival lidocaine or procaine do not decrease the intraocular penetration or antibiotic activity of subconjunctiva penicillin G, methicillin, cephaloridine, or gentamicin.[103] Comparison of the subconjunctival route with continuous intravenous injection of oxacillin shows no benefit to systemic medication with respect to anterior segment drug concentrations.[104] Levels of oxacillin reaching the vitreous were unimpressive from either the intravenous or the subconjunctival route. Subconjunctival injection gave relatively high values in the anterior eye and the choroid and retina.

### Intraocular Injection

The dangers inherent in intraocular injections far outweigh possible benefits in almost all circumstances. Probably the only clear indication for this route is the administration of antibiotics as treatment for severe endophthalmitis during surgery required for correction of an infected laceration or a ruptured surgical wound. Only minute amounts of antibiotic are tolerated within the eye. For example, the maximum safe anterior chamber dose of polymyxin B is 0.1 mg. Even penicillin G is toxic within the eye, which questionably will tolerate only 4,000 units (24 mg).[41]

### Intravenous Injection

It is assumed that continuous intravenous administration of an antibiotic is an effective way of maintaining intraocular levels.[104] Because of the barriers and possible reservoir effects of the eye, however, antibiotics such as ampicillin, chloramphenicol, and erythromycin penetrate into the eye at higher initial levels and maintain at least comparable intraocular levels for 4 hours when given as a single intravenous bolus rather than by continuous infusion.[105]

Inflammation may affect the barrier properties of the eye to permit better penetration of substances from the circulation into the eye.[106] This is demonstrated by the appearance of fluorescein in the vitreous as a result of leakage from the retinal vessels in the presence of inflammation.

The distribution of ampicillin, tetracycline, and dexamethasone in rabbit eye tissues after intravenous administration was studied.[6] Highest levels were found in the sclera and conjunctiva, followed by the iris and ciliary body, cornea, aqueous humor, choroid, and retina. Very low levels appeared in the lens and vitreous. There were no marked differences among the drugs in their distribution. The distribution pattern seems to be determined by the vascularity of the tissue and what barriers occur between the blood and the tissue.

### Delayed-Release Oral Preparations

The practical value of sustained-release preparations should be noted.[48, 107] For example, a single dose of acetazolamide will reduce intraocular pressure for up to 10 hours, whereas a single dose of sustained-release acetazolamide will produce a comparable effect lasting 20 hours. Sustained-release medications offer advantages of a more steady blood level of drug, avoiding marked peaks and valleys, and a reduction in the frequency of administration to give greater convenience to the patient.

## REFERENCES


1. Shell JW: Pharmacokinetics of topically applied ophthalmic drugs, *Surv Ophthalmol* 26:207, 1982.
2. Mishima S, Nagataki S: Conrad Berens Memorial Lecture: pharmacology of ophthalmic solutions, *Contact Intraocular Lens Med J* 4:22, 1978.
3. Mishima S: Clinical pharmacokinetics of the eye, Proctor Lecture, *Invest Ophthalmol* 21:504, 1981.
4. Schoenwald RD: Ocular pharmacokinetics/pharmacodynamics. In Mitra AK, editor: *Ophthalmic drug delivery systems,* Marcel Dekker, New York, 1993.
5. Maurice DM: Kinetics of topically applied ophthalmic drugs. In Saettone MF, Bucci M, Speiser P, editors: *Ophthalmic drug delivery, biopharmaceutical, technological and clinical aspects,* vol 2, New York, 1987, Springer-Verlag, New York, p 19.
6. Maurice DM, Mishima S: Ocular pharmacokinetics. In Sears ML, editor: *Pharmacology of the eye: handbook of experimental pharmacology,* vol 69, New York, 1984, Springer-Verlag New York, p 19.
7. Schoenwald R: Ocular drug delivery pharmacokinetic considerations, *Clin Pharmacokinet* 18:255, 1990.
8. Plazzonet B, Grove J, Durr M, and others: Pharmacokinetics and biopharmaceutical aspects of some anti-glaucoma drugs. In Saettone MF, Bucci M, Speiser P, editors: *Ophthalmic drug delivery, biopharmaceutical, technological and clinical aspects,* vol 1, New York, 1987, Springer-Verlag New York, p 117.
9. Schoenwald R: The control of drug bioavailability from ophthalmic dosage forms. In Smolen VF, Ball LA, editors: *Controlled drug bioavailability,* vol 3, New York, 1985, John Wiley & Sons, p 257.
10. Wagner JG: Kinetics of pharmacologic response: I. proposed relationships between response and drug concentration in the intact animal and man, *J Theoret Biol* 20:173, 1968.
11. Burstein NL, Anderson JA: Review: corneal penetration and ocular bioavailability of drugs, *J Ocul Pharmacol* 1:309, 1985.
12. Chiang CH, Schoenwald RD: Ocular pharmacokinetic models of clonidine-$^3$H hydrochloride, *J Pharmacokinet Biopharm* 14:175, 1986.
13. Schoenwald RD: Ocular drug delivery pharmacokinetic considerations, *Clin Pharmacokinet* 18:225, 1990.
14. Schoenwald RD, Huang HS: Corneal penetration behavior of β-blocking agents: 1. Physiochemical factors, *J Pharm Sci* 72:1266, 1983.
15. Wilson CG: Scintigraphic evaluation of polymeric formulations for ophthalmic use. In Saettone MF, Bucci M, Speiser P, editor: *Ophthalmic drug delivery, biopharmaceutical, technological and clinical aspects,* vol 11, New York, 1987, Springer-Verlag New York, p 143.
16. Fitzgerald P, Hadgraft J, Kreuter J, and others: A γ-scintigraphic evaluation of microparticulate ophthalmic delivery systems: liposomes and nanoparticles, *Int J Pharm* 40:81, 1987.

17. Wagner JG: Half-life and volume of distribution. In *Biopharmaceutics and relevant pharmacokinetics,* Hamilton, Ill, 1979, Drug Intelligence Publishing, p 252.
18. Shell JW, Baker RW: Diffusional systems for controlled release of drugs to the eye, *Ann Ophthalmol* 6:1037, 1974.
19. Shell JW: Ophthalmic drug delivery systems, *Surv Ophthalmol* 29:117, 1984.
20. Holly FJ: Tear film physiology, *Int Ophthalmol Clin* 27:2, 1987.
21. Farris RL, Stuchell RN, Mandel ID: Basal and reflex human tear analysis: I. Physical measurements: osmolarity, basal volumes, and reflex flow rate, *Am Acad Ophthalmol* 88:852, 1981.
22. Stuchell RN, Farris RL, Mandel ID: Basal and reflex human tear analysis: II. Chemical analysis: lactoferrin and lysozyme, *Am Acad Ophthalmol* 88:858, 1981.
23. Mishima S, Gasset A, Klyce Jr. SD, and others: Determination of tear volume and tear flow, *Invest Ophthalmol* 5:264, 1966.
24. Lee VHL, Robinson JR: Review: topical ocular drug delivery: recent developments and future challenges, *J Ocul Pharmacol* 2:67, 1986.
25. Raviola G: The structural basis of the blood ocular barriers: the ocular and cerebrospinal fluids, *Exp Eye Res* 25(suppl):27, 1977.
26. Bito LZ, Klein EM: Transport functions of the blood-retinal barrier system and the micro-environment of the retina. In Cunha-Vaz JG, editor: *The blood-retinal barriers, NATO Advance Study Institutes series,* vol 32, New York, 1980, Plenum, p 133.
27. Bito LZ, Salvador EV: Intraocular fluid dynamics: III. The site and mechanism of prostaglandin transfer across the blood intraocular fluid barriers, *Exp Eye Res* 14:233, 1972.
28. Zaki I, Fitzgerald P, Hardy JG, and others: A comparison of the effect of viscosity on the precorneal residence of solutions in rabbit and man, *J Pharm Pharmacol* 38:463, 1986.
29. Chen KK, Poth EJ: Racial difference of the mydriatic action of ephedrines, cocaine and euphthalmine, *J Pharmacol Exp Ther* 36:429, 1929.
30. Obianwu HO, Rand MJ: The relationship between the mydriatic action of ephedrine and color of the iris, *Br J Ophthalmol* 49:264, 1965.
31. Salazar M, Shimada K, Patil PN: Iris pigmentation and atropine mydriasis, *J Pharmacol Exp Ther* 197:79, 1976.
32. Patil PN: Some factors which affect the ocular drug response, *Trends Pharmacol Sci* 5:201, 1984.
33. Lee VHL, Wulf LW, Kashi SD, and others: Metabolic and permeation barriers to the ocular absorption of topically applied enkephalins in albino rabbits, *J Ocul Pharmacol* 2:345, 1986.
34. Lee VHL, Smith RE: Effect of substrate concentration, product concentration, and peptides on the *in vitro* hydrolysis of model ester prodrugs by corneal esterases, *J Ocul Pharmacol* 1:269, 1985.
35. Lee VHL, Chang SC, Oshiro CM, and others: Ocular esterase composition in albino and pigmented rabbits: possible implications in ocular prodrug design and evaluation, *Curr Eye Res* 4:1117, 1985.
36. Chen CC, Anderson J, Shackleton M, and others: The disposition of bunolol in the rabbit eye, *J Ocul Pharmacol* 3:149, 1987.
37. Ariens EJ: Stereoselectivity, a natural aspect of molecular biology: a blind spot in clinical pharmacology and pharmacokinetics. *Eur J Drug Metab Pharmacokinet* 13:307, 1988.
38. Patil PN, Miller DD, Trendelenburg U: Molecular geometry and adrenergic drug activity, *Pharmacol Rev* 26:323, 1974.
39. DeCamp WH: The FDA perspective on the development of stereoisomers, *Chirality* 1:2, 1989.
40. Martin AN: Buffered systems and the colorimetric determination of pH. In *Physical pharmacy, physical chemical principles in pharmaceutical science,* Philadelphia, 1960, Lea & Febiger, p 260.
41. Havener WH: Pharmacokinetics: routes of administration. In *Ocular pharmacology,* St Louis, 1981, The CV Mosby Co.
42. Ahmed I, Patton TF: Importance of noncorneal absorption route in topical ophthalmic drug delivery, *Invest Ophthalmol Vis Sci* 26:584, 1985.
43. File RR, Patton TF: Topically applied pilocarpine, *Arch Ophthalmol* 98:112, 1980.
44. Patton TF, Francoeur M: Ocular bioavailability and systemic loss of topically applied ophthalmic drugs, *Am J Ophthalmol* 85:225, 1978.
45. Brown C, Hanna C: Use of dilute drug solutions for routine cycloplegia and mydriasis, *Am J Ophthalmol* 86:820, 1978.
46. Chrai SS, Makoid MC, Eriksen SP, and others: Drop size and initial dosing fre-

quency problems of topically applied ophthalmic drugs, *J Pharm Sci* 63:333, 1974.
47. Leibowitz HM, Kupferman A: Drug interaction in the eye, *Arch Ophthalmol* 95:682, 1977.
48. Huang TC, Lee DA: Punctal occlusion and topical medications for glaucoma, *Am J Ophthalmol* 107:151, 1989.
49. Zimmerman TJ, Kooner KS, Kandarakis AS, and others: Improving the therapeutic index of topically applied ocular drugs, *Arch Ophthalmol* 102:551, 1984.
50. Zimmerman TJ, Sharir M, Nardin GF, and others: Therapeutic index of epinephrine and dipivefrin with nasolacrimal occlusion, *Am J Ophthalmol* 114:8, 1992.
51. Zimmerman TJ, Sharir M, Nardin GF, and others: Therapeutic index of pilocarpine, carbachol, and timolol with nasolacrimal occlusion, *Am J Ophthalmol* 114:1, 1992.
52. Fraunfelder FF: Extraocular fluid dynamics: how best to apply topical ocular medication, *Trans Am Ophthalmol Soc* 74:457, 1976.
53. Salminen L: Review: systemic absorption of topically applied ocular drugs in humans, *J Ocul Pharmacol* 6:243, 1990.
54. Van Buskirk EM, Fraunfelder TF: Ocular beta blockers and systemic effects, *Am J Ophthalmol* 98:623, 1984.
55. Lahdes K, Huupponen R, Kaila T, and others: Systemic absorption of ocular cyclopentolate in children, *German J Ophthalmol* 1:16, 1992.
56. Abrams DA, Robin AL, Pollack IP, and others: The safety and efficacy of topical 1% ALO 2145 (ρ-aminoclonidine hydrochloride) in normal volunteers, *Arch Ophthalmol* 105:1205, 1987.
57. Coles WH, Jaros PA: Dynamics of ocular surface pH, *Br J Ophthalmol* 68:549, 1984.
58. Van Ooteghem MM: Factors influencing the retention of ophthalmic solutions on the eye surface. In Saettone MF, Bucci M, Speiser P, editors: *Ophthalmic drug delivery, biopharmaceutical, technological and clinical aspects,* New York, 1987, Springer-Verlag New York, p 7.
59. Benjamin WJ, Hill RM: Human tears: osmotic characteristics, *Invest Ophthalmol Vis Sci* 24:1624, 1983.
60. Snibson GR, Greaves JL, Soper NDM, and others: Ocular surface residence times of artificial tears solutions, *Cornea* 11:288, 1992.
61. Chrai SS, Robinson JR: Ocular evaluation of methylcellulose vehicle in rabbits, *J Pharm Sci* 63:1218, 1974.
62. Larsen NE, Balazs EA: Drug delivery systems using hyaluronan and its derivatives, *Adv Drug Delivery Rev* 7:279, 1991.
63. Patton TF, Robinson JR: Ocular evaluation of polyvinyl alcohol vehicle in rabbits, *J Pharm Sci* 64:1312, 1975.
64. Goldberg I, Ashburn Jr. FS, Kass MA, and others: Efficacy and patient acceptance of pilocarpine gel, *Am J Ophthalmol* 88:843, 1979.
65. Schoenwald RD, Boltralik JJ: A bioavailability comparison in rabbits of two steroids formulated as high-viscosity gels and reference aqueous preparations, *Invest Ophthalmol* 18:61, 1979.
66. Morrison WH: Stability of aqueous solutions commonly employed in the treatment of primary glaucoma, *Am J Ophthalmol* 37:557, 1954.
67. Sieg JW, Robinson JR: Corneal absorption of fluorometholone in rabbits, *Arch Ophthalmol* 92:240, 1974.
68. Saettone MF, Giannaccini B, Guiducci A, and others: Semisolid ophthalmic vehicles: III. An evaluation of four organic hydrogels containing pilocarpine, *Int J Pharm* 31:261, 1986.
69. Lee VHL: Review: new directions in the optimization of ocular drug delivery, *J Ocul Pharmacol* 6:157, 1990.
70. Gurny R, Ibrahim H, Boye T, and others: Latices and thermosensitive gel as sustained delivery systems to the eye. In Saettone MF, Bucci M, Speiser P, editors: *Ophthalmic drug delivery, biopharmaceutical, technological and clinical aspects,* New York, 1987, Springer-Verlag New York, p 27.
71. Fraunfelder FT, Hanna C: Ophthalmic ointment, *Trans Am Acad Ophthalmol Otolaryngol* 77:OP-467, 1973.
72. Robin JS, Ellis PP: Ophthalmic ointments, *Surv Ophthalmol* 22:335, 1978.
73. Fraunfelder FT, Hanna C, Cable M, and others: Entrapment of ophthalmic ointment in the cornea, *Am J Ophthalmol* 76:475, 1973.
74. Scheie HG, Rubenstein A, Katowitz JA: Ophthalmic ointment bases in the anterior chamber, *Arch Ophthalmol* 73:36, 1965.
75. Castroviejo R: Ointment bases in the anterior chamber, *Arch Ophthalmol* 74:143, 1965.
76. Heller J: Controlled drug release from monolithic systems, In Saettone MF, Bucci M, Speiser P, editors: *Ophthalmic drug delivery, biopharmaceutical, technological*

*and clinical aspects,* New York, 1987, Springer-Verlag New York, p 179.

77. Macoul KL, Pavan-Langston D: Pilocarpine Ocusert system for sustained control of ocular hypertension, *Arch Ophthalmol* 93:587, 1975.
78. Quigley HA, Pollack IP, Harbin Jr. TS: Pilocarpine Ocuserts, *Arch Ophthalmol* 93:771, 1975.
79. Drance SM, Mitchell DWA, Schulzer M: The effects of Ocusert pilocarpine on anterior chamber depth, visual acuity and intraocular pressure in man, *Can J Ophthalmol* 12:24, 1977.
80. Stewart RH, Novak S: Introduction of the Ocusert ocular system to an ophthalmic practice, *Ann Ophthalmol* 10:325, 1978.
81. Calabria G, Rathschuler F: Contact lenses as therapeutic systems. In Saettone MF, Bucci M, Speiser P, editors: *Ophthalmic drug delivery, biopharmaceutical, technological, and clinical aspects,* New York, 1987, Springer-Verlag New York, p 67.
82. McDermott ML, Chandler JW: Therapeutic uses of contact lenses, *Surv Ophthalmol* 33:381, 1989.
83. Mondino BJ: Collagen shields, *Am J Ophthalmol* 112:587, 1991.
84. Friedberg ML, Pleyer U, Mondino BJ: Device drug delivery to the eye collagen shields, iontophoresis, and pumps, *Ophthalmology* 98:725, 1991.
85. Mishima S, Mindel JS: Ocular drug bioavailability from topically applied liposomes, *Surv Ophthalmol* 29:335, 1985.
86. Lee VHL, Urrea PT, Smith RE, and others: Ocular drug bioavailability from topically applied liposomes, *Surv Ophthalmol* 29:335, 1985.
87. Schaeffer HE, Krohn DL: Liposomes in topical drug delivery, *Invest Ophthalmol Vis Sci* 21:220, 1982.
88. Kreuter J: Nanoparticles and liposomes in ophthalmic drug delivery. In Saettone MF, Bucci M, Speiser P, editors: *Ophthalmic drug delivery, biopharmaceutical, technological, and clinical aspects,* New York, 1987, Springer-Verlag New York, p 102.
89. Couvreur P, Vauthier C: Polyalkylcyanoacrylate nanoparticles as drug carrier: present state and perspectives, *J Controlled Release* 17:187, 1991.
90. Couvreur P, Kante B, Roland M, and others: Polycyanoacrylate nanocapsules as potential lysosomotropic carriers: preparation, morphological and sorptive properties, *J Pharm Pharmacol* 31:331, 1979.
91. Wood RW, Li VHK, Kreuter J, and others: Ocular disposition of poly-hexyl-2-cyano[3-$^{14}$C]acrylate nanoparticles in the albino rabbit, *Int J Pharm* 23:175, 1985.
92. Diepold R, Kreuter J, Himber J, and others: Comparison of different models for the testing of pilocarpine eyedrops using conventional eyedrops and a novel depot formulation (nanoparticles), *Graefes Arch Clin Exp Ophthalmol* 227:188, 1989.
93. Marchal-Heussler L, Maincent P, Hoffman M, and others: Antiglaucomatous activity of betaxolol chlorhydrate sorbed onto different isobutylcyanoacrylate nanoparticle preparations, *Int J Pharm* 58:115, 1990.
94. Harmia T, Speiser P, Kreuter J: A solid colloidal drug delivery system for the eye: encapsulation of pilocarpin in nanoparticles, *J Microencapsulation* 3:3, 1986.
95. Li VHK, Wood RW, Kreuter J, and others: Ocular drug delivery of progesterone using nanoparticles, *J Microencapsulation* 3:213, 1986.
96. Davis SD, Sarff LD, Hyndiuk RA: Comparison of therapeutic routes in experimental *Pseudomonas* keratitis, *Am J Ophthalmol* 87:710, 1979.
97. Leibowitz HM, Ryan Jr. WJ, Kupferman A: Route of antibiotic administration in bacterial keratitis, *Arch Ophthalmol* 99:1420, 1981.
98. Barza M, Kane A, Baum J: Excretion of gentamicin in rabbit tears after subconjunctival injection, *Am J Ophthalmol* 85:118, 1978.
99. Swan KC, Christman HR, Bailey Jr. PF: Subepithelial versus subcapsular injections of drugs, *Arch Ophthalmol* 56:26, 1956.
100. Hardy Jr. RG, Paterson CA: Ocular penetration of $^{14}$C-labeled chloramphenicol following subconjunctival or sub-Tenon's injection, *Am J Ophthalmol* 71:1307, 1971.
101. Patterson CA: Intraocular penetration of $^{14}$C-labeled penicillin after sub-Tenon's or subconjunctival injection, *Ann Ophthalmol* 5:171, 1973.
102. Wine NA, Cornall AG, Basu PK: The ocular uptake of subconjunctivally injected $C^{14}$ hydrocortisone, *Am J Ophthalmol* 58:362, 1964.
103. Ellis PP, Rendi MA: Effect of local anesthetics on intraocular penetration of subconjunctival antibiotics, *Am J Ophthalmol* 88:160, 1979.
104. Barza M, Kane A, Baum J: Oxacillin for

bacterial endophthalmitis: subconjunctival, intravenous, both or neither? *Invest Ophthalmol* 19:1348, 1980.

105. Goldman JN, Broughton W, Javed H, and others: Ampicillin, erythromycin and chloramphenicol penetration into rabbit aqueous humor, *Ann Ophthalmol* 5:147, 1973.
106. Barza M: Treatment of bacterial infections of the eye. In Remington JS, Swartz MM, editors: *Current clinical topics in infectious diseases,* New York, 1980, McGraw-Hill Book Co, pp 158–193.
107. Rosen E, Tannenbaum P, Ellison T, and others: Absorption and excretion of radioactively tagged dextroamphetamine sulfate from a sustained-release preparation, *JAMA* 194:1203, 1965.

# CHAPTER 3

# Autonomic Drugs

## INTRODUCTION

The autonomic nervous system is also called the visceral, involuntary, or vegetative nervous system. It is widely distributed throughout the body. The autonomic nervous system works through neurohumoral transmission, which is the propagation of nerve impulses across synapses and neuromuscular junctions by specific chemical agents referred to as neurohumoral transmitters. It is imperative to have a clear understanding of the anatomy and physiology of the autonomic nervous system to discuss the pharmacology of the autonomic drugs. The effect of an autonomic agent on the eye can be predicted if the responses to nerve impulses that reach the eye are known. The autonomic drugs, which include the miotic, mydriatic, and cycloplegic agents and β-blockers include many of the most important and most commonly used drugs in ophthalmology.

A discussion of the autonomic innervation of the eye and its effective chemicals is necessary before going into further detail about specific drugs. The main divisions of the autonomic nervous system are the sympathetic and parasympathetic outflow systems.

The sympathetic nervous system is diagrammed in Figs. 3–1 and 3–2. The sympathetic nervous system begins in the hypothalamus and then sends a signal to a

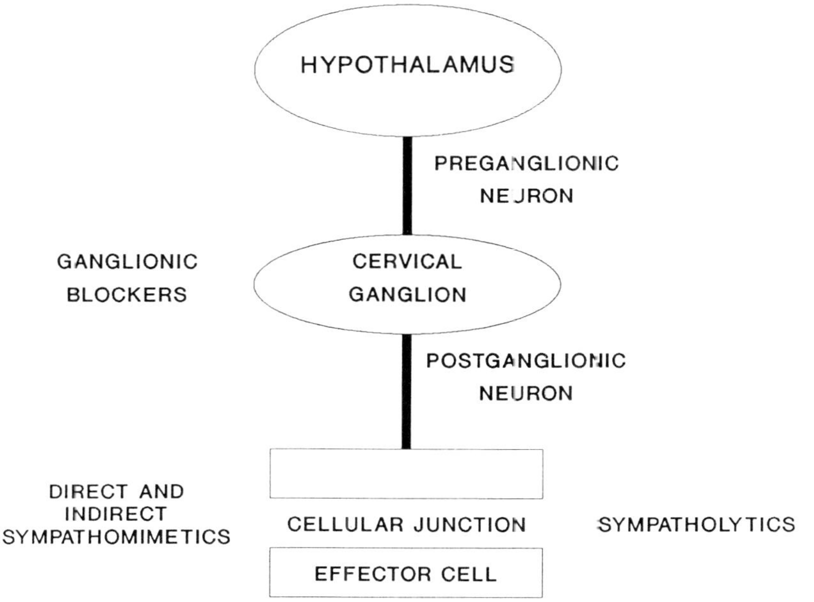


**FIG 3–1.**
Schematic of the sympathetic pathway.

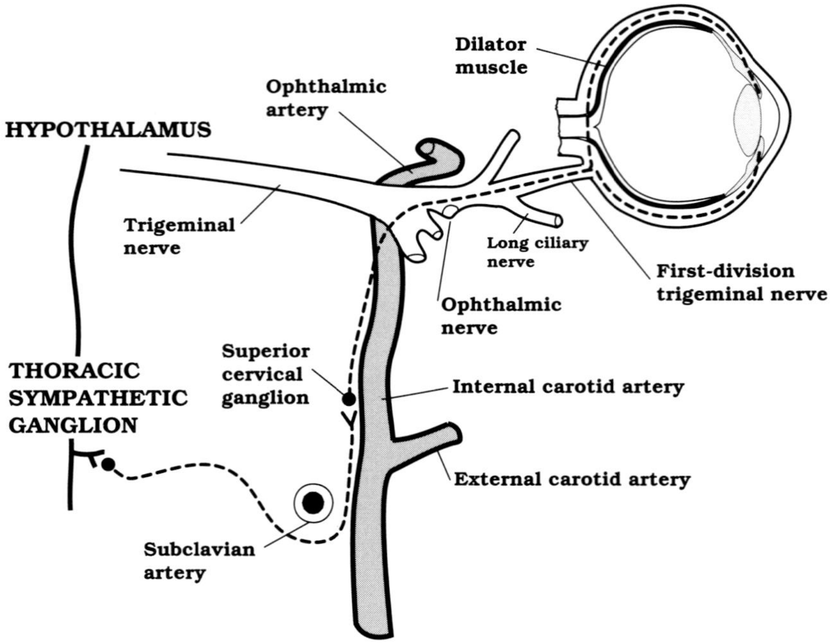


**FIG 3–2.**
Sympathetic pathway to the eye.

descending pathway to the intermediolateral cell columns of the spinal cord. Sympathetic innervation to the eye synapses at cell bodies in C8 to T3. The axons from these cells exit the anterior nerve root through the white ramus communicans and then ascend and synapse in the superior cervical ganglion. From there it is the postganglionic fibers that leave the superior cervical ganglion and run either in the internal carotid plexus or alongside the ophthalmic artery in its periarterial plexus. The nerve fibers that travel with the internal carotid plexus enter the orbit through its superior fissure. After passing through the superior orbital fissure, they form the sympathetic root of the ciliary ganglion. The fibers pass through the ganglion without synapsing and then become incorporated in the seven to 10 short ciliary nerves. Other fibers join the ophthalmic nerve or its nasociliary branch and reach the eye via the two to three long ciliary nerves that supply the dilator muscle of the pupil. Both long and short ciliary nerves contain afferent fibers from the cornea, iris, and choroid. Fibers that are part of the short ciliary nerves pass through a communicating ramus from the ciliary ganglion to the nasociliary nerve. This is called the sensory root of the ciliary ganglion. There are still some other sympathetic fibers from the internal carotid plexus that reach the eye through the ophthalmic periarterial plexus.

The parasympathetic division is outlined in Fig. 3–3. The parasympathetic preganglionic fibers for the eye are the axons of cells in the oculomotor nucleus. They run in the third cranial nerve and exit in the motor root of the ciliary ganglia where they synapse. The postganglionic parasympathetic fibers then travel to the eye in the short ciliary nerves, where they are distributed to the constrictor fibers of the iris, to the ciliary muscle, and to the blood vessels in the coats of the eyeball.

## IRIS

Sympathetic fibers innervate principally the dilator muscle of the iris. They also innervate iris blood vessels and melanocytes. The parasympathetic fibers supply the

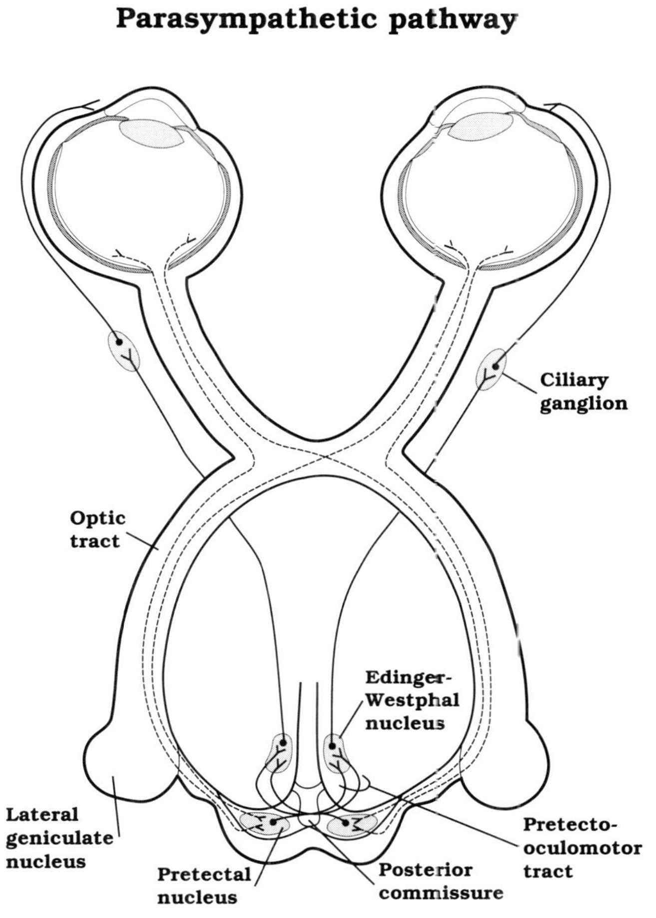


**FIG 3–3.**
Parasympathetic pathway to the eye.

sphincter and to a lesser degree the dilator muscle. To affect the action of the iris, one can stimulate or inhibit the sympathetic or parasympathetic systems.

## CILIARY MUSCLE

The ciliary muscle is affected by the autonomic nervous system. α-Adrenergic stimulation appears to increase outflow via the trabecular meshwork. Both α- and β-adrenergic stimulation diminish aqueous outflow. Studies of aqueous humor dynamics indicate that aqueous humor production is generally decreased by β-antagonistic selective drugs.[1] The probable site of action of these drugs is the ciliary epithelium resulting in decreased aqueous formation and a drop in the intraocular pressure.[2]

## SUMMARY

The autonomic nervous system is intimately involved in the normal function of the eye. We may manipulate the autonomic system using drugs, surgery, and even optics (bifocals for accommodative esotropia). The autonomic drugs may be loosely grouped as follows: adrenergic agonists, α-adrenergic antagonists, β-adrenergic antagonists, cholinergics, and the anticholinergics. The reader will realize that many of these agents are used as either glaucoma drugs or anesthetics. They are included in the section on autonomic drugs to allow organization around their underlying pharmacology.

SECTION ONE

# Adrenergic Agonists (Sympathomimetics)

MARY LOU KACHMER MCGREGOR

## EPINEPHRINE

In ophthalmology, epinephrine is useful because of its vasoconstrictor and ocular hypotensive affects.

### Pharmacology

Epinephrine and norepinephrine are the naturally occurring sympathomimetic effector substances. Epinephrine acts on both α- and β-receptors (Table 3–1). Norepinephrine acts primarily upon α-receptors. Both drugs act directly on the effector cells. Sympathetic denervation blocks sympathetic nerve transmission but induces a cellular supersensitivity to the sympathetic transmitter substances. Epinephrine is produced by the adrenal medulla and acts mainly as a neurohumoral agent. Norepinephrine is the neurotransmitter of the peripheral sympathetic nerves. Epinephrine and norepinephrine cause sympathomimetic effects in extremely mild doses. A concentration as dilute as 0.01 μg/ml will cause demonstrable relaxation of ciliary muscle.[3]

**TABLE 3–1.**
Adrenergic Agonists (Sympathomimetics)

| Direct Acting | Indirect Acting |
|---|---|
| α | Cocaine |
| Norepinephrine | Ephedrine |
| Phenylephrine | Hydroxyamphetamine |
| Apraclonidine | |
| β | |
| Isoproterenol | |
| Salbutamol (albuteral) | |
| Metaproterenol | |
| Terbutaline | |
| Ethylnorepinephrine | |
| Isoetharine | |
| Bitolterol | |
| α and β | |
| Epinephrine | |

The adrenergic neurotransmitter chemicals are catecholamine derivatives. The three sympathomimetically active catecholamines (dopamine, norepinephrine, and epinephrine) all are derived from tyrosine, and the chemical sequence is tyrosine, dopamine, norepinephrine, and then epinephrine. Norepinephrine, the true sympathetic neurotransmitter, is stored in vesicles at the synaptic end of the axon. The release of norepinephrine is accomplished by extrusion of vesical contents. Although norepinephrine may be inactivated by monoamine oxidase or by catechol-O-methyltransferase, inhibition of these enzymes does not greatly potentiate the effects of nerve stimulation.[4] Reuptake by sympathetic neurons is a more important means of norepinephrine removal than either metabolism or diffusion. Sympathetic supersensitivity, as may be produced by cocaine administration or chronic sympathetic denervation, is associated with the significant decrease in norepinephrine uptake by the sympathetic neuron.[5]

### Vasoconstriction

The vasoconstricting effect of epinephrine helps to control bleeding from capillaries and small arterioles but is ineffective against hemorrhage from larger vessels. During most ophthalmic operations it is the oozing from these smaller vessels that obscures surgical details; hence, preliminary use of epinephrine is of considerable value in eye surgery. It may be used in a 1:1,000 solution for surface application to the conjunctiva or wound surface and in a 1:200,000 solution (combined with the anesthetic) for injection at the site of incision. Vasoconstriction occurs within 5 minutes but lasts for less than 1 hour.

Inclusion of a 1:200,000 concentration of epinephrine in solutions of anesthetics for local injection will cause vasoconstriction sufficient to delay the loss of anesthetic effect through absorption. Used in this way, epinephrine reduces possible systemic toxicity by allowing time for detoxification of the slowly absorbed anesthetic and by reducing the amount of anesthetic required for the procedure. No local ischemic damage results from the injection of this concentration of epinephrine about the eye.

Epinephrine enhances intraocular penetration of subconjunctivally injected medications. Presumably vasoconstriction prevents rapid loss of the medication into the general circulation.[6]

Application of epinephrine in a 1:1,000 solution has been suggested as a means of differentiation between superficial and deep inflammation. Epinephrine vasoconstriction primarily affects the superficial conjunctival vessels, but it also has an effect on the deep conjunctival vessels.[7] Repeated application of epinephrine will ultimately also constrict the episcleral vessels. Hence, prompt blanching of a red eye suggests that conjunctivitis is a more likely diagnosis than is iritis. However, epinephrine blanching is a less reliable diagnostic criterion in the evaluation of a red eye than are the physical signs such as pupil size, intraocular pressure (IOP), and opacities of the media.[8]

Because of their vasoconstricting effects, solutions of 1:1,000 and 1:100 epinephrine may be used as decongestants to blanch conjunctival vessels that have become reddened because of nonspecific chronic irritation or allergy. This blanching effect usually lasts for less than 1 hour and may be followed by reactive hyperemia. Hence, the longer-acting sympathomimetic drugs such as phenylephrine are more commonly prescribed as nonspecific decongestants.

The vasoconstricting effects of epinephrine are also useful before the injection of botulinum toxin into an extraocular muscle. The decrease in hyperemia of the conjunctiva allows one to better delineate the location of the muscle and also reduces the chances of a subconjunctival hemorrhage as a result of damage to the conjunctival vessels.

## Mydriasis

Epinephrine in a 1:1,000 concentration is not a very good mydriatic in the normal human eye, probably because of its rapid destruction. When the permeability of the eye is increased by trauma (e.g., during surgery for strabismus), the pupil may become quite dilated from topical application of epinephrine Prolonged contact with the eye (and probably minor trauma) may be achieved by placing a small cotton pack soaked with epinephrine in the lower cul-de-sac. This method of application will result in mydriasis and has been advocated for the breaking of posterior synechiae. The use of epinephrine together with miotics in glaucoma therapy will cause the pupil to be slightly larger than it is with miotics alone.

It is well recognized that mydriatics are less effective in dark-colored eyes than in light-colored ones. Epinephrine, an adrenergic mediator for the dilator system, is destroyed by dihydroxyphenylalanine (dopa), a link in melanin metabolism. Homogenates of dark-colored rabbit irides (but not of light-colored ones) will inactivate epinephrine.[9] Guinea pig irides that are pigmented will bind twice as much norepinephrine as will those that are nonpigmented.[10]

Although cocaine sensitizes the iris dilator muscle to respond to lesser amounts of epinephrine, the sensitization is not synonymous with increased strength of contraction. The strength of a muscle at any given degree of contraction is greater in response to epinephrine alone than to a combination of epinephrine and cocaine.[11] Clearly, cocaine decreases the working capacity of the dilator muscle. Hence, the ancient combination of cocaine and epinephrine is an ineffective approach to dilatation of the pupil.

## Glaucoma

Although it seems paradoxical to use a pupil dilating drug in the treatment of glaucoma, there is sound evidence to support such therapy. Clinicians have long known that sympathomimetic mydriatics are not useful in provocative testing for open-angle glaucoma, because they are more likely to reduce pressure than to cause elevation. Also for this reason, drugs such as phenylephrine and hydroxyamphetamine (Paredrine) have been advocated to aid the general practitioner in ophthalmoscopic examination. They do not cause dangerous pressure elevation in chronic simple glaucoma, produce minimal cycloplegia, and act for only a short period.

It is important to remember that any mydriatic can produce angle closure glaucoma in a susceptible eye. Gonioscopy is advised before use of sympathomimetic mydriatics to avoid precipitation of acute angle-block glaucoma. Particular caution is necessary if the anterior chamber is visibly shallow.

Sympathomimetic mydriatics were originally believed to reduce intraocular pressure by decreasing the rate of aqueous formation. In most patients the coefficient of outflow is at first unchanged by the use of sympathomimetics. Particularly important is the fact that the therapeutically effective increase in the coefficient of outflow produced in human glaucomatous eyes by miotics is not decreased when the pupils are dilated by simultaneous use of sympathomimetics such as phenylephrine.[12] An additive effect is produced by the simultaneous use of miotics and sympathomimetics (and also carbonic anhydrase inhibitors) in the treatment of glaucoma.

Clinical study of a number of sympathomimetic compounds showed that a 1% solution of *l*-epinephrine often helped to control glaucoma.[13] A 10% solution of phenylephrine was slightly more effective than a 1% concentration of *l*-epinephrine but was less effective than a 2% solution of *l*-epinephrine. The 2% solution (Glaucon) was used predominantly in this study of 219 glaucoma patients. It was found to be stable for more than 6 months when refrigerated and was well tolerated by most patients. Topical application of a 2% solution of *l*-epinephrine to 44 glaucomatous eyes caused an average drop in pressure of 13.5 mm Hg (range 3–38 mm Hg). A marked pressure drop was obtained within 1 hour, and pressure continued to fall slightly for 4 hours (Fig. 3–4). A slow rise followed, with a good effect lasting for 12 hours and a slight effect for as long as 24 hours. Eyes most likely to respond well to a 2% solution of *l*-epinephrine were those with a coefficient of outflow better than 0.15, the pressures of which were maintained in the upper twenties with miotics. The pressure in most of these eyes could be dropped to the low twenties or less by instillation of a 2% solution of *l*-epinephrine twice daily. Although in some instances glaucoma could be controlled by a 2% concentration of

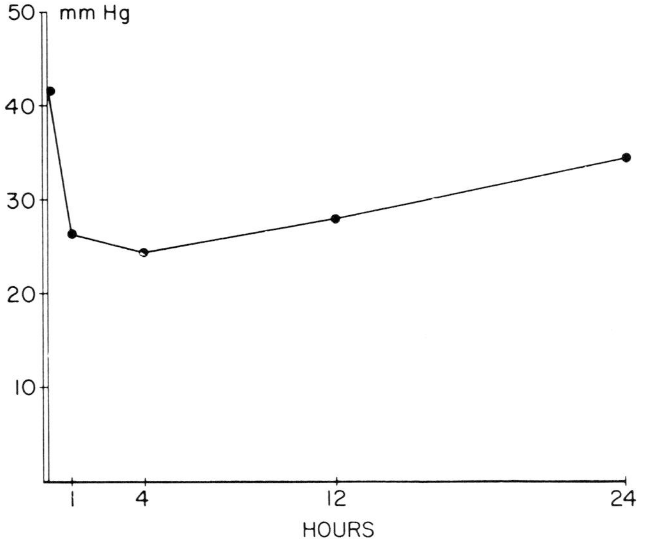


**FIG 3–4.**
Average response of 44 untreated glaucomatous eyes to 1 drop of a 2% solution of *l*-epinephrine. (From Garner LL, and others: *Arch Ophthalmol* 62:230, 1959. Used by permission.)

*l*-epinephrine alone, the best results were obtained when this drug was used in combination with a miotic. Patients with early cataracts were particularly pleased by the improvement in vision resulting from partial dilatation of the pupil. Secondary, absolute, and congenital types of glaucoma were not controlled by a 2% solution of *l*-epinephrine.

A pressure-lowering effect can be demonstrated with epinephrine concentrations as low as 0.125%; however, a substantially greater response occurs to 1%.[14]

There were few significant adverse effects from the topical use of a 2% solution of *l*-epinephrine. Systemic effects such as tachycardia were not troublesome. Blanching of the conjunctival vessels caused the eyes to appear very white, which was cosmetically desirable. Several patients developed reactive hyperemia of the conjunctiva, which appeared about 5 hours after instillation. Two patients suffered intense orbital pain for several hours after treatment. However, the comment that any type of local medication resulted in considerable pain in these same two patients suggests that they were exceptionally sensitive individuals. Mydriasis, with photophobia and blurred vision, resulted from the use of a 2% solution of *l*-epinephrine alone but was eliminated by simultaneous use of a 1% concentration of pilocarpine or some stronger miotic. Three cases of allergy were noted, but all were proved to result from the tetracaine used in the experimental solution.

The side effects of topical epinephrine therapy are quite annoying. In one series of 50 patients, only 20% could continue epinephrine drops for a 4-year period.[15] Reactive hyperemia, irritation, and tearing affected two thirds of the patients. Headaches affected 5 patients, cardiac palpitation 4, blurred vision 10, allergy 6, and conjunctival pigmentation 12. The epinephrine preparations originally available, which were used in this series of patients, were much more irritating than were the later developed commercial preparations. Thus, ocular tolerance to currently dispensed epinephrine drops is better than that indicated by these statistics.

The effect of single drops of three different epinephrine compounds — bitartrate (Epitrate), hydrochloride (Glaucon), and epinephryl borate (Eppy) — on intraocular pressure and outflow facility was evaluated in 24 patients. No significant difference was found.[16]

An additive effect occurs when epinephrine and acetazolamide (Diamox)[17] are used simultaneously to reduce the rate of aqueous secretion. Forty-one glaucomatous eyes treated with 250 mg of acetazolamide every 6 hours showed an average pressure drop of 13 mm Hg (range 5–50 mm Hg). Addition of a 4.5% solution of epinephrine bitartrate at night (only once daily) further lowered intraocular pressure by an average of 6.4 mm Hg (range 1–21 mm Hg). When epinephrine was used initially, the pressure in 20 eyes dropped an average of 13.4 mm Hg (range 4–54 mm Hg). Addition of acetazolamide further lowered the pressure an average of 7 mm Hg (range 2–15 mm Hg). These studies were carried out on known glaucomatous eyes that were continued on their regular miotic therapy throughout the experiment. The facility of aqueous outflow was unchanged by epinephrine or acetazolamide. In many of these patients the addition of epinephrine, acetazolamide, or both made the difference between uncontrolled pressures and a good therapeutic response. These results indicate that aqueous secretion was suppressed approximately 37% by topical application of epinephrine and 50% by acetazolamide. Used together, the drugs have an additive effect, reducing secretion an average of 66%.

What is the mechanism whereby aqueous secretion is decreased by sympathomimetic amines? Manometry and fluorometric measurement of outflow were employed in glaucomatous eyes to evaluate the effect of *l*-epinephrine, *d*-epinephrine, and isoproterenol (a strong β-agonist).[18] (Isoproterenol inhibits smooth muscle and is not a vasoconstrictor.) The average pressure drop after administration of *l*-epinephrine was 8.5 mm Hg, after *d*-epinephrine was 2.5 mm Hg, and after isoproterenol was 10.7 mm Hg. It was concluded that the sympathomimetic pressure-lowering effect is not caused by vasoconstriction, because isoproterenol is not a vasoconstrictor and the pressure-lowering effect lasted for 24 hours or more (longer than the duration of vasoconstriction). Nor is the increased tone of the dilator muscle responsible for the reduced aqueous production, because isoproterenol is not a mydriatic.

The explanation advanced at that time was that some type of β-sympathetic effect on the secretory mechanism resulted in hyposecretion of aqueous. Currently, it is believed that β-stimulation increases the rate of aqueous formation. Isoproterenol will reduce IOP for as long as 8 hours after topical instillation in the rabbit.[19]

A second mechanism of action by which epinephrine reduces IOP, namely, improvement of the facility of outflow, has been suggested. This improved facility is not immediate but may be observed after several months of topical epinephrine therapy. Evidence supporting this mechanism of action consists of a retrospective study of 72 patients and a controlled study of 38 patients.[20] The first group of patients had used a 2% solution of epinephrine topically twice daily for 6 to 24 months. All of the patients had proven open-angle glaucoma. In this series of 121 glaucomatous eyes, 62% showed increased facility of outflow by at least 50% over pretreatment levels at the end of 6 months. Of 55 eyes followed for more than 2 years, 56% still maintained this 50% (or more) improvement in outflow. Side effects forced discontinuance of epinephrine therapy in 27 of these 72 patients. Twenty had reactive hyperemia, and seven developed severe contact allergy of the lids. No corneal or lens opacities or other serious complications have been attributed to epinephrine therapy.

The second group, consisting of 38 patients, used a 2% *l*-epinephrine solution in one eye only, the other eye serving as a control. The topographically more abnormal eye was selected for treatment. At the end of 3 months, the facility of outflow of the treated eyes averaged 145% of the pretreatment level, whereas the average facility of the control eyes was only 98% of the pretreatment value. At 6 months the facility of outflow of treated eyes averaged 163% of pretreatment values compared with outflow facility of control eyes of 106%. The improvement of outflow in the treated eyes is of a statistically significant magnitude and must be accepted as valid evidence of an epinephrine effect.

That the coefficient of outflow in glaucomatous eyes is improved after prolonged *l*-epinephrine therapy has been confirmed by other studies.[21] In a series of 81 eyes with chronic simple glaucoma, 68% were found to attain an increase in outflow facility of at least 50% after *l*-epinephrine therapy. This increase in outflow facility occurred only after prolonged therapy. In 40% of the treated eyes, the response occurred within 1 month, and in 63% it occurred within 1 year. In five eyes improved outflow was first noted only after more than 1 year of epinephrine therapy. Although the improved outflow was maintained by most eyes, it was subsequently lost in ten eyes after intervals of 2 to 9 months. About 10% of this series of patients developed allergy to the epinephrine preparation. It was suggested that this sensitivity might be caused by antioxidants in the solution and not by epinephrine itself.

The outflow-increasing effect of epinephrine was thought to result from its action on the innervation of the trabecular meshwork. Experimental work indicating this as the site of action may be summarized as follows[22]: Cervical sympathectomy in rabbits increased the sensitivity of the outflow response to norepinephrine by about 150 times. (Intracameral injection of 0.02 μg/ml in the denervated eye produced an outflow increase comparable with that produced by 3 μg in normal eyes.) Complete sympathetic blockade (by intravenous phenoxybenzamine) eliminated all outflow response to norepinephrine. The increased facility of outflow is quite marked 1 hour after injection of norepinephrine into the anterior chamber.[23] Other sites of action that were ruled out included episcleral resistance (excluded by dissection away of surface tissue and by a lesser response to subconjunctival injection than to intracameral injection), ciliary muscle stimulation (excluded by lesser response to vitreous injections adjacent to the ciliary muscle), iris (excluded by absence of pupil response at low levels and by absence of aqueous protein alterations), mechanical deepening of the anterior chamber (excluded by control injection of saline solution), nonspecific chemical effect (excluded by phenoxybenzamine block), and vascular responses (excluded by the variation in response to different sites of injection and by absence of aqueous protein changes).

In monkeys, an immediate increase in the true facility of outflow and in pseudofacility can be demonstrated after topical application of epinephrine.[24] Apparently primate eyes can respond to epinephrine by both immediate and delayed improvement of outflow. A comparable immediate increase in outflow facility has been demonstrated in some normal and glaucomatous human eyes.[25]

Topically applied epinephrine may have primarily a β-effect (enhanced uveoscleral outflow) in low concentrations (0.06%–0.50%), whereas higher concentrations (1.0%–2.0%) activate the alpha mechanism (increased outflow facility).[26] However, such a supposition seems incompatible with the extreme sensitivity known to characterize autonomic responses. This study also indicated that epinephrine supplementation of 4% pilocarpine therapy in glaucomatous eyes was of no clinical value in concentrations of less than 0.5% epinephrine. An increasing hypotensive response was reported with epinephrine concentrations ranging from 0.5% to 2%. A 20% to 30% increase in the hypotensive effect was achieved by adding 2% epinephrine to the 4% pilocarpine.

Chemical sympathectomy with 6-hydroxydopamine sensitizes the eye to epinephrine. Subsequent epinephrine therapy (1% three times daily) maintained 29 of 36 eyes at less than 20 mm Hg for up to 29 weeks. This management was most effective in patients who had previously been well controlled with pilocarpine and epinephrine and was not very effective in patients who had not been well controlled medically before use of the 6-hydroxydopamine.[27] Chemical sympathectomy is not likely to supplant conventional medical therapy.

Epinephrine responsiveness may be among the factors that differ between persons with primary open-angle glaucoma and normal individuals. Topical epinephrine 1% decreased IOP by more than 5 mm Hg in 88% of 16 patients with open-angle glaucoma but in only 31% of 16 patients with secondary glaucoma. Epinephrine therapy produced premature ventricular contractions in 69% of the open-angle glaucoma patients but in only 19% of the secondary glaucoma patients.[28] This report does not identify whether the secondary glaucoma eyes responded to other medications.

The use of epinephrine in the treatment of glaucoma is not new but was popular a generation ago.[29–32] Because of the advances in new glaucoma medications, epinephrine is not a frequently prescribed drug; however, its effects and uses are still very important.

## Dose-Response Relationships

Although dose-response studies indicate that 2% epinephrine has a greater pressure-lowering effect than lesser concentrations (Fig. 3–5),[33, 34] continuous delivery eye inserts providing a dose of only 4 μg/hour reduce intraocular pressure as effectively as will a dose of 550 μg (1 drop of 1% epinephrine) given every 12 hours (Fig. 3–6).[35] The therapeutic effect is a function of not only the concentration of the drug used but also the duration of the exposure to the drug.

## Toxicity

### *Sympathomimetic Effect*

**During Surgery.**—Minor systemic side effects commonly occur after injection of solutions of epinephrine and anesthetic. These effects include nervousness and anxiety, tachycardia, tremors, headache, and pallor. Such symptoms may be quite alarming to the patient, who should be reassured that they are without significance and will soon disappear. Conditions such as coronary artery disease, hypertension, and thyrotoxicosis increase the susceptibility of the patient to epinephrine response and contraindicate its use.

The frequency of these side effects is not surprising if one realizes that the average adult therapeutic dose of epinephrine, 0.25 mg, is contained in 12.5 ml of a 1:50,000 solution of epinephrine and anesthetic. Of

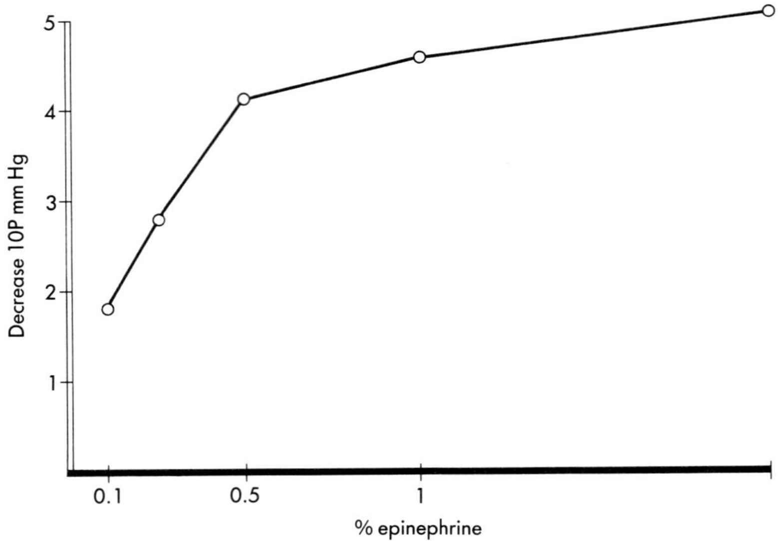


**FIG 3–5.**
Dose-response curve for epinephrine-treated monkey eye. (Modified from Lamble JW, Lamble AP: *Invest Ophthalmol Vis Sci* 16:628, 1977.)

course, this is not all absorbed at once, and the rapid systemic detoxification of the drug helps to reduce the frequency and severity of reactions.

Accidental intravenous injection of epinephrine may cause a transient rise in blood pressure as high as 400/300 mm Hg. To minimize the hazard of intravenous injection, one should aspirate the syringe before

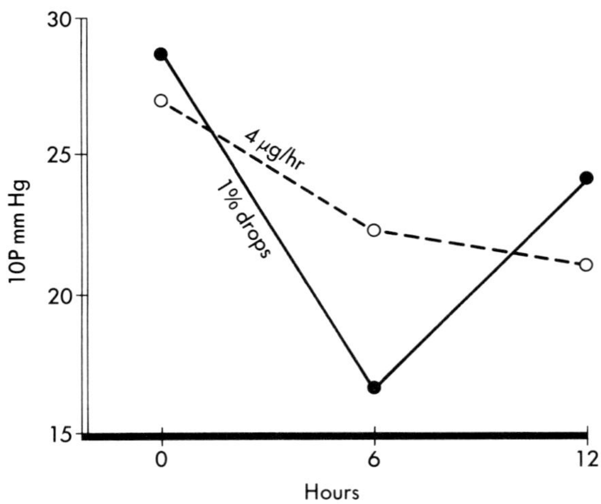


**FIG 3–6.**
Intraocular pressure (IOP) response (rabbit) to epinephrine given as continuous delivery system at 4 µg/hour or as a single eyedrop of 1%. (Modified from Birss SA, and others: *Ann Ophthalmol* 10:1045, 1978. Used by permission.)

injection of solutions of epinephrine and anesthetic.

Pallor, perspiration, and faintness, associated with an increase in blood pressure to 230 mm Hg, were reported in two patients after topical use of 2 drops of 2% epinephrine (2.7 mg), for hemostasis during local surgery in one case and to relieve redness after tonometry in the other.[36] A number of similar reactions were cited in this paper. The toxic effects of epinephrine closely simulate adverse reactions to anesthetic agents. As a result, the local anesthetic is often wrongly blamed for what is really a complication of the vasoconstrictor. Prolonged and severe cardiac palpitations and headaches are almost pathognomonic of toxic reactions to vasoconstrictors. In contrast, topical application of 10% phenylephrine rarely elevated blood pressure. Nevertheless, a subarachnoid hemorrhage associated with a hypertensive episode has been reported to follow a conjunctival pack of 10% phenylephrine.[37]

Excessively large doses of epinephrine may cause cerebral hemorrhage and ventricular fibrillation. Patients with hypertension, hyperthyroidism, coronary artery disease, and advanced cerebral arteriosclerosis are more likely to suffer these serious complications.

During general anesthesia induced by cyclopropane or halothane, the myocardium is more susceptible to stimulation by epinephrine, which may precipitate ventricular fibrillation. The topical use of epinephrine is therefore contraindicated during anesthesia with these agents.

A number of sympathomimetic drugs interact with certain anesthetics to produce cardiac arrhythmias. The mechanisms of action involved are extremely complex.[38] The safe use of catecholamines for local hemostasis during general anesthesia requires minimal doses and avoidance of hypercarbia and hypoxia. The ophthalmologist should obtain the approval of the anesthesiologist before applying epinephrine to the operative field.

**During Glaucoma Therapy.**—The usual systemic dose of epinephrine is 0.1 to 0.5 mg. One drop of 2% epinephrine contains approximately 0.1 mg of drug. Because such drops are usually instilled in both eyes, twice this dosage may be reached during glaucoma therapy. Extrasystoles can be recognized in tonograms as sudden downward deflections of the tonographic tracing. Analysis of tonograms of 535 patients indicated that extrasystoles occurred roughly twice as frequently in patients on epinephrine as in those not receiving this drug. Such objective evidence supports the occasional complaints of palpitations, tachycardia, and faintness encountered after epinephrine therapy. Because of the known cardiotoxic effects of epinephrine in doses comparable with those used in the eye, ophthalmologists should be aware of the cardiac status of patients for whom use of epinephrine is being considered.[39]

Actually, these extrasystoles are enhanced by the stress of tonography. Electrocardiographic monitoring showed that premature ventricular systoles can be induced by tonography or even by Goldmann applanation tonometry.[40]

### *Local Irritation*

The topical use of *l*-epinephrine is accompanied by a number of annoying side effects. Early commercial preparations produced a very severe burning sensation, which was often sufficiently marked to incapacitate the patient for 1 minute or so and required preliminary use of a local anesthetic in some patients. A boric acid and epinephrine complex, epinephryl borate (Eppy 1%), was developed that is much less irritating. Because of improved stability, this preparation can be buffered to pH 7.4 (increase of the pH 3.5 previously necessary), which is more physiologic and may result in better corneal penetration. Refrigeration is not required for preservation of this boric acid and epinephrine complex, because it maintains stability for at least 3 years in closed containers and for at least 1 month when kept open at room temperature.

Forty of 56 patients treated with epinephryl borate once or twice daily found it significantly less irritating than the previously available forms of epinephrine.[41] Its tension-lowering effect over a 10-month period seemed equal to that of other forms of epinephrine. However, as in the past, severe headaches, aching of the eyes, conjunctival hyperemia, and local allergy occur with this form of epinephrine. It was used in two patients with narrow-angle glaucoma, and, as expected, they developed acute angle-closure glaucoma.

Epinephrine inhibits mitosis and migration of corneal epithelial cells and doubles the time required for healing of corneal epithelial defects. Tissue cultures of human corneal epithelium develop vacuolation, granularity, and finally cell death when exposed to 0.001% concentrations of epinephrine. (This is 10 μg/ml, the level at which an antibiotic would inhibit a moderately sensitive microorganism.[42])

Epinephrine has been instilled into the anterior chamber to induce pupillary dilatation at the time of cataract surgery. This practice may result in serious damage to the endothelial cells, causing transitory or irreversible corneal edema and opacification. The endothelial damage results from the toxic action of the 0.1% sodium bisulfite that is used as an antioxidant in commercially available epinephrine solutions. Pure epinephrine, 1:1000, does not cause endothelial damage even after 5 minutes of perfusion.[43] This is often referred to as "cardiac epinephrine." After 2 to 6 years of unilateral epinephrine treatment, the corneal endothelial cell count averaged only 1.5% less for the treated eye than for the fellow eye in nine patients.[44]

### *Allergy*

Prolonged topical use of *l*-epinephrine may rarely cause a local conjunctival allergy but does cause tearing, burning, and ocular discomfort. The conjunctiva is slightly hyperemic (less so than in the usual allergy because of the vasoconstricting properties of epinephrine), follicles appear on the palpebral conjunctiva, and eosinophils may be demonstrated in scrapings. A case is reported in which allergic conjunctivitis caused by epinephrine persisted 7 months before it was diagnosed.[45]

On a statistical basis, allergy to pilocarpine, eserine, and environmental factors should first be suspected and, if present, should be eliminated or treated with corticosteroids. This accounts for the delay in diagnosis, which is unavoidable because the ophthalmologist must evaluate the diagnostic possibilities. The patient in this case was not relieved by corticosteroid therapy but was asymptomatic within 5 days after epinephrine therapy was stopped. To rule out the possibility of reaction to other ingredients of the commercially prepared solution, chlorobutanol and sodium bisulfite were instilled and did not cause ocular irritation. At 2 weeks and 2 months after diagnosis, epinephrine was used and the allergic conjunctivitis returned within 48 and 24 hours, respectively.

That epinephrine "allergy" truly represents a sensitization phenomenon was proved by demonstration of circulating antiepinephrine antibodies in a series of five patients with clinical evidence of epinephrine therapy. No cross-reactivity to phenylephrine or pilocarpine was demonstrated. In these patients the conjunctival allergy was manifested by diffuse vascular engorgement, follicular hypertrophy, and finally chemosis. Slight iritis developed in several cases, with fine deposits on the posterior corneal and lens surface and 1+ aqueous cells and flare. Fine subepithelial infiltrates of the cornea were frequent.[46]

## Epinephrine Pigmentation

The prolonged use of epinephrine drops may result in localized conjunctival deposits of pigment,[47] which are referred to as adrenochrome deposits. One year or more of daily therapy is required for the development of such lesions. Presumably these deposits develop within the translucent conjunctival cysts commonly seen in older patients. Oxidation of the epinephrine results in a slow accumulation of black or dark brown pigment within these cysts.

Pigmented deposits of oxidized epinephrine may also accumulate within roughened and edematous corneal areas. Two such cases of circumscribed, black, nodular, superficial corneal deposits developed after use of a 2% solution of epinephrine three or four times daily for more than 1 year.[48] Epinephrine treatment of a patient with chronic secondary glaucoma for more than 1 year resulted in dense brown-black discoloration of the entire central corneal stroma, much like severe bloodstaining of the cornea.[49]

Corneal pigmentation caused by epinephrine is particularly likely to occur in eyes with a damaged epithelium and is enhanced by the use of old and discolored solutions of oxidized epinephrine.[50] The granules of pigment can be deposited intralamellarly throughout the stroma of a corneal graft.[51] In another patient an elevated, densely black plaque of oxidized epinephrine was deposited between the epithelium and Bowman's membrane, covering half of the corneal surface. This eye was enucleated after the mistaken diagnosis of malignant melanoma.[52]

The prolonged use of epinephrine in patients wearing soft contact lenses may cause the lens to turn almost jet black. Although one might think that such a lens is irreparably damaged, immersion in 3% hydrogen peroxide for 5 hours will bleach it back to its original state. Be sure to rinse out the peroxide in water before using again.[53]

Conjunctival pigmentation somewhat similar in appearance to that produced by epinephrine may follow prolonged use of dark cosmetics applied to the conjunctival side of the eyelash margin. The black cosmetic pigment is deposited as multiple circumscribed dots within the center of conjunctival papillae. The upper margin of the superior tarsal conjunctiva is selectively involved. Although the associated symptom of conjunctival irritation disappears within a few weeks if the cosmetic is kept from the conjunctiva, the pigmentation itself persists as a permanent tattoo.[54]

After 13 years of epinephrine use, a glaucoma patient developed a persistent foreign body sensation and corneal ulceration diagnosed as being a herpetic infection. This lesion was unresponsive to medical therapy for more than 1 month. At that time, an exposed 3-by-1.5-by-1-mm black adrenochrome deposit was found in the upper lid overlying the corneal ulcer. Removal of this black nodule resulted in prompt cure of the corneal defect.[55]

### Epinephrine Maculopathy

Aphakic patients using epinephrine topically as treatment for glaucoma tend to develop a reversible maculopathy.[56] This epinephrine maculopathy affects at least 20% to 30% of aphakic eyes treated with epinephrine. The onset of symptoms may occur within a few weeks to many months after therapy is started. The affected patient complains initially of blurring and distortion of vision and later of progressively decreasing visual acuity. In some patients, visual acuity will drop to as low as 20/400 during prolonged epinephrine use.

Examination of the patient reveals an edematous appearance of the macula, most readily recognized with biomicroscopy. Occasionally small cysts or hemorrhages develop at the posterior pole.

Discontinuance of epinephrine therapy is usually followed by improvement in visual acuity and ophthalmoscopic appearance. Usually visual improvement is detectable within 1 month, but maximum return of vision often requires 6 months or more. If epinephrine maculopathy is unrecognized and continues for many months, some permanent loss of acuity may result. For this reason, the ophthalmologist should be alert to the possibility of epinephrine maculopathy when the aphakic patient with treated glaucoma complains of changes in central vision. Do not immediately assume the condition is an untreatable senile macular degeneration, aphakic cystoid macular edema, or a problem with aphakic glasses.

The existence and characteristics of epinephrine maculopathy have been described in a number of studies of aphakic glaucoma treated with epinephrine. For example, fluorescein angiography of 56 consecutive aphakic glaucomatous eyes treated with epinephrine showed macular edema in 28% compared with 13% of 72 such eyes not currently treated with epinephrine.[57] In seven eyes, epinephrine therapy was discontinued; in six of the seven the edema resolved within 1 year. One eye was reported in which the edema disappeared, recurred, and disappeared again as epinephrine was stopped, started and stopped. No correlation was found between macular edema and the use of other antiglaucoma drugs. Neither was there a relationship between the length of time of epinephrine use and the time required for resolution of edema after epinephrine was discontinued. Unfortunately, the statistics presented do not permit evaluation of whether the predisposition to epinephrine maculopathy is a bilateral characteristic of an individual exhibiting undue reactivity to epinephrine.

Another study attempted to differentiate cystoid macular edema from epinephrine maculopathy by demonstrating disappearance of the edema with epinephrine withdrawal and recurrence with renewal of epinephrine therapy.[58] Of 69 aphakic, glaucomatous, epinephrine treated eyes, only 12 could be followed sufficiently well to establish whether or not epinephrine reversibility of macular edema existed. Of these 12, seven ceased to leak when epinephrine was stopped, and 6 of these redeveloped edema when epinephrine was again used. Overall, of 53 adequately examined aphakic, epinephrine-treated, glaucomatous eyes, 18 had macular edema. In this series, a total of 69 eyes were derived from 49 patients, suggesting that macular edema will affect the second eye in perhaps half of patients with cystoid macular edema or epinephrine maculopathy. These authors advised that visual acuity measurement is an inadequate method of evaluating the status of a leaky macula and urged periodic fluorescein evaluation of any aphakic patient requiring epinephrine for pressure control. Whenever possible, other medications than epinephrine should be used for treatment of aphakic glaucoma unless the pressure cannot be controlled except with epinephrine.

Substitution of another sympathomimetic drug such as 10% phenylephrine does not appear to be helpful. One patient developed maculopathy while using epinephrine only twice weekly and 10% phenylephrine four times daily.

Timolol, miotics, or combination of these drugs will usually be preferable to epinephrine in treatment of aphakic glaucoma. Of course, any medications can be associated with problems.

The clinical and fluorescein photographic appearance of postcataract cystoid macular edema and epinephrine maculopathy are identical.[59, 60] Presumably a similar predisposing factor underlies both conditions. However, there is no question but that alternating use and nonuse of epinephrine can result in correlated exacerbation and remission of maculopathy.[61]

Explanation of the production of epinephrine maculopathy might presume that underlying vascular disease predisposes to vascular leakage. The average age of epinephrine maculopathy patients was 76.5 years (range 57–91 years) compared with an average age of epinephrine users without maculopathy of 68 years (range 30–84 years).[57] Some evidence of epinephrine in the target tissue would be suggestive. Selective catecholamine uptake mechanisms exist in all adrenergically innervated tissues, such as choroid, retina, and optic nerve. Nonspecific uptake of many chemicals, such as catecholamines, occurs wherever melanin exists. The actual presence of labeled epinephrine can be demonstrated in the choroid and retina of an aphakic eye after topical application.[62, 63]

Presence of an intact posterior capsule greatly reduces the amount of epinephrine reaching the choroid. Lesser amounts of labeled epinephrine are found in the retina and optic nerve and also reach the opposite optic nerve via the systemic circulation. Suggested toxic mechanisms include increased rate of prostaglandin synthesis, which is induced by epinephrine; decreased protein biosynthesis resulting from the combination of epinephrine and ultraviolet light (transmitted through aphakic media and capable of inhibiting up to 80% of protein synthesis)[64]; and decreased blood supply. (Subconjunctival injection of 0.002 mg of epinephrine in the rat will decrease choroidal blood volume by 68%.[65]) The α-effect of topical epinephrine can significantly reduce uveal blood flow.[66]

Intravenous injection of 1 mg of epinephrine in rabbits will transiently abolish the C wave of an electroretinogram (ERG). This wave disappears in 1 to 3 minutes and returns to normal in 10 to 20 minutes. Because the C wave originates from the pigment epithelium, this finding apparently indicates that epinephrine is selectively toxic to the pigment epithelium. (The other components of the ERG were unaffected.[48]) Perhaps this C-wave change offers an explanation of the mechanism of epinephrine maculopathy.

### Herpes Simplex Reactivation

Multiple factors alter the equilibrium between latent herpes simplex and active infection. Such physiologic insults as exposure, illness, fever, or corticosteroid application may activate herpes ulcers. Injected intramuscularly in rabbits on 3 consecutive days, 0.5 ml of a 1:500 concentration of epinephrine in oil was reported to reactivate experimental corneal herpes simplex, as judged by virus recovery or corneal staining.[67]

Epinephrine has also been shown to enhance the intracerebral penetration of poliovirus in mice. This finding may explain the relationship between stress and susceptibility to poliomyelitis.[68]

Herpes simplex–infected rabbits harbor latent virus in the trigeminal and superior cervical ganglia. Epinephrine iontophoresis will cause reactivation with viral recovery from tear film possible from 100% of rabbits within 3 days. This epinephrine technique is the most effective way to reactivate the herpes virus after local ocular inoculation.[69]

### Drug-induced Pemphigoid

In a series of 29 cases of ocular pemphigoid, 14 had used epinephrine eye drops.[70] Other drugs causing this syndrome include echothiophate and antiviral medications when used for long periods.

## DIPIVEFRIN (DIPIVALYL EPINEPHRINE)

Dipivefrin is a lipophilic epinephrine derivative that is able to penetrate the intact cornea 17 times as readily as does epinephrine. It is an inactive prodrug, requiring conversion by tissue enzymes to epinephrine. Its onset of hypotensive action appears within 30 minutes, with maximum effect reached by 1 hour.[71]

Dipivefrin is up to 600 times more soluble in organic solvents than is epinephrine. Its penetration into the human eye was studied by an extraordinarily sensitive method of identifying catecholamines.[72] In this technique, radioactive dansyl chloride combines with catecholamines, thereby rendering them detectable by chromatography and radioautography without requiring exposure of the subject to radioactivity. Only 0.1 ml of aqueous humor is required for this method. Thirty minutes after application of 0.5% dipivefrin to the human eye (a dose of $6.45 \times 10^{-7}$ mol), 7% of it ($45.07 \times 10^{-9}$ mol) was present in the aqueous humor. The aqueous humor content then consisted of $9.02 \times 10^{-9}$ mol of dipivefrin and $36.05 \times 10^{-9}$ mol of epinephrine, indicating that 80% of the dipivefrin had already undergone biotransformation to epinephrine within the 30 minutes.

At 120 minutes, only $0.89 \times 10^{-13}$ mol of dipivefrin remained in the aqueous (this is the limit of sensitivity of the procedure, 100 trillionth of 1 mol) and $43.89 \times 10$ mol of epinephrine, indicating that 6.79% of the applied dipivefrin entered the aqueous and essentially 100% of the dipivefrin had undergone biotransformation to epinephrine.

The saline technique used with 2% epinephrine showed only 0.32% of the applied drug to enter the aqueous at 30 minutes and 0.40% at 120 minutes. Proportionately, dipivefrin transcorneal passage was 17 times greater than that of epinephrine.

Actually, the penetration of dipivefrin into the eye must have been far greater than the 7% identified in the aqueous because uptake by the iris occurs rapidly, and 1%/min is lost by aqueous outflow. Despite this, the aqueous content of drug remained almost constant for 1½ hours.

Comparison of a 6-month crossover treatment of 17 glaucoma patients with 0.1% dipivefrin or 2% epinephrine showed an average pressure decrease of 23.7% with dipivefrin and 27.4% with epinephrine.[73] Burning and irritation affected 24% of the epinephrine-treated eyes but only 3% of the dipivefrin-treated eyes. Apparently 0.1% dipivefrin is intermediate in strength between 1% and 2% epinephrine, which would be expected with 17 times greater penetration.

### Combination Therapy

Additive use of dipivefrin and timolol seems to indicate that 0.25% timolol is slightly more effective than 0.1% dipivefrin (Fig. 3–7).[74] Addition of timolol in a group of 17 patients (34 eyes) who had been using dipivefrin showed a modest average drop in IOP of 3 to 4 mm Hg. Addition of dipivefrin in a group of seven patients (14 eyes) who had been using timolol showed an insignificant average drop of about 1 mm Hg. In each group, the combined therapy resulted in a definite drop of both systolic and diastolic blood pressure (142/83 to 129/77). In the dipivefrin-added group, three patients stopped the new drop because of ocular blurring and one because of headache. No patients in the timolol-added group refused to continue. The magnitude of additive response of timolol and dipivefrin in this study was not very impressive; however, all these patients had been under adequate pressure control with the single drug previously used. The study does not establish the response of poorly controlled patients.

Betaxolol, a $\beta_1$-selective $\beta$-blocker, shows a greater drop in IOP with the addition of epinephrine products than timolol. It must be remembered, however, that timolol is associated with a larger drop

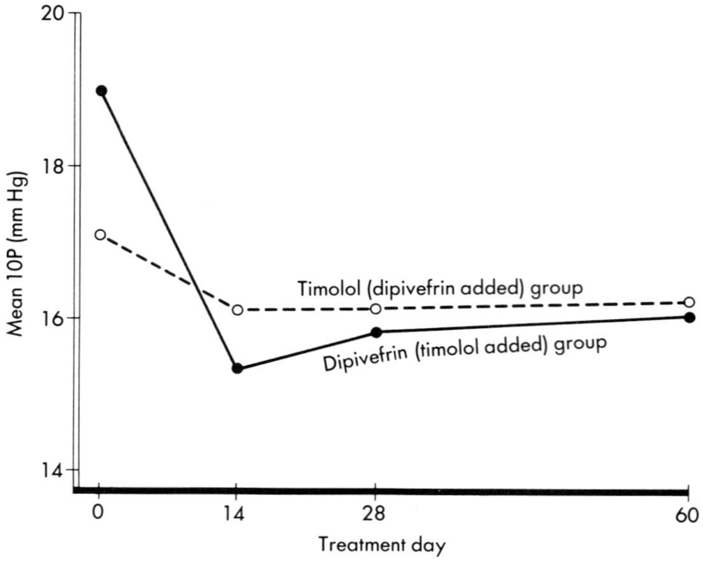


**FIG 3–7.**
IOP response when 0.25% timolol is added to dipivefrin 0.1% *(solid line)* and vice versa *(dotted line)*. (Modified from Keates EU, Stone RA: *Am J Ophthalmol* 91:243, 1981. Used by permission.)

in IOP than betaxolol when used as single agents. The combination of either of the β-blockers with epinephrine shows similar overall IOP lowering (Figs. 3–8 and 3–9).[75, 76] These data become important when a patient with glaucoma is initially controlled with a nonselective β-blocker, has to be switched to a selective β-blocker for pulmonary concerns, and now has poorly or marginally controlled IOP. This patient will probably benefit from the addition of epinephrine or dipivefrin *even if* these drugs were unsuccessful when the patient was on the nonselective β-blocker therapy.

Combined use of dipivefrin and echothiophate in rabbits suggested that cholinesterase inhibition inactivates the enzyme converting dipivefrin to epinephrine.[77] Echothiophate alone reduced IOP 5 mm Hg, dipivefrin alone reduced it 8 mm Hg, echothiophate with added dipivefrin reduced it 5 mm Hg, echothiophate with dipivefrin with added epinephrine reduced it 9 mm Hg, and dipivefrin with added echothiophate reduced it 5 mm Hg. Addition of dipivefrin to echothiophate was of no benefit.

A similar study in 16 human eyes showed that the epinephrine-echothiophate combination was never more effective than the dipivefrin echothiophate combination.[78] In fact, neither drug added much to the echothiophate effect. The average baseline pressure was 15.1 mm Hg, dropping to 10.7 mm Hg with 0.25% echothiophate. Addition of 2% epinephrine gave results at various times averaging 10.2 to 11.5 mm Hg; addition of dipivefrin resulted in an average of 9.4 to 10.9 mm Hg.

## Toxicity

Fourteen glaucoma patients taking 0.1% dipivefrin twice daily were followed for 3 years.[79] Four patients had blepharoconjunctivitis develop, requiring that the drug be stopped after 17 to 26 months. Two of these four had previously been epinephrine intolerant. No patients had systemic cardiovascular side effects or conjunctival pigmentation.

Karyomegaly (abnormally large nuclei) occurs in epinephrine conjunctivitis and in mucosal smears from folic acid–deficient patients. Folic acid transfers methyl groups needed for DNA synthesis. Catechol-O-methyltransferase also uses methyl groups for epinephrine detoxification.[79] Would folic acid benefit epinephrine conjunctivitis?

Of 26 patients on twice daily 0.1% dipiv-

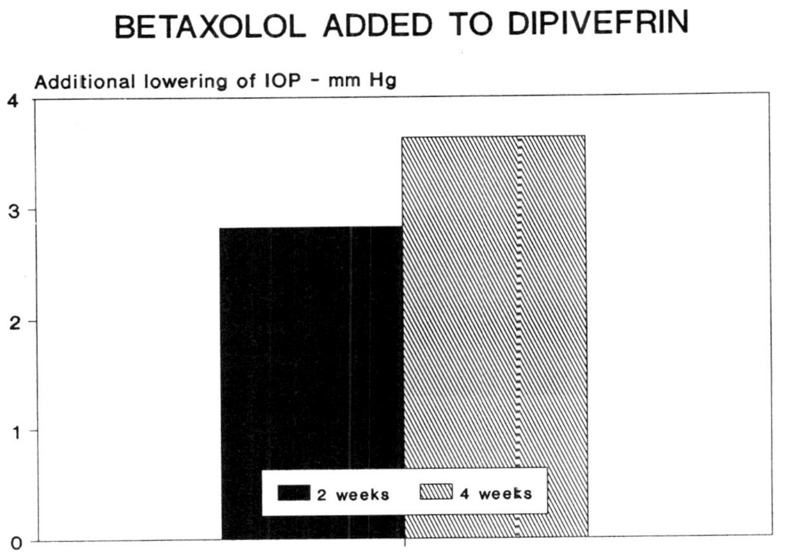


**FIG 3–8.**
Further lowering of IOP with the addition of betaxolol to eyes already on dipvefrin therapy. (From Weinreb RN, Ritch R, Kushner FM: *Am J Ophthalmol* 101:196, 1986. Used by permission.)

efrin therapy, 6 discontinued the medication because of blepharoconjunctivitis occurring after 5 to 22 months of therapy. Four of the six had prior reactions to epinephrine.[80]

In contrast to the marked difference in ocular absorption, the systemic absorption of dipivefrin and epinephrine is about the same.[81] After careful instillation of a 50-μl drop with prevention of blinking, 55% to 65% of the topical dose of either drug was systemically absorbed (radioactive study in rabbits). The drug pathways within the body differ greatly whether given intravenously or topically. By the intravenous route, peak

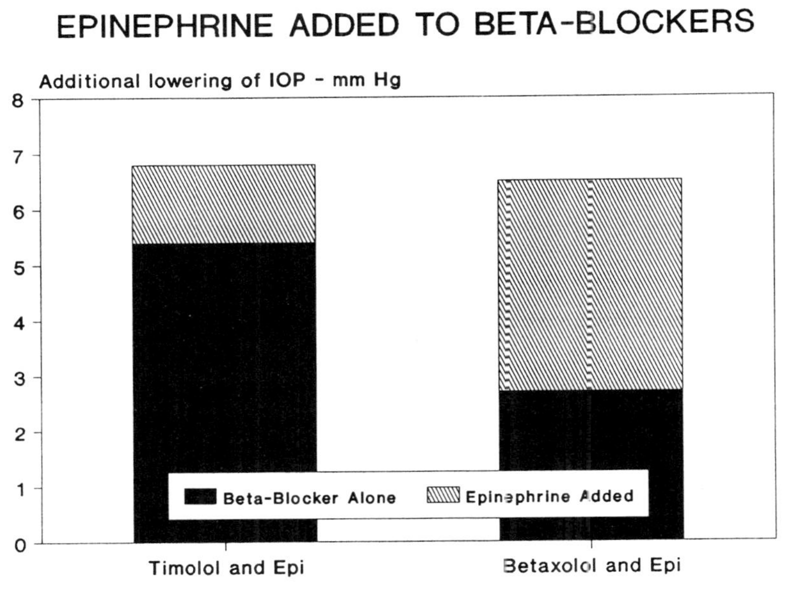


**FIG 3–9.**
Additive effect of epinephrine to either betaxolol or timolol. (From Allen RC, Epstein DL: *Arch Ophthalmol* 104:1178, 1986. Used by permission.)

tissue levels are reached in 15 minutes; they occur in tissues rich in adrenergic nerves such as heart, uvea, lung, and adrenal gland, and 96% of the drug is excreted via the urine. By the topical ocular route, peak general tissue levels are reached in 1 hour. By far the highest levels are in the eye, followed by pituitary gland and intestine. Only 55% is excreted via the urine and 25% in the feces, indicating that a substantial portion of the systemic absorption of ocular drops must be via the gastrointestinal tract. (After all, patients do complain of the taste of eye drops.)

### Lens Discoloration

Five glaucoma patients with soft contact lenses used dipivefrin for up to 84 weeks without developing any lens discoloration.[82]

### Summary

Epinephrine and propine are effective drugs against glaucoma. They do not cause as great a hypotensive effect as do pilocarpine or β-blockers and therefore are effective against a smaller proportion of cases of glaucoma. Epinephrine frequently causes side effects such as local allergy and systemic cardiovascular adrenergic responses. It may cause angle-closure glaucoma and aphakic maculopathy.[83] Epinephrine does not produce the pilocarpine effects of miosis (especially undesirable with cataracts) and breakdown of blood-aqueous barrier.

Norepinephrine 2% has, as would be expected, an effect compatible with that of epinephrine when used in treatment of glaucomatous eyes. Norepinephrine acts on the α-adrenergic system to increase the facility of outflow and produces an effect additive to that of pilocarpine. It is less irritating to the eye than is epinephrine and does not produce β-adrenergic effects such as tachycardia.[84]

## PHENYLEPHRINE

Phenylephrine hydrochloride, 2.5% to 10%, a direct-acting sympathomimetic mydriatic that stimulates α-receptors, is a valuable aid in ophthalmoscopy. It burns transiently on ocular instillation, causes several hours of light sensitivity (as do all dilating drops), may occlude structurally narrow angles, and usually produces no or only minimal systemic side effects after topical application of a few drops.

Phenylephrine pivalate is similar to dipivalyl epinephrine in having increased corneal penetration and therefore effectiveness in lower concentration than the nonconjugated drug.[85]

### Clinical Use

#### *Mydriasis*

Mydriasis from a single instillation of phenylephrine occurs in 60 to 90 minutes. Recovery from mydriasis takes 5 to 7 hours. The dose-response curve for phenylephrine shows an increasing dilatation as concentrations increase to about 5%. Little additional response is achieved by increasing the strength to 10%.[86] Repeated instillations of a mydriatic, either alone or in combination with a cycloplegic, will achieve greater dilatation.

Intense light stimulation, as in indirect ophthalmoscopy or fundus photography, will cause constriction of a pupil that has been dilated with only one instillation of phenylephrine. Cycloplegic drops will prevent this response to illumination.

A combination of 2.5% phenylephrine and 0.75% tropicamide instilled in the right eyes of 100 patients showed an average pupil dilatation to 7.5 mm (Fig. 3–10). The left eyes were dilated with 10% phenylephrine and 1% tropicamide, reaching an average dilatation of 7.6 mm. In both eyes, mydriasis was well maintained during the intense illumination of indirect ophthalmoscopy. These solutions were instilled subsequent to topical anesthesia and tonometry, which considerably enhance corneal penetration by drugs. A single drop of either concentration resulted in good dilatation within 15 minutes and maximal effect by 25 minutes.[87]

Sympathomimetic mydriatics are particularly useful as an aid to ophthalmoscopy. They act rapidly and do not have an excessively long duration. Virtual absence of cycloplegic effect spares the patient the

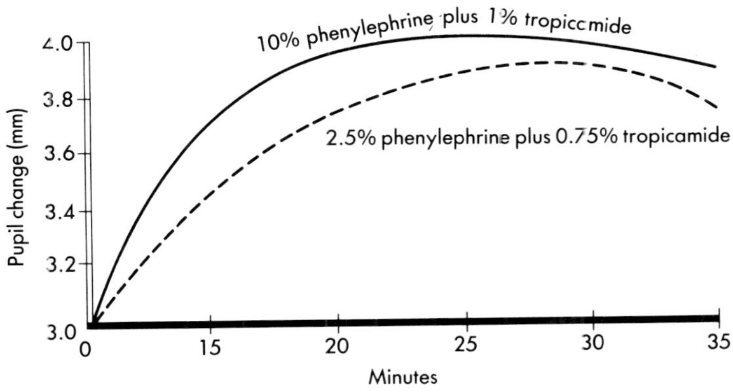


**FIG 3–10.**
Comparison of pupil dilatation induced by 2.5% phenylephrine and 0.75% tropicamide *(dotted line)* or by 10% phenylephrine and 1% tropicamide *(solid line)*. (Modified from Forman AR: *Ophthalmology* 87:213, 1980. Used by permission.)

inconvenience of being unable to read or see near details.

Although the miosis of old age is commonly attributed to mechanical changes of the iris, it is most likely caused by decreased sympathetic tone. Comparison of the effect of 10% phenylephrine in young and old subjects resulted in an equal dilatation of young and old pupils (average pupil diameter 8 mm), although the original pupil size was definitely smaller in the older patients. Hydroxyamphetamine and cocaine drugs with an indirect mechanism of action were not nearly so effective in dilating older patients, indicating the decrease in sympathetic tonus.[88]

Phenylephrine mydriasis is slightly less than that produced by cycloplegic drugs. The comparative effects of these drugs, as measured 40 minutes after instillation of 3 drops of each medication tested, are illustrated in Fig. 3–11.[89] As expected, the eyes of black persons dilate with greater difficulty, especially when phenylephrine, cyclopentolate, and hydroxyamphetamine are used.

The mydriatic effect may be enhanced by use of a phenylephrine pack.[90] After instillation of a topical anesthetic, a small piece of cotton is placed in the lower conjunctival sac and moistened with about 3 drops of 10% phenylephrine. The patient then closes the lids for about 30 minutes.

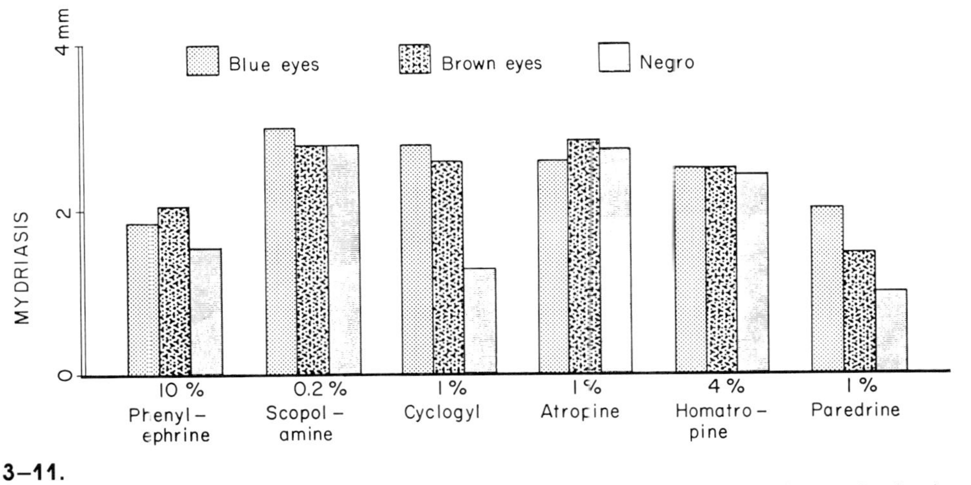


**FIG 3–11.**
Comparison of mydriasis produced by phenylephrine, scopolamine, cyclopentolate (Cyclogyl), atropine, homatropine, and hydroxyamphetamine (Paredrine). (Modified from Barbee RF, Smith WO: *Am J Ophthalmol* 44:617, 1957. Used by permission.)

The temptation to instill additional drops at frequent intervals should be resisted, lest systemic toxicity result from transconjunctival absorption.

Even in concentrations as small as 0.125%, phenylephrine may cause mydriasis. The mydriatic effect is greater if the corneal epithelium is damaged, thereby increasing drug penetration. The effect of 2 drops of 0.125% phenylephrine instilled in one eye of each of ten patients with normal corneas was measured after 45 minutes.[91] In only three patients was the pupil dilated 1 to 1.5 mm greater than its mate. Three eyes were dilated 0.5 mm, and four were unchanged. Similar phenylephrine instillation was done in 10 patients after routine tonography of both eyes. In all these patients who were not receiving miotic therapy, the test pupil was dilated and in several instances attained a diameter of 8 mm (Fig. 3–12).

This study of the mydriatic effect of a 0.125% concentration of phenylephrine was initiated because an attack of narrow-angle glaucoma had been precipitated by use of a solution of 0.125% phenylephrine and 0.25% zinc sulfate. Fourteen years previously the patient had undergone an operation for acute glaucoma in the right eye. A 2% concentration of pilocarpine has been used twice daily in the left eye for 14 years. The zinc and phenylephrine medication had been prescribed for mild conjunctivitis in both eyes (IOP of the left eye was 16 mm Hg). Within 2 hours the left eye was painful. The next day, IOP of the left eye was 57 mm Hg, and the angle was completely occluded. This acute glaucoma developed during use of pilocarpine (last instillation of a 2% solution of pilocarpine was 8 hours before use of phenylephrine) and was not controlled by subsequent pilocarpine administered by the patient. The case history convincingly shows the 0.125% concentration of phenylephrine to be the cause of this attack of angle-closure glaucoma; however, the patient obviously was strongly predisposed to angle closure.

Phenylephrine in a 0.125% concentration is contained in numerous drops designed to produce vasoconstriction and whiten the eye. These medications, usually prescribed freely, are potentially harmful in

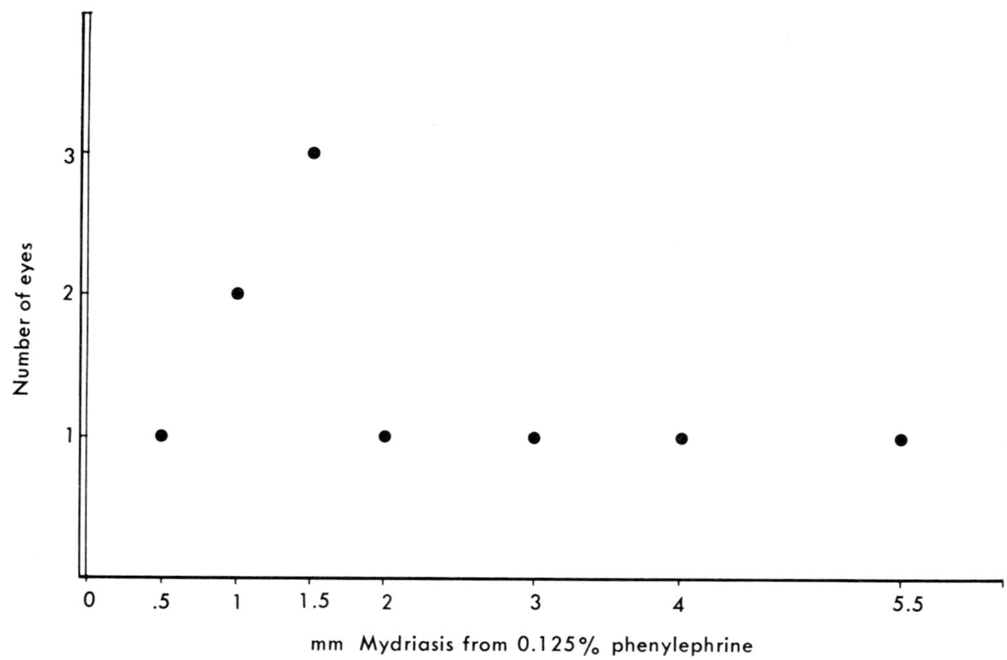


**FIG 3–12.**
Pupillary dilatation produced in 45 minutes by a 0.125% solution of phenylephrine instilled after tonography. (From Weiss DI, Shaffer RN: *Arch Ophthalmol* 68:727, 1962. Used by permission.)

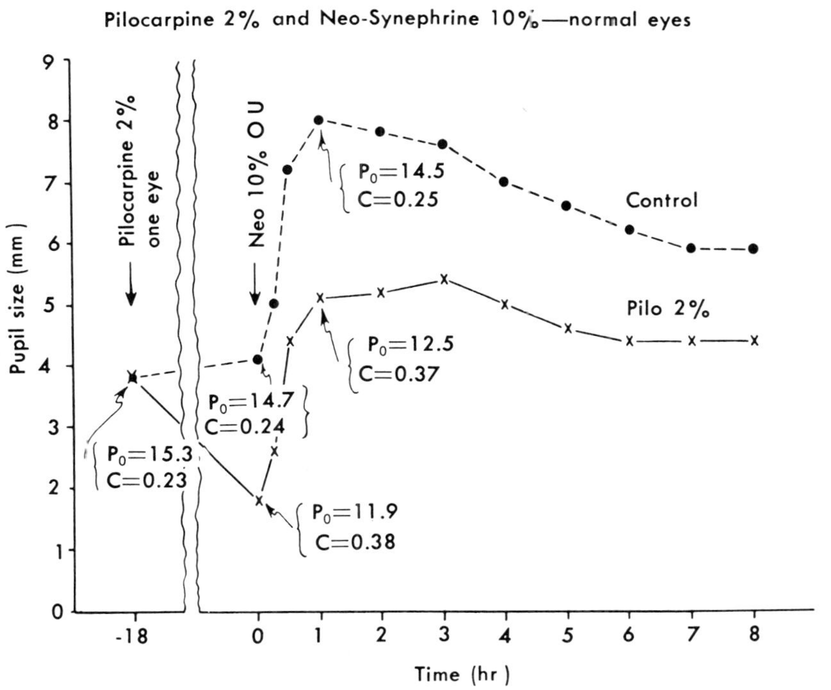


**FIG 3–13.**
Mydriatic effect of phenylephrine, 10% solution. *Solid circles:* response of normal pupil. *Crosses:* response of eye pretreated with 2% solution of pilocarpine. $P_O$, IOP; *C*, facility of outflow. (From Becker B, and others: *Am J Ophthalmol* 48:313, 1959. Used by permission.)

eyes predisposed to angle-closure glaucoma, especially if the corneal epithelium is abraded by tonometry or disease.

### *Competitive Action With Miotics*

The effect of 10% phenylephrine solution on eyes pretreated with 2% pilocarpine solution is illustrated in Fig. 3–13.[1] The untreated pupil dilates in response to phenylephrine, reaching a maximum diameter within 30 to 60 minutes. Maximum dilatation persists for several hours and then gradually decreases. The pilocarpine-treated pupil also dilates in response to phenylephrine, although not as widely as the untreated pupil. Instillation of additional mydriatic or miotic drops would, of course, further alter the size of the pupil in the expected direction.

In a series of 16 patients with chronic simple glaucoma adequately controlled with demecarium, a 10% solution of phenylephrine dilated the pupil nicely (average increase in pupil size 2.4 mm). Both before and after phenylephrine dilatation, the mean coefficient of outflow in these patients was 0.22.[12] These findings imply that phenylephrine will partially overcome the miosis produced by even the strongest miotics and can therefore be used for periodic fundus examination in patients with chronic simple glaucoma. Furthermore, diagnostic dilatation with phenylephrine does not jeopardize the control of open-angle glaucoma. This is in contrast to parasympatholytic dilatation, which does reduce the coefficient of outflow. Phenylephrine is not necessarily safe to use in patients with shallow angles, particularly if subacute angle closure already exists.

Infrequently phenylephrine or epinephrine may increase intraocular pressure in open-angle chronic simple glaucoma.[92] This is less likely to occur if the patient is simultaneously receiving miotic therapy. Because of this occasional pressure increase, it is prudent to recheck the intraocular pressure during the week after prescription of sympathomimetic supplements to glaucoma therapy.

***Ptosis***

Ptosis resulting from sympathetic denervation (Horner's or Raeder's syndrome) may be relieved by topical instillation of a 0.125% concentration of phenylephrine. The frequency of dosage depends on response but is usually three or four times daily. Such treatment will sometimes benefit other types of mild ptosis that are cosmetically undesirable because of the uneven palpebral apertures that accompany the condition. Ptosis seen after enucleation may be reduced by instillation of a 10% solution of phenylephrine if a proper fitting of the prosthesis does not correct it. Apparently the mechanism of response is direct action on Müller's muscle.

The resection of Müller's muscle for ptosis may be selectively advised for patients in whom instillation of 10% phenylephrine will elevate the lid to a normal level.[93]

***Test for Horner's Syndrome***

One percent phenylephrine causes minimal or no dilatation of the normal pupil but will markedly dilate a pupil with postganglionic sympathetic denervation. If 10% phenylephrine is used, both the normal pupil and the Horner's pupil will dilate, but the denervated pupil will respond more rapidly and will tend to be 1 or 2 mm larger during the dilatation process. Although such minimal differences are recognizable in photographs, they may be difficult to assess reliably in clinical practice. Unilateral corneal epithelial abrasions will permit entry of more phenylephrine, resulting in a misleading increase in dilatation on the damaged side, a false-positive.[94]

## Systemic Toxicity

Even a drug as safe as phenylephrine requires some prudence in its use. One may become so preoccupied with the goal of wide mydriasis that one forgets that systemic absorption occurs transconjunctivally and through the nasal mucosa.

Three cases of severe acute hypertension (210/110 mm Hg and higher) were reported after the use of 10% phenylephrine eye drops during surgery.[95] The authors point out that a single drop of a 10% solution contains 3.3 mg of drug. One patient, a 5.4-kg infant, received 6 drops of 10% phenylephrine and responded with a systolic pressure of 230 mm Hg. It was also postulated that systemic absorption may be enhanced by an inflamed or postsurgical eye and that some individuals may be more susceptible to the hypertensive effect.

Acute hypertension so severe as to cause subarachnoid hemorrhage was documented by insertion in the lower cul-de-sac of a cotton wick soaked in 10% phenylephrine.[37]

The National Registry of Possible Drug Induced Ocular Side Effects has reported 33 instances of cardiopulmonary responses after use of phenylephrine eye drops. Fifteen were myocardial infarctions, 11 of which were fatal.[96–98]

Patients with sympathetic denervation are much more susceptible to the hypertensive side effects of phenylephrine. Such conditions include idiopathic orthostatic hypotension.[99] Four such patients averaged a 44 mm Hg increase in systolic blood pressure 20 minutes after placing a single drop of 2.5% phenylephrine in each eye.

Pharmacologic sympathectomy occurs with the use of guanethidine or reserpine, as for treatment of hypertension. After administration of 10% phenylephrine eye drops, a group of 12 such patients averaged a systolic increase of 30 mm Hg.[100]

Diabetic neuropathy is commonly associated with autonomic dysfunction. A group of 14 chronic diabetic patients averaged a systolic increase of 34 mm Hg after administration of 10% phenylephrine every 15 minutes for a total of three doses before cataract extraction. Patients with sympathetic denervation are deprived of the nerve terminal catecholamine uptake mechanism that is the primary method of inactivation of such drugs. Also monoamine oxidase inhibitors interfere with enzymatic destruction of catecholamines.

Of practical clinical significance, such patients are very prone to exhibit a substantial hypertensive response to topical phenylephrine and injected epinephrine (with the anesthetic), both of which are likely to be given before cataract extraction. It is known that cataract patients occasionally have such an overreaction to sympathomimetic drugs and therefore their use should be avoided in these sensitive persons.

On the other hand, the average patient without such a predisposition to sympathetic sensitivity will tolerate topical phenylephrine well. In a study of 100 patients, 1 drop of 10% phenylephrine in each eye caused no change in mean blood pressure or heart rate.[101] One hypertensive patient responded with a blood pressure increase greater than 20 mm Hg. The significance of this finding is obscured by the fact that of 50 patients receiving tropicamide (not a vasopressor), two hypertensive patients responded with a pressure increase greater than 20 mm Hg. Perhaps hypertensive patients simply react to any type of stress, such as an eye examination. Ten percent phenylephrine is contraindicated in premature infants. The dose : weight ratio is enormous.

### Hazard in Acute Glaucoma

Caution is necessary when any dilating drop is used in an eye predisposed to acute angle-closure glaucoma. This precaution applies to the use of sympathomimetic mydriatics, as well as parasympatholytic cycloplegics.

Particular care is necessary if the intraocular pressure is at a borderline level before dilatation or if the eye has had a previous attack of acute glaucoma that was subsequently controlled by miotic therapy without surgery. Under such circumstances, dilatation is justifiable only if the patient's symptoms suggest a melanoma, retinal detachment, or a similar major ocular disorder. A prophylactic laser peripheral iridectomy is clearly indicated in most patients with occludable anterior chamber angles in which dilatation of the pupil is necessary. Before dilatation is started, the patient should be informed that the necessity for fundus examination outweighs the danger of peripheral iridectomy, which may well become necessary as an emergency procedure. Even with the aid of carbonic anhydrase inhibitors, intravenous osmotic agents, and miotics, attacks of acute glaucoma that are medically irreversible can be precipitated by sympathomimetic mydriatics. If dilatation is necessary in the examination of any eye structurally predisposed to angle closure, the patient should remain in the office for several hours until good miosis is reestablished, the pressure has returned to normal, and the eye is comfortable. α-Adrenergic blockers thymoxamine and dapiprazole will reverse sympathomimetic dilatation.

### Miotic Cysts

Miotic cysts of the iris, sometimes the result of ocular drug therapy, can be prevented by the simultaneous administration of phenylephrine.[102] Commercially available phenylephrine solution may be used to dissolve echothiophate powder and thereby both drugs can be dispensed in a single solution. Twenty patients with esotropia received a 0.125% concentration of echothiophate iodide alone in one eye every night. The other eye received a 0.125% solution of echothiophate combined with phenylephrine in solutions of 10%, 5%, or 2.5%. After 1 to 6 weeks of therapy, 11 of the eyes treated solely with echothiophate developed iris cysts,[102] but none of the eyes on combined medication did so. These cysts will disappear in 1 or 2 months if echothiophate is discontinued or if combined echothiophate and phenylephrine therapy is substituted. The 2.5% concentration of phenylephrine was as effective in preventing cyst formation as was the 10% solution. Phenylephrine did not interfere with the therapeutic effect of the echothiophate on the accommodative esotropia. The only undesirable effect of the phenylephrine was the slight burning it caused on application; this was less with the 2.5% solution than with the stronger concentrations.

The mechanism of cyst formation by echothiophate and cyst prevention by phenylephrine is not clearly understood. If a 10% solution of phenylephrine is used each morning and echothiophate is instilled each night, iris cysts will develop. This observation suggests that prevention of the initial intense miosis is a more likely mechanism of action than is parasympathetic-sympathetic interaction.

Addition of a 2.5% solution of phenylephrine to a 0.125% solution of echothiophate iodide is recommended to prevent the development of miotic cysts during the treatment of accommodative esotropia.

### Liberation of Iris Pigment

An interesting side effect of sympathomimetic mydriatics is the release of pigment granules from the iris neuroepithelium. This pigment debris may be confused with the biomicroscopic appearance of iritis, but it is readily differentiated by the absence of other inflammatory signs, including aqueous flare.

In a series of 948 eyes examined with the slit lamp before and after dilatation with a 5% solution of phenylephrine hydrochloride, 44 eyes showed a definite increase in aqueous floaters with dilatation.[103] The subsequent responses of these 44 eyes were evaluated after instillation of solution of 5% phenylephrine, 0.1% epinephrine, 1% atropine, 1% homatropine, 3% cocaine, 1% pilocarpine, and 0.5% eserine. Aqueous floaters in varying numbers were produced in all cases in which phenylephrine and epinephrine were used. The other five drugs caused no floaters at all in most cases and only a few scattered cells in the remainder. Direct stimulation of the dilator muscle (composed of pigmented epithelial cells) by the sympathomimetic drugs was postulated as the cause of rupture of some of these cells, with subsequent release of pigment granules. Microscopic examination of aspirated aqueous revealed these aqueous floaters to be pigment granules from the iris neuroepithelium. This pigmentary response to dilatation was found primarily in older patients and is considered a senile change.

In general, floaters first appear about 30 minutes after instillation of phenylephrine, increase for 1 to 2 hours, and disappear within 12 to 24 hours. Repeated dilatations of the same eye will again produce pigment floaters but not in as great a number. Gonioscopy shows that patients in whom mydriasis produces floaters have trabecular pigmentation considerably greater than normal. No reference was made to the presence or absence of glaucoma in these patients, who might be expected to show a predisposition to chronic trabecular blockage.

Detailed study of the phenylephrine response of 49 patients with pigmentary dispersion syndrome, of whom 31 had pigmentary glaucoma, detected only two patients (both with glaucoma) who showed a pressure increase of more than 2 mm Hg in response to the drug. The highest increase was 7.7 mm Hg. Apparently this biomicroscopically visible pigment liberation is almost always insufficient to result in a measurable rise in pressure.[104]

### Postdilatation Miosis

In older patients, phenylephrine appears to alter the dilator muscle, resulting in a smaller pupil that is less responsive to subsequent dilatation.[86] This change is of such magnitude that the maximally dilated pupil area may be decreased by 30% to 40%. In a series of 12 patients more than 50 years of age, electronic pupillography showed an average increase in pupil diameter of 2 mm 75 minutes after instillation of 2 drops of 10% phenylephrine. Twenty-four hours later the average pupil diameter was 0.73 mm smaller than it was before the use of phenylephrine. Repeated instillation of phenylephrine at this time resulted in a dilatation of only 1.5 mm compared with the previous 2 mm. Whether this miosis and decreased response to mydriatic instillation lasted more than 1 day was not reported. Cyclopentolate dilatation did not cause such a postdilatation miosis.

### Endothelial Toxicity

During the prolonged surgery of vitrectomy, the corneal epithelium may become hazy and the pupil small. One way of dealing with these problems is to scrape off the epithelium and instill 10% phenylephrine. Unfortunately, this results in rapid clouding of the cornea. The reason for this was first thought to be phenylephrine toxicity,[105–107] but it actually is the fault of the vehicle. Commercial preparations of phenylephrine are dispensed at a low pH level to maintain stability. When the epithelium is not present, the penetration of this acid pH is more rapid than can be neutralized by the buffering capacity of the cornea. Detailed pharmacologic and electron microscope studies have shown the consequence to be severe pH-related vacuolation of the endothelial cells.[108] This consequence could occur any time the epithelium is not present.

### Psychotropic Effects

Several cases of hallucinations have been attributed to prolonged excessive use of phenylephrine nose drops.[109]

### Other Sympathomimetics

The itching of allergy, the discomfort of minor irritants, and undesirable redness of the eye motivate people to purchase more than 1 million bottles of vasoconstricting eye drops each month. Because minor causes of ocular redness and irritation are enormously more common than the serious causes (e.g., acute glaucoma or uveitis), lay use of these over-the-counter nonprescription medications only infrequently results in significant delay in seeking necessary medical attention. In the dilute concentration allowed for nonprescription availability, toxic side effects are extremely rare. Sporadic case reports document attacks of acute angle-closure glaucoma when decongestant drops are used in susceptible eyes after corneal epithelial abrasions (e.g., by contact lenses or tonometry).

The commercially available decongestant drops contain naphazoline in concentrations ranging from 0.012% to 0.1%, tetrahydrozoline concentrations of 0.05%, or phenylephrine concentrations of 0.12%. Evaluation of the effectiveness of such vasoconstrictors was done with a test method in which 0.5 μg of histamine was instilled into the pretreated human eye. Optimal response was achieved with a 0.02% concentration of naphazoline. Lesser concentrations were less effective; higher concentrations were not more effective. The other two drugs in specified concentration were less effective than 0.02% naphazoline.[110]

A combination of 0.05% naphazoline (vasoconstrictor) and 0.5% antazoline (antihistaminic) was found to be more effective than either drug alone in preventing histamine-induced symptoms.[111] Redness was more effectively relieved by the vasoconstrictor; itching was more effectively relieved by the antihistamine.

The common belief that use of such eye drops is a necessary part of good eye hygiene is unfortunate and untrue. In fact, the brief application of a cool, moist washcloth to the closed eyelids will provide virtually the same relief to tired and burning eyes as can be obtained by any eye drop. Now, a new nonsteroidal ketorolac tromethamine (Acular, Allergan) has been approved for allergic conjunctivitis. This will decrease some of the side effects seen with corticosteroids and sympathomimetics.

## HYDROXYAMPHETAMINE

Hydroxyamphetamine hydrobromide is an indirect-acting sympathomimetic drug.[112] Its effect is reduced or abolished by pretreatment with guanethidine, which depletes norepinephrine from the adrenergic nerve terminal. In a 1% solution, hydroxyamphetamine is an effective mydriatic when instilled in an eye with normal adrenergic innervation.

The use of 1% hydroxyamphetamine in testing for defective postganglionic sympathetic innervation is more specific and subject to less error than the cocaine or epinephrine tests. Hydroxyamphetamine releases endogenous norepinephrine from the normal nerve terminal. In postganglionic Horner's syndrome, norepinephrine is absent; hence, dilatation cannot occur. Fig. 3–14 summarizes the responses to hydroxyamphetamine of 12 patients with unilateral Horner's syndrome.[94] In central and preganglionic lesions, endogenous epinephrine is present and dilatation occurs. In postganglionic lesions, the affected pupil actually becomes smaller because more light enters the opposite dilated pupil.

In all such tests the drops should be instilled in both eyes to permit comparison of the normal and abnormal pupil responses. The cocaine, epinephrine, and phenylephrine tests are subject to error if

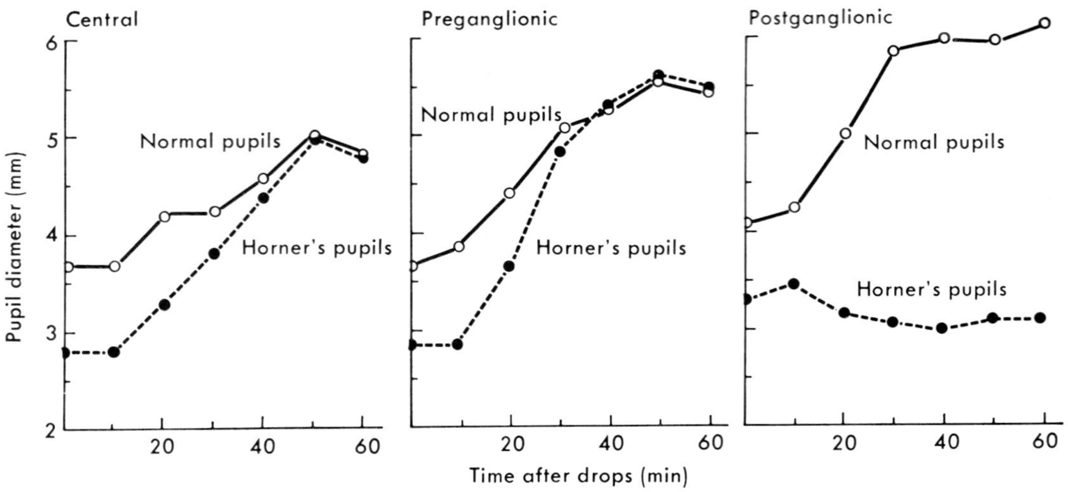


**FIG 3–14.**
Pupil responses to 1% hydroxyamphetamine in unilateral Horner's syndrome. (From Thompson HS, Mensher JH: *Am J Ophthalmol* 72:472, 1971. Used by permission.)

one eye has an epithelial abrasion, permitting entry of a greater amount of drug. The hydroxyamphetamine test is not subject to errors as a result of somewhat uneven administration of drops, because the response depends primarily on the amount of norepinephrine available for release. One possible error should be avoided. Cocaine blocks the uptake of hydroxyamphetamine into the nerve endings; hence, the hydroxyamphetamine test should not be performed within 2 days after a cocaine test. Incidentally, another possible source of error in testing for Horner's pupil occurs in patients with a heavily pigmented iris; cocaine dilatation in such a dark iris is extremely slow and may take as long as 3 hours to become maximal.[94]

Because of the similarity of molecular structure between hydroxyamphetamine and norepinephrine, the possibility of direct action of hydroxyamphetamine on smooth muscle adrenergic receptors has been suggested. If this were to occur, perhaps the differentiation between preganglionic and postganglionic lesions might not be quite as certain as has been suggested.[113]

The reliability of a hydroxyamphetamine (Paredrine) test for differentiating postganglionic from preganglionic lesions is not so great as has been theoretically stated. Injury may damage both preganglionic and postganglionic neurons. In congenital Horner's syndrome, transsynaptic degeneration may occur. The hydroxyamphetamine test localized the lesion in the peripheral neuron in 89 patients. Of these, only 75 (84%) actually did have peripheral lesions. Incorrectly localized central or intermediate lesions were found in 14 (16%). When the test localized the lesion to the central or intermediate neuron (in 72 patients), the test was 97% accurate. The importance of performing this test is that neoplasms causing Horner's syndrome almost always affect the central or intermediate neuron rather than the peripheral neuron. However, of 450 patients with Horner's syndrome, in only 13% this condition was caused by tumors and in only 3% by undetected tumors. The cocaine and epinephrine test are much less reliable than the hydroxyamphetamine test.[114, 115]

### Cocaine

Cocaine was originally used in ophthalmology as an anesthetic (now replaced by less toxic synthetic anesthetics). However, cocaine is also an indirect-acting sympathomimetic drug. Its mechanism of action has been postulated to be prevention of uptake of catecholamines by the adrenergic nerve terminal,[5] thereby prolonging the action of epinephrine and norepinephrine. Because of this indirect sympathomimetic action, cocaine is the only local anesthetic that causes vasoconstriction and mydriasis.

Topical cocaine in a dosage of 1.5 mg/kg was applied to the nasal mucosa before endotracheal intubation before cardiac surgery.[116] In this dosage no sympathomimetic cardiovascular effects were observed.

Studies with radiolabeled cocaine incubated on the guinea pig iris showed that the pigmented iris had an uptake of 18 times as much cocaine as did the nonpigmented iris. Furthermore, the cocaine was firmly bound to the pigmented iris, resisting the washout that easily occurred in the nonpigmented iris. Chemical sympathectomy with 6-hydroxydopamine did not alter cocaine binding by the iris, indicating that the effect was unrelated to sympathetic nerve terminals.[117]

## EPHEDRINE

This indirect-acting sympathomimetic drug causes rapid displacement of norepinephrine from the adrenergic nerve terminal.[118] It is not currently used by ophthalmologists.

The pigmented iris accumulates much more ephedrine than does the nonpigmented iris but is much less responsive to dilatation because of melanin binding and inactivation of the drug.[119]

## APRACLONIDINE

Apraclonidine (Iopidine 1%, Alcon) is an $\alpha_2$-adrenergic agonist approved for the prevention of intraocular pressure increases associated with ophthalmic laser procedures. It is a derivative of clonidine, which was abandoned as a glaucoma drug because of its significant systemic hypotensive effects when given topically.[120] Apraclonidine does not cross the blood-brain barrier. Apraclonidine reduces aqueous formation by acting on $\alpha_2$-receptors on the surface of the nonpigmented epithelium of the pars plicata (of the ciliary body). Gharagozloo and Brubaker[121] hypothesize that β-receptors stimulate and $\alpha_2$-receptors inhibit adenyl cyclase activity, therefore affecting the conversion of adenosine triphosphate (ATP) to cyclic adenosine monophosphate (cAMP) and aqueous production.[121] This similar mechanism of action would explain the lack of effect of adding apraclonidine to timolol therapy in the acute setting[122] and the minimal (but statistically significant) IOP reduction (1.3 mm Hg) with the addition of apraclonidine to an eye chronically treated with timolol.[121, 123] The authors suggest that with chronic timolol use a basal cAMP synthesis exists that can then be suppressed with apraclonidine. This basal cAMP synthesis may not exist in the acute period of β-blockade. Another mechanism of apraclonidine activity may be vasoconstriction of the afferent arterioles of the ciliary body, reducing aqueous flow.

### Prophylactic Use With Laser Procedures

Apraclonidine blunts the IOP rise often seen after ophthalmic laser procedures (Fig. 3–15). Of 28 eyes undergoing peripheral iridectomy with the argon laser, half received apraclonidine and half placebo preoperatively. Only three of 14 apraclonidine eyes developed modest IOP rises (< 11 mm Hg), whereas four of 14 placebo treated eyes had pressure rises of this magnitude and six of 14 had IOP rises greater than 10 mm Hg during the initial 3-hour postoperative period.[124] Similarly, apraclonidine prevented large (≥ 10 mm Hg) pressure spikes after argon laser trabeculoplasty, whereas the eyes randomized to placebo developed IOP rises of 10 mm Hg or greater in 18% (six of 34). Indeed, most eyes had lower pressures after argon laser trabeculoplasty when given apraclonidine preoperatively.[125]

### Prevention of Cycloplegic-Induced Pressure Rises

Apraclonine may be used to blunt IOP spikes with cycloplegia. Tropicamide caused 6–mm Hg IOP rise in eyes with open-angle glaucoma not treated with miotics. A 3.5–mm Hg rise was found in eyes with open-angle glaucoma treated with miotics (see Fig. 3-15). Apraclonidine use was associated with a 2.1– and a 0.5–mm Hg *drop*

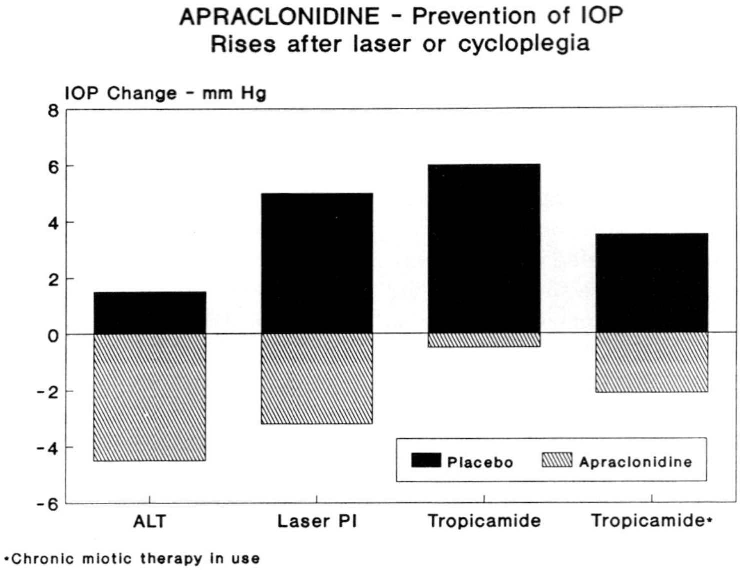


**FIG 3–15.**
Effect of apraclonidine on pressure rises produced by argon laser trabeculoplasty *(ALT)*, laser peripheral iridectomy *(PI)*, and cycloplegia of the glaucomatous eye with and without chronic miotic therapy. (Adapted from Robin AL, and others: *Arch Ophthalmol* 105:1208, 1987; Robin AL, Pollack IP, deFeller JM: *Arch Ophthalmol* 105:646, 1987; Hill RA, Minckler DS, Lee M, and others: *Ophthalmology* 98:1083, 1991.)

in IOP with and without miotic use, respectively.[126]

### Adverse Reactions

The systemic hypotension found with topical clonidine has not been associated with apraclonidine because it does not pass through the blood-brain barrier.[127] Systemic effects cannot be excluded until apraclonidine is used chronically on a large-scale basis. Ocular side effects are uncommon but include irritation, mydriasis, conjunctival blanching or congestion, and upper lid elevation.

SECTION TWO

# α-Adrenergic Antagonists (Sympatholytics)

MARY LOU KACHMER MCGREGOR

## GUANETHIDINE

Guanethidine is a sympatholytic drug that acts by displacing norepinephrine from the sympathetic nerve terminals. For the first few hours after topical ocular administration of 10% guanethidine sulfate, intraocular liberation of norepinephrine occurs. This causes mydriasis and a transitory increase of facility of aqueous outflow. Thereafter the tissue stores of norepinephrine are depleted, resulting in miosis and reduced secretion of aqueous humor. Both of these guanethidine effects lower IOP.[1, 2]

Topical instillation of 10% guanethidine produced significant cosmetic and symptomatic improvement in seven patients with lid retraction associated with thyroid disorder. The dosage was 1 to 4 drops daily. The lid-lowering effect of 1 drop appeared about 6 to 8 hours after instillation and lasted for about 1½ days. Apparently the action of guanethidine is cumulative, because a greater effect is achieved after 2 to 3 days of treatment. Miosis occurs in the treated eye.

Horner's syndrome was produced in human eyes by the topical instillation of 10% guanethidine monosulfate three times daily for 1 week. This chemical syndrome is entirely analogous to postganglionic cervical sympathetic denervation in respect to pupillography and testing with cocaine and epinephrine. Horner's syndrome disappeared 1 week after the guanethidine was discontinued.[3]

### 6-Hydroxydopamine

6-Hydroxydopamine, an isomer of norepinephrine, has the unique capability of causing selective degeneration of adrenergic nerve terminals without affecting other nerves. It can be used to perform chemical sympathectomy.

The technique of treatment is simply subconjunctival injection. Special care should be taken to avoid blood vessels; an operating microscope is advised for this purpose. After injection, a cotton-tipped applicator is used to massage the fluid around the circumference of the limbus. Injection is not made at the 12 o'clock position to avoid ptosis from denervation of Müller's muscle.

Only 0.2 ml of a 2% solution is required. The chemical is unstable and must be freshly dissolved in a 0.045 mol solution of sodium bisulfite at pH 6.9. Oxidation results in a faint pink discoloration, at which time the solution should be discarded.

Epinephrine therapy should be discontinued 2 days before 6-hydroxydopamine injection, because these drugs are competitive for uptake at the sympathetic terminal.

The local reaction to injection is a moderately severe conjunctival hyperemia, sometimes associated with mild chemosis and lid edema, which persists for several days to 1 week. The pupil dilates for 2 or 3 hours and then becomes miotic during the first day.

Systemic side effects do not occur, but enough drug enters the general circulation to cause demonstrable but minimal sympathetic supersensitivity in the other eye.

The day after injection, a hydroxyamphetamine (Paredrine) test is performed to check the completeness of denervation. Five drops of 1% hydroxyamphetamine given over 1 hour should cause less than 0.5-mm dilatation of the pupil if sympathetic denervation is complete. If the sympathectomy is incomplete, glaucoma will not be controlled and another injection need be given.

After 6-hydroxydopamine injection, intraocular pressure dropped within 3 hours of the injection, presumably because of liberation of norepinephrine from the adrenergic terminals. The maximum pressure drop occurred by the third day, suggesting continuing norepinephrine release. Pressure returned to baseline in about 2 weeks, apparently indicating exhaustion of the normal norepinephrine stores.[4, 5]

This return to baseline of IOP after stabilization of the 6-hydroxydopamine sympathectomized eye is an interesting phenomenon of ocular adrenergic physiology. It may indicate that the trabecular outflow mechanism (parasympathetic control) normally governs IOP, quite independently of the sympathetic system. Sympathetic stimulation may activate the uveoscleral unconventional exit of aqueous. This alternate route may predominate in glaucomatous eyes.

Sympathetic denervation does not in itself have any effect on glaucoma control. Its only purpose is to induce sympathetic supersensitivity and thereby enhance the pressure-lowering effect of epinephrine.

As would be expected, sympathetic terminal regeneration occurs. Chemical sympathectomy must be repeated three or four times yearly. The duration of effect varies from a few weeks to 6 months or more.

The effects of treatment in 128 eyes (92 patients) were reported. These patients were selected because their pressures could not be controlled by maximal medical therapy or because they could not tolerate the necessary drugs. The study extended over a 2-year period. Up to 70% of these patients could be controlled (pressures $<20$ mm Hg) after sympathectomy. It must be emphasized that even though topical epinephrine and pilocarpine therapy was still necessary, it resulted in much better control than before 6-hydroxydopamine injection.[6–8]

In another study of 137 eyes treated with 6-hydroxydopamine, only 39% were controlled.[9]

Since the advent of β-blockers and laser surgery for glaucoma, 6-hydroxydopamine therapy has never achieved any real clinical popularity; however, this technique may provide some insight into the autonomic physiology of the human eye. This chemical sympathectomy results in both α- and β-adrenergic supersensitization. Various degrees of pupil dilatation with phenylephrine (α-agonist) occur after sympathectomy in response to drug concentration approximately one tenth that required before sympathectomy. Isoproterenol (β-agonist) does not dilate the pupil significantly either before or after denervation. These results indicate that adrenergic pupil dilatation in the human eye is a pure α-response.

Five percent phenylephrine lowered IOP by 5 mm Hg in the untreated eyes. The same pressure drop occurred with 0.01% phenylephrine in the denervated eyes. A 2.5% concentration of isoproterenol lowered IOP by 5 mm Hg in the untreated eye. The same drop occurred with 0.0001% isoproterenol after sympathetic denervation. In the human eye IOP is lowered by both α- and β-agonists.

Neither phenylephrine nor isoproterenol changed the tonographic facility of outflow either before or after sympathectomy, indicating that adrenergic stimuli do not change facility.[10]

## THYMOXAMINE

Thymoxamine is a competitive antagonist of the α-effect of norepinephrine (the physiologic α- and β-adrenergic effector substance liberated at neural synapses). It has no β-adrenergic blocking effect. Thymoxamine is such a specific α-blocker that it is now the standard against which such pharmacologic action is compared.[11] Other α-blockers are dapiprazole, tolazoline, phenoxybenzamine, phentolamine, and ergotoxine. Of these α-blockers, thymoxamine and dapiprazole are the only ones free of the intolerable side effects that limit clinical use (Table 3–2).

The ophthalmic uses of thymoxamine are derived from the sympathetic innervation of Müller's muscle and the iris dilator muscle and the relative absence of sympathetic innervation of the ciliary muscle. Ophthalmic drops of 0.5% solution are well tolerated by the eye, causing only mild conjunctival hyperemia (loss of vessel tonus) lasting several hours. Ptosis and miosis may occur, as would be expected. Because there is little, if any, effect on the ciliary muscle, facility of outflow is not affected, and IOP

**TABLE 3–2.**
Adrenergic Antagonists (Sympatholytics)

| α-Blockers | | β-Blockers | |
|---|---|---|---|
| Systemic | Topical | Systemic | Topical |
| Tolazoline | Thymoxamine | Nonselective | Nonselective |
| Pentolamine | Dapiprazole | Propranolol | Timolol |
| Labetalol | | Practolol | Levobunolol |
| Dibenamine | | Pronethalol | Carteolol |
| Phenoxybenzamine | | Nadolol | Metipranolol |
| Guanethidine | | Timolol | |
| 6-Hydroxydopamine* | | Carteolol | |
| Bretylium | | Penbutolol | |
| | | Labetalol | |
| | | Pindolol | |
| | | $β_1$-Selective | $β_1$-Selective |
| | | Atenolol | Betaxolol |
| | | Esmolol | |
| | | Betaxolol | |
| | | Metaprolol | |
| | | Acebutolol | |

*6-Hydroxydopamine destroys adrenergic nerve fibers.

does not change in normal or glaucomatous eyes.

Fluorophotometric study of 25 normal human eyes showed no thymoxamine-induced change in rate of aqueous formation, intraocular pressure, blood-aqueous barrier, or anterior chamber volume. There was a 12% greater aqueous humor flow, but the values did not reach statistical significance.[12]

The most obvious use of thymoxamine is to reverse phenylephrine mydriasis. This is an ideal way to examine a glaucomatous fundus, especially in patients with narrow-angle glaucoma. Unlike cycloplegics, phenylephrine does not increase IOP in glaucomatous eyes; however, it may occlude narrow angles if the pupil is allowed to return to its normal size spontaneously. Counteracting the mydriasis with pilocarpine increases the physiologic pupil block and increases the probability of angle-closure glaucoma by shallowing the anterior chamber. Thymoxamine not only nullifies the mydriatic action of phenylephrine but also causes additional miosis (α-block of physiologic norepinephrine) lasting for hours longer than the effect of the phenylephrine. Thymoxamine does not cause shallowing of the anterior chamber. One drop of 0.5% thymoxamine will completely reverse 10% phenylephrine mydriasis within 30 minutes. The mean time for 1% pilocarpine reversal of 10% phenylephrine is 22 minutes. Pilocarpine lasts longer than phenylephrine and will routinely cause accommodative spasm with pain and blurred distant vision.

Theoretically, thymoxamine may also be of value in the treatment of acute angle-closure glaucoma. During mildly increased IOP, the perfusion of the iris sphincter may be less effective than that of the dilator, thereby resulting in the typical pupil dilatation of acute glaucoma. Relaxation of the dilator might be more effective than stimulation of the paralyzed sphincter. Also concepts of vectors of force suggest that sphincter miosis enhances physiologic pupillary block, whereas dilator relaxation miosis does not do so. In practice, four cases of angle-closure glaucoma in the pressure range of 30 to 50 mm Hg responded to treatment with topical thymoxamine alone given as 1 drop of 0.5% solution every 5 minutes for three doses, then every 15 minutes until control of pressure, which was achieved within 1 to 2 hours. Two cases with pressures of 60 mm Hg did not respond to thymoxamine.[13]

A thymoxamine test will differentiate angle-closure glaucoma from open-angle glaucoma with narrow angles.[14] Treatment for the first condition is iridectomy; treatment for the second is medical management. Thymoxamine does not change the intraocular pressure or facility of outflow in open-angle glaucoma but will open the angle and reduce intraocular pressure in angle-closure glaucoma, causing moderate pressure elevations. In 26 patients the exact status of the angle could not be gonioscopically determined. Use of thymoxamine visibly opened eight angles without reducing pressure, thereby diagnosing open-angle glaucoma for which the patient was subsequently satisfactorily treated. In 12 eyes the angle opened and the pressure dropped, thereby diagnosing angle closure for which successful iridectomy was performed. Three angles did not open, and the pressure remained high, indicating angle-closure glaucoma. In three eyes both open- and closed-angle glaucoma were present; both iridectomy and subsequent medical therapy were required.

Sympathetic overactivity of Müller's muscle is believed to contribute to hyperthyroid lid retraction. Of nine such cases, seven were significantly improved with 0.5% thymoxamine. The two failures were in chronic cases of long duration. Improvement appears within 15 minutes and lasts for hours. Guanethidine has a similar therapeutic effect but causes unpleasant side effects.

Brief dilatation and constriction of the pupil may help in repositioning iris-supported intraocular lenses.

## DAPIPRAZOLE

Dapiprazole produces miosis by α-adrenergic receptor blockage in the dilator muscle of the iris. It was introduced as a means of providing safe and rapid reversal of mydriasis and cycloplegia. Many patients complain of inconvenience after cycloplegia and mydriasis for ophthalmic examination. Cholinergic miotic pilocarpine is associated with adverse effects such as pain and blurred vision and therefore is not really applicable in reversing dilatation in cycloplegia. Dapiprazole hydrochloride is a 0.5% sterile ophthalmic solution containing benzalkonium chloride as a preservative. Reversal of mydriasis after use of 2.5% phenylephrine usually occurs within 30 minutes. Reversal of mydriasis when 1% tropicamide is used also occurred within 30 minutes after administration and continued through the 2-hour posttreatment examination. Dapiprazole has also been shown to induce miosis after mydriasis induced by parasympatholytics. A concentration of 0.5% dapiprazole produces a greater and longer-lasting miotic effect than does 0.5% or 1% thymoxamine.[15]

It also appears that dapiprazole is effective in reversal of decreased accommodation after use of 1% tropicamide and phenylephrine. Toxicity and side effects appear to be mild with the use of dapiprazole. They include fluorescein staining of the cornea, significant conjunctival injection, mild ecchymosis, lid erythema, and corneal edema. These findings were rare. There is no apparent systemic toxicity.[15] Dapiprazole is affected by the color of the irides. The rate of pupillary constriction seems to be slightly slower in individuals with darker irides. Because dapiprazole does not have any significant action on the ciliary muscle, it does not significantly change the anterior chamber depth or thickness of the lens. This is important because it adds to the safety of the drug in preventing angle-closure glaucoma.

SECTION THREE

## β-Adrenergic Receptor-Blocking Agents

LOUIS M. DESANTIS, JR.

β-Adrenergic receptors or adrenoceptors in various tissues mediate certain of the physiologic responses to the sympathetic neurotransmitters and adrenal medullary hormones epinephrine and norepinephrine. Three subtypes of β-adrenoceptors, designated $\beta_1$, $\beta_2$, and $\beta_3$, have been discovered. Their distribution and functions vary among tissues. Some tissues contain multiple subtypes of β-adrenoceptors in varying proportions. β-adrenoceptors are cell-surface receptors functionally coupled to membrane-bound adenylyl cyclase enzyme via heterotrimeric guanine nucleotide–binding regulatory protein (i.e., $G_s$-protein), comprising α, β, and γ subunits. The complex consisting of the agonist bound to the receptor catalyzes the dissociation of guanosine diphosphate (GDP) from the α-subunit of the $G_s$-protein, permitting the subsequent binding of guanosine triphosphate (GTP). The α-GTP dissociates from the β and γ subunits and goes on to regulate the activity of the effector, adenylyl cyclase.[1] Thus, the occupation of the β-adrenoceptor by a β-agonist leads to the stimulation of cAMP synthesis by adenylyl cyclase. Constant stimulation of β-adrenoceptors results in a decrease in their number, known as downregulation. Constant blockade results in upregulation, or an increase in the number of receptors and adaptive supersensitivity. Rapidly developed (tachyphylaxis) and delayed tolerance to the IOP lowering effect of β-blockers may be related to this supersensitivity of ocular β-receptors. Supersensitivity of β-adrenoceptors might result in a greater enhancement of aqueous secretion by more effective competition with the β-blocker by endogenous epinephrine. β-Adrenoceptors exhibit stereoselectivity in their affinity toward agonists and antagonists with an asymmetric carbon atom at the β-position of the alkyl side chain in their chemical structure. Most often the levorotatory, or S−(−), isomer of the racemic mixture of isomers has higher receptor affinity compared with the dextrorotatory, or *f* R−(+), isomer; therefore, it exhibits higher potency. However, some isomers of β-blockers, notably timolol, are less different in their potency for reducing IOP than they are for inhibiting other physiologic functions. It is structural conformation rather than the direction of rotation of polarized light that determines adrenoceptor stereoselectivity.

$\beta_1$-Receptors in cardiac tissue mediate positive chronotropic (rate) and inotropic (force) effects. In the heart, the sympathetic and parasympathetic systems are functionally antagonistic; the sympathetic increases rate and force of contraction, and the parasympathetic decreases them. $\beta_1$-Adrenoceptors in fat cells mediate lipolysis, and in the liver they mediate glycogenolysis. Blockade of the hepatic β-adrenoceptors participates in the accentuation of hypoglycemia and prolongation of recovery from it. $\beta_2$-Receptors in the bronchi mediate bronchodilatation, and those in blood vessels mediate vasodilatation. In the bronchioles, sympathetic and parasympathetic input are functionally antagonistic, the former mediating bronchodilatation and the latter bronchoconstriction. When bronchial β-adrenoceptors are blocked, sympathetic bronchodilatory tone is inhibited and parasympathetic bronchoconstrictive tone becomes unopposed. In blood vessels, particularly those located in skeletal muscle, the stimulation of β-adrenoceptors causes relaxation, whereas the stimulation of α-adrenoceptors causes vasoconstriction. Epinephrine stimulates both α- and β-adrenoceptors. Thus, when vascular β-adrenoceptors are blocked in the presence of epinephrine, the vasodilatory response is inhibited, and the α-adrenoceptor-mediated vasoconstrictive effect becomes dominant. $\beta_2$-Adrenoceptors in the pancreas mediate insulin release. $\beta_3$-Receptors, like $\beta_1$, mediate metabolic responses, such as lipolysis. In the eye, the nonpigmented epithelial cells of the ciliary processes and the cells of the trabecular meshwork contain $\beta_2$-receptors that mediate an increase in intracellular cAMP.[2] β-Blockers in general inhibit this response and decrease the formation of aqueous humor, resulting in the reduction of IOP. However, the precise cellular mechanism or mechanisms for the effect of β-blockers on aqueous flow has not been elucidated. The blockade of β-adrenoceptors in the trabecular meshwork can inhibit the aqueous outflow response to epinephrine.

## β-BLOCKER PHARMACOLOGY

β-Adrenergic blockers competitively antagonize the action of β-adrenergic agonists, or stimulants, at β-adrenoceptors. They inhibit the physiologic actions of the adrenergic neurohormones norepinephrine and epinephrine. They exhibit high affinity for β-adrenoreceptors and can competitively displace other ligands that bind to these sites. Thus, their blocking action can be overcome by a sufficiently high concentration of the competing agonist. β-Blockers can vary according to their ancillary pharmacologic properties, the main ones being membrane stabilizing and intrinsic sympathomimetic activities. In addition, some β-blockers are selective for a particular subtype of β-adrenoceptor, whereas others are nonselective and act on multiple subtypes. Recently it was discovered that certain β-blockers have vasorelaxant activity.

### Membrane-Stabilizing Activity

Membrane-stabilizing activity (MSA) produces local anesthetic activity. Some β-blockers and local anesthetics have certain chemical structural features in common: (1) a carbocyclic or heterocyclic ring of the aromatic type (lipophilic part), (2) an intermediate chain, and (3) an amino group (hydrophilic part). Because the corneal epithelium is directly exposed to a topically instilled β-blocker and high concentrations of drug may be reached in this tissue, corneal anesthesia may result from membrane stabilization of the sensory nerves. The membrane-stabilizing potency and lipophilicity of the β-blocker determine the degree to which corneal anesthesia occurs. There are conflicting reports on the occurrence of corneal anesthesia with the individual β-blockers, perhaps because of variation in age- or pathology-related factors among the study populations or to the methodology employed to measure corneal sensitivity.[3–6] In some cases a sensitive measurement technique such as the use of the Cochet-Bonnet anesthesiometer is necessary to demonstrate the effect. The use of β-blockers at the higher concentrations in older patients may have a greater propensity to produce corneal anesthesia.[4] Unless the effect is a strong one, the protective corneal touch response is not diminished to where it poses a risk to the patient. However, subtle effects of MSA on corneal metabolism and physiology may become important in patients with already compromised corneal sensitivity or abnormal corneal physiology. Twenty cases of superficial punctate keratitis, possibly stemming from MSA, were mentioned among 547 reports of adverse ocular reactions to topical timolol.[7, 8]

### Intrinsic Sympathomimetic Activity

Intrinsic sympathomimetic activity (ISA) refers to the ability of a β-blocker to stimulate the β-adrenoceptor and elicit a stimulatory response. This action is also called "partial agonism" because it does not produce the maximum response attainable in the tissue by the full agonist norepinephrine. On the heart, ISA is manifest as tachycardia in an animal that has been depleted of endogenous cardiac catecholamines by reserpinization or sympathectomy. It may attenuate the β-blocking effect of the drug under conditions of low physiologic sympathetic or adrenergic tone. For example, β-blockers with or without ISA can block effectively the stimulation of cardiac β-adrenoceptors and produce bradycardia under conditions of high sympathetic tone, as during stress or exercise. However, under conditions of low sympathetic tone, as in the resting state, those agents with ISA produce tachycardia in contrast to those without it that produce bradycardia. However, the clinical significance of ISA is not clear for ophthalmic β-blockers.

An analogy may be extended to the bronchial response to agents with ISA. An individual with normal bronchial function may not be affected by ophthalmic instillation of a β-blocker either with or without ISA. However, should the individual have compromised bronchial function being treated with a sympathomimetic bronchodilating drug, there may be no benefit from the ISA of the β-blocker. Rather, the β-blocking action of either type of drug may be fully manifest, and the individual could experience ventilatory difficulty. β-Blockers with ISA may be less likely than those without ISA to exacerbate symptoms in patients with intermittent claudication and to reduce high-density lipoprotein (HDL)–cholesterol levels.[9]

### β-Adrenoceptor Selectivity

β-Adrenoceptor selectivity is a result of the β-blocker having a higher affinity for one subtype of β-adrenoceptor over another. Selectivity is relative to the concentration of β-blocker at the receptor and may be nullified when a sufficiently high concentration of drug is reached at the receptor. β-Blockers selective for $\beta_1$-adrenoceptors are referred to as cardioselective because that subtype predominates in cardiac tissue. Both selective and nonselective β-blockers have been found to lower the IOP. Because the predominant subtype of adrenoceptor in the ciliary processes has been characterized as $\beta_2$, it appears that the selectivity of the $\beta_1$-blocker betaxolol is overcome at the concentration reached in the ciliary processes after its topical instillation. Betaxolol and other $\beta_1$-selective blockers can lower the IOP comparably with the nonselective agents.

To extend this discussion of ISA to adrenoceptor selectivity, it is apparent that a β-blocker with $\beta_1$-selectivity will spare to some degree the bronchodilatory $\beta_2$-adrenoceptors and interfere less with compensating adrenergic tone or the action of a sympathomimetic bronchodilator. Thus, the $\beta_1$-selective agent will be less likely than the nonselective one to cause an adverse pulmonary event in the patient with compromised pulmonary function. One must remember, however, that receptor selectivity is relative to dose, and it may be absent if a sufficiently high concentration of β-blocker is reached in the bronchial tissue. Therefore, careful observation must be made of the patient with obstructive pulmonary disease when therapy is instituted with any ophthalmic β-blocker.

$\beta_1$-Selective blockers are less likely to interfere with the vasodilatory actions of endogenous epinephrine that is mediated through vascular $\beta_2$-adrenoceptors. Compared with nonselective β-blockers, with or without ISA, $\beta_1$-selective blockers are found to have the least effect on plasma lipoprotein concentrations.

## OCULAR PHARMACOLOGY

β-Blockers effectively reduce the IOP by decreasing the inflow rate of aqueous humor. This effect on aqueous flow has been measured clinically using the aqueous fluorophotometry technique. By this technique, the reduction of aqueous flow by timolol, betaxolol, carteolol, levobunolol, and others has been demonstrated. The effect of timolol on aqueous humor flow is markedly lessened during sleep when flow rates are reduced to a basal rate compared with the awake state.[10] The mechanism for this physiologic variation in flow rate has not been elucidated. However, epinephrine is a plausible candidate as the endogenous regulator of aqueous flow. Epinephrine increases aqueous humor flow rate during sleep. Flow is depressed during sleep when sympathetic tone is usually low and is enhanced during wakefulness when sympathetic tone is usually higher. However, patients with unilateral Horner's syndrome do not exhibit a difference in aqueous flow rate between affected and unaffected eyes.[11] Perhaps some adaptive response or collateral innervation occurs or supersensitivity to epinephrine enhances aqueous flow in the Horner's eye. Circulating epinephrine from the adrenals may play a role. Should some adrenergic tone to the ciliary processes drive the formation of aqueous humor, it is plausible that β-blockers, by blocking this tone, would decrease the inflow of aqueous humor. Alternate explanations of the mechanism of action of β-blockers for reducing aqueous flow include an effect on anterior ciliary blood flow by the passive vasoconstriction mechanism or the blockade of a chloride channel in the ciliary epithelium.

There is no convincing evidence to support that IOP reduction by β-blockers is significantly mediated through an action on the outflow of aqueous humor, either through the trabecular or uveoscleral outflow routes. However, a slight outflow effect has been observed with both metipranolol and timolol.[12] β-Blockers do not appear to alter episcleral venous pressure.

β-Blockers do not significantly affect accommodation or responses of the pupil. Although there is a small β-adrenergically mediated component to relaxation of the ciliary muscle, β-blockade does not produce clinically meaningful changes of accommodation. Pupillary dilatation is mediated via α-adrenoceptors located in the radial muscles of the iris. Unless the β-blocker has α-blocking activity as well, it will not affect this response. The circular muscle of the iris is predominantly innervated by parasympathetic nerves and contains cholinergic receptors of the muscarinic type. A β-adrenoceptor-mediated relaxation of the iris sphincter, contributing approximately 30% of maximum pupillary dilatation, has been observed.[13] Thus, β-blockade may cause a small miotic effect. The lack of effect of β-blockers on accommodation and the pupil compared with the miotics gives them a significant clinical advantage over those drugs from the standpoint of ocular side effects and patient acceptance and compliance.

## CLINICAL USE

The ability of β-blockers to lower the IOP in humans was discovered in patients receiving propranolol intravenously.[14] Later it was shown that orally and topically administered propranolol also gave this effect.[15] Subsequently this action was described for practolol and atenolol, both of which are $\beta_1$- or cardioselective blockers. A complete review of this early history has been published elsewhere.[16]

Timolol was the first ophthalmic β-blocker to be approved by the U.S. Food and Drug Administration (FDA). It was immediately successful. As a glaucoma drug, timolol's efficacy for reducing IOP was excellent, and the lack of effect on the pupil and accommodation stood out in marked contrast to the side effects of pilocarpine. Betaxolol was next approved and was the first $\beta_1$-selective ophthalmic β-blocker to become available. It was followed, in turn, by levobunolol, metipranolol, and carteolol. All but betaxolol are nonselective β-blockers, and among them only carteolol possesses intrinsic sympathomimetic activity. None requires more than twice daily instillation to be effective. These agents vary according to systemic β-blocking potency and pharmacokinetic behavior, which accounts for differences among them with respect to their propensity to cause side effects. $\beta_1$-Selectivity can offer an advantage for the use of β-blockers in patients with pulmonary problems. Although the IOP-lowering efficacy of β-blockers was immediately apparent on their investigation, a truer perspective on their systemic safety came along after their broad and open use.[8]

## TOLERANCE TO THE INTRAOCULAR PRESSURE EFFECT

Tachyphylaxis, tolerance, escape, and long-term drift are terms used to describe the relative loss of effectiveness of a drug over time. Patients who have never before been treated with an ophthalmic β-blocker may exhibit a sudden diminution of the initial IOP reduction by timolol.[17] Acute tolerance has been reported to occur in as many as one third of patients using timolol.[18, 19] In Canadian multicenter trials, a highly statistically significant but clinically nonmeaningful escape from IOP control by 1 to 2 mm Hg was seen during the first 50 weeks of 0.25% or 0.5% timolol use in 137 out of 227, or 60% of eyes maintained less than 22 mm Hg of pressure for 200 weeks by timolol therapy alone. No further upward trend or drift in IOP was seen over the remaining 150 weeks of the study period. However, the 117 patients participating in this study had previously participated in a 6-week study in which it had been established that their IOP was controlled by either 0.25% or 0.5% timolol alone, 86 by 0.25%, and 31 by 0.5%. After 200 weeks, the IOP was held to less than 22 mm Hg in 52% of each group by the original concentration of timolol. Thus, these patients had already undergone an adjustment in the efficacy of timolol before entering the longer study.[20]

Tolerance and drift are used somewhat interchangeably to describe the loss of ocular hypotensive efficacy with longer-term treatment. It is noteworthy that up to 25% of patients experience loss of IOP control over the long term using timolol.[21, 22] The response to timolol at 1 hour after the initial dose was not useful to predict the drug's continued effectiveness over time in previously untreated ocular hypertensive patients.[23] Possible explanations for these phenomena include the progressive worsening of the patient's disease condition and modifications of the β-adrenoceptor number or coupling to the effector system of the cell. Attempts have been made to prevent the loss of IOP-lowering efficacy by providing for a therapeutic "holiday" of 30 to 60 days during which epinephrine or dipivefrin may be substituted. The success of this maneuver is variable from one patient to the next.[24]

The influence of a 4-week sojourn in timolol treatment during which dipivefrin was substituted for the former drug was studied. Timolol was restarted after 4 weeks of dipivefrin therapy to see whether there was a restoration of the original timolol effect. This maneuver was not associated with a significant change in IOP. Thus, a role for pulsed therapy, alternating between β-blocker and β-agonist, does not seem to influence the long-term drift seen with prolonged timolol therapy.[25]

## SAFETY

The potency of β-blockers is such that systemic side effects and adverse events can occur and pose a significant risk to the patient. During the initial clinical trials with timolol, there were few reports of significant side effects and adverse events. Indeed, the same has been true for many ophthalmic drugs while they have undergone clinical trials before being marketed and used openly. This is probably a result of the nature of controlled clinical trials because many patients with systemic disease are excluded from participating because the safety of the investigational drug has not yet been established under their conditions. It is the rule to establish the safety of a new drug in healthy individuals before exposing patients with disease to the drug. Because timolol was used more openly in large populations of patients, many of whom were aged and had one or more systemic diseases, its potential for causing side effects and adverse events became increasingly apparent. Timolol is not the sole β-blocker to cause systemic effects, and this potential must be borne in mind with both the selective and nonselective β-blockers.

Pharmaceutical companies engage in postmarketing surveillance studies to address the issue of safety of new drug use in patient populations under various systemic disease conditions. Furthermore, the rate of occurrence and type of adverse events, when reported, are monitored and reported to the FDA so there is forewarning when the incidence of adverse events becomes of concern. Approved drugs can be and are withdrawn from the market when it is deemed necessary to do so. Fortunately, although β-blockers can cause adverse events that may be life-threatening, their potential for doing so is becoming well recognized, and steps can be taken to avoid their occurrence.[26] It behooves the ophthalmologist prescribing a β-blocker to know and understand the actions of this class of drugs and to be diligent in reviewing the patient's medical history and evaluating the risk to benefit aspects for a particular patient. The β-blocker with the most favorable risk/benefit ratio or therapeutic index for that patient should be selected.

## ADVERSE REACTIONS

A number of adverse reactions, systemic and ocular, are known to occur with the systemic and ophthalmic use of β-blockers.

Ocular adverse reactions of β-blockers include conjunctivitis, eyelid dermatitis, blepharitis, tearing, photophobia, browache, blurred or cloudy vision, conjunctival hyperemia, conjunctival edema, corneal punctate keratitis, foreign body sensation, dryness of the eyes, erythema, discharge, inflammation, decreased visual acuity, crusting of the eyelashes, stinging and burning, aphakic cystoid macular edema, iridocyclitis, itching, blepharoptosis, diplopia, refractive changes (sometimes related to withdrawal of miotic therapy), decreased corneal sensitivity, ptosis, abnormal corneal staining, ocular pain, and decreased night vision. Not all agents produce all of these adverse reactions.

Systemic adverse reactions include:

1. *Cardiovascular:* abnormal cardiac rhythm, atrial tachycardia, bradycardia, heart block, congestive heart failure, palpitation, hypotension, hypertension, myocardial infarct, cardiac arrest, syncope, cerebral ischemia, cerebral vascular accident, edema, worsening of arterial insufficiency, Raynaud's phenomenon, and vasodilatation.
2. *Digestive:* nausea, diarrhea, weight loss, anorexia, dyspepsia, dry mouth, glossitis.
3. *Nervous system/psychiatric:* vertigo, dizziness, increased signs and symptoms of myasthenia gravis, depression, paresthesia, insomnia, dizziness, anxiety, somnolence, nervousness, fatigue, hallucinations, disorientation, mental confusion, vivid dreams, decreased libido, nightmares, and diminished concentration.
4. *Respiratory:* bronchospasm (predominantly in patients with preexisting bronchospastic disease), rales, respiratory failure, dyspnea, nasal congestion, rhinitis, epistaxis, cough, thickened bronchial secretions, asthma, and respiratory failure.
5. *Skin:* hypersensitivity, localized or general rash, urticaria, alopecia, hives, toxic epidermal necrolysis, pruritus, increased pigmentation, sweating, and cold hands and feet.
6. *Endocrine:* masked symptoms of hypoglycemia in insulin-dependent diabetics, hypoglycemia, and hyperglycemia.
7. *Musculoskeletal:* arthralgia and claudication.

8. *Body as a whole:* asthenia, headache, chest pain, fatigue, and decreased exercise tolerance.

Not all agents cause all adverse reactions, and a causal relationship for all these adverse reactions has not been established.

## CONTRAINDICATIONS

The use of ophthalmic formulations of β-blockers is contraindicated in patients with known hypersensitivity to any of their components. β-Blockers are contraindicated in patients with secondary- or tertiary-degree atrioventricular block, cardiogenic shock, sinus bradycardia, or overt cardiac failure. Nonselective β-blockers are contraindicated in patients with bronchial asthma or with a history of bronchial asthma, or severe chronic obstructive pulmonary disease. The use of β-blockers selective for $\beta_1$-adrenoceptors in these pulmonary conditions must still be used with caution and in consultation with the physician managing the patient's pulmonary disease (Table 3–3).

## DRUG INTERACTIONS AND WARNINGS ON THE USE OF β-BLOCKERS

Caution should be used to avoid additive effects when ophthalmic β-blockers are administered to patients who are taking β-blockers orally. In patients who have impaired cardiac function, the coadministration of an ophthalmic β-blocker and an oral or intravenous calcium channel antagonist raises the possibility for the precipitation of left ventricular failure and hypotension. Using a β-blocker concomitantly with digitalis and calcium channel antagonists may produce prolonged atrioventricular conduction time. β-Blockers should be used with caution in patients receiving adrenergic transmitter–depleting psychotropic drugs. Vertigo, syncope, or postural hypotension may result from hypotension or marked bradycardia in patients receiving β-blockers and catecholamine-depleting drugs such as reserpine. β-Blockers may retard the recovery from insulin- or exercise-induced hypoglycemia and may accentuate and accelerate the fall in blood glucose levels during prolonged and strenuous exercise. Furthermore, β-blockers may mask the signs and symptoms of acute hypoglycemia and certain clinical signs of thyrotoxicosis. Abrupt withdrawal of β-blocker therapy in a patient developing thyrotoxicosis may precipitate a thyroid gland storm. The necessity to withdraw β-blocker therapy before surgery is controversial. Should it be deemed necessary, gradual withdrawal is best. Mydriasis can occur in patients receiving timolol and epinephrine concomitantly, probably because of stimulation of α-receptors in the iris dilator muscle by epinephrine.

**TABLE 3–3.**
Conditions Placing Patients at Higher Risk of Side Effects from β-Blockers

| Condition |
|---|
| Asthma |
| Chronic bronchitis |
| Peripheral vascular disease |
| Duodenal ulcer |
| Bradycardia ($<60$ beats/min) |
| Heart block |
| Renal failure |

## REVERSING THE EFFECTS OF β-BLOCKADE

Should it ever become necessary to reverse the effects of β-blockade, sufficient doses of sympathomimetic agonists such as isoproterenol, dopamine, dobutamine, or levarterenol may be given.

## SYSTEMIC ABSORPTION AND PHARMACOKINETICS

β-Blockers are potent drugs, and for some agents, the ophthalmic dosage delivers a sufficient amount to cause systemic effects after absorption into the circulation. Once absorbed systemically, the systemic pharmacokinetic behavior of the drug comes into play. Unless the amount of drug in the circulation is sufficient to contribute to the action in the eye, the persistence of the drug in the blood has little bearing on the duration of the ocular effect. Thus, the drug with the longest systemic half-life is not necessarily the one with the longest duration of IOP effect. However, the systemic half-life of a drug does influence the steady-state blood level of drug achieved after repeated ocular instillation. A drug with a long half-life tends to accumulate more readily at short interdose intervals than one with a short half-life. Furthermore, it must be recognized that the fate and distribution of drugs absorbed after ocular instillation may differ from that after oral or parenteral administration. For example, drugs absorbed into the circulation within the head region escape first-pass metabolism by the liver before encountering the heart and the lungs. Because these organs contain rather high densities of β-adrenoceptors and are target organs for adverse events, it must be considered that they may acquire sufficient levels of β-blocker to exhibit a response.

Lipophilicity plays an important role in determining the absorption and distribution characteristics of the drug. More lipophilic drugs are better absorbed and distribute more readily across lipophilic barriers, such as the blood-brain and blood-ocular barriers. The same is true for the corneal and conjunctival epithelia and the nasolacrimal mucosae. The volume of distribution of a drug is a useful pharmacokinetic parameter to consider when drugs are compared. A high volume of distribution is reflected in lower plasma levels of drug and indicates the drug may be less likely to reach effective levels in the blood, thereby reducing side effects.

## PUNCTAL OCCLUSION AND DOSAGE VOLUME

A commonly used maneuver intended to limit the systemic absorption of ocularly instilled drugs is punctal occlusion. Mean plasma levels of timolol in patients on chronic therapy with 0.5% timolol were 0.34 ng/ml at baseline and rose to 1.34 ng/ml 1 hour after topical drop instillation. With punctal occlusion, the 1-hour level of timolol was 0.9 ng/ml.[27]

Another approach to diminish systemic absorption is to reduce the total drug dosage by decreasing the volume of the eye drop. This is based on the observation that the cul-de-sac has a finite volume, and when the instilled drop volume exceeds that capacity, the excess drains rapidly into the nasolacrimal duct where it becomes readily available for systemic absorption. By keeping the instilled volume close to that of the cul-de-sac volume, the excess is minimized. The efficiency of absorption of drug into the eye may be improved when the dose of drug is incorporated into a smaller volume. Reflex tearing caused by instilling an irritating or uncomfortable drug further limits ocular bioavailability because the drug is more rapidly diluted and washed away from the corneal absorptive surface. Conjunctival absorption of β-blockers is known to occur and contributes to the amount of drug in the circulation.

The drop size of 0.5% levobunolol was varied among 20, 35, and 50 μl, and the safety of this drug was evaluated in a double-masked, crossover study. When drug or vehicle was instilled 1 hour before exercise on a treadmill, a significantly lower heart rate was observed in subjects using the drug compared with vehicle. No significant difference in the heart rate response to exercise was observed among the subjects receiving the three dose volumes. In another randomized, double-masked, parallel study in 117 ocular hypertensive patients, one of the three previously mentioned dose volumes containing 0.5% levobunolol was instilled twice daily for 3 months. No significant differences among the three groups were seen with respect to (1) heart rate or blood pressure changes and (2) mean IOP decrease. Thus, no advantage was perceived by varying the drop volume between 20 and 50 μl.[28]

## BLOOD FLOW AND β-BLOCKERS

β-Blockers effectively decrease the IOP by reducing the inflow of aqueous humor. Although their therapeutic benefit is believed to be derived primarily from a reduction in IOP, other of their actions, principally those involving ocular blood flow, may either enhance or detract from this primary beneficial effect. Indeed, it may be postulated that β-blockers might exacerbate glaucomatous visual field loss by causing vasoconstriction in the vessels that supply the optic nerve. Such an effect could result if vasodilatory vascular $\beta_2$-adrenoceptors are blocked and α-adrenergic vasoconstrictive tone becomes predominant. Blockade of vascular $\beta_2$-adrenoceptors is less likely to occur with $\beta_1$-selective blockers. Furthermore, the intrinsic vasodilatory action of some β-blockers could prevent marked vasoconstriction from occurring.

The extraocular part of the central retinal artery and the ciliary arteries are sympathetically innervated. The iris, ciliary processes, and choroid receive a rich sympathetic supply. Uveal α-adrenoceptors serve an important physiologic role to assist in the control of ocular blood flow against the threat of elevated systemic blood pressure. Such elevations occur during mental and physical stress as a result of increased sympathetic nervous activity. Contemporaneous systemic hypertension and ocular vasoconstriction, brought about by increased sympathetic tone, prevent overperfusion of ocular vessels that might cause breakdown of the blood-ocular barrier. Little change in retinal blood flow occurs with uveal vasoconstriction because retinal vessels effectively autoregulate the flow.[29]

The presence of β-adrenoceptors on uveal and retinal vessels is much less clear. The permeability of the iridial vessels of the rat is subject to regulation by β-adrenergic drugs. Isoproterenol, a nonselective β-agonist, caused increased vascular permeability, which was inhibited by timolol.[30] The radioiodinated nonselective β-blocker cyanopindolol was used in ligand-binding and autoradiographic experiments to investigate the presence of β-adrenoceptors in choroidal vessels of rabbits. In the same report, the clinical effects in 26 subjects using oral and topical timolol on choroidal vascular tone were compared using the computerized pneumatonometer (ocular blood flow instrument) to measure the pulsatile change in total intraocular blood volume. Specific binding of cyanopindolol was observed in decreasing amount in choroidal vessels, retinal tissue, and retinal pigment epithelium, indicating the presence of β-adrenoceptors there. A total of 20 mg of oral timolol produced a statistically significant reduction in volume amplitude, the difference in intraocular volume between systole and diastole, but topical 0.5% timolol produced a smaller and statistically nonsignificant change. The authors proposed several conclusions from their results: (1) there are β-adrenoceptors in choroidal vessels, (2) there is sufficient choroidal vascular tone so that β-blockade results in vasoconstriction, and (3) systemic but not topical timolol reaches choroidal β-adrenoceptors in sufficient quantity to cause blockade.[31] There have been other reports of the presence of β-adrenergic-binding sites in the choroid.[32, 33] These observations should be kept in mind when one is reading about the individual β-blockers and their effects on ocular blood flow later in this chapter.

An elevation in IOP greater than the normal level causes a corresponding increase in intraocular venous pressure. Because the pressure differential between the arteries entering the eye and the veins at the point just before exiting the eye determines the pressure head for ocular blood perfusion, an increased IOP results in a reduced ocular perfusion pressure. A decrease in arterial blood pressure is associated with decreased perfusion pressure. Thus, an increase in IOP and a decrease in arterial blood pressure have the same effect. When IOP is decreased, there is a corresponding fall in intraocular venous pressure. If systemic blood pressure remains constant, a passive increase in ocular perfusion pressure may occur with a reduction in IOP. When this happens, the myogenic autoregulatory response may be evoked by stretching of the vascular wall, tending to limit the increase in blood flow. The vasculature of the eye responds in this manner to protect the delicate ocular tissues against sudden rapid rises in systemic blood pressure. Autoregulation occurs in the retina and ciliary body but apparently not in the choroid.

It appears that the vasculature tone in the eye is normally rather low because blood flow rates are usually high compared with other tissues in the body. It is not clear what mediates this physiologic vasodilatory tone. Nitric oxide, a gaseous vasodilator produced by the vascular endothelial cells, is one possible candidate. Nevertheless, should the vasodilatory $\beta_2$-receptors in vascular tissue be blocked under conditions of sufficiently high adrenergic tone, there can be a shift in emphasis toward the stimulation of vasoconstrictive α-adrenoceptors, the net effect being vasoconstriction. The source of adrenergic tone is the neurohormones epinephrine and norepinephrine, either released locally from sympathetic nerve terminals or coming from the adrenal medulla via the blood circulation. However, the evidence for the presence of β-adrenoceptors in the retinal and posterior ciliary arteries is controversial. Both vessels exhibit weak relaxation in response to isoproterenol, a drug that stimulates both $\beta_1$- and $\beta_2$-adrenoceptors and causes $\beta_2$-receptor-mediated vasodilation. Recently the presence of $\beta_1$- and $\beta_2$-receptors in the retina and retinal vessels,[34, 35] where they may mediate vasodilation, has been reported. Marked vasodilation of the choroidal vessels may divert blood flow away from the retina and optic nerve head. A so-called steal phenomenon has been described for the brain. Furthermore, a reduction in heart rate and cardiac output by cardiac β-blockade may result in reduced ocular pulsatile blood flow.

It is known that the microvasculature of the retina and optic nerve has the ability to autoregulate. That is, the lumen diameter of the vessels changes in the appropriate direction to maintain constant blood flow. Autoregulation occurs either myogenically or metabolically.[29] When intravascular pressure rises and the vessel wall is stretched, the myogenic autoregulatory response of the smooth muscle surrounding the vessel is to contract, thereby decreasing the lumen diameter to reduce blood flow toward normal.

There is evidence that the pericytes of capillaries can contract and alter the lumen diameter.[36] Furthermore, it appears that β-adrenoceptors are present in pericytes isolated from bovine retinal capillaries. The nonselective β-blocker propranolol was found to block the isoproterenol-induced production of cAMP by these pericytes.[37] It can be speculated that adrenergic tone modulates blood flow at the capillary level. Changes that might occur in microvascular pericytes as they undergo chronic stress of systemic hypertension were studied in spontaneously hypertensive rats. Increased actin filament bundles within the pericytes and capillary constriction were observed. Systemic hypertension is considered to be a risk factor for glaucoma, and such microvascular changes might contribute to the glaucomatous optic neuropathic process.[38]

Increasing the partial pressure of carbon dioxide in the tissue, as may occur under conditions of inadequate blood perfusion, is accompanied by metabolic autoregulation, resulting in a compensatory increase in the lumen diameter and in blood flow. The autoregulatory process is thought to be adversely affected with age and in the presence of vascular pathologic conditions, such as atherosclerosis. Furthermore, the autoregulatory capacity of the ocular blood vessels can be exceeded when IOP is elevated to levels greater than 30 mm Hg. If this IOP value is exceeded or an individual's autoregulatory capacity has been reduced, optic nerve blood flow may be decreased, which could contribute to the occurrence of glaucomatous optic neuropathy. Reduction in IOP per se may improve ocular perfusion pressure. Mean retinal vascular calibers at the optic disc border were measured before and after IOP reduction from mean values of 35.3 to 16.5 mm Hg for 11.2 weeks.[39] A positive correlation between arterial and venous caliber decreases and magnitude of IOP reduction was found. Although the IOP-dependent retinal arterial caliber change was highly significant in the patients 55 years of age and younger, it was not significant in those more than 55 years of age. Thus, age is a more important factor in determining the retinal arterial caliber change than is the degree of IOP reduction itself. The interaction between age-related changes in vascular responsiveness and susceptibility of changes in blood vessel diameter to alteration in IOP level is complex.

The sustained handgrip maneuver produces an elevation of systemic blood pressure that should elicit a decrease in retinal vessel diameter as part of the autoregulatory response. Retinal vessel response to sustained handgrip contraction was investigated in two groups of ten diabetic patients each. The groups were well matched with respect to their mean age, type and duration of diabetes, blood glucose control, and mean resting blood pressures. However, one group exhibited a higher incidence of autonomic dysfunction compared with the other one. The former group displayed significantly greater decreases in mean arteriolar and venular constrictions to sustained handgrip contraction. This was judged to be a sign of impaired autoregulation of the retinal vasculature accompanying hemodynamic alterations associated with the diabetes. It should be recalled that diabetes is considered to be a risk factor for glaucomatous optic neuropathy.[40]

In low or normal tension glaucoma, it is thought that episodic vasospasm of ocular blood vessels may contribute to visual field disturbances.[41–43] The role that β-blockers might play in altering autoregulation, enhancing or diminishing the blood flow to the retina and optic nerve, requires further study.

It has been demonstrated that some β-blockers have a vasorelaxant effect unrelated to their blockade of α- or β-adrenoceptors, membrane stabilization, or intrinsic sympathomimetic activity. This vasorelaxant activity is similar to that of certain of the calcium channel blockers, and the potency for this action varies among β-blockers.[44] This property is observed under in vitro conditions when the isolated blood vessel, such as the posterior ciliary artery, has been precontracted by increasing the concentration of potassium ion in the buffer with substitution for sodium ion by the addition of prostaglandin $F_{2\alpha}$ or a thromboxane mimetic. The rank order of vasorelaxant potency and effectiveness for several ophthalmic β-blockers studied on the porcine posterior ciliary artery was found to be betaxolol, carteolol, and then timolol.[45] The concentrations required for this action are higher than those needed to block β-adrenoceptors but, for betaxolol at least, appear to be within the range of tissue concentrations to be achieved from topical ocular instillation. Thus, under appropriate conditions, a β-blocker that possesses a relatively potent vasorelaxant activity may influence beneficially for the preservation of visual field the vascular tone of ophthalmic blood vessels. It is assumed that the drug could reach the vessels in the posterior segment via the vitreous and uveoscleral pathways, as well as through the circulation. It seems though most likely that the choroidal vessels and anterior uveal ophthalmic vessels are more accessible to the topically instilled drug.

## THERAPEUTIC EFFICACY

Historically, the efficacy of β-blockers, indeed, all modalities of glaucoma therapy, has been measured by the degree of IOP reduction produced. However, true efficacy of an antiglaucomatous drug should be measured by the degree of prevention or arrest of progress of visual field loss. There are few randomized, controlled, prospective clinical trials documenting the true efficacy of glaucoma medications. Nevertheless, β-blockers are considered to be effective for reducing IOP in patients with primary open-angle glaucoma and several other variants of glaucoma or ocular hypertension.

## EFFICACY IN VARIANTS OF GLAUCOMA

In addition to those types of glaucoma in the discussions that follow, timolol has been reported to be effective for lowering IOP in certain conditions: surgical aphakia, neovascular, low-tension, early and late postsurgical, exfoliation syndrome, traumatic, aniridic, and inflammatory glaucoma.[46]

### Angle-Closure Glaucoma

It is considered inappropriate to use drugs that reduce aqueous flow, such as β-blockers, in the long-term management of angle-closure or narrow-angle glaucoma. β-Blockers do not constrict the pupil, so they do not ameliorate the formation of peripheral anterior synechiae. However, β-blockers should not promote the formation of posterior pupillary synechiae as miotics tend to do. Timolol has been used successfully in eyes operated for closed-angle glaucoma.[47] Gonioscopy should be used to determine the state of the angle before β-blocker therapy is instituted.

β-Blockers are useful to treat acute angle-closure glaucoma, lowering pressure and reducing corneal edema, allowing definitive diagnosis and treatment.[48]

Timolol controlled the IOP that was uncontrolled on miotic and carbonic anhydrase inhibitor therapy in 9 out of 13 eyes with secondary angle-closure glaucoma after penetrating keratoplasty.[49]

### Congenital Glaucoma

In 78% of eyes with uncomplicated congenital glaucoma and in 50% of complicated cases, IOP was controlled with timolol.[50] However, surgery is the preferred therapeutic approach for congenital glaucoma.

### Childhood Glaucoma

There have been several studies with timolol in pediatric glaucoma patients.[51–53] One hundred eyes of 67 patients with childhood glaucoma were treated with timolol. Forty percent of the eyes did not require additional surgery or medication over the 6- to 60-month follow-up period. Seventy-eight percent (18) of the eyes exhibited an IOP decrease greater than 10 mm Hg. This study found timolol is effective in childhood glaucoma.[54] However, the labeling of ophthalmic β-blockers states that their efficacy and safety have not been established in children. In one study, the levels of timolol measured in the plasma of children ranged from 3.5 to 34 ng/ml.[27]

### Ghost Cell Glaucoma

Control of IOP in phakic eyes that had experienced vitreous hemorrhage was achieved in one case with medical treatment. Two remaining cases required trabeculectomy.[55]

### Pigmentary Glaucoma

Although β-blockers effectively lower the IOP in cases of pigmentary glaucoma, their use has been argued against. It is reasoned that a diminished rate of clearance of pigment from the trabecular meshwork would result from the decrease in aqueous humor flow caused by the β-blocker, possibly exacerbating the accumulation of pigment in the trabecular meshwork. Furthermore, reduced aqueous humor flow may aggravate the rubbing of the posterior iris surface against the lens zonules from the presumed reverse pupillary block and release more pigment.[56]

## EFFICACY IN CONDITIONS OTHER THAN GLAUCOMA OR OCULAR HYPERTENSION

Spikes in IOP occur after neodymium:YAG laser capsulotomy. One study reported that β-blocker and 2% pilocarpine prevented this postoperative rise in IOP.[57] The mean IOP rise was significantly less in eyes pretreated with 0.5% timolol compared with placebo treatment when measured 1 hour after neodymium:YAG laser capsulotomy. However, at the later time point of 4 hours, there was no significant difference between the timolol and placebo groups. Thus, pretreatment with timolol did not prevent the late pressure rises that occur after capsulotomy.[58]

The effect of timolol on the postoperative IOP rise after extracapsular cataract surgery with an intraocular posterior chamber lens implant was studied in 34 eyes. From a baseline mean IOP of 18.7 mm Hg in both timolol and untreated control patients, IOP rose to 20.0 mm Hg in the timolol group and to 20.7 mm Hg in the untreated group on the first postoperative day. Twenty-six percent of the timolol patients and 33% of untreated patients exhibited a pressure rise to greater than 23.0 mm Hg. Thus, timolol provided no benefit to these patients undergoing cataract surgery.[59]

In patients with mild corneal edema,

such as pseudophakic bullous keratopathy or Fuchs' corneal dystrophy, lowering the IOP with a β-blocker may reduce the edema.

## ADDITIVITY TO DRUGS OTHER THAN β-BLOCKERS

The effect of β-blockers on IOP is generally additive to that of the other glaucoma drugs, particularly the miotics. There is an issue associated with the concomitant use of the nonselective β-blockers and the sympathomimetic agents epinephrine and dipivefrin relative to the potential for antagonism of the latter's effect on aqueous humor outflow. The use of a nonselective β-blocker with epinephrine or dipivefrin can be less than additive, depending on the order and timing of administration of the individual drugs. This occurs because the β-blocker antagonizes the action of the sympathomimetic drug at the $\beta_2$-adrenoceptors in the trabecular meshwork. It was found that epinephrine caused a substantial and rapid increase in cAMP in cultured human trabecular meshwork cells. This effect was completely blocked by $10^{-6}$ mol timolol, with a slow recovery of about 30% to 40% over 9 hours. In contrast, this same concentration of betaxolol produced less than complete blockade, which had recovered by 50% within 15 minutes. This observation provides some explanation for the apparent interference by timolol but not by betaxolol with the facility-increasing effect of epinephrine that has been observed in clinical trials.[60]

## COMBINATION WITH ACETAZOLAMIDE OR METHAZOLAMIDE

The effect of timolol on IOP is less than fully additive to that of the oral carbonic anhydrase inhibitors acetazolamide and methazolamide in patients with primary open-angle glaucoma.[61] Neither drug class alters conventional and uveoscleral aqueous humor outflow or episcleral venous pressure. Betaxolol caused an additional 18.1% decrease of outflow pressure in patients receiving 500 mg of oral acetazolamide every 12 hours. This same dosage regimen of acetazolamide caused an additional mean outflow pressure decrease of 35.1% when added to twice daily 0.5% betaxolol therapy. The safety of chronic use of β-blockers together with the carbonic anhydrase inhibitors acetazolamide and methazolamide and hypothetically the topically active carbonic anhydrase inhibitors currently under investigation has been debated from the standpoint of excessive reduction of aqueous humor flow. It has long been an argument that insufficient aqueous humor secretion could adversely affect the avascular lens and cornea.

## COMBINATION WITH PILOCARPINE, CARBACHOL, OR ECHOTHIOPHATE IODIDE

Of the possible adjunctive drugs to use with β-blockers, the miotics, principally pilocarpine, provide a most logical rationale for their combined use.[62] Because β-blockers lower IOP by decreasing aqueous humor inflow, it makes ultimate sense that the action of miotics to increase aqueous outflow offers a balance of drug mechanisms. Furthermore, because impaired outflow is commonly associated with elevated IOP in glaucoma patients, increasing aqueous outflow addresses the cause of the problem. Of course, β-blockers do little to ameliorate the ocular side effects of the miotics. Conversely, miotics do little to ameliorate the systemic side effects of β-blockers. Pilocarpine in either solution or gel form is frequently used in combination with β-blockers. This has motivated the development of a single formulation combining timolol and pilocarpine. Concurrent administration of timolol with carbachol or echothiophate iodide provides clinically useful efficacy. The combination of pilocarpine and timolol provides added benefit for patients with angle-closure glaucoma.[63] Combinations of other ophthalmic β-blockers with pilocarpine or, perhaps, carbachol are likely to be forthcoming.[64]

A pilot study employed the combination of 0.5% timolol with either 2% or 4% pilocarpine in eyes that were at 22 mm Hg while the patients were using timolol alone to evaluate the added benefit of pilocarpine. The results showed an additional IOP reduction of 1.9 mm Hg after 2 hours and 2.1 mm Hg after 6 hours with the 2% pilocarpine plus timolol combination. For the 4% pilocarpine-timolol combination, an additional 3.0, 3.5, and 2.7 mm Hg were obtained after 2, 6, and 12 hours, respectively. Thus, the two drugs are additive, and the higher concentration of pilocarpine offers a longer duration and increased efficacy over the lower concentration.[65]

Fifty-four patients with ocular hypertension or glaucoma were treated with 2% pilocarpine four times daily and either 0.5% or 1% levobunolol or 0.5% timolol for 3 months. Before this study, all patients had been stabilized on therapy with 2% pilocarpine and 0.5% timolol. Continued IOP stability was achieved in 88% of the patients using levobunolol and pilocarpine and in 83% using timolol and pilocarpine. Thus, both β-blockers are effective along with pilocarpine.[66]

A double-masked, randomized, multicenter study compared the efficacy of 0.5% timolol/2% pilocarpine or 0.5% timolol/4% pilocarpine twice daily and 4% pilocarpine four times daily with 25 patients in each group. The combined drugs produced significant IOP reductions of 7.2 mm Hg, or 25%, and 10.7 mm Hg, or 37%, at the lower and higher pilocarpine concentrations, respectively. Pilocarpine alone lowered the IOP by 5.3 mm Hg, or 19%. Mean IOP was significantly lower at 12 hours after the previous dose in patients receiving the higher concentration of pilocarpine, alone or with timolol, compared with those taking 2% pilocarpine with timolol. These results illustrate the additivity between timolol and pilocarpine and point to the value of this combination to achieve greater IOP control.[67]

Two percent pilocarpine and 0.1% metipranolol in fixed combination produced a greater IOP reduction than either drug alone.[68]

The control of IOP over 12 hours was found to be greater for a solution combining 0.5% timolol with 2% pilocarpine compared with a single dose of 0.5% timolol alone. The combination gave more reduction in the mean diurnal IOP, as well as a decreased frequency of larger pressure peaks.[69]

Paradoxically, it is reported that timolol is not additive to aceclidine, a parasympathomimetic miotic agent expected to act like pilocarpine.[70]

## COMBINATION WITH EPINEPHRINE, DIPIVEFRIN, OR APRACLONIDINE

A comparison was made between apraclonidine and dipivefrin as adjunctive drugs to timolol therapy in a randomized, double-masked, crossover study involving 18 patients with ocular hypertension. Each patient was treated with 1% apraclonidine, 0.1% dipivefrin, or placebo twice daily for 3 weeks, together with twice daily 0.5% timolol. Except for 1 day of the study, apraclonidine produced a greater additive effect to timolol than did dipivefrin.[71]

Seventeen patients on bilateral timolol long-term therapy were given a single dose of apraclonidine in one eye and placebo in the other. Fluorophotometric measurement of aqueous flow indicated it to be 1.39 ± 0.41 μl/min in the apraclonidine-treated eye and 1.66 ± 0.38 μl/min in the placebo-treated eye, being a statistically significant difference. Apraclonidine caused a further 1.3–mm Hg decrease in IOP.[72]

A double-masked prospective study to compare the efficacy of the combination of 0.1% dipivefrin with either 0.5% timolol or 0.5% and 1% levobunolol was conducted in 43 patients whose IOP was being controlled by timolol and dipivefrin. Those patients switched to dipivefrin and either 0.5% or 1% levobunolol continued to be under IOP control over a 3-month period. It was concluded that the combination of dipivefrin with levobunolol performs as well as that of dipivefrin and timolol for controlling IOP in these patients.[73]

In patients with open-angle glaucoma, the combination of 0.5% timolol, 0.5% epinephrine, and 3% guanethidine produced a mean IOP reduction of 10.9 mm Hg compared with 7.6 mm Hg with epinephrine plus guanethidine and 5.8 mm Hg with timolol alone. Side effects may also increase with the use of these three drugs in combination.[74]

Twice daily 0.1% dipivefrin was added to one eye only of 32 patients with open-angle glaucoma or ocular hypertension who were receiving bilateral treatment with nonselective β-blockers. In the dipivefrin-treated eyes, mean IOP decreased from 22.7 to 20.2 mm Hg at week 1 and to 21.0 mm Hg at week 12. Adding dipivefrin resulted in an additional 2 mm Hg or more IOP decrease in 50% of eyes and a 3 mm Hg or more decrease in 19% of eyes for the 12-week duration of the study. The clinician must decide whether dipivefrin provides sufficient IOP reduction to warrant its addition to a regimen employing nonselective β-blockers.[75]

From the results of a study in which either epinephrine or dipivefrin was added to either betaxolol or timolol therapy in a randomized manner to ocular hypertensive patients, it was concluded that it is important to assess the response of the patient individually to determine the benefit of combining either adrenergic agent to the β-blocker.[76]

Eighteen patients with open-angle glaucoma were studied prospectively in a randomized, single-masked, crossover trial to evaluate the efficacy of three treatment regimens, each given for 1 month: 0.5% timolol twice daily, 0.5% timolol and 0.1% dipivefrin twice daily instilled separately at 10-minute intervals, and 0.5% timolol and 0.1% dipivefrin twice daily instilled separately at 4-hour intervals. The addition of dipivefrin to timolol therapy produced a small but statistically significant increment of IOP decrease. There was no difference in effect between the two combination regimens.[77]

Dipivefrin and timolol were found to be partially additive in most patients on long-term treatment; however, the response to this combination varies dramatically among individuals and different categories of diagnosis.[78]

The additivity of open-label epinephrine for 4 weeks to either 0.5% timolol or 0.5% betaxolol was studied in patients who had been receiving the β-blockers in masked fashion. In betaxolol patients, adding epinephrine lowered IOP significantly from 24.5 to 19.4 mm Hg at 1 week and to 20.7 mm Hg at 4 weeks, and outflow facility increased from 0.12 to 0.17 μl/min/mm Hg at 1 week and to 0.18 μl/min/mm Hg at 4 weeks. No significant changes of IOP or outflow facility were seen in the patients on timolol therapy when epinephrine was added to the regimen. These results apparently reflect the sparing of $\beta_2$-adrenoceptors by betaxolol, a $\beta_1$-selective blocker, which mediate the response to epinephrine in the trabecular meshwork, but not by timolol, a nonselective blocker.[79]

A double-masked, crossover study was carried out in 30 newly diagnosed patients with primary open-angle glaucoma, 24 of whom had not received previous medical therapy. First all patients were given 0.1% dipivefrin for 2 weeks; then the group was divided into two, and either carteolol 2% or placebo was added. Mean IOP was reduced from the entry level of 31 to 25.8 mm Hg while patients used dipivefrin. During the first and second periods of the crossover, the mean IOP was 20.6 and 22.1 mm Hg in the carteolol group and 25.3 and 19.6 mm Hg in the placebo group. Comparing the IOP means of the two periods to the baseline mean IOP on dipivefrin therapy alone, the incremental decrease in IOP was 3.8 mm Hg with carteolol and 1.9 mm Hg with placebo. This evaluation continued for 1 year, during which the effect of carteolol was maintained.[80]

## COMBINATION WITH PROSTAGLANDIN $F_{2\alpha}$

Prostaglandin $F_{2\alpha}$ significantly lowers IOP in patients with glaucoma whose pressures are inadequately controlled by timolol alone given twice daily. The absolute difference in mean IOP change between prostaglandin- and placebo-treated groups was 4.5 mm Hg, with a 95% confidence interval of 3.1 to 6.6 mm Hg.[81] Prostaglandins of the F series are believed to lower IOP by increasing the aqueous humor outflow through the uveoscleral route. This route follows a path between the ciliary muscle bundles to the suprachoroidal space, then ultimately crosses the sclera and comes out of the eye. The contraction of the ciliary muscle, for example, as with pilocarpine, appears to interfere with the action of prostaglandins on uveoscleral outflow because fattening of the ciliary muscle bundles as they shorten during contraction would tend to close off the interbundle spaces that comprise the outflow path. Because β-adrenoceptors seem to mediate a mild relaxation of the ciliary muscle when stimulated, their blockade might prevent this. However, it is clear from the previous study that timolol does not interfere with the action of prostaglandin $F_{2\alpha}$ to lower IOP.[82]

## BETAXOLOL

Betaxolol hydrochloride is provided in 0.5% concentration as Betoptic Sterile Ophthalmic Solution and in 0.25% concentration as Betoptic S Sterile Ophthalmic Suspension, which contain the racemic mixture of betaxolol isomers. It is a $\beta_1$-adrenoceptor blocker (cardioselective) that does not have intrinsic sympathomimetic activity or significant membrane stabilizing activity. Based on the human daily oral dose for treating systemic hypertension, betaxolol is five times as potent as propranolol. Betaxolol is relatively highly lipophilic, having a log partition coefficient of 2.73, which contributes to its high corneal penetrability. Equivalency between the 0.5% solution and 0.25% suspension formulations for IOP-reducing efficacy has been demonstrated by clinical trial.[83, 84] Betaxolol is distinguished from the other FDA-approved ophthalmic β-blockers by its $\beta_1$-adrenoceptor selectivity.

### Mechanism of Action

Betaxolol has been shown to reduce aqueous humor flow using the technique of fluorophotometry. In a double-masked study in 24 normal subjects, a single instillation of 1% betaxolol suppressed aqueous flow in all individuals. The range of aqueous flow reduction was from 7% to 51%, with a mean decrease of 32%. No consistent change in tonographic outflow resistance was seen.[85]

### Dose Response

Betaxolol 0.25% produced a significant lowering of IOP in 12 patients with chronic open-angle glaucoma or hypertension under study A 30% to 35% decrease less than baseline IOP was maintained during the 1-year observation period. Visual acuity remained stable, and no corneal anesthesia or alteration of tear secretion was observed.[86]

At the end of a 26-week randomized, double-masked study in 46 patients with primary open-angle glaucoma, the percent reduction of IOP was 28.9% in the group treated with 0.5% betaxolol and 33.2% in the group treated with 0.5% timolol.[87]

### Side Effects and Adverse Reactions

Because the $\beta_1$-selectivity of betaxolol offers the potential of greater safety in patients relative to the blockade of $\beta_2$-adrenoceptors in the bronchi and bronchioles, extensive investigation has been made of it in patients with pulmonary problems. The results of these studies firmly support betaxolol's greater safety in these patients. In many instances, rechallenge of patients has ruled out betaxolol as the causative factor when initially an adverse pulmonary experience had been observed.

Spirometric measurements, respiratory rate, heart rate, and blood pressure were monitored in nine patients with reactive airway disease in a randomized, crossover, double-masked, placebo-controlled study. Either 1% betaxolol or 0.5% timolol was ocularly instilled, with the order of administration balanced for the entire group of patients, and the previously mentioned parameters were monitored over a 4-hour period. Isoproterenol, a sympathomimetic bronchodilator acting on β-adrenoceptors, was administered at the end of the test and the measurements repeated. Timolol produced a significant decrease in airflow, as measured by forced expiratory volume in 1 second ($FEV_1$) and the ratio of $FEV_1$ to vital capacity at each observation time after 15 minutes. Neither betaxolol, at two to four times the usual clinical dosage, nor placebo produced significant diminution of airflow. Furthermore, timolol but not betaxolol or placebo blunted the effect of inhaled isoproterenol to increase the ratio of $FEV_1$ to vital capacity and produced a significant reduction of heart rate.[88]

The effect of betaxolol was evaluated on pulmonary function tests of nine patients with glaucoma and chronic obstructive pulmonary disease. When pretreatment test results were compared with those obtained after 2 weeks of 0.5% betaxolol treatment, it was found that the mean ratio of $FEV_1$ to forced vital capacity was 59.33% at baseline and 57.89% at 2 weeks, with no statistically significant difference present. Neither $FEV_1$ nor forced vital capacity was significantly changed by betaxolol. The results of this rather large prospective study support the potential advantage of the $\beta_1$-selective agent betaxolol for use in patients who are at risk to develop pulmonary side effects from β-blocker therapy.[89]

Betaxolol was well tolerated in a group of nine patients with glaucoma and chronic obstructive airways disease, with no adverse symptoms and without any significant changes in $FEV_1$, mean midexpiratory flow rate, and vital capacity.[90]

Histamine provocation was used in ten patients with glaucoma and coexisting obstructive airway disease to evaluate the pulmonary effect of betaxolol treatment. Pulmonary function tests were done at 90 minutes after instillation of betaxolol or placebo eye drops; then a dose of histamine was given sufficient to elicit a decrease of 15% to 20% in $FEV_1$, and the tests were repeated. The histamine concentration required for this level of response was not significantly different for those patients treated with placebo than for those treated with betaxolol, being 5.60 and 5.25 mg/ml, respectively. There was no apparent pulmonary β-adrenoceptor blockade by betaxolol to interfere with pulmonary function in the patients.[91]

A case of angiographically proven cystoid macular edema related to betaxolol therapy has been reported. The condition resolved upon withdrawal of betaxolol and recurred during a monocular therapeutic trial.[92]

A cardiovascular evaluation was made in 24 normal subjects receiving 1% betaxolol, 0.5% timolol, or placebo in a double-masked, three-way crossover study performed at two centers. Cardiovascular parameters, including electrocardiogram, were measured during 10-minute treadmill exercise periods. No significant differences in heart rate or the product of heart rate times systolic blood pressure (double product) were observed after betaxolol or placebo administration. Timolol produced a significant reduction in these parameters compared with betaxolol and placebo. None of the treatments caused a significant change in mean arterial blood pressure.[93]

A randomized, single-masked, three-way crossover study was conducted in 18 normal subjects to assess the degree of systemic β-blockade after ocular instillation of 0.5% timolol, 2% carteolol, and 0.5% betaxolol. Isoproterenol-induced tachycardia was used to assess cardiac β-blockade. The amount of intravenously infused isoproterenol and the infusion time required to cause a 50% increase in heart rate were measured before and after the instillation of each β-blocker. Timolol produced complete cardiac β-blockade in ten subjects and partial blockade in the remaining eight. Carteolol produced complete cardiac β-blockade in nine subjects and partial blockade in another nine. Betaxolol produced partial blockade in only three subjects, without complete blockade in any subject. The effect on $\beta_2$-vascular adrenoceptors was evaluated by variations in forearm arterial blood flow measured by veno-occlusive plethysmography after ocular instillation of these β-blockers. Timolol produced complete $\beta_2$-blockade in 14 subjects and partial blockade in the remaining 4. Carteolol produced complete blockade in 14 of 8 subjects too. Blockade after betaxolol use was partial in six subjects, complete in three, and absent in the remaining nine subjects. Timolol and carteolol produced a greater degree of blockade of both $\beta_1$- and $\beta_2$-adrenoceptors compared with betaxolol.[94]

### Long-term Efficacy

Nineteen patients with open-angle glaucoma or ocular hypertension were treated with either 0.25% betaxolol or placebo twice daily for 6 weeks in a randomized, double-masked prospective study. Nine patients on betaxolol exhibited a statistically significant IOP reduction of 3.8 mm Hg that persisted throughout the study period. A statistically nonsignificant change of IOP of 0.4 mm Hg was seen in the ten patients receiving placebo. There were no changes observed in mean arterial blood pressure, pupil diameter, corneal sensitivity, and basal tear secretion in either group. Betaxolol caused transient stinging in these patients. A subsequently approved and marketed novel suspension formulation of 0.25% betaxolol (Betoptic S) has largely overcome the stinging problem caused by the original formulation employed in this study.[95]

Forty-one patients with glaucoma or ocular hypertension were treated with either 0.5% betaxolol or 0.5% timolol for 26 weeks in a randomized, double-masked trial. The mean IOP reductions were 6.3 mm Hg with betaxolol and 7.2 mm Hg with timolol over the entire study period without adjunctive medications. No changes were seen in pulse, pupil size, or basal tear secretion in either group. Timolol reduced the mean brachial arterial pressure significantly, but the intergroup difference was not significant.[96]

In a 6-month double-masked, randomized study comparing 0.5% betaxolol and 0.5% timolol twice daily in 29 patients with glaucoma, both drugs were comparably effective. The mean reductions of IOP were 7.6 mm Hg, or 26%, with betaxolol and 8.4 mm Hg, or 29%, with timolol.[97]

A prospective, randomized, double-masked 6-month study in 38 patients with open-angle glaucoma evaluated the efficacy of betaxolol and timolol at 0.25% and 0.5% concentrations. Starting from baselines at or greater than 26 mm Hg off therapy, a lower median IOP was observed in the timolol group compared with the betaxolol group, 20.2 vs. 22.5 mm Hg, respectively. Eight patients on betaxolol therapy required adjunctive medication, whereas one patient on timolol therapy required it.[98]

Twenty-six of 40 patients with primary open-angle glaucoma enrolled completed a 26-week double-masked study to compare 0.5% betaxolol and 0.5% timolol, without requiring adjunctive therapy. Both drugs produced significant reductions in IOP from baseline, being 11.1 mm Hg with betaxolol and 10.6 mm Hg with timolol. The longer-term safety and efficacy of betaxolol was demonstrated in a group of 140 eyes for up to 2.5 years of therapy.[99]

### Efficacy Relative to Changes in the Optic Nerve Head and Visual Field

The effects of 0.5% timolol and 0.5% betaxolol on IOP and retinal sensitivity by automated visual field examination were studied in 20 patients with primary open-angle glaucoma. Reduction in IOP was greater with timolol than with betaxolol. Retinal sensitivity was diminished in the first 6 months in the timolol and betaxolol groups by 0.5 to 0.6 dB and 0.2 to 0.3 dB, respectively. At the first- and second-year visits, retinal sensitivity increased 0.8 to 0.9 dB in the betaxolol group only. Thus, the improvement of retinal sensitivity observed seems to be unrelated to the magnitude of IOP reduction caused by each of these β-blockers.[100]

Forty patients with primary open-angle glaucoma received treatment in both eyes twice daily with betaxolol 0.5% or timolol 0.5% in a randomized, double-masked study of IOP and visual fields. Perimetry was performed with the Octopus G1 program 2 weeks after a washout period and 3, 6, 12, and 18 months after initiation of treatment. A more pronounced but not statistically significant reduction in IOP was seen in the timolol-treated group compared with the betaxolol-treated group. In both treatment groups, there was a trend for visual field improvement during the first 6 months of treatment. Visual fields remained stable or tended to deteriorate thereafter. A better treatment effect on visual field was seen in the betaxolol-treated group compared with the timolol-treated group. Again, an apparent separation between IOP reduction and visual field improvement was observed.[101]

## CARTEOLOL

Carteolol hydrochloride is provided in the concentration of 1% as Ocupress Ophthalmic Solution, which contains the racemic mixture of the drug. It is a $\beta_1$- and $\beta_2$-nonselective β-adrenoceptor blocker that has associated intrinsic sympathomimetic activity and is without significant membrane-stabilizing activity. Relative to propranolol, carteolol is four times more potent on the basis of the total human daily oral dose for antihypertensive efficacy. Carteolol's relatively low lipophilicity probably accounts for its relative lack of discomfort on instillation but also confers on it a lesser corneal penetrability. No doubt that speaks to the higher concentrations required for efficacy compared with its β-blocking potency and with other ophthalmic β-blockers.

### Dose Response

The ocular hypotensive effect of a 50-μl dose of carteolol ophthalmic solution in concentrations of 0.5%, 1%, and 2% was investigated in 13 primary open-angle glaucoma or ocular hypertensive patients in a double-masked, placebo-controlled, crossover study. The 0.5% concentration of carteolol had no effect on IOP. The hypotensive effect of 1% or 2% carteolol was significantly greater than that of placebo.[102, 103]

In a 15-week double-masked, placebo-controlled, crossover study, the reduction of IOP at 12 hours after treatment was significantly less for 2% carteolol compared with 0.5% timolol.[104]

Two percent carteolol was studied in 12 glaucoma suspects and its IOP effect compared with that of placebo in a double-crossover trial lasting 6 weeks. Carteolol decreased IOP by 11% and 14% at 1 and 2 weeks, respectively. This result differed significantly from that of placebo.[105]

### Mechanism of Action

One percent carteolol was found to decrease aqueous humor flow by 16% in five normal subjects using the fluorophotometry technique.[106]

In a clinical study in glaucoma and ocular hypertensive patients, no effect on tonographic facility of outflow was seen 2 hours after instillation of pindolol or timolol eye drops. Pindolol is a nonselective β-blocker with some intrinsic sympathomimetic activity. The ISA may not contribute to an effect on aqueous outflow.[107]

### Long-term Efficacy

One open multicenter study of 1% and 2% carteolol in 178 patients with glaucoma revealed a 3% incidence of side effects and a range of IOP decreases between 5.8 and 18.7 mm Hg in previously untreated patients and between 4.8 and 17.8 mm Hg in pretreated patients.[108]

Another open multicenter study of carteolol involved 768 patients who were receiving medical therapy. Without a washout period, the patients were switched to carteolol. Of the patients (57%) who had been well stabilized on their previous medication, 73% continued to have the same or a greater IOP decrease on carteolol therapy. The IOP remained uncontrolled by carteolol in 19% of cases and was brought to 21 mm Hg or lower in 78% of cases previously uncontrolled by medication. Complaints of burning decreased from 25% on the previous medication to 2% on carteolol therapy.[109]

### Effect on Visual Field Indices

A multicenter, double-masked, 12-month prospective study in open-angle glaucoma patients was conducted to compare the effects of carteolol 2% and timolol 0.5%, given twice daily, on IOP and visual field. Seventy eyes of thirty-five patients using carteolol and 74 eyes of 37 patients using timolol were included in the final statistical analysis. The visual field indices analyzed were the mean defect, square root of the corrected loss variance, and short-term fluctuation. The mean IOP decrease over 12 months ranged from 6.9 to 7.5 mm Hg with carteolol and from 7.8 to 8.7 mm Hg with timolol. The differences between drug-induced IOP responses were significant.

Stable visual fields were seen in the majority of patients, with no difference in any of the three indices observed between the two drug groups. Some patients experienced improvement and some deterioration of visual field. The frequency and intensity of side effects were quite similar for both groups.[110]

### Side Effects and Adverse Reactions

Ninety-eight ocular hypertensive patients previously using timolol were switched to either 0.25% timolol or 1% carteolol twice daily for 1 month after a 1-week washout period. Both drugs were equally effective for decreasing IOP, and there were fewer adverse events, particularly eye irritation, reported by the carteolol group.[111]

Carteolol has been studied in patients with elevated IOP or secondary glaucoma associated with endogenous uveitis. Except for those patients with angle-closure glaucoma, IOP was controlled by carteolol at either 1% or 2% concentration. No exacerbation of the intraocular inflammation was noted.[112]

The pulmonary effects of carteolol and metipranolol were evaluated in two groups of ten patients with asthma and compared with placebo. No change in heart rate, systolic and diastolic blood pressures, vital capacity, and expiratory outflow velocity in 1 second was found with placebo. Atrial sinus bradycardia occurred in 10% of patients using either carteolol or metipranolol. The $FEV_1$ was depressed by up to 32% in three patients using carteolol and in six patients using metipranolol. Although carteolol has ISA and metipranolol does not, both drugs have the ability to cause decreased pulmonary function in asthmatics.[113]

## LEVOBUNOLOL

Levobunolol hydrochloride is provided in concentrations of 0.25% and 0.5% as Betagan Liquifilm Sterile Ophthalmic Solution, which contains the *l*-isomer. It is a $\beta_1$- and $\beta_2$-adrenoceptor (nonselective) blocker that does not have intrinsic sympathomimetic activity. It has a similar potency to that of propranolol for causing direct myocardial depression in dogs, which implies that it has some membrane-stabilizing activity. The package labeling of levobunolol states there is a possibility of decreased corneal sensitivity after prolonged use. Based on the total daily oral dose used to treat systemic hypertension, levobunolol is 50 times more potent than propranolol. It is relatively lipophilic but less so than propranolol, the log partition coefficients being 2.4 for levobunolol and 3.21 for propranolol. Because of its long duration of IOP effect, levobunolol may be used once or twice daily, depending on the patient. The prolonged IOP effect of levobunolol is attributed to its ocular and systemic metabolism to dihydrolevobunolol, which is reported to be similarly potent as a β-blocker.[114]

### Mechanism of Action

As with other β-blockers, the mechanism of action of levobunolol is primarily to reduce aqueous humor flow. Treatment with 0.5% levobunolol in 18 patients with ocular hypertension resulted in a 29% decrease of aqueous humor flow and a 36% decrease of IOP. Total outflow facility and episcleral venous pressure were similar in levobunolol- and placebo-treated eyes.[115]

In 31 open-angle glaucoma patients treated with either 0.5% levobunolol or 0.5% timolol for 1 year in a double-blind, randomized, crossover study, tonographically measured facility of outflow was found to be significantly increased in those patients during treatment with levobunolol but not with timolol.[116]

### Dose Response

A dose-response study of levobunolol employing single-drop instillation was conducted in 48 patients with ocular hypertension. The effect of 0.03% levobunolol was not significant. Concentrations of 0.3% and 0.6% decreased IOP significantly from baseline compared with placebo for up to 4 hours after treatment. With 1% and 2% levobunolol, IOP was decreased from baseline for up to 12 hours after administration.[117]

Patients with mild open-angle glaucoma or ocular hypertension were titrated on concentrations of levobunolol ranging from 0.25% to 1% of timolol and from 0.125% to 0.5%, twice daily, starting with the lowest concentrations. The next higher concentration was used if IOP became uncontrolled. The IOP was controlled in 63% of the patients using 0.25% levobunolol and in 69% using 0.125% timolol, with mean changes from baseline of 6 to 8 mm Hg occurring in both groups. Control was achieved overall in 75% of levobunolol-treated patients and 73% of timolol-treated patients.[118]

Of 30 patients with bilateral open-angle glaucoma, uncontrolled by miotics alone, there was normalization of the IOP in 73.3% of eyes and improvement in the remainder over a 3-month follow-up period, during which they were treated with 0.5% levobunolol twice daily.[119]

The efficacy of once daily levobunolol was evaluated in patients with ocular hypertension or open-angle glaucoma in an open-label trial wherein the patients were titrated from 0.25% once daily for 3 months to 0.5% levobunolol if IOP was uncontrolled. A significant mean reduction in IOP of 24% was observed in 72% of patients while using 0.25% levobunolol. One of six patients inadequately controlled by 0.25% levobunolol had a significant IOP reduction when switched to 0.5% levobunolol. It was concluded that 0.25% levobunolol provided IOP control in a majority of these patients.[120]

### Frequency of Administration

Seventy-one patients with open-angle glaucoma or ocular hypertension participated in a randomized, double-masked and controlled multicenter trial comparing the IOP-lowering efficacy of 0.5% levobunolol when given either once or twice daily. An overall mean IOP decrease of 4.5 mm Hg was observed in the once daily group and of 5.6 mm Hg in the twice daily group, with the difference not being statistically significant.[121]

A comparison was made of the effect of 0.5% levobunolol HCl, instilled once and twice daily, in a two-period, randomized, double-masked, crossover study in 20 patients with elevated IOP.[122] After correction for diurnal variation in IOP, the mean IOP change from baseline ranged from 16% ± 11% to 22% ± 9% with twice daily treatment and 14% ± 10% to 18% ± 8% with once daily treatment. On day 1, patients using twice daily drug had a greater IOP effect than once daily patients. By days 14 and 28, no clinically significant difference between regimens was detected. The authors concluded that once and twice daily treatments with 0.5% levobunolol are equal in effect.

In a randomized, double-masked, parallel group study, the efficacy and safety of 0.5% levobunolol and 0.5% timolol, each given once daily, were evaluated in patients with ocular hypertension, open-angle glaucoma, or closed-angle glaucoma. The IOP was decreased by 23% (5.6 mm Hg) overall and was controlled in 78% of 46 patients in the 0.5% levobunolol group. In the timolol group, the IOP was decreased by 26% (6.7 mm Hg) overall, and 89% were controlled. Both drugs were equally effective and caused similar minimal changes in heart rate and blood pressure.[123]

### Long-term Efficacy

In a 3-month, double-masked, randomized comparison of once daily 0.25% levobunolol and once daily 0.25% timolol in 80 patients with open-angle glaucoma, no significant difference was found in the overall mean decrease of IOP. Both drugs lowered IOP by 22% in this study.[124]

A 1-year, randomized, double-masked study in 78 patients with glaucoma or ocular hypertension was conducted to compare IOP control by twice daily 0.25% levobunolol or 0.25% timolol. When IOP was not controlled by the assigned treatment, the concentration was increased to 0.5% for 3 months. Mean reductions of IOP were 4.6 mm Hg by 0.25% timolol and 5.1 mm Hg by 0.25% levobunolol, and 71% of timolol-treated and 70% of levobunolol-treated patients were controlled at this lower concentration. Of those requiring 0.5% drug, 89% of those using timolol and 75% of those using levobunolol were controlled, but the IOP reduction was not necessarily greater than before. The drugs appeared comparable in all aspects of this study.[125]

Three hundred ninety-one patients with open-angle glaucoma or ocular hypertension participated in a randomized, double-masked, parallel group, 4-year multicenter trial to compare the IOP-lowering efficacy and safety of levobunolol and timolol. Patients were treated twice daily with 0.5% levobunolol, 1% levobunolol, or 0.5% timolol. Mean decreases in IOP over the course of therapy were 7.1, 7.2, and 7.0 mm Hg, respectively. The 4-year failure rate for efficacy was about 30% in all groups, with most failures occurring within the first 2 years. The rate of adverse events was about 10%. The investigators concluded that levobunolol is relatively safe and effective for lowering IOP over a 4-year period.[126]

### Side Effects and Adverse Reactions

Eighty-five percent of the 2,041 patients completing a 3-month, open-label, multicenter, noncomparative trial with twice daily 0.5% levobunolol in Germany had well-controlled IOP, whereas 15% did not and had their treatment discontinued. In 80% of patients, efficacy, ocular tolerance, and systemic safety were judged to be improved.[127]

During a study to evaluate the efficacy of twice daily 0.5% levobunolol in 27 patients with ocular hypertension for comparison to timolol, 1 patient with an undisclosed history of childhood asthma experienced bronchospasm while using levobunolol. The incident was related to an acute infection of the upper respiratory tract. This example underscores the need for diligence in carefully observing patients who are taking ophthalmic β-blockers and who have pulmonary symptoms.[128]

Two patients with chronic open-angle glaucoma developed dendriform corneal epithelial lesions while on levobunolol therapy. Another two patients on betaxolol therapy also developed similar lesions. Thus, dendritic epithelial keratopathy may be associated with topical β-blocker therapy.[129]

A case of recurrent allergic contact eczema, localized periocularly, associated with the use of levobunolol eye drops in a glaucomatous eye, was reported. A positive reaction of the crescendo type was observed on epicutaneous testing with either the eye drop preparation or levobunolol itself. Thus, levobunolol may produce an allergic response.[130]

### Blood Flow Effects

An evaluation was made of the effect of 0.5% levobunolol on IOP, ocular pulse volume amplitude, and ocular pulsatile flow in healthy subjects and in patients with glaucoma.[131] The IOP decreased by 28.3% in glaucomatous eyes and 29.6% in healthy eyes 2 hours after instillation of drug. Ocular pulsatile flow changed from 482.1 ± 133.3 to 548.5 ± 180.3 μl/min after levobunolol treatment in glaucomatous eyes and from 457.6 ± 178.2 to 528 ± 223.8 μl/min in healthy eyes. No implication for glaucoma therapy was suggested by these results. It is unclear whether changes in total pulsatile ocular blood flow, as measured by the instrumentation used in this study, reflect any changes that might be occurring in retinal or optic nerve blood flow. Furthermore, it is possible that the changes in blood flow are the result of an increase in perfusion pressure because of a decrease in IOP rather than because of an effect of the drug on the vasculature.

Although levobunolol treatment lowered the IOP in both the erect and supine positions, it did not alter the relationship for these changes of IOP usually seen with altering body position.[132]

## METIPRANOLOL

Metipranolol hydrochloride is provided in the concentration of 0.3% as OptiPranolol Sterile Ophthalmic Solution, which contains the racemic mixture of isomers of metipranolol. Metipranolol is a $\beta_1$- and $\beta_2$-adrenoceptor (nonselective) blocker that does not have significant intrinsic sympathomimetic activity but does have weak membrane-stabilizing activity. Relative to propranolol, metipranolol is ten times more potent based on the total human daily oral dose needed for antihypertensive efficacy.

Metipranolol is available only in the 0.3% concentration in the United States.

### Dose Response

In double-masked comparative studies lasting up to 4 months, 0.1% to 0.6% metipranolol produced reductions of IOP ranging from 20% to 29% of baseline and comparable with those caused by 0.25% and 0.5% timolol and 0.5% levobunolol.[133]

The results of a double-masked, randomized study comparing the efficacy of single-dose 0.1% and 0.3% metipranolol in glaucoma patients showed both concentrations to be effective, but the effect of 0.1% metipranolol was less and of shorter duration (<9 hours) than 0.3%.[134]

### Efficacy Compared With Other β-Blockers

A randomized, double-masked study of parallel design in 46 patients with open-angle glaucoma or ocular hypertension of 3 months' duration compared the efficacy, safety, and comfort of twice daily 0.5% levobunolol and 0.6% metipranolol. Both drugs produced an overall mean decrease in IOP of about 7 mm Hg and caused slight decreases in heart rate and blood pressure. More patients on metipranolol complained of stinging.[135]

A randomized, masked, crossover trial in ten open-angle glaucoma patients compared the effect of 0.3% metipranolol and 0.25% timolol. There were no significant differences between the treatment effects.[136]

### Long-term Efficacy

In a randomized, double-masked trial in 24 ocular hypertensive patients, twice daily treatment with 0.3% metipranolol, 0.6% metipranolol, and placebo for 6 weeks were compared. Aqueous humor flow rates and IOP were reduced by metipranolol but not by placebo. Mean systolic blood pressure, diastolic blood pressure, and pulse rate were not markedly altered. Mean changes in IOP were from baseline of 25.9 to 18.1 mm Hg with 0.6% metipranolol and from baseline of 27.1 to 21.6 mm Hg with 0.3% metipranolol. A 20% decrease in aqueous flow rate occurred.[137]

Fifty-six patients with IOP between 30 and 49 mm Hg were studied in double-masked manner during a 12-week, three-period crossover study of metipranolol. The mean decrease of IOP after 4 weeks of treatment ranged from 12.8 mm Hg with 0.1% metipranolol to 14.1 mm Hg with 0.6% metipranolol using an average eye approach. The range was from 13.4 mm Hg (0.1%) to 16.7 mm Hg (0.6%) by the worst eye approach. The differences were not significantly different between the concentrations of metipranolol. The incidence of stinging was concentration related, ranging from 19% with 0.1% drug to 63% with 0.6% drug. The authors recommend the use of the lowest concentration, 0.1%, based on its lower incidence of stinging and comparable efficacy to the higher concentration.[138]

### Side Effects and Adverse Reactions

In 26 eyes (15 patients) with glaucoma being treated with 0.3% or 0.6% metipranolol, there were 56 episodes of granulomatous anterior uveitis, all associated with large mutton-fat keratitic precipitates, flare, and cells. During 53.6% of the episodes there was loss of intraocular pressure control. Because of this occurrence, 0.1%, 0.3%, and 0.6% metipranolol eye drops were withdrawn from the market in the United Kingdom. The pathogenesis of this adverse effect is uncertain.[139]

## TIMOLOL

Timolol maleate is provided in concentrations of 0.25% and 0.5% as Timoptic Ophthalmic Solution, which contains the maleate salt of the *l*-isomer, S−(−) timolol. It is also provided as preservative-free Timoptic in Ocudose, 0.25% and 0.5%. Timolol is a $\beta_1$- and $\beta_2$-adrenoceptor (nonselective) blocker that does not have significant intrinsic sympathomimetic activity or membrane-stabilizing activities. Based on the human oral dose for the treatment of systemic hypertension, timolol is seven times more potent than propranolol. It has intermediate lipophilicity, having a log partition coefficient of 1.91. It is marketed in concentrations of 0.25% and 0.5%. Timolol was the first ophthalmic β-blocker to be approved to treat glaucoma in the United States. Because of this and its long history of use, timolol frequently serves as the reference drug in active-controlled clinical studies.

### Efficacy Comparison for Timolol Isomers

Usually one isomer of a racemic β-blocker possesses the greater β-blocking potency of the enantiomeric pair. In the case of timolol, this is the S−(−) isomer. Interestingly, however, the R−(+) isomer of timolol is relatively potent for reducing IOP, even though it is much less potent a β-blocker. An evaluation was made of the effect on IOP of 0.25%, 0.5%, 1%, and 2% R−(+) timolol compared with that of 0.25% S−(−) timolol or placebo in ocular hypertensive patients. Single instillation of R−(+) timolol lowered IOP in the range of 20% to 25% compared with 32% for S−(−) timolol and 8% for placebo. It is unusual for the R−(+) isomer of a drug to be so similar in potency to its S−(−) isomer when β-adrenoceptor blockade is involved in the effect. These results suggest a different pharmacologic mechanism of action on the IOP for R−(+) timolol.[140] Of a number of different β-blockers investigated, timolol, with an isomeric ratio, R−(+):S−(−), of 0.82 for the ciliary process β-adrenoceptor, seemed to be the most likely to exhibit this phenomenon. R−(+) timolol has 1/44th the receptor-blocking potency of S−(−) timolol.[141] This implies that R−(+) timolol might cause fewer systemic side effects compared with S−(−) timolol.

### Mechanism of Action

Increase of the facility of outflow is not the cause of IOP reduction by timolol.[142] No effect on aqueous humor outflow was observed in studies in 38 glaucomatous eyes treated for 14 weeks with timolol.[143]

Aqueous flow, as measured by fluorophotometry in 23 clinically normal subjects, was reduced by a mean of 34%, with a range of 13% to 48%, with timolol treatment. No changes were seen in corneal endothelial permeability, anterior chamber volume, or outflow resistance.[144] In this study no difference was found in the response of light or dark eyes to timolol. In another study, 48% of black glaucoma patients required 0.5% timolol for control of pressure compared with only 27% of white glaucoma patients.[145] The IOP effect of timolol appears to outlast its effect on aqueous flow. In 19 patients who had been treated a mean length of time of 44 months with 0.5% timolol, aqueous flow was found to slowly revert to its normal rate after discontinuing timolol. A significant increase of flow was seen 4 days after discontinuation but IOP did not rise significantly until 14 days later. Two to 6 weeks passed before normal flow rate resumed. It was suggested that lower or less frequent doses of timolol may be acceptable for efficacy.[146] These results have implications for the design of clinical drug trials wherein a sufficient amount of washout time must elapse to avoid interaction between the drugs under study.

The effect of 0.5% timolol on aqueous humor dynamics was investigated in 12 clinically normal subjects. After twice daily instillation for 1 week, timolol reduced IOP by 3.9 mm Hg, decreased fluorometric aqueous flow by 0.84 μl/min, but produced no change in tonographic outflow or calculated uveoscleral outflow.[147]

### Dose Response

The dose-response relationship of timolol treatment was studied in 20 patients with open-angle glaucoma, comparing the percent decrease of IOP from the pretreatment baseline, measured after a single drop of medication. It was found that even a 0.1% solution will maintain a 25% decrease in IOP for 24 hours. A 30% to 40% decrease is maintained for 24 hours by 0.5% or 1% timolol. Near-maximal IOP reduction by timolol occurs at 0.5% concentration, which is considered to be an optimal upper concentration for clinical use.[148] A concentration of timolol as low as 0.008% has been shown to reduce IOP.

### Long-term Efficacy

An analysis of the diurnal IOP curves of 1,178 individuals on timolol treatment was made.[149] The mean range of IOP fluctuation was found to be 5.0 mm Hg in normals, 5.8 mm Hg in open-angle glaucoma patients, and 6.8 mm Hg in ocular hypertensive patients. Patients on timolol therapy exhibited a lower mean range of IOP fluctuation compared with those using other types of glaucoma medication.

The effect of timolol was studied in 82 new open-angle glaucoma patients over 4½ years. Of these patients, 20 of 82 required adjunctive medication or surgical treatment. Of 66 patients remaining at the time, 69.7% were controlled by timolol alone. No significant changes in pupil diameter, Schirmer's test, or corneal sensitivity (Cochet and Bonnet method) were observed. Slight reductions of heart rate and blood pressure occurred.[150]

Of 47 glaucoma patients, observed for an average of 33 months, 20 were failures (<20% reduction of outflow pressure) on therapy with either 1% epinephrine (12 patients) or 0.5% timolol (8 patients). During the first year, the failure rate in the epinephrine group was 35%, whereas that in the timolol group was zero. Later the failure rates became similar.[151]

The long-term benefit of timolol for controlling IOP was evaluated by evaluating 155 patients with open-angle glaucoma or ocular hypertension over a mean follow-up period of 31.6 months. Timolol alone controlled IOP in 63.2% of the patients, with most failures occurring within the first 6 months and being related to higher starting IOP. In another 23.2% of patients, timolol plus adjunctive medication was required for control of IOP; in 13.6% of patients either laser trabeculoplasty or filtering surgery were added to timolol for control of IOP. The rate of transient adverse events was 11.2%, and in three cases, local and systemic side effects were serious enough to terminate timolol therapy.[152]

### Side Effects and Adverse Reactions

Tear secretion and basal tear turnover were measured using fluorophotometry in 13 open-angle glaucoma patients not on any ophthalmic therapy, 24 patients using timolol daily, and 41 healthy subjects as controls. The values obtained from patients, whether on therapy or not, were significantly lower than those from control subjects. The tear film breakup times were significantly shorter in patients using timolol compared with those who were not using timolol and healthy controls.[153]

When the tear film breakup times were compared in individuals who had previously been untreated and those using preserved timolol eye drops and having eye irritation and who were changed to unpreserved timolol solution, a significant prolongation of breakup time was seen. Preservative-free β-blocker eye drops appear to have advantages over preserved drops in irritated eyes on therapy.[154]

In a group of 35 subjects of whom 15 were asthmatics, 10 were nonasthmatics with glaucoma, and 10 were elderly normals, administration of timolol caused sinoatrial bradycardia in 91% and decreased $FEV_1$ in 13 of 15 asthmatics and in two patients with chronic bronchitis.[155]

Hyperkalemia occurred in a patient with radiation pneumonitis and glaucoma who was on prednisone therapy and using ophthalmic timolol. After other possible causes were ruled out, timolol was withdrawn from the patient's therapy. His serum potassium levels returned to normal even with continued prednisone therapy. Rechallenge with timolol resulted again in hyperkalemia, which subsequently normalized on the second withdrawal.[156]

A case of systemic lupus erythematosus was reported in a patient receiving only topical ophthalmic timolol therapy. The patient's fever, malaise, pleurisy, and recurrent sterile pleural effusions while using medication subsided or resolved when timolol was withdrawn.[157]

A case of Raynaud's syndrome has been reported in a 58-year-old patient receiving timolol eye drops for glaucoma. When a thermographic test was applied after exposure to cold water, the warm-up time was prolonged after treatment with timolol. Individuals so predisposed may experience Raynaud's syndrome while taking a nonselective β-blocker such as timolol.[158]

Side by side comparisons of the ocular irritation associated with the instillation of 0.5% betaxolol, 0.5% timolol, and artificial tears in 24 patients with glaucoma showed differences among them. Timolol produced a lower incidence of ocular discomfort in this study compared with betaxolol.[159] However, that study used the original Betoptic solution formulation, which has been supplanted largely by the significantly more comfortable Betoptic S formulation.

Plasma lipids were measured at start and finish in fasting blood samples from 28 subjects who used topical 0.5% timolol twice daily for an average of 76 days. Although mean total cholesterol and low-density lipoprotein (LDL)–cholesterol levels did not change over this period, triglyceride levels increased by 12%, HDL-cholesterol levels decreased by 9%, and the total cholesterol-HDL/cholesterol ratio increased by 8%. A decrease in HDL-cholesterol is considered to increase the risk of coronary artery disease.[160] In another study of topical 0.5% timolol in 19 patients with elevated IOP, no significant change in any of the lipid fractions was found at 5 and 15 weeks of treatment.[161]

### Efficacy Relative to Changes in the Optic Nerve Head and Visual Field

A 5-year randomized, double-masked, clinical trial was conducted in patients with ocular hypertension who were at moderate risk of having open-angle glaucoma develop to determine the effectiveness of timolol therapy in preventing or delaying the onset of visual field loss. Of 65 patients enrolled in the study, 42 completed a minimum of 4 years of follow-up. One eye received timolol twice daily, and the fellow eye received placebo. Timolol-treated eyes exhibited a decrease in IOP by a mean value of 4.9 ± 3.1 mm Hg, whereas placebo-treated eyes showed a 2.9 ± 3.1 mm Hg decrease. The between eye mean difference in IOP was 2.3 ± 2.6 mm Hg. During the study, four timolol-treated eyes and 10 placebo-treated eyes developed visual field loss. The difference in incidence was statistically significant. A statistically significant difference in favor of timolol was observed in the optic disc pallor analyzed by computer image analysis. Both groups showed an increase in optic disc pallor, with that in timolol-treated eyes being 0.86% and that in placebo-treated eyes being 1.80%. Optic disc cupping progressed in four timolol- and eight placebo-treated eyes. These results suggest that timolol therapy prevents or delays the onset of visual field loss and optic disc changes when IOP is decreased in ocular hypertensive subjects.[162]

A prospective randomized clinical trial was conducted in 107 patients with ocular hypertension and normal visual fields and the absence of optic disc damage to compare no treatment vs. treatment with timolol. The average follow-up periods were 56 months for the timolol group and 51 months for the no-treatment group. Endpoints for failure were the development of glaucomatous visual field loss, the presence of progressive optic disc changes, and an IOP greater than 32 mm Hg. Nine patients failed in the timolol-treated group and 17 in the no-treatment group, a difference that was statistically significant. Six failures in the timolol group had discontinued using timolol before the failure. Taking these as being lost to follow-up and considering only disc and field changes, the investigators[163] found timolol treatment to be significantly protective compared with no treatment. In this study, protection was associated with a higher tonographic facility of outflow.

Automated perimetry was used to obtain fine-grid meridional differential light sensitivity data every 4 months from 46 glaucoma suspects who had completed 6 years of follow-up study. Of these, 24 patients were being treated with 0.5% timolol and 22 were untreated. None had developed localized visual field defects or acquired optic disc changes. The long-term fluctuation in differential light sensitivity did not differ significantly between the groups, with no significant intergroup differences in either the number of stable locations or the number of locations where sensitivity either increased or decreased. Thus, long-term IOP reduction by timolol appeared not to influence the differential light sensitivity in the test meridians evaluated in this study.[164]

With endpoints defined as reproducible visual field defects on automated perimetry, disc hemorrhages, or stereographically documented optic nerve head changes, the effect of treatment with timolol or no treatment was studied in 143 patients with ocular hypertension (IOP > 22 mm Hg) but without visual field defects or obvious evidence of optic disc damage over a 6-year period. Of the 42 patients in whom endpoints developed, 20 had and 22 had not been treated. Survival analysis revealed no statistically significant differences between the groups with regard to failure time to any endpoints.[165]

Temporal contrast sensitivity was measured in 26 patients with ocular hypertension and in 22 patients with primary open-angle glaucoma, before and after timolol therapy. All glaucoma patients exhibited sensitivity losses compared with normotensive controls, which did not change with treatment. The ocular hypertensives seemed to fall into three groups: those who did not exhibit abnormal flicker sensitivity even with high IOP, those whose initial sensitivity loss improved with IOP lowering, and those whose sensitivity loss persisted even after IOP reduction.[166]

Pattern ERGs were studied in 21 patients with ocular hypertension who had received unilateral timolol treatment for a minimum of 6 years. There was a 2.4–mm Hg difference in IOP between placebo- and timolol-treated eyes. Statistically significant deficits in the amplitude of steady-state pattern ERGs were seen in 16 eyes of 12 patients (10 receiving placebo and 6 timolol); however, the mean amplitudes did not differ between the two groups. A significant correlation for the IOP differences between the placebo- and timolol-treated groups and the corresponding pattern ERG amplitude differences indicate IOP reduction may provide benefit for preserving ganglion cell function.[167]

## Consensual Intraocular Pressure Effect of Timolol

The bilateral IOP response to unilateral instillation of 0.5% timolol was studied in 30 patients recently diagnosed with open-angle glaucoma. Forty-seven percent (14) of the patients exhibited bilateral IOP reduction, with a small difference between the treated (8.2 mm Hg) and untreated (7.7 mm Hg) eyes. Overall, treated eyes changed from a baseline of 28.5 to 21.0 mm Hg, and untreated eyes went from a baseline of 26.4 to 21.9 mm Hg. These results have implication for the design of therapeutic trials wherein one uses the contralateral eye as a control and bases the effect on the intereye difference of IOP.[168]

The consensual ophthalmotonic reaction involves an alteration of IOP in one eye being accompanied by a like IOP change in the contralateral fellow eye. A consensual decrease of IOP was seen to accompany an IOP decrease induced by 0.5% timolol, 1% epinephrine, or 2% pilocarpine in the fellow eye in 13 normal and 13 ocular hypertensive subjects.[169]

When 5% guanethidine, a drug that interferes with sympathetic nervous transmission, was instilled to the consensual eye, along with saline solution, and the fellow eye was treated with either 0.5% timolol or saline solution, the consensual IOP decrease was blocked. Three of four patients with Horner's syndrome also exhibited a decreased consensual ophthalmotonic reaction when the timolol was instilled to the normal eye. These results implicate the sympathetic nervous system in mediating this consensual reaction.[170]

When instilled unilaterally in eyes of normal subjects, 0.5% timolol did not elicit a decrease of IOP in the contralateral untreated eyes, but a significant IOP mean decrease of 26% was observed in the treated eyes. This result is in contrast to that seen in certain glaucomatous eyes in which timolol produces a significant decrease in the contralateral untreated eye.[171]

## Effects on the Ophthalmic Vasculature and Blood Flow

Pulsatile ocular blood flow was measured in 15 patients with chronic open-angle glaucoma while on or off timolol therapy. The intraocular pulse was evaluated in the supine and erect positions because a significant IOP increase is seen with assumption of the supine position. The IOP was decreased while the patients used timolol, but there was no effect on the postural change in the IOP. Pulsatile ocular blood flow was decreased in the supine position; however, there were no significant differences observed between treated and untreated conditions. Timolol did not improve the postural response of pulsatile ocular blood flow in glaucoma patients.[172]

The effect of treatment with 0.5% timolol on retinal circulation was studied in patients with ocular hypertension using laser Doppler velocimetry. Under a double-masked, randomized design, one eye received timolol and the fellow eye received placebo. Vessel diameter, maximum red blood cell (RBC) velocity, and volumetric blood flow were measured in a major retinal vein of each eye just before the instillation of drops and 2 hours later. Placebo-treated eyes exhibited no significant changes of measured parameters. Timolol-treated eyes exhibited an increase of 12% in RBC velocity and of 8.4% in volumetric blood flow rate. Both changes were statistically significant. There was no significant difference in vessel diameter between groups. Timolol-treated eyes had a significantly higher blood flow compared with baseline than did the placebo-treated eyes.[173]

Early arterial, early venous, and late venous retinal circulation times were measured using fluorescein videoangiography in 19 subjects treated with either 1% pindolol or 0.5% timolol in randomized, double-masked fashion. Pindolol reduced mean IOP from 15.47 to 12.16 mm Hg and increased the arterial, early venous, and late venous circulation times by 0.14 second, 0.72 second, and 0.78 second, respectively. Timolol reduced mean IOP from 14.9 to 10.22 mm Hg and increased the arterial, early venous, and late venous circulation times by 0.13 second, 0.4 second, and 0.86 second, respectively. Arm-retina times increased by 1.56 seconds with pindolol and by 3.55 seconds with timolol, with both effects being statistically significant. The author[174] concluded that pindolol, a β-blocker with ISA, and timolol have similar effects on the circulation times measured in this study. Using blue field entoptoscopy in a parallel study, this author[174] reported an apparent reduction to the paramacular capillaries.

Compression ophthalmodynamometry was used to measure ophthalmic artery diastolic, systolic, and mean blood pressures in 19 healthy subjects, before and 2 hours after unilateral instillation of 0.5% timolol, with placebo used in the fellow eye. No significant changes in the three parameters were observed in timolol- and placebo-treated eyes. However, the changes in mean ophthalmic blood pressure between timolol- and placebo-treated eyes were significantly different, suggesting an asymmetric drug effect.[175] The consensual effect of timolol on IOP has already been described.

After a single-dose instillation of phenylephrine, timolol, or betaxolol to nonpigmented eyes of rabbits, there was localized constriction of the arterioles supplying the ciliary processes. After 7 weeks of daily treatment, timolol continued to produce vasoconstriction of similar magnitude as that after a single dose. However, the vasoconstrictive response to betaxolol was not significant and that to phenylephrine was substantially diminished.[176]

Retinal vessel diameters were measured in normal individuals before and after unilateral instillation of 0.5% timolol twice daily for 1 week. Seventy-five percent of the subjects exhibited a decrease in mean arterial diameter. Arterial diameters were reduced significantly by a mean of 4.1% compared with placebo-treated eyes and baseline values. Venous diameters were unchanged.[177]

Ocular perfusion pressure, systemic blood pressure, and heart rate were measured in 50 healthy subjects before and after ocular instillation of 0.5% timolol, 0.5% betaxolol, 2% carteolol, 2% pilocarpine, or oral administration of 750 mg of acetazolamide. Retinal and ciliary perfusion pressures were obtained in separate and simultaneous recordings using oscilloophthalmodynamography (OODG). Despite a significant decrease of IOP in all groups, no changes in retinal or ciliary perfusion pressures, heart rate, or blood pressure were seen in all except the carteolol-treated subjects. Carteolol produced a small but significant decrease in ocular perfusion pressure in the face of lowered IOP. It was expected that an increase of perfusion pressure would accompany a decrease of IOP as long as blood pressure remains constant.[178]

The amplitude of the visual evoked responses was measured in healthy subjects during the artificial stepwise elevation of IOP to study the autoregulatory response of the optic nerve head circulation. It has been observed that glaucomatous eyes do not show a normal autoregulatory response compared with healthy eyes under these conditions. When pretreatment and posttreatment values were compared for the 20 eyes receiving 0.5% timolol for 3 days, only perfusion pressure showed a slight but insignificant decrease, whereas blood pressure and autoregulation did not change.[179]

SECTION FOUR

# Cholinergic Agents

ROBERT J. DERICK

## ACETYLCHOLINE

Acetylcholine is a chemical mediator that transfers nerve impulses from one neuron to another or from neurons to effector cells. It is formed at parasympathetic nerve endings, at skeletal muscle-nerve junctions (Fig. 3–16),[1] and at ganglion synapses. The actions of acetylcholine are classified as muscarinic and nicotinic.

### Pharmacology

Muscarinic action is the stimulation of smooth muscle and glands that are innervated by postganglionic parasympathetic nerves. The muscarinic action of acetylcholine is blocked by atropine but not by curare.

The nicotinic action of acetylcholine entails its stimulation of skeletal muscle and autonomic ganglia. (The former is antagonized by decamethonium and the latter by hexamethonium.[2]) A practical application of this information is the simultaneous administration of prostigmine and atropine in testing for myasthenia gravis. Atropine blocks the undesirable muscarinic side effects of acetylcholine (e.g., bradycardia), and yet it does not alter the desired response to skeletal muscle.

Acetylcholine is destroyed by cholinesterase, which is strategically located in the end-plate region. Within a few milliseconds after release of acetylcholine by the nerve impulse, this effector chemical is hydrolyzed, thereby permitting the end plate to repolarize and become receptive to the next impulse.[3]

The classic concepts of the effects of autonomic drugs have been confirmed by bathing isolated strips of cat ciliary muscle with these drugs (Table 3–4).[4] These experiments provide quantitative data as to the sensitivity of the ciliary muscle to drug stimulation. A concentration of acetylcholine of 1 μg/ml causes abrupt contraction of the ciliary muscle. Physostigmine (1 μg/ml), a reversible cholinesterase inhibitor, poten-

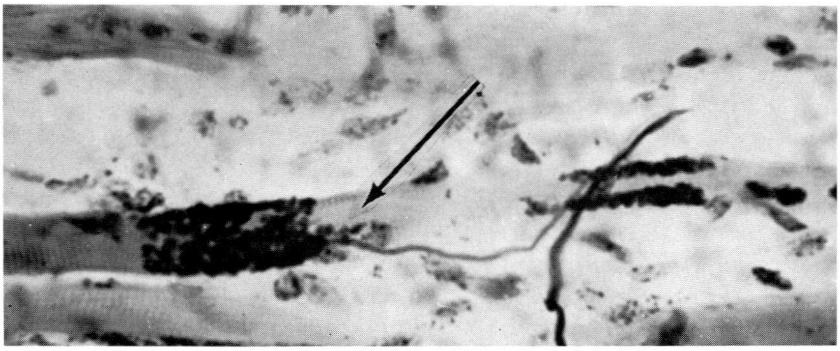

**FIG 3–16.**
Dense accumulation of cholinesterase (special enzyme stain of frozen section) distributed about ending of single nerve axon *(arrow)* on fiber of human extraocular muscle. (From Wolter JR, O'Keefe NT: *Invest Ophthalmol* 2:558, 1963. Used by permission.)

**TABLE 3–4.**
Cholinergic Agents

| |
|---|
| Direct acting |
| Acetylcholine |
| Methacholine |
| Pilocarpine |
| Carbachol* |
| Aceclidine |
| Indirect acting |
| Reversible |
| Physostigmine |
| Neostigmine |
| Edrophonium |
| Carbachol* |
| Irreversible |
| Isoflurophate |
| Echothiophate |
| Demecarium |

*The carbachol molecule has portions of the acetylcholine and the physostigmine molecules, giving it both direct and indirect actions.

tiates the effect of acetylcholine by about 100 times, so that 0.01 μg/ml of acetylcholine will cause contraction of the ciliary muscle.

Physostigmine sensitization of the iris sphincter to acetylcholine is quite different from cocaine sensitization of the dilator to epinephrine.[5] Whereas cocaine decreases the absolute strength of the muscle, physostigmine enhances the strength of contraction. Fig. 3–17 shows the response to maximum effective concentrations of physostigmine and acetylcholine (1:50,000 for each drug) by a sphincter muscle supporting a heavy load (sufficient so that almost no shortening response occurred). Addition of acetylcholine to the strip pretreated with physostigmine produced a much stronger contraction than the maximal response obtained by either drug alone.

## Clinical Use

Despite the extreme sensitivity of the iris to acetylcholine, topical ocular instillation causes no useful response. This is because cholinesterase destroys the molecule more rapidly than it can penetrate the cornea. Accelerated corneal transfer, as by iontophoresis, will produce miosis, as will direct application on the iris.

Instillation of a 1:100 concentration of acetylcholine directly on the iris will cause prompt, marked (2-mm) miosis.[6] The miotic action of acetylcholine is very brief, lasting for only about 10 minutes. Use of acetylcholine at the time of surgery may be preferable to instillation of pilocarpine or physostigmine, because the prolonged miosis caused by these latter drugs is one of the principal causes of postoperative pain.

## Toxicity

Because acetylcholine is so rapidly destroyed, its toxicity is low and its therapeutic effects are very transient. As much as 100 mg/min intravenously can be tolerated by adult humans. There is no evidence of cumulative action. As much as 1 g of acetylcholine has been given intravenously during a 10-minute period with only transient cholinergic effects. Intramuscular or subcutaneous injection of 500 mg does not alter pulse rate or blood pressure.[7]

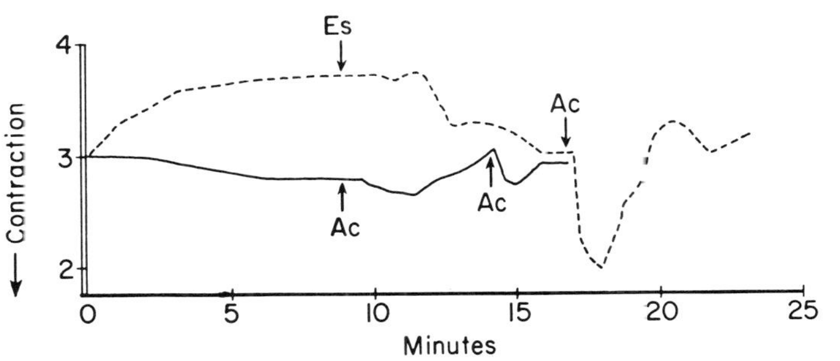


**FIG 3–17.**
Response of sphincter of albino rabbit to repeated applications of acetylcholine *(solid line)* and of the same preparation (after washing) to eserine *(broken line)* and then to acetylcholine *(broken line)*. (Modified from Sachs E, Heath P: *Am J Ophthalmol* 23:1376, 1940. Used by permission.)

A systemic reaction occurred after injection into the anterior chamber of 20 mg of acetylcholine (Miochol) subsequent to cataract extraction.[8] The patient's blood pressure immediately dropped to 75 mm Hg systolic and the pulse rate slowed to 48 beats/min. The cardiac monitor showed transient ventricular bigeminy and sinus bradycardia. Intravenous atropine in two doses of 0.6 and 0.8 mg did not change the heart rate. The hypotension and bradycardia lasted for about 20 minutes. There were no untoward consequences of this episode.

### Intraoperative Miotics

One percent acetylcholine and 0.01% carbachol (Miostat) are each used to achieve transient, intraoperative miosis. Miochol is a sterile solution containing mannitol (3%) as a lyophilizing agent. Miostat is a sterile balanced salt solution. This buffered salt solution makes Miostat less toxic to cultured bovine endothelial cells.[9] One percent acetylcholine has been shown to cause transient lens opacities in both humans and rabbits.[10] These opacities were thought to be an osmotic phenomenon and not related to acetylcholine.[11] These studies serve as reminders to instill in the anterior chamber the smallest amount necessary to obtain the therapeutic effect. Many drugs instilled into the anterior chamber can be removed at the conclusion of the procedure, limiting their exposure time.

## METHACHOLINE (MECHOLYL)

Methacholine bromide has pharmacologic properties quite similar to those of acetylcholine,[12] except that it is considerably more resistant to cholinesterase and therefore has a more prolonged effect. It has been given by retrobulbar injection in an attempt to induce vasodilation and by iontophoresis to constrict the pupil. It has also been used in the diagnosis of Adie's pupil.

### Clinical Use

#### *Diagnosis of Adie's Pupil*

Miosis usually is not produced by topical application of methacholine in concentrations lower than 10%. However, individual variations in sensitivity occur, and infrequently patients become miotic with a 1% solution. Miosis will result from lesser concentrations of methacholine if the corneal epithelium is abraded or if a wetting agent is used.

Breakdown of the corneal epithelium (e.g., in keratitis sicca or after anesthesia and tonometry) allows greater penetration of topical medications such as 2.5% methacholine, which under such circumstances may cause constriction of a normally innervated pupil.[13]

Partial parasympathetic denervation, as from Adie's pupil or in some cases of traumatic mydriasis, sensitizes the iris to cholinergic drugs. Such pupils can be made to constrict by a 2.5% aqueous solution of methacholine (without a wetting agent). Comparison of the drug response of the normal pupil with that of suspected Adie's pupil makes the diagnosis more valid.

The original patient with Adie's syndrome, on whom the observation of methacholine sensitization was first made, still showed the classic hypersensitivity to methacholine when observed 25 years later.[14]

Although hypersensitivity to 2.5% methacholine has been considered characteristic of Adie's tonic pupil syndrome, such hypersensitivity may be absent at the onset of this disorder. Only after periods of 8 and 11 months did two patients have typical sluggish pupillary reaction and the expected methacholine hypersensitivity develop.[15] A positive methacholine test result also occurs in familial dysautonomia, a condition characterized by partial parasympathetic denervation.[16]

Because methacholine is not easily available and is quite expensive, clinical testing for parasympathetic denervation is more easily performed with dilute solutions of pilocarpine.

## CARBACHOL (CARCHOLIN)

Carbachol is a combination of portions of the molecules of acetylcholine and physostigmine. Carbachol is not destroyed by cholinesterase; therefore, its action is not

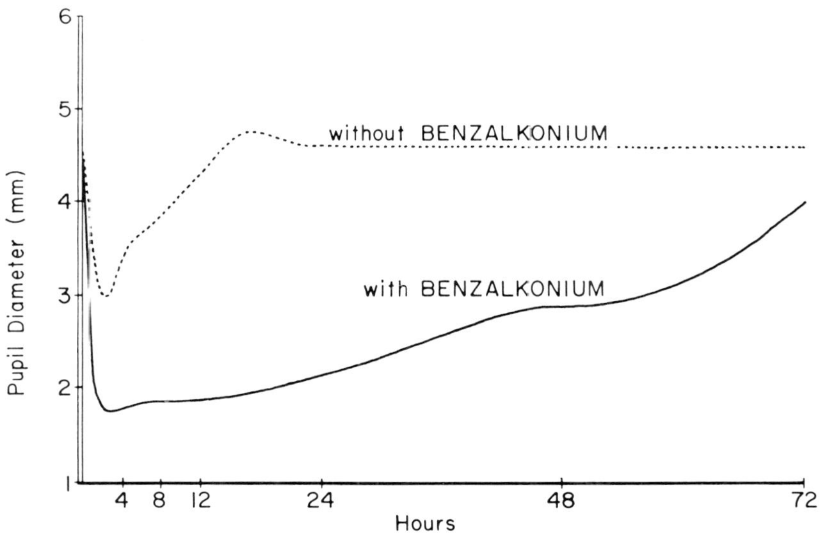


**FIG 3–18.**
Average degree and duration of miosis produced in ten normal adult eyes by a single instillation of a 1.5% solution of carbachol, with and without a 0.03% concentration of benzalkonium. (Modified from O'Brien CS, Swan KC: *Arch Ophthalmol* 27:253, 1942. Used by permission.)

increased by anticholinesterase drugs. In addition to its direct parasympathomimetic action, carbachol is also believed to have an indirect mechanism of action by inhibition of acetylcholinesterase. Carbachol is stable in solution.[17] Unlike the alkaloids used in ophthalmology, carbachol is not lipid soluble at any pH; hence, it penetrates the intact corneal epithelium poorly. To be clinically useful, carbachol must be dispensed in combination with a wetting agent such as 0.03% benzalkonium chloride.[18] The marked enhancement of carbachol action by benzalkonium is illustrated in Fig. 3–18. This enhanced action is not a result of potentiation of drug action by the benzalkonium but of increased corneal penetration. Wetting agents do not greatly enhance the action of pilocarpine or other drugs that readily penetrate the cornea. Systemic toxicity is not caused by ocular use of carbachol in recommended dosages.

## Clinical Use

### *Glaucoma*

Carbachol in a 1.5% solution produces more intense and considerably more prolonged miosis than does a 2% solution of pilocarpine. As shown in Fig. 3–19, a single instillation of carbachol in a normal eye causes miosis lasting more than 2 days.[19] Because of its prolonged action, carbachol is usually prescribed for use only two or three times daily.

A 1.5% solution of carbachol used three times daily has been reported to be more effective than a 2% solution of pilocarpine given four times daily in the control of pressure in chronic simple glaucoma (Fig. 3–20).[19] In another series of 26 patients with glaucoma who were switched to carbachol from pilocarpine, no significant difference in the IOP was found between the two groups, but the patients had more side effects using carbachol.[20]

## Disadvantages

Carbachol causes more severe headache and accommodative spasms of the eye than does pilocarpine, but these symptoms tend to decrease after several days of treatment.[21]

## Intracameral Administration

When used intracamerally, carbachol (Miostat, 0.01%) is an intensely powerful miotic. It is 100 times more effective than acetylcholine, and it is 200 times more

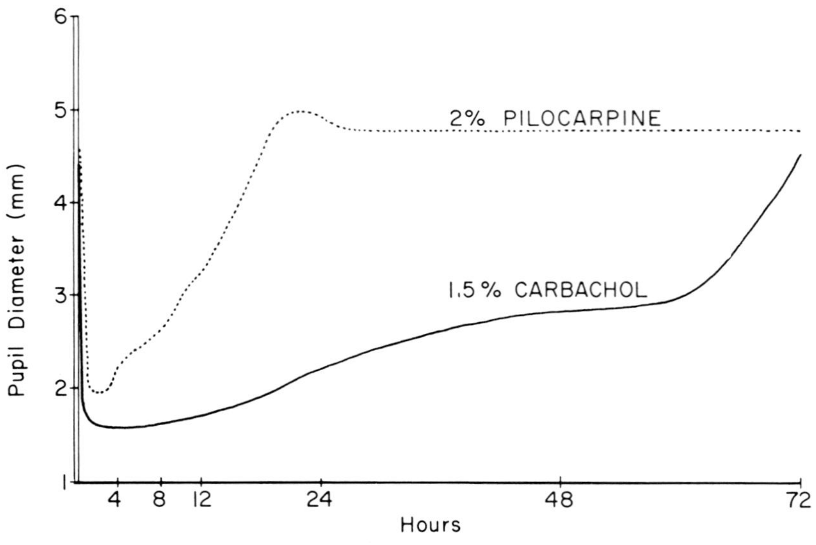


**FIG 3–19.**
Average degree and duration of miosis in ten normal adults after single instillations of pilocarpine and of carbachol. (Modified from O'Brien CS, Swan KC: *Arch Ophthalmol* 27:253, 1942. Used by permission.)

effective than pilocarpine. For example, 0.01% carbachol instilled directly on the rabbit iris produced greater miosis than did 1% acetylcholine or 2% pilocarpine. Maximal miosis is achieved within 5 minutes.[22] In addition, it is longer lasting than acetylcholine. Intraocular carbachol administered at the conclusion of cataract surgery has been shown to be more protective against early postsurgical IOP elevation than acetylcholine.[23, 24]

## PILOCARPINE

### Pharmacology

Pilocarpine is a direct-acting parasympathomimetic drug. Because it acts directly

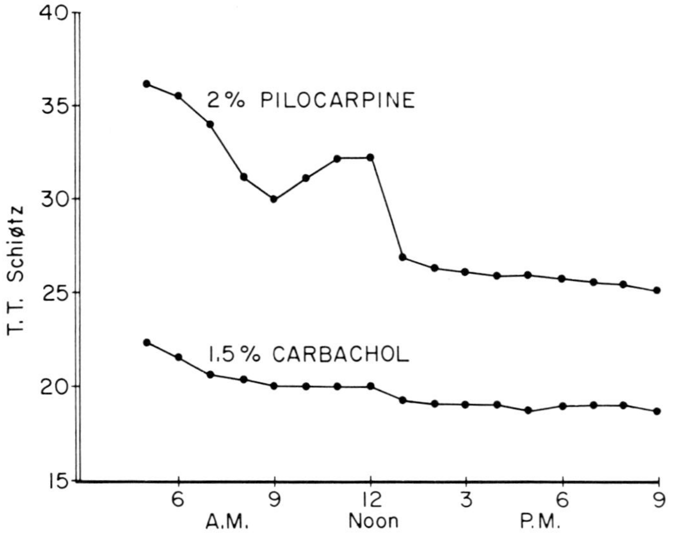


**FIG 3–20.**
Average diurnal tension curves of 34 eyes with chronic simple glaucoma when treated with a 2% solution of pilocarpine four times daily and with a 1.5% solution of carbachol three times daily. (Modified from O'Brien CS, Swan KC: *Arch Ophthalmol* 27:253, 1942. Used by permission.)

on the receptors, it is effective even on denervated structures. Specifically, pilocarpine will constrict the pupil after retrobulbar anesthesia. (Because retrobulbar anesthesia blocks acetylcholine liberation, the indirect-acting miotics such as physostigmine and isoflurophate will not constrict the anesthetized pupil.) In addition to its direct effect, pilocarpine may also have an indirect effect by activating synthesis of acetylcholine.[25]

Pilocarpine duplicates the muscarinic effect of acetylcholine but not its nicotinic effects; hence, it will stimulate smooth muscle and secretory glands but has no effect on striated muscle. It will cause lacrimation, salivation, sweating, vomiting, and diarrhea.[26]

### Ocular Penetration

Pilocarpine is absorbed into the eye primarily through the cornea after topical application. A pilocarpine concentration of 0.2% was found in human aqueous humor 20 minutes after topical instillation of 2 drops of a 2% solution.[27, 28]

Radioactive tracer studies in monkey eyes revealed the aqueous concentrations of pilocarpine shown in Fig. 3–21.[29] Regardless of concentration, the maximum aqueous concentrations were found at the 5-minute paracentesis. As expected, higher drug concentrations resulted in higher aqueous concentrations. The aqueous concentrations decreased rapidly with time. Chromatographic and colorimetric measurements found that topical instillations of pilocarpine could not result in greater than 5 μg/ml aqueous concentrations.[30] Pilocarpine is degraded in the cornea so that only a small portion of the administered dose reaches the anterior chamber.[29–31]

The dose-response curve of the effect of intramuscularly injected pilocarpine on accommodation in monkeys is shown in Fig. 3–22.[32] Systemic effects occurred within the same general range. Salivation began after 0.1 mg of pilocarpine/kg and became profuse with 0.5 mg/kg. Vomiting, defecation, and urination resulted after administration of doses between 1 and 5 mg/kg. Topical pilocarpine causes half maximal miosis in doses about 100 times smaller than those necessary to produce half maximal accommodative change.[33, 34]

A pilocarpine concentration of 1 μg/ml (0.001%) will cause contraction of the ciliary

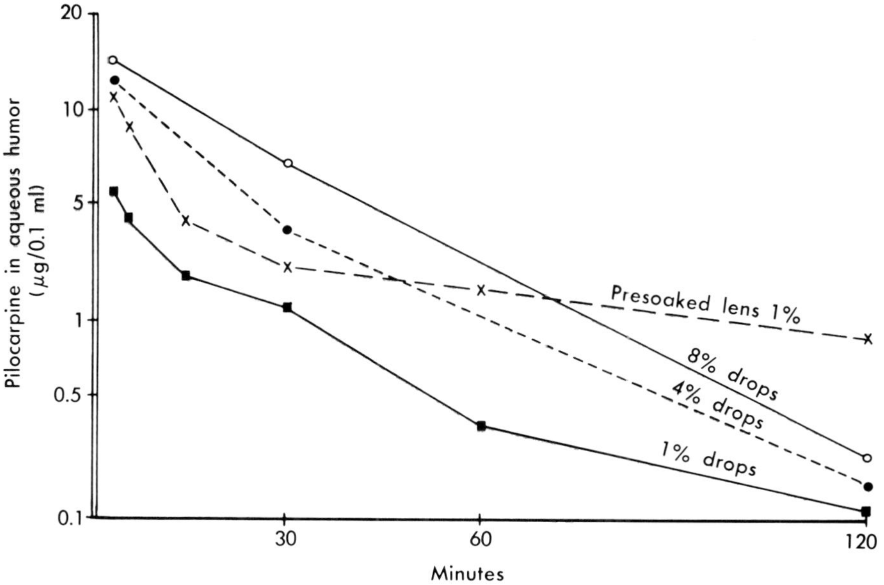


**FIG 3–21.**
Aqueous pilocarpine concentrations after the designated method of administration. (Modified from Asseff CF, and others: *Am J Ophthalmol* 75:212, 1973. Used by permission.)

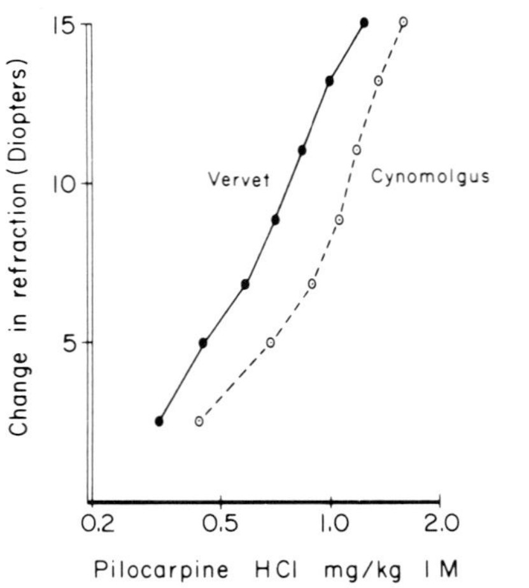


**FIG 3–22.**
Mean curves of dioptric increase of myopia with varying pilocarpine dosage in vervet and cynomolgus species of monkey. (From Törnqvist G: *Invest Ophthalmol* 4:211, 1965. Used by permission.)

muscle. The response to pilocarpine is different from that of acetylcholine in several respects. As seen in the top curve in Fig. 3–23, pilocarpine induces a slowly increasing muscular contraction, which requires several minutes to reach its peak. This contrasts with the second curve (acetylcholine), which rises abruptly to a maximum within a few seconds. The effect of pilocarpine could not be reversed simply by washing it out of the muscle bath. This sustained ciliary contraction is produced by persistent adherence of pilocarpine to the muscle receptors. Unlike pilocarpine, the acetylcholine effect promptly disappears when it is washed from the bath. Pretreatment with physostigmine reduces the response of cat ciliary muscle to pilocarpine (whereas as previously mentioned, physostigmine potentiates acetylcholine).

Pupillographic studies of the effect of a 1% solution of pilocarpine (Fig. 3–24) illustrate the progressive miosis that begins about 10 minutes after instillation, peak miosis within 30 minutes, a gradual decrease over 6 hours, and the pupillary response to light at various stages of miosis.[35] The time relationships of the miotic response to a 0.1-second flash of light are unaltered, but the amount of change in pupillary diameter is greatly reduced by miosis.

### Inactivation

Human serum contains a heat-labile component capable of inactivating pilocarpine. Incubation of 500 mg of pilocarpine with 0.5 ml of human serum at 37° C for 1 hour will inactivate 40% of the pilocarpine. Similar incubation with 0.2 ml of human secondary aqueous inactivates 10% of the pilocarpine.[36] The amount of this human pilocarpine hydrolyzing enzyme is not changed by prolonged pilocarpine use by glaucoma patients, nor is it greater in patients poorly controlled by glaucoma therapy.[37] A remarkably potent pilocarpine esterase activity has been inferred to be present in the cornea of pigmented rabbits.

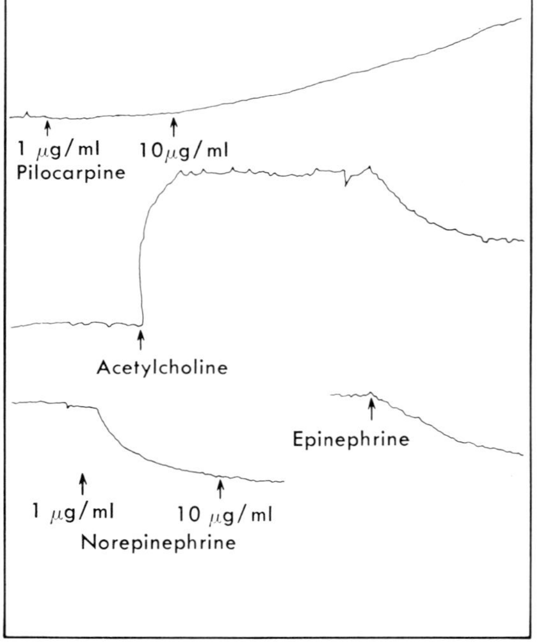


**FIG 3–23.**
Drug-induced responses of eserinized cat ciliary muscle. Small horizontal bar measures 20 seconds; small vertical bar, 20 mg of contraction (ciliary muscle strip was 6 mm wide). Upper curve shows effect of 1 and 10 μg of pilocarpine/ml. Middle curve shows rapid contraction produced by 0.1 μg of acetylcholine/ml. Relaxation of muscle after 1 and 10 μg of norepinephrine/ml is shown. Arrow represents the time of application of epinephrine, 1 μg/ml, with subsequent muscle relaxation. (Modified from van Alphen GW, and others: *Arch Ophthalmol* 68:81, 1962. Used by permission.)

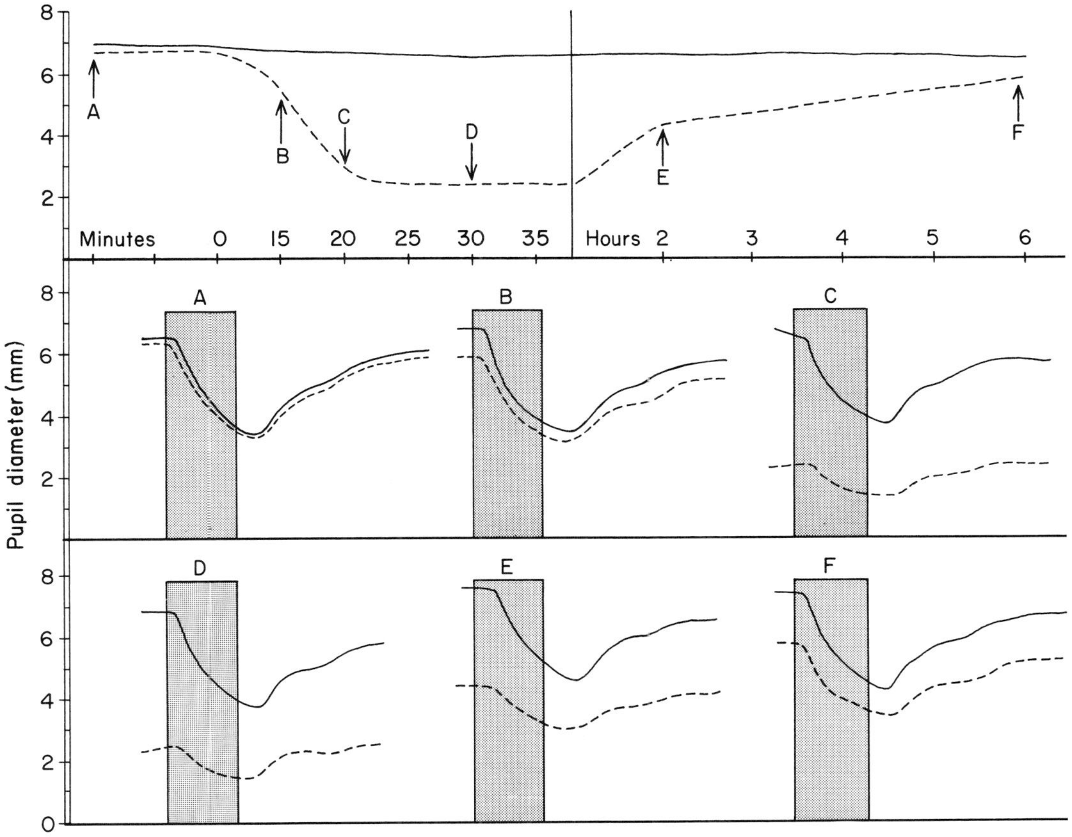


**FIG 3–24.**
Pupillographic study of pilocarpine miosis. *Solid lines:* size of normal pupil. *Broken lines:* pupil size after instillation of a 1% solution of pilocarpine. *A* to *F*, Response to a 0.1-second light flash at the designated times after pilocarpine instillation. (Modified from Lowenstein O: *Am J Ophthalmol* 42:105, 1956. Used by permission.)

In these animals the corneal breakdown of pilocarpine is 100 times greater than in albino rabbits.[38]

## Ocular Responses

### *Iris, Ciliary Body, and Trabeculum*

The structural changes of the iris and ciliary body resulting from miosis and mydriasis have been studied in monkey eyes.[39] As would be expected, the iris is much thicker during mydriasis, whereas the ciliary body is thicker during miosis (circular muscle contraction). The posterior pigment layer of the iris becomes four times as thick during the change from miosis to mydriasis. This increase in thickness is achieved by marked elongation of the cuboidal cells (Fig. 3–25).

The state of contraction or relaxation of the iris does not necessarily affect outflow facility. Rather, it is the ciliary body that primarily determines the facility of outflow. These anatomic facts are in accord with the following pharmacologic responses. Parasympathomimetic stimulation of the ciliary muscle increases outflow, the pupil being coincidentally miotic. Addition of a sympathomimetic drug (e.g., phenylephrine) dilates the pupil but does not alter ciliary innervation and therefore does not reverse the parasympathomimetic enhancement of outflow. However, a parasympatholytic drug (e.g., homatropine) blocks contraction of the ciliary muscle and decreases outflow, the pupil being coincidentally mydriatic. There is no direct relationship between pupil size and outflow facility in open-angle glaucoma.

However, by relieving pupillary block, miosis helps to improve the facility of outflow in angle-closure glaucoma. Contraction of the ciliary muscle relaxes the lens zonules, allowing a forward displacement of the lens-iris diaphragm. In certain instances, this forward movement of the lens can aggravate angle-closure glaucoma.[40]

### *Facility of Outflow*

The main mechanism by which pilocarpine causes IOP reduction is enhanced aqueous outflow. A detailed study of the pilocarpine-induced reduction of outflow resistance has been carried out in monkeys.[41] Within 3 minutes after an anterior chamber injection of 1.5 μg of pilocarpine, the facility of outflow has already measurably increased (Fig. 3–26). A rapid atropine reversal of the pilocarpine effect occurred (Fig. 3–27), almost completely blocking the pilocarpine effect within 10 minutes. All parasympathomimetic drugs stimulate the longitudinal fibers of the ciliary muscle to contract and thus exert a tractional force on the scleral spur. Several studies have shown that this mechanical effect improves aqueous outflow. Voluntary accommodation, ten-

A

B

C

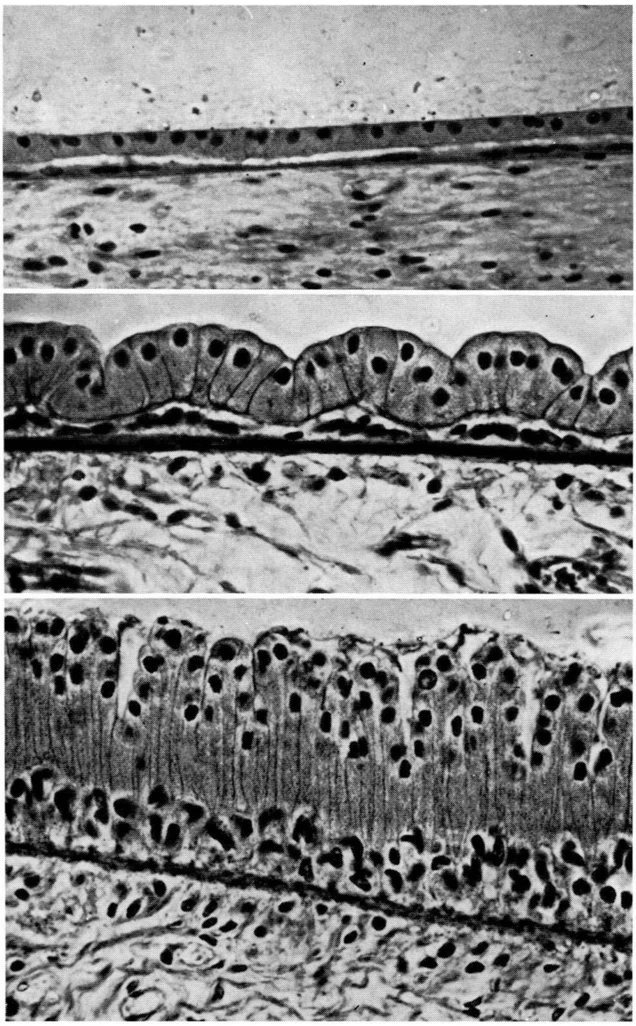

**FIG 3–25.**
Posterior pigment epithelium layer of iris. **A,** During miosis using isoflurophate (DFP). **B,** During dilatation with atropine. **C,** During dilatation with atropine and phenylephrine. (From van Alphen GW: *Arch Ophthalmol* 69:802, 1963. Used by permission.)

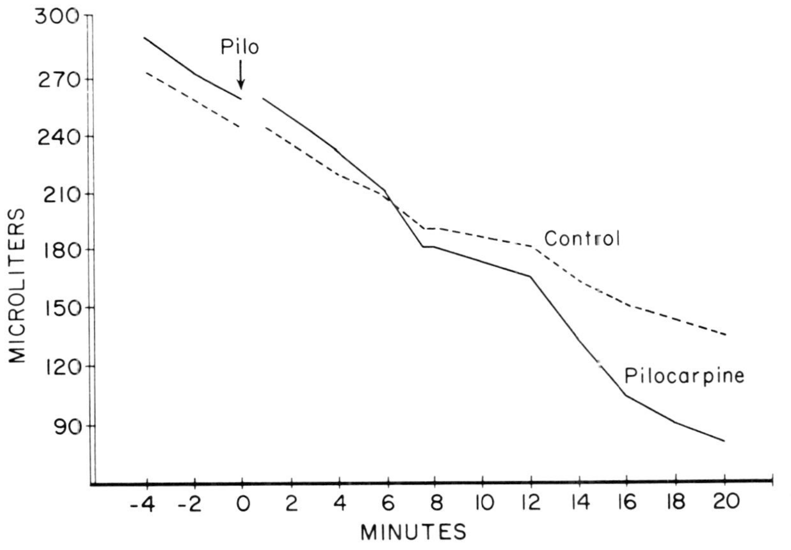


**FIG 3–26.**
Increased outflow facility after infusion of anterior chamber with 1.5 μg of pilocarpine. Ordinate represents microliters of saline solution remaining in perfusion reservoir; slope of fall, therefore, is related to outflow facility. (Modified from Bárány EH: *Invest Ophthalmol* 1:712, 1962. Used by permission.)

sion on the choroid, and traction on the iris root (all conditions that place a tractional force on the scleral spur) improve the facility of outflow.[42–44] An increase in the number of giant vacuoles in the endothelium of Schlemm's canal occurs after the application of pilocarpine, implying improved outflow of aqueous humor.[45] The intravenous administration of pilocarpine causes an immediate drop of resistance to aqueous outflow, reaching a maximum effect within 2 minutes. At this time the aqueous concentration of pilocarpine is too low to cause any outflow change. This finding is interpreted as excluding any direct action on the trabecular tissue or canal of Schlemm as the mechanism of action. Of course, the intravenous route delivers the pilocarpine to the ciliary body, the contraction of which is responsible for the reduction of outflow resistance.[46] Further evidence for the mechanism of action of miotics comes from studies of ciliary muscle disinsertion in monkey eyes. After disinsertion of the ciliary muscle from the scleral spur, the effect of miotics on the facility of outflow was abolished.[47]

Although the conventional trabecular meshwork pathway accounts for most of the

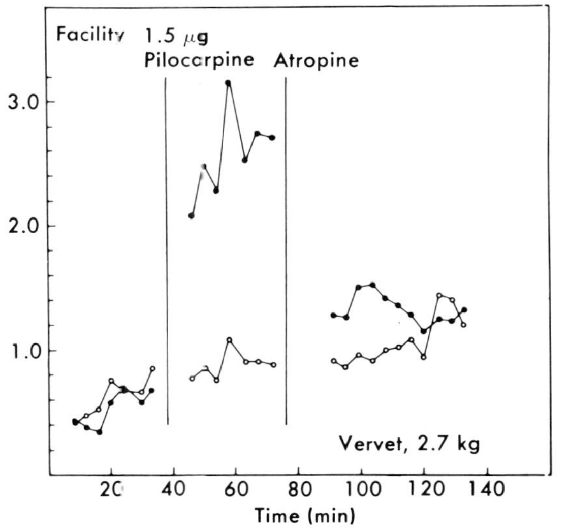


**FIG 3–27.**
Atropine reversal of pilocarpine-increased outflow facility. Facility of outflow is shown during constant pressure perfusion experiment. *Open circles:* control eyes show gradually increased facility attributed to slow trabecular damage from perfusion. Pilocarpine in anterior chamber rapidly and markedly increases outflow facility. Intravenous administration of 1 mg of atropine/kg rapidly blocks most of the pilocarpine effect. A slower component of atropine action requires about 30 minutes to return the outflow facility to that of the untreated control eyes. (From Bárány EH: *Invest Ophthalmol* 1:712, 1962. Used by permission.)

aqueous flow in humans, perhaps 4% to 20% of total aqueous outflow is via the uveoscleral pathway. Cholinergic agents reduce uveoscleral outflow. A carefully studied case of severe angle-recession glaucoma had a tonographic coefficient of outflow of only 0.06.[48] In this patient, three separate trials with 2% pilocarpine increased IOP by 10 mm Hg, presumably because of interference with uveoscleral flow. A 0.125% concentration of echothiophate also caused a pressure increase. Repeated trials with 2% cyclopentolate, 1% atropine, and 2% epinephrine reduced the IOP to normal levels and permitted medical control.

#### *Intraocular Pressure*

Topical pilocarpine reduces IOP that begins 1 hour after administration, is maximal at 2 hours, and lasts for 5 to 8 hours. In a single-dose study, the IOP response to pilocarpine was dose related in concentrations up to 4% and resulted in IOP reductions of 20%.[49] Although pilocarpine is generally administered every 6 hours, recent studies suggest that nasolacrimal occlusion after administration increases the duration of action sufficient to allow for every 12 hours of use.[50] The effect of pilocarpine is influenced by the color of the iris. A study of the response of patients with chronic simple glaucoma to pilocarpine indicated that comparable hypotensive effects were obtained with 1% pilocarpine in blue-eyed patients and with 4% pilocarpine in brown-eyed patients.[51] Concentrations greater than 4% have been reported to cause additional pressure reductions in darkly pigmented eyes, and higher concentrations may extend the duration of action. Thirty-minute incubation of pigmented and albino rabbit irides in pilocarpine solution results in the absorption of 8 μg of pilocarpine/mg of pigmented iris but of only 3.9 μg of pilocarpine/mg of albino iris.[52] Such melanin binding affects not only pilocarpine but also ephedrine, timolol maleate, atropine, cocaine, and cyclopentolate. For example, the binding of cocaine by the pigmented iris is 18 times greater than by the nonpigmented iris.[53] Ephedrine mydriasis is three times greater in albino than in pigmented irides.[54]

#### *Lens and Anterior Chamber*

Ultrasonic measurements of axial length indicate that pilocarpine increases the thickness of the lens. This is a dose-related response, averaging 0.11-mm increased thickness with 1% pilocarpine and 0.39-mm increased thickness with 4% pilocarpine in 20-year-old volunteers. The duration of this effect is longer with higher concentrations of pilocarpine, as is true of all its other pharmacologic effects (pupil, facility of outflow, IOP changes). This lens change is the basis of the myopia induced by pilocarpine.[55]

#### *Secretory Inhibition*

Although the IOP-regulating effect of parasympathomimetic drugs is usually considered to occur via a change in outflow facility, the existence of a possible additional effect of secretory inhibition is questionable. A technique of determining secretion by measuring the rate of decrease in the volume of the ciliary process has been devised[56] and is used to study the effect of various autonomic drugs on aqueous secretion.[57] In vitro secretory inhibition was achieved by a concentration of $10^{-9}$M pilocarpine, $10^{-7}$M physostigmine, $10^{-7}$M atropine, $10^{-6}$M acetazolamide, $10^{-5}$M carbachol, $10^{-5}$M acetylcholine, and $10^{-4}$M epinephrine. The effect of 4% pilocarpine in seven normal young volunteers was to reduce pressure by 3.3 mm Hg, to increase the coefficient of outflow by 0.16, and to decrease aqueous formation by 0.55 μl/min (normal trabecular outflow rate is 2.75 μl/min).[58] Further evidence of the effect of pilocarpine on the metabolism of the ciliary epithelium is obtained by study of the spontaneous movement of iodide from the surrounding medium into the ciliary epithelium. This iodide accumulation is inhibited by $10^{-7}$M pilocarpine. However, fluorophotometric studies in humans fail to show a reduction in aqueous flow after pilocarpine administration.[59]

### Stability

When maintained in a buffered, slightly acid solution, pilocarpine is indefinitely stable, retaining full activity at 6 months. Its effectiveness is maintained across a broad temperature range.[12]

## Commercial Preparations

Pilocarpine is derived chiefly from the plant *Pilocarpus microphyllus.* As an ophthalmic solution, pilocarpine is available in either the hydrochloride form or the nitrate salt in concentrations ranging from 0.25% to 10%. Preparations are also available in ointments and a controlled-release system (Ocusert). Pilocarpine gel 4% (Pilopine) used once daily was found to be as effective as pilocarpine 4% solution used four times daily.[60] The gel preparation is associated with less local side effects; however, in some patients, IOP cannot be adequately controlled for 24 hours. In addition, chronic therapy is associated with a 20% incidence of a diffuse superficial corneal haze.[61] Although the haze produced no symptoms, it can persist after discontinuation of therapy. Another alternative delivery system, pilocarpine Ocuserts, uses polymeric membranes for constant drug release into the conjunctival cul-de-sac. The 20 μg/hour device (Ocusert P-20) releases 20 μg of pilocarpine/hour and provides pressure control similar to 0.5% to 1% pilocarpine four times daily for 7 days. The 40 μg/hour device (Ocusert P-40) has efficacy similar to 2% to 4% pilocarpine.[62] The constant rate of drug release enables delivery of ⅕th of the amount that would be used with a conventional delivery system and substantially reduces the ocular side effects. Disadvantages include problems with retention of the device in the cul-de-sac and the increased side effects associated with an episodic increased drug release from the device. This sudden burst phenomenon generally occurs immediately after the insertion of a new device, and the side effects may be minimized with insertion at bedtime. The duration of action should be determined on an individual basis for both pilocarpine ointment and the Ocusert device.[63]

## Toxicity

Systemic reactions after the ocular use of pilocarpine are rare. Symptoms include salivation, lacrimation, sweating, nausea, vomiting, and diarrhea. Bronchiolar spasm and pulmonary edema may cause death. A 2% pilocarpine solution was instilled every 10 minutes in the treatment of a patient with acute glaucoma.[64] After about 30 drops, the patient began to sweat profusely and to salivate. He was nauseated and vomited. Severe muscular tremor and twitching developed. His blood pressure dropped, and the patient appeared to be in shock. The symptoms disappeared within 7 hours after the intensive administration of pilocarpine was discontinued. Although at the time these symptoms were attributed to the acute glaucoma, in retrospect it was evident that they were caused by pilocarpine toxicity.

If one assumes that 20 drops contain 1 ml of pilocarpine, a solution of 2% pilocarpine contains 1 mg/drop. The diaphoretic (subcutaneous) dose of pilocarpine is 5 mg.

## Ocular Side Effects

The most common adverse reactions to pilocarpine, and to all miotic agents, relate to stimulation of cholinergic receptors in the eye. Similar to the systemic side effects, the ocular side effects of the miotics are more common and severe with the anticholinesterase agents. Miosis, resulting from stimulation of the iris sphincter, can lead to decreased vision in low illumination. Miosis resulting from pilocarpine therapy produces significant declines in threshold sensitivities that can simulate progression of glaucomatous visual field loss.[65] Supraorbital and temporal headaches result from tonic contraction of the ciliary muscle. These headaches tend to be worse at the onset of therapy and can be less troublesome if the physician informs the patient of this side effect and therapy is initiated at a low concentration and low frequency (e.g., 0.5% at bedtime). An induced myopia can occur as a result of the ciliary muscle contraction. Two percent pilocarpine was reported to produce a myopia of 5.8 diopters in patients between the ages of 20 and 40 years. Similar to the headaches associated with pilocarpine, the induced myopia tends to be worse at the onset of therapy. Pilocarpine allergy not uncommonly follows its prolonged use for glaucoma.[66] Miotic cysts may follow long-term use of pilocarpine but are practically never of clinical significance. Retinal detachment has been implicated to occur as a result of pilocarpine therapy, although the evidence is indirect.[67–69] The permeability of the blood-aqueous barrier is considerably increased by miotics.[70] Fig. 3–28 shows the increased penetration of fluorescein into the anterior chamber of rabbits after instillation of solutions of 2% pilocarpine nitrate, 0.5% physostigmine salicylate, and 1% atropine sulfate three times daily for 2 days. Atropine does not significantly reduce the permeability of the normal blood-aqueous barrier, but it does restore toward normal the permeability of an inflamed eye.[71] The miotic-induced increase in permeability of the blood-aqueous barrier has also been demonstrated in humans by the use of the laser flare-cell meter. Pilocarpine was found to increase the permeability of the blood aqueous barrier in a dose-related fashion, whereas tropicamide stabilized the barrier. [72]

## ACECLIDINE

Aceclidine is a synthetic cholinergic drug that acts directly on muscarinic end plates in a manner comparable with pilocarpine. In human eyes with open angles, the pressure-lowering effect of 4% aceclidine was found to be comparable with that of 2% pilocarpine. This drug is currently available only in Europe.[72]

Aceclidine produces far less accommodative spasm than does pilocarpine and could be the drug of choice for most glaucoma patients with considerable remaining accommodation. In patients ranging in age from 26 to 49 years, an average induced myopia of 2.96 D was present 45 minutes after instillation of 2% pilocarpine. At 45 minutes after 2% aceclidine, the induced myopia was only 0.34 D.[73]

## PHYSOSTIGMINE (ESERINE)

Physostigmine is an indirect parasympathomimetic. Because it acts by preserving acetylcholine, physostigmine has no effect on denervated structures. For instance, physostigmine will not constrict the pupil during the period of retrobulbar anesthesia.

### Pharmacology

Physostigmine does not destroy cholinesterase but inactivates it by forming a temporary chemical combination. In vivo,

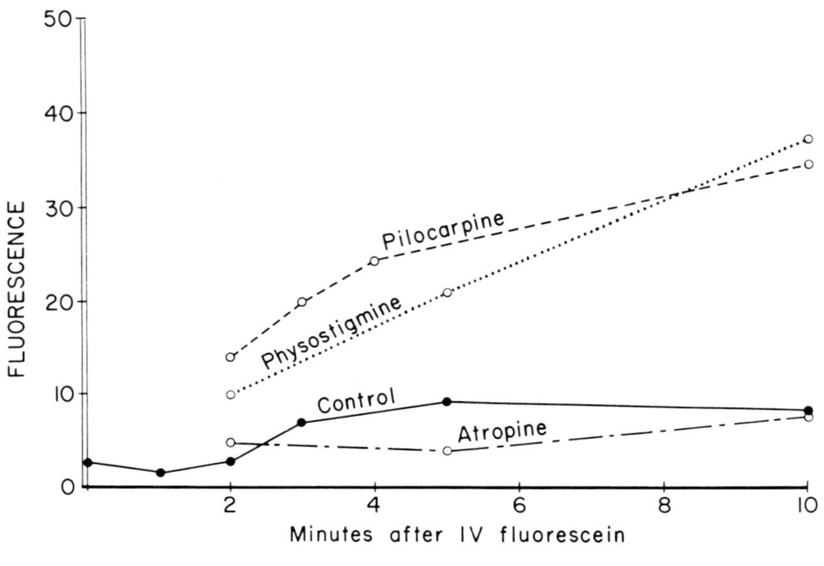


**FIG 3–28.**
Miotic and atropine effects on fluorescein penetration of blood-aqueous barrier. (Modified from Stocker FW: *Arch Ophthalmol* 37:583, 1947. Used by permission.)

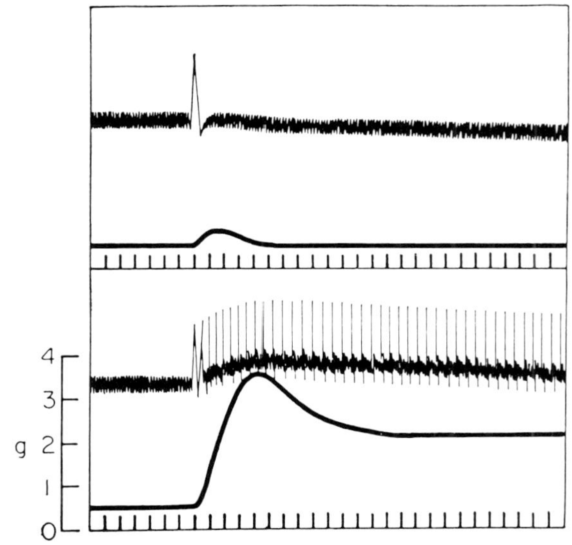


**FIG 3–29.**
Electrical action potential and myogram *(solid line)* of inferior oblique muscle of cat showing response to a single stimulus before *(top)* and after *(bottom)* administration of eserine. Vertical scale represents grams of muscular pull. (From Moses RA: *Adler's physiology of the eye,* ed 5, St Louis, 1970, The CV Mosby Co. Used by permission.)

physostigmine is gradually destroyed, thereby liberating the cholinesterase. Physostigmine is therefore classified as a reversible cholinesterase inhibitor. Neostigmine is a similar synthetic drug.

Because some acetylcholine is constantly present in the normally innervated iris and ciliary body, miosis and accommodation result from physostigmine even when the eye is at rest. In response to the accommodative effort, additional acetylcholine is formed. Preservation of this acetylcholine results in the accommodative spasms typical of indirect parasympathomimetic drugs.

The electrical and motor activity of extraocular muscles are greatly enhanced by physostigmine. Fig. 3–29 shows the grams of force (solid line) exerted by the inferior oblique muscle of a cat and its electrical activity (oscillating line). The upper portion shows the activity without physostigmine, and the lower portion shows the activity after physostigmine administration. In each instance the nerve to the inferior oblique muscle received a single electric stimulus. The normal response to such a stimulus is a single tetanic contraction, followed by relaxation. When acetylcholine destruction is prevented by physostigmine, however, a single stimulus causes prolonged and forceful muscular contraction. Convergence-accommodation studies also demonstrate a similar effect of physostigmine on the ciliary muscle. Physostigmine enhances ciliary contraction and therefore alters the accommodative convergence : accommodation (AC : A) ratio, as shown in Fig. 3–30.[74]

## Clinical Use

### *Glaucoma*

A 0.5% concentration of physostigmine ointment causes intense miosis within 30 minutes. This miosis lasts for 12 to 36 hours. During this period, the facility of outflow is increased. The combined use of both pilocarpine and physostigmine, although theoretically additive in effect, is probably competitive.[75]

### *Myasthenia Gravis*

Although physostigmine may be used as a diagnostic test for myasthenia, neostigmine is more effective. Subcutaneous injection of 0.5 mg of neostigmine will relieve

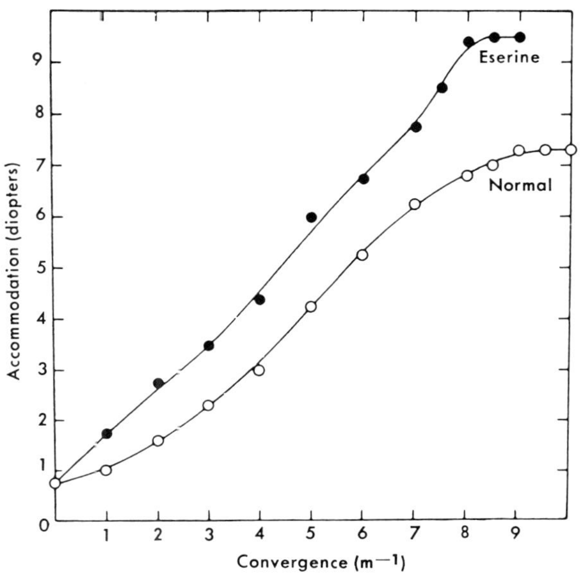


**FIG 3–30.**
Effect of a 0.05% solution of eserine on accommodative convergence/accommodation ratio of 30-year-old patient. (From Fincham EF: *J Physiol* 128:99, 1955. Used by permission.)

myasthenic symptoms within 15 minutes in a high percentage of cases. Diplopia and ptosis, as well as general muscular strength, may be greatly improved by such a diagnostic test. Simultaneous injection of 0.5 mg of atropine blocks the undesirable muscarinic effect of neostigmine (e.g., bradycardia) but does not impair the therapeutic response.

#### *Antidote for Anticholinergic Toxicity*

The potent anticholinergic drugs used in ophthalmology (e.g., atropine, scopolamine, and cyclopentolate) may cause central nervous system (CNS) toxicity with symptoms such as delirium, confusion, hallucinations, agitation, ataxia, and somnolence. Comparable anticholinergic effects may occur from a variety of antihistaminic, hypnotic, antidepressant, and tranquilizing agents. Overdosage of such drugs may occur during clinical use.

One to 4 mg of physostigmine salicylate given subcutaneously or intravenously will inhibit cholinesterase throughout the body, including the CNS. Physostigmine readily crosses the blood-brain barrier and hence is effective against CNS anticholinergic toxicity.[76] Within minutes, such an injection will reverse the anticholinergic toxicity. Because physostigmine is destroyed within 1½ to 2 hours, repeated doses may be necessary in the treatment of severe anticholinergic toxicity.

### Toxicity

Twitching of the eyelids is commonly noted after ocular use of the indirect parasympathomimetic agents. This minor but annoying side effect is caused by percutaneous absorption of the drugs and inactivation of the orbicularis cholinesterase.

Chronic conjunctival irritation is not uncommon after the use of physostigmine. Typical contact allergic dermatitis may develop after prolonged use.

The systemic parasympathomimetic toxicity resulting from physostigmine was the basis for its use as an ordeal poison in ancient Africa.[77, 78]

A rather unusual toxic response is the depigmentation of lid skin in black patients allergic to physostigmine ointment.[79] This depigmentation was noted in four patients and occurred 10 months to 5 years after the beginning of physostigmine treatment. The characteristic itching and irritation of allergic blepharitis were present in two of these patients. The depigmentation gradually disappears when physostigmine is discontinued, but recognizable changes have persisted for as long as 3 years.

Physostigmine gradually oxidizes to a pink or rust color. Because the decomposition products are quite irritating and are therapeutically ineffective, discolored preparations should be discarded.

## EDROPHONIUM (TENSILON)

Edrophonium chloride has both anticholinesterase- and direct neuromuscular-stimulating effects. Its effect is much greater at the neuromuscular junction than at other cholinergic sites; hence, its undesirable muscarinic side effects are minimal and do not ordinarily require symptomatic reversal by atropine. Edrophonium does not increase the strength of normal muscle contraction, but it does counteract the effect of curare and improves the contraction of myasthenic muscles. In excess, edrophonium reverses its action and has a muscle-relaxing effect. This paralyzing action is particularly likely to occur in patients with myasthenia gravis. The side effects of edrophonium are those of cholinergic hyperactivity and include tearing, salivation, gastric distress, lid fasciculations, and bradycardia. Bronchiolar spasm may follow its use in asthmatic patients.

The only ophthalmic use of edrophonium is a test for myasthenia gravis, for which it is the drug of choice. Its effect is transient; therefore, the drug-induced symptoms are brief, and, if necessary, the test may be repeated during the same office visit. Edrophonium will evoke a positive response in some myasthenic patients whose condition is not detected by the neostigmine test.

The technique of the edrophonium test is as follows: A tuberculin syringe containing 1 ml (10 mg) of endrophonium is prepared; 2 mg is injected intravenously during a

15-second period, and the needle is flushed with 1 ml of saline solution. The remaining 8 mg are injected only if there is no response within 60 seconds after administration of the first 2 mg. If a cholinergic reaction occurs after 2 mg, the test should be discontinued.[80] Atropine, 0.4 mg, should be available for intravenous administration if undesirable cardiac or pulmonary symptoms develop.

## ISOFLUROPHATE (DIISOPROPYL FLUOROPHOSPHATE [DFP], FLOROPRYL)

Isoflurophate was useful in the management of chronic simple glaucoma that was uncontrolled by the shorter-acting miotics and in the management of accommodative esotropia. Its use has been replaced by echothiophate, however, because it produces more intense ciliary spasm.

### Pharmacology

#### *Mechanism of Action*

The parasympathomimetic effect of isoflurophate is caused by cholinesterase inactivation. Isoflurophate has no direct effect on the iris muscle itself and causes no miosis in an experimentally denervated iris.

#### *Duration of Action*

Isoflurophate-induced miosis has rapid onset and prolonged duration.[81] In normal human eyes, miosis begins within 5 to 10 minutes and is maximal within 15 to 20 minutes. The duration of miosis is from 2 to 4 weeks. Solutions of a 0.05% concentration produce maximum miosis, whereas solutions of less than 0.01% are ineffective miotics. Isoflurophate reduces the IOP of the normal eye; the maximal reduction is achieved within 24 hours. The return of normal IOP requires about 1 week. Isoflurophate-induced myopia is maximal in 1 hour and lasts for 3 to 7 days. The pain accompanying the ciliary spasm is worse with close work because of the greater production of acetylcholine during accommodation.

The duration of action of isoflurophate may be measured by analyzing the cholinesterase activity of rabbit irises and ciliary bodies after the single instillation of 1 drop of a 0.2% solution of isoflurophate.[82] Within the first half hour, the cholinesterase activity drops to less than 15% of normal (Fig. 3–31).

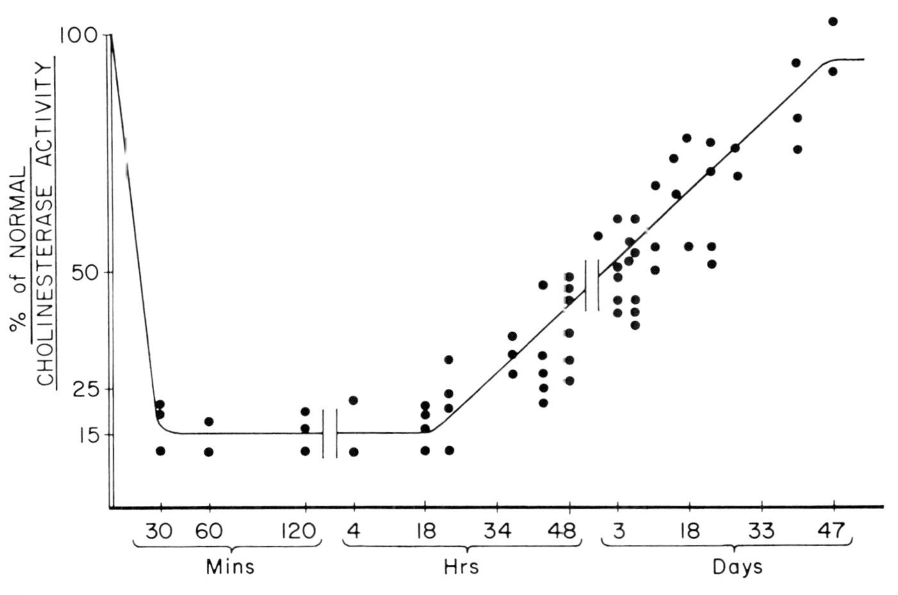


**FIG 3–31.**
Recovery of cholinesterase activity of iris and ciliary body of rabbit after instillation of 1 drop of a 0.2% solution of isoflurophate (DFP). (Modified from de Roetth Jr A: *Am J Ophthalmol* 34:120, 1951. Used by permission.)

Activity remains at this level for 18 hours and then gradually rises. Fifty percent of normal activity returns within the first week, but full recovery takes up to 2 months. The miotic effect of isoflurophate is maximal for 18 hours in rabbits and is gone in 48 hours.

### *Effect on Blood-Aqueous Barrier*

Topical ocular application of anticholinesterase drugs causes a breakdown of the blood-aqueous barrier, permitting protein and cells to enter the aqueous humor. The protein concentration in normal aqueous humor is about 50 mg/100 ml. Isoflurophate increases the protein concentration to as high as 1,200 mg/100 ml.[83] Physostigmine causes a much lower increase in aqueous protein (maximum 120 mg/100 ml) than do the organic phosphates. The increased levels of protein in primary aqueous humor persist for at least 2 weeks after isoflurophate therapy is stopped. There is considerable individual variation in the response of the blood-aqueous barrier to anticholinesterase drugs. (Aqueous protein values after isoflurophate may vary from 35 to 2,253 mg/100 ml.)

### *Systemic Absorption*

The systemic absorption of anticholinesterase drugs applied topically to the eye is rapid and of surprising magnitude. Systemic anticholinesterase activity is detectable within a few minutes of ocular instillation and approaches the levels produced by intravenous administration. The amount of cholinesterase inhibition resulting from ocular instillation of a single drop of a 10% concentration of Dipterex in rabbits is shown in Fig. 3–32.[84] (Dipterex is an anticholinesterase insecticide about 100 times less toxic than isoflurophate.) This single drop reduced cholinesterase levels of the ciliary body to 26% of normal, RBC levels to 38%, brain levels to 48%, and serum levels to 58%. The therapeutic use of related medications (e.g., isoflurophate) causes a similar marked drop of systemic cholinesterase.

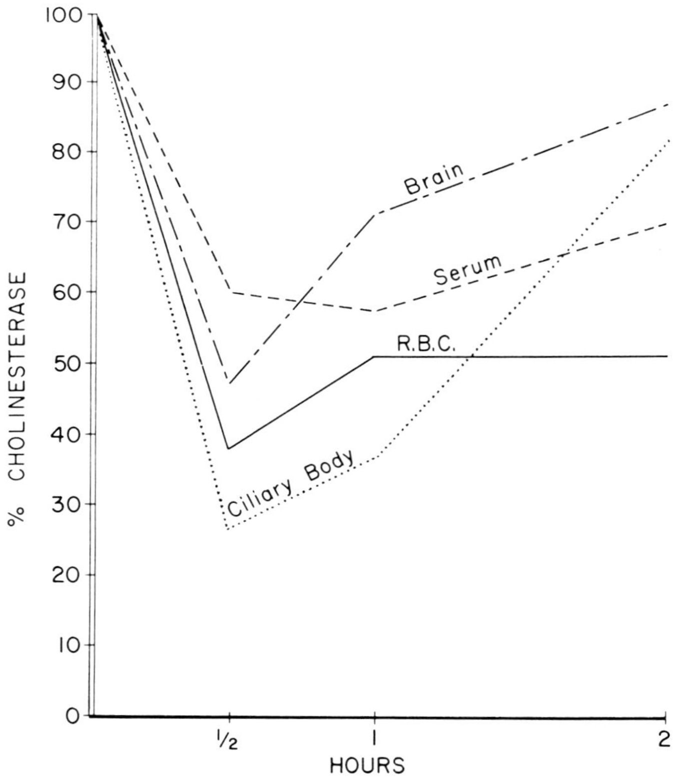


**FIG 3–32.**
Percent of normal cholinesterase activity remaining in various tissues after ocular instillation in rabbits of 1 drop of a 10% solution of Dipterex. (From Kadin M: *Am J Ophthalmol* 53:512, 1962. Used by permission.)

Fortunately, the physiologic margin of safety in this enzyme is so great that toxic symptoms do not occur until more than half of the systemic cholinesterase activity has been inhibited. (The dose of Dipterex lethal to 50% of rabbits is 60 mg/kg and is approximately 1,000 times greater than that contained in 1 drop of a 10% solution.)

Similar reductions of erythrocyte cholinesterase levels have been demonstrated in glaucomatous patients receiving topical therapy with the irreversible cholinesterase inhibitors.[85] The greatest systemic effect resulted from demecarium and the smallest from isoflurophate. The effect of echothiophate was intermediate.

### Stability

Aqueous solutions of isoflurophate deteriorate rapidly, having no effect within 1 week. In contrast, a solution in peanut oil will maintain maximum potency for more than 3 months. Contamination of the bottle with water (e.g., from tears or washing the dropper) rapidly inactivates the isoflurophate. This possibility should be considered when previously well-controlled glaucoma suddenly fails to respond to isoflurophate. An ointment containing a 0.025% concentration of isoflurophate is more stable and less irritating than the drops.

### Clinical Use

#### *Glaucoma*

Tonography indicates that isoflurophate increases aqueous outflow facility in both glaucomatous and normal human eyes, thereby reducing IOP.[86] A single daily instillation of a 0.1% solution of isoflurophate is suggested as the average starting dosage but should be adjusted as necessary to control individual cases of glaucoma. Bedtime use is recommended to minimize the severity of accommodative spasm. Instillation more than twice daily does not usually provide additional glaucoma control, may be toxic, and should rarely be prescribed.

#### *Accommodative Esotropia*

The accommodative component of esotropia may be identified by the use of isoflurophate.[87] The nightly use for 2 weeks of a 0.025% solution (commercial strength solution diluted with anhydrous peanut oil) or ointment will eliminate the accommodative part of the deviation. A diagnostic trial of isoflurophate should be considered even for patients without a significant refractive error, because an occasional emmetropic patient is benefitted, presumably because of a change in the AC:A ratio.

In the treatment of accommodative esotropia with isoflurophate, the smallest effective amount should be used. Dosage is reduced by giving the medication less frequently rather than by decreasing the concentration. (In lower concentrations, isoflurophate becomes so unstable as to be clinically unreliable.) A dosage frequency of every other night, every third night, or even less often may maintain alignment of the eyes.

Thirty-three of a series of 145 patients with esotropia were satisfactorily controlled by isoflurophate.[87] Eight other patients benefitted by the use of this medication after surgery.

Iris cysts, the main complication of isoflurophate therapy in children, may be avoided by reducing the frequency of dosage or by the concomitant use of a 10% solution of phenylephrine.

### Complications

#### *Discomfort*

Ciliary spasm is the most common and annoying side effect encountered in the use of all miotics. The indirect-acting miotics (and particularly the irreversible ones) produce a more severe ciliary spasm than does pilocarpine. Younger persons are more severely affected by this ciliary spasm and may be totally disabled for several days by a single drop of a 0.1% solution of isoflurophate. The conjunctiva of the treated eye typically appears inflamed. Discomfort may occur from ciliary spasm, and vision may be affected by induced myopia. Fortunately, the older glaucoma patient is less likely to experience such severe side effects. Aphakic patients often have no such complaints at all. Use of lower concentrations of miotic and instillation at bedtime will minimize discomfort. With prolonged usage, the glaucomatous patient develops a tolerance to these initially troublesome side effects.

### *Iris Cysts*

Although miotic cysts of the pupillary pigment margin may occur in adults, they are much more frequent in children. Isoflurophate and echothiophate are more likely to cause these cysts than are the weaker miotics. Less frequent miotic use greatly reduces the incidence of cysts. Because cysts are particularly likely to develop in children, it is suggested that isoflurophate be instilled every other night or even less frequently for treatment of accommodative strabismus.

Apparently prolonged and intense miosis is required to produce these cysts. The daily use of isoflurophate caused 42 of 66 children (average age 7 years) to have such cysts develop during an average of 10 weeks. In all patients the cysts disappeared when isoflurophate therapy was stopped, although they persisted for more than 2½ months in eight eyes. The cysts re-formed rapidly if isoflurophate was again used.[88] Occurrence of isoflurophate cysts during treatment of accommodative esotropia may be minimized by the simultaneous use of phenylephrine.[89]

### *Systemic Poisoning*

Generalized parasympathomimetic toxicity is much more likely to complicate the use of echothiophate and demecarium than treatment with isoflurophate and is discussed in the consideration of these drugs.

### *Retinal Detachment*

As previously noted, retinal detachments have been associated with the use of miotics.

### *Cataract*

A particularly serious consequence of the use of strong anticholinesterase drugs such as isoflurophate is the development of cataract. A detailed description of such cataract formation is presented in the section on echothiophate.

## Toxicity

Isoflurophate is a derivative of a class of chemicals used as insecticides and war gases. These drugs are extremely poisonous. The contents of a bottle of eye drops could easily kill a child.

Manifestations of cholinergic poisoning such as diarrhea, epigastric cramps, nausea and vomiting, cold sweats, and salivation are rarely observed under conditions of clinical usage. Although such symptoms may be reduced in severity by the administration of atropine, they indicate serious systemic depletion of cholinesterase and dictate a reduced frequency of medication or complete discontinuance. The specific cause of these symptoms may be confirmed by laboratory testing of the patient's cholinesterase levels. A fairly simple test strip method for determining plasma cholinesterase activity has been devised.[90] This method is suitable for use in glaucomatous patients suspected of having anticholinesterase poisoning.

A specific antidote exists for poisoning by cholinesterase inhibitors (Fig. 3–33).[91] Pyridine-2-aldoxime methyl iodide ($P_2AM$) promptly separates the bound cholinesterase from physostigmine and neostigmine (Prostigmin) and also from the irreversible inhibitors isoflurophate and echothiophate. It is a relatively nontoxic compound. By itself, $P_2AM$ produces no effect on the pupil or on the outflow facility. Topical ocular application is relatively ineffective, but subconjunctival injection of 0.2 ml of a 4% solution of $P_2AM$ will neutralize echothiophate or isoflurophate miosis within 1 hour.[86] Systemic anticholinesterase poisoning is also effectively counteracted by $P_2AM$. Either topical or systemic use of atropine is a quite effective antidote to poisoning by the strong miotics. However, atropine action is purely symptomatic, whereas $P_2AM$ is a specific chemical antidote against phosphoryl inactivation of cholinesterase.[92] It is believed that hydrolysis of acetylcholine results in an intermediate formation of an acetylcholinesterase molecule that is highly unstable and breaks down rapidly, thereby freeing the cholinesterase for further enzymatic action. Phosphate inhibitors such as isoflurophate bind the enzyme in a stable phosphoryl-cholinesterase com-

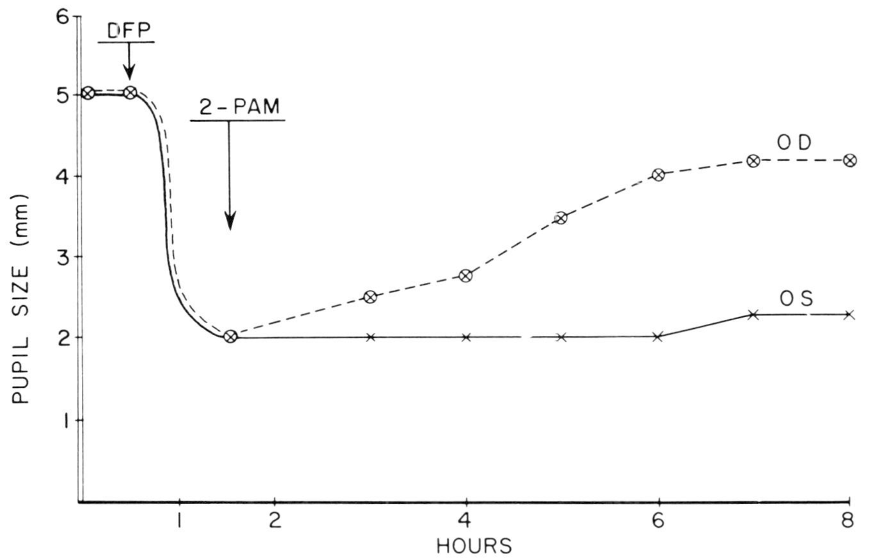


**FIG 3–33.**
Response of rabbit pupil to a 0.1% solution of isoflurophate (DFP) in both eyes and to $P_2AM$, 1% solution, every 10 minutes six times in the right eye. (Modified from Mamo JG, Leopold IH: *Am J Ophthalmol* 46:724, 1958. Used by permission.)

pound. Within minutes $P_2AM$ will reactivate phosphoryl-inhibited cholinesterase. Given in doses of 75 mg/kg of body weight, $P_2AM$ will protect all animals against an $LD_{100}$ dose of cholinesterase inhibitor. The minimal lethal dose of $P_2AM$ is 100 mg/kg.

## ECHOTHIOPHATE (PHOSPHOLINE)

Echothiophate iodide is a relatively irreversible cholinesterase inhibitor. Its clinical characteristics and the indications for its use are similar to those of isoflurophate.

Echothiophate is indefinitely stable when dry; however, it must be kept in tightly sealed containers because the powdered form is hygroscopic. Assay of refrigerated aqueous solutions of echothiophate shows a drop to 90% of the original potency within 4 weeks. At room temperature this drop is to 83% of the original potency within 4 weeks and to 76% in 8 weeks.[93] Solutions should probably be discarded after 2 months at room temperature.

Echothiophate is destroyed by autoclaving. Benzalkonium is incompatible with iodides and may not be used as a preservative. A 0.5% solution of chlorobutanol is a satisfactory and compatible preservative.

Echothiophate is marketed as a powder and accompanied by a diluent sufficient to prepare a 0.125% solution (the strength most commonly employed for treatment of chronic simple glaucoma and accommodative esotropia). In many instances a 0.06% solution gives satisfactory therapeutic results and causes less irritation. Pure echothiophate powder *should not* under any circumstances be applied directly to a patient's eye. Transconjunctival absorption is rapid, and serious systemic poisoning will result.

### Ocular Penetration

The entry of the organophosphorus anticholinesterase agents into rabbit eyes was studied by histochemical demonstration of cholinesterase inhibition by echothiophate.[94] Within 2 hours after the topical application of 2 drops of 0.06% echothiophate, profound inhibition of cholinesterase staining was observed over almost the entire anterior segment of the eye. Cholinesterase activity was abolished in the cornea and conjunctiva, greatly reduced throughout the iris, abolished in the subcapsular lens epithelium in the region of the pupil, and reduced in the lens equator.

Cholinesterase inhibition of the ciliary body appeared to penetrate through the sclera, being most marked near the sclera.

### Pharmacology

Two types of cholinesterase exist. The true cholinesterase, acetylcholinesterase, is extracellular, comprises only 10% to 20% of the total tissue cholinesterase activity, and is the enzyme pool involved in regulating responses to cholinergic drugs. The pseudocholinesterase or nonspecific cholinesterase butyrylcholinesterase is intracellular, comprises 80% to 90% of total tissue cholinesterase activity, and has no pharmacologic role in the cholinergic responses to the various cholinesterase inhibitors. Human eyes contain true cholinesterase, whereas pseudocholinesterase is found in human serum.[95]

True acetylcholinesterase inhibition can be achieved by echothiophate in concentrations as weak as $10^{-8}$ M, whereas no detectable inhibition results from isoflurophate at concentrations less than $10^{-6}$ M. It should be noted that 100% of enzyme inhibition is not produced by echothiophate concentrations as strong as $10^{-3}$M. True cholinesterase inhibition by such concentrations of echothiophate may be reversed within 15 minutes by $10^{-3}$M pralidoxime. Pralidoxime has poor lipid solubility, does not penetrate all membranes, and does not reactivate the inhibited intracellular pseudocholinesterase.

It is a prevalent misconception that there are strong and weak miotics. A response of maximum contractile strength can be obtained from an iris sphincter strip with a cholinergic drug, providing a sufficiently high dose is used. Echothiophate is not a "stronger" miotic and does not, in fact, cause any contraction of the iris sphincter at all. However, by inhibition of cholinesterase, echothiophate renders the affected muscle sensitive to lower concentrations of cholinergic drugs. Another concept of strength may be related to duration. The clinical effect of echothiophate is, indeed, of long duration.[96]

Dose-response analysis of echothiophate with respect to IOP and outflow facility indicates that little additional pharmacologic response is obtained by increasing the drug concentration to more than 0.06% (Fig. 3–34).[97] A 0.03% concentration of echothiophate iodide has been shown to have similar effect of 1% to 2% pilocarpine, and 0.06% echothiophate has a potency similar to 4% pilocarpine.[98, 99] Echothiophate has a duration of action signifi-

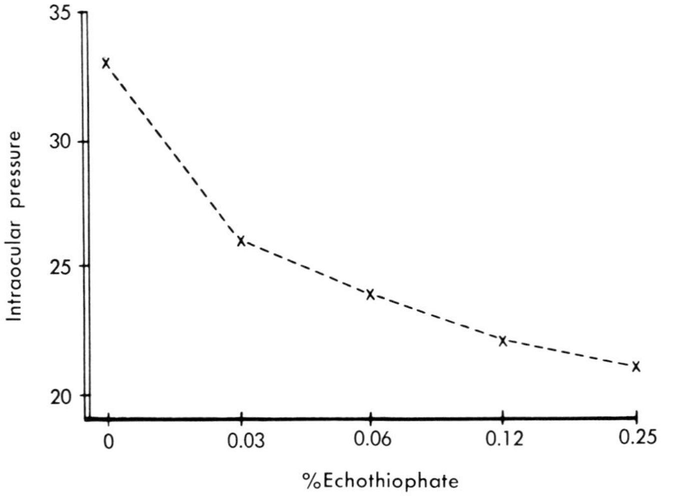


**FIG 3–34.**
Mean IOP in 15 patients with open-angle glaucoma treated with the specified concentrations of echothiophate. (From Harris LS: *Arch Ophthalmol* 86:502, 1971. Used by permission.)

cantly longer than pilocarpine, with a maximal effect in 4 to 6 hours and a substantial effect maintained after 24 hours.

Marked pilocarpine subsensitivity results from topical echothiophate treatment. In untreated monkey eyes, maximum accommodation is produced by 0.5 mg of topical pilocarpine (1 drop of 1%). After several weeks of topical echothiophate treatment, monkey eyes are subsensitive to pilocarpine, being almost nonresponsive to 25 mg of topical pilocarpine (50 times the supramaximal dose in untreated eyes.)[100]

## Clinical Use

### *Open-angle Glaucoma*

Echothiophate lowers IOP by increasing the facility of outflow.[101] An average improvement in outflow facility of 127% was achieved in 28 glaucomatous eyes with a 0.25% or 0.1% solution of echothiophate.

The effect of a 4% solution of pilocarpine given four times daily compared with that of a 0.06% solution of echothiophate iodide given twice daily was studied in 20 glaucomatous eyes in 13 patients.[102]

The clinically used concentrations of echothiophate and of pilocarpine individually maximally saturate the available acetylcholine receptors. No additional effect can be theoretically expected from simultaneous use of both drugs, nor can such enhanced effect be demonstrated in clinical usage for glaucoma management.

Prescription of both echothiophate and pilocarpine together for a glaucoma patient is irrational and can result only in greater toxicity.[103]

### *Accommodative Esotropia*

A 0.1% solution of echothiophate gives results comparable with those of a 0.025% concentration of isoflurophate in the treatment of accommodative esotropia.[104]

A weaker concentration (0.06%) of echothiophate was found to be of benefit in 23 of 32 cases of accommodative esotropia.[105] Medication was required nightly or every other night. Iris cysts developed in only three patients, in contrast to the much higher incidence when stronger concentrations of miotics are used.

## Complications

### *Systemic Toxicity*

The use of long-acting anticholinesterase drugs for the treatment of glaucoma may result in systemic toxicity. The incidence of such toxicity is particularly high with echothiophate iodide. Of 24 patients taking echothiophate, nine had systemic symptoms.[106] Frequency of dosage is an important factor in toxicity. All nine patients with symptoms were using 4 drops/day, whereas the asymptomatic patients were receiving medication less frequently.

The systemic toxic effects caused by echothiophate drops include diarrhea, nausea, abdominal cramps, and general fatigue and weakness. One patient required hospitalization for evaluation of severe, persistent diarrhea of undetermined cause. Respiratory symptoms simulating pulmonary infection may be caused by anticholinesterase poisoning but are more characteristic of the inhalation route of absorption (e.g., by persons using insecticide sprays). Anticholinesterase toxic symptoms may simulate an acute gastrointestinal upset or an upper respiratory tract infection.

If such symptoms appear in a patient receiving echothiophate therapy, determination of the cholinesterase values in RBCs may indicate whether the symptoms can be attributed to this drug. The normal range of cholinesterase in RBCs is between 0.6 and 1.1 units. Values less than 0.4 are usually associated with moderately severe exposure to anticholinesterase chemicals. The nine symptomatic patients using 4 drops of echothiophate/day had an average cholinesterase value of 0.26 in their RBCs.

Low cholinesterase values were also found in 12 asymptomatic patients using 2 drops of echothiophate/day. Their average value was 0.38, but some individual values were much lower. A cholinesterase value of 0.68 was found in two patients receiving only 1 drop of echothiophate/day. Apparently low cholinesterase values do not necessarily mean that the symptoms are drug induced, whereas normal values do rule out drug toxicity.

Plasma and RBC cholinesterase levels were measured in glaucoma patients after the use of 1 drop of echothiophate in both

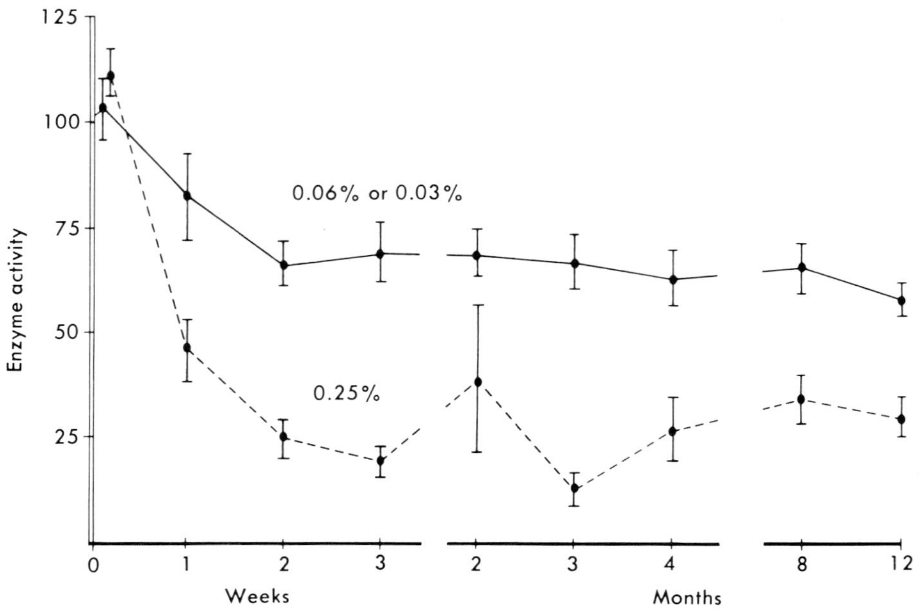


**FIG 3–35.**
Plasma cholinesterase activity measured after use of echothiophate in both eyes two times daily for specified times and drug concentrations. (Modified from de Roetth Jr A, and others: *Am J Ophthalmol* 62:834, 1966. Used by permission.)

eyes twice daily. Within 1 month, 75% to 80% inhibition of the enzyme resulted from the use of 0.25% echothiophate. From 35% to 40% inhibition resulted from the use of 0.06% to 0.03% concentrations (Fig. 3–35).[107]

Although adverse local symptoms may be decreased by the use of 0.0625% echothiophate iodide (instead of 0.25%), RBC cholinesterase values were less than normal in all patients receiving 0.0625% drops once daily for longer than 2½ months, and more than half of these patients had systemic side effects (gastrointestinal disorders, sweating, salivation, nasal congestion, and weakness).[108] The same precautions against systemic toxicity are necessary with either concentration of this potent drug.[109]

Because long-acting anticholinesterase drugs may reduce RBC cholinesterase for as long as 4 months, treatment with a specific antidote may be desirable in patients with severe toxicity. A total of 25 mg of $P_2AM$/kg may be given intravenously in 500 ml of a 5% solution of dextrose and water over a 2-hour period. Both the systemic toxicity and the ocular therapeutic effect are neutralized by $P_2AM$.

Because plasma cholinesterase hydrolyses succinylcholine and procaine, patients with low blood cholinesterase levels resulting from anticholinesterase therapy for glaucoma are more susceptible to the toxic effects of these depolarizing muscle relaxants. Death has been reported from the use of succinylcholine during anesthesia in a patient with low blood cholinesterase levels.[110] It is wise to inform both the patient and the patient's general physician about this important drug interaction.

### *Cornea*

In excessive dosage, echothiophate is toxic to the cornea. In two patients receiving 0.25% echothiophate four times daily, pain, corneal bedewing, and fine endothelial deposits developed. These abnormalities disappeared when the dosage was reduced.[111]

### *Iritis*

Three patients are reported to have had severe fibrinous iritis develop after several days of echothiophate therapy.[112] This iritis was prolonged, despite use of mydriatics, corticosteroids, and $P_2AM$ and the cessation of echothiophate and resulted in formation of posterior synechiae.

***Iris Cysts***

Iris cysts may result from the excessive use of either echothiophate or isoflurophate. Similarly, either drug in a smaller dosage can control accommodative esotropia without extensive cyst formation, especially when phenylephrine is used simultaneously. Use of a 2.5% to 10% solution of phenylephrine in combination with echothiophate in treatment of accommodative esotropia will prevent the formation of miotic cysts and will not impair the therapeutic effect.

A combination of 0.125% echothiophate solution and 2.5% phenylephrine solution was used in 22 patients with esotropia for varying periods (average 3.25 months). In most patients, instillation was nightly, but some patients required treatment twice daily. Iris cysts occurred in only four of these 44 eyes. Fourteen of the 22 patients benefitted from miotic treatment.[113]

***Cataract***

The most serious ocular complication of echothiophate therapy appears to be cataract formation.

Evidence that clinical use of the strong anticholinesterase agents (echothiophate, isoflurophate, and demecarium) causes cataract seems conclusive.[114–116] The typical anticholinesterase cataract begins in the form of anterior subcapsular vacuoles, which are characteristic but not pathognomonic (Fig. 3–36).[112] Typical anterior subcapsular vacuoles were found in 51% of anticholinesterase-treated eyes, in 16% of pilocarpine-treated eyes, and in 15% of the cataracts in nonglaucomatous eyes. The prevalence of cataract formation is greater with treatment of longer duration, with use of higher drug concentration, with greater frequency of dosage, and in older eyes, especially those with preexisting early cataractous changes. Once established, the cataract can progress even if the drug is discontinued. In one prospective study, 35 previously untreated patients with ocular hypertension were given various concentrations of echothiophate in one eye twice daily for 3 years. The fellow eyes served as untreated controls. In another group of patients, one eye was treated with 4% pilocarpine four times daily for 3 years.[117] Half of the patients receiving 0.25%, 0.125%, or 0.06% echothiophate showed progressive visual deterioration in the treated eyes. This visual loss was attributed to anterior and posterior subcapsular opacities. No such vision loss occurred in the eyes treated with

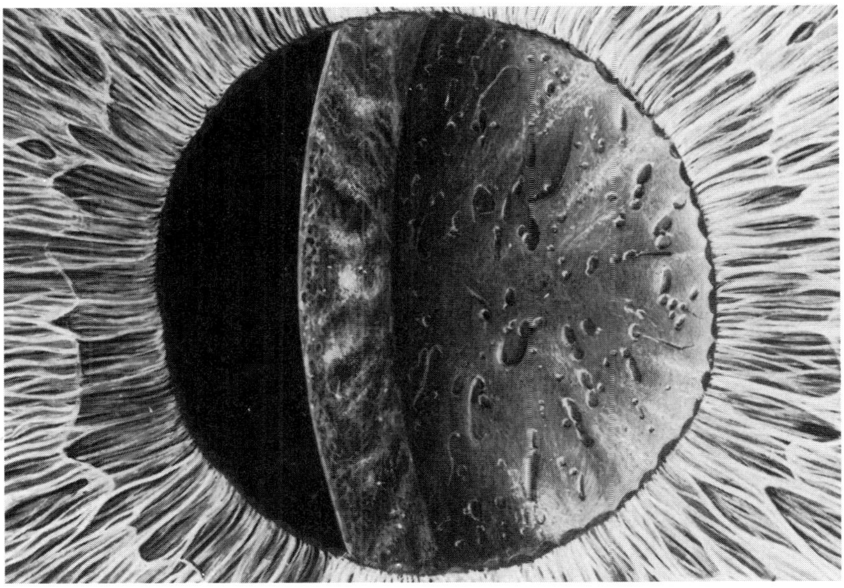

**FIG 3–36.**
Anterior subcapsular vacuoles characteristic of anticholinesterase cataract. (From Shaffer RN, Hetherington JM: *Am J Ophthalmol* 62:613, 1966. Used by permission.)

0.03% echothiophate or 4% pilocarpine. In two patients the visual loss gradually improved during the 6-month period after discontinuance of echothiophate therapy.

In another prospective study group of 10 patients using 0.25% echothiophate twice daily, five had early posterior subcapsular cataracts develop after 4 months of therapy.[118] In the same study, no lens opacities were found in children treated for accommodative esotropia with echothiophate (dose unspecified) for as long as 6 years.

Reversible miotic-induced cataract has been described in two patients. A 13-year-old patient with esotropia developed an anterior subcapsular cataract after 3 months of daily instillation of 0.025% isoflurophate. In another reported case, a 59-year-old glaucoma patient who had used isoflurophate daily for several weeks developed cataracts that disappeared 3 weeks after the miotic therapy was discontinued.[119]

#### Experimental Anticholinesterase Cataract

Intracarotid injection of near-lethal doses of isoflurophate in guinea pigs causes rapidly developing and often irreversible cataracts.[120]

If a relationship exists between the use of anticholinesterase agents and cataract, one would expect to find cholinesterase activity in the lens. Analysis reveals that the lens capsule does have a true cholinesterase activity comparable in amount with that of the iris.[121] Cholinesterase enzymatic activity is demonstrable in the lens epithelium by histochemical and biochemical methods.[116] The complete elimination of this cholinesterase activity by topical instillation of anticholinesterase drugs (e.g., echothiophate) in clinical dosage has been demonstrated in humans and animals. In vitro incubation of the calf and rabbit lens in $10^{-3}$ M concentrations of echothiophate will cause cataract.[115]

Under experimental in vitro conditions, demecarium bromide ($10^{-4}$M) and echothiophate iodide ($10^{-3}$ M) cause a marked increase in lens permeability to positive cations.[122] Similar alterations of lens permeability occur with ionizing irradiation and corticosteroid treatment, which also may cause subcapsular lens vacuoles. Additional studies confirm this in vitro cataractogenesis, which is related to the concentration of anticholinesterase drug in the culture medium.[123] The mechanism of cataract formation is not established and could be mechanical (although ciliary muscle disinsertion from the scleral spur does not prevent it), cholinergic (although not caused by carbachol),[124] or a direct toxic effect of echothiophate.

#### Implications of Anticholinesterase Cataractogenesis

The strong anticholinesterase drugs should not be used in the management of glaucoma in phakic patients.

#### Retinal Detachment

As previously noted, retinal detachments have been associated with the use of miotics.

## DEMECARIUM (HUMORSOL)

Demecarium bromide is an extremely potent long-acting cholinesterase inhibitor synthesized by connecting two neostigmine molecules with a carbon chain. It is water soluble and indefinitely stable in solution. Demecarium is the most toxic of the clinically available anticholinesterase drugs.

### Pharmacology

Pharmacologically, demecarium bromide differs from isoflurophate in that it inactivates both true cholinesterase (found in erythrocytes) and pseudocholinesterase (found in plasma).[125] (Isoflurophate inactivates primarily pseudocholinesterase. Physostigmine inhibits both true cholinesterase and pseudocholinesterase.)

Within 45 to 60 minutes, a single instillation of demecarium in human eyes produces miosis that becomes maximal within 2 to 4 hours. Miosis persists for 3 to 10 days. Rarely, slight miosis may persist for as long as 3 or 4 weeks. The rapidity of onset and duration of miosis are directly related to the

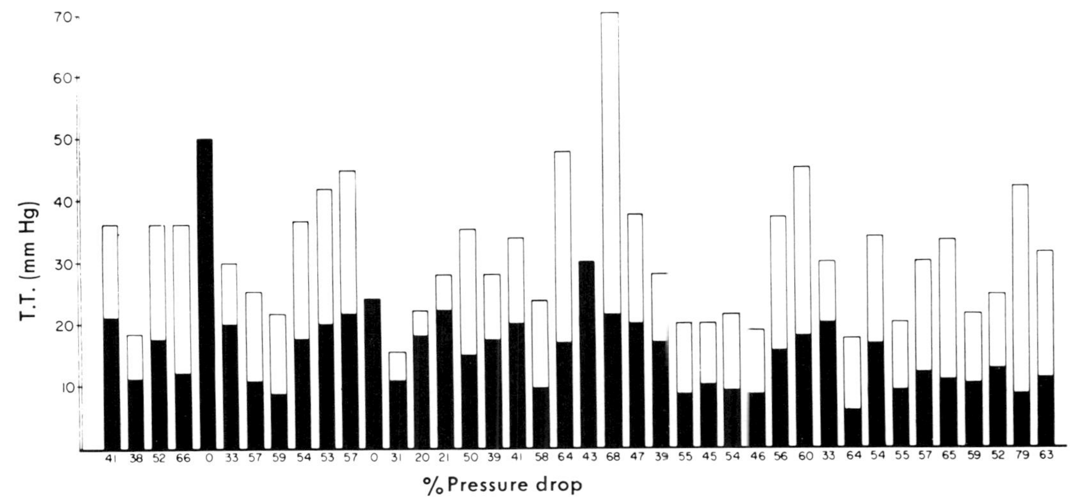


**FIG 3–37.**
Drop in IOP after demecarium treatment. *Solid black bars:* pressures after treatment. (Modified from Drance SM: *Arch Ophthalmol* 62:673, 1959. Used by permission.)

concentration used (0.1% or 0.25%). Reduction of IOP by 3 to 11 mm Hg occurs in normal eyes, is first recorded in about 30 minutes, is maximal at 24 hours, and persists for 9 days or more after a single instillation. This pressure lowering is achieved by increasing the facility of outflow.[126]

### Toxic Effects

After instillation of demecarium in normal eyes, the unpleasant side effects of ciliary spasm are uniformly encountered. These include browache and blurred vision caused by the induced myopia of accommodative spasm. Superficial and deep vascular congestion lasting 1 to 3 days affects almost all eyes. These local side effects rarely persist beyond the first week.

Histologic sections of rabbit eyes after demecarium treatment showed vascular congestion not only in the conjunctiva but also in the iris and ciliary body. Apparently because of this vascular congestion, several human eyes showed transient rises of IOP during the first hour. Permeability of the blood-aqueous barrier is increased. Two of eight patients were nauseated by 2 drops of a 0.5% solution of demecarium instilled on the eyes.

Systemic side effects include nausea, vomiting, diarrhea, salivation, sweating, and bradycardia. Systemic parasympatholytic medication (e.g., atropine) may provide prompt relief. To minimize toxicity, the patient should be instructed to instill only 1 drop (not multiple drops, as some patients are prone to do) and not to use the medication more frequently than advised.

### Clinical Use

#### *Glaucoma*

Use of demecarium in 40 eyes with chronic open-angle glaucoma, uncontrolled by other unspecified miotics, caused a satisfactory pressure reduction in 38 eyes (Fig. 3–37).[127] The average pressure reduction in these eyes was 48%. An average time of 34 hours was required for the maximal fall of IOP to occur. The average increase in facility of outflow was 121%.

## ANTICHOLINESTERASE ANTIDOTES

### Pralidoxime (Protopam)

The oximes are of ophthalmologic interest because of their ability to neutralize anticholinesterase activity. The action of isoflurophate, echothiophate, demecarium, and physostigmine may be reversed by pralidoxime.[128]

***Pharmacology***

**Mechanism of Action.**—Physiologically, acetylcholine and its specific enzyme cholinesterase form a bond that lasts for only a few microseconds. This evanescent compound then hydrolyses into free intact cholinesterase and broken remnants of the acetylcholine molecule. When cholinesterase inhibitors such as organic phosphates (e.g., isoflurophate) react with cholinesterase, a nonhydrolyzable phosphorylated enzyme results. This molecular combination does not destroy the cholinesterase structure but effectively inhibits its enzymatic function.

The effect of the organic phosphates can be reversed by $P_2AM$. The oximes act by separating the phosphoryl group from the enzymes, releasing the cholinesterase molecule intact. Within 1 minute, $P_2AM$ in a $10^{-5}M$ concentration may reactivate 80% of phosphate-inhibited cholinesterase.[129] If isoflurophate is chosen as the enzyme inhibitor, its reversibility slowly decreases with time because of the gradual formation of a more stable chemical bond. This phenomenon of gradually developing resistance to the antidotal effect of oximes is particularly characteristic of the anticholinesterase war gases and is known as "aging" of the chemical bond between the war gas and its receptors.

Pralidoxime does not have a parasympatholytic effect, and its mechanism of action is not like that of atropine. Atropinization of a pupil that is miotic because of use of isoflurophate results in a dilated and nonreactive pupil. Intravenous injection of pralidoxime abolishes the miosis, leaving a pupil of normal size and with intact light reaction.

As would be expected, pralidoxime inactivation of echothiophate nullifies the therapeutic effect of the miotic on the facility of aqueous outflow.[86]

**Administration.**—Because topical ocular instillation of oxime solutions is ineffective, subconjunctival injection is advocated. The dose is 0.1 to 0.2 ml of a 5% aqueous solution of pralidoxime. This is an effective antidote to the otherwise prolonged ocular effects of isoflurophate or echothiophate.

Actually, the failure of topical pralidoxime to neutralize the action of cholinesterase inhibitors on the iris sphincter is a result of inadequate transcorneal penetration. Preparation of the drug in a 1:10,000 concentration of benzalkonium enhances penetration, making its topical administration clinically effective (Fig. 3–38).[130] The neutralizing action against isoflurophate is greatest when the oxime is used within 30 minutes after miotic instil-

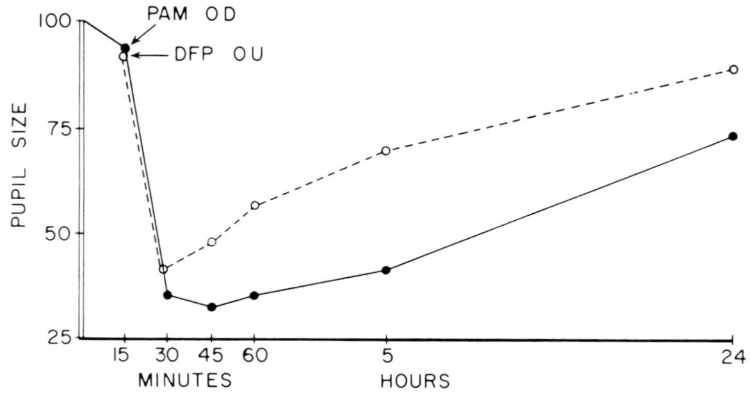


**FIG 3–38.**
Pupil size (expressed as percent of initial size) after bilateral instillation of isoflurophate (DFP) in rabbit eyes. Five percent pyridine-2-aldoxime in a 1:10,000 solution of benzalkonium was instilled in the right eye only. The oxime effect occurs when it is used within 30 minutes before isoflurophate instillation or anytime subsequent to isoflurophate. (Modified from Hunter WS, McCulloch C: *Am J Ophthalmol* 52:841, 1961. Used by permission.)

lation but is demonstrable after a longer period. The neutralizing action of oximes does not wear off and does not permit recurrent miosis from the original instillation of isoflurophate.[131]

### *Stability*

As a dry powder, pralidoxime is indefinitely stable at room temperature if the room is kept dark. Aqueous solutions remain effective for 2 weeks at room temperature and for several months under refrigeration.

### *Clinical Use*

Pralidoxime may be used to reverse the ocular effects of cholinesterase inhibitors and as an antidote to systemic poisoning by these parasympathetic agents.

**Neutralization of Ocular Anticholinesterase Effects.**—The prolonged discomfort resulting from accidental instillation of isoflurophate, echothiophate, and demecarium may be promptly relieved by pralidoxime. Ophthalmoscopic examination of the glaucomatous patient is desirable at periodic intervals or when symptoms referable to the posterior segment of the eye develop. Such fundus examination is aided by miotic neutralization.

Although parasympatholytic drugs such as atropine will also relieve ciliary spasm and mydriasis, these drugs have the disadvantage of causing prolonged cycloplegia and impairing facility of outflow.

**As Antidote for Systemic Anticholinesterase Poisoning.**—Because accidental swallowing of eye drops (e.g., by children) could easily be lethal, a brief outline of treatment is in order.[66, 132] Comparable therapy is appropriate for insecticide poisoning.

1. Gastric lavage will prevent further absorption of any chemical remaining in the stomach. Because percutaneous absorption occurs, contaminated skin should be washed with water.

2. In severe poisoning, artificial respiration and maintenance of an open airway are essential. Nasopharyngeal and bronchial secretions are increased by parasympathomimetic stimulation and may require removal by suction.

3. Atropine should be given intravenously in the dosage of 2 mg every 5 minutes until the symptoms of parasympathomimetic overdosage disappear and should be repeated whenever such symptoms recur. As much as 50 mg of atropine may be required the first day. Full dilatation of the pupils may be used as a criterion for achieving an optimum dose of atropine.

4. Pralidoxime chloride, 1,000 mg, should be given slowly intravenously, in not less than 2 to 5 minutes. An additional 500 mg may be given in 30 minutes if muscular weakness is not relieved. Pralidoxime is effective orally, but this route is usually not feasible because of vomiting. In the case of insecticide poisoning, pralidoxime *is not* an effective substitute for atropine.

5. If convulsions block respiration, intravenous administration of diazepam (Valium) may be even more effective than barbiturates and is recommended as the drug of choice. Diazepam is generally helpful for all the CNS symptoms of anticholinesterase poisoning.

6. Morphine, theophylline, and aminophylline should not be used; these drugs accentuate symptoms.

### *Toxicity*

Intravenous injection of as much as 1,800 mg of pralidoxime in normal human adults results in only minor and transient side effects such as dizziness, blurred vision and diplopia, headache, and nausea. These symptoms last for less than 45 minutes. Within 1 hour after intravenous injection, half of the pralidoxime has already been eliminated, mostly via the urine. Because these doses far exceed the amount used in ocular therapy, no systemic toxicity need be feared after local ophthalmologic use.

The minimal lethal dose of $P_2AM$ is about 100 mg/kg. The $LD_{50}$ dose is 137 mg/kg.[126]

No local toxicity results from subconjunctival injection of 0.2 ml of a 5% solution of pralidoxime chloride other than the expected mechanical trauma.

SECTION FIVE

# Anticholinergic Agents (Parasympatholytics)

MARY LOU KACHMER MCGREGOR

## ATROPINE

Atropine is useful in the management of iridocyclitis and in the refraction of children with accommodative esotropia.

### Pharmacology

#### *Mechanism of Action*

Atropine acts directly on the smooth muscles and secretory glands innervated by postganglionic cholinergic nerves. It blocks the response to acetylcholine and related parasympathomimetic drugs at these sites. This blockage is relative and can be overcome by use of pilocarpine, physostigmine, isoflurophate, and the like if these drugs are applied in sufficient concentration and frequency relative to the amount of atropine used.

The quantitative nature of atropinization is well illustrated by the response of a ciliary muscle, which was contracted by 1 μg of acetylcholine/ml, to different concentrations of atropine.[1] Contraction was not blocked by 0.01 to 0.1 μg of atropine/ml, was diminished by 1 μg/ml, was strongly reduced by 10 μg/ml, and was completely blocked by 100 μg/ml. Peculiarly, washing the atropine out of the muscle bath restored the responsiveness of the muscle to 1 μg of acetylcholine/ml. (Because of the clinically recognized long duration of atropine, one would have expected it to remain fixed to the muscle receptor.)

An alternate explanation of the duration of ocular atropinization could invoke the presence of a nearby atropine depot, as in iris melanin, from which a continuing supply of atropine is released to maintain cycloplegia.

#### *Mydriatic and Cycloplegic Action*

Atropine produces both mydriasis and cycloplegia. Additional mydriasis occurs if sympathomimetic drugs such as phenylephrine are used simultaneously. In clinical usage, such synergistic combinations are commonly prescribed to attain maximal dilatation of the pupil. Cycloplegia is not enhanced by the simultaneous use of sympathomimetic drugs, because they have insignificant cycloplegic action.

The response of individual eyes to cycloplegic drugs varies greatly. Within 30 to 40 minutes, atropine produces maximal mydriasis, which lasts for as long as 12 days. Atropine cycloplegia is attained within a few hours and may last 2 weeks or longer.[2] In comparison, maximal mydriasis from homatropine is attained in 10 to 30 minutes, with recovery in 6 hours to 4 days. Maximal homatropine cycloplegia (from a single instillation) is reached in 30 to 90 minutes, with recovery in 10 to 48 hours (Fig. 3–39).

#### *Other Responses*

The systemic administration of many drugs, including atropine, evokes multiple responses. For instance, atropine inhibits salivation, increases heart rate (by vagus block), and decreases accommodation. Because the rate at which these responses change (in relationship to increasing atropinization) is essentially the same for all systems,[3] this indicates a similar mechanism of action on all systems. However, the sensitivity of these different bodily functions to atropinization varies considerably. A 70% inhibition of salivation has already occurred at a dosage that reduces accommodation by only 10%. It is evident that a 0.5-mg dose of atropine used as preanesthetic medication will effectively reduce secretions and yet cause only minimal ocular response.

Tear secretion is substantially reduced by atropine. Oral doses of 1 and 2 mg will reduce tear secretion from 15 μl/min to 3 and 0.8 μl/min.[4] Because formation of tear protein and lysozyme is unchanged, this reduction in flow rate substantially increases the concentration of these tear constituents.

#### *Absorption and Excretion*

Atropine is readily absorbed transconjunctivally and is distributed throughout the body. It is hydrolyzed in the liver or excreted in the urine. In humans, 50% of an intra-

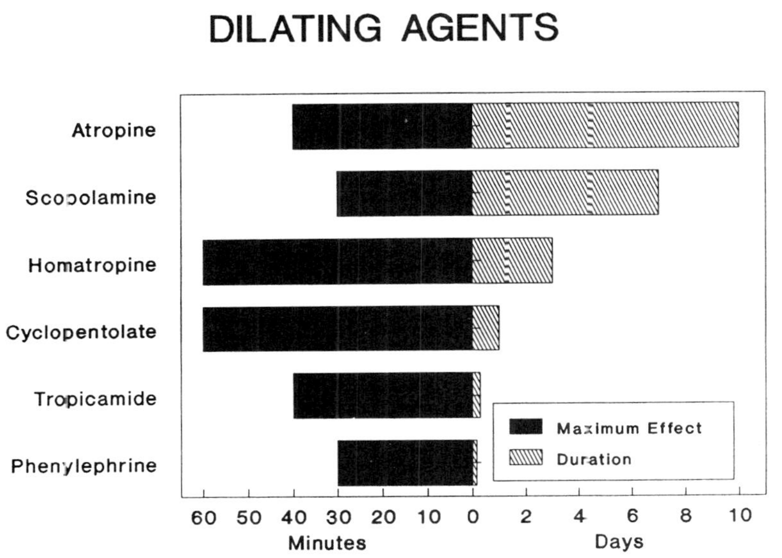


**FIG 3–39.**
Time to maximum effect and duration of common dilating agents.

muscular dose of atropine is excreted in the urine within 24 hours.[5]

### *Effect of Pigment*

When applied to a heavily pigmented eye, atropine exhibits an unusually slow onset of cycloplegic effect. Paradoxically, the same eye that responds only partially and slowly to atropine will then show a quite prolonged duration of cycloplegia. Specifically, the eyes of black patients will not dilate well, even with repeated doses of cycloplegic drugs; thereafter, they will complain of much longer-lasting inability to read and persistent dilatation of the pupils. The explanation for this is the binding effect of melanin on many types of drugs. (For example, miotics are bound just as are cycloplegics, as is phenothiazine, accounting for the well-known ocular toxic effects of this type of drug compound.) Initially the melanin binding of atropine slows attainment of a therapeutic drug level in the iris. Later the melanin-bound drug reservoir slowly releases atropine, resulting in the prolonged cycloplegia.

The hypothesis that the duration of effect of atropine is related to an atropine reservoir in pigment is attractive. However, if melanin binding is the mechanism of prolonged atropine effect, there should be a demonstrable difference in the duration of pigment binding of various cycloplegic drugs, such as atropine, cyclogyl, and tropicamide.

Apparently this stipulated difference in pigment binding of cycloplegic drugs does occur. The time required for washout recovery from half of the blockade against $10^{-5}$ mol carbachol by $2 \times 10^{-7}$ mol atropine is greater than 105 minutes for pigmented atropinesterase–positive rabbit irises. The time required for washout recovery from half the blockade against $10^{-5}$ mol carbachol by $3 \times 10^{-7}$ mol tropicamide is 30 minutes for pigmented rabbit irises.[6] In nonpigmented irises, tropicamide washout is extremely rapid, with full carbachol response restored in less than 15 minutes. In nonpigmented irises, atropine washout permits recovery from half the blockade in 54 minutes. These findings suggest that the shorter duration of tropicamide cycloplegia is related to the much greater ease with which it is washed out of both nonpigmented and pigmented irises in comparison with atropine.

Atropine uptake, washout, and parasympatholytic effect correlate well with pigmentation and can be measured accurately. Corresponding measurements with cyclopentolate and tropicamide are needed to confirm this melanin-binding hypothesis for the duration of atropine cycloplegia.

## Clinical Use

### *Iridocyclitis*

Atropine has long been one of the favorite drugs for the treatment of inflammation of the anterior segment of the eye. The mechanism of its anti-inflammatory effect probably includes the following actions.

Atropinization reduces the pain characteristic of iridocyclitis, presumably because of relaxation of the inflamed musculature of the ciliary body and iris. Quite dramatic relief of severe ocular pain characteristically accompanies the onset of cycloplegia in the treatment of acute iritis; however, this is not a local anesthetic effect and will relieve the pain of a corneal abrasion only to the extent that it is compounded by iritis.

Among the most serious complications of iridocyclitis are those associated with posterior synechiae: seclusion of the pupil with subsequent iris bombe and acute glaucoma, occlusion of the pupil with loss of sight, and cataract formation. If started early enough, atropinization will break these adhesions and decrease the possibility of serious complications resulting from synechiae. The peripheral lens is slightly farther back than the central portion, and the iris-lens contact is less intimate when the pupil is dilated. Furthermore, the greater circumference of a dilated pupil is less likely to be secluded, and its diameter is less likely to be occluded.

The eye with iridocyclitis is much more resistant to atropinization than is a normal eye. If posterior synechiae are present when the eye is first evaluated, an intensive effort should be made to break them while the patient is still in the office. This requires repeated instillation of atropine and phenylephrine or of similar drugs. If synechiae have been present for as long as 1 week, the iris may continue to break away from the lens for several days or more. During active inflammation, instillation of a 1% solution of atropine three times daily, supplemented by a 10% solution of phenylephrine three times daily, may be required to maintain good mydriasis. Less severe inflammation, as follows cataract extraction, may be controlled by atropine administered once daily.

Slit-lamp evaluation of aqueous flare and cells is the best guide to atropinization of the inflamed eye. The red-eyed patient without flare and cells will usually not benefit from cycloplegia and will be handicapped by the paralysis of accommodation. One mistake commonly made by emergency room interns is to treat an eye with a minor corneal abrasion with atropine. This is an unnecessary nuisance to the patient. Cycloplegic therapy of iridocyclitis should not be discontinued until flare and cells have disappeared from the aqueous humor.

The effectiveness of atropine in reducing abnormal vascular permeability may be observed experimentally by the use of a fluorescein marker. In normal cat eyes, intravenous fluorescein does not leak from the ciliary processes. A marked leakage of fluorescein into the aqueous humor occurs if as little as 0.01 μg of acetylcholine/ml bathes the eserinized ciliary processes. Acetylcholine is believed to affect the blood-aqueous barrier by dilating blood vessels. Atropinization of the ciliary processes with 10 μg of drug/ml will completely block the acetylcholine-induced permeability increase.[7]

### *Refraction*

Because accurate measurement of hyperopia is necessary to correct accommodative esotropia and to avoid a blurring of distance vision that will cause a child to refuse to wear glasses, maximum cycloplegia is important. This may be more reliably achieved by the 3-day routine of atropinization than by shorter courses with other medications. The parent is instructed to instill atropine three times daily in both eyes for the 3 days immediately preceding the next office visit unless toxicity occurs. This routine also has the practical advantage of the drops being instilled elsewhere; the child need not wait unhappily in the office.

Actually, this is more atropine than is really necessary for most patients. Repeated refraction during the course of atropine instillation indicates that the maximum cycloplegia is usually reached during the second day, after the patient has received only 4 of the 9 drops.[8] The excess medication ensures that even the most resistant eyes will be completely cycloplegic and allows for the omission of one or more instillations, which so often happens.

Refraction of orthotropic children does not require atropine. Because of its long duration, atropine is not useful for refraction of adults.

Atropine cycloplegia is said to uncover about 0.4 D more hyperopia than is detected by cyclopentolate cycloplegia.[9] The physician's decision as to whether to use atropine or a shorter-acting cycloplegic will depend on the importance of identifying the entire amount of hyperopia. Except in cases of accommodative strabismus, this does not matter.

The patient population in whom recognition of the full hyperopic error is most important clinically is the group of children less than 6 years of age with accommodative esotropia. Refractions were done in 120 such patients with 1% cyclopentolate repeated in 5 minutes with retinoscopy after 45 to 60 minutes and also with 1% atropine given three times daily for 3 days. The mean difference between the two drugs was 0.34 D more hyperopia detected by the atropine refraction (always done second). Of greater importance than the mean difference is the existence of a subgroup of patients in whom the atropine refraction uncovered +1.00 D or more of hyperopia not detected by the cyclopentolate refraction.

This finding occurred in 22% of the patients, almost all of whom showed cyclopentolate hyperopia of +2.00 D or more. Atropine refraction is therefore recommended for all esotropic children who show +2.00 diopters or more of hyperopia.[10]

### *Occlusion*

In the treatment of suppression amblyopia, atropine may be useful if cycloplegia will reduce the acuity of the good eye below that of the amblyopic one and thus force fixation with the amblyopic eye. Because the patient will have a strong inclination to continue using the preferred eye, observation must confirm that the method used (other than occlusion, the effect of which is certain) does, indeed, result in the desired change in fixation. Occlusion is still the method of choice for severe amblyopia. Atropinization has the advantages of avoiding skin irritation by the patch, cosmetic and psychologic problems occasioned by the patch, and the problems of enforcing occlusion upon an uncooperative child. Atropinization will not worsen latent nystagmus, as happens with occlusion.

In a series of 16 patients with mild amblyopia (20/100 or better), nine responded to atropinization with improvement of visual acuity of two lines or more. A single patient with 20/400 and eccentric fixation regained 20/30 vision. (The conventional wisdom that occlusion will not benefit amblyopia associated with eccentric fixation is evidently not always true.) Another situation well suited to atropine use occurs when standard occlusion methods have achieved good vision in each eye but relapse into amblyopia happens after patching is stopped. Of 13 such patients, atropinization maintained vision within one line of best vision in 10 cases.[11]

Unilateral atropinization seems so easy and effective and harmless that nothing can go wrong. This is not true. Infants are highly susceptible to visual deprivation, this potential existing until 5 years of age. In three reported cases, children ranging in age from 10 months to 2½ years had amblyopia develop in the previously good eye subsequent to its atropinization. Prompt recognition of the problem and appropriate patching of the previously amblyopic eye restored normal vision to both eyes.[12]

The danger of inducing amblyopia might not occur to us if the reason for monocular atropinization was treatment of severe iridocyclitis or trauma in a child or perhaps an attempt to permit better vision around an axial congenital monocular cataract.

### *Hyphema*

Use or nonuse of topical atropine was the only variable in treatment of 115 patients with traumatic hyphema. There was no difference between the two groups in rate of absorption of hemorrhage, incidence of secondary hemorrhage, or visual outcome. Poor visual outcome after secondary hemorrhage was attributed to the greater severity of injury more common in such cases. Cycloplegia is useful in examination of such patients and may contribute to the comfort of the eye. In any event, no harmful effect of atropinization was demonstrable.[13]

### *Oculocardiac Reflex*

The oculocardiac reflex can cause marked slowing of the pulse, hypotension, faintness, and nausea. A number of such episodes were encountered during various types of eyelid surgery, and patients did not respond well to increased sedation or local anesthesia. Premedication with 0.4 mg of atropine and more careful lid retraction and manipulation reduced such symptoms to only two patients of 41 eyelid operations. The oculocardiac reflex is ordinarily associated with strabismus surgery, but these reports described it as a response to entropion surgery and ptosis surgery as well.[14]

### *Reversal of Muscle Relaxants*

Atropine, 1.2 mg, is given as part of the procedure to reverse the general anesthetic use of pancuronium bromide, a muscle relaxant. The specific reversing agent is 2.5 mg of neostigmine, which results in cholinergic side effects. The atropine is used as an anticholinergic drug. Pupil dilatation of up to 1.5 mm may result from such combined use of atropine and neostigmine. A patient was reported to suffer an angle-closure glaucoma attack 3 hours after such a muscle relaxant reversal technique.[15]

### *Treatment of Myopia*

Fifty years ago, Walter Lancaster believed that atropinization would arrest the progress of myopia. There has been a general tendency to scoff at this, but periodically poorly controlled studies report such facts as that after 3 years untreated patients average a 1.22-D increase in myopia compared with a 0.07-D average decrease in myopia in eyes treated with 1 drop of 1% atropine every night.[16] Because of uncertainties of selection of these patients and considerable variation in the duration or treatment, it is hard to interpret the validity of such studies. Bilateral instillation of 1% atropine daily for an average of 4 years was said to result in 24% of eyes being more than 3.00-D myopic compared with 67% of a control group.[17] The criteria for selection of these patients cannot be determined and the disclaimer is offered that it was "not a carefully controlled prospective study."

Another uncontrolled study of atropinization for 1 year concluded that no progression of myopia occurred during atropinization, rapid progression of myopia resulted as soon as the atropine was discontinued, and the psychologic problems of bifocals and large pupils were major deterrents to such therapy.[18, 19]

## Toxicity

### *Systemic Reactions*

The fatal dose of atropine is about 100 mg for adults and 10 mg for children. Because 1 drop of 1% atropine solution contains about 0.5 mg of drug (the usual preoperative dose for controlling secretions), simple calculation will reveal that an ordinary ophthalmic bottle of atropine may contain enough drug to kill several children. Patients should be warned to keep drugs such as atropine and isoflurophate safely out of the reach of children.

Only 10 mg of atropine will kill a 4.5-kg child. A fatal dose for a child is contained in 20 drops of atropine; that is 1 drop in each eye for ten doses. In fact, that is only one more set of drops than given in the routine three times daily for 3 days for cycloplegic refraction. The reason that there are not fatalities among children is that humans excrete 50% of an atropine dose within 24 hours and most of the instilled eye drop is washed harmlessly down the face by reflex lid squeezing and tearing. I stress this because cycloplegic and mydriatic drops are not harmless to children. The milligram dose per kilogram of body weight increases rapidly with decreasing body size. Infants are highly vulnerable to eye drop toxicity. Examination of premature infant eyes is the extreme case. Thoughtless use of routine eye drops for dilatation as we examine for retinopathy of prematurity will also routinely poison the child 100% of the time. Repeating the drops because the eyes are hard to examine is flirting with disaster. In the National CRYO-ROP Study, Cyclomydril (2% cyclopentolate and 1% phenylephrine) was used. It is given two times in 15-minute intervals. Excellent dilatation occurs approximately 1 hour after instillation.

Minor but alarming toxic reactions commonly follow the use of atropine for refraction in children. Systemic absorption may be decreased by using ointment rather than drops, by wiping excess solution or ointment from the eye immediately after instillation, or by using 0.5% rather than 1% solutions. Parents should be instructed to skip the drops in the atropine refraction routine if toxic symptoms are present at the time the medication is due. These symptoms include dryness of skin and mouth, fever (because of the inability to perspire), irritability or delirium (caused by stimulation of the CNS), tachycardia (resulting from vagal block), and flushing of the face (caused by cutaneous vasodilation in the blush area). Such symptoms have been misdiagnosed as scarlet fever or other childhood infections.

The exact mechanism of the atropine flush is unclear, but a dramatic picture of a 13-month-old infant with congenital Horner's syndrome shows absence of the parasympatholytic flush on the denervated side of the face.[20] The demarcation line is as sharp as if a paintbrush had been drawn across the face on the normal side. One could reason that the anticholinergic flush is a release of adrenergic tonus, resulting in vasodilation, and that the absence of adrenergic tone on the affected side precludes a response. Exactly how all anticholinergic drug would accomplish this is not evident. A better explanation suggests that the physiologic vasodilation is a result of central relaxation of vasomotor tonus, perhaps induced in an attempt to dissipate the heat resulting from loss of perspiration. The pallor on the Horner's side would then be an active blanching of the skin caused by denervation hypersensitivity to circulating catecholamines.

In this instance, the anticholinergic flush resulted from use of 0.5% cyclopentolate (Cyclogyl) for fundus examination and was recognized because of its unilaterality. Usually such a toxic flush reaction would be misinterpreted as being caused by the crying of an obnoxious infant who is in reality hallucinating from the cycloplegic drug. In view of this, 2 drops of 1% cyclopentolate for refraction of premature infants runs the risk of toxicity.[21]

Should severe atropine poisoning occur, the patient may be treated with subcutaneous injection of 1 mg of physostigmine. Repeated 0.25-mg doses may be given every 15 minutes until salivation occurs or symptomatic relief is obtained.

Subcutaneous injection of 5 mg of methacholine has been suggested as a diagnostic test for parasympatholytic poisoning. This dose normally causes parasympathomimetic symptoms, which will be blocked if the patient has been poisoned by atropine.

Delirium and hallucinations have been reported to occur with use of all cycloplegic drugs. Consider a situation that could easily be misdiagnosed. An elderly patient has just had his cataract operation, is patched on the operated side and sees poorly with the other eye, is in unfamiliar surroundings with no relatives or friends, and has been given analgesics and sedatives for postoperative pain. He now begins to move about aimlessly, talks somewhat incoherently about something the listener does not understand, and thinks he is at his daughter's house. This scenario may be the result of preoperative and postoperative atropinization, which might be easily overlooked during the diagnostic work-up of sudden dementia. The specific antidote for anticholinergic toxicity is physostigmine.[22]

***In Glaucoma***

Parasympatholytic drugs such as atropine will increase IOP in eyes with chronic simple glaucoma and should not be used to dilate such eyes. An IOP elevation of 6 mm Hg or more occurred in response to cycloplegia in 23% of 40 patients with known open-angle glaucoma but in only 2% of 100 nonglaucomatous patients.[23] Hence, such a hypertensive response to cycloplegia is strongly indicative of chronic simple glaucoma. All of the potent cycloplegic agents produced this hypertensive response, which was not caused by noncycloplegic mydriatic drugs.

Eyes predisposed to acute glaucoma (shallow angle and shallow anterior chamber) may develop an acute attack if they are treated with atropine. Atropine is strongly contraindicated in such eyes.

Although atropine is advocated in the management of glaucoma secondary to acute anterior segment inflammation, an eye with old inflammatory scars may have enough trabecular damage to simulate chronic simple glaucoma and require miotic therapy.[24] Atropinization of such eyes may increase IOP.

Will preoperative atropinization in general surgery be harmful to patients with chronic simple glaucoma? This question frequently causes concern. The answer clearly is no for three reasons. First, the sensitivity of the eye to systemic atropine is relatively low. Second, the local effects of miotic therapy are far greater than can be overcome by systemic atropinization. Third, even if the IOP were slightly elevated for 1 or 2 days, no perceptible damage would result. However, in the unlikely event that a patient with untreated subacute angle-closure glaucoma is given atropine preoperatively, complete angle closure might well ensue. When ophthalmologists are treating patients with unilateral acute glaucoma, they must not neglect the other eye, which may also be at risk.

#### *Allergic Reactions*

Contact dermatitis confined to the lids of the treated eye is not uncommonly caused by atropine. This is recognized by the characteristic itching and by the reddened, swollen, weeping texture of the skin. Conjunctival redness, although present, is less conspicuous.

No treatment is satisfactory except discontinuance of the offending drug. Corticosteroids only postpone this necessary step. Fortunately, many effective atropine substitutes are readily available and usually do not cause sensitivity. These include scopolamine, cyclopentolate, and oxyphenonium (Antrenyl).

Even years later the use of atropine usually causes a prompt return of the allergic blepharitis.

#### *In Subluxated Lens*

A rare contraindication to mydriasis is subluxation of the lens, which may occur after injury, in megalocornea, or in Marfan syndrome. Although most such eyes may be dilated without consequence, several instances have been reported in which the lens slipped into the anterior chamber and caused acute pupillary block glaucoma.[25] However, dilatation is clearly indicated in complete examination of an injured eye or of the periphery of an eye with Marfan syndrome and should not be foregone because of the slight risk of anterior lens displacement.

Permanent mydriasis secondary to the use of strong mydriatic agents such as atropine after keratoplasty for keratoconus was first recognized by Castroviejo. This idea has been propagated for many years. Recently studies have been done to refute this hypothesis. Atropine was given immediately after keratoplasty in 83 eyes with keratoconus. No instances of permanent dilation were found.[26]

## HOMATROPINE

Homatropine is a parasympatholytic drug quite similar to atropine except that it is weaker and has a much shorter duration of action. It is used primarily in cycloplegic refraction.

Maximum cycloplegia, induced by a 2% solution of homatropine, is reached within 1 hour after initial drug instillation.[27] The cycloplegic effect is maintained for about 3 hours and then gradually decreases; some effect remains for more than 24 hours. The average recovery time from 2% homatropine solution is 32 hours, varying from 12 to 49 hours in a series of 23 eyes. The residual accommodation averages 1.00 D, varying from 0.50 to 2.00 D. These results were obtained after the instillation of 6 drops of a 2% solution of homatropine at 10-minute intervals in patients ranging from 17 to 39 years of age (average age 22 years).

During the onset and disappearance of cycloplegia, as caused by homatropine, the AC:A ratio changes. The practical implication of this change is that reliable measurements of muscle balance should be made before or after but not during cycloplegia.

In both the normal and glaucomatous

human eyes the resistance of the trabecular meshwork may be reduced by parasympathomimetic tonus and increased by parasympatholytic drugs. The average increase in outflow resistance 45 minutes after instillation of 2 drops of a 5% solution of homatropine in 64 normal human eyes and in 29 eyes with open-angle glaucoma is shown in Fig. 3–40.[28] As illustrated, the glaucomatous eyes showed a greater susceptibility to a cycloplegic-induced rise of outflow resistance than did the normal eyes.

The effect of a 5% concentration of homatropine hydrobromide on IOP was studied in 140 normal eyes and in 70 eyes with chronic simple glaucoma.[29] Forty-five minutes after medication instillation, the IOP had decreased in 50% of the normal eyes, had remained the same in 30%, and had increased in only 20%. In contrast, the pressure of 73% of the glaucomatous eyes increased, 10% remained the same, and 17% decreased. The pressure increase was because of a reduction in the facility of aqueous outflow, which dropped by an average of 28% in the glaucomatous eyes and by 15% in the normal eyes. There was no definite relationship between the amount of mydriasis and the decrease in outflow.

These findings have two clinically important implications. First, routine tonometric screening is more likely to detect increased IOP after parasympatholytic medication, and therefore tonometry should be done on the dilated eye, as well as before dilatation. (Recall that sympathomimetic dilatation does not regularly increase IOP but, rather, decreases it.) Second, because dilatation commonly increases IOP in chronic simple glaucoma, a dilatation-provocative test result for angle-closure glaucoma is not to be interpreted as positive (requiring iridectomy) unless the angle is gonioscopically closed at the time of pressure elevation.

## SCOPOLAMINE

Except for a much shorter duration of action, scopolamine is similar to that of atropine. A 0.25% concentration will achieve a comparable (but shorter duration) effect as 1% atropine. Scopolamine may be substituted for atropine when a shorter duration of action is required or in the presence of an atropine allergy. Systemic side effects, including psychosis, have been reported with topical use.[30]

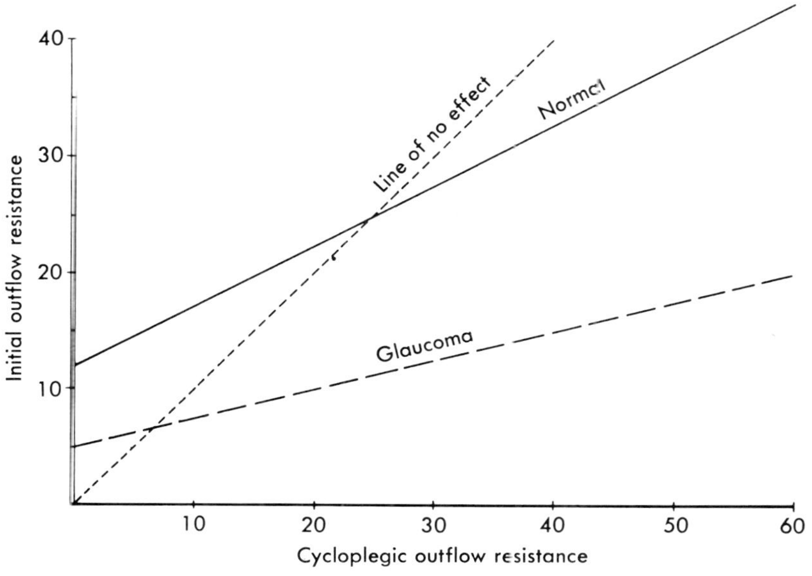


**FIG 3–40.**
Average change of outflow resistance after homatropine in normal and glaucomatous human eyes. Lines represent slopes of the least squares calculations to fit results in 64 normal and 29 glaucomatous eyes. (Modified from Bárány E, Christensen RE: *Arch Ophthalmol* 77:757, 1967. Used by permission.)

## CYCLOPENTOLATE

### Clinical Use

Cyclopentolate is a potent parasympatholytic drug of great value in inducing cycloplegia and wide mydriasis. Its cycloplegia effect is superior to that of homatropine, having a more rapid onset, shorter duration, and greater intensity. A concentration of 0.5% cyclopentolate, instilled two times 10 minutes apart, will produce maximum cycloplegia in 40% of white patients in 15 minutes or less (Fig. 3–41). However, 22% of the eyes treated with cyclopentolate did not attain the maximum effect until 45 minutes or more after instillation. Note that 1.00 D or more of residual accommodation remains in many eyes. It is important to measure this remaining accommodation at the time of refraction; an anisometropic error in prescription may occur if an unequal cycloplegic effect in the two eyes is not recognized. The cycloplegic effect of a 0.5% solution of cyclopentolate is usually dissipated within 24 hours. However, some mydriasis may last for several days.

For comparison, the response of opposite eyes of the same patients to instillation of a 5% solution of homatropine and a 1% solution of hydroxyamphetamine (Paredrine), repeated after 10 minutes, is shown in Fig. 3–42. The eyes treated with homatropine and hydroxyamphetamine attained the same levels of cycloplegia as did the eyes treated with cyclopentolate, but more slowly. The homatropine cycloplegia often lasted more than 24 hours, and the patients were able to read with the cyclopentolate-treated eye sooner than with the opposite eye.

A single drop of a 1% solution (or 2 drops of a 0.5% solution, separated by a 5-minute interval) will provide sufficient cycloplegia for most refractive purposes. Within 1 hour, instillation of 3 drops at 10-minute intervals will give retinoscopic values comparable with those obtained by atropinization for 3 days in children. The eyes of darkly pigmented patients are resistant to cyclopentolate, just as they are to other cycloplegics, and may require repeated instillation of a 2% solution and a longer than usual time for dilatation (Fig. 3–43).[31] As much as 5.00 to 6.00 D of accommodation may remain after two instillations of cyclopentolate in the eye of a darkly pigmented individual.

Excellent mydriasis is produced by cyclopentolate. Pupils dilated with this drug do not constrict even when exposed to the prolonged, intense light of the indirect ophthalmoscope or during fundus photography. Dilatation with the combination of

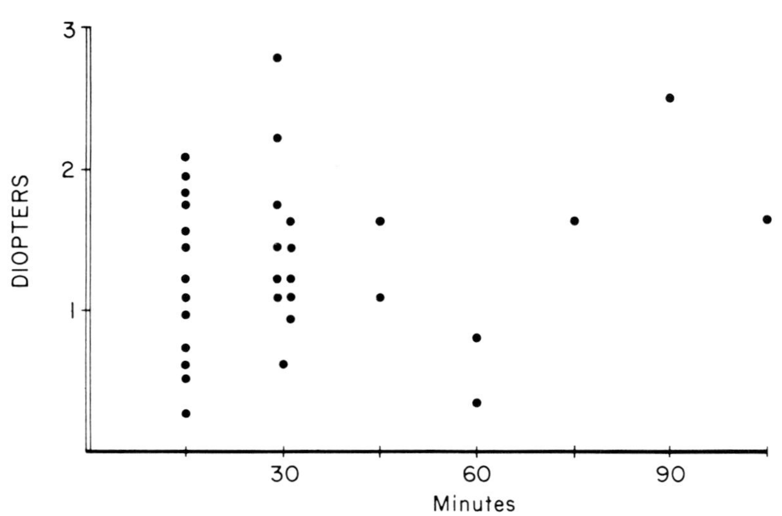


**FIG 3–41.**
Time of onset of maximum cycloplegia and residual accommodation at that time after 2 drops of a 0.5% solution of cyclopentolate in white patients. (Modified from Milder B, Riffinburgh RS: *Am J Ophthalmol* 36:1724, 1953. Used by permission.)

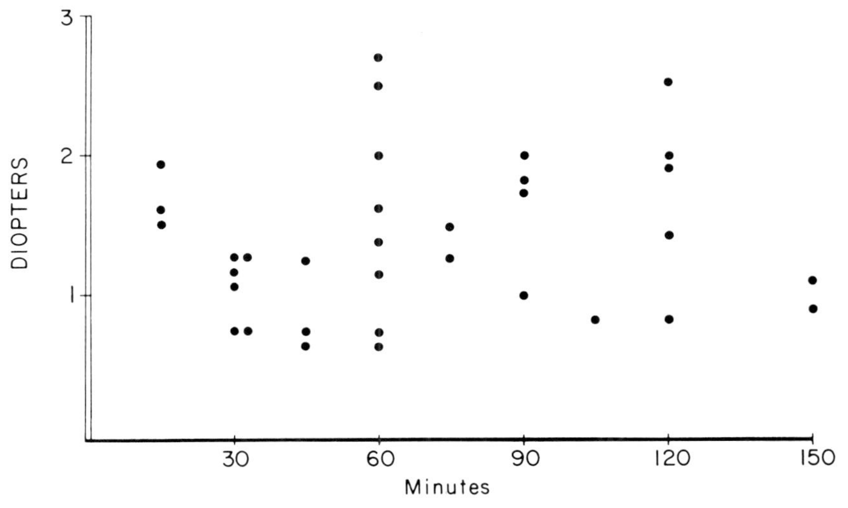


**FIG 3–42.**
Time of onset of maximum cycloplegia and residual accommodation at that time after instillation of 2 drops of a 5% solution of homatropine and of a 1% solution of hydroxyamphetamine (Paredrine) in white patients. (Modified from Milder B, Riffinburgh RS: *Am J Ophthalmol* 36:1724, 1953. Used by permission.)

cyclopentolate and phenylephrine provides maximal mydriasis, which, for instance, is of great value during the examination of patients with retinal detachment. Good mydriasis can be achieved within 20 minutes with cyclopentolate.

Search for a combination of medications that would give maximum mydriasis with minimal toxicity suggested a preliminary drop of proparacaine about 1 minute before the dilating drop.[32] This seems to enhance corneal penetration. The reported protocol did not include tonometry at this time, but an efficient routine could do so. The additional trauma of tonometry should greatly enhance the subsequent drug penetration. Excellent mydriasis at 30 minutes, maximal at 60 minutes, was obtained by use of a combination solution of 2.5% phenylephrine with either 0.5% cyclopentolate or 0.5% tropicamide. This drop was instilled by the "pouch" technique, whereby the lower lid is pulled out to create a space in the lower cul-de-sac, into which the drop is instilled. The patient then looks down and closes the lids gently, without squeezing, and maintains gentle lid closure for 1 minute. This technique of eye drop instillation maintains

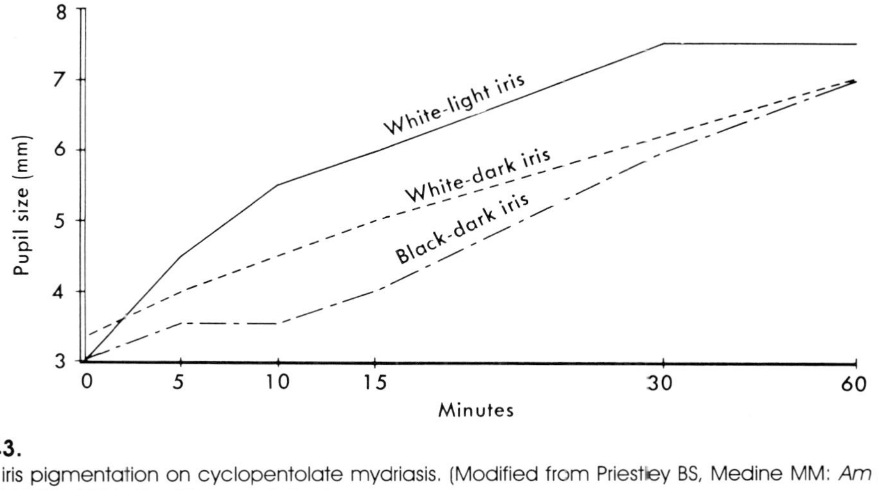


**FIG 3–43.**
Effect of iris pigmentation on cyclopentolate mydriasis. (Modified from Priestley BS, Medine MM: *Am J Ophthalmol* 34:572, 1951. Used by permission.)

the entire drop in contact with the eye for a prolonged time in contrast to the immediate squeezing out of two thirds of the drop that ordinarily occurs. Also, when both drugs are combined in 1 drop, a second different drop dose not wash out the first medication.[29]

Cyclopentolate in a 0.5% solution is a more potent mydriatic and cycloplegic than a 5% solution of homatropine. In 100 patients the average residual accommodation 1 hour after instillation of 2 drops of a 0.5% solution of cyclopentolate was 1.25 D compared with 2.00 D for 2 drops of a 5% solution of homatropine.[31]

Twenty patients with contact allergy to atropine were successfully treated with cyclopentolate, with no cross-sensitivity.[33] If iridocyclitis is severe, it may be necessary to instill cyclopentolate as often as every 3 hours because its duration of action is not as long as that of atropine.

## Toxicity

A considerable burning sensation results from instillation of a 1% or 2% solution of cyclopentolate. The 0.5% solution is definitely less irritating. This burning sensation is transient, and the patient should be assured that it is to be expected and will rapidly disappear. Children are especially distressed by such discomfort.

As is true of all parasympatholytic drugs, cyclopentolate will increase the IOP of most patients with chronic simple glaucoma.[34] Dilatation with any drug, including cyclopentolate, may precipitate an attack of acute glaucoma in patients predisposed to this disorder because of the narrow angles.[35]

Even after prophylactic peripheral iridectomy, a few eyes with narrow angles may develop quite marked pressure elevations after cyclopentolate dilatation.[36] This may be caused by the presence of plateau iris configuration closing the anterior chamber angle with pupil dilatation. Cycloplegia may raise IOP without closing the anterior chamber angle. One percent cyclopentolate caused a rise in IOP of 8 mm Hg or more in 5% of 431 eyes with open-angle glaucoma.[37] Gonioscopy confirmed that the angle remained open during the pressure rise. Some iris pigment granules were liberated by the cyclopentolate in 32% of the eyes. Such pigment within the aqueous is usually associated with phenylephrine mydriasis but obviously is also common with cyclopentolate use, although less marked. Of the six eyes with very profuse pigment liberation, five showed 8 mm or greater rise in pressure, presumably because of transient pigment blockade of the trabeculum.

### *Disturbances of Central Nervous System*

Ocular instillation of cyclopentolate may cause disturbances of the CNS in children. After instillation of 4 drops of a 1% solution of cyclopentolate, an 8-year-old child developed marked ataxia, visual hallucinations, and incoherent speech. Some days later the same child was given 6 drops of a 1% concentration of cyclopentolate during a 15-minute period. Twenty minutes later the previously described symptoms reappeared and persisted for 4 hours. There was no flushing or dryness of skin or mucous membranes. Temperature, pulse, and respiration were normal. One is reminded that each drop of a 1% solution contains 0.5 mg of the medication.[38]

Psychiatric evaluation of 40 children before and after use of a 2% solution of cyclopentolate for refraction detected an acute psychotic reaction in five of these children.[39] Symptoms develop about 30 to 45 minutes after instillation of the drops and include restlessness, aimless wandering, irrelevant talking, hallucinations, memory loss, and faulty orientation as to time and place. A solution of 1% cyclopentolate is much less likely to cause such reactions. Solutions of 1% homatropine and 1% hydroxyamphetamine (Paredrine) did not cause psychotic symptoms. Cyclopentolate contains a dimethylated group that is also found in some hallucinogenic drugs.

Hallucinations and amnesia lasting 3 hours were produced in a 9-year-old boy by 1 drop of a 1% solution of cyclopentolate in each eye, followed in 15 minutes by 1 drop of a 2% solution of the same drug in both eyes.[40]

Rarely, adults may have a comparable reaction. After the instillation of 1 drop of 2% cyclopentolate in each eye, the 27-year-old wife of a physician had an episode of hallucination lasting for 1 hour.[41]

Apparently the rarity of such reactions depends on whether you ask. Direct questioning regarding adverse physical and emotional changes after 1 drop of 2% cyclopentolate in each eye revealed 10 instances of adverse reactions in 66 patients.[42] Nausea, weakness, dizziness, depression, and loss of coordination were the commonest symptoms. Nine of the 10 patients were female, perhaps because their smaller size results in a larger dose per kilogram. Two percent cyclopentolate is unnecessary for ocular response and should not be used because of the frequency of these systemic effects.[37]

***Allergy***

A characteristic type of severe allergic response may follow the repeated use of cyclopentolate. Because of the circumstances of the drug's use and the unusual appearance of this allergy, the ophthalmologist almost always fails to recognize its presence.

The history includes persistent irritation developing within minutes of instillation, rather severe watering, and stringy discharge. Vision is blurred and the eyes are red, whereas itching, the classic sign of allergy, is not a significant complaint. Comparable symptoms occur at each office visit, the allergic reaction sometimes extending over 6 months or more.

In the presence of allergy the eyes are diffusely red after instillation of cyclopentolate. If only one eye is involved, the physician misinterprets the problem as being an exacerbation of whatever condition is under treatment, for example, usually persistent redness after surgery. An annoying amount of stringy white mucus is present, enough to move over the cornea with blinking and to distort the image of the indirect ophthalmoscope. Such mucus is not uncommon in surface infection, so the physician simply wipes it away and continues with the examination. However, if within a few minutes the mucus strands have reformed, this is the first indication of cyclopentolate allergy. Such rapid mucous secretion does not occur in the usual conjunctival infections.

The fundus view is diffusely hazy, not really bad but enough to be annoying. The indistinctness is comparable with any opacity of the media, such as a moderate nuclear cataract or a diffuse vitreous condensation, except that it is a result of corneal changes.

Typically biomicroscopy reveals innumerable tiny superficial punctate epithelial lesions scattered uniformly across the entire corneal surface.

Not only is the acute stage annoying and uncomfortable, but after numerous insults, the lacrimal drainage system may become occluded.

## TROPICAMIDE

Tropicamide is a rapidly acting parasympatholytic drug useful in producing cycloplegia and mydriasis of short duration. It exists as two optical isomers that are present in equal amounts in the commercial preparation. As is usually the case in racemic mixtures, the *l*-isomer has much greater pharmacologic activity.[43] The anticholinergic effect of *l*-tropicamide is 75 times greater than that of the *d*-isomer. Tropicamide does not bind to tissue as firmly as does atropine. The washout time for half recovery of carbachol responsiveness was less than 15 minutes for nonpigmented irises and 30 minutes for pigmented irises.

The diopters of residual accommodation at various times after instillation of a single drop of a 1% solution of tropicamide are shown in Fig. 3–44. Assuming that residual accommodation should not exceed 2.00 D for a satisfactory cycloplegic refraction, it is evident that one instillation of tropicamide in a 1% solution is generally inadequate for such refraction. Even at the time of maximum effect, from 20 to 25 minutes after instillation, only half the patients were adequately cycloplegic. Because of the transient period of cycloplegia, by the time the second eye was examined, its accommodation was frequently as much as 3.0 D greater than that of the first eye. Obviously a disparity of this magnitude may contribute to erroneous refractive findings.

Considerably better cycloplegia was obtained by a second instillation of a 1% solution of tropicamide 5 to 25 minutes after

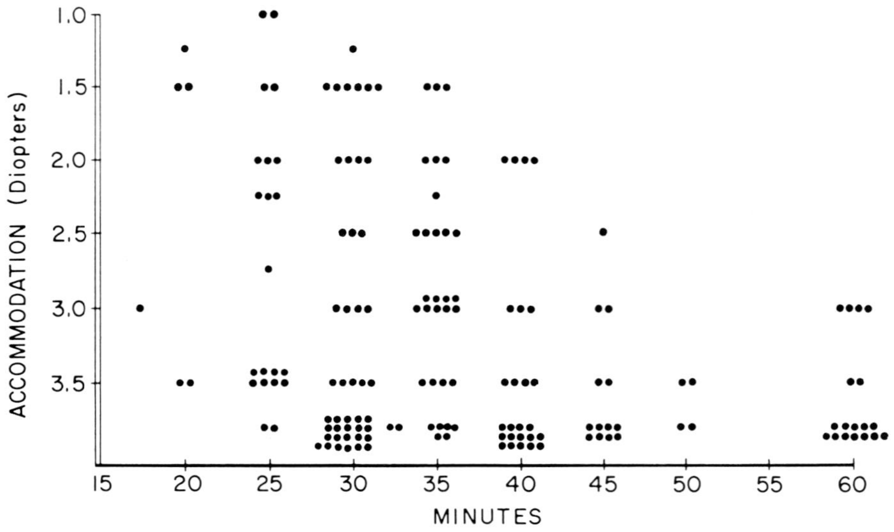


**FIG 3–44.**
Residual accommodation after instillation of 1 drop of a 1% solution of tropicamide. (Modified from Gettes B: *Arch Ophthalmol* 65:632, 1961. Used by permission.)

the first (Fig. 3–45).[44] All patients had 2.00 D or less residual accommodation within 20 to 25 minutes after instillation of the second drop. After 35 minutes, cycloplegia was no longer reliable. All patients were able to read within 2 to 4 hours, with complete return of accommodation within 6 hours.

The mydriatic effect of a 0.5% solution of tropicamide was found to be more rapid than and at least as great as that of a 10% concentration of phenylephrine. Tropicamide in a 0.5% solution is not effective for cycloplegic examination.

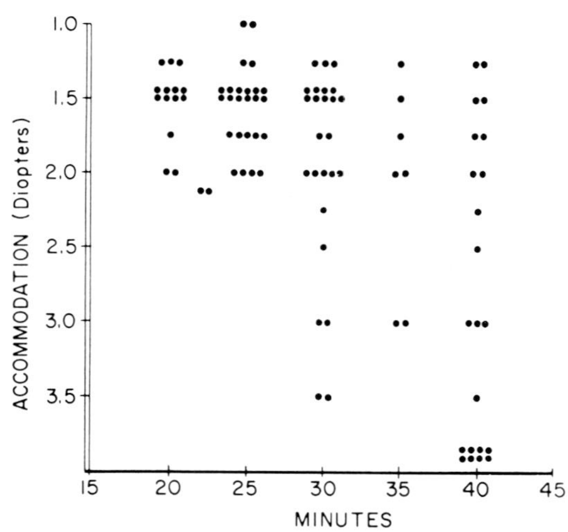


**FIG 3–45.**
Residual accommodation after instillation of a second drop of a 1% solution of tropicamide, instilled 5 to 25 minutes after the first. (Modified from Gettes B: *Arch Ophthalmol* 65:632, 1961. Used by permission.)

Tropicamide tends to have a greater mydriatic than cycloplegic effect. This is clinically important because the presence of tropicamide-induced mydriasis does not necessarily indicate adequate cycloplegia. This mydriatic-cycloplegic dissociation is more characteristic of tropicamide than of cyclopentolate.

The effect of various mydriatics has been particularly accurately studied using the infrared electronic pupillograph. The mydriasis resulting from single instillations of 0.5% tropicamide, 2% homatropine, 1% hydroxyamphetamine, and 10% phenylephrine is compared in Fig. 3–46.[45] The charted lines represent the computer-derived curves of the pupillographic values. Any given reading is the difference in size of the treated pupil and the fellow control pupil at the moment of peak response to a standard light flash. The subjects of this study were 15 white men and women ranging from 12 to 38 years of age (average age 26 years). The method of measurement used in this study probably is the most accurate clinical determination available.

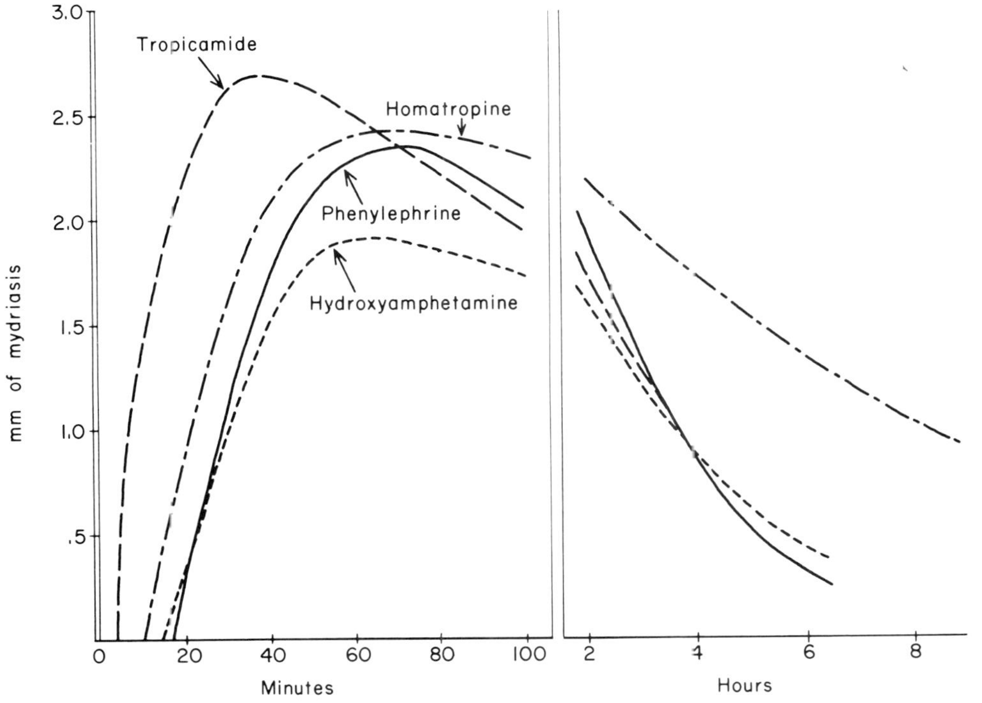


**FIG 3–46.**
Onset, intensity, and duration of mydriasis as measured by electronic pupillograph. (From Gambill HD, Ogle KN, Kearns TP: *Arch Ophthalmol* 77:740, 1967. Used by permission.)

Although tropicamide is the shortest acting of our cycloplegic drugs, it also shares the capability of transiently increasing the IOP of open-angle glaucoma eyes. Used in 50 patients with open-angle glaucoma, 2 drops of 1% tropicamide caused varying pressure elevations, one of which was as great as 10 mm Hg.[46] However, in most of these patients, there was less than a 5-mm Hg elevation of pressure after 40 minutes. The effect is so small as to be clinically insignificant.

Because of its short duration of action, tropicamide rarely causes any systemic symptoms.

## COMPARISON OF CYCLOPENTOLATE, TROPICAMIDE, AND HOMATROPINE

The three short-acting cycloplegic drugs most commonly used for refraction are cyclopentolate hydrochloride (1% solution), tropicamide (1% solution), and homatropine (4% solution). The effectiveness of these cycloplegics is compared in Fig. 3–47. Tropicamide is the most rapidly acting of the three and has the shortest duration of cycloplegia. Because of the very short duration of tropicamide's effect, it is necessary to instill a second drop 5 minutes after the first one. (The comparisons in Fig. 3-47 are of two instillations of tropicamide, 1 drop of cyclopentolate, and two instillations of homatropine.) After two instillations of tropicamide, excellent cycloplegia is obtained within 20 to 35 minutes. After 35 minutes, accommodation returns rapidly. Only 60% of 193 patients could be examined during the interval between 20 and 35 minutes after instillation.[47] The authors[47] emphasized the difficulty of maintaining a schedule of such precision. In clinical practice a third drop of tropicamide must be instilled if examination is delayed beyond 35 minutes. However, tropicamide has the advantage of permitting the patient to recover from cycloplegia within 2 to 6 hours.

Cyclopentolate was found to be an effective cycloplegic between 25 and 75 minutes after a single drop. Recovery time varied from 6 to 24 hours. The slowest acting

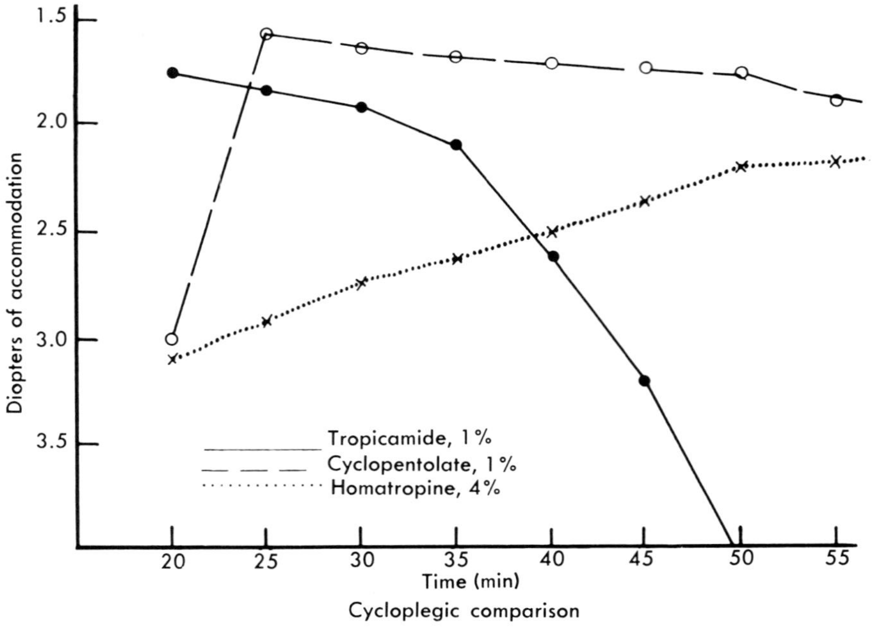


**FIG 3–47.**
Duration and effectiveness of cycloplegia induced by two instillations of tropicamide, 1% solution; 1 drop of cyclopentolate, 1% solution; and two instillations of homatropine, 4% solution. (From Gettes B, Belmont O: *Arch Ophthalmol* 66:336, 1961. Used by permission.)

of the three drugs, homatropine, required two instillations and was effective within 40 to 90 minutes, with residual cycloplegia lasting 36 to 48 hours. Less than 2.50 D of residual accommodation was achieved in 79% of white patients and 69% of black patients receiving tropicamide, in 83% of white patients receiving cyclopentolate, and in 59% of patients (racial breakdown unspecified) receiving homatropine.

In a series of 50 consecutive refractions, tropicamide (1% solution instilled twice, 5 minutes apart) was placed in one eye and compared with solutions of 5% homatropine and 1% cyclopentolate instilled in the other eye twice, 10 minutes apart.[48] Better cycloplegia was produced by homatropine in 20 of 25 patients and by cyclopentolate in 23 of 25 patients. In only seven patients was better cycloplegia attained by tropicamide. The amount of residual accommodation remaining at the time of maximum effect of these drugs is recorded in Table 3–5. It is evident that tropicamide is a relatively inadequate cycloplegic drug, because an average of 6.00 D of accommodation remains in children younger than 10 years and 3.60 D in patients 10 to 14 years of age. The residual accommodation in the patients 10 to 14 years of age with cyclopentolate was 1.60 D and with homatropine, 2.60 D. However, the mydriatic effect of tropicamide was said to be equal to or better than any other available drug in terms of rapidity of onset, size of pupil, and brevity of duration.

In the search for an ideal mydriatic that would after a single instillation produce

**TABLE 3–5.**
Residual Accommodation at Specific Time After Two Instillations of Cycloplegic Drug

| | | Residual Accommodation (D) | |
|---|---|---|---|
| Age (yr) | No. of Cases | Tropicamide at 30 min | Homatropine or Cyclopentolate at 60 min |
| ≤9 | 6 | 6.25 | 2.50 |
| 10–14 | 20 | 3.65 | 2.40 |
| 15–19 | 7 | 3.20 | 1.40 |
| 20–29 | 7 | 3.10 | 1.40 |
| 30–39 | 7 | 2.60 | 2.00 |
| >40 | 3 | 1.70 | 1.10 |

From Milder B: *Arch Ophthalmol* 66:70, 1961. Used by permission.

prompt, maximal, but transient mydriasis that would be maintained despite the intense light of indirect ophthalmoscopy, the combination of 0.8% tropicamide with 5% phenylephrine was found to dilate successfully 98% of eyes, including those with dark irides. Lesser concentrations of either drug (e.g., 0.5% tropicamide or 2.5% phenylephrine) or the use of only one or the other drug did not produce consistent and maintained mydriasis in pigmented eyes. Greater concentrations of tropicamide resulted in its precipitation from the combined solution.[44]

This 0.8% plus 5% combination produces excellent mydriasis within 20 to 30 minutes yet permits the patient to read within 2 to 4 hours. Mydriasis with 1% cyclopentolate and 10% phenylephrine required 30 minutes of action and persisted for 1 day or longer but was not greater in amount at 30 minutes. A second instillation of the 0.8% plus 5% combination instilled 10 minutes later did not give better dilatation except in a small percentage of glaucomatous eyes on long-term miotic therapy. No systemic reactions were observed during the study, and the use of a single drop was considered to minimize the possibility of toxicity.

When preliminary studies had selected the optimal combination of 0.8% tropicamide with 5% phenylephrine, a single drop of this was used in the routine clinical examination of 627 patients. Of these, only 8 (1.2%) required additional mydriatic.[49]

Topical presurgical treatment with a nonsteroidal, anti-inflammatory drug that inhibits prostaglandin synthesis has proved an effective method to maintain intraoperative mydriasis after the use of adrenergic or anticholinergic drugs.[50]

Extemporaneous mixing of commercially available solutions is discouraged because of possible drug and preservative incompatibilities.

## OXYPHENONIUM (ANTRENYL)

Oxyphenonium is a synthetic, potent, long-acting anticholinergic drug. The effect of a 1% solution of oxyphenonium bromide in a 1:5,000 concentration of benzalkonium chloride is comparable in degree and duration to that of a 1% solution of atropine.[51] These two drugs may be used interchangeably in ophthalmic therapy. The structure of oxyphenonium differs from that of atropine much more than does that of scopolamine. It is unusual to see patients with atropine allergy have a cross-sensitivity to oxyphenonium. Oxyphenonium mydriasis is quite resistant to the effect of pilocarpine and isoflurophate.

Oxyphenonium is dispensed commercially as an antispasmodic for gastrointestinal use. A solution suitable for ophthalmic use may be made by preparing a 1% concentration in a 1:5,000 solution of benzalkonium chloride. Rabbit eyes dilate much better with oxyphenonium than with atropine.

## REFERENCES

### INTRODUCTION AND SECTION ONE


1. Becker B, Gage T, Kolker AE, and others: The effect of phenylephrine hydrochloride on the miotic-treated eye, *Am J Ophthalmol* 48:313, 1959.
2. Neufeld AH: Experimental studies on the mechanism of action of timolol, *Surv Ophthalmol* 23:363, 1979.
3. van Alphen GWHM, Robinette SL, Marcri FJ: Drug effects on ciliary muscle and choroid preparations in vitro, *Arch Ophthalmol* 68:81, 1962.
4. Nickerson M: Adrenergic mediators, *Invest Ophthalmol* 4:1085, 1965.
5. Kopin I: Biosynthesis and metabolism of catecholamines, *Anesthesiology* 29:654, 1968.
6. Swan KC: Ocular penetration of procaine following subconjunctival injection, *Arch Ophthalmol* 52:774, 1954.
7. Feldman LA, Sherman H: Hypersensitiveness of mucous membranes: slit lamp studies of conjunctival reactions induced in normal and in atopic persons with histamine, ethylmorphine, and atopens, *Arch Ophthalmol* 29:989, 1943.
8. Havener WH: Differential diagnosis of the red eye, *Ohio Med J* 52:836, 1956.
9. Angenent W: Destruction of epinephrine by the dopa-oxidase system of ocular tissue, *Science* 116:543, 1953.
10. Patil PN, Jacobowitz D: Unequal accumu-

lation of adrenergic drugs by pigmented and nonpigmented iris, *Am J Ophthalmol* 78:470, 1974.
11. Sachs E, Heath P: The pharmacological behavior of the intraocular muscles, *Am J Ophthalmol* 23:1376, 1940.
12. Becker B, Gage T, Kolker AE, and others: The effect of phenylephrine hydrochloride on the miotic-treated eye, *Am J Ophthalmol* 48:313, 1959.
13. Garner LL, Johnstone WW, Ballintine E, and others: Effect of 2% levorotary epinephrine on the intraocular pressure of the glaucomatous eye, *Arch Ophthalmol* 62:230, 1959.
14. Obstbaum SA, Kolker AE, Phelps CD: Low-dose epinephrine, *Arch Ophthalmol* 92:118, 1974.
15. Becker B, Morton WR: Topical epinephrine in glaucoma suspects, *Am J Ophthalmol* 62:272, 1966.
16. Criswick FG, Drance SM: Comparative study of four different epinephrine salts on intraocular pressure, *Arch Ophthalmol* 45:639, 1958.
17. Becker B: Additive effect of epinephrine and acetazolamide in control of intraocular pressure, *Am J Ophthalmol* 45:639, 1958.
18. Weekers R, Dilmarcelle Y, Gustin J: Treatment of ocular hypertension by adrenaline and diverse sympathomimetic amines, *Am J Ophthalmol* 40:666, 1955.
19. Bietti G, Virno M, Pecori-Giraldi J, and others: Possibility of isoproterenol therapy with soft contact lenses: ocular hypertension without systemic effects, *Ann Ophthalmol* 8:819, 1976.
20. Becker B, Pettit TH, Gay AJ: Topical epinephrine therapy of open-angle glaucoma, *Arch Ophthalmol* 66:219, 1961.
21. Ballintine EJ, Garner L: Improvement of the coefficient of outflow in glaucomatous eyes, *Arch Ophthalmol* 66:314, 1961.
22. Sears ML, Sherk TE: The trabecular effect of noradrenalin in the rabbit eye, *Invest Ophthalmol* 3:157, 1964.
23. Sears ML, Sherk TE: The trabecular effect of noradrenalin in the rabbit eye, *Invest Ophthalmol* 3:157, 1964.
24. Barany EH: Topical epinephrine effects on true outflow resistance and pseudofacility in vervet monkeys studies by a new anterior chamber perfusion technique, *Invest Ophthalmol* 7:88, 1968.
25. Krill AE, Newell FW, Novak M: Early and long-term effects of levo-epinephrine, *Am J Ophthalmol* 59:833, 1965.
26. Harris LS, Mittag TW, Galin MA: Aqueous dynamics of pilocarpine-treated eyes, *Arch Ophthalmol* 86:1, 1971.
27. Kitazawa Y, Nose H, Horie T: Chemical sympathectomy with 6-hydroxydopamine in the treatment of primary open-angle glaucoma, *Am J Ophthalmol* 79:98, 1975.
28. Becker B, Montgomery SW, Kass MA, and others: Increased ocular and systemic responsiveness to epinephrine in primary open-angle glaucoma, *Arch Ophthalmol* 95:789, 1977.
29. Green J: Two percent epinephrine solutions as substitutes for levo-glaukosan, *Arch Ophthalmol* 5:350, 1931.
30. Post LT: Levo-glaukosan and epinephrine bitartrate in the treatment of glaucoma, *Arch Ophthalmol* 11:187, 1934.
31. Howell SC: Action of epinephrine on the normal human eye, *Arch Ophthalmol* 12:833, 1934.
32. Howell SC: Action of epinephrine on the diseased human eye, *Arch Ophthalmol* 16:1018, 1936.
33. Harris LS, Galin MA, Lerner R: The influence of low dose L-epinephrine on intraocular pressure, *Ann Ophthalmol* 2:253, 1970.
34. Lamble JW, Lamble AP: Effects of catecholamines on the intraocular pressure of conscious owl monkeys, *Invest Ophthalmol Vis Sci* 16:628, 1977.
35. Birss SA, Longwell A, Heckbert S, Keller N: Ocular hypotensive efficacy of topical epinephrine in normotensive and hypertensive rabbits: continuous drug delivery vs eyedrops, *Ann Ophthalmol* 10:1045, 1978.
36. Lansche RK: Systemic reactions: to topical epinephrine and phenylephrine, *Am J Ophthalmol* 61:95, 1966.
37. McReynolds WU, Havener WH, Henderson JW: Hazards of use of sympathomimetic drugs in ophthalmology, *Arch Ophthalmol* 56:176, 1956.
38. Katz RL: The interaction of anesthetic agents and adrenergic drugs to produce cardiac arrhythmias, *Anesthesiology* 29:763, 1968.
39. Ballin N, Becker B, Goldman M: Systemic effects of epinephrine applied topically to the eye, *Invest Ophthalmol* 5:125, 1966.
40. Lichter PR, Bergstrom TJ: Premature ventricular systole detection by applanation tonometry, *Am J Ophthalmol* 81:797, 1976.
41. Vaughan D, Shaffer R, Riegelman S: A new stabilized form of epinephrine for the treatment of open-angle glaucoma, *Arch Ophthalmol* 66:232, 1961.

42. Krejci L, Harrison R: Epinephrine effects on corneal cells in tissue culture, *Arch Ophthalmol* 83:451, 1970.
43. Hull DS, Chemotti T, Edelhauser HF, and others: Effect of epinephrine on the corneal endothelium, *Am J Ophthalmol* 79:245, 1975.
44. Waltman SR, Yarian D, Hart W, and others: Corneal endothelial changes with long-term topical epinephrine therapy, *Arch Ophthalmol* 95:1357, 1977.
45. Byron HM: Conjunctival reaction due to l-epinephrine bitartrate (Epitrate), *Arch Ophthalmol* 63:567, 1960.
46. Aronson SB, Yamamoto EA: Ocular hypersensitivity to epinephrine, *Invest Ophthalmol* 5:75, 1966.
47. Corwin ME, Spencer WH: Conjunctival melanin depositions, *Arch Ophthalmol* 69:317, 1963.
48. Reinecke RD, Kuwabara T: Corneal deposits secondary to topical epinephrine, *Arch Ophthalmol* 70:170, 1963.
49. Donaldson DD: Epinephrine pigmentation of the cornea, *Arch Ophthalmol* 78:74, 1967.
50. Krejci L, Harrison R: Corneal pigment deposits from topically administered epinephrine, *Arch Ophthalmol* 82:836, 1969.
51. Madge GE, Geeraets WJ, Guerry III D: Black cornea secondary to topical epinephrine, *Am J Ophthalmol* 71:402, 1971.
52. Ferry AP, Zimmerman LE: Black cornea: a complication of topical use of epinephrine, *Am J Ophthalmol* 62:162, 1967.
53. Miller D, Brooks SM, Mobilia E: Adrenochrome staining of soft contact lenses, *Ann Ophthalmol* 8:65, 1976.
54. Zuckerman BD: Conjunctiva pigmentation due to cosmetics, *Am J Ophthalmol* 62:672, 1966.
55. Pardos GJ, Krachmer JH, Mannis MJ: Persistent corneal erosion secondary to tarsal adrenochrome deposit, *Am J Ophthalmol* 90:870, 1980.
56. Kolker AE, Becker B: Epinephrine maculopathy, *Arch Ophthalmol* 79:552, 1968.
57. Thomas JV, Gragoudas ES, Blair NP, and others: Correlation of epinephrine use and macular edema in aphakic glaucomatous eyes, *Arch Ophthalmol* 96:625, 1978.
58. Mackool RJ, Muldoon T, Fortier A, and others: Epinephrine-induced cystoid macular edema in aphakic eyes, *Arch Ophthalmol* 95 791, 1977.
59. Irvine AR: Cystoid maculopathy, *Surv Ophthalmol* 21:1, 1976.
60. Obstbaum SA, Galin MA, Poole TA: Topical epinephrine and cystoid macular edema, *Ann Ophthalmol* 8:455, 1976.
61. Michels RG, Maumenee AE: Cystoid macular edema associated with topically applied epinephrine in aphakic eyes, *Am J Ophthalmol* 80 379, 1975.
62. Kramer SG: Aphakic eyes, *Trans Am Ophthalmol Soc* 78:947, 1980.
63. Zimmerman TJ: Consideration on epinephrine therapy in glaucoma, *Ann Ophthalmol* 10:1077, 1978.
64. Matuk Y, Lou P, Parker JA: Biosynthesis of proteins by the retina. Inactivation by near-ultraviolet light and the effects of tryptophan, epinephrine and catalase, *Invest Ophthalmol* 16:1104, 1977.
65. Matsusaka T, Morimoto K, Kikkawa Y: $^3$H-Dextran method for measurements of the blood volume in the rat choroid, *Jpn J Ophthalmol* 24:429, 1980.
66. Namba H, Takase M: Studies on the blood flow in the anterior uvea of rabbits using heated thermocouple, *Jpn J Ophthalmol* 22:437, 1978.
67. Laibson PR, Kibrick S: Reactivation of herpetic keratitis by epinephrine in rabbit, *Arch Ophthalmol* 75:254, 1966.
68. Sellers MI: *Medical tribune*, July 14, 1961.
69. Kwon BS, Gangarosa LP, Burch KD, and others: Induction of ocular herpes simplex virus shedding by iontophoresis of epinephrine into rabbit cornea, *Invest Ophthalmol* 21:442, 1981.
70. Norn MS: Pemphigoid related to epinephrine treatment, *Am J Ophthalmol* 83:138, 1977.
71. Kaback MB, Podos SM, Harbin Jr TS, and others: The effects of dipivalyl epinephrine on the eye, *Am J Ophthalmol* 81:768, 1976.
72. Mandell AI, Stentz F, Kitabchi AE: Dipivalyl epinephrine: a new prodrug in the treatment of glaucoma, *Trans Am Acad Ophthalmol Otolaryngol* 85:268, 1978.
73. Kohn AN, Moss AP, Hargett NA, and others: Clinical comparison of dipivalyl epinephrine and epinephrine in the treatment of glaucoma, *Am J Ophthalmol* 87:196, 1979.
74. Keates EU, Stone RA: Safety and effectiveness of concomitant administration of dipivefrin and timolol maleate, *Am J Ophthalmol* 91:243, 1981.
75. Allen RC, Epstein DL: Additive effect of betaxolol and epinephrine in primary open angle glaucoma, *Arch Ophthalmol* 104:1178, 1986.
76. Weinreb RN, Ritch R, Kushner FH: Effect

of adding betaxolol to dipivefrin therapy, *Am J Ophthalmol* 101:196, 1986.

77. Abramovsky I, Mindel JS: Dipivefrin and echothiophate: contraindications to combined use, *Arch Ophthalmol* 97:1937, 1979.
78. Mindel JS, Yablonski ME, Tavitian HO, and others: Dipivefrin and echothiophate, *Arch Ophthalmol* 99:1583, 1981.
79. Wandel T, Spinak M: Toxicity of dipivalyl epinephrine, *Ophthalmology* 88:259, 1981.
80. Theodore J, Leibowitz HM: External ocular toxicity of dipivalyl epinephrine, *Am J Ophthalmol* 88:1013, 1979.
81. Anderson JA: Systemic absorption of topical ocularly applied epinephrine and dipivefrin, *Arch Ophthalmol* 98:350, 1980.
82. Newton MJ, Nesburn AB: Lack of hydrophilic lens discoloration in patients using dipivalyl epinephrine for glaucoma, *Am J Ophthalmol* 87:193, 1979.
83. Podos SM: Epinephrine, *Ophthalmology* 87:721, 1980.
84. Pollack IP, Rossi H: Norepinephrine in treatment of ocular hypertension and glaucoma, *Arch Ophthalmol* 93:173, 1975.
85. Mindel JS, Shaikewitz ST, Podos SM: Is phenylephrine pivalate a prodrug? *Arch Ophthalmol* 98:2220, 1980.
86. Haddad NJ, Moyer NJ, Riley Jr FC: Mydriatic effect of phenylephrine hydrochloride, *Am J Ophthalmol* 70:729, 1970.
87. Forman AR: A new low-concentration preparation for mydriasis and cycloplegia, *Ophthalmology* 87:213, 1980.
88. Korczyn AD, Laor N, Nemet P: Sympathetic pupillary tone in old age, *Arch Ophthalmol* 94:1905, 1976.
89. Barbee RF, Smith WO: A comparative study of mydriatic and cycloplegic agents, *Am J Ophthalmol* 44:617, 1957.
90. De Ocampo G, Lim-Catipon P: Phenylephrine pack for flat anterior chamber following cataract extraction, *Am J Ophthalmol* 66:881, 1968.
91. Weiss DI, Shaffer RN: Mydriatic effects of one-eighth percent phenylephrine, *Arch Ophthalmol* 68:727, 1962.
92. Lee PF: The influence of epinephrine and phenylephrine on intraocular pressure, *Arch Ophthalmol* 60:863, 1958.
93. Putterman AM, Urist MJ: Muller muscle-conjunctiva resection, *Arch Ophthalmol* 93:619, 1975.
94. Thompson HS, Mensher JH: Adrenergic mydriasis in Horner's syndrome, *Am J Ophthalmol* 72:472, 1971.
95. Solosko D, Smith RB: Hypertension following 10 percent phenylephrine ophthalmic, *Anesthesiology* 36:187, 1972.
96. Fraunfelder FT: Interim report: national registry of possible drug-induced ocular side effects, *Trans Am Acad Ophthalmol* 86:126, 1979.
97. Fraunfelder FT, Scafidi A: Possible adverse effects from topical ocular 10% phenylephrine, *Am J Ophthalmol* 85:447, 1978.
98. Leopold IH: The phenylephrine saga—a drug dilemma, *Am J Ophthalmol* 85:572, 1978.
99. Robertson D: Contraindication to the use of ocular phenylephrine in idiopathic orthostatic hypotension, *Am J Ophthalmol* 87:819, 1979.
100. Kim JM, Stevenson CE, Mathewson HS: Hypertensive reactions to phenylephrine eyedrops in patients with sympathetic denervation, *Am J Ophthalmol* 85:862, 1978.
101. Brown MM, Brown GC, Spaeth GL: Lack of side effects from topically administered 10% phenylephrine eyedrops, *Arch Ophthalmol* 98:487, 1980.
102. Chin NB, Gold AA, Breinin G: Iris cysts and miotics, *Arch Ophthalmol* 71:611, 1964.
103. Mitsui Y, Takage Y, Machi K: Nature of aqueous floaters due to sympathomimetic mydriatics, *Arch Ophthalmol* 65:626, 1961.
104. Epstein DL, Boger WP, Grant WM: Phenylephrine provocative testing in the pigmentary dispersion syndrome, *Am J Ophthalmol* 97:937, 1979.
105. Edelhauser HF, Hine JE, Pederson H, and others: The effect of phenylephrine on the cornea, *Arch Ophthalmol* 97:937, 1979.
106. Staatz WD, Edelhauser HF, Lehner R, and others: Cytotoxicity of pivalylphenylephrine and pivalic acid to corneal endothelium, *Arch Ophthalmol* 98:1279, 1980.
107. Cohen KL, Van Horn DL, Edelhauser HF, and others: Effect of phenylephrine on normal and regenerated endothelial cells in cat cornea, *Invest Ophthalmol* 18:242, 1979.
108. Edelhauser H, Van Horn D: Personal communication.
109. Escobar JI, Karno M: Chronic hallucinosis from nasal drops, *JAMA* 247:1859, 1982.
110. Abelson MB, Yamamoto GK, Allansmith MR: Effects of ocular decongestants, *Arch Ophthalmol* 98:856, 1980.
111. Abelson MB, Allansmith MR, Friedlaender MH: Effects of topically applied ocular decongestant and antihistamine, *Am J Ophthalmol* 90:254, 1980.
112. Sneddon JM, Turner P: The interactions

of local guanethidine and sympathomimetic amines in the human eye, *Arch Ophthalmol* 81:622, 1969.

113. Mindel JS: Hydroxyamphetamine test in Horner's syndrome, *Am J Ophthalmol* 79:523, 1975.
114. Maloney WF, Younge BR, Moyer NJ: Evaluation of the causes and accuracy of pharmacologic localization in Horner's syndrome, *Am J Ophthalmol* 90:934, 1980.
115. Thompson HS: Pharmacologic localization in Horner's syndrome, *Am J Ophthalmol* 91:416, 1981.
116. Barash PG, Kopriva CJ, Langou R, and others: Is cocaine a sympathetic stimulant during general anesthesia? *JAMA* 243:1437, 1980.
117. Patil PN: Cocaine binding by the pigmented and the nonpigmented iris and its relevance to the mydriatic effect, College of Pharmacy, The Ohio State University (experimental work), Columbus, Ohio.
118. Koelle GB: Functional anatomy of synaptic transmission, *Anesthesiology* 29:643, 1968.
119. Seidehamel RJ, Patil PN: An analysis of ephedrine mydriasis in relationship to iris pigmentation in the guinea pig eye, *J Pharmacol Exp Ther* 171:205, 1970.
120. Harrison R, Kaufmann CS: Clonidine: effect of a topically administered solution on intraocular pressure and blood pressure in open angle glaucoma, *Arch Ophthalmol* 95:1368, 1977.
121. Gharagozloo NZ, Brubaker RF: Effect of apraclonidine in long-term timolol users, *Ophthalmology* 98:1543, 1991.
122. Koskela T, Brubaker RF: Apraclonidine and timolol: combined effects in previously untreated normal subjects, *Arch Ophthalmol* 109:804, 1991.
123. Taldo M, Shin DH, Parrow KA, and others: Additive effect of 1% apraclonidine hydrochloride to nonselective beta-blockers, *Ophthalmology* 98:1075, 1991.
124. Robin AL, Pollack IP, de Faller JM: Effects of topical ALO 2145 (p-aminoclonidine hydrochloride) on the acute intraocular pressure rise after argon laser iridotomy, *Arch Ophthalmol* 105:1208, 1987.
125. Robin AL, Pollack IP, House B, and others: Effects of ALO 2145 on intraocular pressure following argon laser trabeculoplasty, *Arch Ophthalmol* 105:646, 1987.
126. Hill RA, Minckler DS, Lee M, and others: Apraclonidine prophylaxis for postcycloplegic intraocular pressure spikes, *Ophthalmology* 98:1083, 1991.
127. Coleman AL, Robin AL, Pollack IP, and others: Cardiovascular and intraocular pressure effects and plasma concentrations of apraclonidine, *Arch Ophthalmol* 108:1264, 1990.

## SECTION TWO

1. Bonomi L, DiComite P: Outflow facility after guanethidine sulfate administration, *Arch Ophthalmol* 78:337, 1967.
2. Bonomi L, DiComite P: Effect of guanethidine and other sympatholytic drugs, *Am J Ophthalmol* 59:544, 1965.
3. Riley FC, Moyer NJ: Experimental Horner's syndrome: a pupillographic evaluation of guanethidine-induced adrenergic blockage in humans, *Am J Ophthalmol* 69:442, 1970.
4. Diamond JG: 6-Hydroxydopamine in treatment of open-angle glaucoma, *Arch Ophthalmol* 94:41, 1976.
5. Talusan E, Schwartz B, Mandell AI, and others: 6-Hydroxydopamine in the treatment of open-angle glaucoma, *Am J Ophthalmol* 92:792, 1981.
6. Holland MG, Wei CP, Gupta S: Review and evaluation of 6-hydroxydopamine (6HD): chemical sympathectomy for the treatment of glaucoma, *Ann Ophthalmol* 5:539, 1973.
7. Holland MG: Treatment of glaucoma by chemical sympathectomy with 6-hydroxydopamine, *Trans Am Acad Ophthalmol Otolaryngol* 76:437 1972.
8. Holland MG, Mims JL: Anterior segment chemical sympathectomy by 6-hydroxydopamine, *Invest Ophthalmol* 10:130, 1971.
9. Watanabe H, Levene RZ, Berstein MR: 6-Hydroxydopamine therapy in glaucoma, *Trans Am Acad Ophthalmol Otolaryngol* 83:69, 1977.
10. Holland MG, Wei C: Chemical sympathectomy in glaucoma therapy: an investigation of alpha and beta adrenergic supersensitivity, *Ann Ophthalmol* 5:783, 1973.
11. Wand M, Grant WM: Thymoxamine hydrochloride: an alpha-adrenergic blocker, *Surv Ophthalmol* 25:75, 1980.
12. Lee DA, Brubaker RF, Nagataki S: Effect of thymoxamine on aqueous humor formation in the normal human eye as measured by fluorophotometry, *Invest Ophthalmol* 21:805, 1981.
13. Halasa AH, Rutkowski PC: Thymoxamine therapy for angle-closure glaucoma, *Arch Ophthalmol* 90:117, 1973.

14. Wand M, Grant WM: Thymoxamine test, *Arch Ophthalmol* 96:1009, 1978.
15. Allinson RW, Gerber DS, Bieber S, and others: Reversal of mydriasis by dapiprazole, *Ann Ophthalmol* 22:131, 1990.

## SECTION THREE

1. Graziano MP, Gilman AG: Guanine nucleotide-binding regulatory proteins: mediators of transmembrane signaling, *Trends Pharmacol Sci* 8:478, 1987.
2. Nathanson JA: Human ciliary process adrenergic receptor: pharmacological characterization, *Invest Ophthalmol Vis Sci* 21:798, 1981.
3. Vogel R, Clineschmidt CM, Hoeh H, and others: The effect of timolol, betaxolol, and placebo on corneal sensitivity in healthy volunteers, *J Ocular Pharmacol* 6:85, 1990.
4. Weissman SS, Asbell PA: Effects of topical timolol (0.5%) and betaxolol (0.5%) on corneal sensitivity, *Br J Ophthalmol* 74:409, 1990.
5. Draeger J: Local anesthetic effects of beta blockers. In Draeger J, Ackerman M, Buhr-Unger M, and others, editors: *Corneal sensitivity: measurement and clinical importance,* New York, 1984, Springer-Verlag New York, p 78.
6. Spinelli D, Vigasio F, Montenari P: Short-term and long-term timolol maleate effects on corneal sensitivity, *Doc Ophthalmol* 56:385, 1984.
7. Levine L: Clinical implications of reported timolol-induced side effects, *Am J Optometry Physiol Optics* 59:523, 1982.
8. Van Buskirk EM: Adverse reactions from timolol administration, *Ophthalmology* 87:447, 1980.
9. Goldberg M, Fenster PE: Clinical significance of intrinsic sympathomimetic activity of beta blockers, *Drug Ther* 21:35, 1991.
10. Topper JE, Brubaker RF: Effects of timolol, epinephrine and acetazolamide on aqueous flow during sleep, *Invest Ophthalmol Vis Sci* 26:1315, 1985.
11. Wentworth WO, Brubaker RF: Aqueous humor dynamics in a series of patients with 3rd neuron Horner's syndrome, *Am J Ophthalmol* 92:407, 1981.
12. Airaksinen PJ: The long-term hypotensive effect of timolol maleate compared with the effect of pilocarpine in simple and capsular glaucoma, *Acta Ophthalmol* 57:425, 1979.
13. Patil PN, Weber PA: *In vivo* functional implications of isoproterenol-mediated relaxation of isolated human iris sphincter, *J Ocular Pharmacol* 7:297, 1991.
14. Phillips CI, Howitt G, Rowlands PJ: Propranolol as ocular hypotensive agent, *Br J Ophthalmol* 51:222, 1967.
15. Bucci MG, Giraldi JP, Missiroli A, and others: La somministrazione locale del propranololol nella terapia del glaucoma, *Bol Ocul* 47:51, 1968.
16. Boger WP: Beta adrenergic blocking agents and glaucoma, *JCE Ophthalmol* 14:14, 1978.
17. Boger III WP: Shortterm "escape" and longterm "drift." The dissipation effects of the beta adrenergic blocking agents, *Surv Ophthalmol* 28(suppl): 235, 1983.
18. Oksala A, Salminen L: Tachyphylaxie bei timolol behandlung des chronischen, *Klin Monatsbl Augenheilkd* 177:451, 1980.
19. Boger III WP: The treatment of glaucoma: role of β-blocking agents, *Drugs* 18:25, 1979.
20. LeBlanc RP, Saheb NE, Krip G: Timolol: long-term Canadian multicentre study, *Can J Ophthalmol* 20:128, 1985.
21. Boger III WP, Puliafito GA, Steinert RF, and others: Long-term experience with timolol ophthalmic solution in patients with open angle glaucoma, *Ophthalmology* 85:259, 1978.
22. Steinert RF, Thomas JV, Boger III WP: Long-term drift and continued efficacy after multi-year timolol therapy, *Arch Ophthalmol* 99:100, 1981.
23. Krupin T, Singer PR, Perlmutter J, and others: One-hour intraocular pressure response to timolol: lack of correlation with long-term response, *Arch Ophthalmol* 99:840, 1981.
24. Gandolfi SA: Restoring sensitivity to timolol after long-term drift in primary open angle glaucoma, *Invest Ophthalmol Vis Sci* 31:354, 1990.
25. Batterbury M, Harding SP, Wong D: Long-term drift and timolol therapy: possible role for pulsed therapy, *Int Ophthalmol* 16:321, 1992.
26. Fraunfelder FT, Meyer SM: Systemic adverse reactions to glaucoma medications, *Int Ophthalmol Clin* 29:143, 1989.
27. Passo MS, Palmer EA, Van Buskirk EM: Plasma timolol in glaucoma patients, *Ophthalmology* 91:1361, 1984.
28. Charap AD, Shin DH, Petursson G, and

others: Effect of varying drop size on the efficacy and safety of a topical beta blocker, *Ann Ophthalmol* 21:351, 1989.
29. Bill A: Ocular circulation. In Moses RA, editor: *Adler's physiology of the eye. Clinical applications,* St Louis, 1981, Mosby, p 184.
30. Szalay J, Fliegenspan J, Zaager A, and others: Effect of beta adrenergic agents on blood vessels of the rat iris: I. Permeability to carbon particles, *Exp Eye Res* 31:289, 1980.
31. Grajewski AL, Ferrari-Dileo G, Feuer WJ, and others: Beta-adrenergic responsiveness of choroidal vasculature, *Ophthalmology* 98:989, 1991.
32. Elena PP, Kosina-Boix M, Moulin G, and others: Autoradiographic localization of beta-adrenergic receptors in rabbit eye, *Invest Ophthalmol Vis Sci* 28:1436, 1987.
33. Bruinink A, Dawis S, Niemeyer G, and others: Catecholaminergic binding sites in cat retina, pigment epithelium and choroid, *Exp Eye Res* 43:147, 1986.
34. Ferrari-Dileo G: $\beta_1$ and $\beta_2$ adrenergic binding sites in bovine retina and retinal blood vessels, *Invest Ophthalmol Vis Sci* 29:695, 1988.
35. Kobayashi H, Iwasaki T, Izumi F, and others: Adrenergic receptors in bovine retinal microvessels: presence of $\alpha_2$ and $\beta$ but not $\alpha_1$ receptors, *Neuroscience* 24:237, 1988.
36. Ramachandran E, Frank RN, Kennedy A: Effects of endothelin on cultured bovine retinal microvascular pericytes, *Invest Ophthalmol Vis Sci* 34:586, 1993.
37. Ferrari-Dileo G, Davis EB, Anderson DR: Effects of cholinergic and adrenergic agonists on adenylate cyclase activity of retinal microvascular pericytes in culture, *Invest Ophthalmol Vis Sci* 33:42, 1992.
38. Wallow IHK, Bindley CD, Reboussin DM, and others: Systemic hypertension produces pericyte changes in retinal capillaries, *Invest Ophthalmol Vis Sci* 34:420, 1993.
39. Shin DH, Tsai CS, Parrow KA, and others: Intraocular pressure-dependent retinal vascular change in adult chronic open-angle glaucoma patients, *Ophthalmology* 98:1087, 1991.
40. Lanigan LP, Clark CV, Allawi J, and others: Impaired autoregulation of the retinal vasculature and microalbuminuria in diabetes mellitus, *Eye* 4:174, 1990.
41. Gasser P: Ocular vasospasm: a risk factor in the pathogenesis of low-tension glaucoma, *Int Ophthalmol* 13:281, 1989.
42. Guthauser U, Flammer J, Mahler F: The relationship between digital and ocular vasospasm, *Graefes Arch Ophthalmol* 226:224, 1988.
43. Gasser P, Flammer J: Influence of vasospasm on visual function, *Doc Ophthalmol* 66:3, 1987.
44. Bessho H, Suzuki J, Tobe A: Vascular effects of betaxolol, a cardioselective β-adrenoceptor antagonist, in isolated rat arteries, *Jpn J Pharmacol* 55:351, 1991.
45. Hester K, Chen Z, Becker EJ, and others: The vascular relaxant effects of betaxolol, carteolol and timolol on potassium-induced tone in the porcine long posterior ciliary artery, *Invest Ophthalmol Vis Sci* 33:809, 1992.
46. Wilson RP, Kanal N, Spaeth GL: Timolol: its effectiveness in different types of glaucoma, *Ophthalmology* 86:43, 1979.
47. Phillips CI: Timolol in operated closed-angle glaucoma, *Br J Ophthalmol* 64:240, 1980.
48. Kramer P, Ritch R: The treatment of acute angle-closure glaucoma revisited, *Ann Ophthalmol* 16:1101, 1984.
49. Lass JH, Pavan-Langston D: Timolol therapy in secondary angle-closure glaucoma post penetrating keratoplasty, *Ophthalmology* 86:51, 1979.
50. Morgan KS, Black B, Ellis FD, and others: Treatment of congenital glaucoma, *Am J Ophthalmol* 92:799, 1981.
51. Zimmerman TJ, Kooner KS, Morgan KS: Safety and efficacy of timolol in pediatric glaucoma, *Surv Ophthalmol* 28(suppl):262, 1983.
52. Boger III WP: Timolol in childhood glaucoma, *Surv Ophthalmol* 28(suppl):259, 1983.
53. McMahon CD, Hetherington Jr J, Hoskins Jr HD, and others: Timolol and pediatric glaucomas, *Ophthalmology* 88:249, 1981.
54. Hoskins Jr HD, Hetherington Jr J, Magee SD, and others: Clinical experience with timolol in childhood glaucoma, *Arch Ophthalmol* 103:1163, 1985.
55. Frazer DG, Kidd MN, Johnston PB: Ghost cell glaucoma in phakic eyes, *Int Ophthalmol* 11:51, 1987.
56. Ritch R: Treatment of pigmentary glaucoma, *J Glaucoma* 2:44, 1993.
57. Pham Duy T, Wollensak J, Becker U: Elevation of intraocular pressure following Nd-YAG laser capsulotomy, *Klin Monatsbl Augenheilkd* 191:270, 1987.
58. Migliori ME, Beckman H, Channell MM: Intraocular pressure changes after

neodymium-YAG laser capsulotomy, *Arch Ophthalmol* 105:473, 1987.
59. Tomoda T, Tuberville AW, Wood TO: Timolol and postoperative intraocular pressure, *J Am Intra-Ocular Implant Soc* 10:180, 1984.
60. Polansky JR: Beta-adrenergic therapy for glaucoma, *Int Ophthalmol Clin* 30:219, 1990.
61. Berson FG, Epstein DL: Separate and combined effects of timolol maleate and acetazolamide, *Am J Ophthalmol* 92:788, 1981.
62. Kass MA: Efficacy of combining timolol with other antiglaucoma medications, *Surv Ophthalmol* 28(suppl):274, 1983.
63. Steinbach PD, Gruia DG: Long-term study of chronic glaucoma treated with beta blockers (timolol), *Klin Monatsbl Augenheilkd* 190:534, 1987.
64. Soderstrom MB, Wallin O, Granstrom PA, and others: Timolol-pilocarpine combined vs timolol and pilocarpine given separately, *Am J Ophthalmol* 107:465, 1989.
65. Schnarr KD, Merte HJ: Effectiveness and tolerance of an active combination of timolol and pilocarpine, *Klin Monatsbl Augenheilkd* 191:436, 1987.
66. David R, Ober M, Masi R, and others: Treatment of elevated intraocular pressure with concurrent levobunolol and pilocarpine, *Can J Ophthalmol* 22:208, 1987.
67. Airaksinen PJ, Valkonen R, Stenborg T, and others: A double-masked study of timolol and pilocarpine combined, *Am J Ophthalmol* 104:587, 1987.
68. Scharrer A, Ober M: Metipranolol 0.1% and pilocarpine 2% as a fixed combination compared to each substance alone in the treatment of glaucoma. A controlled, randomized clinical study comparing the intraindividual effects and tolerance, *Klin Monatsbl Augenheilkd* 189:450, 1986.
69. Lofors KT, Hovding G, Viksmoen L, and others: Twelve-hour IOP control obtained by a single dose of timolol/pilocarpine, *Acta Ophthalmol* 68:323, 1990.
70. van der Pol BA, Wattel E: Timolol and aceclidine. A clinical study of interaction in the eye, *Acta Ophthalmol* 63:411, 1985.
71. Morrison JC, Robin AL: Adjunctive glaucoma therapy. A comparison of apraclonidine to dipivefrin, *Ophthalmology* 96:3, 1989.
72. Gharagozloo NZ, Brubaker RF: Effect of apraclonidine in long-term timolol users, *Ophthalmology* 98:1543, 1991.
73. Allen RC, Robin AL, Long D, and others: A combination of levobunolol and dipivefrin for the treatment of glaucoma, *Arch Ophthalmol* 106:904, 1988.
74. Pfeiffer N, Grehn F: Treatment of glaucoma chronicum simplex with a combination of 0.5 percent timolol with 0.5 percent adrenaline plus 0.3 percent guanethidine, *Klin Monatsbl Augenheilkd* 194:161, 1989.
75. Parrow KA, Hong YJ, Shin DH, and others: Is it worthwhile to add dipivefrin HCl 0.1% to topical beta 1-, beta 2-blocker therapy? *Ophthalmology* 96:1338, 1989.
76. Clark JB, Brooks AM, Harper CA, and others: A comparison of the efficacy of betaxolol and timolol in ocular hypertension with or without adrenaline, *Aust NZ J Ophthalmol* 17:173, 1989.
77. Tsoy EA, Meekins BB, Shields MB: Comparison of two treatment schedules for combined timolol and dipivefrin, *Am J Ophthalmol* 102:320, 1986.
78. West RH, Gillies WE, Brooks AM: Therapeutic response interactions between timolol maleate and dipivefrin hydrochloride, *Aust NZ J Ophthalmol* 15:131, 1987.
79. Allen RC, Epstein DL: Additive effect of betaxolol and epinephrine in primary open angle, *Arch Ophthalmol* 104:1178, 1986.
80. Longstaff S, Benson MT, Rennie IG: A controlled study of the combined effect of carteolol and dipivefrin in glaucoma patients. In Khoo CY, Ang BC, Cheah WM, and others, editors: *New frontiers in ophthalmology,* New York, 1991, Elsevier North Holland, 1038.
81. Villumsen J, Alm A: The effect of adding prostaglandin $F_2$ alpha-isopropylester to timolol, *Arch Ophthalmol* 108:1102, 1990.
82. Lee PY, Shao H, Camras CB, and others: Additivity of prostaglandin $F_2$ alpha-1-isopropyl ester to timolol, *Ophthalmology* 98:1079, 1991.
83. Weinreb RN, Caldwell DR, Goode SM, and others: A double-masked three-month comparison between 0.25% betaxolol suspension and 0.5% betaxolol ophthalmic solution, *Am J Ophthalmol* 110:189, 1990.
84. Weinreb RN, Jani R: A novel formulation of an ophthalmic beta-adrenoceptor antagonist, *J Parenter Sci Technol* 46:51, 1992.
85. Reiss GR, Brubaker RF: The mechanism of betaxolol, a new ocular hypotensive agent, *Ophthalmology* 90:1369, 1983.

86. Berrospi AR, Leibowitz HM: Betaxolol. A new beta-adrenergic blocking agent for treatment of glaucoma, *Arch Ophthalmol* 100:943, 1982.
87. Berry DP, Van Buskirk EM, Shields MB: Betaxolol and timolol: a comparison of efficacy and side effects, *Arch Ophthalmol* 102:42, 1984.
88. Schoene RB, Abuan T, Ward RL, and others: Effects of topical betaxolol, timolol and placebo on pulmonary function in asthmatic bronchitis, *Am J Ophthalmol* 97:86, 1984.
89. Ofner S, Smith TJ: Betaxolol in chronic obstructive pulmonary disease, *J Ocular Pharmacol* 3:171, 1987.
90. Brooks AM, Gillies WE, West RH: Betaxolol eye drops as a safe medication to lower intraocular pressure, *Aust NZ J Ophthalmol* 15:125, 1987.
91. Bleckmann H, Dorow P: Treatment with betaxolol and placebo eyedrops in patients with glaucoma, *Klin Monatsbl Augenheilkd* 191:199, 1987.
92. Hesse RJ, Swan JL: Aphakic cystoid macular edema secondary to betaxolol therapy, *Ophthalmol Surg* 19:562, 1988.
93. Atkins JM, Pugh BR, Timewell RM: Cardiovascular effects of topical beta-blockers during exercise, *Am J Ophthalmol* 99:173, 1985.
94. LeJeunne C, Munera Y, Hugues F-C: Systemic effects of three β-blocker eyedrops: comparison in healthy volunteers of $\beta_1$- and $\beta_2$ adrenoceptor inhibition, *Clin Pharmacol Ther* 47:578, 1990.
95. Feghali JG, Kaufman PL: Decreased intraocular pressure in the hypertensive human eye with betaxolol, a beta 1-adrenergic antagonist, *Am J Ophthalmol* 100:777, 1985.
96. Feghali JG, Kaufman PL, Radius RL, and others: A comparison of betaxolol and timolol in open angle glaucoma and ocular hypertension, *Acta Ophthalmol* 66:180, 1988.
97. Stewart RH, Kimbrough RL, Ward RL: Betaxolol vs timolol. A six-month double-blind comparison, *Arch Ophthalmol* 104:46, 1986.
98. Allen RC, Hertzmark E, Walker AM, and others: A double-masked comparison of betaxolol vs timolol in the treatment of open angle glaucoma, *Am J Ophthalmol* 101:535, 1986.
99. Levy NS, Boone L, Ellis E: A controlled comparison of betaxolol and timolol with long-term evaluation of safety and efficacy, *Glaucoma* 7:54, 1985.
100. Collignon-Brach J: Long-term effect of ophthalmic beta-adrenoceptor antagonists on intraocular pressure and retinal sensitivity in primary open angle glaucoma, *Curr Eye Res* 11:1, 1992.
101. Messmer C, Stumpfig D, Flammer J: Influence of betaxolol and timolol on the visual fields of patients with glaucoma, *Am J Ophthalmol* 112:678, 1991.
102. Kitazawa Y, Horie T, Shirato S: Efficacy and safety of carteolol hydrochloride: a new beta-blocking agent for the treatment of glaucoma. In Henkind P, Shimizu K, Blodi FC, and others, editors: *Acta International Congress of Ophthalmology,* vol 1, Philadelphia, 1982, JB Lippincott, p 683.
103. Kitazawa Y, Azuma I, Takase M, and others: Ocular hypotensive effects of carteolol hydrochloride in primary open-angle glaucoma and ocular hypertensive patients. A double-masked cross-over study for the determination of concentrations optimal for the clinical use, *Nippon Ganka Gakkai Zasshi* 85:798, 1981.
104. Duff GR, Newcombe RG: The 12-hour control of intraocular pressure on carteolol 2% twice daily, *Br J Ophthalmol* 72:890, 1988.
105. Duff GR, Graham PA: A double-crossover trial comparing the effects of topical carteolol and placebo on intraocular pressure, *Br J Ophthalmol* 72:27, 1988.
106. Araie M, Takase M, Komuro Y: Effects of various antiglaucomatous eye drops on human aqueous humor dynamics: a fluorophotometric study. In Henkind P, editor: *Acta International Congress of Ophthalmology,* vol 1, Philadelphia, 1983, JB Lippincott, p 708.
107. Diestelhorst M, Krieglstein GK: The effect of betablockers with and without ISA on tonographic outflow facility, *Int Ophthalmol* 13:63, 1989.
108. Schnaudigel OE, Becker H, Fuchs HB: Carteolol: general practice-oriented assessment of the effectiveness and tolerance of a new beta-blocker in the treatment of glaucoma, *Klin Monatsbl Augenheilkd* 192:248, 1988.
109. Schnarr KD: Comparative multicenter study of carteolol eyedrops with other beta blockers, *Klin Monatsbl Augenheilkd* 192:167, 1988.
110. Flammer J, Kitazawa Y, Bonomi L, and others: Influence of carteolol and timolol

on IOP and visual fields in glaucoma: a multi-center, double-masked, prospective study, *Eur J Ophthalmol* 2:169, 1992.

111. Scoville B, Mueller B, White BG, and others: A double-masked comparison of carteolol and timolol in ocular hypertension, *Am J Ophthalmol* 105:150, 1988.
112. Ohno S, Ichiishi A, Matsuda H: Hypotensive effect of carteolol on intraocular pressure elevation and secondary glaucoma associated with endogenous uveitis, *Ophthalmologica* 199:41, 1989.
113. Hugues FC, Le Jeunne C, Munera Y, and others: Comparison of the effects of carteolol and metipranolol eyedrops on the ventilatory and cardiovascular functions in asthmatics, *J Fr Ophthalmol* 10:485, 1987.
114. Novack GD: Ophthalmic beta blockers since timolol, *Surv Ophthalmol* 31:307, 1987.
115. Yablonski ME, Novack GD, Burke PJ, and others: The effect of levobunolol on aqueous humor dynamics, *Exp Eye Res* 44:49, 1987.
116. Calugaru M: The effect of levobunolol eyedrops on trabecular outflow of aqueous humor, *Klin Monatsbl Augenheilkd* 194:164, 1989.
117. Partamian LG, Kass MA, Gordon M: A dose-response study of the effect of levobunolol on ocular, *Am J Ophthalmol* 95:229, 1983.
118. Long D, Zimmerman T, Spaeth G, and others: Minimum concentration of levobunolol required to control intraocular pressure, *Am J Ophthalmol* 99:18, 1985.
119. Szymankiewiczowa S: Vistagan-Liquifilm in the treatment of simple glaucoma, *Klin Oczna* 91:163, 1989.
120. Wandel T, Fishman D, Novack GD, and others: Ocular hypotensive efficacy of 0.25% levobunolol instilled once daily, *Ophthalmology* 95:252, 1988.
121. Rakofsky SI, Melamed S, Cohen JS, and others: A comparison of the ocular hypotensive efficacy of once-daily and twice-daily levobunolol treatment, *Ophthalmology* 96:8, 1989.
122. Derick RJ, Robin AL, Tielsch J, and others: Once-daily versus twice-daily levobunolol (0.5%) therapy. A crossover study, *Ophthalmology* 99:424, 1992.
123. Rakofsky SI, Lazar M, Almog Y, and others: Efficacy and safety of once-daily levobunolol for glaucoma therapy, *Can J Ophthalmol* 24:2, 1989.
124. Rose A, Stoecker J, Kelley E, and others: Evaluation of once-daily levobunolol 0.25% and timolol 0.25% therapy for increased intraocular pressure, *Am J Ophthalmol* 112:56, 1991.
125. Boozman FW, Carriker R, Foerster R, and others: Long-term evaluation of 0.25% levobunolol and timolol for therapy for elevated intraocular pressure, *Arch Ophthalmol* 106:614, 1988.
126. Levobunolol. A four-year study of efficacy and safety in glaucoma, *Ophthalmology* 96:642, 1989.
127. Novack GD, Kelley EP, Lue JC: A multicenter evaluation of levobunolol (Vistagan) in Germany, *Ophthalmologica* 197:90, 1988.
128. Seamone C, LeBlanc R, Saheb N, and others: Efficacy of twice-daily levobunolol in the treatment of elevated intraocular pressure, *Can J Ophthalmol* 23:168, 1988.
129. Wilhelmus KR, McCulloch RR, Gross RL: Dendritic keratopathy associated with beta-blocker eyedrops, *Cornea* 9:335, 1990.
130. Schultheiss E: Hypersensitivity to levobunolol, *Derm Beruf Umwelt-Occupat Environ Derm* 37:185, 1989.
131. Bosem ME, Lusky M, Weinreb RN: Short-term effects of levobunolol on ocular pulsatile flow, *Am J Ophthalmol* 114:280, 1992.
132. Smith DA, Trope GE: Effect of a beta-blocker on altered body position: induced ocular hypertension, *Br J Ophthal mol* 74:605, 1990.
133. Battershill PE, Sorkin EM: Ocular metipranolol. A preliminary review of its pharmacodynamic and pharmacokinetic properties, and therapeutic efficacy in glaucoma and ocular hypertension, *Drugs* 36:601, 1988.
134. Demailly P, Lecherpie F: Metipranolol 0.1%: effect of a single dose on the nycthemeral pressure, *J Fr Ophtalmol* 10:447, 1987.
135. Krieglstein GK, Novack GD, Voepel E, and others: Levobunolol and metipranolol: comparative ocular hypotensive efficacy, *Br J Ophthalmol* 71:250, 1987.
136. Mills KB, Wright G: A blind randomised cross-over trial comparing metipranolol 0.3% with timolol 0.25% in open-angle glaucoma: a pilot study, *Br J Ophthalmol* 70:39, 1986.
137. Serle JB, Lustgarten JS, Podos SM: A clinical trial of metipranolol, a noncardioselective beta-adrenergic antagonist, in ocular hypertension, *Am J Ophthalmol* 112:302, 1991.
138. Hickey-Dwyer M, Campbell SH, Harding S: Doubled-masked three-period crossover

investigation of metipranolol in control of raised intraocular pressure, *J Ocular Pharmacol* 7:277, 1991.

139. Akingbehin T, Villada JR: Metipranolol-associated granulomatous anterior uveitis, *Br J Ophthalmol* 75:519, 1991.
140. Mills KB, Jacobs NJ, Vogel R: A study of the effects of four concentrations of D-timolol, 0.25%, 0.25% L-timolol, and placebo on intraocular pressure on patients with raised intraocular pressure, *Br J Ophthalmol* 72:469, 1988.
141. Nathanson JA: Stereospecificity of beta adrenergic antagonists: R-enantiomers show increased selectivity for beta-2 receptors in ciliary process, *J Pharmacol Exp Ther* 245:94, 1988.
142. Zimmerman TJ, Harbin R, Pett M, and others: Timolol and outflow facility, *Invest Ophthalmol* 16:623, 1977.
143. Sonntag JR, Brindley GO, Shields MB: Effect of timolol on outflow facility, *Invest Ophthalmol* 17:293, 1978.
144. Coakes RL, Brubaker RF: The mechanism of timolol in lowering intraocular pressure, *Arch Ophthalmol* 96:2045, 1978.
145. Katz IM, Berger ET: Effects of iris pigmentation on response of ocular pressure to timolol, *Surv Ophthalmol* 23:395, 1979.
146. Schlecht LP, Brubaker RF: The effects of withdrawal of timolol in chronically treated glaucoma, *Ophthalmology* 95:1212, 1988.
147. Schenker HI, Yablonski ME, Podos SM, and others: Fluorophotometric study of epinephrine and timolol in human subjects, *Arch Ophthalmol* 99:1212, 1981.
148. Zimmerman TJ, Kaufman HE: Timolol, dose response and duration of action, *Arch Ophthalmol* 95:605, 1977.
149. David R, Zangwill L, Briscoe D, and others: Diurnal intraocular pressure variations: an analysis of 690 diurnal curves, *Br J Ophthalmol* 76:280, 1992.
150. Maclure GM: Chronic open angle glaucoma treated with Timolol. A four year study, *Trans Ophthalmol Soc UK* 103:78, 1983.
151. Alexander DW, Berson FG, Epstein DL: A clinical trial of timolol and epinephrine in the treatment of primary open angle glaucoma, *Ophthalmology* 95:247, 1988.
152. Uusitalo RJ, Palkama A: Long-term evaluation of timolol, *Acta Ophthalmol* 67:573, 1989.
153. Kuppens EV, Stolwijk TR, de Keizer RJ, and others: Basal tear turnover and topical timolol in glaucoma patients and healthy controls by fluorophotometry, *Invest Ophthalmol Vis Sci* 33:3442, 1992.
154. Marquardt R, Schubert T: Modification of tear film break-up time by beta blocker eyedrops without preservatives, *Klin Monatsbl Augenheilkd* 199:75, 1991.
155. Hugues FC, Le Jeunne C, Munera Y, and others: Evaluation of the systemic effects of timolol maleate in eye drops, *J Fr Ophtalmol* 8:389, 1985.
156. Swenson ER: Severe hyperkalemia as a complication of timolol, a topically applied beta adrenergic antagonist, *Arch Int Med* 146:1220, 1986.
157. Zamber RW, Starkebaum G, Rubin RL, and others: Drug induced systemic lupus erythematosus due to ophthalmic timolol, *J Rheumatol* 19:977, 1992.
158. Meuche C, Heidrich H, Bleckmann H: Raynaud syndrome following timolol-containing eyedrops, *Fortschr Ophthalmol* 87:45, 1990.
159. Kendall K, Mundorf T, Nardin G, and others: Tolerability of timolol and betaxolol in patients with chronic open-angle glaucoma, *Clin Ther* 9:651, 1987.
160. Coleman AL, Diehl DLC, Jampel HD, and others: Topical timolol decreases plasma high-density lipoprotein cholesterol level, *Arch Ophthalmol* 108:1260, 1990.
161. West J, Longstaff S: Topical timolol and serum lipoproteins, *Br J Ophthalmol* 74:663, 1990.
162. Kass MA: Timolol treatment prevents or delays glaucomatous visual field loss in individuals with ocular hypertension: a five-year, randomized, double-masked, clinical trial, *Trans Am Ophthalmol Soc* 87:598, 1990.
163. Epstein DL, Krug Jr JH, Hertzmark E, and others: A long-term clinical trial of timolol therapy versus no treatment in the management of glaucoma suspects, *Ophthalmology* 96:1460, 1989.
164. Chauhan BC, Drance SM, Douglas GR: The effect of long-term intraocular pressure reduction on the differential light sensitivity in glaucoma suspects, *Invest Ophthalmol Vis Sci* 29:1478, 1988.
165. Schulzer M, Drance SM, Douglas GR: A comparison of treated and untreated glaucoma suspects, *Ophthalmology* 98:301, 1991.
166. Tytla ME, Trope GE, Buncic JR: Flicker sensitivity in treated ocular hypertension, *Ophthalmology* 97:36, 1990.
167. Nesher R, Trick GL, Kass MA, and others: Steady-state pattern electroretinogram fol-

lowing long term unilateral administration of timolol to ocular hypertensive subjects, *Doc Ophthalmol* 75:101, 1990.
168. Kwitko GM, Shin DH, Ahn BH, and others: Bilateral effects of long-term monocular timolol therapy, *Am J Ophthalmol* 104:591, 1987.
169. Gibbens MV: The consensual ophthalmotonic reaction, *Br J Ophthalmol* 72:746, 1988.
170. Gibbens MV: Sympathetic influences on the consensual ophthalmotonic reaction, *Br J Ophthalmol* 72:750, 1988.
171. Martin XD, Rabineau PA: Intraocular pressure effects of timolol after unilateral instillation, *Ophthalmology* 95:1620, 1988.
172. Trew DR, Smith SE: Postural studies in pulsatile ocular blood flow: II. Chronic open angle, *Br J Ophthalmol* 75:71, 1991.
173. Grunwald JE: Effect of timolol maleate on the retinal circulation of human eyes with ocular hypertension, *Invest Ophthalmol Vis Sci* 31:521, 1990.
174. Weber RG: The effect of the beta blockers timolol and pindolol on retinal blood flow in the human eye, *New Trends Ophthalmol* 2:71, 1987.
175. Grunwald JE, Furubayashi C: Effect of topical timolol maleate on the ophthalmic artery blood pressure, *Invest Ophthalmol Vis Sci* 30:1095, 1989.
176. Van Buskirk EM, Bacon DR, Fahrenbach WH: Ciliary vasoconstriction after topical adrenergic drugs, *Am J Ophthalmol* 109:511, 1990.
177. Martin XD, Rabineau PA: Vasoconstrictive effect of topical timolol on human retinal arteries, *Graefes Arch Klin Exp Ophthalmol* 227:526, 1989.
178. Pillunat L, Stodtmeister R: Effect of different antiglaucomatous drugs on ocular perfusion pressures, *J Ocular Pharmacol* 4:231, 1988.
179. Pillunat LE, Stodtmeister R, Wilmanns I, and others: Effect of timolol on optic nerve head autoregulation, *Ophthalmologica* 193:146, 1986.

## SECTION FOUR

1. Wolter JR, O'Keefe NT: Localization of nerve endings in relation to cholinesterase deposits in normal human eye muscles, *Invest Ophthalmol* 2:558, 1963.
2. Gilman AG, Goodman LS, Gilman A: *Goodman and Gilman's: the pharmacologic basis of therapeutics,* ed 6, New York, 1980, MacMillan, p 83.
3. Leopold IH: Cholinesterase, *Am J Ophthalmol* 62:771, 1966.
4. Van Alphen GWHM, Robinette SL, Macri FJ: Drug effects on ciliary muscle and choroid preparations in vitro, *Arch Ophthalmol* 68:81, 1962.
5. Kronfeld PC: Early effects of single and repeated doses of L-epinephrine in man, *Am J Ophthalmol* 72:1058, 1971.
6. Barraqer JI: Acetylcholine as a miotic agent for use in surgery, *Am J Ophthalmol* 62:484, 1967.
7. Goodman L, Gilman A: *The pharmacological basis of therapeutics,* ed 4, New York, 1970, Macmillan.
8. Babinski M, Smith RB, Wickerham EP: Hypotension and bradycardia following intraocular acetylcholine injection, *Arch Ophthalmol* 94:675, 1976.
9. Yee RW, Wallace G, Yu M: Effects of the components of miochol and miostat on bovine corneal endothelial cells. in vitro, *Invest Ophthalmol Vis Sci* 30(suppl):335, 1989.
10. Lazar M, Rosen N, Nemet P: Miochol-induced transient cataract, *Ann Ophthalmol* 9:1142, 1977.
11. Rosen N, Lazar M: The mechanism of the miochol lens opacity, *Am J Ophthalmol* 86:570, 1978.
12. Morrison WH: Stability of aqueous solution commonly employed in the treatment of primary glaucoma, *Am J Ophthalmol* 37:391, 1954.
13. Gay AJ: Comments, *Arch Ophthalmol* 81:601, 1969.
14. Laties AM, Scheie HG: Adie's syndrome: duration of methacholine sensitivity, *Arch Ophthalmol* 74:458, 1965.
15. Hedges Jr TR: The tonic pupil, *Arch Ophthalmol* 80:21, 1968.
16. Smith AA, Dancis J, Breinin G: Ocular responses to autonomic drugs in familial dysautonomia, *Invest Ophthalmol* 4:358, 1965.
17. Velhagen IL: Die grundlager der okularen pharmakologie und toxicologie des carbaminocholins, *Arch Augenheilkd* 107:319, 1933.
18. Smolen VF, Clevenger JM, Williams EJ, and others: Biophasic availability of ophthalmic carbachol: I. Mechanism of cationic polymer and surfactant-promoted miotic activity, *J Pharm Sci* 62:958, 1973.
19. O'Brien CS, Swan KC: Carbaminoylcholine

chloride in the treatment of glaucoma simplex, *Arch Ophthalmol* 27:253, 1942.
20. Reichert R, Sheilds MB, Stewart WC: Intraocular pressure response to replacing pilocarpine with carbachol, *Am J Ophthalmol* 106:747, 1988.
21. Francois J, Goes F: Ultrasonic study of the effect of different miotics on the eye components, *Ophthalmologica* 175:328, 1977.
22. McDonald TO, Beasley C, Borgmann A, and others: Intraocular administration of carbamylcholine chloride, *Ann Ophthalmol* 1:232, 1969.
23. Ruiz RS, Rhem MN, Prager TC: Effects of carbachol and acetylcholine on intraocular pressure after cataract extraction, *Am J Ophthalmol* 107:7, 1989.
24. Linn DK, Zimmerman TJ, Nardin GF, and others: Effect of intracameral carbachol on intraocular pressure after cataract extraction, *Am J Ophthalmol* 107:133, 1989.
25. Mindel JS, Kharlamb AB: Alteration of acetylcholine synthesis by pilocarpine, *Arch Ophthalmol* 102:1546, 1984.
26. Goldstein AM, dePalau A, Botelho SY: Inhibition and facilitation of pilocarpine-induced lacrimal flow by norepinephrine, *Invest Ophthalmol* 6:498, 1967.
27. Potts A: Physiological chemistry of the eye, *Arch Ophthalmol* 66:578, 1961.
28. Muller HK, Hockwin O, Kleifeld O: Die Bestimmung von Pilocarpin in Menschlichen Kammerwasser mit Hilfer der Polarographie, *Graefes Arch Klin Exp Ophthalmol* 162:107, 1960.
29. Asseff CF, Weisman RL, Podos SM, and others: Ocular penetration of pilocarpine in primates, *Am J Ophthalmol* 75:212, 1973.
30. Krohn DL, Breitfeller JM: Transcorneal flux of topical pilocarpine to the human aqueous, *Am J Ophthalmol* 87:50, 1979.
31. Chrai SS, Robinson JR: Corneal permeation of topical pilocarpine nitrate in the rabbit, *Am J Ophthalmol* 77:735, 1974.
32. Tornqvist G: Effect of refraction of intramuscular pilocarpine in two species of monkey (*Cercopithecus aethiops* and *Macaca irus*), *Invest Ophthalmol* 4:211, 1965.
33. Tornqvist G: Accommodation in monkeys, *Acta Ophthalmol* 45:429, 1967.
34. Tornqvist T: Comparative studies of the effect of pilocarpine on the pupil and on the refraction in two species of monkey (*Cercopithecus ethiops* and *Macaca irus*), *Invest Ophthalmol* 3:388, 1964.
35. Lowenstein O: The Argyll Robertson pupillary syndrome, *Am J Ophthalmol* 42:105, 1956.
36. Schonberg SS, Ellis PP: Pilocarpine inactivation, *Arch Ophthalmol* 82:351, 1969.
37. Ellis PP, Littlejohn K: Pilocarpine hydrolysis: clinical significance, *Invest Ophthalmol* 12:931, 1973.
38. Lee BH, Hui EW, Robinson JR: Corneal metabolism of pilocarpine in pigmented rabbits, *Invest Ophthalmol Vis Sci* 19:210, 1980.
39. Van Alphen GWHM: The structural changes in miosis and mydriasis of the monkey eye, *Arch Ophthalmol* 69:802, 1963.
40. Abramson DH, Coleman DJ, Forbes M, and others: Pilocarpine: effect on the anterior chamber and lens thickness, *Arch Ophthalmol* 87:615, 1972.
41. Barany EH: The mode of action of pilocarpine on out flow resistance in the eye of a primate (*Cercopithecus ethiops*), *Invest Ophthalmol* 1:712, 1962.
42. Armaly MF, Burian HM: Changes in the tonogram during accommodation, *Arch Ophthalmol* 60:60, 1968.
43. Moses RA, Grodzki WJ: Choroid tension and facility of aqueous outflow, *Invest Ophthalmol Vis Sci* 16:1062, 1977.
44. Cairns JE: Goniospasis: a method designed to relieve canalicular blockade in primary open angle glaucoma, *Ann Ophthalmol* 8:1417, 1976.
45. Holmberg A, Barany EH: The effect of pilocarpine on the endothelium forming the inner wall of Schlemm's canal: an electron-microscope study in the monkey *Cercopithecus aethiops*, *Invest Ophthalmol* 5:53, 1966.
46. Barany EH: The immediate effect on outflow resistance of intravenous pilocarpine in the vervet monkey, *Cercopithecus ethiops*, *Invest Ophthalmol* 6:373, 1967.
47. Kaufman PL, Barany EH: Loss of acute pilocarpine effect on outflow facility following surgical disinsertion and retrodisplacement of the ciliary muscle from the scleral spur in the cynomologous monkey, *Invest Ophthalmol Vis Sci* 15:793, 1976.
48. Bleiman BS, Schwartz AL: Paradoxical intraocular pressure response of pilocarpine, *Arch Ophthalmol* 97:1305, 1979.
49. Drance SM, Nash PA: The dose response of human intraocular pressure to pilocarpine, *Can J Ophthalmol* 6:9, 1971.
50. Zimmerman TJ, Sharir M, Nardin GF, and others: Therapeutic index of pilocarpine,

carbachol, and timolol with nasolacrimal occlusion, *Am J Ophthalmol* 114:1, 1992.
51. Harris LS, Galin MA: Effect of ocular pigmentation on hypertensive response to pilocarpine, *Am J Ophthalmol* 72:923, 1971.
52. Lyons JS, Krohn DL: Pilocarpine uptake by pigmented uveal tissue, *Am J Ophthalmol* 75:885, 1973.
53. Patil PN: Cocaine binding by the pigmented and nonpigmented iris and its relevance to the mydriatic effect, *Invest Ophthalmol* 11:739, 1972.
54. Seidehamel RJ, Tye A, Patil PN: An analysis of ephedrine in relationship to iris pigmentation in the guinea pig eye in vitro, *J Pharmacol Exp Ther* 171:205, 1970.
55. Abramson DH, Chang S, Coleman J, and others: Pilocarpine-induced lens changes, *Arch Ophthalmol* 92:464, 1974.
56. Berggren L: Effect of composition of medium and of metabolic inhibitors on secretion in vitro by the ciliary processes in the rabbit eye, *Invest Ophthalmol* 4:91, 1965.
57. Berggren L: Effect of parasympathomimetic and sympathomimetic drugs on secretion in vitro by the ciliary process of the rabbit eye, *Invest Ophthalmol* 4:91, 1965.
58. Kupfer C: Drugs and glaucoma, *Trans Am Acad Ophthalmol Otolaryngol* 85:233, 1978.
59. Nagataki S, Brubaker RF: Effect of pilocarpine on aqueous humor formation in human beings, *Arch Ophthalmol* 100:818, 1982.
60. March WF, Stewart RM, Mandell AI, and others: Duration of effect of pilocarpine gel, *Arch Ophthalmol* 100:1270, 1982.
61. Stewart RH, Kimbrough RL, Smith JP, and others: Long acting pilocarpine gel: a dose response in ocular hypertensive subjects, *Glaucoma* 6:182, 1984.
62. Quigley HA, Pollack IP, Harbin Jr TS: Pilocarpine ocuserts. Long-term clinical trials and selected pharmacodynamics, *Arch Ophthalmol* 93:771, 1975.
63. Worthen DM, Zimmerman TJ, Wind CA: An evaluation of the pilocarpine ocusert, *Invest Ophthalmol Vis Sci* 13:296, 1974.
64. Epstein E, Kaufmann I: Systemic pilocarpine toxicity from overdosage, *Am J Ophthalmol* 59:109, 1965.
65. Rebolleda G, Munoz FJ, Fernandez Victorio JM, and others: Effect of pupillary dilation on automated perimetry in glaucoma patients receiving pilocarpine, *Ophthalmology* 99:418, 1992.
66. Nardia GF, Zimmerman TJ, Zalta AM, and others: Ocular cholinergic agents. In *The glaucomas*, St Louis, 1989, Mosby, p 517.
67. Alpar JJ: Miotics and retinal detachment, *Ann Ophthalmol* 11:395, 1979.
68. Pape LG, Forbes M: Retinal detachment and miotic therapy, *Am J Ophthalmol* 85:558, 1978.
69. Beasley H, Fraunfelder FT: Retinal detachments and topical ocular miotics, *Trans Am Acad Ophthalmol* 86:95, 1979.
70. Stocker FW: Experimental studies on the blood-aqueous barrier, *Arch Ophthalmol* 37:583, 1947.
71. Colasanti BK, Barany EH: Potentiation of the mydriatic effect of norepinephrine in the rabbit after monoamine oxidase inhibition, *Invest Ophthalmol* 18:200, 1979.
72. Drance SM, Fairclough M, Schulzer M: Response of human intraocular pressure to aceclidine, *Arch Ophthalmol* 88:394, 1972.
73. Fechner PU, Teichmann KD, Weyrauch W: Accommodative effects of aceclidine in the treatment of glaucoma, *Am J Ophthalmol* 79:104, 1975.
74. Fincham EF: The proportion of ciliary muscular force required for accommodation, *J Physiol* 128:99, 1955.
75. Kronfeld PS: The efficacy of combinations of ocular hypotensive drugs. A tonographic approach, *Arch Ophthalmol* 78:140, 1967.
76. Hussey HH: Physostigmine: value in treatment of central toxic effects of anticholinergic drugs, *JAMA* 231:1066, 1975.
77. Rodin FH: Eserine: its history in the practice of ophthalmology, *Am J Ophthalmol* 30:19, 1947.
78. Levensohn JE: The first miotic, *Am J Ophthalmol* 55:657, 1963.
79. Jacklin HN: Depigmentation of the eyelids in eserine allergy, *Am J Ophthalmol* 59:89, 1964.
80. Osserman KE, Teng P: Studies in myasthenia gravis—a rapid diagnostic test, *JAMA* 160:153, 1956.
81. Leopold IH, Comroe Jr JH: Effect of diisopropyl fluorophosphate (DFP) on the normal eye, *Arch Ophthalmol* 36:17, 1946.
82. de Roetth AJ: Further studies on cholinesterase activity in ocular tissues, *Am J Ophthalmol* 34:120, 1951.
83. Kadin M: Studies of total protein and radio-iodinated serum albumin (Risa) content of primary aqueous humor, *Am J Ophthalmol* 55:512, 1962.

84. Kadin M: Studies on the toxicity and effect of Dipterex in rabbits, *Am J Ophthalmol* 53:512, 1962.
85. Leopold IH, Krishna N, Lehman RA: The effects of anticholinesterase agents on the blood cholinesterase levels of normal and glaucoma subjects, *Trans Am Ophthalmol Soc* 57:63, 1959.
86. Becker B, Pyle GC, Drew RC: The tonographic effects of echothiophate (Phospholine) iodide: reversal by pyridine-2-aldoxime methiodide ($P_2AM$), *Am J Ophthalmol* 47:635, 1959.
87. Wheeler MD: Isoflurophate (DFP) in the handling of esotropia, *Arch Ophthalmol* 71:298, 1964.
88. Abraham SV: Intraepithelial cysts of the iris, *Am J Ophthalmol* 37:327, 1954.
89. Newell FW: Editorial, *Am J Ophthalmol* 56:311, 1963.
90. Wang RIH: Determining cholinesterase activity in human plasma, *JAMA* 183:792, 1963.
91. Mamo JG, Leopold IH: Oximes in ophthalmology, *Am J Ophthalmol* 46:724, 1958.
92. Kewitz H, Wilson IB: A specific antidote against lethal alkylphosphate intoxication, *Arch Biochem* 60:26, 1956.
93. Lawlor RC, Lee P: Use of echothiophate (phospholine iodide) in the treatment of glaucoma, *Am J Ophthalmol* 49:808, 1960.
94. Laties MM: Localization in cornea and lens of topically-applied irreversible cholinesterase inhibitors, *Am J Ophthalmol* 89:49, 1973.
95. Leopold IH, Furman M: Cholinesterase isoenzymes in human ocular tissue homogenates, *Am J Ophthalmol* 72:460, 1971.
96. Harris LS, Shimmyo M, Mittag TW: Cholinesterase and contractility of cat irides, *Arch Ophthalmol* 89:49, 1973.
97. Harris LS: Dose-response analysis of echothiophate iodide, *Arch Ophthalmol* 86:502, 1971.
98. Barsam PC: Comparison of the effect of pilocarpine and echothiophate on intraocular pressure and outflow facility, *Am J Ophthalmol* 73:742, 1972.
99. Harris LS: Comparison of pilocarpine and echothiophate iodide in open angle glaucoma, *Ann Ophthalmol* 4:736, 1972.
100. Kaufman PL: Anticholinesterase-induced cholinergic subsensitivity in primate accommodative mechanism, *Am J Ophthalmol* 85:622, 1978.
101. Drance SM, Carr F: Effects of phospholine iodide (217 MI) on intraocular pressure in man, *Am J Ophthalmol* 49:470, 1960.
102. Pratt-Johnson JA, Drance SM, Innes R: Comparison between pilocarpine and echothiophate for chronic simple glaucoma, *Arch Ophthalmol* 72:485, 1964.
103. Kini MM, Dahl AA, Roberts CR, and others: Echothiophate, pilocarpine, and open-angle glaucoma, *Arch Ophthalmol* 89:190, 1973.
104. Miller JE: A comparison of miotics in accommodative esotropia, *Am J Ophthalmol* 49:1350, 1960.
105. Abrahamson Jr IA, Abrahamson Sr IA: Preliminary report on 0.06 percent phospholine (echothiophate) iodide in the management of esotropia, *Am J Ophthalmol* 57:290, 1964.
106. Humphreys JA, Holmes JH: Systemic effects produced by echothiophate iodide in treatment of glaucoma, *Arch Ophthalmol* 69:834, 1966.
107. de Roetth Jr A, Wong A, Dettbarn WD, and others: Blood cholinesterase activity of glaucoma patients treated with phospholine iodide, *Am J Ophthalmol* 62:834, 1966.
108. Wahl JW, Turner GS: Echothiophate iodide, *Am J Ophthalmol* 60:419, 1965.
109. de Roeth Jr A, Dettbarn WD, Rosenberg P, and others: Effect of phospholine iodide on blood cholinesterase levels of normal and glaucoma subjects, *Am J Ophthalmol* 59:586, 1965.
110. Ellis PP: Systemic effects of locally applied anticholinesterase agents, *Invest Ophthalmol* 5:146, 1966.
111. Klayman J: Use of long-acting cholinesterase agents in glaucoma, *Invest Ophthalmol* 5:136, 1966.
112. Becker B, Pyle GC, Drew RC: The tonographic effects of echothiophate (Phospholine) iodide: Reversal by pyridine-2-aldoxime methiodide ($P_2AM$) *AM J Ophthalmol* 47:635, 1959.
113. Abraham SV: The use of a echothiophate phenylephrine formulation (echophenyline-b-3) in the treatment of convergent strabismus and amblyopia—with special emphasis on iris cysts, *J Pediatr Ophthalmol* 1:68, 1964.
114. Axelsson U, Holmberg A: The frequency of cataract after miotic therapy, *Acta Ophthalmol* 44:421, 1966.
115. Shaffer RN, Hetherington JM: Anticholinesterase drugs and cataract, *Am J Ophthalmol* 62:613, 1966.
116. de Roetth Jr A: Lens opacities in glaucoma

patients on phospholine iodide therapy, *Am J Ophthalmol* 62:619, 1966.
117. Morton WR, Drace SM, Fairclough M: Effect of echothiophate iodide on the lens, *Am J Ophthalmol* 68:1003, 1969.
118. Pietsch RL, Bobo CB, Finklea JF, and others: Lens opacities and organophosphate cholinesterase-inhibiting agents, *Am J Ophthalmol* 73:236, 1972.
119. Harrison R: Bilateral lens opacities, *Am J Ophthalmol* 50:153, 1960.
120. Diamant H: Cataract due to cholinesterase inhibitors in the guinea pig, *Acta Ophthalmol* 32:357, 1954.
121. Michon Jr J, Kinoshita JH: Cholinesterase in the lens, *Arch Ophthalmol* 79:611, 1968.
122. Michon Jr J, Kinoshita JH: Experimental miotic cataract, *Arch Ophthalmol* 79:611, 1968.
123. Michon Jr J, Kinoshita JH: Experimental miotic cataract, *Arch Ophthalmol* 70:70, 1968.
124. Albrecht M, Barany E: Early lens changes in *Macaca fascicularis* monkeys under topical treatment with echothiophate or carbachol studied by slit-image photography, *Invest Ophthalmol Vis Sci* 18:179, 1979.
125. Terner II, Lin J, Goldstrohm R: Clinical experiences with demecarium bromide (BC-48) in the treatment of glaucoma, *Am J Ophthalmol* 52:533, 1961.
126. Krishna N, Leopold IH: The effect of BC-48 (demecarium bromide) on normal rabbit and human eyes, *Am J Ophthalmol* 49:270, 1960.
127. Drance SM: Effect of demecarium bromide (BC-48) on intraocular pressure in man, *Arch Ophthalmol* 62:673, 1959.
128. Krishna N, Leopold IH: Effect of protopam on the rabbit pupil, *Am J Ophthalmol* 52:565, 1961.
129. Kewitz H, Wilson IB, Nachmansohn D: A specific antidote against lethal alkyl phosphate intoxication: II. Antidotal properties, *Arch Biochem* 64:456, 1956.
130. Hunter WS, McCulloch C: The neutralization of cholinesterase inhibition by various oximes and by atropine, *Am J Ophthalmol* 52:841, 1961.
131. Harris G, McCulloch C: Neutralization of the action of diisopropyl fluorophosphate by an oxime (monosionitrosoacetone), *Am J Ophthalmol* 50:414, 1960.
132. Grob D, Johns RJ: Use of oximes in the treatment of intoxication by anticholinesterase compounds in normal subjects, *Am J Med* 24:497, 1958.

## SECTION FIVE

1. Van Alphen GWHM, Robinette SL, Macri FJ: Drug effects on ciliary muscle and choroid preparations in vitro, *Arch Ophthalmol* 68:81, 1962.
2. Wolfe AV, Hodge HC: Effects of atropine sulfate, methylatropine nitrate (Metropine) and homatropine hydrobromide on adult human eyes, *Arch Ophthalmol* 36:293, 1946.
3. Riker WF: Contributions to medicine by research in pharmacology, *JAMA* 179:355, 1962.
4. Crandall DC, Leopold IH: The influence of systemic drugs on tear constituents, *Trans Am Acad Ophthalmol* 86:115, 1979.
5. Goodman LS, Gilman A: *The pharmacologic basis of therapeutics,* ed 4, New York, 1970, MacMillan.
6. Patil PN: Antimuscarinic effects of stereoisomers of tropicamide on rabbit iris sphincter, *Invest Ophthalmol Vis Sci* 17:65, 1978.
7. Van Alphen GWHM, Macri FJ: Entrance of fluorescein into aqueous humor of cat eye, *Arch Ophthalmol* 75:247, 1966.
8. Marron J: Cycloplegia and mydriasis by use of atropine, scopolamine, and homatropine-paredrine, *Arch Ophthalmol* 23:340, 1940.
9. Fultron AB, Dobson V, Salem D, and others: Cycloplegic refractions in infants and young children, *Am J Ophthalmol* 90:239, 1980.
10. Rosenbaum AL, Bateman JB, Bremer DL, and others: Cycloplegic refraction in esotropic children, *Ophthalmology* 88:1031, 1981.
11. Von Noorden GK, Milam JB: Penalization in the treatment of amblyopia, *Am J Ophthalmol* 88:511, 1979.
12. Von Noorden GK: Amblyopia caused by unilateral atropinization, *Ophthalmology* 88:131, 1981.
13. Gilbert HD, Jensen AD: Atropine in the treatment of traumatic hyphema, *Ann Ophthalmol* 5:1297, 1973.
14. Anderson R: Blepharocardiac reflex, *Arch Ophthalmol* 96:1419, 1978.
15. Schwartz H, Apt L: Mydriatic effect of anticholinergic drugs used during reversal of nondepolarizing muscle relaxants, *Am J Ophthalmol* 88:609, 1979.
16. Gimbel HV: The control of myopia with atropine, *Can J Ophthalmol* 8:527, 1973.
17. Dyer JA: Role of cycloplegics in progressive myopia, *Trans Am Acad Ophthalmol* 86:692, 1979.
18. Sampson WG: Role of cycloplegia in the

management of functional myopia, *Trans Am Acad Ophthalmol* 86:695, 1979.

19. Bedrossian RH: The effect of atropine on myopia, *Trans Am Acad Ophthalmol* 86:713, 1979.
20. Weinstein JM, Zweifel TJ, Thompson HS: Congenital Horner's syndrome, *Arch Ophthalmol* 98:1074, 1980.
21. Dobson V, Fulton AB, Manning K, and others: Cycloplegic refractions of premature infants, *Am J Ophthalmol* 91:490, 1981.
22. Summers WK, Reich TC: Delirium after cataract surgery: review and two cases, *Am J Psychiatry* 136:386, 1979.
23. Harris LS: Cycloplegic-induced intraocular pressure elevations, *Arch Ophthalmol* 79:242, 1968.
24. Gorin G: Glaucoma induced by prolonged use of atropine, *Am J Ophthalmol* 56:639, 1963.
25. Hilding AC: Pupillary blockage by a subluxated lens, causing glaucoma, *Am J Ophthalmol* 57:33, 1957.
26. Geyer O, Rothkoff L, Lazar M: Atropine in keratoplasty for keratoconus, *Cornea* 10:372, 1991.
27. Thorne FH, Murphey HS: Cycloplegics, *Arch Ophthalmol* 22:274, 1939.
28. Barany E, Christensen RE: Cycloplegia and outflow resistance in normal human and monkey eyes in primary open-angle glaucoma, *Arch Ophthalmol* 77:757, 1967.
29. Christensen RE, Pearce I: Homatropine hydrobromide, *Arch Ophthalmol* 70:376, 1963.
30. Doczy L: A comparison of the action of atropine and scopolamine producing cycloplegia, *Klin Monatsbl Augenheilkd* 138:398, 1961.
31. Priestley BS, Medine MM: A new mydriatic and cycloplegic drug, *Am J Ophthalmol* 34:572, 1951.
32. Apt L, Henrick A: Pupillary dilatation with single eyedrop mydriatic combinations, *Am J Ophthalmol* 89:553, 1980.
33. Gettews BC: Three new cycloplegic drugs, *Arch Ophthalmol* 51:467, 1954.
34. Schimek RA, Lieberman WJ: The influence of Cyclogyl and Neo-Synephrine on tonographic studies of miotic control in open-angle glaucoma, *Am J Ophthalmol* 51:871, 1961.
35. Gartner S, Billet E: Mydriatic glaucoma, *Am J Ophthalmol* 43:975, 1957.
36. Lipisch MP: Effect of cyclopentolate on the aqueous dynamics of iridectomized eyes, *Am J Ophthalmol* 66:543, 1968.
37. Valle O: The cyclopentolate provocative test in suspected or untreated open-angle glaucoma: III. The significance of pigment for the result of the cyclopentolate provocative test in suspected or untreated open-angle glaucoma, *Acta Ophthalmol* 54:653, 1976.
38. Simcoe CW: Cyclopentolate (Cyclogyl) toxicity, *Arch Ophthalmol* 67:406, 1962.
39. Binkhorst RD, Weinstein GW, Baretz RM, and others: Psychotic reaction induced by cyclopentolate (Cyclogyl), *Am J Ophthalmol* 55:1243, 1963.
40. Beswick JA: Psychosis from cyclopentolate, *Am J Ophthalmol* 53:879, 1962.
41. Awan KJ: Systemic toxicity of cyclopentolate hydrochloride in adults following topical ocular instillation, *Ann Ophthalmol* 8:803, 1976.
42. Awan KJ: Adverse systemic reactions of topical cyclopentolate hydrochloride, *Ann Ophthalmol* 8:695, 1976.
43. Patil PN: Antimuscarinic effects of stereoisomers of tropicamide on rabbit iris sphincter, *Invest Ophthalmol Vis Sci* 17:65, 1978.
44. Gettes B: Tropicamide, a new cycloplegic mydriatic, *Arch Ophthalmol* 65:632, 1961.
45. Gambill HD, Ogle KN, Kearns TP: Mydriatic effect of four drugs determined with pupillograph, *Arch Ophthalmol* 77:740, 1967.
46. Portney GL, Purcell TW: The influence of tropicamide on intraocular pressure, *Ann Ophthalmol* 7:31, 1975.
47. Gettes B, Belmont O: Tropicanide: comparative cycloplegic effects, *Arch Ophthalmol* 66:336, 1961.
48. Milder B: Tropicamide as a cycloplegic agent, *Arch Ophthalmol* 66:70, 1961.
49. Bonomi L, Perfetti S, Bellucci R, and others: Prevention of surgically induced miosis by diclofenac eye drops, *Ann Ophthalmol* 19:142, 1987.
50. Havener WH, Falls HF: Oxyphenonium (Antrenyl), *Arch Ophthalmol* 52:515, 1954.

CHAPTER 4

# Glaucoma Therapy

SECTION ONE

## Carbonic Anhydrase Inhibitors

ROBERT J. DERICK

The carbonic anhydrase inhibitors (CAI) are the only systemic agents used in the long-term treatment of patients with glaucoma (Table 4–1). Because these agents work by reducing the production of aqueous humor, they are useful in essentially all forms of glaucoma. Unfortunately, the systemic side effects of the oral CAIs are severe enough in 40% to 50% of patients to require discontinuation of therapy (Table 4–2).[1–3] Improved topical formulations are currently being evaluated in clinical trials. These agents may be able to provide intraocular pressure (IOP) reduction without producing the disabling side effects associated with the oral preparations.

### MECHANISM OF ACTION

The combination of carbon dioxide with water to form carbonic acid, as well as the reversal of this process, is catalyzed by carbonic anhydrase[4, 5]:

$$CO_2 + H_2O \xleftrightarrow{CA} H_2CO_3 \longleftrightarrow HCO_3^- + H^+$$

Acetazolamide, like all CAIs, reversibly blocks this process. The carbonic anhydrase enzyme is ubiquitous—present in many tissues of the body, including the kidney, pancreas, central nervous system, red blood cells (RBCs), and lung. In addition, it is present in many parts of the eye, including the corneal endothelium, the nonpigmented and pigmented ciliary epithelia, the Müller cells, and retinal pigment epithelium.[6, 7]

Bicarbonate ions are transported actively into the posterior chamber from the cytoplasm of the nonpigmented ciliary epithelium. Sodium cations are actively transported into the posterior chamber at a rate linked to bicarbonate secretion and fluid follows at a similar rate by the osmotic gradient that is produced.[8, 9] The CAIs inhibit the rapid interconversion of bicarbonate and $CO_2$ and therefore inhibit the movement of bicarbonate and sodium ions that are most likely to underlie the movement of fluid. In addition, the creation of a local acidic environment through the inhibition of carbonic anhydrase may reduce the production of aqueous humor.[10]

Several lines of evidence support the concept that CAIs lower IOP by reducing aqueous humor production.[11–22] Although substantial lowering of IOP follows treatment with acetazolamide, the facility of outflow does not change.[23]

In both humans and rabbits, tonographic studies indicate a 50% to 60% inhibition of aqueous flow by acetazolamide.[12, 14] No further decrease in secretion occurs with even a tenfold increase in acetazolamide dosage. This suggests that the uncatalyzed hydration of carbon dioxide in the ciliary processes is sufficiently rapid to permit 40% of normal secretion in the absence of carbonic anhydrase. Fluoropho-

**TABLE 4–1.**
Carbonic Anhydrase Inhibitors

| Agent | Dose |
|---|---|
| Acetazolamide | Up to 1 g daily in divided doses<br>125-, 250-, 500-mg tablets<br>500-mg sustained-release capsule<br>250–500 mg, parenteral |
| Methazolamide | 25–100 mg q8–12h orally |
| Dichlorphenamide | 50 mg q8–12h orally |

tometry may be used to determine the rate of disappearance of fluorescein from the anterior chamber of the normal human eye. In normal human subjects, 500 mg of acetazolamide will reduce the rate of fluorescein disappearance by 38%.[13] In very large doses (100 mg/kg intravenously), acetazolamide is capable of inhibiting aqueous flow by as much as 75% in dogs.[24] Another method of measuring aqueous flow, the fluorescein appearance time, also indicates that acetazolamide inhibits the rate of aqueous flow by slightly more than 50%.[25]

Demonstrable blocking of aqueous secretion occurs in the presence of acetazolamide concentrations as small as $10^{-6}$ M. This effect was demonstrated by photographic measurement of the rate of shrinkage of isolated rabbit ciliary processes.[26] Metabolic acidosis is known to reduce IOP and has been proposed as a possible mechanism of action for CAIs[27]; however, the hypotensive effect of the CAIs has been shown to be unrelated to blood or aqueous pH.[28–30]

**TABLE 4–2.**
Side Effects of Carbonic Anhydrase Inhibitors

| |
|---|
| Transient myopia |
| Cross allergenicity with sulfa drugs |
| Paresthesia |
| Tinnitus |
| Metallic taste |
| Anorexia |
| Nausea/vomiting/diarrhea |
| Hepatic necrosis |
| Diuresis |
| Nephrolithiasis/renal colic |
| Fatigue |
| Malaise |
| Confusion |
| Coma |
| Metabolic acidosis |
| Agranulocytosis |
| Aplastic anemia |

The rate of exchange of carbon dioxide between plasma and aqueous is rapid. Within less than 1 minute after intravenous injection of radioactive carbon-labeled bicarbonate, the concentration of labeled carbon dioxide in posterior chamber aqueous has already become 20% greater than the plasma concentration. (It is estimated that the half-life of carbon dioxide in the posterior chamber aqueous is less than 10 seconds.) In the acetazolamide-treated rabbit, 5 minutes elapse before the posterior chamber aqueous labeled carbon dioxide reaches a similar excess over plasma carbon dioxide. The anterior chamber aqueous does not reach its equilibrium with the plasma for about 15 minutes; this time lag accounts for the time lapse between intravenous administration of acetazolamide, its virtually instantaneous inhibition of ciliary body carbonic anhydrase, and a clinically recognizable drop of IOP.[15]

The molecular dimensions of carbonic acid and of the active end of CAI molecules are virtually identical. This leads to the supposition that the carbonic anhydrase enzyme may have a shape complementary to these molecules.[31] Of course, obstruction of the enzyme surface with the inhibitor would block its catalytic availability. The same active configuration exists in the molecules of the clinically useful CAIs acetazolamide, methazolamide, and ethoxzolamide. A double-active configuration exists in the dichlorphenamide molecule.

The relatively prolonged action of acetazolamide on the eye is best explained by the concept of a preferential affinity for certain tissues. Intravenous injection of radioactive sulfur-labeled acetazolamide into rabbits, with subsequent autoradiography of sections of the eye (frozen 2 hours after injection), shows a considerably higher concentration of acetazolamide to exist in the iris and ciliary processes than in other portions of the eye.[32] The drug is not distributed solely on the basis of random diffusion into the body fluids.

Histochemical localization of enzymes within the body demonstrates where their actions can be expected to take place. Carbonic anhydrase is found in high concentrations in the cytoplasm of the corneal endothelium but not in the trabecular meshwork. Intense staining occurs at the lateral and apical cell membranes of the nonpigmented ciliary epithelium and the pigmented iris epithelium. The pigment epithelium of the retina and the ciliary processes show intense staining, indicating that in both locations the cells derived from the outer layer of the optic cup have a very active metabolism designed to support the overlying cells derived from the inner layer.[7]

The enzyme exists in several isoforms, with type II being the most important in the eye.[33–36] Radioimmunosorbent techniques permit precise qualitative and quantitative evaluation of ciliary process carbonic anhydrase. Only the type II isoenzyme was found to be present in human ciliary processes. RBCs have two types of carbonic anhydrase isoenzymes, I and II. Acetazolamide and other CAIs inhibit the type II isoenzyme much more effectively that type I. Acetazolamide could not reduce the IOP in a patient with carbonic anhydrase type II deficiency.[37] Also, RBCs contain 100 times as much carbonic anhydrase as do the ciliary processes. These facts indicate that the ciliary processes might be relatively more vulnerable to inhibition than would be the blood.[33, 34]

In dogs, adrenalectomy reduces the ocular hypotensive action of acetazolamide. Ocular instillation of β-adrenergic blocking agents will also reduce the effect of acetazolamide. These findings suggest that the adrenergic system is in some way related to the mechanism of action of acetazolamide.[38–40]

### Diuretic-Hypotensive Relationship

The hypotensive effect of acetazolamide is not a result of its diuretic action. No such response follows the use of other diuretics.[41–44] Acetazolamide will reduce IOP in nephrectomized rabbits; hence, its action cannot be mediated by a diuretic effect.[23] Hydrochlorothiazide (Esidrix), a potent diuretic with a mechanism of action more closely related to mercurial diuretics than to carbonic anhydrase inhibition, has been evaluated in 45 normal and 37 glaucomatous patients.[45] The resulting drop of IOP was not clinically significant. Diuretics that are not CAIs are not clinically useful in the treatment of glaucoma.

The dose response curve for CAIs is steep, and aqueous humor production is not significantly lowered until greater than 99% of the enzyme is inhibited.[46–48] Conversely, if the dosage in use exceeds maximum inhibition, systemic side effects become more frequent. Metabolism of the CAIs depends on the specific agent. Eighty percent of acetazolamide is recovered unchanged in the urine, unlike methazolamide, in which 75% is metabolized in the liver before renal clearance.[47, 49–51] The commercially available CAIs are administered orally, intramuscularly, or intravenously.

### Intracranial Pressure Reduction

Such CAIs as acetazolamide reduce cerebrospinal fluid formation by 20% to 30%.[52] In treatment of pseudotumor cerebri, acetazolamide is used to reduce ICP. Dosages may vary from 500 mg of acetazolamide every other day to 4 g daily when necessary.[53]

## SPECIFIC CARBONIC ANHYDRASE INHIBITORS

### Acetazolamide

Acetazolamide was the first CAI to be commonly used in the treatment of glaucoma.

#### *Oral Administration*

Orally administered acetazolamide is rapidly absorbed; plasma levels of the drug reach near maximum levels by 2 hours (Fig. 4–1), persist for 4 to 6 hours, and then rapidly drop because of urinary excretion of acetazolamide. The effect of acetazolamide may be prolonged by dispensing it in a coated granule form (Diamox Sequels). This sustained-release acetazolamide not only maintains more prolonged plasma levels and therapeutic effect but also is better tolerated because of the less severe side effects. The rate of release of acetazolamide

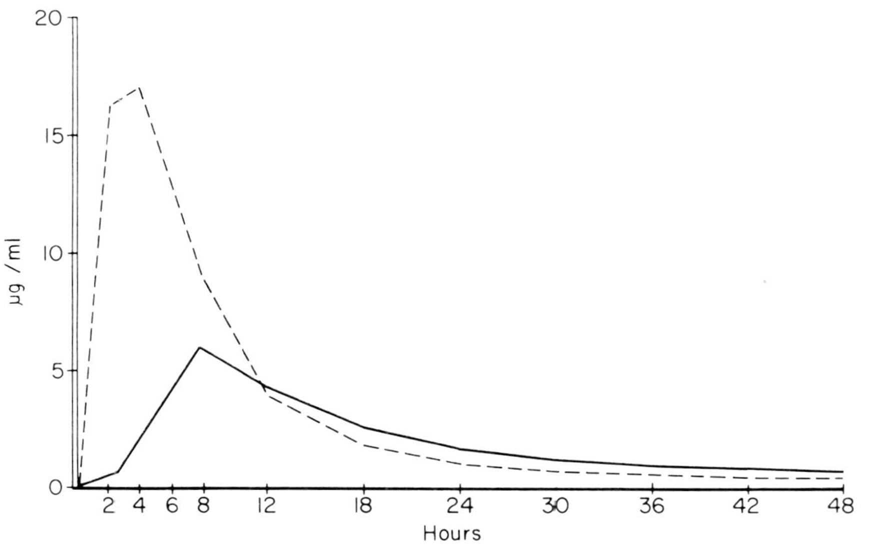


**FIG 4–1.**
Plasma levels of acetazolamide. *Broken line:* levels after oral administration of 500 mg of acetazolamide. *Solid line:* levels after administration of 500 mg of sustained-release acetazolamide. (Modified from Lederle Laboratories: Research data, Pearl River, NY.)

from these coated granules is shown in Fig. 4–2.

#### *Intravenous Injection*

The intravenous injection of acetazolamide (50 mg/kg) in cats causes a decrease of IOP that is already recognizable 1 minute after injection.[54] Intravenous administration may occasionally be necessary and results in a peak IOP effect in 15 minutes and a duration of action for 4 to 6 hours. The recommended dose is 250 to 500 mg intravenously.

#### *Intracameral Injection*

The intracameral injection of 0.1 ml of a 1% acetazolamide solution does not reduce IOP. Intracameral injection of a 10% solution causes acute pain and acute cornea edema that persist for approximately 7 days.[55]

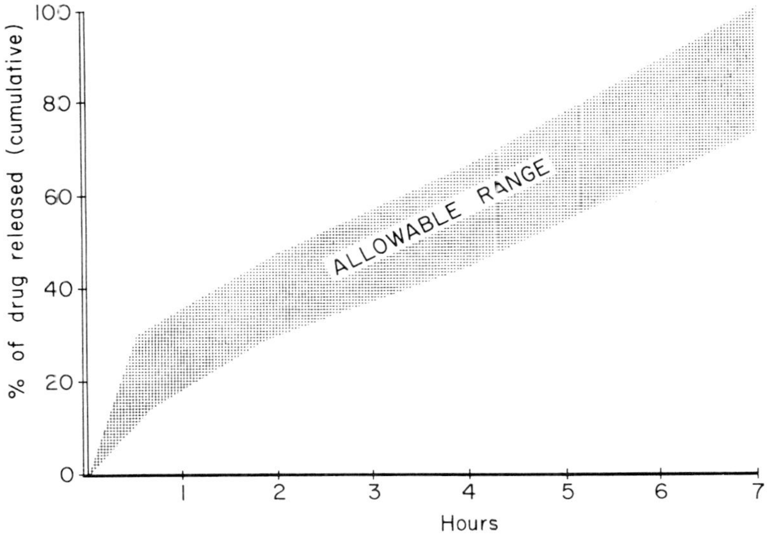


**FIG 4–2.**
Rate of release of coated form of acetazolamide. (From Lederle Laboratories: Research data, Pearl River, NY.)

#### *Hypotensive Response*

Dose-response relationships are relatively complex in the case of enzyme-inhibiting drugs. Specifically, acetazolamide causes only insignificant lowering of IOP until given a sufficient dosage to inhibit at least 99% of carbonic anhydrase activity. Furthermore, when two thirds of aqueous secretion is inhibited, the remaining one third is unaffected by virtually unlimited increase in the dosage of acetazolamide.[46] This is because the reaction $CO_2 + H_2O \rightarrow H_2CO_3$ proceeds at a considerable velocity even in the complete absence of carbon anhydrase.

The ocular hypotensive effect of acetazolamide parallels its plasma concentration. The maximum effect of a single oral dose is attained within 2 hours and is maintained for 2 to 6 hours after administration. The effect of a single capsule of the sustained-released form of acetazolamide may extend over a 24-hour period. Although the traditional dose is 250 mg every 6 hours or 500-mg sustained-release capsules twice daily, a single-dose study showed that 63 mg gave the maximum effect on IOP and 250 mg had only a slightly longer duration of action.[56] To minimize side effects, patients should use the minimally effective dose and start with a relatively low dose. Acetazolamide sustained-release capsules used twice daily have been shown to be better tolerated by patients than either 50 mg of methazolamide four times daily, 250-mg acetazolamide tablets, 125 mg of ethoxzolamide, or 50 mg of dichlorphenamide.[57] Oral acetazolamide can be administered to infants and children in a dose of 5 to 10 mg/kg every 6 hours.

### Methazolamide (Neptazane)

Methazolamide is a CAI chemically similar to acetazolamide. Its use in the control of glaucoma is comparable with that of acetazolamide.

#### *Pharmacology*

Because methazolamide more readily penetrates the blood-aqueous and blood-brain barriers (as much as 50 times higher concentration of methazolamide than acetazolamide can be attained in human cerebrospinal fluid) and because it is a more potent CAI (in vitro RBC enzyme inhibition is 60% greater than that with acetazolamide), it is effective in a lower dosage than is acetazolamide.[58] The suggested dosage is 50 to 100 mg two or three times daily; however, it is probably best to initiate therapy at a lower dose and to increase this dose as required to limit side effects. A dose of 50 mg of methazolamide twice daily is slightly less effective than a dose of 250 mg of acetazolamide four times daily or 500-mg sustained-release capsules twice daily.[59] Almost complete carbonic anhydrase inhibition is attained by 5 mg of methazolamide/kg, and little additional therapeutic effect results from increasing the dose to as much as 100 mg/kg.

Both methazolamide and acetazolamide are stable, are absorbed from the intestinal tract within 2 hours, produce comparable plasma levels that are virtually gone in hours (Fig. 4–3), and are selectively concentrated in RBCs (although methazolamide concentrations in RBCs are double those of acetazolamide at 24 hours; 20% of the administered dose is retained in RBCs compared with 10%). Within 24 hours, 90% of a dose of acetazolamide can be recovered from the urine in contrast to 15% of methazolamide. Methazolamide is metabolized primarily in the liver and only 20% to 50% of methazolamide is excreted unchanged.[49, 50] Because of its good lipid solubility and low plasma protein binding, methazolamide diffuses into tissues and fluids much more readily than does acetazolamide.[47]

### Dichlorphenamide (Daranide)

#### *Pharmacology*

Dichlorphenamide contains within its molecule two configurations (sulfamyl groups) resembling carbonic acid. Very probably this dual structure is the reason for its considerably greater CAI potency and resulting smaller dosage. Only 50 mg of dichlorphenamide is the therapeutic equivalent of 250 mg of acetazolamide. The maintenance dosage is 25 to 100 mg three times daily. This must be adjusted to the needs of the individual patient.

Unlike the other CAIs, dichlorphena-

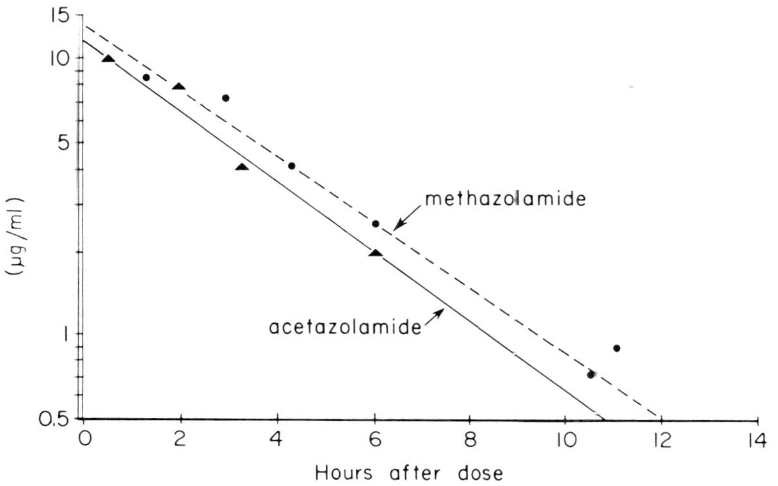


**FIG 4–3.**
Rate of disappearance of methazolamide and acetazolamide from plasma after intravenous dose of 5 mg/kg in dog. (From Lederle Laboratories: Research data, Pearl River, NY.)

mide increases chloride excretion (in addition to increased sodium, potassium, and bicarbonate excretion). As a result, metabolic acidosis is less frequent and less marked after dichlorphenamide than after other CAIs. The decreased likelihood of acidosis is associated with a more persistent diuresis. This is in contrast to acetazolamide, chronic administration of which usually does not cause a persistent diuresis.

Dichlorphenamide is readily water soluble and is promptly absorbed after oral administration. Within 30 minutes after dichlorphenamide ingestion, IOP drops, is at its lowest within 2 to 4 hours, and returns to normal in 6 to 12 hours. In a series of 30 normal and 20 glaucomatous eyes, a single oral dose of 200 mg of dichlorphenamide reduced aqueous humor formation by an average of 40%.[60]

### Ethoxzolamide (Cardrase)

The mechanism of action, therapeutic results, and side effects of ethoxzolamide are essentially the same as those for acetazolamide.

The IOP of normal and glaucomatous eyes is reduced by ethoxzolamide. The average dose used is 125 mg every 6 hours. After 125 mg, the IOP is reduced within 2 hours, the fall is maximal at 5 hours, and pressure has returned to normal in 12 hours. At the time of maximum effect, this dosage reduces aqueous formation by 40%. Facility of outflow is unaffected. In a series of 36 glaucomatous eyes inadequately controlled by miotics, addition of ethoxzolamide caused an average drop in pressure of 43%.[61]

## SIDE EFFECTS

Side effects are frequent with the CAIs particularly among elderly patients (Table 4–3). Gastrointestinal upsets are one of the more frequent causes of CAI intolerance severe enough to force discontinuance of treatment. Symptoms may range from vague abdominal discomfort and a peculiar metallic taste to severe nausea and diarrhea. Frequency of urination may be annoying to some patients but usually decreases with time. Paresthesias commonly affect the

**TABLE 4–3.**

| Contraindications to Carbonic Anhydrase Use |
|---|
| Hyponatremia |
| Hypokalemia |
| Kidney dysfunction |
| Liver dysfunction/cirrhosis |
| Known sulfa allergy |
| Pulmonary obstruction or emphysema (may aggravate acidosis) |
| Concomitant use of high-dose aspirin |

hands and feet and the circumoral region. This numbness and tingling may be so severe as to interfere with dexterity. Drowsiness and malaise affect some patients. In a masked crossover trial, 90 mEq/day of sodium acetate caused improvement of malaise and fatigue in 15 of 28 patients receiving acetazolamide. Placebo therapy benefitted only five of the same patients. The symptomatic relief correlated with improvement in the carbon dioxide combining power, which was interpreted to confirm the theory that the symptoms were caused by metabolic acidosis and would be benefitted by supplemental alkalization.[1, 62] Metabolic acidosis can be especially severe in patients with renal failure, hepatic insufficiency, adrenocortical insufficiency, hyponatremia or hypokalemia, or severe obstructive pulmonary disease.

Replacement therapy of 2 g of potassium chloride/day has been claimed to decrease the side effects and enhance the hypotensive action of acetazolamide.[63] However, long-term use of acetazolamide is generally not associated with potassium depletion. Fifteen patients with glaucoma receiving a daily dose of 500 to 750 mg acetazolamide for an average of 2 years were not found to have a depletion of total body potassium.[64] This is in contrast to the characteristic potassium loss occurring in the first few weeks of treatment, a loss that is replaced spontaneously despite continuing therapy. Significant hypokalemia can result in patients receiving diuretics, adrenocorticotropic hormone, or corticosteroids or in patients with hepatic insufficiency.

Because acetazolamide is a sulfonamide derivative (but has no antibacterial action), it may cause the various toxic responses associated with other sulfonamides. These include agranulocytosis,[65] thrombocytopenia,[66] exfoliative dermatitis, hypersensitivity nephropathy,[67] renal calculi, and transient myopia.

### Acetazolamide-induced Myopia

Uncommonly acetazolamide will cause rapidly developing transient myopia. The amount of this myopia in eight cases varied from 1.00 to 7.00 D.[68] Accommodative spasm is not the mechanism responsible for this myopia because it persists despite cycloplegia and does not change accommodative amplitudes. Presumably as in diabetes, an increase in the refractive power of the lens is responsible for this transient myopia. Transient myopia has been reported with other sulfonamide derivatives, including ethoxzolamide[69, 70] and hydrochlorothiazide.[71]

Although high concentrations of carbonic anhydrase activity are demonstrable in the lens,[72] cataract formation has not been reported to follow prolonged treatment with acetazolamide.

### Renal Stones

Of 148 patients receiving chronic acetazolamide therapy (mean duration 40.9 months), 12 developed one or more episodes of renal stones. Of these, 75% developed during the first year of treatment. Five of these patients developed a second stone a mean of 29 months after the first. The rate of developing stones per year was 15 times greater in the acetazolamide patients than in 367 non-acetazolamide-treated patients recruited from the same practices. The rate for 1,000 individuals developing stones per year was 2.2 in the control group, 1.6 in the acetazolamide group before therapy, and 23.8 in the acetazolamide group after therapy.[73]

Urinary calcium deposits occur in animals given acetazolamide. The acetazolamide-induced predisposition to the formation of renal calculi results from the 60% to 90% reduction in urinary citrate after use of this drug. (Urinary citrate improves calcium solubility.) Because acetazolamide, methazolamide, and dichlorphenamide equally decrease urinary citrate, the problem of renal calculus formation cannot be avoided by substituting another CAI for acetazolamide.[74] Methazolamide was said not to interfere with urinary excretion of citrate and therefore to be less likely to cause renal calculi than is acetazolamide. However, calcium phosphate renal stones have been reported after methazolamide therapy.[75]

### Blood Dyscrasias

Similar to other drugs in the sulfonamide group, the CAIs have been linked to various hematologic reactions, including leukopenia, aplastic anemia, agranulocytosis, and thrombocytopenia. Fatal aplastic anemia occurred in a 69-year-old man receiving 116 g of acetazolamide over 4½ months for treatment of glaucoma. This was believed to be a sulfonamide-induced hematopoietic suppression.[76] In the evaluation of causes of drug-induced blood dyscrasias, acetazolamide was believed to account for 10 of 652 case of agranulocytosis and for 3 of 266 cases of aplastic anemia. All of the sulfonamide drugs, including the CAIs, may cause aplastic anemia.[77] Sulfonamides are the second most common cause of drug-induced aplastic anemia (phenothiazine tranquilizers are first). Glaucoma therapy resulted in the deaths from aplastic anemia of a 72-year-old man taking acetazolamide and a 71-year-old woman taking methazolamide.[78]

The incidence of CAI-related fatal aplastic anemia appears to be less than 1:15,000. Most cases have been reported to occur within the first 6 months of therapy.[79] Routine screening complete blood cell counts at baseline and every 6 months thereafter have been suggested to detect cases at an early stage; however, most clinicians do not currently follow this recommendation.[80] Blood dyscrasias can be either dose related or idiosyncratic. Although discontinuation of a CAI is advised if a blood dyscrasia develops, the effect of early drug discontinuation on the prognosis of patients with aplastic anemia is unknown. The value of routine complete blood cell counts is unproved.

### Teratogenicity

About one third of the offspring of rats given acetazolamide during early pregnancy have malformation of the forepaw usually characterized by absence of the fourth and fifth digits. The dosage required would be comparable with 0.5 to 1.5 g/day in humans. Mice and hamsters develop a comparable defect, but monkeys do not. Ophthalmologists are cautioned against giving CAIs to women during the first trimester of pregnancy.[81] A fatal sacrococcygeal teratoma half as large as the infant was delivered by a mother using 750 mg of acetazolamide daily for glaucoma.[82]

## COMPARATIVE TOLERANCE

Patients differ in their tolerance of the various CAIs. All of the drugs cause similar side effects, but the severity may vary. The individual with acetazolamide intolerance may do well with another CAI. Listed in order of increasing frequency of side effects, these drugs are sustained-release acetazolamide, dichlorphenamide, acetazolamide, methazolamide, and ethoxzolamide.[83]

In another study, 10 glaucomatous patients were given acetazolamide (250 mg), ethoxzolamide (125 mg), and dichlorphenamide (50 mg), each for 10-day periods.[84] The purpose of this triple-blind study was to determine adequacy of IOP control and the relative incidence of systemic side effects. All drugs achieved essentially the same IOP control. Side effects were greatest with dichlorphenamide and the least with ethoxzolamide In another study, sustained-release acetazolamide (Sequels) was found to be tolerated the best, followed by methazolamide, ethoxzolamide, acetazolamide tablets, and dichlorphenamide.[57] Although the side effects of ethoxzolamide are similar to those of acetazolamide, patients who cannot tolerate acetazolamide may tolerate ethoxzolamide and vice versa.[85]

## TOPICAL CARBONIC ANHYDRASE INHIBITORS

Clinical evaluations of the commercially available CAIs for topical use have been undertaken but these agents have not had a significant ocular hypotensive effect. Several new topical CAIs are in the final phases of clinical evaluation and are expected for release in the near future. These agents differ from the currently available CAIs primarily by virtue of enhanced corneal penetration. Three CAIs have been demonstrated to reduce IOP after topical administration. MK-927 (R,S-5,6-dihydro-4-[2-methylpropyl] amino-4H-thieno-[2,3b]thiopyran-2-sulfonamide-7,7-dioxide hydrochloride) is a water-soluble topical CAI that significantly reduces the IOP in rabbits, monkeys, and humans with elevated IOP.[86–88] In patients with ocular hypertension, administration of 2% MK-927 has resulted in IOP reductions of 27% to 33%.[89, 90] Two percent MK-927 reportedly has only a minimally significant effect 12 hours after dosing.[91] MK-417 is the more active S-enantiomer of MK-927 and has been shown to produce greater and longer IOP reductions than MK-927.[92] A twice daily study of 1.8% MK-417 and 2% MK-927 with a placebo control for 14 days was performed in 48 ocular hypertensive patients. Maximum IOP reductions occurred 2 hours after the morning dose and were 20%, 18%, and 2%, respectively.[93] MK-507 is structurally related to MK-927 but has been shown to be more potent than either MK-927 or MK-417 in in vitro studies.[94] In monkeys with elevated IOP, MK-507 produced a significantly greater and longer reduction in IOP than MK-927.[95] In clinical studies, 2% MK-507 and 1.8% MK-417 produced comparable peak IOP reductions in patients with elevated IOP (26.2% vs. 22%, respectively).[96] Addition of MK-507 to patients already receiving 0.5% timolol produces significant reductions in IOP.[97] All three topical CAIs have been well tolerated. Side effects have been minor and include transient burning and stinging and a bitter taste.

SECTION TWO

# Osmotic Agents

ELSON L. CRAIG

Osmotic agents, substances that can increase the osmotic pressure of the plasma relative to that of aqueous and vitreous, can reduce IOP. Such osmotherapy is very effective for the short-term treatment of acute elevations of IOP, but has no role in the treatment of chronic glaucoma.

An ideal agent for altering the plasma-ocular osmotic gradient to reduce IOP should have a low molecular weight, be nontoxic, and have relatively poor ocular penetrance. For example, sodium chloride meets the first two requirements, but because it diffuses into the aqueous rapidly, it cannot maintain the plasma hypertonic to intraocular fluids. Sucrose and sorbital penetrate the eye poorly and can maintain an osmotic differential, but because of high molecular weight, they cause renal damage and in addition require very large doses to obtain the desired osmotic effect. Glycerin, isosorbide, mannitol, and urea generally have desirable characteristics, will effectively reduce acutely elevated IOP, and are clinically useful for that purpose.

The basic principles of osmotherapy have been derived from experiments using a number of different drugs. Their primary modes of action are to decrease the intraocular fluid volume through a blood-ocular osmotic gradient and to cause osmotic diuresis by elevating the osmolarity of the glomerular filtrate hindering tubular reabsorption of water. The pharmacologic characteristics and clinical application of the osmotic agents used in ophthalmology are discussed in this section.

## UREA

Although urea is no longer commonly used as a hyperosmotic agent in the treatment of acute elevation of IOP, a number of important principles in osmotherapy were developed from its use. For this reason it is appropriate to review some of the characteristics of this drug here. A prompt and marked drop of IOP can be achieved in most cases of increased IOP by the intravenous infusion of urea. The mechanism of the pressure drop results entirely from its osmotic effect. Urea penetrates ocular tissue poorly, and this has been attributed to low lipid solubility and high nitrogenous content. Because urea is a small molecule, it causes a strong osmotic effect across a semipermeable membrane. Osmotic effect is a function of the number of molecules, not of their molecular weight. As indicated in Table 4–4, a 70-g dose of urea contains 1,165.5 mOsm compared with only 204.52

**TABLE 4–4.**
Osmotic Characteristics of Urea and Sucrose

| | Molecular Weight | mOsm/70 g |
|---|---|---|
| Urea | 60.06 | 1165.5 |
| Sucrose | 342.30 | 204.52 |

mOsm in 70 g of sucrose; therefore weight for weight, urea has more than five times the osmotic effect of sucrose.

The relationship between blood and aqueous urea levels has been studied after intravenous urea administration in humans.[1] Aqueous was obtained at the time of surgery with simultaneous drawing of a blood sample. In all patients the aqueous urea concentrations were lower than the blood urea concentrations. Blood and aqueous urea levels at different time intervals after cessation of urea infusion are shown in Fig. 4–4. Blood levels had a rapid rise but dropped within a few hours and were essential normal within 24 hours. Because urea is slow to pass the blood-aqueous barrier, aqueous urea levels were still low when the infusion was terminated and required 1 to 2 hours to reach maximum concentration. The greatest differential in urea concentration occurred in the first 30 to 45 minutes after starting the infusion, which coincides with the clinically observable IOP drop that usually occurs in about the same time.

The hypotensive effect of urea is produced not only by its effect on the aqueous humor but also by osmotic alteration of the vitreous body. The urea concentrations in rabbit blood, aqueous, and vitreous after the rapid intravenous injection of 1 g of urea/kg of body weight are shown in Fig. 4–5. The vitreous concentration of urea changes slowly and is proportionately below that of the blood for 4 to 5 hours. The hypotensive effect of urea continues during this time, which is considerably longer than the several hours during which the blood/aqueous ratio is altered. Approximately 5 to 7 hours after intravenous injection the vitreous concentration of urea becomes proportionately higher than the normal ratio with blood concentration and remains elevated for many hours. During this time the blood-vitreous osmotic relationship may actually cause an increase in IOP.

The volume of the vitreous body changes after urea administration. Vitreous volume is least when its osmotic pressure is lower than that of blood and greatest when its osmotic pressure is higher. Because of osmotic-induced reduction in vitreous volume, the anterior chamber may deepen by as much as 0.2 mm after urea treatment, a result important in the treatment of angle-

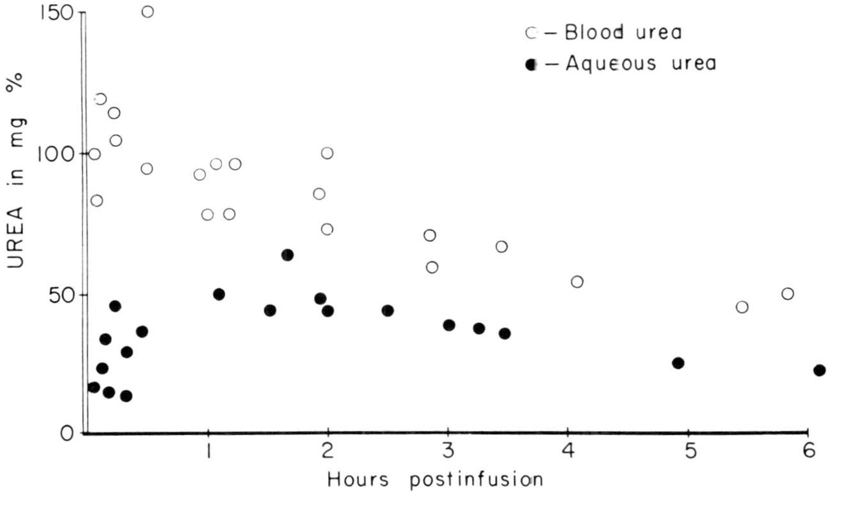


**FIG 4–4.**
Blood and aqueous urea values determined in human subjects immediately after intravenous administration of urea, 1 g/kg, given as a 30% solution at rate of 3 ml/min. (Modified from Galin MA, Nano HL, Davidson R: *Arch Ophthalmol* 65:805, 1961. Used by permission.)

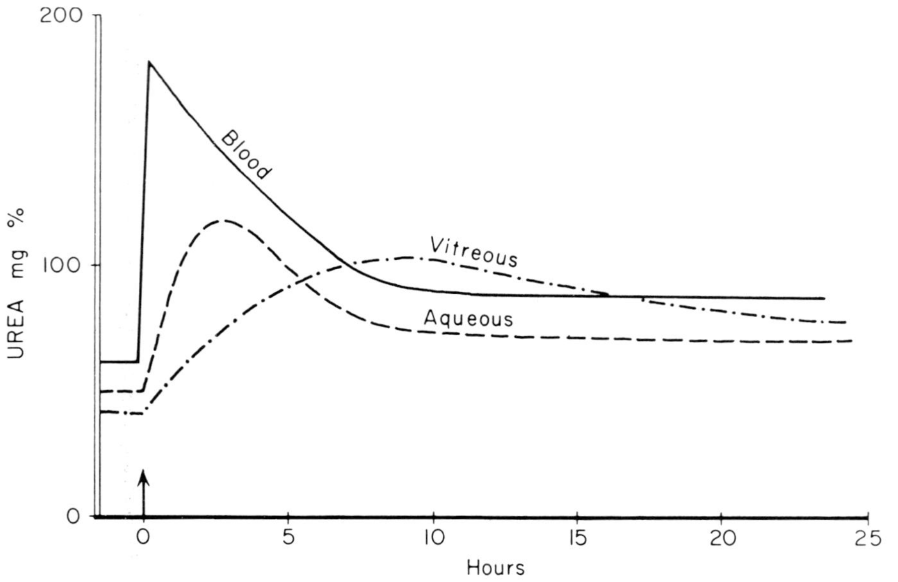


**FIG 4–5.**
Urea concentration in blood, aqueous, and vitreous after 1 g of urea/kg given intravenously within 10 minutes. (Modified from Bleeker GM, Haeringen NJ, Glasius E: *Am J Ophthalmol* 56:561, 1963. Used by permission.)

closure glaucoma. A decrease in rabbit vitreous weight of 3% to 4% occurs subsequent to osmotherapy with urea, as well as with other osmotic agents such as mannitol or glycerol. These experimental data are compatible with the clinical observation that the vitreous volume can be reduced by osmotherapy.[2] It is probable that vitreous dehydration is a primary mechanism whereby hyperosmotic agents lower IOP.

Measurements of the localization of radioactive carbon–labeled urea in rabbit eyes are in agreement with the already cited biochemical determinations.[3] Two hours after intravenous infusion of radioactive carbon–labeled urea, its aqueous concentration was 36% of that in the plasma. Audioradiographs of these eyes showed a relatively high concentration of labeled urea in the ciliary processes and the anterior surface of the iris. The therapeutic significance, if any, of this localization is not evident.

The possibility that "osmoreceptors" in the brain have neural regulatory effect on the IOP has been suggested by the observation that small intravenous doses of hyperosmotic agents will cause a small drop (2 or 3 mm Hg) in IOP in the normal eye but not in an eye with a transected optic nerve.[4–7]

### Preparation and Administration

For intravenous administration, a 30% solution of urea is used. This must be freshly prepared because stale solutions decompose to ammonia, which is toxic. Urea for intravenous use is supplied as a powder in a 40-g vial. The urea is desolved in a 10% invert sugar solution to prevent hemolysis of erythrocytes. When urea is dissolved, an endothermic reaction occurs and the solution becomes extremely cold. For this reason it may be necessary to warm the solution before intravenous administration, but warming it to nearly 50° C will cause ammonia formation and should be avoided. To prepare 135 ml of a 30% solution of urea, mix 40 g of urea with 105 ml of the diluent.

The average adult dosage of urea is 1.0 to 1.5 g/kg of body weight. The usual rate of infusion is 90 to 120 drops/min and should not exceed 4 ml/min; the total daily dosage should not exceed 120 g. A marked diuretic effect occurs within 30 to 45 minutes after administration and may persist for 5 to 6 hours. When administered orally, urea is also effective in reducing IOP. A dosage of 1.5 to 2.0 g/kg will cause a substantial drop in pressure within 2 hours. In approximately 7 hours IOP returns to pretreatment levels. However, the nausea that generally occurs with an acute glaucoma attack will often interfere with oral administration of urea. Urea is unpalatable and must be disguised by some other liquid such as cherry syrup on ice before being given orally.

The ocular hypotensive effects of urea is additive to that of other types of antiglaucoma medications. Fig. 4–6 shows the drop of pressure produced in 14 patients with acute angle-closure glaucoma by the use of acetazolamide, pilocarpine or carbachol, eserine, and in some cases epinephrine.[8] This group of patients did not respond sufficiently to therapy with these drugs, although the average drop in pressure was 35 mm Hg before administration of urea. Routine medical treatment with these drugs was continued for an average of 17.5 hours (3–24 hours) before urea was started. Within 30 minutes after administration of urea, IOP in all the patients dropped rapidly to normal levels. Of particular interest is the still further reduction of pressure achieved by the injection of a retrobulbar anesthetic and ocular massage, which is another mechanism of lowering IOP.

In practice, miotics and CAIs are used concomitantly with osmotherapy in the management of acute increases in IOP. If the pressure can be brought under control with this combination therapy and can be maintained at a lower level after the effect of the osmotic agent is lost, surgery can usually be delayed to bring the patient to optimal physical condition.

The complications associated with the intravenous use of urea, in general, apply to all parenterally administered osmotic agents. Foremost is the rapid and massive diuresis that occurs in nearly 100% of patients. If the patient has genitourinary problems, an indwelling catheter must be

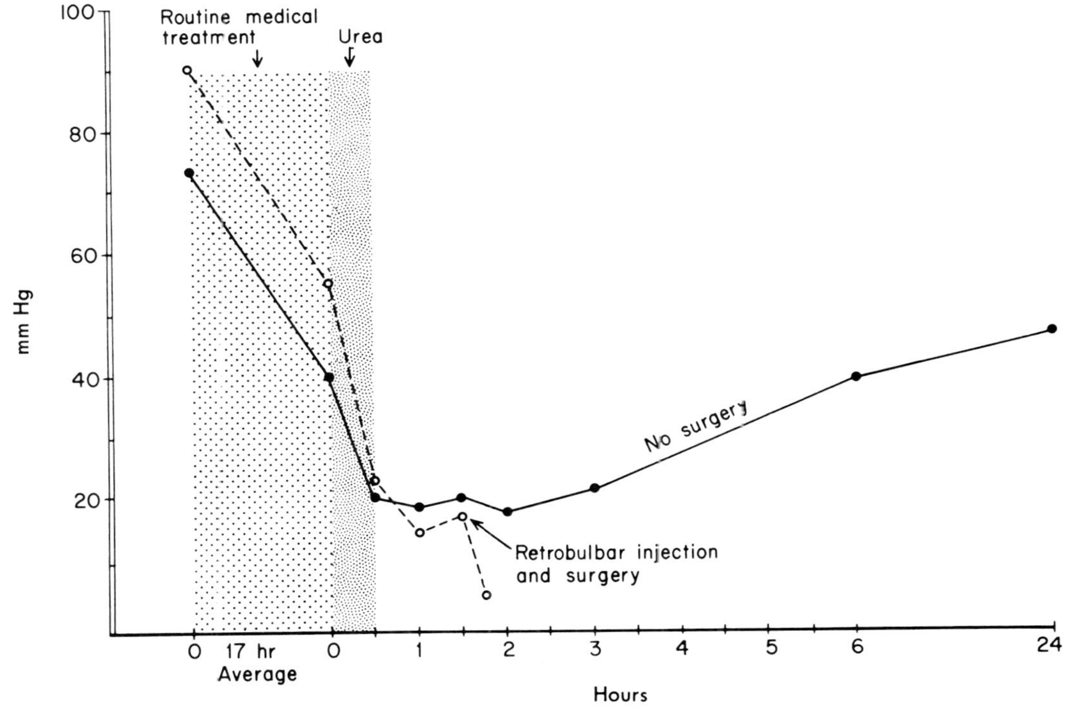


**FIG 4–6.**
Additive hypotensive effects of acetazolamide and miotics, urea infusion, and retrobulbar anesthesia with massage are illustrated in a series of 14 patients with acute glaucoma. Note that in patients not operated on, pressure returned to preurea levels within 6 hours despite continuing miotic therapy. (Modified from Tarter RC, Linn JG: *Am J Ophthalmol* 52:323, 1961. Used by permission.)

inserted and may be necessary for up to 3 hours. Serious distention of the bladder may occur in an anesthetized, noncatheterized patient during urea administration. The rapid shift of fluid into the extracellular space can exacerbate chronic heart failure, possibly leading to pulmonary edema. Rapid intravenous infusion of urea may cause hemolysis. Urea should not be administered through the same tubing through which blood is being infused. Urea has a direct effect on the cerebral vasomotor centers, which may result in increased capillary bleeding. This can be avoided by not exceeding an infusion rate of 4 ml/min. A more severe bleeding, a subdural hematoma, has been reported as a rare complication of urea-induced dehydration.[9]

Extravasation of a 30% urea solution will cause local tissue reactions that can range from mild to severe necrosis and sloughing and is a major reason that this drug is not used frequently. When the drug is used, care should be taken to assure that the needle is securely within an adequate-size vein, and the site of administration should be checked frequently to be certain that the needle does not accidentally become dislodged. If at all possible, urea should not be infused in veins of the lower extremities, particularly in elderly patients, because phlebitis and thrombosis may occur. Table 4–5 lists the adverse reactions that can occur with the intravenous use of hyperosmotic agents.

**TABLE 4–5.**
Adverse Reactions from the Use of Osmotic Agents*

| |
|---|
| Diuresis |
| Dehydration, thirst, dryness of mouth |
| Nausea and vomiting |
| Central nervous system (headaches, confusion, syncope, convulsions) |
| Pulmonary congestion and edema |
| Fluid and electrolyte imbalance, electrolyte loss |
| Acidosis |
| Tachycardia, angina-like chest pain |
| Hypotension, hypertension |
| Osmotic nephrosis |
| Thrombophlebitis, thrombosis |
| Blurred vision |
| Arm pain, skin necrosis (more common with urea) |

*Adverse reactions occur more frequently in elderly patients.

**TABLE 4–6.**
Hyperosmotic Agents Used in Ophthalmology

| Name | Trade Name | Preparation |
|---|---|---|
| Mannitol | Osmitrol | 5%–20% solution |
| Urea | Ureaphil | 40 g (powder) |
| Glycerin | Glyrol | 75% solution |
| | Osmoglyn | 50% solution |
| Isosorbide | Ismotic | 45% solution |

It should be remembered that elderly patients are more likely to have an adverse reactions to medications, particularly those that affect the cardiovascular system. In addition, elderly patients are frequently taking multiple medications for various chronic systemic conditions with increased risk of drug interaction.[10] This, coupled with the recognized morphologic and physiologic changes that occur in the elderly,[11] may make them even more prone to have adverse reactions when osmotherapy is used. Another factor to consider is that when any patient is given an osmotic agent by oral or intravenous route, complications caused by the agent given or possibly resulting from drug interaction can have a delayed onset. For this reason these patients should be monitored for at least 3 hours after administration.

As previously discussed, considerable experimental and clinical data have been obtained from the use of urea, but because of undesirable side effects, it has been replaced by other osmotic agents. Table 4–6 lists the parenteral osmotic agents currently in use in ophthalmology. Urea (Ureaphil) is listed because this drug is available and is occasionally used.

## MANNITOL

Mannitol is one of the more commonly used osmotic agents for the reduction of IOP and fluid volume. The mannitol molecule is three times larger than that of urea, but it exerts a comparable osmotic effect. This can best be explained by the fact that mannitol is concentrated in the extracellular fluid compartments, which contain only one third of the total body water, whereas urea diffuses more freely throughout the body water.

Mannitol is only slightly metabolized and is rapidly excreted by the kidneys. Approximately 80% of the parenterally administered dose is excreted into the urine in 3 hours. Mannitol induces diuresis by increasing the osmolarity of the glomerular filtrate hindering tubular reabsorption of water. As with urea, the mannitol-induced pressure-lowering effect coincides with the increase in serum osmotic pressure. This ocular hypotensive effect occurs in 30 to 60 minutes, depending on the rate of infusion, and persists for approximately 6 hours. Similar to urea, intravenous infusion of mannitol causes vitreous dehydration and deepening of the anterior chamber.

For maximum osmotic effect, the dosage of mannitol is 2 g/kg of a 20% solution given intravenously. For a 50-kg adult, this would be 500 ml of a 20% solution. The rate of administration may vary from 20 to 45 minutes but is usually given over a 30-minute period. The osmotic effect of mannitol depends not only on the amount given but also on the rate that it is infused. When given rapidly, a marked reduction in IOP may occur, causing an eye with a very high pressure to suddenly become soft. This can lead to a number of undesirable side effects but most likely intraocular hemorrhaging.

Because mannitol is soluble only to a 15% concentration in cold water, to assure a 20% preparation, warm the solution in a water bath, then cool it to body temperature before administration. This will also eliminate the crystals that may be present in a cold solution. Administration of the mannitol solution through a blood filter will also eliminate entry of crystals into the bloodstream. Mannitol is stable in solution and can therefore be heat sterilized and stored without the risk of deterioration. Mannitol is commercially available in ready-mixed vials in various concentrations and volumes. Because mannitol is not absorbed from the intestinal tract, it has no osmotic effect on the eye when given orally.

Mannitol is not metabolized to a significant degree and therefore may be used in diabetic patients without creating metabolic problems. Mannitol is the reduced form of mannose and does not give a positive Benedict reaction for urine sugar.

Renal disease does not contraindicate the use of mannitol, although in patients with severe impairment of renal function, a test dose of mannitol should be tried and if there is an inadequate response the medication should not be used. In high concentrations, mannitol decreases renal blood flow and glomerular filtration rate. This may seriously compromise the function of an already damaged kidney. Renal failure traps the mannitol in the extracellular space together with the water that has been drawn from the intracellular space. This dilutes the extracellular sodium, causing hyponatremia. Hyponatremia can cause lethargy and may lead to coma. Continuing the mannitol infusion further compromises the brain by maintaining plasma hyperosmolarity and cerebral dehydration. Because renal failure makes the condition irreversible, extracorporeal hemodialysis is the most effective way to remove the mannitol. Peritoneal hemodialysis is less effective. If, on the other hand, water loss is in excess of electrolyte loss, an imbalance can occur, leading to hypernatremia. Electrolytes, particularly sodium and potassium, should be determined before and after intravenous use of mannitol. Urine output should be closely monitored; if the output is low or declines during mannitol infusion, the patient's status should be reviewed and, if necessary, the infusion discontinued.

Mannitol is less toxic than urea and hence produces fewer side effects. One of the major advantages of mannitol over urea is the freedom from tissue damage at the site of infusion if the solution extravasates. Approximately 100 ml of a 20% mannitol solution extravasated in one reported case had no harmful effects except transient swelling. Thrombophlebitis is less likely to occur with mannitol than with urea. Thrombosis and local irritation have been reported, but these reactions are rare. The headaches caused by decreased intracranial pressure as a result of cerebral dehydration do occur and may be minimized by bed rest. Occasionally patients may experience chills during mannitol infusion. An acute allergic reaction to mannitol can occur, and the physician should be alert to this possibility.

## OSMOTIC STRESS

The magnitude of osmotic force can be great. A single milliosmole of difference on the two sides of a semipermeable membrane can result in 18 mm Hg of pressure. Relating this to the eye, a pressure gradient of 13 mm Hg is thought to be normally present between the vitreous and the choroid. This gradient is a composite of hydrostatic and osmotic forces. Normal retinal apposition is securely maintained by this pressure.[12] Marmor[13] reported that an injection of hyperosmotic solution into the vitreous cavity draws fluid from the choroid and rapidly induces a nonrhegmatogenous retinal detachment. Negi and Marmor[14] later showed that an intravenous injection of hyperosmotic solution facilitates fluid resorption from the subretinal space into the choroid. These investigators suggested that conditions that dehydrate the subretinal space are likely to help keep the retina closely apposed, possibly by keeping the interphotoreceptor matrix compact and viscous. A second mechanism may be that the hyperosmolarity caused by the mannitol creates an outward flow that exerts pressure against the retina, keeping it in apposition to the retinal pigment epithelium. Another study was conducted in which pigmented rabbits were given mannitol intravenously; at various times the blood osmolarity was measured, the eyes enucleated, and the retinal adhesiveness to the retinal pigment epithelium measured.[15] A measurable increase in retinal adhesion was found as early as 10 minutes and as late as 4 hours after mannitol injection. Again, changes in the adhesive properties of the interphotoreceptor matrix were thought to be the cause for this increased adhesiveness. These authors speculated that mannitol use could have clinical application in the management of retinal detachments. They clearly pointed out, however, that the data obtained from their studies in rabbits may not be applicable to humans and that more study is needed before any use in humans for this purpose could be considered.

From these and other studies it is clear that solutions containing osmotically active molecules when used about the eye can have significant effects, depending on their hypertonicity or hypotonicity. Cellular mechanisms for volume regulation to nonphysiologic solutions are dependent on a complex process involving primarily movement of sodium and potassium ions across the cell membrane.[16] Excessively high or low osmolarity can overcome this mechanism and cause cellular damage as well. Intravitreal injection of hyperosmotic solutions can cause not only an osmotically induced retinal detachment but also permanent structural damage to the retina.

## GLYCEROL (GLYCERIN)

Glycerol may be used as an osmotic agent to reduce IOP. Similar to other osmotic agents, glycerol works by increasing serum osmolarity. Glycerol is a naturally occurring component of body fats (1,2,3-propanetriol), usually representing about 1% of body weight. Glycerol may be used as a carbohydrate and apparently may cause no harmful effect even when its use represents as much as 40% of the total dietary intake.[17] Glycerol given orally is relatively free of side effects. It usually does not cause gastrointestinal side effects or diuresis. If the 75% solution is used, a smaller volume is required. Approximately 2 g/kg has been given to human patients three times daily for 50 days without ill effects. Hyperglycemia and glycosuria can result from oral administration of glycerol.

Glycerol has the advantage of being an effective osmotic agent when taken orally and of being relatively nontoxic. The oral dosage is 1 to 1.5 g of a 50% solution/kg dissolved in 0.9% saline solution. One milliliter of a 50% glycerol solution contains 0.62 g of glycerol. The addition of lemon or orange juice and chilling the solution make it more palatable. Glycerol is for oral use only and should not be given intravenously. When given intravenously, glycerol in saline solution causes hematuria in both rabbits and humans. The hematuria has been shown to be caused by severe vasoconstriction of the glomerular arterioles. This vasoconstriction may persist for 30 to 40 minutes, with subsequent vasodilation lasting 5 to 8 hours.

When glycerol is given orally, a drop in IOP usually begins within 10 minutes and is maximum at 30 minutes. In about 5 hours IOP may rise again to pretreatment levels unless other pressure lowering medications are used. A second dose 5 hours after the first will again cause a pressure drop. Because glycerol is the most easily used osmotic agent, it is most suitable for office use in the initial treatment of an acute glaucoma attack. However, its pressure-lowering effect is inferior to that of mannitol and urea. Because of uncertain absorption, the hypotensive response to glycerol is quite variable.

Glycerol aqueous levels are appreciably higher in the inflamed eye than in the normal eye, suggesting that a decreased osmotic effect will occur. Ocular inflammation induced by the injection of 0.1 ml of 0.0M sodium hydroxide into the rabbit anterior chamber did not significantly alter aqueous mannitol concentration from those in the uninflamed eye.[18] This would suggest that mannitol is a more effective osmotic agent than glycerol in the treatment of an inflamed eye as can occur in acute glaucoma. Therefore, if the administration of glycerol in the office does not control the pressure in a case of acute glaucoma, subsequent administration of mannitol in the hospital is indicated.

Adverse reactions to glycerol are similar to other osmotic agents and include occasional nausea, vomiting, diarrhea, headaches, cardiac arrhythmia, pulmonary edema, and central nervous system symptoms. Headaches resulting from decreased intracranial pressure seem to be the major annoying side effect of glycerol when given orally.

Glycerin is commonly used as a hypertonic (hyperosmolar) agent to clear fluid from an edematous cornea, restoring transparency so that gonioscopic and ophthalmoscopic examinations can be performed. The hypertonic solution when applied to the corneal surface creates an osmotic gradient across the corneal epithelium, drawing fluid out of the corneal tissues. Because the topical application of glycerol is painful, its use should be preceded by a topical anesthetic. Concentrations ranging from 50% to the pure anhydrous 100% glycerol are effective in clearing the cornea of edema usually within 1 to 2 minutes after application. Commercially available glycerin ophthalmic solution for topical use (Ophthalgan) is glycerin with 0.5% chlorobutanol in 7.5-ml bottles (Table 4–7). Additional glycerol can be used as the gonioscopic contact solution to prolong the clearing effect. No corneal damage results from glycerol application. In fact, glycerol dehydration is desirable before tonometry, because the dehydration may collapse any epithelial blebs, thereby preventing their mechanical rupture by the tonometer footplate.

Hypertonic sodium chloride can be used for topical osmotherapy of corneal edema. It can also be used as a contact solution for gonioscopy and biomicroscopy. Preparations of sodium chloride in 2% and 5% concentrations are available in solution and ointment forms. Hypertonic solutions of glucose (40% solution) can be used in a similar manner to clear the cornea of edema.

Unfortunately, osmotic dehydration is too transient to be of therapeutic value in diseases causing corneal edema. Measurements made with the vapor pressure osmometer have shown that after instillation of 0.2 ml of a 2.5% salt solution into the lower cul-de-sac, the tears bathing the eye return to normal osmotic pressure (average

**TABLE 4–7.**
Hypertonic (Hyperosmolar) Agents for Corneal Deturgescence*

| Name | Trade Name | % | Preparation |
|---|---|---|---|
| Sodium chloride | Adsorbanac | 2% or 5% | Solution |
| | AK-NACL 5% | 5% | Solution/ointment |
| | Muro-128 | 5% | Solution/ointment |
| Glycerin | Ophthalgan | | Solution/ointment |
| Glucose | Glucoso 40% | 40% | Solution |

*For topical use only.

values 0.91–1.14 mm Hg) within only 90 seconds. Sodium chloride in 2% to 5% solution has been used in the treatment of mild cases of stromal and epithelial edema caused by endothelial damage. Again, the effect is transient (90 seconds) and is not effective in severe cases.[19, 20] Used in combination with a bandage soft lens, 5% saline solution may be instilled into the eye four times daily or more frequently if needed in the treatment of bullous keratopathy. When used with a soft bandage lens on a damaged cornea, the saline solution should contain a preservative to prevent contamination.

## ISOSORBIDE

Isosorbide is a hyperosmotic agent that resembles mannitol in chemical structure and can be given orally. The commercial form (Ismotic) is a 45% solution of isosorbide in a vanilla-mint-flavored vehicle. It is readily absorbed from the gastrointestinal tract, and 95% of the dose given is excreted unchanged in the urine. Isosorbide is not metabolized and provides no calories as does glycerol. It does enter the aqueous but at a slower rate than plasma levels are attained, therefore creating an effective osmotic gradient. The maximum hypotonic effect is achieved 1 hour after ingestion.

Compared with glycerol, isosorbide seems to cause less nausea and vomiting. Minimal nausea followed isosorbide administration in two of 10 patients. Four of these patients had previously been unable to tolerate glycerol treatment because of nausea and vomiting.

With suitable doses, the fall of IOP after oral isosorbide is comparable with that after oral glycerol, intravenous mannitol, or urea. A dose of 1.5 to 2.0 g/kg of isosorbide given as a 45% solution is comparable with 1 to 1.5 g/kg of glycerol. Isosorbide causes the same side effects as all other hyperosmotic agents. Cardiac or renal disease may be a contraindication for its use. Isosorbide dinitrate (Isordil) is a vasodilator used for angina pectoris and should not be confused with the osmotic agent.[21]

## DEXTRAN

Collidal osmotic agents such as dextran may be used in storage solutions to help reduce corneal thickness and maintain clarity of corneas used for transplantation. The osmotic pressure within the normal cornea is the sum of the ions and the collidal molecules within the cornea, and if they exceed the ion and collidal molecule concentration outside the cornea, swelling will occur. Compromise of the membrane ion pump also contributes to corneal swelling, both in corneal storage and in surgery. Including colloidal osmotic agents in the storage fluid containing the corneas reduces the amount of work the membrane must do to maintain corneal dehydration. In 1974 McCary recommended an improved storage medium for corneas to be used for transplantation (M-K medium).[22] This solution was formulated using a modified tissue culture medium (M-199) to maintain cellular function and 5% dextran (400,000 kD) to reduce corneal swelling. Corneas are stored in M-K medium at 4° C, and for a number of years this was the most common method employed to store human corneas. In 1985, Kaufman et al.[23] recommended a modification of the M-K medium, called K-Sol.[24] In this solution dextran was replaced by 2.5% chondroitin sulfate, which was treated to remove small molecular weight components. This formulation was thought to allow longer storage time compared with the M-K medium.[25–28] More recently Dexsol has been introduced and is formulated using minimum essential medium (MEM) culture medium, 1.35% chondroitin sulfate, and 1% dextran. Corneas stored in this medium for up to 12 days showed good endothelial cell viability and minimum swelling and, when compared with those in other storage solutions, were found to be superior, at least for the first 6 days.[29]

## SUMMARY

Hyperosmotic agents can be used topically or given by oral or intravenous routes, and they have a number of important uses in clinical ophthalmology and during ophthalmic surgery. The mechanism of action of all these compounds is to create an osmotic gradient between the blood and ocular tissues, causing fluid to be drawn out of the tissues. When they are given intravenously or orally, the major effect on the eye is to reduce vitreous volume, the net effect of which is to deepen the anterior chamber and lower IOP. Hyperosmotic agents are critical for the management of acute glaucoma and in many cases may be sight saving. They are important in any condition in which it is advantageous to have a soft eye. Systemic side effects from the use of hyperosmotic agents are common but are usually mild, such as nausea and vomiting. The most important severe side effect is massive diuresis. This can lead to a number of serious complications, such as cerebral dehydration, producing syncope and even coma, electrolyte imbalance, cardiac, pulmonary, and renal complications. Care should be taken when these agents are used, and patients should be monitored for at least 3 hours after administration.

SECTION THREE

# Medical Therapy of Glaucoma

PAUL A. WEBER

The role of medical therapy for primary open-angle glaucoma is currently undergoing intense discussion and evaluation. The purpose of this section is not to discuss the merits and place of medical therapy but to provide some practical guidelines in the use of medical treatment for primary open-angle and the other glaucomas once it has been decided to institute this modality.

## GENERAL GUIDELINES

Among the reasons the role of medical therapy is being reevaluated are patient compliance and side effects of the medications. There are several general concepts of medical therapy worth keeping in mind any time medical treatment is being contemplated to help address these problems:

1. Use the weakest medication that has a reasonable chance of working to maximize the risk/benefit ratio for the patient.
2. Prescribe the medication in the lowest frequency necessary. This helps to maximize the risk/benefit ratio, as well as improve patient compliance.[1]
3. When multiple medications are required, keep them to a minimum. Too many times when one medication has been ineffective a second, third, or even fourth medication is added when the first medication should have been discontinued and a new one substituted.
4. Instruct all patients using topical medications in nasolacrimal occlusion or eyelid closure. Nasolacrimal occlusion has been shown to decrease by nearly 60% the systemic absorption of topical drugs while increasing their therapeutic efficacy.[2] Many patients, even when properly instructed, perform nasolacrimal occlusion improperly. Eyelid closure for 3 to 5 minutes after the instillation of eye drops is simpler for many patients and nearly as effective as nasolacrimal occlusion.
5. Educate patients about their disease and the importance of medical treatment being prescribed. Although we tend to blame noncompliance on patients, many times it is physicians who are at fault. If patients have never been adequately educated about their disease, they cannot be expected to be totally compliant.
6. Warn patients of potential side effects of the medication being prescribed before therapy is instituted. If a patient experiences side effects from a medication and has not been warned of their potential occurrence, anger and loss of confidence in the physician frequently result. No matter how much explanation is given after the fact, the patient's comfort with and confidence in the physician may not be restored.
7. Communicate either directly or through the patient with the primary care physician any time medical therapy is begun or altered.

## ANTIGLAUCOMA MEDICATIONS

The various agents currently available to treat glaucoma are listed in the following outline:

- I. Topical
    - A. β-Adrenergic blocker
        - 1. Selective
            - a. Betaxolol
        - 2. Nonselective
            - a. Timolol
            - b. Levobunolol
            - c. Metipranolol
            - d. Carteolol
    - B. Cholinergic
        - 1. Pilocarpine
        - 2. Carbachol
        - 3. Echothiophate
        - 4. Demecarium bromide
    - C. Sympathomimetic
        - 1. Epinephrine
        - 2. Dipivalyl epinephrine
    - D. $\alpha_2$-Agonist apraclonidine
- II. Oral
    - A. CAI
        - 1. Acetazolamide
        - 2. Methazolamide
    - B. Osmotic
        - 1. Glycerol
        - 2. Isosorbide
- III. Intravenous
    - A. CI
        - 1. Acetazolamide
    - B. Osmotic
        - 1. Mannitol

## INITIATION OF MEDICAL THERAPY

Several factors need to be considered in selection of the initial antiglaucoma drug for the patient:

1. Type of glaucoma
2. Age of patient
3. Medical history
4. Ocular status
    - a. Cataract
    - b. Narrow angle
    - c. Retinal pathologic condition
5. Severity of glaucoma

### Type of Glaucoma

The type of glaucoma being treated will partially dictate which medications to consider. Miotics will be ineffective in eyes with total synechial closure of the angle because their mechanism of action is via improving outflow. The miotics also cause a breakdown in the blood-aqueous barrier; therefore, they are to be used with caution in the secondary inflammatory glaucomas and in neovascular glaucoma.

### Age of Patient

Because of the effects miotics have on the ciliary muscles, they are seldom tolerated in the younger age group. Intense pain, visual blurring, nontolerance, and noncompliance frequently result.

Although the β-blockers have not been approved by the U.S. Food and Drug Administration (FDA) for use in children, they have been shown to be effective.[3–5] However, caution is indicated. A case of cardiopulmonary arrest in a child has been reported with the use of timolol.[6] If they are needed in this age group, begin with a selective β-blocker in the lowest concentration with nasolacrimal occlusion.

In women of child-bearing age, the physician needs to discuss with the patient potential effects of topical and oral antiglaucoma medications on the fetus and newborn. Although there are few data to suggest fetal malformation from topical β-blockers and miotics, minimizing exposure, especially in the first trimester, seems prudent. There is more evidence that these drugs are excreted into breast milk and may have adverse effects on the nursing infant. The β-blockers have been associated with neonatal depression, bradycardia, and hypoglycemia. Pilocarpine has been associated with seizures, diaphoresis, and hyperthermia in the newborn. The topical anticholinesterases have been reported to cause muscular weakness.

There is more suggestive evidence of potential fetal problems from the epinephrine drugs with reports of cataracts in animals and suggestions of possible fetal hypoxia and inguinal hernia causation. The meager evidence available, then, would support the use of β-blockers and miotics over epinephrine in pregnancy.

Oral CAIs should probably be avoided in pregnancy because of a case of teratoma in one fetus exposed to acetazolamide in the first trimester and because of teratogenic effects in animal studies.[7]

### Medical Status

Because of the systemic absorption of topical medications and the systemic effects of oral medications, it is imperative that a thorough medical history be obtained before any new medical therapy is instituted for glaucoma management. In high-risk cases it may be necessary to obtain more detailed medical information from the patient's primary care physician along with additional diagnostic testing as indicated to determine the potential danger or safety of a medication.

Because of their tendency to cause potassium loss, CAIs need to be used with caution in patients taking other potassium-depleting diuretics, especially if they have concurrent cardiac disease that may be aggravated by hypokalemia.

CAIs must also be cautiously prescribed in patients with (1) pulmonary disease because of potential acidosis, (2) a history of nephrolithiasis, (3) allergy to sulfonamides, and (4) anemias and bone marrow abnormalities.

Every side effect attributed to oral β-blockers has been described with topical β-blockers. A cardiovascular history is imperative to rule out any contraindications. Reactive airway disease should lead one away from the nonselective β-blockers. Although betaxalol, a selective $\beta_1$-agent, has not been shown to adversely affect pulmonary function parameters in several studies,[8–10] clinical experience of many physicians suggests caution is still needed in these patients.[11, 12]

As a general rule, epinephrine drugs should not be a first-line drug in patients with hypertension or unstable coronary artery disease. If a hypertensive patient is begun on an epinephrine drug, he or she should have blood pressure monitored more closely for a period after initiation of therapy. Dipivalyl epinephrine, because of its lower concentration and increased corneal penetration, causes fewer extraocular side effects while being as effective in lowering the IOP as epinephrine itself.

### Ocular Status

Although there is some controversy concerning whether or not miotics cause retinal detachments, caution is necessary in those eyes at risk. Miotics should probably not be a first-line agent in these eyes. A dilated peripheral retinal examination should be performed before miotics are instituted in these cases to rule out preexisting retinal faults.

Miotics, although not contraindicated, may be poorly tolerated in eyes with cataracts, especially posterior subcapsular opacities.

The status of the lens (phakic, pseudophakic, or aphakic) will dictate medical decision making. The anticholinesterases are contraindicated in phakic eyes because of their cataractogenic potential.

Epinephrine agents can cause macular edema in up to 20% of aphakic eyes.[13, 14] This does not mean that these drugs are absolutely contraindicated in the aphake. It does, however, mean that if you place an aphakic patient on epinephrine, you are obligated to watch for epinephrine maculopathy and to discontinue it if this is documented or suspected because the macular edema is reversible if caught early. Although no good studies have been performed to look at epinephrine maculopathy in the pseudophakic eye, on a theoretical basis, if the posterior capsule is intact, the risk should be low; if the capsule is disrupted, the risk may approach the 20% seen in the aphake.

In eyes with narrow angles, the epinephrine agents, especially when combined with a β-blocker,[15, 16] may cause pupillary dilatation and precipitate either chronic or acute angle-closure glaucoma. Initial and follow-up gonioscopy is mandatory in such eyes.

Strong miotics may also precipitate angle closure by increasing pupillary block.

### Severity of Glaucoma

The more severely damaged the optic nerve is, the more aggressively we need to lower the IOP. Because there are eyes in which a nonselective β-blocker lowers the IOP more effectively than a selective β-blocker, it is reasonable to prescribe a nonselective β-blocker in the more advanced cases.

## PRIMARY OPEN-ANGLE GLAUCOMA

Depending on the various considerations discussed earlier, any one of the topical glaucoma medications and, rarely, oral CAIs may be used as initial therapy.

The β-blockers are the most commonly prescribed medication for primary open-angle glaucoma. When therapy is initiated, recent studies suggest the nonspecific β-blockers may be equally effective when used once daily compared with twice daily. When prescribed on a once daily regimen, they should be administered in the morning, because there is evidence that aqueous production decreases to a baseline level during sleep, below which the β-blockers cannot suppress aqueous production further.[17]

Although most patients will obtain a similar decrease in IOP when using a nonspecific vs. a $\beta_1$-selective agent, a small but definite percentage of individuals will have a significantly greater effect from the nonspecific agents. Thus, if a patient's IOP is inadequately controlled using a selective β-blocker, switching to a nonspecific agent may be worthwhile.

When pilocarpine is selected, three forms are available: solution, ointment, and controlled-release system.

Pilocarpine solution is the most commonly used form. Because ocular, especially iris, pigmentation affects the availability of this drug, it is useful to think of pilocarpine in low and high dose according to iris color, respectively, 1% and 2% in blue eyes and 2% and 4% in brown eyes. General guidelines for pilocarpine solutions are to (1) begin with the lowest concentration, (2) prescribe application every 6 to 8 hours, (3) consider an initial unilateral trial, and (4) always discuss the potential side effects before initiating therapy. On this last point, if the patient is not warned ahead of time of these potential side effects, numerous telephone calls to the physician will result. Even more important, the patient's confidence in you as his or her physician may be severely damaged. No matter how much you explain after the fact, the patient is frequently skeptical thereafter.

The Ocusert controlled–delivery system is meant to minimize side effects through a low-dose continuous release of the drug. Two strengths are available, Ocusert 20 and Ocusert 40. In most patients they remain effective for 7 days. However, there is individual variation, so the IOP should be measured at the beginning and end of the 7-day cycle to determine if more frequent changing is required. There is commonly a surge of release of the pilocarpine after instillation into the cul-de-sac, so it is wise to have the patient exchange the device at nighttime so that this surge and its accompanying side effects are gone by morning.

Pilopine HS Gel is a 4% compound whose effects last approximately 24 hours. Again, application at bedtime is preferable to minimize the blurred vision from the gel itself.

Carbachol is far less commonly prescribed than pilocarpine and is usually used when patients are allergic to pilocarpine. As noted previously, phospholine iodide should not be used in phakic eyes but should not be forgotten in pseudophakic or aphakic eyes. Its twice daily regimen is more convenient and more feasible for some individuals.

When epinephrine is prescribed, the preferred agent is dipivefrin (Propine). By use of this prodrug rather than epinephrine itself, better ocular tolerance and fewer systemic side effects result. Twice daily application of this 0.1% solution is the recommended frequency.

It appears that fewer and fewer ophthalmologists are prescribing oral CAIs for the control of primary open-angle glaucoma unless other modalities have failed. The reasons for this are probably twofold: the very high incidence of systemic side effects and medicolegal concerns.

Gastrointestinal upset, general malaise, paresthesias, and renal stone formation are the most common reasons for discontinuing these agents. Even when the patient denies any side effects from CAIs, the physician should question family members because a large number of patients will have experienced personality changes they themselves have not recognized. Many patients who thought they were tolerating these agents well will recognize only the subtle but significant effects on discontinuing the drug.

Because of the potentially fatal blood dyscrasias that can be caused by the CAIs, medicolegal concerns are significant. This issue has resulted in debate about the necessity and advisability of hematologic testing of patients prescribed these agents. Because these drug-induced blood dyscrasias are believed to be idiosyncratic and not dose related, the majority of ophthalmologists surveyed do not routinely obtain hematologic evaluation. The reader is referred to the references for a more detailed discussion of this debate.[18–20]

If CAIs are prescribed, studies have shown that acetazolamide sequels were best tolerated, followed by methazolamide, with ethoxzolamide, acetazolamide tablets, and dichlorphenamide being least tolerated.

## COMBINATION DRUG THERAPY

All of the classes of drugs previously discussed can be used in combination therapy with a few caveats.

When deciding that the initial therapy is inadequate, think seriously about whether adding a second or third agent is appropriate as opposed to discontinuing one drug and substituting a new agent. Too frequently drugs are added when the first drug has had no or limited effect, subjecting the patient to needless expense and potential side effects and aggravating the compliance issue.

Although the additive effects of miotics, β-blockers and CAIs are well documented and accepted, there is conflicting literature concerning the effectiveness of combination therapy of epinephrine and the β-blockers[15, 16, 21–27] In practice, dipivefrin is frequently ineffective when added to the β-blockers. However, there are numerous individuals in whom there is a significant additive effect to warrant a trial. Again, keep in mind the need to discontinue one of the agents if no significant benefit is being gained from simultaneous usage.

## SECONDARY OPEN-ANGLE GLAUCOMAS

### Exfoliation Glaucoma

Medical therapy of glaucoma associated with the exfoliation syndrome is essentially the same as for primary open-angle glaucoma. Studies suggest, however, that exfoliation glaucoma is more difficult to control medically than is primary open-angle glaucoma.[28]

### Pigmentary Glaucoma

Although the principles of medical therapy of pigmentary glaucoma are similar to primary open-angle glaucoma, the fact that these patients are frequently in the younger age group means that pilocarpine solutions are usually not tolerated or, if prescribed, not used by the patient. Ocuserts find their greatest use in some practices for this entity.

α-Blocking agents, which cause pupillary constriction by inhibiting the pupillary dilator muscle, offer a theoretical treatment for pigmentary glaucoma.

## OTHER SECONDARY OPEN-ANGLE GLAUCOMAS

To formulate a rational medical regimen for the other open-angle glaucomas, one needs to consider the mechanism for the elevated IOP. In many instances, aqueous suppressants are the agents of choice. In open-angle glaucoma associated with intraocular inflammation, recall that the miotics can aggravate the breakdown of the blood-eye barrier. This does not necessarily preclude miotics in these cases; however, low concentrations should be used to minimize potential aggravation of the underlying inflammation.

## PRIMARY ANGLE-CLOSURE GLAUCOMA

In most instances, medical management of primary angle-closure glaucoma should be the initial modality. Although acute angle-closure glaucoma can be broken with laser surgery, if the laser is not situated in the facility where the patient is first treated, any delay in getting the patient to a laser can be deleterious. In addition, prior medical treatment, if fully or partially successful, usually results in the laser surgery being more easily and successfully completed by virtue of a clearer cornea and a more comfortable, and therefore, more cooperative patient.

The goals of medical treatment are twofold: protect the optic nerve and vascular supply to the retina and optic nerve through rapid reduction of the IOP and break the pupillary block.

Reduction of the IOP is achieved by a combination of hyperosmotic agents, CAIs, and topical β-blockers.

### Hyperosmotic Agents

If the patient is not nauseated or vomiting, oral hyperosmotic agents isosorbide or glycerol are given. They are generally better tolerated if given over ice. Isosorbide is not metabolized to the same extent as glycerol and thus is safer in diabetics.

Because many of these patients are nauseated or vomiting, intravenous mannitol is frequently needed.

### Carbonic Anhydrase Inhibitors

Acetazolamide can be given orally, intramuscularly, or intravenously in a 500-mg dose.

### β-Blockers

After a careful history, a selective or nonselective topical β-blocking agent may be used to suppress aqueous production.

Apraclonidine, the $\alpha_2$-agonist, has an aqueous suppressant action and is frequently instilled during an acute attack of angle-closure glaucoma. It has not been formally approved at this time for use in acute angle closure but can be used in these instances in anticipation of laser iridotmy, a use for which FDA approval has been given.

The agents mentioned thus far do not by themselves break the attack of angle closure but are necessary components. Pilocarpine is used to break the pupillary block. However, the pupillary sphincter on which pilocarpine acts becomes ischemic from an acute increase in IOP and cannot respond to this direct-acting parasympathomimetic. The lowering of the IOP by the other agents is therefore necessary before the pilocarpine can act on the sphincter muscle.

In the heat of the battle it is not uncommon to have the physician instill pilocarpine drops rather frequently, sometimes to the point of causing pilocarpine toxicity. One to three drops of a 1% to 2% solution given over 15 minutes is adequate to saturate the receptors in the sphincter muscle.

The α-adrenergic blocking agents (thymoxamine and dapiprazole) inhibit the pupillary dilator, which is more resistant to ischemia. In addition, by acting by a different mechanism, this class of drugs may offer improved success in the medical therapy of breaking the pupillary block.

## SECONDARY ANGLE-CLOSURE GLAUCOMAS

The mainstay of medical management of secondary angle-closure glaucomas (i.e., synechial angle closure secondary to uveitis, flat anterior chamber glaucoma, or neovascular glaucoma) is the aqueous suppressants. One of the most common mistakes in glaucoma management is the use of miotics in an eye with total synechial angle closure. Not only are the miotics ineffective in lowering the IOP, but they frequently cause discomfort and increase the breakdown of an already compromised blood-eye barrier present in many of these eyes.

## CILIARY BLOCK (MALIGNANT) GLAUCOMA

As in angle-closure glaucoma, the medical therapy of ciliary block, or malignant, glaucoma may be in preparation for more definitive laser surgical or conventional surgical treatments. In many cases, however, the ciliary block attack may be successfully managed entirely by medical treatment.

In this form of glaucoma there appears to be a posterior misdirection of aqueous into the vitreous cavity. The goals of medical treatment are again twofold: reduction of the IOP and disruption of the posterior misdirection of aqueous.

As in acute angle-closure glaucoma, oral or parenteral hyperosmotic agents and CAIs, along with topical β-blockers and possibly apraclonidine, are used to lower the IOP. The aqueous suppressants may also assist in breaking the ciliary block by reducing the amount of aqueous flowing posteriorly.

Cycloplegics and mydriatics are employed to disrupt the posterior aqueous misdirection and to pull the lens back by tightening the zonules and rotating the ciliary body. One percent atropine and 2.5% to 10% Neo-Synephrine are given four times daily. If definitive surgical treatment is not performed, the atropine may need to be continued indefinitely once daily. If the cycloplegic is discontinued, the ciliary block may recur and may not respond to reinstitution of medical management.[29]

If the patient develops an allergy to the atropine, scopolamine may be successfully substituted.

Keep in mind that miotics are contraindicated in the management of malignant glaucoma because they can precipitate an attack of malignant glaucoma and worsen an existing malignant glaucoma episode.

The response to medical therapy in malignant glaucoma is frequently not immediate and may, in fact, take several days to have its maximum effect.

## REFERENCES

### SECTION ONE


1. Epstein DL, Grant WM: Carbonic anhydrase inhibitor side effects, *Arch Ophthalmol* 95: 1378, 1977.
2. Lichter PR: Reducing side effects of carbonic anhydrase inhibitors, *Ophthalmology* 88:266, 1981.
3. Lichter PR, Newman LP, Wheeler NC, and others: Patient tolerance to carbonic anhydrase inhibitors, *Am J Ophthalmol* 85:495, 1978.
4. Maren TH: The rates of movement of $Na^+$, $CL^-$, and $HCO_3^-$, from plasma to posterior chamber: effect of acetazolamide and relation to the treatment of glaucoma, *Invest Ophthalmol* 15:356, 1976.
5. Richardson KT: Cellular responses to drugs affecting aqueous dynamics, *Arch Ophthalmol* 89:65, 1973.
6. Green H, Bocher CA, Calnan AF, and others: Carbonic anhydrase and the maintenance of intraocular tension, *Arch Ophthalmol* 53:463, 1955.
7. Lutjen-Drecoll E, Lonnerholm G: Carbonic anhydrase distribution in the rabbit eye by light and electron microscopy, *Invest Ophthalmol Vis Sci* 21:782, 1981.
8. Maren TH: Carbonic anhydrase: general perspectives and advances in glaucoma research, *Drug Dev Res* 10:255, 1987.
9. Zimmerman TJ, Garg LC, Vogh BP, and others: The effect of acetazolamide on the movement of sodium into the posterior chamber of the dog eye, *J Pharmacol Exp Ther* 199:510, 1976.
10. Bergren L: Effect of composition of medium and of metabolic inhibitors on secretion in vitro by the ciliary processes of the rabbit eye, *Invest Ophthalmol* 4:83, 1965.
11. Becker B: Decrease in intraocular pressure in man by a carbonic anhydrase inhibitor, Diamox, *Am J Ophthalmol* 37:13, 1954.
12. Becker B, Constant MA: Experimental tonography, *Arch Ophthalmol* 54:321, 1955.
13. Bloom JN, Levene RZ, Thomas G, and others: Fluorophotometry and the rate of aqueous flow in man: I. Instrumentation and normal values, *Arch Ophthalmol* 94:435, 1976.
14. Becker B: The effect of acetazolamide on ascorbic acid turnover, *Am J Ophthalmol* 41:522, 1956.
15. Kinsey BE, Reddy DBN: Turnover of total carbon dioxide in the aqueous humor and the effect thereon of acetazolamide, *Arch Ophthalmol* 62:78, 1959.

16. Becker B: The measurement of aqueous flow with iodide, *Invest Ophthalmol* 1:52, 1962.
17. Constant MA, Falch J: Phosphate and protein concentrations of intraocular fluids: I. Effect of carbonic anhydrase inhibition in young and old rabbits, *Invest Ophthalmol* 2:332, 1963.
18. Garg LC, Opplet WW: The effect of ouabain and acetazolamide on the transport of sodium and chloride from the plasma to the aqueous humor, *J Pharmacol Exp Ther* 175:237, 1970.
19. Holm O, Wiebert O: The effect of systemically given acetazolamide on the formation of aqueous humor in the human eye measured with a new photogrammetric method, *Acta Ophthalmol* 46:1243, 1968.
20. Linner E, Friedenwald JS: The appearance time of fluorescein as an index of aqueous flow, *Am J Ophthalmol* 44:225, 1957.
21. Macri FJ, Dixon RL, Rall DP: Aqueous humor turnover rates in the cat: I. Effect of acetazolamide, *Invest Ophthalmol* 4:927, 1965.
22. Oppelt WW: Measurement of aqueous humor formation rates by posterior-anterior chamber perfusion with inulin. Normal values and the effect of carbonic anhydrase inhibition, *Invest Ophthalmol* 6:76, 1967.
23. Becker B: The mechanism of the fall in intraocular pressure induced by the carbonic anhydrase inhibitor, Diamox, *Am J Ophthalmol* 39:177, 1955.
24. O'Rourke J, Macri FJ, Berghoffer B: Studies in uveal physiology, *Arch Ophthalmol* 81:526, 1969.
25. Friedenwald JS: Carbonic anhydrase inhibition and aqueous flow, *Am J Ophthalmol* 39:59, 1959.
26. Berggren L: Direct observation of secretory pumping in vitro of the rabbit eye ciliary processes, *Invest Ophthalmol* 3:266, 1964.
27. Bietti G, Virno M, Pecori-Giraldi J, and others: Acetazolamide, metabolic acidosis, and intraocular pressure, *Am J Ophthalmol* 80:360, 1975.
28. Benedikt O, Zirm M, Harnoncourt K: Relations between metabolic acidosis and intraocular pressure after inhibition of carbonic anhydrase with acetazolamide, *Graefes Arch Ophthalmol* 190:247, 1974.
29. Friedman Z, Krupin T, Becker B: Ocular and systemic effects of acetazolamide in nephrectomized rabbits, *Invest Ophthalmol* 23:209, 1982.
30. Mehra KS: Relationship of pH of aqueous and blood with acetazolamide, *Ann Ophthalmol* 11:63, 1979.
31. Becker B: Carbonic anhydrase and the formation of aqueous humor, *Am J Ophthalmol* 47:342, 1959.
32. Goren SB, Newell FW, O'Toole JJ: The localization of Diamox-$S^{35}$ in the rabbit eye, *Am J Ophthalmol* 51:87, 1961.
33. Wistrand PJ, Garg LC: Evidence of a high-activity C type of carbonic anhydrase in human ciliary processes, *Invest Ophthalmol Vis Sci* 18:802, 1979.
34. Dobbs PC, Epstein DL, Anderson PJ: Identification of isoenzyme C as the principal carbonic anhydrase in human ciliary processes, *Invest Ophthalmol Vis Sci* 18:867, 1979.
35. Kumpulainen T: Immunohistochemical demonstration of carbonic anhydrase C in the epithelium of the human ciliary process, *Histochemistry* 77:281, 1983.
36. Wistrand PJ, Schenholm M, Lonnerholm G: Carbonic anhydrase isoenzymes CA I and CA II in the human eye, *Invest Ophthalmol* 27:419, 1986.
37. Krupin T, Sly WS, Whyte MP, and others: Failure of acetazolamide to decrease intraocular pressure in patients with carbonic anhydrase II deficiency, *Am J Ophthalmol* 99:396, 1985.
38. Thomas PR, Riley MW: Acetazolamide and ocular tension, *Am J Ophthalmol* 60:204, 1965.
39. Dailey RA, Brubaker RF, Bourne WM: The effects of timolol maleate and acetazolamide on the rate of aqueous formation in normal human subjects, *Am J Ophthalmol* 93:232, 1982.
40. Flammer J, Drance SM: Effect of acetazolamide on the differential threshold, *Arch Ophthalmol* 101:1378, 1983.
41. Stepanik J: The effect of chlorothiazide (Diuril, Chlotride) on ocular tension in humans, *Ophthalmologica* 138:361, 1959.
42. Henry MM, Lee PF: Clinical comparison of diclorphenamide, chlorothiazide, and sulocarbilate with acetazolamide in control of glaucoma, *Am J Ophthalmol* 47:199, 1959.
43. Schimek RA, Balian JV, Lepley FJ, and others: Evaluation of dichlorphenamide as an ocular hypotensive agent, *Arch Ophthalmol* 60:1054, 1958.
44. Gonzales-Jiminez ER, Leopold IH: Chlorothiazide and ocular pressure, *Arch Ophthalmol* 60:70, 1958.
45. Fajardo RB, Hamilton R, and Leopold IH: The effect of hydrochlorothiazide (Esidrex)

in intraocular pressure in man, *Am J Ophthalmol* 49:1321, 1960.
46. Friedenwald JS: Current studies on acetazolamide (Diamox) and aqueous humor flow, *Am J Ophthalmol* 40:139, 1955.
47. Maren TH, Haywood JR, Chapman SK, and others: The pharmacology of methazolamide in relation to the treatment of glaucoma, *Invest Ophthalmol Vis Sci* 16:730, 1977.
48. Wistrand PJ, Rawls JA, Maren TH: Sulfonamide carbonic anhydrase inhibitors and intra-ocular pressure in rabbits, *Acta Pharmacol Toxicol* 17:377, 1960.
49. Maren TH: Carbonic anhydrase: chemistry, physiology and inhibition, *Physiol Rev* 47:595, 1967.
50. Bayne WF, Tao FT, Rogers G, and others: Time course and disposition of methazolamide in human plasma and red blood cells, *J Pharmacol Sci* 70:75, 1981.
51. Dahlen K, Epstein DL, Grant WM, and others: A repeated dose-response study of methazolamide in glaucoma, *Arch Ophthalmol* 96:2214, 1978.
52. Kister S: Carbonic anhydrase inhibition: The effect of acetazolamide on cerebral spinal fluid flow, *J Pharmocol Exp Ther* 117:402–405, 1956.
53. Gucer G, Viernstein L: Long-term intracranial pressure recording in the management of pseudotumor cerebri, *J Neurosurg* 49: 256, 1978.
54. Macri F, Brown J: The constrictive action of acetazolamide on the iris arteries of the cat, *Arch Ophthalmol* 66:570, 1961.
55. Foss RH: Local application of Diamox, *Am J Ophthalmol* 39:366, 1955.
56. Friedland BR, Mallonee J, Anderson DR: Short-term dose response characteristics of acetazolamide in man, *Arch Ophthalmol* 95:1809, 1977.
57. Lichter PR, Newman LP, Wheeler NC, and others: Patient tolerance to carbonic anhydrase inhibitors, *Am J Ophthalmol* 85:495, 1978.
58. Lederle Laboratories: Research data, Pearl River, NY.
59. Stone RA, Zimmerman TJ, Shin DH, and others: Low-dose methazolamide and intraocular pressure, *Am J Ophthalmol* 83:674, 1977.
60. Gonzales-Jiminez E, Leopold IH: Effect of dichlorphenamide on the intraocular pressure of humans, *Arch Ophthalmol* 60:427, 1958.
61. Drance SM: The effects of ethoxzolamide (Cardrase) on intraocular pressure, *Arch Ophthalmol* 62:679, 1959.
62. Arrigg CA, Epstein DL, Giovanoni R, and others: The influence of supplemental sodium acetate on carbonic anhydrase inhibitor-induced side effects, *Arch Ophthalmol* 99:1969, 1981.
63. Harrison R: Annual review—glaucoma, *Arch Ophthalmol* 70:842, 1963.
64. Spaeth GL: Potassium acetazolamide, and intraocular pressure, *Arch Ophthalmol* 78:578, 1967.
65. Pearson JR, Binder CI, Neber J: Agranulocytosis following Diamox therapy, *JAMA* 157:339, 1955.
66. Reisner Jr. EH, Morgan MC: Thrombocytopenia following acetazolamide (Diamox) therapy, *JAMA* 160:206, 1956.
67. Glushien AS, Fisher ER: Renal lesions of sulfonamide type after treatment with acetazolamide (Diamox), *JAMA* 160:204, 1956.
68. Muirhead J, Scheie H: Transient myopia after acetazolamide, *Arch Ophthalmol* 63:315, 1960.
69. Beasley FJ: Transient myopia—ethoxzolamide, *Arch Ophthalmol* 68:490, 1962.
70. Halpern AE, Kulvin MM: Transient myopia, *Am J Ophthalmol* 48:354, 1959.
71. Beasley FJ: Transient myopia and retinal edema during hydrochlorothiazide (Hydrodiuril) therapy, *Arch Ophthalmol* 65:212, 1961.
72. Reich T: Anhydrase activity of bovine lenses, *Am J Ophthalmol* 36:500, 1953.
73. Kass MA, Kolker AE, Gordon M, and others: Acetazolamide and urolithiasis, *Ophthalmology* 88:261, 1981.
74. Constant MA, Becker B: The effect of carbonic anhydrase inhibitors on urinary excretion of citrate by humans, *Am J Ophthalmol* 49:929, 1960.
75. Sheilds MB, Simmons RJ: Urinary calculus during methazolamide therapy, *Am J Ophthalmol* 81:622, 1976.
76. Lubeck J: Aplastic anemia following acetazolamide therapy, *Am J Ophthalmol* 69:684, 1970.
77. Gangitano JL, Roster SH, Contro RM: Nonfatal methazolamide-induced aplastic anemia, *Am J Ophthalmol* 86:138, 1978.
78. Wisch N, Fischbein FI, Siegel R, and others: Aplastic anemia resulting from the use of carbonic anhydrase inhibitors, *Am J Ophthalmol* 75:130, 1973.
79. Fraunfelder FT, Meyer SM, Bagby GC, and others: Hematologic reactions to carbonic

anhydrase inhibitors, *Am J Ophthalmol* 100:79, 1985.

80. Mogk LG, Cyrlin MN: Blood Dyscrasias and the carbonic anhydrase inhibitors, *Ophthalmology* 95:768, 1988.
81. Maren TH: Teratology and carbonic anhydrase inhibition, *Arch Ophthalmol* 85:1, 1971.
82. Worsham GF, Beckman EN, Mitchell EH: Sacrococcygeal teratoma in a neonate, *JAMA* 240:251, 1973.
83. Garner LL, Carl EF, Ferwerda JR: Acetazolamide in glaucoma, Exhibit, Sixty-Sixth Annual Convention, *Am Acad Ophthalmol Otolaryngol* 1961.
84. Garrison L, Roth A, Rundle H, and others: A clinical comparison of three carbonic anhydrase inhibitors, *Trans Pac Coast Otoophthalmol Soc* 51:137, 1967.
85. Drance SM: Ethoxzolamide (Cardrase) in the management of chronic simple glaucoma, *Arch Ophthalmol* 64:433, 1960.
86. Maren TH, Bar-Ilan A, Conroy CW, and others: Chemical and pharmacological properties of MK-927, a sulfonamide carbonic anhydrase inhibitor that lowers intraocular pressure by the topical route, *Exp Eye Res* 50:27, 1990.
87. Wang RF, Serle JB, Podos SM, and others: The effect of MK-927, a topical carbonic anhydrase inhibitor, on IOP in glaucomatous monkeys, *Curr Eye Res* 9:163, 1990.
88. Higgingbottom EJ, Kass MA, Lipps EA, and others: MK-927: A topical carbonic anhydrase inhibitor: dose response and duration of action, *Arch Ophthalmol* 108:65, 1990.
89. Pfeiffer N, Hennekes R, Lippa EA, and others: A single dose of the carbonic anhydrase inhibitor MK-927 decreases IOP in patients, *Br J Ophthalmol* 74:405, 1990.
90. Bron AM, Lippa EA, Hoffman H, and others: MK-927: A topically effective carbonic anhydrase inhibitor in patients, *Arch Ophthalmol* 107:1143, 1989.
91. Higgingbottom EJ, Kao SF, Kass M, et al: Once-daily and twice-daily treatment with the topical carbonic anhydrase inhibitor MK-927, *Invest Ophthalmol* 30(suppl):23, 1989.
92. Bron AM, Lippa EA, Gunning F, and others: Multiple dose efficacy comparison of the two carbonic anhydrase inhibitors sezolamide and MK-927, *Arch Ophthalmol* 109:50, 1991.
93. George J-L, Sirbat D, Lesure P, and others: MK-417 vs MK-927: multiple dose efficacy comparison of two topical carbonic anhydrase inhibitors, *Invest Ophthalmol* 30(suppl):98, 1989.
94. Lippa EA, Schuman JS, Higgingbottom EJ, and others: MK-507 vs sezolamide, *Ophthalmology* 98:308, 1991.
95. Sugrue MF, Mallorga P, Schwam H, and others: A comparison of L-671,152 and MK-927, two topically effective ocular hypotensive carbonic anhydrase inhibitors, in experimental animals, *Curr Eye Res* 9:607, 1990.
96. Lippa EA, Carlson L-E, Ehinger B, and others: Dose response relationship of the novel topical CAI MK-507, *Invest Ophthalmol* 32(suppl):946, 1991.
97. Nardin G, Lewis R, Lippa EA, and others: Activity of topical CAI MK-507 bid when added to timolol bid, *Invest Ophthalmol* 32(suppl):989, 1991.

## SECTION TWO

1. Galin MA, Davidson R: Aqueous and blood urea nitrogen levels after intravenous urea administration, *Arch Ophthalmol* 65:805, 1961.
2. Robbins R, Galin MA: Effects of osmotic agents on the vitreous body, *Arch Ophthalmol* 82:694, 1969.
3. Gorne SB, Newell F: The autoradiographic localization of urea C-14 in the rabbit eye, *Am J Ophthalmol* 54:63, 1962.
4. Podos SM, Krupin T, Becker B: Effects of small-dose hyperosmotic injections on intraocular pressure of small animals and man when optic nerves are transected and intact, *Am J Ophthalmol* 71:989, 1971.
5. Krupin T, Podos SM, Lehman RAW, and others: Effect of optic nerve transection on intraocular pressure in monkeys, *Arch Ophthalmol* 84:668, 1970.
6. Podos SM, Krupin T, Becker B: Mechanism of intraocular pressure after optic nerve transection, *Am J Ophthalmol* 72:79, 1971.
7. Krupin T, Podos SM, Becker B: Effect of optic nerve transection on osmotic alterations of intraocular pressure, *Am J Ophthalmol* 70:214, 1970.
8. Tarter RC, Linn JC: A clinical study of the use of intravenous urea in glaucoma, *Am J Ophthalmol* 52:323, 1961.
9. Marshall S, Hinman F: Subdural hematoma following administration of urea for diagnosis of hypertension, *JAMA* 182:233, 1962.
10. Cadieux RJ: Drug interaction in the elderly, *PostGrad Med* 86:179, 1989.

11. Wei JY: Mechanisms of disease: age and the cardiovascular system, *N Engl J Med* 327:1735, 1992.
12. Marmor MF, Martin LJ, Tharpe S: Osmotically induced retinal detachment in the rabbit and primate, *Invest Ophthalmol Vis Sci* 19:1016, 1980.
13. Marmor RF: Retinal detachment from hyperosmotic intravitreal injection, *Invest Ophthalmol Vis Sci* 18:1237, 1979.
14. Negi A, Marmor MF: Effects of subretinal and systemic osmolality on the rate of subretinal fluid resorption, *Invest Ophthalmol Vis Sci* 25:616, 1984.
15. Yao XY, Moore KT, Marmor MF: Systemic mannitol increase retinal adhesiveness measured in vitro, *Arch Ophthalmol* 109: 275, 1991.
16. Farahbakhsh NA, Gordon LF: Volume regulation of non-pigmented cells from ciliary epithelium, *Invest Ophthalmol Vis Sci* 28: 934, 1987.
17. Thomas R: Glycerin, *Arch Ophthalmol* 70:625, 1963.
18. Galin MA, Diaidson R, Shachter N: Ophthalmological use of osmotic therapy, *Am J Ophthalmol* 62:629, 1966.
19. Marisi A, Aquavella JV: Hypertonic saline solution in cornea edema, *Ann Ophthalmol* 7:229, 1975.
20. Green K, Downs S: Reduction of corneal thickness with hypertonic solutions, *Am J Ophthalmol* 75:507, 1973.
21. Buckley EG, Shields MB: Isosorbide and isosorbide dinitrate, *Am J Ophthalmol* 89:457, 1980.
22. McCarey BE, Kaufman HE: Improved corneal storage, *Invest Ophthalmol* 13:165, 1974.
23. Kaufman HE, Varnell ED, Kaufman S, and others: K-Sol corneal preservation, *Am J Ophthalmol* 100:299, 1985.
24. Yau CW, Kaufman HE: A medium-term cornea preserving medium (K-Sol), *Arch Ophthalmol* 104:598, 1986.
25. Bourne WM: Endothelial cell survival on transplanted human corneas preserved at 4° C in 2.5% chondroitin sulfate for one to 13 days, *Am J Ophthalmol* 102:382, 1986.
26. Smith RM, Bourne WM, Campbell RJ: Chondroitin sulfate for corneal preservation at 4° C, *Arch Ophthalmol* 104:1358, 1986.
27. Walkenbach RJ, Corwin JG, Guo-Sui Y: Corneal function after storage in commercial eye bank media, *Invest Ophthalmol Vis Sci* 32:1551, 1991.
28. Keates RH, Rabnin BR: Extending corneal storage with 2.5% chondroitin sulfate (K-Sol), *Ophthalmic Surg* 19:817, 1988.
29. Lass JH, Reinhart WJ, et al: An in vitro and clinical comparison of corneal storage with chondroitin sulfate corneal storage medium with and without dextran, *Ophthalmology* 97:96, 1990.

## SECTION THREE

1. Kass MA, Gordon M, Morley RE, and others: Compliance with topical timolol treatment, *Am J Ophthalmol* 103:188, 1987.
2. Zimmerman TJ, Kooner KS, Kandarakis AS, and others: Improving the therapeutic Index of topically applied ocular drugs, *Arch Ophthalmol* 102:551, 1984.
3. McMahon CD, Hetherington Jr. J, Hoskins Jr. HD, and others: Timolol and pediatric glaucomas, *Ophthalmology* 88:249, 1981.
4. Boger III WP, Walton DS: Timolol in uncontrolled childhood glaucomas, *Ophthalmology* 88:253, 1981.
5. Zimmerman TJ, Kooner KS, Morgan KS: Safety and efficacy of timolol in pediatric glaucoma, *Surv Ophthalmol* 28(suppl):262, 1983.
6. Burnstine RA, Felton JL, Ginther WH: Cardiorespiratory reaction to timolol maleate in a pediatric patient. A case report, *Ann Ophthalmol* 14:905, 1982.
7. Samples JR, Meyer SM: Use of ophthalmic medications in pregnant and nursing women, *Am J Ophthalmol* 106:616, 1988.
8. Schoene RB, Abuan T, Ward RL, and others: Effects of topical betaxolol, timolol, and placebo on pulmonary function in asthmatic bronchitis, *Am J Ophthalmol* 97:86, 1984.
9. Van Buskirk EM, Weinreb RN, Berry DP, and others: Betaxolol in patients with glaucoma and asthma, *Am J Ophthalmol* 101:531, 1986.
10. Ofner S, Smith TJ: Betaxolol in chronic obstructive pulmonary disease, *J Ocular Pharmacol* 3:171, 1987.
11. Harris LS, Greenstein SH, Bloom AF: Respiratory difficulties with betaxolol, *Am J Ophthalmol* 102:274, 1986.
12. Roholt PC: Betaxolol and restrictive airway disease, *Arch Ophthalmol* 105:1172, 1987.
13. Kolker AE, Becker B: Epinephrine maculopathy, *Arch Ophthalmol* 79:552, 1968.
14. Michels RG, Maumenee AE: Cystoid macular edema associated with topically applied epinephrine in aphakic eyes, *Am J Ophthalmol* 80:379, 1975.

15. Goldberg I, Ashbum FS, Palmberg PF, and others: Timolol and epinephrine, a clinical study of ocular interactions, *Arch Ophthalmol* 98:484, 1980.
16. Ohrstrom A, Pandolfi M: Regulation of intraocular pressure and pupil size by beta-blockers and epinephrine, *Arch Ophthalmol* 98:2182, 1980.
17. Topper JE, Brubaker RF: Effects of timolol, epinephrine, and acetazolamide on aqueous flow during sleep, *Invest Ophthalmol Vis Sci* 26:1315, 1985.
18. Fraunfelder FT, Meyer SM, Bagby Jr. GC, and others: Hematologic reactions to carbonic anhydrase inhibitors, *Am J Ophthalmol* 100:79, 1985.
19. Lichter PR: Carbonic anhydrase inhibitors, blood dyscrasias, and standard-of-care, *Ophthalmology* 95:711, 1988.
20. Mogk LG, Cyrlin MN: Blood dyscrasias and carbonic anhydrase inhibitors, *Ophthalmology* 95:768, 1988.
21. Thomas JV, Epstein DL: Timolol and epinephrine in primary open angle glaucoma. Transient additive effect, *Arch Ophthalmol* 99:91, 1981.
22. Thomas JV, Epstein DL: Study of the additive effect of timolol and epinephrine in lowering intraocular pressure, *Br J Ophthalmol* 65:596, 1981.
23. Cyrlin MS, Thomas JV, Epstein DL: Additive effect of epinephrine to timolol therapy in primary open angle glaucoma, *Arch Ophthalmol* 100:414, 1982.
24. Korey MS, Hodapp E, Kass MA, and others: Timolol and epinephrine. Long-term evaluation of concurrent administration, *Arch Ophthalmol* 100:742, 1982.
25. Knupp JA, Shields MB, Mandell AI, and others: Combined timolol and epinephrine therapy for open angle glaucoma, *Surv Ophthalmol* 28(suppl):280, 1983.
26. Weinreb RN, Ritch R, Kushner FH: Effect of adding betaxolol to dipivefrin therapy, *Am J Ophthalmol* 101:196, 1986.
27. Allen RC, Epstein DL: Additive effect of betaxolol and epinephrine in primary open angle glaucoma, *Arch Ophthalmol* 104:1178, 1986.
28. Olivius E, Thorburn W: Prognosis of glaucoma simplex and glaucoma capsulare. A comparative study, *Acta Ophthalmol* 56:921, 1978.
29. Chandler PA, Grant WM: Mydriatic-cycloplegic treatment in malignant glaucoma, *Arch Ophthalmol* 68:353, 1962.

CHAPTER 5

# Anesthesia

Elson L. Craig

## LOCAL ANESTHESIA

The majority of ocular diagnostic and surgical procedures may be performed with the patient under local anesthesia. Minor manipulations of the cornea, conjunctiva, or eyelids may require only topical instillation of a surface-active anesthetic. When more extensive procedures are to be undertaken, injection anesthesia is necessary. This may consist of infiltration of a localized area, a nerve block for regional anesthesia, retrobulbar or peribulbar injection for anesthesia and akinesia of the orbit and globe, or the regional infiltration of the facial nerve for orbicularis akinesia. Indications for general anesthesia in ophthalmic surgery vary but are usually reserved for more extensive surgical procedures or for patients who cannot tolerate local injection anesthesia. Understanding the principles and procedures for obtaining good anesthesia is essential for the success of any ocular surgery. Equally as important is a thorough knowledge of the pharmacology of the various drugs employed.

### Mechanism of Action

The drugs suitable for use as local anesthetics cause a reversible block of conduction through nerve fibers. The potency of a local anesthetic parallels its affinity for the nerve receptor protein when both are isolated in solution.[1] Tetracaine and related local anesthetics are similar in structure to acetylcholine. Procaine differs from acetylcholine only in the substitution of an aniline ring for a methyl group. The acetylcholine system is ordinarily thought of as mediating neural impulses at synapses only. Actually it also controls the ion movements within nerve fibers, as well as at synapse and junctional complexes.

As the concentration of a local anesthetic increases, the various activities of a nerve are progressively blocked. The amplitude of the nerve action potential and its rate of rise are decreased. Conduction velocity slows, and the refractive period lengthens. The firing threshold rises until finally the nerve becomes inexcitable. All these changes occur in a reversible manner, without damage to the neural membrane or axon.

Impulse propagation along a nerve axon is characterized by a rapid passage along the nerve membrane of an increase in membrane permeability to sodium ions. The nerve membrane is lipoidal and resists passage of cations except at pores known as transmembrane sodium channels. A local anesthetic is believed to act by impeding sodium access to the axon, probably by blocking transmembrane sodium channels. This channel blockade occurs on the inner aspect of the channel, not on the outside of the nerve membrane. The actual block may result from the binding of the cationic portion of the local anesthetic to the phospholipid membrane that surrounds the inner openings of the sodium channels. This results in a physical occlusion of the channels, which bars sodium entry and prevents axon depolarization (a nondepolarization block).[2]

Local anesthetic agents have properties similar to those of drugs that readily traverse the cornea. They must be capable of existing alternately in ionized (water-soluble) and nonionized (lipid-soluble) form. During their lipoid-soluble phase they traverse the nerve membrane to its interior. Becoming ionized, the anesthetic cation then binds to the inner end of the transmembrane sodium channel.

In aqueous solutions, the anesthetic cation and the nonpolar base exist in an equilibrium that is pH dependent. The amount of base (and therefore the membrane-penetrating capability of the anesthetic) is increased by alkalinity (pH increase). The pH adjustment of local anesthetic solutions with sodium bicarbonate may shorten onset time and improve spread of neural blockade.[3] The use of bicarbonate-buffered anesthetic solutions may also reduce pain during tissue infiltration. Higher pH increases the nonionized fraction of an acid anesthetic. The nonionized form has better nerve sheath penetration, a shorter onset of nerve blockade, and perhaps less effect on pain receptors.[4] This pH dependency is the reason that local anesthetics are less effective in inflamed tissue, which has a more acid pH than normal; there is a lesser proportion of membrane-penetrating base.

## Duration of Action

The duration of the anesthetic effect is determined by the length of time the drug remains bound to the nerve protein. This varies with the chemical structure of the drug, its concentration, and the rate of removal by diffusion and circulation. The rapidity of onset and the duration of anesthesia increase in proportion to the logarithm[5] of the concentration of a given drug until a maximal concentration is reached.[6] No further increase in duration results when the maximal effective concentration is exceeded. Hence, using more than the maximal effective concentration achieves nothing but greater systemic toxicity. The maximal effective concentrations of tetracaine, cocaine, and proparacaine are 1%, 20%, and 0.5%, respectively. In the interest of safety and practical efficiency of anesthesia, the optimal concentration of a drug may be less than the maximal effective concentration. Less than maximal concentrations (e.g., 0.5% tetracaine) may be less irritating to the eye, for instance, and therefore better suited to clinical practice. Combination of two or more local anesthetic drugs does not enhance activity beyond that which would be obtained by an equivalent concentration of the stronger drug. Because the toxic systemic effect of multiple drugs is additive, the therapeutic index is not improved by using mixtures of anesthetic agents. An exception to the preceding statement occurs with mixtures of injection anesthetics having a different duration of action. Characteristically a long-acting anesthetic such as bupivacaine or etidocaine has a slow onset of anesthesia, perhaps requiring as long as ½ hour for development of an adequate effect. A mixture of bupivacaine and lidocaine will result in the rapid and predictable onset of lidocaine anesthesia, combined with the much longer duration of action of bupivacaine.[7]

Although vasoconstrictors retard the absorption of injected anesthetic solutions, they do not influence the systemic absorption of anesthetics applied topically to normal mucous membranes, nor do they materially prolong the duration of action of topical anesthetics. For instance, the duration of anesthesia of the tip of the tongue was 53 minutes after application of a 1% tetracaine solution with a 1:10,000 concentration of epinephrine.[6] A similar test of tetracaine on the tongue using a methylcellulose vehicle to increase contact time was found not to prolong the duration of anesthesia. Comparable tests using viscous anesthetic solutions on the conjunctiva have not been performed.

## Toxicity

Fortunately in ophthalmology it is not necessary to use large quantities of topical anesthetics. Indeed, excessive amounts are not retained in the cul-de-sac but run harmlessly down the cheek. One should be aware, nevertheless, that these drugs are extremely toxic. For instance, 100 mg of tetracaine is considered to be a potentially lethal dose. This is only 5 ml of a 2% solution. Fatal reactions are rarely a result of idiosyncrasy or an allergy but occur from the use of excessive quantities of anesthetic. Because generalized reactions to the topical application of anesthetic solutions result from systemic absorption of excessive quantities of drug, such reactions are virtually nonexistent after topical ocular anesthesia because of the small quantities required.

The rate of drug absorption across mucous membranes is extremely rapid and is comparable with intravenous administration. The blood levels in dogs after 30 mg of tetracaine was administered by rapid (30 seconds) intravenous injection, slow (20 minutes) intravenous injection, and pharyngeal and tracheal instillation, and subcutaneous injection revealed that absorption across the mucous membranes was far more rapid than that after subcutaneous injection or slow intravenous administration (Fig. 5–1). Regardless of the concentration used, the maximum blood level attained after topical application was only a fraction of the level attained from rapid intravenous administration. Because a minimal lethal dose of a local anesthetic is destroyed by the liver within 20 to 60 minutes,[8] recovery from local anesthetic poisoning is rapid, provided the patient can be kept alive by emergency measures. For instance, toxic reactions to tetracaine are often characterized by a sudden onset of cardiac and respiratory collapse and may quickly prove fatal. Convulsions usually do not occur, and in this respect tetracaine toxicity differs from that of cocaine and most other topical anesthetics. Cocaine reactions usually begin with excitement, apprehension, and convulsions. Treatment of these serious complications may require cardiopulmonary resuscitation, which should be instituted immediately and must be continued until the patient recovers. Intravenous administration of barbiturates is of value in controlling convulsions only and should not be given to the collapsed patient, because depression of vital functions is only made worst. Intravenous administration of pressor agents may help hypotension and when given in high doses, may make resuscitation from cardiac arrest more effective (high-dose epinephrine).[9] Respiratory stimulants are considered to be ineffectual. Further details concerning the management of anesthetic reactions can be found in the discussion of local anesthesia by injection.

### Anesthetic Effects on Tear Flow

In a study of 466 eyes anesthetized with 0.5% proparacaine, the Schirmer paper strip wetting length was reduced by 40%. If the tear lake was blotted dry after instillation of

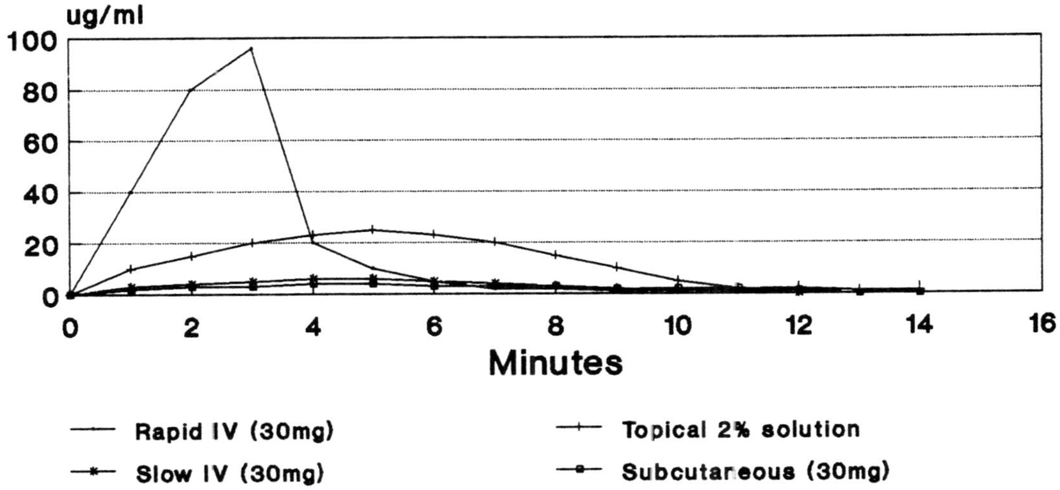


**FIG 5–1.**
Blood levels of tetracaine by different routes of administration in dogs. (Modified from Adriani J, Campbell D: *JAMA* 162:1527, 1956. Used by permission.)

**TABLE 5–1.**
Topical Anesthetic Agents Commonly Used in Ophthalmology

| Name | Trade Name | Concentration |
|---|---|---|
| Cocaine hydrochloride | | 1%–4% |
| Proparacaine hydrochloride | Ak-Taine | 0.5% |
| | Alcaine | 0.5% |
| | Ophthaine | 0.5% |
| | Ophthetic | 0.5% |
| Tetracaine | Pontocaine | 0.5% |

Modified from *PDR for ophthalmology*, ed 22, Montvale, NJ, 1994, Medical Economics Data. Used by permission.

the anesthetic drop, 15% of normal volunteers had Schirmer values up to 3 mm.[10] The lid margins and cilia remain sensitive despite conjunctival anesthesia, and stimulation of these areas will increase tear flow by as much as 300%. Because of many sources of error such as this, the Schirmer test gives variable results and correlates poorly with symptoms of dryness. The test is virtually impossible to interpret in an anesthetized eye, because tear secretion decreases in proportion to the loss of sensory stimulation.[11]

## TOPICAL ANESTHETICS

Surface-active anesthetics available for topical use in ophthalmology are listed in Table 5–1. These drugs have many characteristics in common; they all act readily on mucosal surfaces and are relatively ineffective when applied on less permeable surfaces such as skin. Because surface-active anesthetics are relatively toxic, they should not be injected. Furthermore, the application of excessive amounts of topical anesthetic to mucosal surfaces may result in the absorption of enough drug to cause systemic reactions.

### Tetracaine Hydrochloride

Tetracaine is one of the most popular topical anesthetics used in ophthalmology. Solutions of 0.5% to 2% may be instilled directly into the conjunctival cul-de-sac. The majority of patients will complain of a burning sensation that lasts about 30 seconds, but this is not of clinical significance except in some children and apprehensive patients who may become frightened and uncooperative. The initial discomfort is less severe if the eyes are closed after instillation. A peculiar numb sensation persists for 10 to 20 minutes, depending on the number of drops used. Usually patients will attempt to rub their eyes. Because the corneal epithelium can be injured in this manner, patients should be instructed to gently pat away the tears from the closed eyelids.

Within 20 seconds after instillation of a single drop of 0.5% tetracaine solution, anesthesia is ordinarily adequate for most procedures, such as tonometry. When additional or more involved procedures are required, repeated application of the anesthetic solution at 30-second intervals should be used. Probing the nasolacrimal duct of an adult may require irrigation of the lacrimal sac with 0.25 ml of a 0.5% tetracaine solution. Tetracaine instillation on the conjunctival surface usually fails to achieve effective scleral anesthesia. For example, surface cautery of intrascleral nerve loops was said to be painful when only topical tetracaine anesthetic was employed.[12]

#### *Corneal Toxicity*

As every biomicroscopist knows, transitory superficial corneal epithelial lesions are commonly seen after tetracaine anesthesia. Repeated and prolonged anesthesia will intensify this epithelial damage. This is one of several reasons that it is unwise to prescribe topical anesthetics for patients to use at home. Healing is significantly retarded by such medication, and normal corneal epithelium may be damaged by both chemical toxicity and the patient's rubbing of the anesthetized eye. Intentional abuse of topical anesthetics has been reported, and in two cases the anesthetic was stolen from the ophthalmologist's office.[13] This would emphasize the need to closely monitor topical anesthetics in examination areas. Corneal staining occurred in 60% of 74 subjects after the sequential instillation of fluorescein and proparacaine. The use of the topical anesthetic seemed to enhance a nonuniform penetration of fluorescein into the epithelium in specific regions of the cornea of some of the subjects studied. The authors[14] suggested that some patients may respond clinically with an increase in epithelial permeability or breakdown after the instillation of a topical anesthetic.

Experimental proof of the deleterious effects of topical anesthetics on epithelial regeneration is readily obtained. Both mitosis and cellular migration are inhibited.[15] Regeneration of the anesthetized rat corneal epithelium damaged by experimentally produced minute puncture wounds has been studied. One drop of each anesthetic solution used was instilled every 15 minutes for 3 hours, at which time the rat was killed and the eyes fixed and studied microscopically. No healing occurred during this 3-hour period with solutions of 2% butacaine (Butyn), 4% cocaine benoxinate (Dorsacaine), 1% phenacaine (Holocaine), 0.1% dibucaine (Nupercaine), and 0.5% proparacaine (Ophthaine).[16] Only partial healing was noted in patients treated with a 0.5% solution of tetracaine. Almost complete healing, with only slight distortion of the restored epithelium, occurred within 3 hours in the controls and with the use of solutions of 2% piperocaine (Metycaine) and 2% lidocaine.

Tetracaine seriously impairs the ability of the corneal epithelium to oxidize glucose and pyruvate. In the presence of a 0.0003M concentration of tetracaine, corneal epithelium oxidation of carbohydrates was reduced by more than 80%.[17] During tetracaine anesthesia the oxygen uptake of the cornea is inhibited (17% inhibition with 0.0001M tetracaine, 62% with 0.002M tetracaine, and 75% with 0.004M tetracaine), and lactic acid concentration increases within the tissue.[18] Although the mechanism for corneal epithelial damage by topical anesthetics is unknown, metabolic, toxic, and immune causes have been postulated.[19–21]

Clinical evidence of anesthetic-induced failure of epithelial healing has been provided by a number of reports.[22–24] In one report a series of six patients had sought relief of pain through the home use of tetracaine.[23] The sequence of events was similar. Initially the tetracaine was instilled every few hours for the relief of pain. Gradually the discomfort became more annoying, and the tetracaine was required at more frequent intervals. Within several days the pain became more severe and could not be relieved by tetracaine, which several patients used as often as every 10 minutes. Duration of the tetracaine use varied from several days to as long as 2 weeks. The corneas of these patients showed extensive erosions of the epithelium and were insensitive to touch. In several, grayish stromal infiltrates were present. Healing was slow in all patients and required several months in those patients who had used tetracaine for 2 weeks. Epithelial cell growth was delayed and in every case was further retarded by faulty adherence to Bowman's membrane. Loose flaps of epithelium about the borders of the cornea were subject to recurrent erosion, and these repeated breakdowns greatly prolonged the healing time. Infectious crystalline keratopathy associated with topical anesthetic abuse has been reported in two patients.[25] In both patients the corneas showed large epithelial defects and multiple stromal crystalline infiltrates. Characteristically, these lesions were caused by *Streptococcus viridans*, and there was an absence of inflammatory cells associated with the bacterial infiltrates.

In rabbit experiments the same effect of topical anesthesia has been duplicated (with tetracaine, cocaine, and dibucaine), accompanied by epithelial erosion, stromal infiltration, prolonged insensitivity, and delayed healing. It seems evident that there are a number of reasons that topical anesthetics should not be routinely prescribed for prolonged use.

#### *Allergy*

Although local allergy to tetracaine may develop because of repeated use, as in patients with glaucoma, these reactions are extremely uncommon. The ophthalmologist should suspect tetracaine allergy when the patient complains of itching, persistent redness, and swelling of the eyelids.

#### *Effect on Microorganisms*

Whenever possible, material to be cultured should be obtained without the prior instillation of an anesthetic. Not only are most commercial topical anesthetic preparations compounded with added preservatives, but the anesthetic drugs themselves are often toxic to microorganisms as well. Tetracaine, 0.5%, without added preservatives, completely inhibited all subsequent growth of *Staphylococcus albus, Pseudomonas,* and *Candida albicans* when the drug and the organisms were incubated together for 24 hours. In contrast, 0.5% proparacaine did not significantly inhibit growth of any of these organisms. In commercial preparations proparacaine contains 0.2% chlorobutanol, which partially inhibits these organisms in a 24-hour culture. Chlorobutanol, 0.4%, is a more effective preservative, completely inhibiting all three organisms first mentioned for 24 hours. Benoxinate, 0.4%, inhibited *Staphylococcus* and *Candida* but not *Pseudomonas.* Cocaine hydrochloride, 2.5%, inhibited all organisms.[26] In this study the practical effect of instillation of anesthetic drops for a brief period was not evaluated; certainly less than 24 hours of incubation is required for a corneal scraping. No doubt considerably less inhibition would occur in a shorter period; regardless, corneal scraping is impossible without an anesthetic.

Another study was designed to simulate the clinical conditions of anesthetic use. The amount of growth inhibition resulting from a 2-minute exposure and a subsequent 10 times dilution of the anesthetic was determined.[27] Under these circumstances the growth of *S. albus* was inhibited by both tetracaine and proparacaine. Proparacaine also inhibited the growth of *C. albicans.* Cocaine and benoxinate did not inhibit the growth of bacteria or fungi.

In vitro exposure of herpes simplex virus to commercial proparacaine reduced the amount of recoverable virus by more than 99%. However, the rate of recovery of virus from infected rabbit corneas was not reduced after 1 minute of exposure to 1 drop of topical proparacaine.[22]

### Proparacaine Hydrochloride

Proparacaine is a synthetic topical anesthetic with characteristics essentially similar to those of tetracaine. Proparacaine is supplied as a 0.5% solution with 0.2% chlorobutanol and 1:10,000 benzalkonium chloride added. Topical instillation of a 0.5% proparacaine and of tetracaine produced similar anesthetic effects. The time of onset of anesthesia after tetracaine instillation ranged from 9 to 26 seconds (average 14.7 seconds); that of proparacaine ranged from 6 to 20 seconds (average 12.9 seconds). The duration of action of tetracaine ranged from 9 to 24 seconds (average 15.2 seconds). Ocular instillation of proparacaine is considerably more comfortable than the use of tetracaine. Rated on a 4+ pain scale, discomfort with tetracaine averaged 1.5+ compared with 0.5+ for proparacaine used in the fellow eye.[28]

### Benoxinate Hydrochloride

Benoxinate has clinical characteristics that are essentially similar to those of proparacaine. Both drugs are less irritating than tetracaine and cause less punctate epithelial damage. A concentration of 0.4% benoxinate produces corneal anesthesia essentially identical in intensity, time of onset, and duration to that of a 0.5% proparacaine solution. In a series of 86 patients receiving benoxinate in one eye and tetracaine in the other, no irritation was reported by 22 persons receiving benoxinate and 13 receiving tetracaine.[29] In patients reporting discomfort, the duration of benoxinate burning and stinging averaged 9.8 seconds compared with 23 seconds for tetracaine.

In a series of more than 1,000 patients anesthetized with benoxinate, no toxic effects were encountered locally or systemically.[30] Six of these patients who were allergic to other topical anesthetics (tetracaine, butacaine, and cocaine) had no reaction to benoxinate. Chemical analysis demonstrated ready penetration of benoxinate into the eye. Within 3 minutes after the application of a 1% solution to the intact cornea, concentrations of 70 mg/100 ml existed in the corneal epithelium and 7.5 mg/100 ml in the stroma. Rapid diffusion occurred, and within 15 minutes the corneal concentrations dropped to one third of their initial value. For this reason effective anesthesia did not last for more than 10 to 15 minutes. Benoxinate hydrochloride is no longer available for use as a topical anesthetic only but is used as the anesthetic agent in a commonly used product, Fluress (0.25% fluorescein sodium 0.4% benoxinate hydrochloride).

### Cocaine Hydrochloride

Cocaine, a naturally occurring alkaloid, was the first drug to be used successfully as a local anesthetic.[31–33] Excellent surface anesthesia is obtained by the use of 1% to 4% solutions, concentrations usually employed in ophthalmology. The anesthesia produced is adequate to allow painless grasping of the eye with forceps for about 10 minutes. Incomplete anesthesia persists for another 5 to 10 minutes. The indications and the procedure for the use of cocaine are essentially the same as those described previously for tetracaine. For ophthalmologic use, the newer synthetic anesthetics have replaced cocaine because of its deleterious effect on the cornea, its sympathomimetic properties, and its addicting potential. The rate of onset and the duration of anesthesia after 1 drop of a 2% solution was placed on the cornea have been reported. Within 30 seconds the cornea is insensitive, adequate to allow tonometry. The depth of anesthesia rapidly increases during the first minute, reaches a maximum at 2 minutes, and begins to decline by 3 minutes. After 8 minutes the anesthetic effect rapidly decreases.

The use of 2 or more drops of a higher drug concentration substantially increased the duration of anesthesia. A persistent clinical myth represents cocaine as having extraordinarily superior anesthetic properties that permit painless force duction tests[34] or minor surgical procedures. Proparacaine, 0.5%, anesthetizes the cornea and conjunctiva as well as or better than 4% cocaine and with much less corneal damage. Cocaine potency is dose related, as is true of all anesthetics. A 20% cocaine solution was reported to be necessary to match the anesthetic potency of 1% tetracaine.[11]

#### *Epithelial Damage*

The epithelial damage resulting from corneal anesthesia appears in its most exaggerated form when cocaine is used. Grossly visible grayish corneal pits and irregularities are readily produced by cocaine. Loosening of the epithelium may result in large erosions. In fact, this characteristic of cocaine proves useful in the treatment of dendritic ulcers, where it is used to remove the epithelium. Repeated instillation of cocaine over a period of several minutes will produce excellent anesthesia. It is then possible to dislodge the intact epithelium with an iodine-impregnated swab. Inasmuch as cocaine iodide is an insoluble precipitate, the previous cocainization affords some protection against stromal damage by the iodine. Care should be taken to avoid excessive chemical cauterization to prevent scar formation.

When cocaine is used for topical anesthesia, the sympathomimetic effects on the pupil should be recognized. Approximately 15 minutes after the instillation of cocaine on the eye the pupil will begin to dilate, reaching maximum size within the first hour and returning to normal size within several hours. This effect is caused by the indirect action of cocaine on actively functioning sympathetic nerves in the ocular sympathetic pathway. Cocaine should not be used for topical anesthesia in ocular surgery if the surgeon does not wish the pupil to be dilated or if good visualization of the fundus is necessary.

Considerable central nervous system (CNS) stimulation results from systemic absorption of cocaine. Because cocaine potentiates catecholamines, it is particularly dangerous in patients with hypertensive cardiovascular disease or in simultaneous use with sympathomimetic drugs.[35] Stimu-

**TABLE 5–2.**
Regional Anesthetic Agents Used in Ophthalmic Surgery

| Name | Maximum Concentration | Onset of Action (min) | Duration of Action |
|---|---|---|---|
| Procaine (Novocaine) | 1%–4%/500 mg | 7–8 | 30–45 min (with epinephrine) |
| Tetracaine | 0.25% | 5–9 | 120–140 min (with epinephrine) |
| Hexylcaine | 1%–2% | 5–10 | 60 min |
| Bupivacaine (Marcaine) | 0.25–0.75% | 5–11 | 8–12 hr (with epinephrine) |
| Lidocaine (Xylocaine) | 1%–2%/500 mg | 4–6 | 40–60 min |
| Mepivacaine (Carbocaine) | 1–2%/500 mg | 3–5 | 120 min |
| Etidocaine | 1% | 3 | 5–10 hr |

Modified from *PDR for ophthalmology*, ed 22, Montvale, NJ, 1994, Medical Economics Data. Used by permission.

lation of the CNS with excitement, anxiety, convulsions, and circulatory and respiratory collapse characterizes cocaine toxicity. Severe reactions have followed doses as low as 20 mg (1 ml of a 2% solution) of cocaine. Doses in excess of 1 g are considered to be fatal.

## INJECTION AGENTS

The majority of ophthalmic operations can be performed using regional or nerve block anesthesia obtained with one of the available injection anesthetics (Table 5–2). In most cases this is clearly the method of choice. Uncooperative patients, children, or an extremely anxious person would be the exception. The advantage to the patient is avoiding the many potential complications of a general anesthetic, as well as the personal discomforts it can cause. Postanesthetic morbidity after a general anesthetic may last for weeks.

The ease and apparent safety with which local anesthesia can be achieved with current injection techniques should not lead to a false sense of security. Although complications from the injection of local anesthetics are rare, when they occur they may lead to serious ocular or even life-threatening events. A carefully taken preoperative history and medical examination are essential. Fortunately, most ophthalmic surgery is elective, and generally the patients are healthy (class I or II, Table 5–3).[36] This allows the surgeon adequate time to obtain all necessary information before the operation. In those cases where systemic disease exists, a more detailed evaluation is required, particularly when the cardiopulmonary system is involved. Local anesthetic injections should not be used unless the physician has immediately available an effective method for performing cardiopulmonary resuscitation. The physician should also be aware of the various complications that can occur to the globe and periocular tissues from the injection of a local anesthetic and be able to take appropriate action. These same precautionary measures should be followed when any medication is injected into ocular or periocular tissues.

### Procaine Hydrochloride

This potent and relatively nontoxic anesthetic achieved wide popularity in injection anesthesia. Procaine penetrates poorly and is unsatisfactory for topical application to mucous membranes. When injected, procaine is only one fourth as toxic as cocaine[8] and furthermore is detoxified

**TABLE 5–3.**
Classification of Physical Status of Preoperative Patients by the American Society of Anesthesiologists

| Class | Description |
|---|---|
| I | Healthy patient |
| II | Systemic disease—mild, no functional limitations |
| III | Systemic disease—severe, functional limitations |
| IV | Systemic disease—severe, threat to life |
| V | Moribund |

more rapidly by the body. If caution is exercised to avoid intravenous injection, 0.5 g of procaine is considered to be a safe dose. This is the equivalent of 50 ml of a 1% solution, far more than is necessary in ophthalmic surgery. A further margin of safety is gained by simultaneous injection of epinephrine, thus retarding absorption.

Procaine may be used in concentrations varying from 0.5% to 4.0%. There is rarely a need to use a solution stronger than 1% for ophthalmologic anesthesia. Obviously stronger concentrations introduce a greater amount of potentially toxic drug. Toxic reactions are similar to those described for other injectable anesthetics.

### Lidocaine Hydrochloride

Lidocaine is one of the most popular drugs for local injection anesthesia. Although similar to procaine in its anesthetic effect, lidocaine diffuses more readily through tissue and therefore produces a wider area of anesthesia. Its duration is longer than that of procaine. Reliable surgical anesthesia from lidocaine can be expected for 45 minutes to 1 hour. Postoperative discomfort usually takes several hours to occur. As would be expected from its greater potency, lidocaine is about 50% more toxic than procaine. Reactions to lidocaine are similar to those observed with other local anesthetic agents and involve the CNS and the cardiovascular system. The excitatory reactions because of CNS effects may be brief or not occur at all, in which case the first signs of a toxic reaction may be drowsiness, rapidly progressing to unconsciousness and respiratory arrest.

A 1% lidocaine solution is adequate for most ophthalmic uses. Although most often used as a 2% solution, for practical purposes, this does not further increase the anesthetic effect but doubles the dosage and increases the potential for a toxic reaction. Not more than 0.5 g of lidocaine should be given to a patient during a single surgical procedure. This is 50 ml of a 1% solution. Because most ophthalmic procedures rarely require more than 10 to 15 ml of solution, a large margin of safety exists for the use of this anesthetic.

### Mepivacaine Hydrochloride

Mepivacaine is a synthetic anesthetic administered by injection.[37] Its toxicity and tissue tolerance are comparable with those of procaine and lidocaine. Although adequate, its anesthetic potency (in dosages of 1.5 ml of a 2% solution) seems slightly less than other commonly used anesthetics when evaluated in terms of akinesia of extraocular muscles or reduction of intraocular pressure.[38] The average duration of sensory anesthesia after retrobulbar injection of 1.5 ml of a 2% solution was 2 hours. This was measured by grasping the conjunctiva of human subjects with forceps every 10 minutes until sensation returned. An indication for the use of mepivacaine would be a history of allergy to other anesthetic agents.

### Bupivacaine Hydrochloride

Bupivacaine is another of the synthetic aminoacyl anesthetics similar to lidocaine in its therapeutic and toxic effects. Bupivacaine is approximately four times more toxic than lidocaine; therefore, a 0.5% concentration of bupivacaine is comparable with 2% lidocaine. The maximum safe dose of bupivacaine in adults is 250 mg (50 ml of a 0.5% solution). Bupivacaine is available in concentrations of 0.25%, 0.5%, and 0.75%.

The great advantage of bupivacaine is its prolonged duration of anesthesia. The primary disadvantage is a slow and unpredictable rate of onset of anesthesia, which may be delayed for as long as 30 minutes. Solutions of 0.5% bupivacaine produce globe anesthesia that lasts for approximately 5 hours and akinesia that lasts for 6 to 10 hours.[39] The duration of anesthesia of 0.75% bupivacaine was 8 to 12 hours, producing profound anesthesia and akinesia. Partial paralysis of extraocular muscles may persist for 1 to 2 days. Histopathologic changes induced in these muscles have been studied to determine if bupivacaine has increased myotoxicity.[40, 41] Maximum myotoxic response was observed at 14 days after injection, and pathologic changes were resolved by 27 days. The authors found similar changes when lidocaine was injected and concluded that these effects are a property common to the entire class of aminoacyl anesthetics. Carlson et al.[42] reported that retrobulbar injections of humans and monkeys with 0.75% bupivacaine, 2.0% mepivacaine, or 2.0% lidocaine with 1:100,000 epinephrine most often caused a complete degeneration of a thin rim of superficial muscle fibers in the extraocular muscles, but this was not considered adequate to cause changes in contractile properties. Massive destruction of large numbers of fibers within the muscle body was thought to be caused by direct injection of the anesthetic solution into the muscle.

Transient strabismus, caused by either hemorrhage into the affected muscle or myotoxicity of the anesthetic agent, may occur after retrobulbar anesthesia. Most often when strabismus does occur, it results from restriction of the inferior rectus muscle.[43] Fortunately, this restriction, in most cases, resolves spontaneously without permanent contracture requiring surgical correction. Similarly, blepharoptosis occurring after local anesthesia is of great concern to the patient and the surgeon but seems to resolve spontaneously in the majority of patients.

Several authors who conducted studies comparing a 0.5% with a 0.75% bupivacaine solution concluded that the weaker solution has a slower onset of anesthesia and incomplete akinesia and is therefore not adequate for use alone as a retrobulbar block in ocular surgery.[44, 45] On the other hand, 0.75% bupivacaine was found to produce adequate anesthesia and akinesia, and the addition of hyaluronidase potentiates its effect.[46] The addition of epinephrine to the bupivacaine block solution did not increase the duration of anesthesia. Unless epinephrine is needed for hemostasis, the prolonged period of anesthesia obtained with bupivacaine allows the surgeon to avoid the use of this potential dangerous drug. Combinations of bupivacaine with lidocaine or similar short-acting anesthetics produce an anesthesia with the prompt and reliable onset of the short-acting anesthetic and the long duration of bupivacaine.

In a randomized series of 126 retinal detachment cases, a 3:2 mixture of 0.75% bupivacaine with 1:200,000 epinephrine and 4% lidocaine was chosen. Retrobulbar injection of 3 to 5 ml of this mixture gave adequate anesthesia for 2 or more hours of surgery in most cases, failing in 10 cases of the mixture and in 21 cases of the control (4% lidocaine alone). Postoperatively, 30% of bupivacaine-lidocaine patients required no narcotics for pain compared with 10% of lidocaine patients. These surgeons were pleased with the quality of anesthesia obtained with the combination and advocated it in preference to general anesthesia.[47]

In practice bupivacaine alone or in combination with other anesthetic agents is widely used. Adequate anesthesia and akinesia for most ocular surgery are obtained. The complication rate seems to be very low if bupivacaine is used in small volumes, and if lidocaine is added, the concentration does not exceed 2%. Some surgeons believe that a combination of 0.75% bupivacaine and hyaluronidase alone may be adequate for most ophthalmic surgical procedures.

A study of 3,123 retrobulbar injections given by different surgeons at one institution was performed to determine the incidence of respiratory arrest and to identify possible risk factors. In 2,235 patients the anesthetic agent consisted of 2% lidocaine and 0.75% bupivacaine (50:50 mixture totaling 10 ml) with 150 USP (TR) units of hyaluronidase. The remaining 888 patients received a similar agent prepared with 4% lidocaine. Respiratory arrest occurred in 0.79% of patients who received 4% lidocaine mixed with bupivacaine compared with 0.09% who received the mixture made with 2% lidocaine. The authors concluded that 4% lidocaine increased the risk of respiratory arrest and that the mechanism was probably not direct intravascular or CNS injection but rapid absorption of the more concentrated drug.[48]

## Associated Medication

### *Epinephrine*

The desired effects of local anesthetics such as procaine and lidocaine can be enhanced by the concomitant use of a 1:200,000 solution of epinephrine. Use of epinephrine may be desirable in highly vascular areas as exist in periocular tissues, and the resulting vasospasm also slows drug absorption from the injected area, thereby prolonging anesthesia. In addition, this decreased rate of systemic absorption allows more time for the anesthetic drug to be detoxified or excreted, reducing the chance of a toxic reaction. Infiltration-type injection of an anesthetic at the operative site usually causes considerable hemorrhaging, which can be greatly reduced if epinephrine is added to the block solution. This is particularly true in lid surgery. Although dacryocystorhinostomy is ordinarily performed with the patient under general anesthesia, if the operative site is infiltrated with a local anesthetic containing epinephrine, excellent hemostasis can be obtained.

The patient with hypertension, cardiovascular disease, or thyrotoxicosis should, in general, have local anesthesia without epinephrine. If a patient is under general anesthesia, it is important to inform the anesthesiologist of your intent to inject epinephrine or to use it intraocularly, because it elevates blood pressure and may cause cardiac fibrillation when agents such as cyclopropane and halothane are being used. Some surgeons warn the patient that after local injection of epinephrine they may experience tachycardia, palpitations, nervousness, and apprehension. Such symptoms are transient and do not interfere with subsequent surgery. Undue restlessness should be allowed to subside before beginning surgery; the patient will be quieter, a toxic anesthetic reaction can be ruled out, and it is less likely that the patient will have unexpected and undesirable reactions resulting from apprehension. Epinephrine does cause tremor, apprehension, pallor, and tachycardia but does not result in convulsions, twitching, or disorientation. Epinephrine reactions produce marked elevation of blood pressure in contrast to the cardiovascular collapse and hypotension of anesthetic toxicity.

### *Hyaluronidase*

Hyaluronic acid is a mucopolysaccharide found in the interstitial spaces of tissue, as well as in the vitreous body. Hyaluronidase is an enzyme that depolymerizes this polysaccharide. Removal of hyaluronic acid from tissues greatly increases their permeability to injected fluids. The permeability returns to normal within 24 to 48 hours because of the formation of new hyaluronic acid. Hyaluronidase is nontoxic and does not damage or inflame tissues. Because there is no hyaluronic acid in the wall of capillaries, hyaluronidase does not affect capillary permeability.

Hyaluronidase is measured in turbidity-reducing units (TRU). Within 30 minutes 1 TRU will reduce the turbidity of a 0.2-mg hyaluronic acid suspension in serum to that of a 0.1-mg suspension. The enzyme is marketed in 150-TRU vials and may be added to 20 ml of lidocaine before injection. As little as 7 TRU/ml will effectively dissolve hyaluronic acid barriers. More than 2 million TRU/kg can be tolerated intravenously by mice.[49]

Mechanical pressure is needed to spread hyaluronidase through tissue. The extent of fluid spread is more closely proportional to the amount of injected fluid than to the dosage of hyaluronidase. Hyaluronidase will not promote the passage of fluids across fascial barriers such as Tenon's capsule or through fibrin clots. For this reason hyaluronidase does not increase the intraocular penetration of medications injected periocularly or subconjunctivally.

Hyaluronidase is useful in enhancing the effect of local injection anesthesia and in increasing the hypotony resulting from retrobulbar anesthesia. Hyaluronidase may increase the effective area of an injected anesthesia by as much as 40%.[50] When used, the time of onset of local anesthesia is shortened, but the duration of anesthesia will also be shortened by hyaluronidase alone. The simultaneous use of epinephrine will help maintain the usual duration of the anesthetic. In addition to ensuring better sensory and motor nerve blockade, the use of hyaluronidase in the anesthetic solution will produce a softer eye than will a similar retrobulbar injection without hyaluronidase. Because retrobulbar injection of hyaluronidase alone has no effect on intraocular pressure, the hypotony must result from enhancement of the anesthetic effect,[51] probably on the extraocular muscles.[52] The effects of the Honan intraocular pressure reducer (Lebanon Corp. Inc., Lebanon, Ind.) were studied in 48 patients undergoing cataract surgery. After retrobulbar injection of a 50:50 mixture of 2% lidocaine without epinephrine and 0.5% bupivacaine with hyaluronidase, 7.5 TRU/ml, the Honan device was placed on the protected eye and the pressure maintained at 30 mm Hg. After 7 to 10 minutes mean intraocular pressure in the study group decreased 6.2 mm Hg. In the control group, who received 4 ml retrobulbar injection but no application of the pressure device, the decrease was 0.7 mm Hg.[53] Clearly the soft eye obtainable by the addition of hyaluronidase to the injected anesthetic solution, followed by the use of the Honan pressure reducer or some other means of ocular pressure, is an extremely important safeguard for anterior segment surgery.

## TECHNIQUES OF LOCAL INJECTION

Local injection anesthesia for ophthalmic surgery may involve the general technique of regional infiltration or the specialized techniques of orbicularis block and peribulbar or retrobulbar injections. Regional infiltration is simply the injection of the anesthetic agent into the area to be operated on, for example, the lid for chalazion surgery. This technique is too obvious to require further description.

Before intraocular surgery, adequate anesthesia and akinesia are necessary to prevent the serious complications that may result from squeezing or eye movement. Such injections should precede intraocular surgery, even if the patient is under general anesthesia, to help prevent problems should the patient become partially awake and move at a critical stage of the operation.

### Orbicularis Block

Orbicularis paralysis can be achieved by blocking the facial nerve at any point along its course. Most commonly a vertical injection is made about 1 cm lateral to the orbital rim (Atkinson block).[54] Four to 6 mm of anesthetic solution may be injected as the needle advances deep to skin and muscle. Injection in this area gives excellent orbicularis paralysis and does not cause lid edema, which could interfere with surgical exposure. Some surgeons prefer the Van Lint akinesia. This involves the injection of the anesthetic solution inferior and superiorly along the orbital rim in the region of the terminal branches of the facial nerve, producing a more local effect. This technique may cause lid swelling, may increase chances for hemorrhage, and produces greater postoperative pain.

An alternate method of blocking the facial nerve below the ear (O'Brien technique) is less convenient, may cause weakness of the entire face, and is more likely to cause prolonged nerve damage. When orbicularis paralysis is achieved by the injection of an anesthetic about the facial nerve as it exits the skull through the stylomastoid foramen (Nadbath block), prolonged facial paralysis may ensue. In 4 of 150 patients receiving such an injection the paralysis lasted for up to 3 months, and tarsorrhaphy was necessary to protect the cornea. The prolonged facial paralysis was not caused by the toxic effects of the anesthetic but by needle injury of the nerve, which is fixed in unyielding surrounding tissue at the site of the injection and therefore cannot roll away from the needle.[55] Dysphagia and respiratory distress developed in three patients after a Nadbath block. The distress was thought to result from paresis of the vagus, glossopharyngeal, and spinal accessory nerves, causing aspiration of oral secretion.[56]

A comparison of the effectiveness of 2% lidocaine, 2% mepivacaine, and 0.75% bupivacaine in producing lid akinesia was made using a force-sensitive lid speculum.[57] Subjects, who had not received premedication, were injected by a modified O'Brien facial nerve block after which voluntary lid closure was measured over a 240-minute period. All three agents were equal in the rapidity of onset and the completeness of akinesia. Duration of effect varied; however, the force of lid closure returned to 60% in 45 minutes with 2% lidocaine and 180 minutes with 2% mepivacaine, and there was no return of closure force at 360 minutes with bupivacaine 0.75%. The authors concluded that because all three agents were similar in effect when equal volumes of injection were used (10 ml), it is unnecessary to mix different agents to achieve a more rapid or more complete lid block. This is in contrast to other reports in which bupivacaine alone has been found to have a slower onset of akinesia compared with mepivacaine and lidocaine.[7, 47]

The ability to obtain adequate lid akinesia in most patients from a well-placed periocular or retrobulbar block alone has been recognized and is being used with greater frequency. Usually a large volume of anesthetic solution (4–6 ml), followed by pressure on the orbital contents, is recommended, although effective anesthesia and akinesia have been reported in one series using only 2.0 ml of retrobulbar injection.[58] The mechanism of a lid block from an injection into the orbit is not clear, but in addition to the effect on the nerves in the orbit, diffusion of the solution into lid tissue and into the lateral canthal area most likely is sufficient to produce paralysis of the orbicularis oculi. Any lid movement that occurs when akinesia is obtained from the retrobulbar block seems to be minimal and does not interfere with the surgery. When this technique is used, most ophthalmic surgery, including vitreoretinal and retinal detachment surgery, can be performed without patient discomfort or unwanted movement or pressure from lids. In situations where the orbit is shallow and the globe is very proptotic, supplemental lid injection may be advisable, however, because of the greater possibility of lid pressure on the globe.

### Retrobulbar and Peribulbar Injections

The technique of injection used will determine the portion of the orbit that is anesthetized. A retrobulbar injection may be intended to produce sensory anesthesia alone or a combination of sensory and motor anesthesia. An anterior retrobulbar injection is placed in the relatively avascular region just behind the globe. A small quantity of solution (e.g., 1 ml) in this anterior retrobulbar position will cause only sensory anesthesia. In contrast, a posterior (or apical) retrobulbar injection will produce both sensory and motor anesthesia to include sensory block of the optic nerve. Because the vessels in the apex of the orbit are larger and more fixed in position and cannot be readily displaced by a needle, they are much more likely to be pierced with a posterior injection than with an anterior one. This may be the reason that retrobulbar hemorrhages are more frequently encountered after posterior injections. Slicing movements of the needle in the deep orbit may further increase the changes for a hemorrhage.

Because no tissue barriers exist between the anterior and posterior portions of the retrobulbar space, motor anesthesia of a posterior block may be achieved simply by injecting a larger volume of solution anteriorly. Four to 6 ml of an anesthetic solution with hyaluronidase may be safely injected into the anterior space. After 5 to 10 minutes of pressure from digital massage or the Honan device, total muscular akinesia and ocular anesthesia will be produced. The slight proptosis that often occurs with the larger volume of anesthetic actually facilitates cataract surgery, especially if the patient has deeply sunken eyes. If the eye is sunkened into an atrophic orbit, as much as 6 ml may be injected to raise the eye to a more surgically accessible position. As much as 8 ml can be injected into the orbit without operative complications, provided that hyaluronidase is used.[59]

The distinction between anterior and posterior retrobulbar injection is particularly important when alcohol injections are given for the relief of pain. Such an injection must be given anteriorly to produce a sensory block hopefully without causing paralysis of the extraocular muscles. The alcohol should be confined within the retrobulbar space, because if it leaks anteriorly, severe chemosis and pain result.

Retrobulbar injections for delivering medications to the orbit and for anesthesia have, for many years, been a common procedure in ophthalmology, and serious complications are rarely encountered. Despite the frequency of use by large numbers of physicians, techniques still vary, and although infrequent, complications continue to occur. The most serious of these involve systemic or CNS toxicity from the injected medications because of either excessive absorption or inadvertent intravascular injection, perforation of the globe, intraocular injection of medication, and retrobulbar hemorrhage.[60–62] All techniques require the blind insertion of a relatively sharp needle into the orbital space, where many delicate vascular and neurologic structures are located. Because they become more closely spaced as the orbital apex is approached, as the sharp needle is passed toward the orbital apex, the chance for accidental damage to these structures or the globe increases. A study using computed tomography (CT) scanning of a cadaver as the retrobulbar needle was introduced into the orbit showed that in the upward and inward gaze position (the Atkinson position), the optic nerve, the superior orbital artery and its branches, and the posterior pole of the globe are very close to the tip of the needle.[63] Also, in this position the optic nerve appeared stretched and displaced downward and outward, making it more susceptible to being punctured by a sharp needle. Placing the globe in either a straight ahead position or even slightly downward and outward was thought to reduce the chances for injury to the optic nerve and the globe.

A number of modifications to the standard method of giving a retrobulbar injection have been developed to reduce the possibility of causing damage to structures in the orbit.[64] The ultrasharp, small-bore needle used to give the retrobulbar injections is important for patient comfort but, on the other hand, greatly increases the chance of perforating orbital vessels and the globe. The use of a blunt-tipped 23-gauge needle was thought to reduce the occurrence of these types of complications.[60, 65, 66] Perforation of the globe during the injection of the eyelids with local anesthesia using a blunt-tipped needle has been reported.[67] In 23 cases of ocular penetration during injection for ocular anesthesia, 16 (70%) were from sharp (22-, 23-, and 25-gauge) needles, and 7 (30%) were from blunt (23- and 25-gauge) needles.[68] In 12 cases of ocular perforation where the injection was performed by nonophthalmologist, five were caused by blunt needles and seven by sharp needles.[69] The relative safety of blunt-tipped needles compared with sharp needles remains uncertain. All complications of retrobulbar injections with sharp-tipped needles have been reported with blunt-tipped needles, although the frequency seems to be less with the latter.

The placement of a soft, flexible catheter into the muscle cone to allow repeated injection of an anesthetic agent where the operation time is anticipated to be prolonged was first suggested by Scheie[70] in 1956 and more recently by Tamai.[71] This procedure involves introducing a catheter on a blunted needle into the muscle cone. The needle is pulled out and the catheter remains in place. During the surgery it is then possible to reinject anesthetic solutions as required. A similar procedure can be used to give the initial periocular injection, or, if desired, the surgeon can leave the catheter in place for subsequent injection of anesthetic solution as needed. A small skin wheal of short-acting anesthetic is made in the lid skin at the site of the injection. The angiocath needle is then passed through the lid skin and the orbital septum, at which point the passage of the needle is stopped and the catheter is advanced further into the orbit. Anesthetic solution is then injected, and after orbital pressure and sufficient time to allow for the spread of the anesthetic, both akinesia and anesthesia are obtained. The use of bupivacaine with its long period of effect would seem to make these techniques unnecessary purely for anesthesia. However, this may provide a safer method of introducing the anesthetic solution into the orbit.

The standard use of a 35-mm Atkinson needle and the depth to which it is inserted into the orbit in retrobulbar injections have been reported to influence the chances for complications. The orbital depth and the position of orbital structures in relation to the length of needles used for retrobulbar anesthesia were measured in 120 humans. The distance from the inferior temporal orbital rim to the nasal entrance of the optic foramen ranged from 42 to 54 mm. Taking into account the size of the optic nerve, the authors reported that a 38-mm retrobulbar needle could perforate the optic nerve where it is fixed in front of the optic foramen in more than 11% of the population.[72] Regardless of the length of the needle used, the surgeon must recognize the anatomic variations that exist in the orbit and the globe and not insert the needle any more deeply than is absolutely necessary.

Peribulbar injection techniques for anesthesia have gained popularity among ophthalmic surgeons as a means of reducing the complications of retrobulbar injections.[73–76] In peribulbar anesthesia the anesthetic solution is placed in the anterior or posterior orbital space outside the muscle cone. The needle is directed parallel to the floor of the orbit and more toward the lower part of the superior orbital fissure rather than toward the orbital apex. The major disadvantages of this procedure are that a larger volume of anesthetic is usually needed, maximum anesthesia from the block takes longer, and the incidence of incomplete akinesia and anesthesia is higher.

Ten patients undergoing cataract surgery were given a local anesthetic of lidocaine solution mixed with iohexol contrast medium. The location of the needle and the substance injected were determined by CT after retrobulbar or periocular injection. The retrobulbarly inserted needles were in the muscle cone, directed toward the optic foramen. The periocular needles were outside the muscle cone, tangentially along the orbital floor or pointing slightly upward. After the retrobulbar injection the contrast medium was seen within the muscle cone immediately and outside the cone as soon as 3 minutes. With the periocular injection, diffusion of the contrast medium into the muscle cone was rapid, occurring within 2 minutes. The authors[77] concluded that retrobulbar-like anesthesia can be readily induced by an appropriate periocular technique.

Several authors[78] have suggested that adequate anesthesia for cataract surgery can be obtained with subconjunctival injections of anesthetic. Friedberg et al.[79] placed local anesthetic into sub-Tenon's space posteriorly using a blunt irrigating cannula in a series of 100 patients undergoing vitreoretinal surgery. They reported that this technique was effective in 98% of the patients and with no associated morbidity.

The use of topical anesthetics alone for cataract surgery has been recommended as a safe and effective alternative to either retrobulbar or peribulbar anesthesia. Fichman[80] reported performing phacoemulsification on 75 eyes with the use of 0.5% tetracaine hydrochloride drops and mild systemic sedation. Only 5% of the patients reported feeling pain. Similar results were obtained by Fenzl,[81] who performed cataract and glaucoma surgery with topical tetracaine and topical 4%, nonpreserved injectable lidocaine hydrochloride.[81] Both surgeons found that they had good results with topical anesthesia but cautioned that the patient should be well prepared to gain good cooperation. Some pain occurred when sutures were placed in the sclera or when instruments touched the iris. With the current use of small or self-sealing incisions, small anterior capsulotomies, and phacoemulsification of lens material, in a well-sedated patient, the use of topical anesthetics may be possible in selected cases.

Excellent surgical anesthesia and akinesia with a rapid onset can be obtained in the majority of patients with a single injection of 4 to 6 ml of a 50:50 mixture containing 2% lidocaine and 0.75% bupivacaine with 7.5 TRU of hyaluronidase/ml. Such an injection is adequate for nearly all ophthalmic surgical procedures. The ability to perform surgery with the patient completely comfortable and with the surgical area fully anesthetized seems ideal. In addition, the prolonged anesthesia that occurs will allow the patient to be comfortable for a long period postoperatively.

## Hypotony

One of the truly important milestones in the development of cataract surgery was the recognition of the importance of a soft eye, which can be achieved with a combination of retrobulbar anesthetic, hyaluronidase, and external pressure. The factors responsible for hypotony are multiple.

Immediately after retrobulbar injection of an anesthetic, intraocular pressure drops rapidly and spontaneously, generally reaching a minimum level within 5 minutes.[82] A pressure drop comparable with that after retrobulbar anesthesia accompanies thiopental general anesthesia. Retrobulbar anesthesia given during thiopental general anesthesia caused only an insignificant additional drop in pressure (averaging 1.4 mm Hg in 10 patients). Because of the similar magnitude of the pressure drop with general and local anesthesia and because there is no significant additive effect, one possible mechanism of action for producing hypotony could be relaxation of the extraocular muscles that occurs with both types of anesthesia.

### Complications From Injection Anesthesia

The complications can be separated into those caused by drug toxicity and those caused by the mechanical process of introducing a needle into the orbit and injecting an anesthetic solution without direct visualization.

Orbital hemorrhage after injection anesthesia is the most common complication and has been reported to occur in 1% to 3% of surgical cases.[83, 84] Most of these involve minor hemorrhaging and do not prevent continuing the surgical procedure. When the hemorrhage involves the arterial system, severe proptosis, ecchymosis, and subconjunctival injection may occur. Usually the surgeon will note that the patient will have immediate paralysis of ocular movement (giving the false impression of a perfect block). As the orbital pressure increases, the optic nerve and the retinal vessels may become compressed.[85, 86] In most cases the patient will have a sudden loss of vision, but occasionally the eye will be anesthetized or for other reasons the vision will be impaired and the patient will be unable to report vision changes. Klien et al.[87] reported a case of central retinal artery occlusion without retrobulbar hemorrhage after retrobulbar anesthesia presumably from orbital pressure. If the retinal vessels are compromised, immediate orbital decompression must be performed. An equally serious complication is a central retinal artery or vein occlusion or even a combined central retinal artery and central retinal vein occlusion occurring after direct injection into the optic nerve.[88]

Accidental perforation of the globe may occur during attempted retrobulbar and peribulbar anesthesia, periocular injection, or even eyelid injection.[89] The reported incidence from several large series (mostly retinal detachment procedures) was 0.075% of cases.[90–92] This rate may be high for patients with normal axial length receiving a single injection. Patients at increased risk for ocular perforation are uncooperative patients, myopic eyes with increased axial lengths and thin sclera, posterior staphyloma, an enophthalmic globe, and patients who have had previous surgery such as scleral buckling. Other factors include injections given by nonophthalmologist and the use of repeated injections.[65, 91] Duker et al.[92] presented strong support to the hypothesis that axial myopia is a very high risk factor for globe perforation in injection anesthesia. In their 20 cases 45% occurred in patients with eyes that had an axial length of 26 mm or greater. They concluded that because 1.5% of the general population has been reported to have an axial length of this magnitude, and by taking their 45% occurrence rate, the risk of perforation in these eyes was approximately 30 times greater than in the average patient. They further concluded that by using conservative estimates of globe perforations from peribulbar blocks, the risk factor for perforation in eyes 26 mm or longer was 1 in 140 injections. The ophthalmologist should be alert to the possibility that a needle perforation of the globe has occurred and be prepared to manage the complications. Visual prognosis seems to be worst in patients who develop a retinal detachment.[91]

Toxicity of the CNS from injected anesthetics produces symptoms involving the respiratory and cardiovascular systems. Initially the patient may become agitated and develop slurred speech and tremors of the hands or face muscles. Respiratory depression, even apnea, may follow, and the patient may quickly become unresponsive. Unless the patient is closely monitored, these events may progress unnoticed, particularly in patients who are already sedated. Toxicity may occur because of one of a number of mechanisms: an allergic or other idiosyncratic reaction to the drug, by absorption of toxic levels into the blood stream or CNS tissues, by direct injection of the anesthetic into the optic nerve sheath, or by injection into the orbital vessels with retrograde flow of anesthetic to the brain.

When injection into the optic nerve sheath allows the anesthetic agent to gain entrance into the subdural space, causing brainstem anesthesia, most often delayed but in some cases even sudden respiratory arrest can occur. (Unilateral or bilateral sudden visual loss can also develop.) Accidental injection into the sheath of the optic nerve with intracranial extension during contrast orbitography has been documented by subsequent x-ray studies.[93] Rapid-sequence radiography during retrobulbar injection of a radiopaque dye on a fresh cadaver was performed. A 25-gauge, 38-mm needle was introduced into the orbit in the same relative orientation as for a retrobulbar block. After 3 ml of contrast material was injected, progression of the dye along the subdural space of the optic nerve, into the chiasm, and into the subdural space of the midbrain was demonstrated. The author[94] concluded that it was not only technically feasible but relatively likely that a dural sheath penetration could occur if the needle was introduced deeply enough and with sufficient force. Because the optic nerve sheath has been demonstrated to be in continuity with the intracranial subarachnoid space, anesthetic injected into the nerve sheath can gain access to the cranial nerve roots, midbrain, and spinal cord. Lidocaine and bupivacaine were found in the cerebral spinal fluid of a patient 10 minutes after he became unresponsive and apneic after a retrobulbar injection.[95] Javitt et al.[62] in their report of eight cases of brainstem anesthesia after retrobulbar block suggested four mechanisms by which anesthetic solution could possibly reach brain tissue. Two of these were related to excessive absorption or paradoxical response to the anesthetic; the other two were mechanical—inadvertent injection into vessels or into the subarachnoid space. Symptoms in their patients developed within 2 to 5 minutes after injection, progressed for 10 minutes, and then resolved within 60 to 90 minutes. The delayed onset of symptoms suggested that the primary mechanism involved was an inadvertent injection of anesthetic into the subarachnoid space. Intravascular injection of an anesthetic would most likely cause a rapid rise in blood levels and a concomitantly rapid onset of systemic symptoms. For instance, the intravascular injection of bupivacaine has been reported to cause immediate cardiovascular collapse with inadequate time for respiratory arrest to develop.

Serum levels of lidocaine and bupivacaine from seven patients who experienced respiratory arrest after retrobulbar anesthesia were compared with 20 controls; all patients were from a series of 3,123 retrobulbar injections.[48] The authors[48] reported that disorientation and decreasing responsiveness preceded apnea. The period of apnea ranged from 5 to 55 minutes. Serum levels of lidocaine and bupivacaine in both groups of patients studied were well below the level reported to cause CNS toxicity (lidocaine 0.5 μg/ml, bupivacaine 2.1–4.5 μg/ml). The blood level rise occurred between 5 and 15 minutes after injection and declined over 2 to 3 hours. They did not believe that there was an intravascular injection of the anesthetic because of the delayed onset of respiratory distress. Four percent lidocaine was found to be more likely to cause symptoms than a 2% solution. This suggested that absorption was greater with the stronger concentration or that some patients are more susceptible to the drugs at the higher concentration.

A rapid onset of symptoms, particularly cardiovascular symptoms, would suggest that an intravascular injection of anesthetic has occurred. With delayed onset of symptoms, for instance, several minutes, CNS symptoms characterized by progressive unresponsiveness with respiratory depression or apnea can be expected. Regardless, a full support system must be available at all times when injection anesthesia is attempted, and the patient should be monitored by trained personnel for at least 2 to 3 hours after the injection is given. Clearly, with more than 1,000,000 retrobulbar injections delivered annually in the United States alone,[92] the incidence of any type of complication is remarkably low. The progressive refinement of injection technique, the availability of the services of standby anesthesia personnel, and the use of highly sophisticated monitoring and life support equipment in the perioperative area and the operating suite all are essential for the overall safety of the patient. Any patient who is given injection anesthesia deserves these support measures.

### Periocular Anesthesia for Pain Control

The use of injection anesthetics such as lidocaine or bupivacaine for pain relief has been used in a number of different situations.[96] In a prospective, randomized, double-masked clinical trial, where retrobulbar bupivacaine irrigation for postoperative pain after scleral buckling surgery was evaluated, 12% receiving bupivacaine irrigation required parenteral pain relief in the first 24 hours after surgery compared with 72% of the controls.[97] Pain and nausea were relieved within 5 minutes in patients with angle-closure glaucoma after receiving retrobulbar anesthesia. This allowed for therapy to be conducted with much less discomfort for the patients.[98]

## PREANESTHETIC PREPARATION

Psychologic preparation of the patient can greatly reduce preoperative apprehensions and should be undertaken with every patient undergoing any surgical procedure no matter how minor. As much time as necessary should be taken to give a clear explanation of the surgical procedure, expected results, and the anesthesia to be used. A discussion of the possible side effects of the anesthesia should be given in as much detail as possible. This discussion not only will reduce anxiety but will increase the patient's confidence in the surgeon.

Preoperative history and physical examination and appropriate laboratory tests are an essential part of the surgical procedure. The history and physical examination should be directed toward uncovering factors that might interfere with surgery or the postoperative period. When a minor ophthalmic surgical procedure is performed with topical anesthesia on a healthy patient, a brief medical history, determination of any drug allergies, and a baseline blood pressure are adequate. A complete preoperative evaluation should be performed if injection anesthesia or general anesthesia is planned. If the history or the physical examination uncovers major health problems, surgery should be delayed until a complete evaluation can be conducted. Most institutions have established guidelines for preanesthetic evaluation generally based on the patient's age and health status (Table 5–4). Patients with major health problems such

**TABLE 5–4.**
Minimum Requirements of Preoperative Laboratory Testing*

| $<40$ yr | $\geq 40$ yr | Regional Anesthesia |
|---|---|---|
| CBC† count | Hemoglobin/hematocrit or CBC count<br>Sodium, potassium levels<br>Chest x-ray film<br>Electrocardiogram | PT†<br>PTT†<br>Platelet count (may be required of some patients) |

*All laboratory and radiologic tests must be performed within 30 days of surgical procedure and electrocardiogram within 12 months. Perform additional tests as needed for appropriate conditions (e.g., glucose). Requirements vary in different hospitals.
†*CBC count*, Complete blood cell count; *PT*, prothrombin time; *PTT*, partial thromboplastin time.

as cardiovascular or pulmonary diseases, bleeding tendency, diabetes, hypertension, renal disease, or musculoskeletal or neurologic defects may require approval for surgery by the staff anesthesiologist. Diabetic patients present a particular problem both preoperatively and intraoperatively because they may have some degree of autonomic neuropathy that can mask symptoms and may even allow sudden death to occur. Determining the physical status classification of the patient (see Table 5-3) will help determine the preoperative work-up necessary.

## PREOPERATIVE MEDICATIONS

Preoperative medications are given to decrease pain, relieve anxiety, counteract possible toxic effects of injection anesthesia, reduce secretions (in the case of general anesthesia), and minimize postoperative nausea and vomiting. The commonly used drugs include narcotics, barbiturates, parasympatholytics, and tranquilizers. Representatives of each group are discussed.

### Meperidine Hydrochloride

Meperidine is one of the more popular analgesics for use in ocular surgery. Probably the most common error in the use of meperidine is giving it too late. Usually the injection is given just before the orderly arrives to take the patient to surgery. The patient is therefore fully awake and unsedated during this journey, which is feared by most persons. After intramuscular administration of meperidine, its analgesic effect appears within 15 minutes, but the maximum effect may not be reached for as long as 1 hour. Therefore, meperidine should be given 45 to 90 minutes before the start of surgery. Actually, the time of greatest need for analgesia is at the beginning of surgery, when the various local or intravenous injections are being given. Because the duration of the narcotic effect is 2 to 6 hours, depending on the size of the dose, the surgeon need not fear loss of the meperidine effect if the start of surgery is delayed. Furthermore, if meperidine is given at least 1 hour before the operation, any untoward effect such as vomiting or confusion will become evident before the surgical incision is started.

Because the sedative effect of meperidine is relatively slight, it is usually accompanied by a barbiturate for preanesthetic medication. Solutions of meperidine hydrochloride and sodium phenobarbital cannot be mixed in the same syringe, because the phenobarbital will precipitate, making the mixture unsuitable for administration. Hence, it is necessary that each drug be given separately.

Meperidine may be administered intravenously preceding or during intraocular surgery. Prompt drowsiness and relaxation occur. This procedure is of value in the management of a patient who is unduly apprehensive or restless before or during cataract surgery under local anesthesia.[99] The injection should be given slowly, over 1 to 2 minutes, and the patient should be titrated with small doses, perhaps 10 mg or less at one time. Such intravenous use is not superior to adequate premedication with meperidine but has the advantage of quickly relaxing the patient who has received insufficient premedication. Nausea and vomiting may follow intravenous administration of meperidine, especially if the injection has been rapid. This can obviously cause serious problems if the eye is surgically open.

For preoperative medication the usual dosage is 0.5 to 1 mg/kg intramuscularly, most commonly in the average adult, a total of 75 to 100 mg. Elderly patients tend to require proportionately less drug, particularly if they are frail and underweight. Conversely, higher dosage is tolerated and desirable for young, muscular, or heavy apprehensive persons. When given orally, meperidine acts within 20 to 60 minutes.

## BARBITURATES

For the purposes of preoperative medication, the effects of barbiturates almost perfectly complement those of meperidine. Barbiturates are effective sedatives but have no significant analgesic power. Hence the combination of meperidine and a barbiturate induces both sedation and analgesia.

### Pentobarbital Sodium

Pentobarbital is rapidly absorbed when given orally or by injection. It is destroyed by the liver and therefore has an unduly prolonged effect in patients with hepatic disease. A hypnotic dose will induce sleep in 20 to 60 minutes if the patient is undisturbed. Because the effect of pentobarbital will last 3 hours or more, the drug should be given 1 hour or more preoperatively. Considerable individual variations in response exist, however, 100 mg in the average-size adult seems to be well tolerated. Infrequently barbiturates will cause delirium and confusion rather than sedation, particularly in elderly patients. Such a response may be detected if a test dose of the drug is given on the evening preceding surgery.

Premedication with barbiturates is thought to increase the threshold of toxic reactions to injected local anesthetics. Some authorities have indicated that the usual 100-mg dose is inadequate and that 300 to 500 mg is required to counteract such toxicity. Actually only the convulsive component of an anesthetic reaction is alleviated by barbiturates. Barbiturate overdosage will worsen respiratory and cardiac depression; therefore, not more than 300 to 500 mg of pentobarbital should be given intravenously to control anesthetic-induced convulsions, and no barbiturates should be given if convulsions are not present. Regardless of whether premedication with pentobarbital increases resistance to the toxic effect of local injection anesthetics, such premedication strikingly reduces the incidence of apprehension, fainting, and shocklike responses that are commonly encountered when local anesthetic procedures are performed without such premedication.

## NONBARBITURATE SEDATIVES

### Benzodiazepine Derivatives

#### *Diazepam*

Diazepam is effective in both the short- and long-term management of anxiety disorders. Moderate anxiety such as that which occurs in the average patient preoperatively can be controlled with 2 to 5 mg of diazepam (Valium) given either intramuscularly or intravenously. When it is administered, care must be taken to assure that the medication is given into a large vein or a well-placed intravenous infusion line and the medication should be given slowly, approximately 1 ml/min. Too rapid of an infusion can cause apnea or cardiac arrest. When given in conjunction with a narcotic analgesic, consideration should be given to reducing the narcotic dose to one third or less. Diazepam was used in combination with meperidine and local injection anesthesia in 160 eye operations.[100] The medication was given intravenously in variable dosages titrated to meet the patients' needs. Most patients received less than 10 mg of diazepam and 15 mg of meperidine. In addition, premedication with up to 100 mg of pentobarbital or 1 g of chloral hydrate was given. Good patient cooperation was achieved in 91% of these 160 patients. Four patients were restless and uncooperative and could not be controlled by the medication. Half of the patients had complete amnesia for the operation, and one fourth had only slight recall of the procedure.

Diazepam is one of the most frequently prescribed drugs in the United States.[101] It is prescribed for anxiety, pain, insomnia, muscular discomfort, alcohol abuse, and a variety of emotional disorders. Habituation and impaired coordination and psychomotor skills, as well as reduced alertness and responsibility, are undesirable side effects of this benzodiazepine drug. If the drug history reveals that the patient is a chronic user of diazepam, the frequency and actual amount taken should be determined as best as possible.

#### *Lorazepam*

When given in the recommended dosage of 2 to 4 mg intramuscularly or intravenously, lorazepam causes sedation (sleepiness or drowsiness), relief of anxiety, and amnesia in most patients. The clinical sedation obtained with this drug is such that patients are generally able to respond to verbal commands despite the appearance of being asleep. The effects of the normal adult dose of lorazepam persist for 6 to 8 hours. Recommended dosage does not seem to alter the sensitivity of the patient to respiratory stimulants and does not enhance the respiratory depressant effects of meperidine, even at levels of 100 mg.

#### *Midazolam Hydrochloride*

Midazolam is a water-soluble benzodiazepine and a short-acting sedative. It is supplied with 5 mg/ml of solution. When given intravenously, the usual dose is 0.5 ml, or 2.0 to 2.5 mg, and should be given very slowly. Sedation after intravenous administration occurs within 3 to 5 minutes. The time of onset is affected by the total dosage and the concurrent administration of other narcotic premedications. Midazolam was reviewed by a panel of expert consultants, and they concluded that this drug will probably replace diazepam for perioperative use because of its lack of tissue irritation, its faster onset of action, and its more rapid elimination.[102]

#### *Methohexital Sodium*

Brevital differs chemically from other barbiturates in that it contains no sulfur, important if the patient is allergic to sulfur. Intravenous dosage has a rapid onset and an ultrashort duration. The drug must be mixed with a diluent, either sterile water, dextrose, or sodium chloride solution, and is not compatible with lactated Ringer's solution. Intravenous dose is 50 to 120 mg (5–12 ml of a 1% solution).

## NARCOTIC ANALGESICS

The increased use of ambulatory surgery and local injection anesthesia has shortened the time the patient spends in the surgical unit both preoperatively and postoperatively. Preoperative medications with a more rapid time of onset have become a necessity. Analgesics such as meperidine that may not have a maximum effect for 1 hour or more when given intramuscularly is not adequate. Other short-acting, potent narcotic analgesics are being used more frequently.

### Fentanyl Citrate

Fentanyl citrate is a potent narcotic analgesic. A dose of 0.1 mg (2 ml) is equivalent in analgesic effect to 10 mg of morphine or 75 mg of meperidine. The onset of action after an intravenous dose is immediate to several seconds, and the duration of effect is 30 to 60 minutes. Onset time after intramuscular injection is 7 to 8 minutes, and the duration of effect is 1 to 2 hours. Respiratory depressant effect may persist longer than the analgesic effect, and the patient should be continuously monitored. Commonly fentanyl is given simultaneously with a sedative such as midazolam (Versed).

### Nalbuphine Hydrochloride

Nalbuphine is a synthetic narcotic agonist-antagonist analgesic of the phenanthrene series and is a potent analgesic. When it is given intravenously, its onset of action is 2 to 3 minutes, and the duration of effect is 3 to 6 hours. When it is used for either preoperative or postoperative pain control, the usual adult dosage is 10 mg. This dosage is equivalent to 10 mg of morphine, 40 mg of pentazocine (Talwin), and 75 mg of meperidine hydrochloride (Demerol). The reported benefit of nalbuphine is the low incidence of side effects, the most frequent one being nausea.[103] Lorazepam and nalbuphine were used for 30 local anesthesic ophthalmic surgery cases with the desired effects of rapid onset of action, long duration, excellent sedation, potent analgesia, and amnesia. Unwanted side effects were uncommon.[104]

## CHLORPROMAZINE

Psychotropic drugs continue to be among the most widely used prescription medications.[105] Chlorpromazine was the first of the large number of phenothiazine derivatives to be recognized for its tension-relieving, antiemetic, and anesthetic-potentiating effects. Knowledge of the phenothiazines is important to the ophthalmologist because their therapeutic effect is valuable in the treatment of surgical eye patients and because their toxic complications may involve the eyes.

### Antiemetic Effect

The incidence of postoperative nausea, vomiting, and retching was studied in 554 patients receiving 50 mg of chlorpromazine, placebo, 100 or 150 mg of pentobarbital, or 100 mg of dimenhydrinate (Dramamine).[106] These medications were administered as unknown units in a random sequence and were given intramuscularly 10 to 30 minutes before conclusion of nitrous oxide and ether anesthesia. The occurrence of symptoms was verified by constant observation by special technicians. The problem of placebo reaction was eliminated, because all patients were completely unaware of the medication or the study. Interestingly, most patients when questioned later were unaware of nausea or vomiting that was observed to occur during the first 4 hours postoperatively, a fact that may account for the lower incidence of vomiting in a series of cases studied by questioning the patient rather than by continuous observation.

Chlorpromazine is effective in reducing the frequency of postanesthetic nausea, vomiting, and retching. However, this drug also prolongs recovery time from anesthesia by an average of almost 1 hour and caused a 30% incidence of disturbing hypotension. The potential danger of aspiration and vascular instability is sufficiently great that routine prophylactic use of chlorpromazine may not be advisable. Pressor amines, including levarterenol, are not effective against chlorpromazine-induced arterial hypotension, which usually improves spontaneously in 2 to 4 hours without long-term complications. Similar conclusions were reached in a study of 725 patients where particular caution was advised in patients with labile blood pressure, especially if systolic pressure was greater than 160 or less than 100 mm Hg.[107]

Some anesthesiologists consider the intensified and prolonged sedation and the hypotensive effects of the phenothiazine tranquilizers to be so disturbing that they advocate discontinuing such medications for at least 10 days before surgery.[108] Because it is estimated that as many as one person in seven may at some time use these tranquilizers, inquiry as to the routine use of these drugs is in order before medications are prescribed.

Because phenothiazine antiemetics are effective even after severe vomiting has started, the routine prophylactic use of such drugs is not ordinarily justified and may subject patients to the hazards of a drug they do not need. However, in a series of 2,230 patients, 23% had retching and temporary vomiting after general anesthesia without the use of tranquilizers, and only 3.5% who were premedicated with a phenothiazine drug had persistent and severe vomiting.[109] Currently most ophthalmic surgeons reserve the use of these drugs for their antiemetic effects once they occur, and this can be achieved equally as well with any of the phenothiazine drugs. The frequency of side effects, particularly hypotension, makes these medications less desirable. If used, however, hypotension is less likely with 12.5 or 25 mg of promethazine (Phenergan) than with chlorpromazine.

### Analgesics

Minor to moderate pain associated with injuries or disorders requiring surgery or caused by the surgery itself is often treated with aspirin, acetaminophen (Tylenol), propoxyphene (Darvon), or medications containing narcotic. Such medications are generally considered to be innocuous. However, microscopic gastrointestinal bleeding may be a complication of aspirin ingestion. Analgesic overuse (aspirin, phenacetin, and acetaminophen) has been reported to be the cause of 20% to 25% of cases of interstitial nephritis and the cause of 13% of cases of chronic renal failure. Usually six or more tablets daily for several years are required to cause severe renal damage.[110] Propoxyphene is one of the most commonly prescribed analgesics, and each year nearly 2,000 deaths are caused by this drug, mostly suicides. This is second only to barbiturates as a cause of death. A total of eight capsules daily is a sufficient dose to result in physical and psychologic dependence.[111] Patients who have significant postoperative pain would probably be expected to take as much pain medication as necessary to be comfortable and in some cases even take more than recommended by their physician. A review of 526 medical records of surgical patients at the University of Rochester School of Medicine and Dentistry found that patients received on the average 30% less pain medication than the maximum prescribed. In some cases the patients did not request the medication, and in other cases the nurses did not give it.[112] The use of postoperative medication should be carefully monitored by the surgeon. Any analgesic given to the patient for postoperative pain has the potential to be abused or to cause unexpected side effects. Careful instructions to the patient as to the proper use of the drug, careful control of the quantity of the drug given, and an awareness of potential side effects are an equally important part of the postoperative care of the patient.

## GENERAL ANESTHESIA

The decision to use general anesthesia should be tempered with the knowledge that a number of complications, including primary anesthetic death, can occur. Lesser complications such as pneumonia, thrombophlebitis, pressure damage to peripheral nerves, exposure keratopathy, and prolonged nausea and vomiting are not rare. The prolonged convalescence that occurs after general anesthesia is often unnoticed or disregarded but is nevertheless real.[113, 114] For 1 month or more after anesthesia, many patients do not feel well, have no endurance, and generally feel as if they are recovering from a severe case of influenza. In the elderly patient, this period of debility may be prolonged, lasting many months. These late aftereffects of general anesthesia cannot be lightly disregarded in the decision as to the type of anesthesia the ophthalmologist recommends as best for the patient. General anesthesia is necessary, however, when one is dealing with a potentially uncooperative patient such as a child, a deaf person, an emotionally unstable and apprehensive patient, or a psychotic person. Long and uncomfortable procedures (retinal detachments) or emotionally unpleasant operations (enucleation) are better done with the patient asleep.

A combination of local anesthesia with light general anesthesia is another option. If a normal depth of general anesthesia is contraindicated by the health of the patient, relief of pain with a local anesthetic will permit carrying the patient with relatively light general anesthesia. This decision will require consultation with the anesthesiologist.

Currently most ophthalmic surgery is being performed either with local anesthesia or, more commonly, with local standby anesthesia. Local standby anesthesia has a number of advantages in that the patient is spared the unpleasant aftereffects of a general anesthetic, very adequate local anesthesia and akinesia can be obtained, and the patient is monitored by a member of the anesthesia staff. An additional benefit is having the ability to request supplemental sedation in the event the patient becomes restless or apprehensive during the procedure. The current monitoring techniques used by anesthesiologists are highly sophisticated and offer the patient maximum safety.

Even if the surgery is done with the patient under general anesthesia, supplemental injection of a local anesthetic may be desirable for the following reasons:

1. A lighter plane of anesthesia is possible without the hazard of the patient moving in response to occasional painful stimuli.
2. Postoperative pain will be less during the first few hours, which are the most likely to be uncomfortable.
3. Squeezing of the eyelids during the immediate postoperative period is prevented by the local anesthesia.
4. Oculocardiac reflexes may be decreased.
5. If epinephrine is contained in the local injection, bleeding is decreased.

### Effects on Intraocular Pressure

Anesthesia produced by intravenous administration of thiopental sodium (Pentothal) causes a significant drop of intraocular pressure in both normal and untreated glaucomatous eyes. The mechanism of this pressure decrease was postulated in one study to be improved facility of outflow. The aqueous humor dynamics in 20 patients with chronic simple glaucoma (not operated on for glaucoma and not given miotics within 48 hours before anesthesia) were studied before and after thiopental anesthesia.[115] Preanesthetic pressure in these patients varied from a low of 29 mm Hg to a high of 66 mm Hg. Within 20 minutes after the start of anesthesia, a marked drop of pressure (average 19 mm Hg) occurred in all patients. This decrease in intraocular pressure was accompanied in all but one patient by an increase facility of outflow. Cardiovascular changes could not have been responsible for the intraocular pressure drop, because the systolic blood pressure dropped an average of only 9 mm Hg in contrast to the 19–mm Hg intraocular pressure drop.

General anesthesia with any of the commonly used agents also causes a 5– to 7–mm Hg drop of intraocular pressure in normal eyes. The drop increases to maximum as deeper levels of anesthesia are obtained[116] and is produced equally by cyclopropane, diethyl ether, thiopental sodium, and vinyl ether.[117] After anesthesia, the intraocular pressure rapidly returns to normal. Tonography findings in these patients suggested that the mechanism of the pressure drop was an increase in the facility of outflow. Intraocular pressure correlates closely with the depth of anesthesia, being lowest in deep anesthesia and rising when the anesthesia is lightened.

Relaxation of the extraocular muscles is another attractive explanation for the reduced intraocular pressure resulting from anesthesia.[118] Clearly, respiratory disturbances such as coughing or straining cause increased intraocular pressure that persists for some minutes. A marked rise of intraocular pressure results from intubation if the patient is not relaxed. The implication of these findings in respect to the diagnosis of congenital glaucoma (a disease in which tonometry is often done with the patient under anesthesia) deserves comment. Elevated readings during the early stages of anesthesia, even several minutes after struggling and breath holding, may be artifactual and cannot be relied on as being indicative of glaucoma. Elevated readings taken during deep anesthesia several minutes after any muscular activity has ceased represent a genuine elevation of intraocular pressure. Any reading taken during deep general anesthesia is probably lower than the patient's normal intraocular pressure; therefore, a borderline pressure under these conditions probably represents an abnormal elevation. The average pressure of 140 eyes taken while the patients were under general anesthesia was only 10 to 12 mm Hg. The intraocular pressure of an infant less than 2 years of age is approximately 5 mm Hg less than that of an adult.[119]

### Autonomic Effects

The parasympathetic stimulation resulting from general anesthesia is well known to manifest itself as pupillary miosis. In a study of 36 patients, general anesthesia was found to cause varying degrees of accommodation, reaching values as high as 5 D.[120] Children were particularly likely to accommodate strongly during anesthesia. The practical implication of this finding is that adequate cycloplegia is essential in obtaining an accurate refraction with the patient under anesthesia. This fact should be remembered if a pediatric examination with the child under general anesthesia is to include a refraction.

The accommodation convergence/accommodation (AC/A) ratio may also be altered by drugs that act on the CNS (presumably, the convergence center). Barbiturates decrease convergence and amphetamines enhance convergence.[121] This effect explains why a convergence strabismus may disappear completely when the patient is anesthetized before surgery.

### Effect on Intraocular Gases

The laws of diffusion and partial pressure of gases require that equilibration of concentration will occur whenever a new gas is introduced into a biologic system. Specifically, if 60% nitrous oxide is used as an anesthetic, nitrous oxide will enter every gas-filled space in the body until it equilibrates with a content of 60% nitrous oxide. If the eye contains a bubble of air, sulfur hexafluoride, or a perfluorcarbon gas, the gas within the eye cannot escape and to it is added 60% nitrous oxide to establish equilibrium. The only possible consequence is a precipitous rise of pressure, actually measured at 101 mm Hg in a detachment operation involving the intravitreal injection of a large air bubble during nitrous oxide anesthesia.[122, 123] The practical consequence is that a gaseous anesthetic must not be given to a patient with a large volume of intraocular air or gas, or the intraocular pressure will rise, probably to a dangerous levels.[124] The solubility of the gas will determine its expansion potential and the safe volume that can be placed in the eye.[125–127] Simone and Whitacre[128] derived a set of mathematical equations describing the relationship between intraocular pressure, atmospheric pressure, the coefficient of scleral rigidity, intraocular gas, and intraocular fluid volumes in an ideal eye. The data provided were thought to be useful in understanding the various parameters related to increased intraocular pressure in eyes with intraocular gases. In addition, it was suggested that these data could be used to determine the amount of gas to be removed from the eye to reduce the pressure to a safe level postoperatively. If any gas is to be used intraocularly during surgery, this should be communicated to the anesthesia personnel preoperatively so that the agents used for general anesthesia can be selected.

### Effects on Tear Production

Schirmer measurement of tear production showed baseline levels averaging about 19 mm before surgery on 20 patients. After premedication with diazepam and atropine, the tear flow was still 18 mm. After induction of general anesthesia with halothane, enflurane, or nitrous oxide, the tear flow dropped to less than 1 mm of wetting. This decrease persisted throughout the duration of the anesthesia.[129] It is well known that the eyes must be protected from desiccation during general anesthesia.

### Succinylcholine Chloride

Succinylcholine, an acetylcholine competitor, blocks the myoneural junction through depolarization, thereby causing temporary paralysis of skeletal muscles. It is widely used to attain muscular relaxation during general anesthesia. Initially the extraocular muscles react to succinylcholine with increased activity. Intravenous injection of succinylcholine produces a steep rise in intraocular pressure resulting from this demonstrable contraction of the extraocular muscles.[130, 131] The duration of elevated intraocular pressure is sufficiently short (only a few minutes) so that use of succinylcholine for intubation will not cause difficulty during the surgical procedure.

When the patient is deeply anesthetized, succinylcholine has no pressure-elevating effect on the eye. This has been confirmed in a series of 82 patients.[132] This difference in response of anesthetized and nonanesthetized extraocular muscles accounts, at least partially, for the conflicting reports as to the safety of succinylcholine in ocular surgery. Apparently general anesthesia paralyzes the extraocular muscles sufficiently to prevent their contraction when succinylocholine is administered. Without anesthesia there is an initial stage of contraction, after which the extraocular muscles are paralyzed by succinylcholine and may be maintained in this relaxed state by continuous administration of the drug. It is therefore safe to use succinylcholine during intraocular surgery if it is started well in advance of opening the eye and if effective levels are maintained throughout the operation. It has been generally assumed that succinylcholine should not be started after the eye has been opened because of the possible hazard of losing intraocular contents from increased intraocular pressure from contraction of extraocular muscles. Further, its administration is thought to be contraindicated if the anesthesia becomes light during the operation and the patient begins to move, because in this light anesthetized state the extraocular muscles will contract strongly in initial response to the drug. If the eye is already open at the start of anesthesia (because of a laceration, iris prolapse, incision disruption, or other causes), the use of succinylcholine may be extremely dangerous. Before intubation of such a patient's airway, the level of anesthesia should be sufficiently deep to achieve complete relaxation. Bucking of the patient during intubation is similar to the effects created by a Valsalva maneuver, which may induce venous back pressure sufficient to raise intraocular pressure to as high as 50 mm Hg. Such a danger to the eye from succinylcholine is not only theoretical but was proved in the case of a 70-year-old patient who coughed on the endotracheal tube after cataract extraction had been uneventfully concluded.[133] Fifty milligrams of succinylcholine was given intravenously to stop the coughing and was immediately followed by an expulsive hemorrhage and ultimate evisceration. On the other hand, Moreno et al.[134] studied the effects of succinylcholine on the intraocular contents of open globes in the cat eye. Thirty anterior traumas were produced consisting of 6 mm penetrating keratoplasties, corneal incisions with a trephine, linear corneal incisions, and corneal incisions with removal of lens and vitreous humor. Eight posterior traumas consisted of making a 3 by 3 mm scleral opening and removing the exposed choroid. Succinylcholine was administered intravenously at a dose of 0.1 mg/kg. The only observable effect of the succinylcholine administration was forward displacement of the lens and iris. No intraocular contents were lost in any of the surgically produced events. The authors believe that this study supports the argument that succinylcholine may be used when the globe is open without fear of losing intraocular contents. Currently there is no absolute contraindications for the use of succinylcholine during general anesthesia for ophthalmic surgical procedures even with an open globe. Succinylcholine is never used as a supplement to local anesthesia, because it paralyzes respiration.

Succinylcholine causes a sustained contraction of the extraocular muscles that interferes with the performance of a forced duction test for as long as 20 minutes. An alternative muscle relaxant, pancuronium, does not cause such a muscle spasm.[135] However, the amount of muscle deviation of patients with strabismus was not changed by succinylcholine.[136]

Unlike curare, succinylcholine is not antagonized by anticholinesterase drugs. Cholinesterase inhibitors such as neostigmine or physostigmine prolong the action of succinylcholine and are therefore contraindicated in the treatment of succinylcholine overdose. Succinylcholine is destroyed in 3 to 4 minutes by pseudocholinesterase; hence, the paralysis it induces is of short duration. Chronic systemic intoxication with the long-acting anticholinesterase drugs as may be used in the treatment of glaucoma or strabismus can greatly prolong the effect of succinylcholine. The ophthalmologist should make the anesthesiologist aware of prior use of such drugs. A genetic deficiency of pseudocholinesterase also exists. Such patients may remain apneic for 4 to 8 hours after a single dose of succinylcholine.[137, 138]

As would be expected, succinylcholine initiates the relaxation of accommodation, beginning within 20 seconds after intravenous administration, reaching a maximal level from 45 to 210 seconds, and disappearing after 300 seconds. This was determined by ultrasonic measurement of lens thickness and anterior chamber depth.[139]

## CARDIAC ARREST

The entire staff of the surgical unit should be capable of recognizing that a patient is having cardiac problems. When the heart stops pumping blood, the brain can survive for approximately 3 to 4 minutes. Regardless of whether the heart is in asystole or in fibrillation, two problems face the physician initiating emergency treatment:

1. Restoration of blood flow (including oxygenation)
2. Restoration of the normal heartbeat

Steps toward cardiac resuscitation should be started immediately whenever the pulse and blood pressure are lost and should be continued until an effective and spontaneous heartbeat has been restored.

There is no time to take an electrocardiogram. Do not give artificial respiration and wait! Medication cannot be given by any route, including intravenously, because the circulation has stopped. There is no time to experiment or to look up directions; therefore, the surgeon and all operating room personnel should know what to do. Despite reports that resuscitation measures have been found to be successful in nearly 70% of cases of cardiac arrest, the eventual outcome is less optimistic. Of 50 patients with cardiac arrest who were resuscitated at Johns Hopkins, only five (10%) eventually left the hospital.[140] Killip[141] reviewed a series of six articles published in the *Journal of the American Medical Association* in which the perioperative risk of cardiac complications in patients undergoing general anesthesia for noncardiac surgery was presented. The conclusion from these studies was that general anesthesia is a safe procedure with no intraoperative deaths occurring in the 474 male patients studied. Although no deaths occurred during surgery, intraoperative and postoperative myocardial ischemia could be predicted from preoperative findings such as general physical status, cardiovascular status, coronary artery disease, left ventricular hypertrophy, hypertension, diabetes treated with drugs, and treatment with digoxin. Monitoring with a two-lead Holter monitor was effective, and ventricular arrhythmias were a frequent finding (44%) but did not correlate with cardiac morbidity or death occurring postoperatively.

## Oculocardiac Reflex

With respect to the numbers of patients involved, prevention of cardiac arrest is more important than its treatment. Anesthesiologists are responsible primarily for establishing and maintaining a good airway that will prevent anoxia and accumulation of carbon dioxide, both of which are precursors of cardiac arrest. Furthermore, they are responsible for avoiding dangerously deep levels of anesthesia. It has been proposed that the ophthalmologist can help prevent cardiac arrest by blocking the oculocardiac reflex.

The oculocardiac reflex is a trigeminovagal reflex that causes cardiac slowing or standstill.[142] This reflex may be elicited by pressure on the globe, traction on extraocular muscles or optic nerve, or direct pressure on the orbital contents that remain after enucleation. These cardiac responses may occur during either light or deep anesthesia. In a series of 50 eye operations, muscle traction produced significant bradycardia in 15 patients (30%).[143] Retrobulbar injection of lidocaine or procaine was given to 12 of these patients, and in each instance the oculocardiac reflex was abolished.

The findings from different clinical studies do not agree as to whether intravenous administration of atropine or retrobulbar injection of an anesthetic is the most effective agent in preventing cardiac irregularities resulting from the oculocardiac reflex. In a series of 50 consecutive eye operations performed with the patient under local anesthesia, attempts were made to induce cardiac slowing by applying pressure or traction on ocular structures.[144] Reproducible cardiac changes occurred in 5 of the first 25 patients and in 4 of the next 25. The first five were treated with a retrobulbar injection of 2 ml of a 2% solution of lidocaine, which abolished the oculocardiac reflex in all five patients. Atropine, 0.5 mg administered intravenously, was used in the group of four patients, and it prevented the recurrence of the abnormalities in only two of these patients. Subsequent lidocaine retrobulbar block abolished the oculocardiac reflex in one instance of atropine failure. In the fourth patient, atropine injection was followed by tachycardia to 240 beats/min, which was attributed to atropine sensitivity. The authors recommended routine retrobulbar anesthesia in all cases of eye surgery whether a local or general anesthetic is used.

Another study suggested that atropine was considerably more effective than retrobulbar anesthesia in preventing the oculocardiac reflex.[145] In a group of 28 patients, cardiac slowing of 10% to 50% occurred in 82% of the patients during surgery on the extraocular muscles. This bradycardia occurred despite premedication with 0.1 to 0.4

mg of atropine or scopolamine. However, intravenous administration of atropine (0.1–0.2 mg) during surgery did prevent bradycardia for as long as 30 minutes in all but one of 17 patients. (Two to 3 mg of atropine is required to produce a complete vagal block in an adult.) In 17 other patients, retrobulbar block with a 1% solution of lidocaine, 1 to 2 ml injected into the anterior portion of the retrobulbar space, did not significantly decrease bradycardia in 12 of the patients. In a series of 14 patients who developed bradycardia from a marked oculocardiac reflex during strabismus surgery, intravenous administration of atropine 0.003 mg/lb abolished the cardiac slowing within 1 minute.[146]

Knowledge that the oculocardiac reflex is more likely to occur when there is a combination of apnea and eye stimulation leads to another effective treatment.[147] Nothing more than artificial respiration will often promptly relieve the bradycardia resulting from ocular stimulation. To be effective, the respiratory exchange must inflate the lungs widely. Immediately on detection of dangerous cardiac slowing during eye surgery, the ophthalmologist should discontinue surgical manipulation and the patient should be made to breathe deeply. It should be noted, however, that the oculocardiac reflex may in some cases occur without anoxia or hypercapnia.

A study of 810 patients receiving various types of anesthesia supported the conclusion that assisted or controlled respiration during reflex stimulation was the simplest and most useful method for routine control of the oculocardiac reflex. Such respiratory control does not eliminate reflex activity but does terminate reflex-induced bradycardia and respiratory depression.[148]

Should retrobulbar anesthesia be used routinely to supplement general anesthesia for the purpose of preventing the oculocardiac reflex is unclear. Actually, the bradycardia and marked cardiac arrhythmias that commonly occur (47% of cases)[149] during the process of intubation exceed the cardiac response usually resulting from ocular surgery. The hazard of such minor arrhythmias induced by the surgery without a retrobulbar block is slight, possibly less than the dangers associate with a retrobulbar injection.[150] Indeed, of three cardiac arrests during eye surgery over a 20-year period at one hospital, two occurred within 5 minutes after retrobulbar injection for cataract extraction with the patients under local anesthesia. The incidence of cardiac arrest is very low despite demonstrable oculocardiac reflexes in 30% to 80% (depending on whose statistics you choose) of patients undergoing ocular surgery under general anesthesia.

## MALIGNANT HYPERTHERMIA

This condition is so rare that no case has ever occurred during eye surgery in our hospital. The incidence is 1 in 50,000 administrations of anesthetics in adults and 1 in 15,000 in children. Malignant hyperthermia is an autosomal dominantly transmitted disorder of the muscle membranes. When exposed to agents such as succinylcholine, halothane, or any other inhalation anesthetics, muscles become rigid and hyperthermic because of hypermetabolism, and the patient develops tachycardia and uncontrollable temperature elevation. The condition may be predicted to exist if a family history is present or if the serum creatine phosphokinase level is elevated.

Tetracaine, procaine, pentothal, and morphine apparently do not provoke malignant hyperthermia. Almost everything else used in anesthesia may do so, including atropine, meperidine, lidocaine, nitrous oxide, and digitalis glycosides. If possible, identify susceptible patients and avoid use of these drugs. If necessary, pretreat susceptible patients with dantrolene.

## REFERENCES

1. Nachmanshon D: Basic aspects of nerve activity explained by biochemical analysis, *JAMA* 179:145, 1962.
2. DeJong RH: Neural blockade by local anesthetics, *JAMA* 238:1383, 1977.
3. Zahl K, Jorrdan A, McGroarty J, and others: Peribulbar anesthesia—effect of bicarbonate on mixtures of lidocaine,

bupivacaine, and hyaluronidase with or without epinephrine, *Ophthalmology* 98:239, 1991.

4. Eccarius SG, Gordon ME, Parelman, JJ: Bicarbonate-buffered lidocaine-epinephrine hyaluronidase for eyelid anesthesia, *Ophthalmology* 97:1499, 1990.
5. Matsumoto S, Hayashi K, Tsuchisaka H, and others: Pharmokinetics of surface anesthesia in the human cornea, *Jpn J Ophthalmol* 25:335, 1981.
6. Adriani J, Zepernick, R: Clinic effectiveness of drugs used for topical anesthesia, *JAMA* 188:711, 1964.
7. Kennerdell JS, Rydze D, Robertson M: Comparison of retrobulbar marcaine and combined marcaine-carbocaine in ophthalmic surgery, *Ann Ophthalmol* 8:1236, 1976.
8. Goodman LS, Gilman A: *The pharmacological basis of therapeutics*, ed 4, New York, 1970, Macmillan.
9. Koscove EM, Paradis NA: Successful resuscitation from cardiac arrest using high-dose epinephrine therapy—report of two cases, *JAMA* 259:3031, 1988.
10. Lamberts DW, Foster CS, Perry HD: Schirmer test after topical anesthesia and the tear meniscus height in normal eyes, *Arch Ophthalmol* 97:1082, 1979.
11. Jordan A, Baum J: Basic tear flow does it exist? *Ophthalmology* 87:920, 1980.
12. Stevenson TC: Intrascleral nerve loops, *Am J Ophthalmol* 55:935, 1963.
13. Rosenwasser GOD, Holland S, Pflugfelder SC, and others: Topical anesthetic abuse, *Ophthalmology* 97:967, 1990.
14. Josephson JE, Caffery BE: Corneal staining after instillation of topical anesthetic, *Invest Ophthalmol* 29:1096, 1988.
15. Gundersen T, Liebman SD: Effect of local anesthetic on regeneration of corneal epithelium, *Arch Ophthalmol* 31:29, 1944.
16. Marr WG, Wood R, Senterfit L, Singleman S: Effects of topical anesthetics, *Am J Ophthalmol* 43:606, 1957.
17. Kinoshita JH: Some aspects of the carbohydrate metabolism of the cornea, *Invest Ophthalmol* 1:78, 1962.
18. Hermann H, Moses S, Friedenwald JS: Influence of pontocaine hydrochloride and chlorobutanol on respiration and glycolysis of cornea, *Arch Ophthalmol* 28:652, 1942.
19. Behrendt T: Experimental study of corneal lesions produced by topical anesthesia, *Am J Ophthalmol* 41:99, 1956.
20. Willis WE, Laibson PR: Corneal complications of topical anesthetic abuse, *Can J Ophthalmol* 5:239, 1970.
21. Rosenwasser GOD: Complications of topical anesthetics, *Int Ophthalmol Clin* 29:157, 1989.
22. Weinberg RJ, Oh JO: The effect of topical anesthetic on the recovery of herpes simplex virus, *Ann Ophthalmol* 9:977, Aug 1977.
23. Behrendt T: Experimental secondary effects of topical anesthesia of the cornea, *Am J Ophthalmol* 44:74, 1957.
24. Linn JG, Vey EK: Topical anesthesia in ophthalmology, *Am J Ophthalmol* 40:697, 1955.
25. Kintner JC, Grossniklaus HE, Lass JH, and others: Infectious crystalline keratopathy associated with topical anesthetic abuse, *Cornea* 9:77, 1990.
26. Kleinfeld J, Ellis PP: Effects of topical anesthetic on the growth of microorganisms, *Arch Ophthalmol* 76:712, 1966.
27. White JH, Corotti AA: The inhibition of growth of microorganisms by anesthetics, *Eye Ear Nose Throat Dig* 49:22, 1970.
28. Boozan CW, Cohen IJ: Ophthaine, *Am J Ophthalmol* 36:1619, 1953.
29. Emmerich R, Carter GZ, Berens C: An experimental clinical evaluation of dorsacaine hydrochloride (benoxinate, novesine), *Am J Ophthalmol* 40:841, 1955.
30. Schlegel HE, Swan KC: Benoxinate (Dorsacaine) for rapid corneal anesthesia, *Arch Ophthalmol* 51:633, 1954.
31. Koller C: Preliminary report on local anesthesia of the eye, *Arch Ophthalmol* 12:473, 1934.
32. Bloom S, Koller C: Cocaine, *Arch Ophthalmol* 31:344, 1944.
33. Koller K: On the use of cocaine to anesthetize the eye, *Arch Ophthalmol* 13:404, 1884. (Translated by Knapp H: On cocaine and its use in ophthalmolmic and general surgery, *Arch Ophthalmol* 68:31, 1962.)
34. Grove Jr AS: New diagnostic techniques for the evaluation of orbital trauma, *Trans Am Acad Ophthalmol Otolaryngol* 83:P-626, 1977.
35. Meyers EF: Cocaine toxicity during dacryocystorhinostomy, *Arch Ophthalmol* 98:842, 1980.
36. Bartley GB, Narr BJ: Preoperative medical examination for patients undergoing ophthalmic surgery, *Am J Ophthalmol* 112:725 Dec. 1991.
37. Council on Drugs: New drugs and devel-

opments in therapeutics, *JAMA* 183:178, 1963.
38. Vey EK, Finlay J, Everett WG: A clinical evaluation of mepivacaine, *Am J Ophthalmol* 53:827, 1962.
39. Laaka V, Nikki P, Tarkanen A: Comparison of bupivacaine with and without adrenalin and mepivacaine with adrenaline in intraocular surgery, *Acta Ophthalmol* 50:229, 1972.
40. Porter JD, Edney DP, McMahan EJ, and others: Extraocular myotoxicity of the retrobulbar anesthetic bupivacaine hydrochloride, *Invest Ophthalmol Vis Sci* 29:163, 1988.
41. Rainin EA, Carlson BM: Postoperative diplopia and ptosis: a clinical hypothesis based on the myotoxicity of local anesthetics, *Arch Ophthalmol* 103:1337, 1985.
42. Carlson BM, Emerick S, Komorowski TE, and others: Extraocular muscle regeneration in primates-local anesthetic-induced lesions, *Ophthalmology* 99:582, 1992.
43. Hamed LM, Mancuso A: Inferior rectus muscle contracture syndrome after retrobulbar anesthesia, *Ophthalmology* 96:1506, 1991.
44. Gills JP, Rudisill JE: Bupivacaine in cataract surgery, *Ophthalmic Surg* 5:67, 1974.
45. Smith RB, Linn Jr JG: Retrobulbar injection of bupivacaine (Maracaine) for anesthesia and akinesia, *Invest Ophthalmol* 13:157, 1974.
46. Chin GN, Almquist HT: Bupivacaine and lidocaine retrobulbar anesthesia, *Ophthalmology* 90:369, 1983.
47. Holekamp TLR, Arribas NP, Boniuk I: Bupivacaine anesthesia in retinal detachment surgery, *Arch Ophthalmol* 97:109, 1979.
48. Wittpenn JR, Rapoza P, Sterberg Jr P, and others: Respiratory arrest following retrobulbar anesthesia, *Ophthalmology* 93:867, 1986.
49. Seifter J, Baeder DH, Begany AJ: Influence of hyaluronidase and steroids on permeability of synovial membrane, *J Proc Soc Biol Med* 72:277, 1949.
50. Moore DC: An evaluation of hyaluronidase in local and nerve block analgesia: a review of 519 cases, *Anesthesiology* 11:470, 1950.
51. De Roeth A, Carroll FD: Effect of retrobulbar procaine injection on aqueous humor dynamics, *Arch Ophthalmol* 53:399, 1955.
52. Losada F, Wolontz AH: Bell's palsy: a new ophthalmologic sign, *Ann Ophthalmol* 5:1093, 1973.
53. Jay WM, Harvey C, Williams B, and others: Effect of applying the Honan intraocular pressure reducer before cataract surgery, *Am J Ophthalmol* 100:523, 1985.
54. Atkinson WS: Observations on anesthesia for ocular surgery, *Trans Am Acad Ophthalmol* 60:376, 1956.
55. Atkinson WS: Facial nerve block, *Am J Ophthalmol* 57:144, 1964.
56. Koenig SB, Snyder RW, Jonathan K: Respiratory distress after a Nadbath block, *Ophthalmology* 95:1285, 1988.
57. Parrish RK, Spaeth GL, Poryzees BS, and others: Evaluation of local anesthesia agents using a new force-sensitive lid speculum, *Ophthalmic Surg* 14:575, 1983.
58. Zauberman H: Controlled retrobulbar anesthesia for ECCE and IOL implantation, *Ophthalmic Surg* 16:560, 1985.
59. Atkinson WS: Large retrobulbar injections, *Am J Ophthalmol* 57:328, 1964.
60. Lichter PR: Editorial, Avoiding complications from local anesthesia, *Ophthalmology* 95:565, 1988.
61. Morgan CM, Schatz H, Andrew K, and others: Ocular complications associated with retrobulbar injections, *Ophthalmology* 95:660, 1988.
62. Javitt JC, Addiego R, Friedberg HL, and others: Brain stem anesthesia after retrobulbar block, *Ophthalmology* 94:718, 1987.
63. Unsöld R, Stanly JA, DeGroot J: The CT-topography of retrobulbar anesthesia: anatomic-clinical correlation of complications and suggestions of a modified technique, *Graefes Arch Klin Opthalmol* 217:125, 1981.
64. Feibel RM: Current concepts in retrobulbar anesthesia: diagnostic and surgical techniques, *Surv Ophthalmol* 30:102, 1985.
65. Bettman JW: A retrospective look at twenty-two medicolegal claims. How they might have been avoided, *Surv Ophthalmol* 28:56, 1983.
66. Callahan A: Ultrasharp disposable needles, *Am J Ophthalmol* 62:173, 1966.
67. Zaturansky B, Hyams S: Perforation of the globe during the injection of local anesthesia, *Ophthalmic Surg* 18:585, 1987.
68. Hay A, Flynn HW, Hoffman JI, and others: Needle perforation of the globe during retrobulbar and peribulbar injections, *Ophthalmology* 98:1017, 1991.
69. Grizzard WS, Kirk NM, Pavan PR, and others: Perforating ocular injuries caused by anesthesia personnel, *Ophthalmology* 98:1011, 1991.
70. Scheie HG: Continuous retrobulbar anes-

thesia, *Trans Am Acad Ophthalmol* 60:389, 1956.
71. Tamai M: A retained retrobulbar catheter for repetitive injection of anesthetics during ophthalmic surgery, *Ophthalmic Surg* 14:579, 1983.
72. Katsev DA, Drews RC, Rose BT: An anatomic study of retrobulbar needle path length, *Ophthalmology* 96:1221, 1989.
73. Bloomberg LB: Administration of peribulbar anesthesia, *J Cataract Refract Surg* 12:677, 1980.
74. Davis II DB, Mandel MR: Posterior peribulbar anesthesia: an alternative to retrobulbar anesthesia, *Geriat Ophthalmol* 3:27, 1987.
75. Weiss JL, Deichman CB: A comparison of retrobulbar and peribulbar anesthesia for cataract surgery, *Arch Ophthalmol* 107:96, 1989.
76. Davis II DB, Mandel MR: Periocular anesthesia: a review of technique and complications, *Ophthalmol Clin North Am* 3:101, 1990.
77. Ropo A, Nikki P, Ruusuvaara P, and others: Retrobulbar anesthesia, peribulbar anesthesia, *Br J Ophthalmol* 75:417, 1991.
78. Peterson WC, Yanoff M: Subconjunctival anesthesia: an alternative to retrobulbar and peribulbar techniques, *Ophthalmic Surg* 22:199, 1991.
79. Friedberg MA, Spellman FA, Pikerton AR, and others: An alternative technique of local anesthesia for vitreoretinal surgery, *Arch Ophthalmol* 109:1615, 1991.
80. Fichman RA: Topical eye drops replace injection for anesthesia-by Darvon Harr, Ocular Surgery News staff writer, *Ocular Surgery News* 10:1, March 1992.
81. Fenzl RE: Indications for use of topical anesthesia in cataract surgery, *Ocular Surg News* 10:4, 1992 (guest commentary).
82. Everett WG, Vey EK, Veenis CY: Factors in reducing ocular tension prior to intraocular surgery, *Trans Am Acad Ophthalmol* 63:286, 1959.
83. Linn Jr JG, Smith RB: Intraoperative complications and their management, *Int Ophthalmol Clin* 13:149, 1973.
84. Cionni RJ, Osher RH: Retrobulbar hemorrhage, *Ophthalmology* 98:1153, 1991.
85. Goldsmith MO: Occlusion of the central retinal artery following retrobulbar hemorrhage, *Ophthalmologica* 153:191, 1967.
86. Sullivan KL, Brown GC, Forman AR, and others: Retrobulbar anesthesia and retinal vascular obstruction, *Ophthalmology* 90:373, 1983.
87. Klein ML, Jampol LM, Condon PI, and others: Central retinal artery occlusion without retrobulbar hemorrhage after retrobulbar anesthesia, *Am J Ophthalmol* 93:573, 1982.
88. Paulter SE, Gizzard WS, Thompson LN, and others: Blindness from retrobulbar injection into the optic nerve, *Ophthalmic Surg* 17:334, 1986.
89. Zaturansky B, Hyams S: Perforation of the globe during the injection of local anesthesia, *Ophthalmic Surg* 18:585, 1987.
90. Cibis PA: General discussion opening remarks. In Schepens CL, Regan CDJ, editors: *Controversial aspects of the management of retinal detachments,* Boston, 1965, Little, Brown, p 222.
91. Ramsay RC, Knobloch WH: Ocular perforation following retrobulbar anesthesia for retinal detachment surgery, *Am J Ophthalmol* 86:61, 1978.
92. Duker JS, Belmont JB, Benson WE, and others: Inadvertent globe perforation during retrobulbar and peribulbar anesthesia—patient characteristics, surgical management, and visual outcome, *Ophthalmology* 98:519, 1991.
93. Reed JW, MacMillan Jr AS, Lazenby GW: Transient neurologic complication of positive contrast orbitography, *Arch Ophthalmol* 81:508, 1969.
94. Drysdale DB: Experimental subdural retrobulbar injection of anesthetic, *Am Ophthalmol* 16:715, 1984.
95. Kobet KA: Cerebral spinal fluid recovery of lidocaine and bupivacaine following respiratory arrest subsequent to retrobulbar block, *Ophthalmic Surg* 18:11, 1987.
96. Knopf HLS: Periocular anesthesia for relief of pain, *Ann Ophthalmol* 19:181, 1987.
97. Duker JS, Nielsen J, Vander JF, and others: Retrobulbar bupivacaine irrigation for postoperative pain after scleral buckling surgery, *Ophthalmology* 98:514, 1991.
98. Lewis RA, Landers MB: The use of a retrobulbar anesthetic in managing pain and nausea from elevated intraocular pressure, *Ophthalmic Surg* 18:523, 1987.
99. Fishof F: Meperidine in cataract surgery, *Am J Ophthalmol* 53:672, 1962.
100. McTique JW, Urweider HA: The use of diazepam (Valium) in ophthalmic surgery, *Trans Am Acad Ophthalmol Otolaryngol* 73:78, 1969.
101. Hascay JD, Karch FE: Benzodiazepine prescribing in a family medicine center, *JAMA* 246:1321, 1981.

102. Abromowicz M: Midazolam, *Med Lett Drugs Ther* 28:73, 1986.
103. Elliott HW, Navarro G: A double-blind controlled study of the pharmacologic effects of nalbupine, *J Med* 1:74, 1970.
104. Hofmann RF, Weiler HH: Lorazepam and nalbuphine as local anesthetic ophthalmic surgery premedication, *Ann Ophthalmol* 15:64, 1983.
105. Dorsey R, Ayd Jr FJ, Cole JR, and others: Psychopharmacological screening criteria development project, *JAMA* 241:1021, 1979.
106. Knapp MR, Beecher HK: Postanesthetic nausea, vomiting, and retching, *JAMA* 160:376, 1956.
107. Weiss WA, McGee JP, Branford J, and others: Value of chlorpromazine in preoperative medication, *JAMA* 161:812, 1956.
108. Papper EM: The proper use of tranquilizers in surgical patients, *Trans Am Acad Ophthalmol* 64:689, 1960.
109. Adriani J, Arens J, Anthony SO: Postanesthetic vomiting, *JAMA* 175:666, 1961.
110. From the NIH: Analgesic-associated nephropathy—an underrecognized but preventable renal disorder, *JAMA* 246:729, 1981.
111. Fatalities due to propoxyphene, *FDA Drug Bull* 9:2, 1979.
112. Sriwatanakul K, Weis OF, Alloze JL, and others: Analysis of narcotic analgesic usage in the treatment of postoperative pain, *JAMA* 250:926, 1983.
113. Ewards H, Rose EA, Schorow M, and others: Postoperative deterioration in psychomotor function, *JAMA* 245:1342, 1981.
114. Neuhaus RW, Meyer KT: Chest pain in the postoperative ophthalmic patient, *Ophthalmology* 88:445, 1981.
115. De Roetth A, Schwartz H: Aqueous humor dynamics in glaucoma, *Arch Ophthalmol* 55:755, 1956.
116. Magora F, Collins V: The influence of general anesthetic agents on intraocular pressure in man, *Arch Ophthalmol* 66:806, 1961.
117. Kornblueth W, Aladjemoff L, Magora F, and others: Influence of general anesthesia on intraocular pressure in man, *Arch Ophthalmol* 61:84, 1959.
118. Self WG, Ellis PP: The effect of general anesthetic agents on intraocular pressure, *Surv Ophthalmol* 21:494, 1977.
119. Sampaolesi R, Reca R, Carro A, and others: Intraocular pressure in children up to six years of age with and without general anesthesia; importance for the early diagnosis of congenital glaucoma, *Perspect Ophthalmol* 1:197, 1977.
120. Burch PG: Accommodation during general anesthesia, *Arch Ophthalmol* 81:202, 1969.
121. Westheimer G: Amphetamine, barbiturates, and accommodation-convergence, *Arch Ophthalmol* 70:830, 1963.
122. Smith RB, Carl B, Linn Jr JG, and others: Effect of nitrous oxide on air in vitreous, *Am J Ophthalmol* 78:314, 1974.
123. Smith RB: Nitrous oxide anesthesia with gas in the vitreous cavity, *Am J Ophthalmol* 80:779, 1975.
124. Aronowitz JD, Brubaker RF: Effect of intraocular gas on intraocular pressure, *Arch Ophthalmol* 94:1191, 1976.
125. Lincoff H, Mardirossian J, Lincoff A, and others: Intravitreal longevity of three perfluorocarbon gases, *Arch Ophthalmol* 98:1610, 1980.
126. Crittenden JJ, de Juan Jr E, Tiedeman J: Expansion of long-acting gas bubbles for intraocular use: principles and practice, *Arch Ophthalmol* 103:831, 1985.
127. Miller B, Lean JS, Miller H, and others: Intravitreal expanding gas bubble: a morphologic study in the rabbit eye, *Arch Ophthalmol* 102:1708, 1984.
128. Simone JN, Whitacre MM: The effect of intraocular gas and fluid volumes on intraocular pressure, *Ophthalmology* 47:238, 1990.
129. Krupin T, Cross DA, Becker B: Decreased basal tear production associated with general anesthesia, *Arch Ophthalmol* 95:107, 1977.
130. Lincoff HA, Ellis CH, Devoe AG, and others: The effect of succinylcholine on intraocular pressure, *Am J Ophthalmol* 40:501, 1955.
131. Lincoff HA, Breinin GM, DeVoe AG: The effect of succinylcholine on extraocular muscles, *Am J Ophthalmol* 43:404, 1957.
132. Lewallen WM, Hicks BL: The use of succinylcholine in ocular surgery, *Am J Ophthalmol* 61:985, 1966.
133. Norskov K: Expulsive hemorrhage caused by succinylcholine, *Acta Ophthalmol* 38:285, 1960.
134. Moreno RJ, Kloess P, Carlson DW: Effect of succinylcholine on the intraocular contents of open globes, *Ophthalmology* 98:636, 1991.
135. France NK, France TD, Woodburn JD, and others: Succinylcholine alteration of the forced duction test, *Ophthalmology* 87:1282, 1980.
136. Mindel JS, Raab EL, Eisenkraft JB, and

others: Succinyldicholine-induced return of the eyes to the basic deviation, *Ophthalmology* 87:1288, 1980.

137. Alfano JE: Pseudocholinesterase, cholinesterase and congenital glaucoma, *Am J Ophthalmol* 61:985, 1966.

138. Lessell S, Kuwabara T, Feldman RG: Myopathy and succinylcholine sensitivity, *Am J Ophthalmol* 68:789, 1969.

139. Abramson DH: Anterior chamber and lens thickness changes induced by succinylcholine, *Arch Ophthalmol* 86:643, 1971.

140. Taylor GJ, Rubon R, Tucked M, and others: External cardiac compression, a randomized comparison of mechanical and manual techniques, *JAMA* 240:644, 1989.

141. Killip T: Anesthesia and major noncardiac surgery, *JAMA* 268:252, 1992 (editorial).

142. Gay AJ, Jaoffe WS, Barnet R: The afferent course of the oculorespiratory reflex of the third, fourth, and sixth cranial nerves, *Invest Ophthalmol* 3:451, 1964.

143. Kirsch RE, Samet P, Kugel V, and others: Electrocardiographic changes during ocular surgery and their prevention by retrobar injection, *Arch Ophthalmol* 58:348, 1957.

144. Mendelblatt F, Kirsch R, Lemberg L: A study of comparing methods of preventing the oculocardiac reflex, *Am J Ophthalmol* 53:506, 1962.

145. Bosomworth PP, Ziegler CH, Jacoby J: The oculocardiac reflex in eye muscle surgery, *Anesthesiology* 19:1, 1958.

146. Welhaf WR, Johnson DC: The oculocardiac reflex during extraocular muscle surgery, *Arch Ophthalmol* 73:43, 1965.

147. Aserinsky E, DeBias A: Suppression of oculocardiac reflex by artificial respiration, *Arch Ophthalmol* 86(suppl):1, 1966.

148. Pontinen PJ: The importance of the oculocardiac reflex during ocular surgery, *Acta Ophthalmol* 86(suppl):1, 1966.

149. Landers PH, Moyer JK: Electrocardiographic observations, *Am J Ophthalmol* 60:71, 1965.

150. Beler DK: The oculocardiac reflex, *Am J Ophthalmol* 56:954, 1963.

# CHAPTER 6

# Antimicrobials

Thomas F. Mauger

SECTION ONE

## Antibacterials

Our antibiotic choices have a staggering impact on health care economics. Decisions as to whether antibiotics are needed at all and, if so, which particular antibiotic would be most appropriate equate into millions of dollars every day. Compare the cost of amikacin vs. gentamicin in Fig. 6–1. Amikacin dosed at 5 mg/kg/day costs $118.53 and gentamicin dosed at 1 to 1.5 mg/kg/day costs the hospital almost $17.00. Let us assume that we consistently use amikacin instead of gentamicin on 1,000 patients with 10-day courses of parenteral medication. The cost to the hospital of the gentamicin would be $169,800.00, whereas the cost of the amikacin would be $1,185,300. The difference in cost would be more than $1 million.[1] It is easy to see why hospital administrators, pharmacists, insurance companies, and governmental agencies are quite concerned with our use of antibiotics. Cost containment committees and antibiotic usage review committees are in place in almost every hospital. Fig. 6–2 shows the effect of the institution of physician education programs at the Ohio State University Hospitals during recent years. A 29% ($607,000) savings occurred. This significant cost saving can be achieved only when physicians are made aware of the efficacy and price issues associated with antibiotic use.[2]

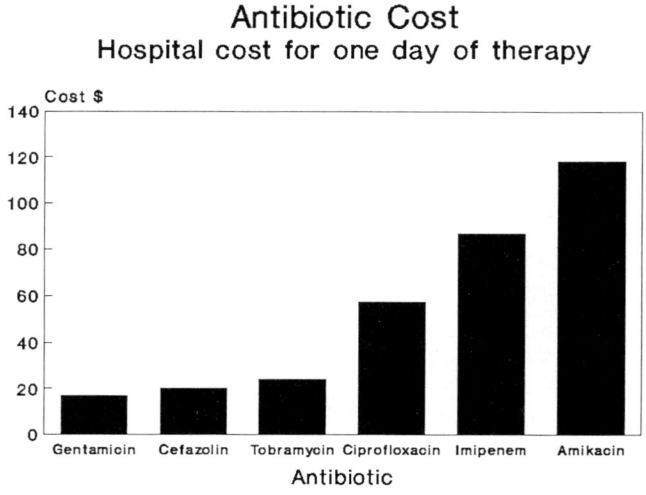


**FIG 6–1.**
Cost of single day of antibiotic therapy. (Data from the *Guide to choice of antibiotic therapy*, Riverside Methodist Hospitals, Columbus, Ohio, 1992. Used by permission.)

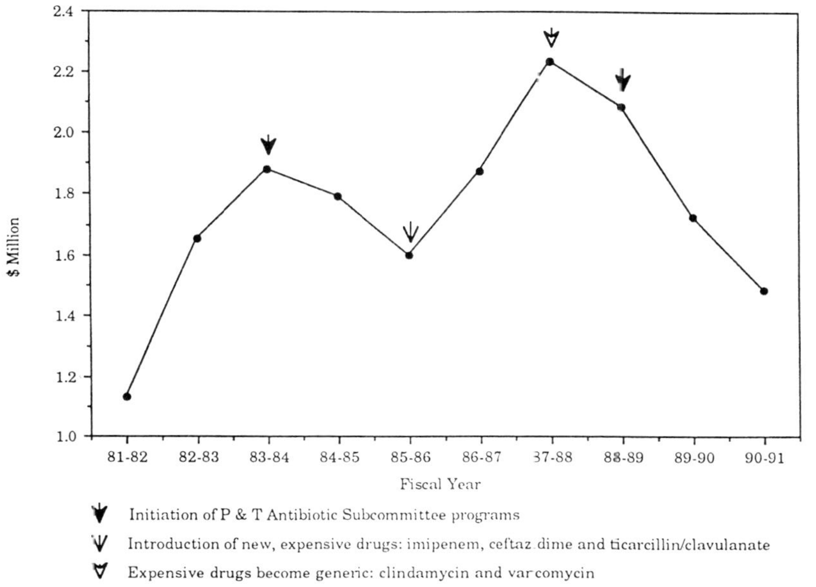


**FIG 6–2.**
Ohio State University Pharmacy costs 1981–1991 for parental antibacterial agents. (From Fass RJ: Report of the pharmacy and therapeutic antibiotics subcommittee, 1991, Ohio State University Hospitals, Columbus, Ohio. Used by permission.)

The Joint Commission on Accreditation of Hospitals now requires a regular review of clinical usage of antibiotics. This ruling is based on the belief that physician prescribing habits are less than ideal and directly contribute to a large number of adverse reactions to antibiotics (perhaps 4.5% of hospitalized patients), the cost (one third or more of a hospital pharmacy budget is consumed by antibiotics), and the development of resistant bacteria and infections. Yeast and fungal superinfections may follow antibiotic therapy (0.7% of 14,077 patients).[3]

## PROPHYLAXIS

Antibiotic prophylaxis is of no value in routine clean general surgery performed on healthy patients with normal resistance. Should topical antibiotics be used prophylactically before intraocular surgery? To answer this question intelligently, the surgeon must know the origins and characteristics of the intraocular infection, as well as the antibacterial spectrum of the antibiotic being considered (Table 6–1).

Certainly it is possible to introduce organisms from the environment into the eye, and for this reason, meticulous aseptic surgical techniques must be rigidly followed. I know of a small epidemic in which three eyes were lost because *Pseudomonas* infection developed after cataract surgery. The same strain of bacteria, as judged by sensitivity characteristics, was isolated from each of the three eyes and from the interior of a rubber irrigating bulb that had been used in each of the three operations. The bulb had not been autoclaved but had been ineffectively soaked in sterilizing solution before being used on the next patient. Many other instances are known in which an infection originated from an external source.

Exogenous infection should always be suspected when clusters of infection appear. In a series of more than 23,000 cataract operations performed in India, 9 separate clusters, accounting for 41% of all infections, occurred. Only one cluster was encountered in a second series of more than 25,000 cataract operations. The infection rate in the first series was 2.9 : 1,000; in the second series, it was 1.01 : 1,000.[4] The authors attributed this decrease in infection rate to prophylaxis with combined penicillin, chloramphenicol, and sulfadimidine treatment. Another interpretation of this infor-

**TABLE 6–1.**
Susceptibilities (Percent) of Important Organisms to Selected Antibiotics

| | Ami-kacin | Genta-micin | Tobra-micin | Cipro-floxacin | Cefti-zoxime | Vanco-mycin | Imi-penem | Trimethoprim-sulfa |
|---|---|---|---|---|---|---|---|---|
| *Staphylococcus aureus* | — | 91 | — | 81 | 83 | 100 | 83 | 98 |
| *Staphylococcus epidermidis* | — | 52 | — | 76 | 25 | 99 | 25 | 69 |
| *Streptococcus viridans* | — | — | — | — | 95 | 100 | 95 | 85 |
| *Haemophilus influenzae* | — | 100 | — | 100 | 100 | — | 100 | — |
| *Klebsiella pneumoniae* | 100 | 91 | 92 | 96 | 99 | — | 100 | 89 |
| *Serratia marcescens* | 100 | 91 | 89 | 96 | 99 | — | 100 | 97 |
| *Proteus mirabilis* | 100 | 96 | 96 | 99 | 100 | — | 99 | 96 |
| *Pseudomonas aeruginosa* | 96 | 77 | 96 | 83 | — | — | 84 | — |

Modified from Antimicrobial sensitivities, 1990, 1991, Clinical Microbiology, The Ohio State University Hospitals, Columbus, Ohio. Used by permission.

mation is that the earlier series (starting in 1963) differed from the second series (starting in 1973) in that facilities became available for better sterile technique during the second decade of the study. This is a particularly nice illustration of the invalidity of comparing consecutive groups of cases. You will note that most of the advocates of prophylactic antibiotic therapy for eye surgery base their advice on such comparisons of series of before and after cases.

Antibiotic usage by general surgeons was considered to be inappropriate in 66% of the patients as reviewed retrospectively.[5] Prophylaxis is the most controversial area. Doubtful critics state that preventive use of antibiotics simply ensures that subsequent infections will be resistant to the antibiotics used.[6] All surgeons (not only ophthalmologists) seem convinced that their particular specialty is so critical as to justify antibiotic prophylaxis, even though prophylaxis demonstrably does not work. In thoracic surgery, for example, postoperative infection developed in 17.2% of 29 placebo-treated patients and in 17.8% of 28 antibiotic-treated patients.[7] In 265 sutured hand lacerations, 1.1% of the placebo-treated patients and 2.5% of the antibiotic-treated patients developed infections.

Nearly 40% of all antibiotic use is for prophylactic treatment.[8, 9] Of course the cost of prophylactic antibiotic use in ophthalmology must be exceedingly small because we rarely use parental antibiotics. Wrong! If we used only $20 of antibiotics for prophylaxis in each of 1 million cataract surgeries, the total bill for prophylaxis could be $20 million/year for cataract surgery alone. Our choices of prophylaxis for ophthalmic surgery are important in terms of cost, adverse reactions, and development of resistance because of the enormous numbers of patients that are involved.

Most investigations on the development of postsurgical infections and the role of prophylactic antibiotics are limited by the rarity of the event, the ancillary changes in perioperative management that may have occurred during the duration of the study, and the presence of retrospective controls in the study. The incidence of postoperative endophthalmitis after ophthalmic surgery ranged from 0.66% to 3.16% before the use of prophylactic antibiotics. More recent studies involving use of prophylactic antibiotics show rates up to 0.57% and as low as 0% (Fig. 6–3).[10]

The goal of prophylaxis is to prevent postoperative infection. The source of bacterial contamination is from the lids, lashes, and conjunctiva of the patient and also from poorly sterilized ophthalmic instruments. Conjunctival flora varies from day to day and week to week; therefore, preoperative cultures can be misleading and counterproductive in the selection of prophylactic antibiotics. Even the trauma of the culture itself can change the bacterial flora.[11] Organisms that may otherwise be considered normal flora or contaminants such as *Staphylococcus epidermidis* are potential pathogens to the eye. The use of preoperative topical antibiotics may decrease or eliminate bacterial flora from the conjunctiva[12]; however, such use will not prevent intraoperative contamination of the wound or anterior chamber. A recent study found 43% of 30 patients to have culture positive anterior chamber aspirates after uncomplicated cataract surgery.[13] These patients were treated with topical gentamicin antibiotic, as well as a chlorhexidine facial scrub, the night before surgery. Just before surgery the eyelids were scrubbed with both hexachlorophene and 5% povidone-iodine. Povidone-iodine was placed topically on the cornea, and then the eye and skin were irrigated with sterile saline solution. After surgery, aqueous humor was aspirated through the surgical wound and cultured. Thirteen of 30 eyes grew bacteria. Of 13 culture-positive eyes, *S. epidermidis* was found in 8. Despite the presence of organisms, no clinical infections were found, probably because of the small inoculant size and the presence of an intact posterior capsule. Subconjunctival gentamicin was placed in the inferior fornix after each operation. The aqueous humor provides a limited antimicrobial effect when small inoculants are involved. This is overwhelmed when large inoculants are presented. Bacterial contamination of the vitreous appears to be relatively resistant to current prophylactic measures. All 25 rabbit eyes given subconjunctival gentamicin and cefazolin after vitreous injection of *Pseudomonas* went on to develop clinical endophthalmitis.[14]

The choice of antibiotic cannot be determined based on antibiotic sensitivities alone. Locatcher-Khorazo[12] showed that despite apparently good sensitivities of bacteria to chloramphenicol and Terramycin, the medications had little effect on bacterial colony counts when applied to the living eye. Intraocular antibiotic concentrations found when topical medications are used are usually insufficient to be bactericidal for possible pathogenic bacteria. Subconjuncti-

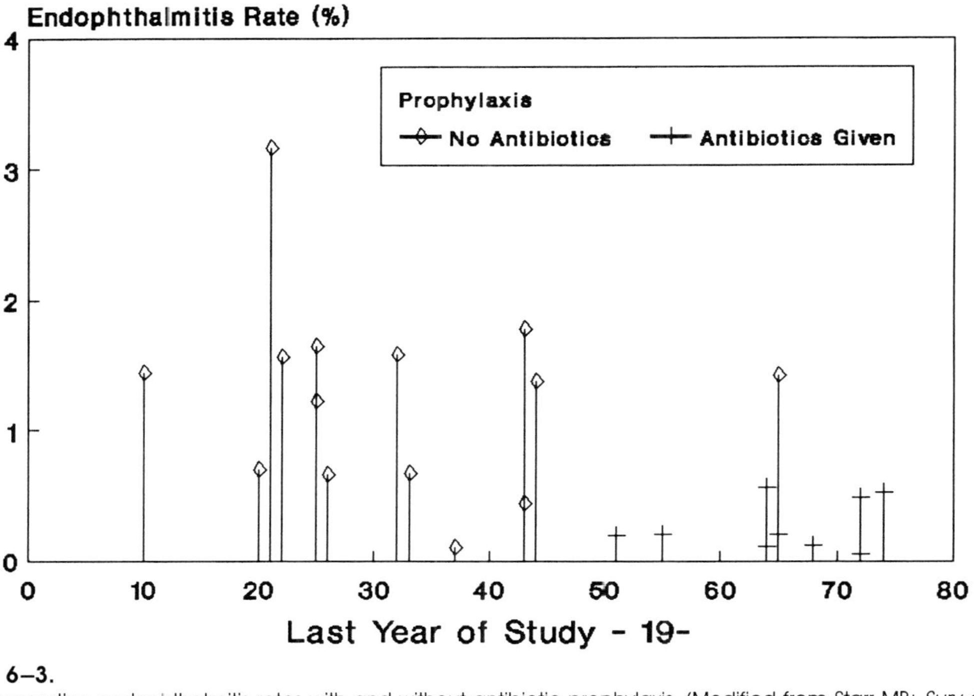


**FIG 6–3.**
Postoperative endophthalmitis rates with and without antibiotic prophylaxis. (Modified from Starr MB: *Surv of Ophthalmol* 27:353, 1983. Used by permission.)

val injections before or after surgery may give bactericidal levels of antibiotics in the anterior chamber at least for a short period. A prospective, controlled study investigating the role of subconjunctival antibiotic prophylaxis in 974 patients undergoing ocular surgery was performed in 1967.[15] Untreated controls had intraocular infections develop in 1.42% of cases compared with only 0.21% of the treated group. Treatment consisted of subconjunctival penicillin and streptomycin. The controls were given no antibiotics. Neither group of patients was given preoperative or postoperative topical or systemic antibiotics. The sevenfold decrease in the postoperative endophthalmitis rate was assumed to be the result of the subconjunctival penicillin and streptomycin used. A concern with the use of subconjunctival antibiotic use is the possibility of masking an early infection, allowing it to manifest later in the postoperative course when it has become well advanced with a poorer prognosis. This issue is of questionable significance when compared with the vast improvement in postoperative infection rates associated with the prophylactic use of subconjunctival antibiotics.

A small prospective study comparing topical and subconjunctival postoperative antibiotics with cataract surgery was reported in 1992. Sixty patients were randomized to receive either 2 mg of the corticosteroid betamethasone (Betnesol) and 20 mg of gentamicin subconjunctival or 0.1% betamethasone and 0.5% neomycin topically. Increased conjunctival injection and anterior chamber reaction were found with subconjunctival injection. The small study numbers allow no conclusions concerning the prevention of postoperative endophthalmitis. Cultures were not performed from either the aqueous humor or the conjunctiva. The study did not differentiate between the effects of subconjunctival corticosteroids compared with antibiotics. This study simply reports the relative safety of both methods of surgical prophylaxis but provides no meaningful finding about relative efficacy.[16]

Systemic antibiotic use has not been advocated because of the poor risk/benefit ratio. Recently oral ciprofloxacin has been found to produce vitreous levels in the bactericidal range for many important bacteria. Doses of 750 mg of ciprofloxacin given as a single dose 4 to 8 hours before surgery or as multiple doses 24 and 12 hours before surgery were found to give bactericidal vitreous levels.[17] Cost effectiveness, risk/benefit ratio, and development of resistance to organisms have not been evaluated for the possible use of this modality of prophylaxis in routine ophthalmic surgery. It does seem to make clinical sense, for instance, in the case of an intraocular foreign body penetrating to the vitreal cavity. It may also have a role as a postoperative medication when the vitreous has been disturbed during ocular surgery, for example, after unplanned posterior capsule rent and anterior vitrectomy during cataract surgery.

Intraocular antibiotics have been used as prophylaxis in cataract surgery either as a single injection or as an infusion. Both modalities are rational in the sense that decreasing or eliminating intraocular organisms will probably reduce cases of endophthalmitis. The risk of intraocular toxicity are much higher than with topical or subconjunctival antibiotics, and this has not been properly evaluated in a large group of patients.[18]

Other than antibiotic toxicity, the other objection to prophylactic treatment is the possibility of development of resistant organisms. Most evidence indicates that resistant organisms occur with the systemic administration of antibiotics over long periods. There is little evidence indicating that topical antibiotics delivered over a short period contribute to development of resistant organisms. The magnitude of their use in ophthalmic surgery, however, demands attention to this possibility. It is not rational to use the newest and most expensive antibiotics for prophylactic treatment in routine ocular surgery when a less expensive, established antibiotic will be equally effective. We must, however, remain cognizant of the development of resistant organisms with any antibiotic and evaluate the sensitivity of these organisms in our community so that our use of prophylaxis may be adjusted. Particular attention should be given to the development of resistance with

*Staphylococcus* organisms, because these are a common cause of postoperative endophthalmitis.[10, 19]

Aseptic preparation of the eye before surgery is important in reducing endophthalmitis postoperatively. Silver protein solution has been used during the preoperative preparation of the eye but has been shown to have little antimicrobial effect. It is useful in staining mucus and therefore ensuring adequate irrigation at the end of the preparation. Caldwell et al.[20] reported a 9.6% postoperative positive culture rate after the use of half-strength povidone-iodine solution applied to the lids, brows, and conjunctival cul-de-sac. This study also included an intensive 1½ days' use of gentamicin eye drops given every 2 hours. This positive culture rate is much lower than previously reported, but this study is flawed because of the absence of controls.[20]

Another study reported 7 years later compared the effect of dilute povidone-iodine preparation on mean colony counts.[21] The conjunctiva was cultured before and after conjunctival preparation. The study also compared ½-day vs. 3-day antibiotic preparation. Although the povidone-iodine preparation did eliminate all fungal cultures, the overall incidence of positive bacterial culture after preparation *increased* from 2.33 to 4.95 colonies per patient. This difference was not significant statistically. The authors believed the preparation and possibly the initial culturing freed bacteria from crevices in the conjunctival fornices, increasing the colony counts. The study did show a significant difference between 3-day gentamicin treatment and ½-day treatment, showing a 1.88 colony count per patient after 3-day treatment and a 5.42 colony count with ½-day treatment.[21] How should we assimilate these two studies into a rational preoperative preparation? One study indicates that povidone-iodine conjunctival preparation decreases the incidence of postoperative cultures, and the other study indicates that povidone-iodine preparation of the eye increases conjunctival colony counts. A third study reported in 1991 goes a long way in answering this question. Two operating suites in the New York Eye Infirmary were used to compare a dilute povidone-iodine preparation against silver protein solution during the 11-month period between April 1989 and February 1990. During a similar period before initiation of the study, 0.18% of cases from suite A and 0.16% cases from suite B developed culture-proven postoperative endophthalmitis. During the study only 0.06% of patients from suite A, using povidone-iodine preparation, had postoperative, culture-proven endophthalmitis develop compared with 0.24% cases from suite B using silver protein solution. During this time, 3,384 operations were performed in suite A and 3,289 were performed in suite B. It is interesting to note that in suite B (with the higher infection rate) a much higher percentage of cases were noncataract procedures. A similar percentage of noncataract surgery procedures were performed during the retrospective control period before initiation of the study. Therefore, the difference in infection rates probably results from the different preparation regimens. Concomitant conjunctival culturing was not performed during this study. Nine of the 31 cases of postoperative endophthalmitis involved cases of cataract extraction with vitrectomy, suggesting that disturbance of the vitreous cavity increases the risk of endophthalmitis. Cataract cases involving disturbed vitreous may deserve special attention for prevention of endophthalmitis, such as the use of intravitreal antibiotic injections, antibiotics added to the infusion fluid, or systemic antibiotics (Table 6–2).[22]

It would seem that an adequate preparation before ocular surgery should include preoperative topical antibiotics with a spectrum of action similar to the suspected pathogens. The topical antibiotic should be used 1 to 3 days before surgery to decrease colony counts. The skin preparation should be a meticulous scrub with 5% to 10% povidone-iodine. This solution should be allowed to remain in contact with the skin for at least 2 minutes. Special attention should be directed to the lid margins and base of the cilia, removing all matter from these areas. A solution of 5% povidone-iodine should be used as a conjunctival irrigation. I personally swab the conjunctival fornices with a cotton swab soaked in this

**TABLE 6–2.**
Systemic and Ophthalmic Dosage of Selected Antibiotics for Adults

| Drug | Topical | Subconjunctival (in 0.25–0.75 ml) | Intravitreal (in 0.1 ml) | Systemic Daily Dose* |
|---|---|---|---|---|
| Amikacin | 10–50 mg/ml | 25–50 mg | 400 ug | 15 mg/kg IM, IV |
| Gentamicin | 8–20 mg/ml | 20 mg | 100–200 ug | 3–5 mg/kg IM, IV |
| Tobramycin | 8–20 mg/ml | 20 mg | 100–200 ug | 3–5 mg/kg IM, IV |
| Ciprofloxacin | 3 mg/ml | — | 100 ug | 0.5–1.5 g po |
| Cefazolin | 33–66 mg/ml | 50–100 mg | 2.25 mg | 1–6 g IM, IV |
| Cefamandole | 50 mg/ml | 50–100 mg | 2.0 mg | 1.5–12 g IM, IV |
| Clindamycin | 10 mg/ml | 15–40 mg | 1.0 mg | 0.6–3.6 g IM, IV |
| Vancomycin | 50 mg/ml | 25 mg | 1.0 mg | 0.5–2 g po 2 g IV |
| Penicillin G | 100,000 units/ml | 0.5–1 million units | — | 1.2–24 million units IM, IV |
| Imipenem | 5 mg/ml | — | — | 1–4 g IV |

**IM*, Intramuscularly; *IV*, intravenously; *po*, orally.

solution, allowing the solution to remain in the cul-de-sacs for several minutes. The nasolacrimal systems can be a source of bacterial contamination, and these areas, including the caruncle, should be prepared at the same time as the conjunctiva. Povidone-iodine should be irrigated liberally from the conjunctiva so that intraocular instillation does not occur. The povidone-iodine may then be reapplied to the skin surface to allow continued antimicrobial action. If the eye is obviously infected at the time of elective surgery, the surgery should be delayed. It is virtually impossible to sterilize a clinically infected eye. The eye should be cultured, broad-spectrum topical antibiotics started, and the surgery delayed 2 to 4 weeks. Conjunctival cultures should be negative before surgery is considered after a recent ocular infection.

Several conclusions can be made in regard to the large body of literature on prophylaxis for ophthalmic surgeries. First, postoperative infections result from either periocular flora or contaminated surgical instrumentation. The reduction or elimination of periocular flora should reduce the incidence of postoperative endophthalmitis. Second, intensive preoperative topical treatment with antibiotics is an effective way to reduce the periocular flora. Preoperative cultures do not add significant information to antibiotic selection because of their variability. The antibiotic should be able to deliver bactericidal levels to the common causes of postsurgical infection (e.g., *Staphylococcus* species). Third, periocular and conjunctival preparation with dilute povidone-iodine solution decreases the incidence of postoperative endophthalmitis. Fourth, subconjunctival antibiotics either immediately preoperatively or after closing of the incision can achieve bactericidal levels in the anterior chamber, presumably decreasing the bacterial colony counts. Finally, the role of prophylactic systemic and intraocular antibiotics is still unclear, and the risk/benefit ratio needs to be determined through study of large numbers of patients with appropriate controls.

### Donor Cornea Management

Antibiotic treatment of donor eyes for corneal transplantation is a special kind of prophylaxis. Despite sterile technique in removal and handling, up to 100% of donor eyes are culture positive after removal.[23] Washing with antibiotics significantly reduces the bacterial counts on the donor eyes. One report[24] showed that there were no clinical infections present even though 25 cases out of 200 consecutive keratoplasties grew bacteria and three grew new fungi from the corneal scleral rims. A number of host infections have been reported that can be linked to donor disease. Among these include *Cryptococcus neoformans, Strepto-*

*coccus pneumoniae* in a patient with bronchial pneumonia,[25] *Pseudomonas* in a patient with septicemia,[26, 27] Creutzfeld-Jacob disease,[28] and rabies. Streptococcal contamination of donor eyes is not uncommon. *Streptococcus viridans* was recovered in 2.3% of the cultures of 4,167 donor eyes.[29] *Propionibacterium acnes* has been cited as a cause of endophthalmitis after penetrating keratoplasty and also a source of contamination in donor corneas and corneal storage medium.[30] Both *P. acnes* and *Streptococcus* species are organisms that are frequently resistant to gentamicin, which is the current antibiotic additive to corneal preservation solution. Gentamicin had little bactericidal effect at the low (4° C) storage temperature used with intermediate-term storage medium but becomes effective when the tissue is returned to room temperature during corneal transplantation. It is reasonable to assume that broadening the antimicrobial spectrum by adding another antibiotic to the corneal preservation solution will decrease the frequency of postpenetrating keratoplasty infections. Recent studies have indicated that vancomycin in a dosage of 100 μg/ml can be tolerated by the donor cornea for intermediate storage.[31] Other studies have indicated the efficacy of adding either vancomycin or streptomycin to intermediate corneal storage medium to enhance the antimicrobial spectrum of the solutions. These studies indicate that the addition of vancomycin does enhance the spectrum and increases the antimicrobial activity of the solution at 4° C.[32, 33] Ciprofloxacin has also been found to be a useful adjuvant or alternative to gentamicin in the intermediate-storage solution, significantly increasing its antimicrobial spectrum, particularly against gentamicin-resistant *Pseudomonas aeruginosa.*[33]

These modifications of corneal storage solutions with antibiotics do not take the place of meticulous handling of tissue and evaluation of the tissue before its use. The use of tissue from donors with known sepsis or other systemic transmittable infections is contraindicated. Obvious ocular trauma or infection is also an absolute contraindication. Aseptic technique in surgery, just as in other ophthalmic operations, is essential in preventing postoperative endophthalmitis.

### Contact Lens Management

The use of a "bandage" contact lens in the short-term management of an acute corneal defect may create a difficult situation. In a series of 278 patients wearing soft contact lenses for protective purposes, 4 developed corneal infections.[34] Frequent observation of such patients to permit early detection of an infection was advised. Several days of antibiotic usage when a beginning infection is suspected is reasonable.

Both *P. aeruginosa* and *Staphylococcus aureus* have been shown to adhere to soft and rigid contact lenses. This adherence is not related to protein deposits, and bacteria will adhere to new, unworn contact lenses.[35, 36] A large percentage (34.5%[37]) of soft contact lens wearers do not adequately disinfect their lenses. Longer exposure (extended wear) and underlying disease (bullous keratopathy) increase the risk of infectious keratitis. Meticulous care, limited wearing time, attention to preexisting problems (blepharitis), and maximizing fitting characteristics are keys to successful therapeutic contact lens wear.

Another circumstance in which prophylaxis might be considered is the continuous wearing of a hydrophilic contact lens on a normal eye. What happens if a drop of neomycin-polymixin B-gramicidin solution (Neosporin) is instilled four times daily for 3 months? Apparently nothing happens, except the development of bacterial resistance.[38] In this study 17 volunteers were fitted with a continuous-wear soft lens in only one eye. The Neosporin drops were randomly assigned to the eye with or without the contact lens. At the end of the 12-week period, the normal flora had not been displaced from any of the treated eyes, nor had secondary invaders appeared. With *S. epidermidis* used as an indicator, resistance appeared in 2 weeks in the treated eyes and in 4 weeks in the opposite, untreated eyes. Quite clearly prophylactic antibiotics are not indicated for routine use with continuous-wear cosmetic contact lenses.

### Orbital Fractures

Should prophylactic antibiotics be used in fractures that cause communications between the paranasal sinuses and the orbit or the intracranial cavity? Case reports suggest this,[39, 40] but adequate controls do not exist.

A rationale approach includes the use of a broad-spectrum oral antibiotic (e.g., a cephalosporin) and the avoidance of retrograde flow of material from the nares and sinuses to the orbit during "nose blowing."

### Foreign Body Management

How about management of intraocular foreign bodies with prophylactic antibiotics? Again, we do not have controlled series of cases and must rely on clinical prejudices. My personal prejudice is to treat vigorously and immediately every patient with an intraocular foreign body. Why? We know that intraocular infections do develop in some such cases, that the sight of the eye is almost invariably lost if an overt infection develops, and that antibiotic treatment will sterilize most such severely infected eyes (not fungus infections) even though sight is lost. I interpret these facts to indicate that early and vigorous treatment with intraocular, systemic, and topical antibiotics of an eye destined to be lost (if untreated) to a susceptible microorganism will prevent development of the infection and will save the eye. Vitreous and aqueous taps, followed by intraocular injection of gentamicin, clindamycin, and dexamethasone, have been recommended as prophylaxis in the case of an intraocular foreign body.[41] Not all injured eyes develop infection, and routine prophylaxis will certainly treat many patients who would have healed just as well without treatment. Unfortunately, there is no way to differentiate these patients before infection develops; hence, I treat them all.

Iatrogenic foreign bodies are often inserted at the time of retinal detachment surgery. If smooth, as in the case of silicon rubber, infection is unlikely. Silicone sponges, with thin multiple cavities, represent a much greater hazard of infection. Saturating such a sponge with antibiotic before implantation can reduce the incidence of infection to as low as 2% or 3%[42] compared with frequencies as high as 18%. However, the postoperative use of penicillin, 4 million units daily for 5 days, and topical antibiotics for 3 weeks did not further reduce the rate of infection.

## ALTERATION OF MICROFLORA

Proof of the inhibitory effect of one microorganism by another was provided by a study of 24,389 strains isolated from eye patients.[43] Forty-seven percent of the organisms provided antibiotics effective against the test organism *(Corynebacterium pseudodiphtheriticum)*. The frequency of this inhibitory ability indicates that elimination of one microorganism with antibiotic treatment may permit an overgrowth of other microorganisms.

Severely burned patients provide a dramatic illustration of microflora alteration.[44] Burn patients combine susceptibility to infection with antibiotic therapy. In a study of conjunctival skin flora of 53 severely burned patients, a dramatic change to gram-negative organisms occurred at about the fifth to sixth day. *Pseudomonas* was found in 34% of the eyes but remarkably caused no infection as long as the corneal epithelium was intact. Every effort must be made to protect against exposure keratopathy in such patients. Their hospital course is prolonged and difficult, and their attendants are not oriented toward the importance of eye care. As a consultant, the ophthalmologist must stress the absolute necessity of avoiding exposure keratopathy. Despite the prophylactic use of Neosporin ointment four times daily (or maybe because of it) in 16 eyes, *Pseudomonas* was cultured from 62% of these treated eyes. A false sense of security resulting from the knowledge of antibiotic "prophylaxis" is unwarranted and dangerous. Prophylactic antibiotic use should be avoided in these debilitated patients and reserved for use when active ocular infection is diagnosed. Otherwise, the topical antibiotic with its concomitant ocular toxicity will confuse the clinical picture and contribute to the development of resistance.

A report of an outbreak of methicillin-resistant *S. aureus* infections in a burn unit is an excellent example of the impact of resistant organisms on a hospital. This study, conducted from 1979 through 1981, showed the development of a serious endemic of resistant *S. aureus*.[45] The infection appeared to be transmitted to the burn unit via the plastic surgery service. During the subsequent 2 years colonization and infection rate with this tetracycline-resistant strain of methicillin-resistant *S. aureus* rose from 0.03% and 0.2% to 0.16% and 0.28% respectively. Hundreds of patients were colonized with this bacteria. By 1981, 53% of all *S. aureus* infections were caused by methicillin-resistant strains compared with a 16% rate in 1979. Twenty-four percent of 41 personnel caring for colonized or infected burn unit patients had transient carriage of methicillin-resistant *S. aureus* compared with only 7% of personnel caring for nonburn patients. This outbreak of infections required permanent closure of the burn unit, resulting in decreased incidents of methicillin-resistant *S. aureus* colonization and infection among nonburn unit patients. Burn units and intensive care units may serve as reservoirs for resistant organisms in a hospital. These organisms were most probably transferred into this unit through hospital personnel. The authors point out the importance of hand washing in preventing transmission of resistant organisms. Hand washing is the single most important procedure in reducing the incidence of nosocomial infections. In the United States, 1.5 million suffer from nosocomial infections. Care of these patients adds $1 billion to medical expenses. Even in the age of human immunodeficiency virus (HIV) infections and stringent Occupational Safety and Health Administration (OSHA) regulations, proper hand washing is not exercised in a consistent fashion in health care facilities.[45, 46]

## Fungus Overgrowth

Oral administration of the broad-spectrum antibiotics (notably the tetracyclines) significantly alters the normal intestinal microflora. A most common consequence is the uninhibited multiplication of the remaining resistant species, notably the yeasts, such as *Candida albicans*. Such infection usually remains confined to the intestinal tract but may rarely disseminate systemically.

Direct potentiation of fungi by antibiotics has been suspected but cannot be regarded as established. The concept of antibiotic potentiation of fungus growth is based on suggestive experimental work. In one such experiment, both corneas of 11 young rabbits were infected by intrastromal injection of *C. albicans*.[47] A 1% solution of oxytetracycline (Terramycin) was added to the inoculum of the right eyes, and the left eyes remained untreated as controls. Corneal perforation occurred in eight treated eyes and in one control eye. Although on first glance this 8:1 ratio appears to indicate fungus potentiation by antibiotics and has frequently been referred to as providing such proof, this is not necessarily the case. Intralamellar injection of tetracyclines is irritating, and this nonclinical method of application may have caused enough damage to the thin corneas of these young rabbits to account for the higher incidence of perforation. Furthermore, this experimental result was obtained only in infection with *C. albicans* and after treatment with oxytetracycline by intralamellar injection. Infection of adult rabbits with other types of fungi (including *Aspergillus*) treated with chlortetracycline (Aureomycin) showed no increased growth resulting from the presence of the antibiotic. These experiments, characterized by the author as "exploratory," certainly cannot be interpreted as a rational contraindication to the clinical use of antibiotics in ocular therapy.

The effect of chlortetracycline on fungus infections has been evaluated in mice infected with *C. albicans*.[48] Intraperitoneal injection of 2 mg of chlortetracycline in 17 mice and of 320 million *Candida* cells in 17 other mice resulted in no deaths. However, when 3 doses of chlortetracycline and *Candida* were combined and injected simultaneously, 16 of 17 mice died of *Candida* infection. In a variation of this experiment, incubation of *Candida* with chlortetracycline and subsequent washing away of the antibiotic did not enhance virulence. Inactivation of chlortetracycline solutions by boiling or by being allowed to stand at room temperature destroyed its fungus-enhancing properties. Chlortetracycline did not alter *Candida* growth in vivo.

This experiment indicates that chlortetracycline interferes, for at least 1 day, with the normal defense mechanisms of the animals studied. However, chlortetracycline given 8 to 24 hours after infection does not enhance *Candida* growth. Whether these experiments indicate that chlortetracycline is a biologic activator of fungus infections or simply damages resistance as a nonspecific irritant cannot be determined from the facts available.

A claim for possible neomycin potentiation of *Candida* keratitis was based on a study of seven rabbits, four of which were made somewhat worse with neomycin treatment, whereas three were not.[49] Such a finding is statistically insignificant, and it remains to be confirmed that antibiotics potentiate the ocular growth of the fungi commonly encountered in mycotic keratitis.[50] Furthermore, a high proportion of corneal infections are caused by bacteria and a very small proportion by fungi. To withhold antibiotic therapy in a patient with a corneal infection of unknown cause would not be clinically prudent.

Is fungus growth potentiated by topical antibiotic therapy in clinical practice? Fungus cultures were taken twice, at intervals of 3 to 6 weeks, from the eyes of 245 Indian children.[51] Of these children, 102 had trachoma and were treated with topical erythromycin or tetracycline ointments or with parenteral triple sulfonamides. Negative fungus cultures were obtained both before and after treatment in 70% of the antibiotic-treated patients and in 61% of the nontrachomatous, untreated controls. In 30% of the treated patients, the initial tests were fungus negative but became fungus positive after antibiotic treatment. However, an even higher proportion of untreated patients, 39%, developed ocular fungus contamination during the same period. Hence, this study fails to show any potentiation of ocular fungus infection by antibiotic therapy.

Although many of these Indian children had fungi on their lids or conjunctivae, in only 7 of the 245 children was the same type of fungus found at both sites. This indicates that fungal contamination of the extraocular tissues is transient and presumably of environmental origin, in contrast to the true carrier state of infection characteristic of bacteria.

## ADVERSE RESPONSES

The effect of topical antibiotics on the healing of corneal epithelial wounds is of obvious practical importance, because these drugs are commonly used in the prophylactic treatment of eyes with epithelial defects. Even the preservatives in the antibiotic formulation can affect epithelial healing. Slight delays in corneal healing occur even with artificial tears containing polyvinyl alcohol, povidone, and chlorobutanol. In the absence of the masking effects of preservatives, significant delays in healing occurred with fortified gentamicin (10 mg/ml), neomycin (8 mg/ml), and bacitracin (10,000 units/ml) but not with the lower doses that are commercially available.[52, 53] Dose-related metabolic depression and microvillus loss and blunting have been reported with the aminoglycoside antibiotics.[54]

The relative safety with which antibiotics can be prescribed for adults apparently does not extend to treatment of the infant or unborn fetus. As examples, colistimethate sodium causes abnormalities of infantile renal tubular cells, the eighth nerve of the newborn is particularly sensitive to streptomycin, tetracycline may cause pseudotumor cerebri and dental defects, pyrimethamine damages cerebral development, novobiocin increases the chance of developing kernicterus, and chloramphenicol may kill a newborn child. Obviously this means that the ophthalmologist should use systemic antibiotics in the treatment of pregnant women or of infants only when clearly required[55] and with the consultation of the primary care physician.

The usual treatment of intraocular infection consists of intensive use of intraocular as well as systemic and topical routes of antibiotic administration. Intra-

**TABLE 6–3.**
Amount of Antibiotic Tolerated on Injection into Anterior Chamber

| Agent | Dosage |
|---|---|
| Amikacin | 0.25 mg |
| Bacitracin | 500–1,000 units |
| Chloramphenicol | 1–2 mg |
| Clindamycin | 1.0 mg |
| Colistin | 0.1 mg |
| Erythromycin | 1–2 mg |
| Neomycin | 2.5 |
| Penicillin G | 1,000–4,000 units |
| Methicillin | 1 mg |
| Polymyxin B | 0.1 mg |
| Streptomycin | 0.5–5 mg |
| Tetracycline | 2.5–5 mg |
| Tobramycin | 0.5 mg |

Adapted from Leopold IH: *Invest Ophthalmol* 3:504, 1964; and Strainer GA, Peymar GA, Meisels M, and others: *Ann Ophthalmol* 9:615, 1977

cameral injection of antibiotics may lead to operative complications and drug irritation but has the advantage of rapidly achieving a very high intraocular antibiotic concentration. The risks and benefits of such injection must be weighed in each case. Presumably intracameral antibiotic injection would be particularly suitable to the treatment of infected conditions that necessitate surgery (e.g., closure of a ruptured operative wound or repair of a contaminated laceration). Antibiotic dosages tolerated in the anterior chamber are listed in Table 6–3.

Irrigation of the anterior chamber with an excessive amount of antibiotic, even penicillin, can destroy the endothelium, result in dense corneal opacity, produce destructive iritis with neovascularization, and induce cataract. Be reasonably certain that the alternative is worse than taking the risk of injecting any type of antibiotic into the anterior chamber. Most of the eyes that exhibit alarming redness and flare during the first few days after cataract surgery will do very well without any additional surgical ventures and certainly do not warrant prophylactic intracameral injections. If endophthalmitis is clearly present, aqueous and vitreous taps for cultures should be followed by intravitreal antibiotic injection (Table 6–4).

**TABLE 6–4.**
Maximum Tolerated Intravitreal Antibiotics

| | Intravitreal Injection (mg) | Intravitreal Infusion (μg/ml) |
|---|---|---|
| Amikacin | 0.4 | 10.0 |
| Gentamicin | 0.4 | 8.0 |
| Tobramycin | 0.4 | 10.0 |
| Clindamycin | 1.0 | 9.0 |
| Cefazolin[167] | 2.25 | — |
| Cephaloridine | 0.25 | — |
| Moxalactam | 1.0 | — |
| Vancomycin | 1.0 | — |
| Chloramphenicol | 2.0 | 10 |
| Imipenem[176] | — | 16 |

From Peyman GA, Schulman JA: *Jpn J Ophthalmol* 33:392, 1989.

## SERUM CONCENTRATIONS

Obviously a pharmacokinetic relationship must exist between the dose of an antibiotic given, the route of administration, the entry and retention of drug within the eye, and time. A detailed compilation of the serum levels achieved by various antibiotics and dosages has been prepared.[56] Reproduction of pages of these data is of little practical value to the ophthalmologist, but a generalization may be helpful. After 1 hour, 1 ml of serum will contain perhaps 1/10,000 of the antibiotic dose. For example, 1 hour after 2 g of carbenicillin was given intravenously, a serum concentration was 100 μg/ml.

## TOXIC CONJUNCTIVITIS

Not uncommonly chronic keratoconjunctivitis will develop after topical antibiotic treatment of a surface ocular infection. Although it is caused by the antibiotic, this inflammation is often misinterpreted as being a continuing infection. Neomycin is a particularly frequent cause of allergic reactions, as is the preservative thimerosal. Such a toxic keratoconjunctivitis may gradually become more severe during prolonged treatment. When this diagnosis is suspected, all medications should be discontinued and treatment limited to cold compresses. Often it will be difficult to convince these patients that treatment should be stopped, particularly because a latent period of some days may precede improvement. Conjunctival scrapings of toxic keratoconjunctivitis characteristically show mononuclear cells with typical basophilic granules.[57]

## MECHANISMS OF ACTION

Antibacterial drugs are historically designated as either bacteriostatic or bactericidal. This is inexact and dependent on the concentration of drug present. Many otherwise bacteriostatic drugs will become bactericidal when used in high concentrations as may occur with ophthalmic topical application. Bacteriostatic drugs are erythromycin, tetracycline, chloramphenicol, and sulfonamides. Bactericidal agents are aminoglycosides, penicillins, and cephalosporins (Table 6–5).

Penicillins act through inhibition of peptidoglycan (mucopeptide) synthesis in the bacterial cell wall. Penicillins bind to target enzymes in the cell wall called penicillin-binding proteins (PBPs), which vary among bacterial species, accounting for a different spectrum of activity that cannot be predicted on the basis of β-lactamase production. Cephalosporins, imipenem, bacitracin, and vancomycin act through similar mechanisms. Polymyxin B and gramicidin affect the bacterial osmotic barrier through a detergent-like action.

**TABLE 6–5.**
Mechanisms of Action

Cell wall function
- Inhibition of peptidoglycan synthesis
  - Penicillins
  - Bacitracin
  - Cephalosporins
  - Vancomycin
  - Imipenem
- Alteration of the osmotic barrier
  - Aminoglycosides
  - Tetracyclines
  - Erythromycin
  - Clindamycin
  - Chloramphenicol

Inhibition of nucleic acid synthesis
- Sulfonamides
- Trimethoprim
- Pyrimethamine
- Rifampin

Aminoglycosides are examples of action through inhibition of bacterial protein synthesis. Aminoglycosides *irreversibly* bind to the 30-S ribosomal subunit. They are bactericidal to susceptible bacteria. Chloramphenicol, erythromycin, and clindamycin bind to the 50-S ribosomal subunit. Tetracyclines *reversibly* bind to the 30-S ribosomal subunit.

Sulfonamides interfere with the biosynthesis of the reduced form of folic acid (tetrahydrofolic acid) through interference with the utilization of *p*-aminobenzoic acid (PABA). Later stages of folic acid synthesis are inhibited by pyrimethamine and trimethoprim, which therefore act synergistically with sulfonamides.[58]

## MECHANISMS OF RESISTANCE

Bacteria may produce enzymes that destroy the antimicrobial drug. β-Lactamases are best known enzymes in this category. β-Lactamases are produced by a wide variety of organisms and affect a large spectrum of penicillin-like drugs. Penicillinase-resistant analogs have been created to overcome this form of resistance. Enzymatic resistance to other antimicrobials, including chloramphenicol and the aminoglycosides, has occurred. Bacterial resistance via enzymatic production may be transferred between organisms through plasmids (extrachromosomal DNA).

Absence of target enzymes in the cell wall will cause relative resistance to penicillins, whereas the lack of binding sites on the ribosomes induces resistance to aminoglycosides, erythromycin, and clindamycin. Permeability changes in the bacterial cell wall are yet another mechanism of resistance preventing buildup of bactericidal concentrations of antibiotics within the bacteria.

The development of antibiotic resistance with ophthalmic antimicrobial drug use is not well understood. Assuming that the enormous volume of topical antimicrobials in use have a commensurate impact, it is rational to follow these principles to limit the development of resistance. First, limit antimicrobial use to diagnosed infections caused by susceptible organisms. For instance, it is unnecessary to use a broad-spectrum antibiotic in the treatment of a viral conjunctivitis. Second, avoid chronic use of antibiotics. Third, use newer antibiotics only when necessary for treatment of infection resistant to traditional therapy. Finally, completely treat all clinical infections and consider using a second agent to prevent emergence of resistant organisms.

## SPECIFIC AGENTS

### Aminoglycosides

Aminoglycosides are one of the most commonly used group of antibiotic drugs in ophthalmic practice. They comprise a group of antibiotics and semisynthetic antibiotic derivatives, including streptomycin, amikacin, gentamicin, kanamycin, neomycin, netilmicin, paromomycin, and tobramycin. They contain one or two amino sugars glycosidically linked to an aminocyclitol. Aminoglycosides bind irreversibly to the 30-S ribosomal subunit inhibiting protein synthesis in susceptible bacteria, resulting in a bactericidal action. They are active against aerobic gram-negative and some gram-positive bacteria. They are inactive against anaerobic bacteria. Amikacin, gentamicin, netilmicin, and tobramycin are active against most strains of *P. aeruginosa,* whereas kanamycin, neomycin, paromomycin and streptomycin are generally inactive against this organism. Amikacin has a slightly broader antimicrobial spectrum against some aerobic gram-negative bacteria than either gentamicin or tobramycin. However, there are some amikacin-resistant strains of bacteria that are susceptible to gentamicin, tobramycin, or both. Aminoglycosides have little activity against *Streptococcus* but are active against many strains of *S. aureus* and *S. epidermidis.* Resistance may be conveyed to a bacteria to modify the drug enzymatically. Amikacin is resistant to many of these aminoglycoside-modifying enzymes. Resistance may also occur because of decreased permeability of the bacterial cell wall or alterations in the ribosomal binding site. This type of resistance is effective against all aminoglycosides and is fortunately rare. Streptomycin is active against *Microbacterium tuberculous, Microbacterium marinum,* and some strains of *Microbacterium kansasii, Microbacterium intracellulare,* and *Microbacterium avium.* Ototoxicity and renal toxicity are the most serious adverse reactions to aminoglycoside therapy. Renal toxicity is more likely in dehydrated patients or patients with preexisting renal failure. Risks of toxicity increase with duration of therapy and in the elderly. Ototoxicity occurs by damage of the eighth cranial nerve and may include both auditory and vestibular symptoms. Renal toxicity is usually reversible on discontinuation of the drug, but uremic death may rarely occur. Aminoglycosides can produce neuromuscular blockade, causing peripheral neuropathy or encephalopathy, including numbness, paresthesias, seizures, and myasthenia gravis–like syndromes. Optic neuritis has been reported with aminoglycoside use.

Antibacterial activity of aminoglycosides may be additive or synergistic with β-lactam antibiotics and vancomycin. It appears that penicillin, by inhibiting bacterial cell wall synthesis, allows the aminoglycosides to have greater access to the ribosomal binding site. Penicillins have been shown to inactivate aminoglycosides in vitro and may result in falsely low aminoglycoside concentrations on serum assays. Tobramycin is the most susceptible to in vitro inactivation by β-lactam antibiotics. Penicillinase may be added to serum before the drug assay to correct for this effect.[59]

### Amikacin

Gentamicin, tobramycin, and kanamycin may be inactivated by at least nine distinct bacteria-produced enzymes, the presence of which confers resistance on the organism. Amikacin is acetylated kanamycin. This semisynthetic additive prevents enzymatic destruction except by the acetyltransferase bacterial enzyme. In a challenge against 319 resistant bacterial strains, amikacin was effective against 80% compared with 40% for tobramycin, 30% for gentamicin, and 11% for kanamycin. These percentages illustrate that cross-resistance to aminoglycosides commonly occurs and is found especially in *Pseudomonas* species.

Amikacin was used intravenously in patients receiving systemic cancer therapy who were granulocytopenic. This was reported in 315 patients treated in a 13-month period from 1979 through 1980. Resistance of gram-negative bacteria to amikacin and gentamicin dropped during the course of the study. Amikacin resistance dropped from 1.8% of organisms in 1970 to 0.3% in 1982. Organisms resistant to gentamicin only dropped from 5.4% in 1977 to 1.2% in 1982, and organisms resistant to both amikacin and gentamicin dropped from 3.6% to 2.5%. This study does indicate that decrease in the use of gentamicin over time also decreased the instance of resistant organisms. Resistant organisms, however, were not found to develop against amikacin during the short period of this study. Ongoing surveillance for the development of resistant organisms in a hospital setting is obviously necessary to allow proper antibiotic selection in very ill patients, as reported in this study.[60]

Amikacin is ineffective orally and is given intravenously or intramuscularly in adults in a dosage of 15 mg/kg daily in divided doses every 8 to 12 hours. Doses should be adjusted in renal failure. Peak blood levels reach 18 to 25 μg/ml in ½ to 1 hour. The plasma half-life is 2 hours. After 8 hours, levels may fall to less than 2 μg/ml. More than 90% of sensitive microorganisms are inhibited by 2 to 4 μg/ml. Aqueous humor concentrations of amikacin were measured after a single intramuscular injection of 7.5 mg/kg given before cataract surgery. Aqueous humor concentrations ranged from 0.15 to 3.10 mg/L, with an average value of 1 mg/L between 2 and 10 hours after injection. This level is approximately that which should be bactericidal for many bacteria. The systemic administration of this drug, however, does not seem to offer any distinct advantages over prophylaxis with subconjunctival aminoglycosides, such as gentamicin or tobramycin. The subconjunctival delivery gives bactericidal anterior chamber concentrations without subjecting the patient to systemic toxicity.[61] Even lower levels are found in the tears after intravenous administration of gentamicin, tobramycin, amikacin, and netilmicin. Mean peak of two concentrations after intravenous administration were not in the range of the minimum inhibitory concentrations for *Pseudomonas,* and this mode of treatment would certainly not be recommended in the treatment of routine bacterial keratitis.[62] Indeed, aminoglycosides in the tear film seem to inhibit the body's natural protective mechanism furnished by lysozyme.[63]

Within 24 hours 98% of a dose of amikacin is excreted unchanged in the urine. In the presence of renal failure, retention of amikacin leads to excessively high drug levels and serious toxicity, including additional nephrotoxicity. As with all aminoglycosides, renal and ototoxicities are major hazards. In one series, three of 15 patients suffered hearing loss.[64] Patients receiving aminoglycosides should be questioned daily about hearing loss, tinnitus, fullness in the ears, vertigo, and unsteadiness.

Penicillin derivatives and aminoglycosides act synergistically; therefore, carbenicillin and amikacin, for instance, may be combined in the treatment of resistant gram-negative organisms. Do not mix the two drugs in a common injection, because this may physically inactivate the aminoglycoside. This physical inactivation may also contribute to artificially low measured serum levels of aminoglycosides. Penicillinase should be added to the serum before measurement of aminoglycoside levels if a penicillin derivative is given concurrently.

Simultaneous use of different aminoglycosides causes additive toxicity, as also occurs in combination with colistin, vancomycin, streptomycin, or diuretics, such as furosemide and ethacrynic acid.

Although amikacin is the aminoglycoside least frequently inactivated by bacterial enzymes, principles of good antibiotic usage indicate primary usage of gentamicin, next tobramycin, and last amikacin to reduce the rate of development of resistant organisms. None of these valuable and toxic drugs should be used except when clearly indicated by the severity and danger of an infection caused by susceptible gram-negative organisms.[65]

Ophthalmic use of amikacin includes its use as an intravitreal antibiotic for the treatment of postoperative bacterial endophthalmitis. Intravitreal amikacin use is recommended in combination with vancomycin or a cephalosporin. We rationalize its use over that of gentamicin and tobramycin because of the possibility of the presence of a resistant organism, which, if not covered, could destroy the eye before cultures and antibiotic sensitivities were available. Intravitreal concentration of 400 μg in 0.10 ml of solution has been recommended. This has been shown to be nontoxic to the retina. Retinal toxicity is found with a dose of 1,500 μg of amikacin compared with only 400 μg of gentamicin or 800 μg of tobramycin. Therefore, in the case of severe sight-threatening endophthalmitis, amikacin offers a broader spectrum of action along with lower toxicity.[66, 67] Reinjection of intravitreal antibiotic at 48-hour intervals did show an increase in toxicity. However, even in these cases, amikacin appeared to be less toxic than similarly administered gentamicin or tobramycin.[68]

Topical use of amikacin in the treatment of bacterial keratitis should be limited to culture-proven organisms resistant to gentamicin or tobramycin. The recommended dose of amikacin is 10 to 50 mg/ml compared with 8 to 20 mg/ml of gentamicin and tobramycin.[69] Corneal epithelial toxicity to this dosage is similar to that, as measured by metabolic and morphologic means, found with tobramycin. Both of these show less toxicity than that found after topical application of gentamicin.[54]

### Gentamicin

Gentamicin is obtained from cultures of *Micromonospora purpura*. Its mechanism of action is similar to the other aminoglycosides and seems to convey bactericidal activity via inhibition of protein synthesis through binding of the 30-S subunit of the ribosomal protein. The recommended systemic dose is 3 mg/kg/day in divided doses at 8-hour intervals, given intramuscularly or intravenously. This dose may be increased to 5 mg/kg/day in life-threatening infections and raised to 6 to 7.5 mg/kg/day in children and 7.5 mg/kg for infants given intravenously. This recommended dose should be altered after obtaining serum levels of the drug. As with all aminoglycosides, the drug is nephrotoxic, and renal function should be monitored during usage. Dosage in patients with renal failure should be decreased appropriately. Gentamicin is very active against many aerobic gram-negative rod-shaped organisms. Diffusion of gentamicin through tissue may be limited because of its positive charge. Therefore, gentamicin and other aminoglycosides may be inactivated by such negatively charged polymers as heparin. They are inactive against anaerobes that lack oxidative phosphorylation and an active transport system, which is necessary for the aminoglycoside to penetrate into the bacteria. Resistance to gentamicin is produced by the presence of inactivating or modifying enzymes. This may be plasmid mediated. A second type of resistance involves a decrease in the active transport system for the drug. This type of resistance affects all aminoglycosides nonspecifically. Fortunately, this type of resistance is rare. At Ohio State University, 77% of *P. aeruginosa* is sensitive to gentamicin compared with 96% sensitivity to tobramycin and amikacin. Gram-positive effectiveness of gentamicin is variable, with 91% of *S aureus* organisms sensitive compared with only 52% of *S. epidermidis* organisms.[70] Multiple-drug therapy, combining an aminoglycoside with a penicillin derivative or a cephalosporin, is often recommended to prevent the emergence of resistant organisms. Synergism between β-lactam antibiotics and aminoglycosides has been demonstrated in the laboratory, and this translates into clinical benefit by allowing greater penetration of the aminoglycoside into the bacteria.[71]

#### *Prophylactic Treatment Before Ocular Surgery*

A large volume of data concerns the use of gentamicin as prophylaxis before eye surgery.[10] Gentamicin was compared with chloramphenicol in 40 consecutive patients undergoing cataract surgery. Five drops of antibiotic were given over 4 minutes between pretreatment and posttreatment conjunctival cultures. Complete elimination of bacteria was achieved in 68.75% of the cases by use of gentamicin compared with only 25% with chloramphenicol use.[72] Other studies comparing gentamicin with sulfacetamide, neomycin-polymyxin B–gramicidin solution, oxytetracycline, and polymixin β–bacitracin-neomycin ointment, show that gentamicin is consistently more effective at decreasing bacterial counts and eliminating bacteria from the eye before surgery.[73, 74]

### *Ocular Penetration*

Whether instilled topically as drops or ointment or given intramuscularly, gentamicin penetrates very poorly into normal rabbit eyes. Aqueous levels as high as 0.8 μg/ml may be achieved by subconjunctival injection of 0.5 ml of 0.3% gentamicin solution. Aqueous levels as high as 1.6 μg/ml may be achieved in mechanically abraded or chemically burned rabbit eyes by topical instillation of a 0.3% solution or ointment.[75] No measurable vitreous levels of gentamicin were achieved in any of the eyes. Of 53 strains of *Pseudomonas,* 45 were inhibited by 1.6 μg/ml of gentamicin. This concentration will also inhibit growth of many penicillin-resistant staphylococci. Topical concentrations will greatly exceed this level on the ocular surface with 0.3% solution, whereas fortified concentrations may be necessary to achieve therapeutic levels consistently in the anterior chamber. Gentamicin should therefore be a useful drug for treatment of anterior segment infections caused by *Pseudomonas* or *Staphylococcus.* Do not expect any vitreous penetration from topical or subconjunctival gentamicin.

The diffusion of a compound from the serum into the aqueous humor is inversely proportional to its insolubility in lipid, its degree of protein binding, and its molecular weight. Gentamicin is relatively insoluble in lipids, is 25% to 30% protein bound, and has an intermediate molecular weight of 425 daltons; hence, it would be expected to meet considerable resistance at the blood-eye barriers. In rabbits, subconjunctival injection of 4 mg of gentamicin produced average primary aqueous levels of 3 μg/ml lasting for several hours. Increasing the subconjunctival dose to 10 mg (in 0.5-ml volumes) raised the aqueous level to 4 μg/ml. In secondary aqueous, gentamicin levels were about twice as high as in the primary aqueous and approximated ½,₀₀₀ of the concentration in the subconjunctival space. The aqueous levels achieved by subconjunctival injection were sufficient to inhibit sensitive gram-negative microorganisms.[76]

Diffusion into other ocular tissues has also been evaluated. One hour after subconjunctival injection of 20 mg of gentamicin in the rabbit eye, the following levels (in micrograms per milliliter) were achieved: aqueous, 12; vitreous, 1.3; cornea, 11.5; iris, 6.5; lens, 0.5; retina, 12; sclera, 74; and conjunctiva, 185. Levels of 0.2 to 0.6 μg/ml persisted at 24 hours. Much greater levels were achieved in an inflamed eye, for example, 20 μg/ml in the retina at 1 hour.[77]

In rabbit eyes inflamed by experimentally induced *Pseudomonas* corneal ulcers, very high aqueous levels of gentamicin can be achieved simply by topical instillation. Use of 4 drops of 2% gentamicin solution every 15 minutes gave aqueous levels averaging 9.5 μg/ml at 30 minutes and 32μg/ml at 1 hour.[78] (Four drops of 2% solution contain 5 mg of drug. If given every 15 minutes, 80 mg is administered in 4 hours. The allowable daily dose of gentamicin is 1 mg/kg. Toxic systemic levels could be approached by generous topical instillations of gentamicin.)

Inundation of the eye with gentamicin by combined intramuscular, subconjunctival, and topical routes resulted in rabbit posterior vitreous gentamicin concentrations as high as 4 μg/ml in phakic, uninfected eyes.[79] These levels were much higher than those resulting from any of the routes used alone. The clinical implication is that endophthalmitis should be treated by all three routes to maximize antibiotic entry to the posterior vitreous. The highest vitreous levels are obtained by direct intravitreal injection.

Before cataract surgery, 15 patients received subconjunctival injection of 10 mg of gentamicin in 0.25-ml volumes. Aqueous drug levels were determined at varying time intervals and ranged from 2 to 7 μg/ml at 1 hour and from 1 to 9 μg/ml at 2½ hours.[80]

The question of the efficacy of postcataract extraction prophylaxis by the subconjunctival injection of 20 mg of gentamicin immediately after surgery was evaluated by a series of experiments in 57 rabbits.[81] One-hour aqueous levels up to 100 μg/ml were attained, remaining at 20 μg/ml at 4 hours. An interesting indication of the systemic absorption of this subconjunctival dose was the attainment of 1 μg/ml of gentamicin in the aqueous of the *opposite* eye. Introduction of 5,000 *S. aureus* organisms into the gentamicin-treated operated eyes resulted in no infections, although this inoculum resulted in a 90% infection rate in eyes not receiving prophylactic gentamicin. Inocula of 10,000 to 19 million *S. epidermidis* organisms resulted in clinically recognizable infection in only five of 32 eyes, even without antibiotic therapy. In only three eyes could this organism be recovered by paracentesis and only on the first postoperative day. (Perhaps this explains the appearance of a mildly inflamed eye after human cataract surgery.)

### *Intravitreal Use*

Intravitreal antibiotics represent the most effective way of treating endophthalmitis caused by susceptible bacteria. Other routes of administration achieve only minimal intravitreal levels of antibiotic. A representative study inoculated the vitreous with approximately 1,000 *Pseudomonas* organisms in both eyes of 17 rabbits.[82] All rabbits were treated for 5 days with intramuscular gentamicin 5 mg/kg/day in three divided doses. The control left eyes received no other treatment, and all were destroyed by the infection. The usual course was redness of the eye by 3 hours, vitreous haze by 6 hours, corneal haze by 24 hours, massive fibrinous exudate by 48 hours, and complete opacity with secondary glaucoma by 72 hours. The contralateral eyes, treated 6 hours after infection with intravitreal gentamicin in doses of 500, 250, or 125 μg, were free of inflammation and appeared grossly normal at 72 hours. Only one injection was given. The half-life of intravitreal gentamicin in phakic rabbit eyes was found to be 32

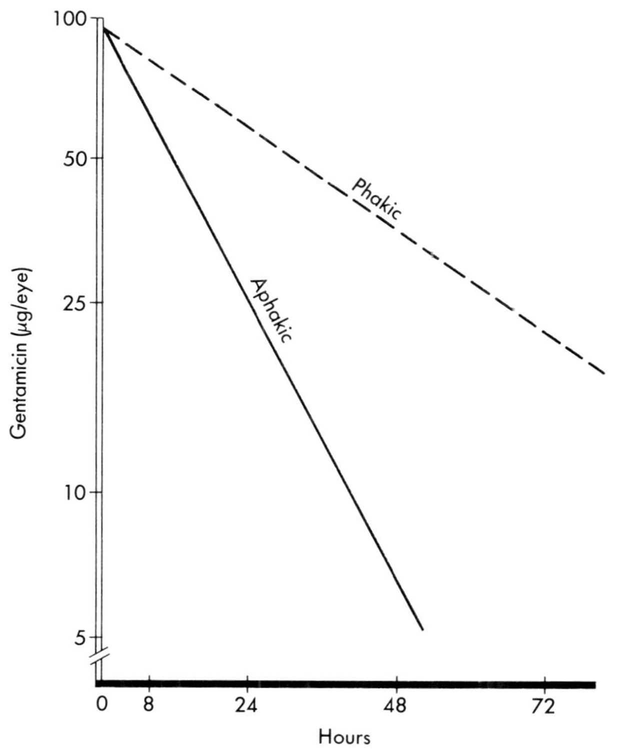


**FIG 6–4.**

Clearance rate of 100 mg of intravitreal gentamicin from phakic and aphakic eyes. (Modified from Cobo LM, Forster RK: *Am J Ophthalmol* 92:59, 1981. Used by permission.)

hours, compared with only 12 hours in aphakic eyes (Fig. 6–4).[83] The half-life decreased with inflammation down to 19 hours in phakic and 14 hours in aphakic eyes. In most cases of bacterial endophthalmitis, a single injection of antibiotic is sufficient to sterilize the eye; however, in persistent infections, reinjection may be appropriate in 48 hours. Initial culturing is vitally important in these persistent cases to modify the antibiotic regimen for the second dose.

### *Topical Use*

Topical gentamicin is clinically effective in the treatment of many external eye infections. In a series of 101 patients, all but one were clinically cured from their external eye infection after 1 to 2 weeks of treatment with gentamicin. Thirty percent of the patients had persistent bacterial flora, indicating that complete bacterial eradication is not clinically necessary or realistic. Currently, commercially available topical gentamicin sulfate is in a concentration of 3 mg/ml. Fortified doses can be formulated from the intravenous preparation in doses of 8 to 20 mg/ml. These high doses of gentamicin are toxic to the corneal epithelium, delay corneal epithelial healing, and should be reserved for sight-threatening eye infections with susceptible organisms. Fortified gentamicin or tobramycin in combination with a cephalosporin or vancomycin are recommended as the initial empiric treatment of bacterial corneal ulcers after culturing is performed. Initial treatment includes multiple dosing every 5 minutes during the first 30 minutes and then application every 30 to 60 minutes. Fortified gentamicin ointment showed comparable reduction in colony counts in an animal model of *Pseudomonas* keratitis compared with gentamicin solution. Ophthalmic ointments are thought to be less effective than solutions from a theoretical standpoint because of binding of the drug to the ointment vehicle, decreasing the available antibiotic. Use of fortified ointments may allow extended dosing intervals and improved compliance.[84] Corneal levels of gentamicin associated with topical and systemic administration were determined in patients undergoing penetrating keratoplasty. They were given either fortified gentamicin (13.6 mg/ml) or 1 mg of gentamicin/kg intramuscularly in four separate injections every 8 hours before surgery. With topical administration, corneal gentamicin levels averaged 16.2 μg/g, and aqueous levels were 0.3 μg/ml. Corneal and aqueous levels with parenteral administration were 6.1 μg/g and 0.4 μg/ml, respectively. Parenteral antibiotics are a poor choice for the treatment of a corneal infection because topical antibiotics may achieve high tissue levels without the risk of systemic adverse reactions associated with parenteral administration.[85]

Hydrophilic contact lenses and collagen shields may be used to modify drug delivery in corneal ulcers. The amount of drug delivered by hydrogel lenses is dependent on the initial concentration of the soaking solution and also the water content and thickness of the lens. Thicker, higher water content lenses will deliver more drug than thinner, lower water content lenses.[86] High antibiotic levels with constant exposure may lead to increased corneal epithelial toxicity.

Transscleral iontophoresis of gentamicin performed in monkeys produced therapeutic vitreal levels. Iontophoresis was performed in monkeys over a 2-week period. Five treatments were given over this period. The vitreal level averaged 28 μg/ml after the first treatment and 12 μg/ml after the fifth treatment. Retinal and pars plana burns over the area where the electrode was applied were found to be the only adverse reactions of the treatment. This treatment may offer a less invasive alternative to introduce intravitreal antibiotics compared with the currently accepted injection method.[86a]

### *Toxicity*

Toxicity of aminoglycoside antibiotics can occur near their therapeutic range. Although a number of systemic dosing methods have been developed to initiate therapy, there is a wide interpatient variability in final serum concentrations after standard dosage with aminoglycosides in patients with similar renal function. Most probably this is because of variable tissue retention of the aminoglycoside. Peak and trough serum concentrations are necessary to adjust systemic dosage. Nephrotoxicity and ototoxicity are the most serious side effects of aminoglycosides. These happen more commonly in the elderly, dehydrated patients with renal impairment, and patients receiving high doses over long periods. Both auditory and vestibular symptoms may occur with aminoglycoside ototoxicity. The vestibular symptoms are more common with streptomycin, gentamicin, and tobramycin, whereas auditory symptoms are more often associated with amikacin, kanamycin, neomycin, and paromomycin. Gentamicin accumulates selectively within lysosomes and causes a reduction of sphingomyelinase activity. As a result, phospholipid storage occurs within the cells in the form of concentric, lamellar structures, similar to the whirl inclusions of Niemann-Pick disease. Nephrotoxicity includes tubular necrosis, increase in blood urea nitrogen (BUN) and serum creatinine levels, and decreases in urine specific gravity and creatinine clearance. Proteinuria and metabolic acidosis may also occur. Aminoglycosides may produce neuromuscular blockade, resulting in respiratory paralysis or a myasthenia gravis type of syndrome. Peripheral neuropathy and encephalopathy may occur. Pupillary mydriasis and conjunctival paresthesias have been reported after topical and subconjunctival use of gentamicin.[87] A causal relationship between these symptoms and the medication could not be directly ascertained with the mydriasis; however, in the patient with conjunctival paresthesias, the symptoms were relieved after discontinuation of the drops and reappeared again when the eye drops were readministered. No such symptoms developed when the medication was changed to chloramphenicol eye drops.[87]

The corneal and conjunctival epithelium can show characteristic concentric lamellar structures associated with gentamicin use because of accumulation of the drug in lysosomes, causing phospholipid storage. These changes do not seem to have clinical significance. Topical gentamicin does cause corneal epithelial wound healing delays. Commercially available gentamicin (3 mg/ml) did not significantly retard normal epithelial wound healing in the rabbit, but higher doses (10 mg/ml) did. Reductions in oxygen uptake indicative of metabolic depression and changes in the corneal epithelial microvilli can be demonstrated with single and multiple dosing of aminoglycosides. Gentamicin causes greater changes in microvilli than similar doses of tobramycin.[52–54] Obviously the lowest possible concentration of antibiotic used at low frequency is desirable when an infection is treated. It must be remembered, though, that using minimal doses of antibiotics may suppress the infection without totally clearing it, leading to a confusing clinical picture.

***Summary***

Gentamicin is highly effective against many gram-negative organisms, as well as some resistant staphylococci. It has a narrow therapeutic range; therefore, monitoring of serum levels is essential with parenteral use. It is a first-line aminoglycoside for treatment of serious systemic infections. Gentamicin has a well-documented ability to decrease bacterial colony counts of the eye before ocular surgery. Because of its poorer gram-positive coverage and possibility of the development of resistant organisms, it is not indicated in the treatment of routine bacterial conjunctivitis. Other antibiotics that do not have such important systemic indications should be the first-line treatment of such routine infections.

## Neomycin

Neomycin is an aminoglycoside antibiotic obtained from *Streptomyces fradiae*. It is a complex of neamine and neomycin B and C. The commercially available drug is the sulfated form of neomycin B. Its antibacterial spectrum is broader than that of bacitracin, penicillin, or streptomycin. The drug is very stable at room temperature and is not inactivated by body fluids.

Neomycin is used clinically either orally or topically. Intramuscular and intravenous use are contraindicated because of nephrotoxicity and ototoxicity. Approximately 3% of an oral dose is absorbed from the normal gastrointestinal (GI) tract; however, increased absorption may occur with abnormal GI motility. It may be given as a retention enema in patients who cannot take oral medication. It is indicated in the treatment of hepatic encephalopathy and preoperative intestinal antisepsis. It is also useful in the treatment of diarrhea caused by *Escherichia coli.*

Its ophthalmic use is primarily in combination with other medications as a topical antibiotic. It is used in combination with polymyxin B and gramicidin as a broad-spectrum antibacterial combination solution. Its spectrum encompasses most causes of bacterial eye infections. Neomycin is bactericidal for many gram-positive and gram-negative organisms. Neomycin is used in combination with polymyxin B and bacitracin as an ointment.

The question has been raised as to whether neomycin causes allergy with undue frequency. It was rated among the top ten sensitizers in dermatology clinics in 1972. However, in a study of 2,175 young adults, skin patch testing showed only two to be allergic to neomycin.[88] Of 98 children with chronic dermatitis, patch testing showed only one to be allergic to neomycin. Patients who use a combination antibiotic containing neomycin for long periods for treatment of chronic infections will frequently develop an allergic reaction. Long-term use of any antibiotic is usually not recommended and may result in colonization with resistant microorganisms.

### Streptomycin

Streptomycin is obtained from cultures of *Streptomyces griseus.* Because of its limited bacterial spectrum when compared with other aminoglycosides, its use in bacterial infections has largely been supplanted by gentamicin, tobramycin, and amikacin. Streptomycin is used in combination with at least one other agent in the treatment of tuberculosis. It may also be used in the treatment of tularemia, plague, brucellosis, glanders, lymphogrannuloma inguinale, and chancroid. Prolonged peaks in serum concentrations of streptomycin greater than 40 μg/ml may be associated with increased risk of ototoxicity and nephrotoxicity. Aminoglycosides should be used with caution in patients with myasthenia gravis, Parkinson's syndrome, or other neuromuscular disorders. These drugs may aggravate muscular weakness due to neuromuscular blockade and cause respiratory paralysis. This effect can occur even in people handling the drug, and proper precautions should be taken. Streptomycin should not be given alone in the treatment of tuberculosis. It is usually used for only the first few months of therapy until the bacteriologic studies become negative. The other agents used in the combination treatment are continued for a full year. Streptomycin is given in a dosage of 15 mg/kg/day in adults being treated for tuberculosis. Smaller doses should be given in geriatric patients or patients with renal failure or eighth cranial nerve abnormalities.

### Tobramycin

Tobramycin is obtained from cultures of *Streptomyces tenebrarius.* Like other aminoglycosides, it is bactericidal through inhibition of protein synthesis and susceptible bacteria because of binding of the 30-S subunit of the ribosome. Its bacterial spectrum is similar to gentamicin. It is active against 96% of *P. aeruginosa* compared with only 77% activity of gentamicin.[70] Tobramycin use should be restricted to those infections not responding to gentamicin or with antibacterial sensitivity showing resistance to gentamicin. It may also be used in the case of a life-threatening or sight-threatening infection that has a high probability of being caused by *P. aeruginosa* because of the differential sensitivities of the two drugs and the importance of optimum initial empiric drug selection.

#### *Clinical Use*

The usual intravenous dosage is 3 mg/kg daily given in three divided doses at 8-hour intervals. This dosage may be increased to 5 mg/kg for life-threatening infections. Peak serum concentrations are vital in adjusting the dosage to maintain optimum levels and limit toxicity. This is particularly important in patients with renal impairment. Renal function should be monitored throughout the course of treatment (BUN and serum creatinine levels).

Topical tobramycin sulfate is available commercially in a 0.3% solution. This solution does contain a preservative and is not appropriate for intraocular injection. Fortified topical preparations may be prepared from the intravenous solution. Sterile parenteral tobramycin can be obtained in concentrations of 10, 20, 40, 60, and 80 mg/ml. Fortified concentrations for topical use in severe keratitis range from 8 to 20 mg/ml.[69] Subconjunctival injection of 20 mg in 0.5 ml may be used. Tobramycin in doses of 0.1 to 0.4 mg in 0.1 ml may be used intravitreally and in the vitreous infusion fluid at a dose of 10 μg/ml.[89] Tobramycin may be applied via a collagen shield. Care must be taken in the concentration used because prolonged corneal epithelial toxicity and sloughing may result if the highest fortified dosage is used.

Very low levels of aqueous and vitreous tobramycin are detected after systemic administration. These peak at 1 to 2 hours after administration. Cornea and tear levels are even lower at 0.2 and 0.5 μg/ml, respectively. This compares with minimum inhibitory concentrations of tobramycin in the range of 2 to 4 μg/ml.[90] Much higher levels of tobramycin are found in the aqueous after subconjunctival injection, exceeding 15 μg/ml 2 hours after administration of a 10-mg dose and reaching nearly 25 μg/ml with a 20-mg subconjunctival dose.[91] Adequate tear and corneal levels may be sustained over 1 hour with fortified topical solutions. A corneal and conjunctival reservoir of solution appears to be present, allowing this persistence of tear drug levels. The tear levels of the drug may be increased by occlusion of the lacrimal puncta with intracanalicular collagen plugs.[92] Multiple applications of the drug result in dramatic increases of corneal tear levels. Drops given every 15 minutes will increase initial tear levels from 20 to more than 50 μg/ml in 4 hours. Similarly, corneal levels will increase from 10 to 50 μg/ml. One must remember with these frequent topical instillations and also with subconjunctival injections that significant serum levels may be obtained.[91, 93] Ionophoresis has been used experimentally to provide vitreous levels of tobramycin without injection.[94]

## Penicillins

Penicillin is a generic term often used without the realization that a number of natural and synthetic derivatives of 6-aminopenicillanic acid exist. All of the clinically useful penicillins effectively inhibit certain bacteria, resist inactivation by human tissues, and are remarkably nontoxic. Considerable variations exist in solubility, stability, and resistance to destruction by penicillinase.[95]

Do not overestimate the power of antibiotics or underestimate the resistance of the host as factors in the control of infection. Even when microorganisms are susceptible to antibiotics, prolonged treatment may not eradicate the organism. In a study of the effect of penicillin V on group A streptococcal pharyngitis, a dosage of 20 mg/kg/day was given orally in three divided doses. After 7 days of therapy, streptococci could be recovered from 31% of patients, after 10 days from 18%. Compliance in taking the medication was checked by measuring penicillinuria. Only two thirds of the 10-day patient urine test results were positive for penicillin, but there was no correlation between the microbiologically cured patients and their penicillinuria. Clinical cure occurred despite continuing presence of microorganisms.[96, 97]

### *Types*

*Potassium penicillin G* is water soluble and is ideal for attaining high plasma concentrations rapidly. This form of penicillin is absorbed and excreted rapidly; therefore, it must be administered intramuscularly at least every 6 hours to maintain satisfactory blood levels. As much as 100 million units/day may be given intravenously for overwhelming or resistant infections. Intramuscular doses greater than 500,000 units may be very painful.

Although potassium penicillin G may be given orally, its absorption is limited because of its instability in gastric acid. Only about 15% of the orally administered drug can be recovered in urine. To avoid destruction of the drug oral doses should always be given at least 1 hour before or 2 hours after meals. For treatment of infections caused by sensitive bacteria, the minimal recommended oral dose is 400,000 units four times daily.

*Procaine penicillin G* is less soluble in water and is therefore absorbed more slowly than potassium penicillin G. Intramuscular doses of 600,000 units every 24 hours will maintain demonstrable plasma concentrations comparable with those attained by oral administration of 250 mg of phenoxymethyl penicillin or potassium phenethicillin four times daily. If higher blood levels are desired, large injections of potassium penicillin G should be used. Giving doses of procaine penicillin G larger than 600,000 units and more often than every 12 hours is an inefficient method of achieving high plasma concentrations.

*Benzathine penicillin G* is only slightly water soluble and produces very low blood levels, which may last for several weeks. A single injection of 2,400,000 units will cure early syphilis in most cases. The longer-acting forms of penicillin are more likely to produce hypersensitivity reactions.

*Phenoxymethyl penicillin* (penicillin V) is much more acid stable than is penicillin G; hence, it is well suited for oral use. As much as 75% of an oral dose may be recovered in the urine, indicating absorption two to five times that of oral penicillin G. Phenoxymethyl penicillin may be given without regard to the time of meals. An oral dose of 250 mg four times daily is adequate for most infections. The oral route may be considerably more economical than the parenteral route (and more comfortable). *Phenoxyethyl penicillin* is pharmacologically comparable with phenoxymethyl penicillin.

All types of penicillin described to this point differ in solubility and stability. Their antibacterial effect, however, is essentially the same, as all are effective against most gram-positive cocci (with the noteworthy exception of penicillinase-producing and therefore resistant staphylococci), gonocci, enterococci, *Haemophilus, Clostridium,* and spirochetes. Most gram-negative bacteria (specifically *Pseudomonas*) are resistant to these forms of penicillin.

*Sodium methicillin* is resistant to destruction of penicillinase and is a first-choice agent against resistant staphylococci (unless the patient is allergic to penicillin). Minimal dosage is 1 g intramuscularly every 6 hours. Serious infections may require 2 g every 4 hours, given by continuous intravenous drip. The renal excretion of methicillin is rapid, half being excreted within 2 hours after intramuscular injection and 1 hour after intravenous administration.

Methicillin is extremely unstable in even slightly acid solutions and therefore should be dissolved just before use. When added to infusion fluids, it may be inactivated within several hours.

*Sodium oxacillin* is pharmacologically comparable with methicillin except that it is more acid stable and may therefore be given orally (500 mg every 2 hours). Frequent dosage is necessary because of the rapid excretion of the drug.[98] Oxacillin is not excreted in sweat and thus is not effective against skin-surface infections.

*Ampicillin* is an acid-stable, orally absorbed synthetic penicillin with broad-spectrum antibacterial activity. It is effective against a variety of gram-negative bacteria, particularly *E. coli* and *Proteus.*[99] The drug is administered orally, 0.75 g every 6 hours. It is indicated chiefly for the treatment of infections caused by tetracycline-resistant, gram-negative bacteria. Being inactivated by penicillinase, ampicillin is ineffective against penicillin G–resistant staphylococci. Minimal inhibitory concentrations of ampicillin for the common gram-positive organisms range from 0.01 to 0.05 μg/ml.[100] *Amoxicillin* is comparable with ampicillin. *Azlocillin* is an acylaminopenicillin with expanded gram-negative activity. It is comparable to piperacillin and mezlocillin.

*Carbenicillin* is a semisynthetic penicillin that acts against gram-negative pathogens. Inhibition of most strains of *Pseudomonas* requires doses of up to 50 μg/ml. *Proteus* and *E. coli* may respond to carbenicillin therapy. Penicillinase-producing staphylococci are resistant. Gentamicin and carbenicillin are incompatible in solution; however, they are synergistic against gram-negative microorganisms. The drug has low toxicity and may be used in doses of 20 to 40 g/day. Because of acid instability, carbenicillin must be given parenterally. The intravenous route is ordinarily used. Fig. 6–5 shows the aqueous levels achieved after subcon-

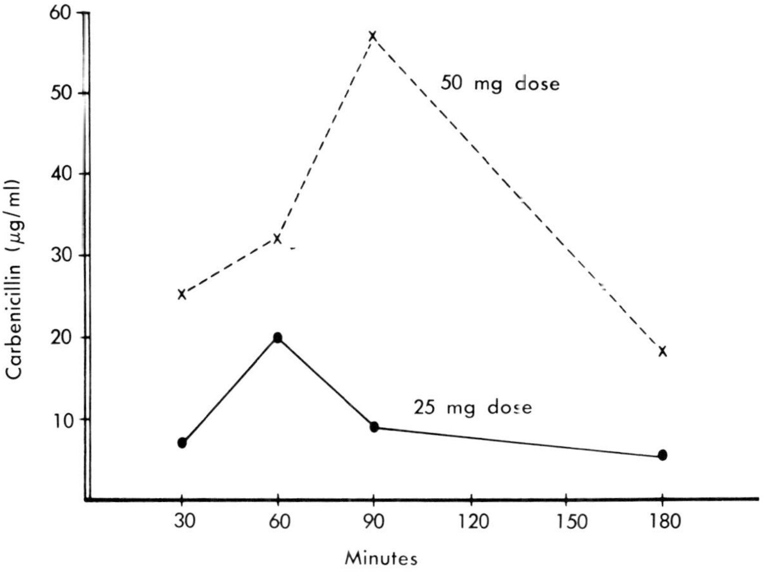


**FIG 6–5.**
Primary aqueous levels (rabbit) obtained after subconjunctival injection of carbenicillin in 25- and 50-mg dosage. (Modified from Rich AM, Dunlap WA, Partridge JR: *Am J Ophthalmol* 75:490, 1973. Used by permission.)

junctival injection.[101] *Ticarcillin* is comparable with carbenicillin.

### *Ocular Penetration*

The blood-aqueous and blood-vitreous barriers severely limit passage of nonlipid-soluble drugs such as penicillin into the vitreous, aqueous, and lens. A comparable barrier separates the healthy vitreous from the aqueous.[102] A common error is to think of the entire eye as being within the blood-aqueous barrier; this is not true. The uveal tract is freely accessible to blood-borne medications.

The semisynthetic penicillin derivatives vary considerably in their intraocular penetration. Methicillin, carbenicillin, cloxacillin, and amoxicillin do not penetrate nearly as well as does ampicillin.[103–105]

When an ointment containing 100,000 units/ml of penicillin is applied to the surface of the healthy rabbit eye, aqueous drug levels will reach only about 4 units/ml and will have dropped to 1 unit/ml in 2½ hours (Fig. 6–6).[106] Similar low levels are obtained in the intact sclera, cornea, and uveal tract. Fortunately, the common infections of the corneal surface either are outside the blood-aqueous barrier or destroy it and are therefore more than normally accessible to penicillin therapy. Purified crystalline penicillin is virtually nontoxic to the exterior of the eye and can

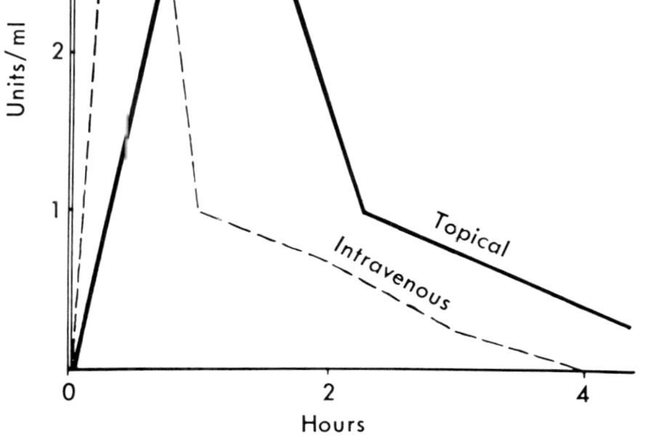


**FIG 6–6.**
Penicillin in rabbit aqueous (units/milliliter) after topical application of ointment, 100,000 units/ml, and intravenous administration of 50,000 units. (Modified from Sorsby A, Ungar J: *BMJ* 114:4480, 1946. Used by permission.)

be used in very high concentrations without ocular irritation. Topical application achieves much higher concentrations on the corneal surface than the systemic routes of administration. For these reasons, topical penicillin therapy is effective against keratitis but is ineffective against endophthalmitis.

Subconjunctival injection of 1 million units of crystalline penicillin G produces effective intraocular levels of penicillin.[107] These levels persist for as long as 48 hours. Smaller amounts of penicillin without epinephrine produce substantially lower intraocular levels. As noted in Figs. 6–7 and 6–8, an intramuscular injection of penicillin results in much lower intraocular concentrations than those obtained by subconjunctival injection of an equal amount of drug. Intraocular concentrations of penicillin obtained by retrobulbar injection were higher than those achieved by intramuscular injection but lower than those after subconjunctival injection. As a specific example, 24 hours after treatment, 16 units/ml of drug persisted in the aqueous after the subconjunctival injection compared with less than 0.1 unit/ml after intramuscular injection. One should realize that these figures were obtained in normal rabbits and that a comparable intramuscular dose for humans would require many millions of units. The penetration of the subconjunctival dose should be less directly related to the size of the body. These penicillin levels were ob-

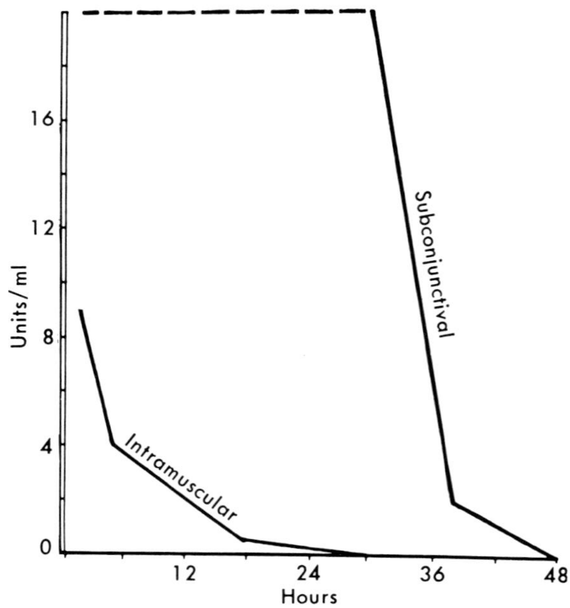


**FIG 6–7.**
Penicillin in rabbit aqueous (units/milliliter) after injection of 1 million units in a 1 : 1,000 solution of epinephrine by subconjunctival and intramuscular routes. (Modified from Sorsby A, Ungar J: *Br J Ophthalmol* 32:964, 1948. Used by permission.)

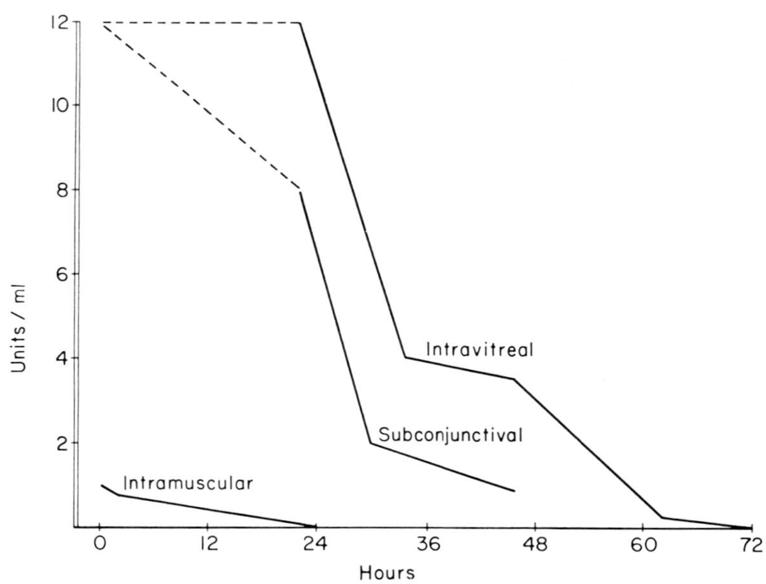


**FIG 6–8.**
Penicillin in rabbit vitreous (units/milliliter) after injection of 1 million units in a 1 : 1,000 solution of epinephrine by subconjunctival and intramuscular routes. Intravitreal injection was 5,000 units. (Modified from Sorsby A, Ungar J: *Br J Ophthalmol* 32:864, 1948. Used by permission.)

tained in healthy rabbit eyes, and higher values should result in inflamed eyes with damaged blood-aqueous barriers.

Twenty-four hours after subconjunctival injection of 1 million units of penicillin in an epinephrine solution, the corneal concentration was more than 500 units/g of tissue and the posterior uveal concentration more than 300 units/g. The lens had the lowest level of all eye tissues, only 4 units after 24 hours. Vitreous levels are lower than those of the aqueous, for instance, 8 units/ml after 24 hours (see Fig. 6-8). It is noteworthy that by the second day similar vitreous levels are produced by subconjunctival injection of 1 million units in epinephrine and by 5,000 units injected intravitreally. This is a most practical point, because subconjunctival injection is far more convenient and safer than intravitreal injection. In view of the effective levels of penicillin obtained by the two routes, intravitreal injections can be justified only when the vitreous cavity is already opened, as by trauma or in the case of postoperative endophthalmitis when aqueous and vitreous taps are performed and vitreal injection is needed to immediately sterilize the eye. Even under these circumstances, manipulation of the remaining vitreous may have undesirable effects. Although intravitreal injection of 5,000 units of crystalline penicillin (this amount is toxic to the retina) produces good levels within the vitreous cavity for up to 48 hours, it diffuses poorly to the anterior segment of the eye.[107] At 24 hours the vitreous penicillin concentration is more than 32 units/ml, at 48 hours it is 16 units/ml, and at 64 hours it remains as only a trace. At 24 hours only 4 units/ml are in the aqueous.

After systemic administration, penicillin levels are far higher in the vascular tissues of the eye than in the internal fluids. Two hours after intramuscular injection of penethamate (a synthetic penicillin ester) in rabbits, the following concentrations in units per gram of wet tissue were measured: blood, 0.38; cornea, 0.12; aqueous, 0.04; anterior uvea, 3.8; lens, less than 0.01; vitreous, 0.09; posterior uvea, 1.82; and sclera, 0.39. Note that aqueous levels are not representative of concentrations in the surrounding tissues and that this particular compound was selectively concentrated in the uveal tract in concentrations higher than in the blood.[102]

Selective concentration also occurs on the surface of susceptible microorganisms. Although radioisotope studies show ion exchange within living tissues to proceed with almost unbelievable rapidity, this does not necessarily mean that particles of medication diffuse freely away from their target tissues. By the use of radioisotope-labeled penicillin, it has been shown that within 60 seconds of treatment time the penicillin may become firmly absorbed to the surface of the cell wall of *Bacillus subtilis.*[108]

The application of penicillin by iontophoresis (2 mA for 5 minutes) increased the aqueous concentrations to levels eight times higher than those attained by simply bathing the cornea in the same concentration of penicillin.[109]

Plasma levels of penicillin may be increased by blocking renal excretion. Each hour, approximately 60% of the circulating penicillin is excreted. Probenecid and carinamide will increase penicillin plasma levels from 2 to 10 times.[110] Dosage of probenecid is 500 mg four times daily and of carinamide, 2 g every 3 hours. In practice, these tubule-blocking drugs are rarely used, because the same effect can be achieved just as economically by giving more penicillin. Furthermore, these drugs may cause allergy or renal stones, and their action is inconsistent.

An active transport system removes organic anions from the vitreous. This mechanism can be blocked by probenecid, just as renal excretion is blocked. A dosage of 150 mg of probenecid intravenously twice daily was given to rabbits to evaluate whether methicillin levels resulting from intravitreal injection could be prolonged. The untreated half-life of intravitreal methicillin was 3.5 hours; the half-life with probenecid was 4.25 hours. This was not of great clinical significance, because the duration of inhibitory concentration of intravitreal methicillin was 39 hours for the control and 43 hours for the probenecid-treated rabbits.[111]

The differences in antibiotic concentrations in various parts of the eye were evaluated using both radioactive and bioassay techniques.[112] The inadequacy of aqueous levels as a measure of the antibiotic concentration within the eye was emphasized. For example, after systemic administration of penicillin, the iris concentrations averaged 2.5 times those of the aqueous, whereas vitreous levels were less than 0.1 of the aqueous levels. Choroid and retina levels approximated aqueous levels.

#### *Methicillin*

A therapeutic concentration of methicillin (sodium dimethoxyphenyl penicillin) will penetrate into the normal rabbit aqueous after subconjunctival injection of 20 mg (Fig. 6–9).[113] Intraocular penetration is less effective when the route of administration is intramuscular.

In an evaluation of the penetration of antistaphylococcal antibiotics into rabbit aqueous, methicillin dosage of 30 mg/kg intramuscularly every 6 hours for five doses resulted in aqueous drug levels ranging from 0.8 to 4.2 μg/ml. This was the only antistaphylococcal drug that achieved therapeutic aqueous levels by the intramuscular route, with nafcillin, cephalothin, cefazolin, and gentamicin failing to do so.[114]

The intraocular penetration of methicillin in humans was studied by bioassay of aqueous obtained at cataract surgery.[115] Continuous intravenous infusion of 8 g of methicillin (with oral probenecid) over a 24-hour period achieved an average serum concentration of 45 μg/ml but an aqueous level of only 0.46 μg/ml. A concentration of 4 μg/ml inhibits growth of most gram-positive organisms. In an eye with iridocyclitis, the aqueous concentration was 6 μg/ml. Two diabetic eyes with cataracts but otherwise clinically normal demonstrated aqueous concentrations of 6.5 μg/ml, presumably indicating abnormal vascular permeability in the diabetic eye. These data indicate that therapeutic concentrations of methicillin do not enter the normal human eye but may be achieved when the blood-aqueous barriers are broken down by inflammation or disease.

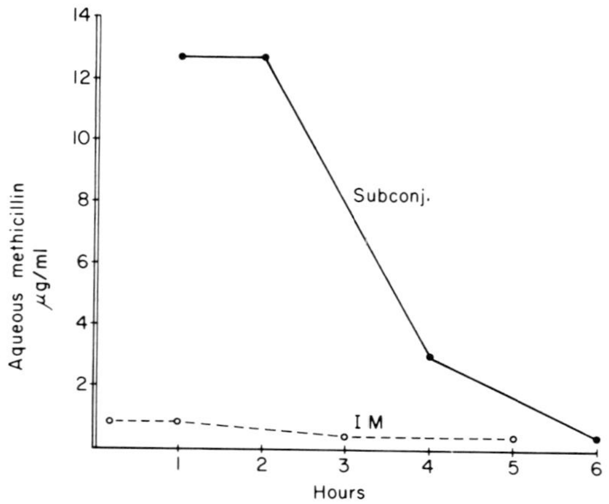


**FIG 6–9.**
Aqueous concentrations (milligrams/milliliter) of methicillin after subconjunctival injection of 20 mg and intramuscular injection of 40 mg/kg. (Modified from Green WR, Leopold IH: *Am J Ophthalmol* 60:800, 1965. Used by permission.)

#### *Oxacillin*

No measurable levels of oxacillin could be detected in aqueous humor obtained from 40 patients during cataract extraction. The drug had been administered by intramuscular injection before surgery, resulting in serum levels as high as 5.7 μg/ml at the time of surgery. In humans, approximately 93% of the oxacillin in the blood is bound to plasma protein. The protein-bound oxacillin is completely blocked from entry into the aqueous. Clearly, oxacillin is not likely to be an effective drug in the treatment of intraocular infection. Indeed, oxacillin does not penetrate even into the inflamed animal eye.[116]

#### *Ampicillin*

Ampicillin is reported to produce aqueous humor levels approximately twice as high as those achieved with comparable doses of aqueous penicillin G.[117] Blockage of renal tubular excretion by oral probenecid (35 mg/kg given 30 minutes before ampicillin injection) resulted in aqueous humor levels two to five times greater than those achieved without probenecid. There was considerable variation in the format and the results of experimental determination. Fig. 6–10 shows an even greater ampicillin penetration compared with penicillin G.[118]

The aqueous levels shown in Fig. 6–11 resulted from a single, intramuscular ampicillin dosage of 50 mg/kg, which would be

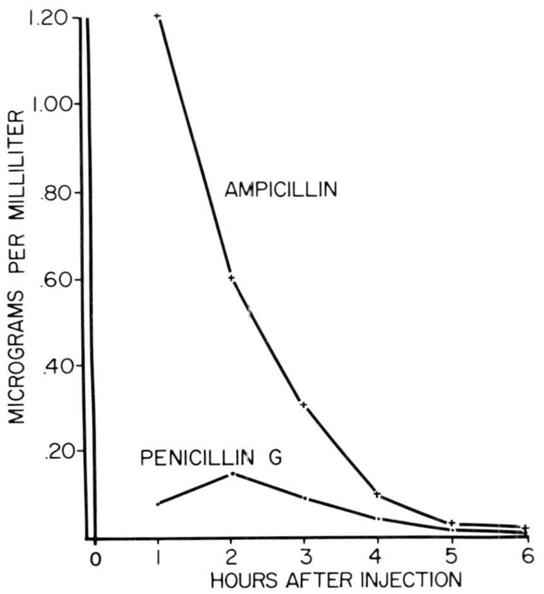


**FIG 6–10.**
Aqueous drug concentrations (rabbit) after intramuscular injection of 21 mg of antibiotic/kg. (Modified from Goldman JN, Klein JO: *Ann Ophthalmol* 2:35, 1970. Used by permission.)

3,500 mg for a 70-kg man.[117] A titer of 2 μg/ml will inhibit most gram-positive cocci.

Subconjunctivally injected ampicillin penetrates the anterior chamber with remarkable rapidity. After a subconjunctival injection of 100,000 units (62.5 mg) of ampicillin in a 0.25-ml solution, bacteriostatic concentrations of antibiotic are demonstrable in the rabbit aqueous within 30 seconds. Peak levels are reached in 30 minutes, declining to zero in about 12 hours (Fig. 6–12).[119] Incidentally, it was noted in this study that if antibiotic levels are of value during and after cataract surgery, it is more rational to give a subconjunctival injection before rather than after the operation.

Topical application of 2 mg of ampicillin on rabbit corneas resulted in the concentrations shown in Fig. 6–13.[100]

Human aqueous concentrations of ampicillin were measured by securing aqueous samples at the time of cataract extraction.[100] The aqueous levels achieved by different oral doses are shown in Fig. 6–14. These data suggest that an oral dosage of 1 g of ampicillin every 4 hours should maintain antibiotic concentrations in the anterior segment of the eye sufficient to inhibit the common gram-positive organisms. Consistent aqueous levels effective against relatively resistant gram-negative organisms cannot be maintained with reasonable dosage schedules.

Plasma protein binding of antibiotics

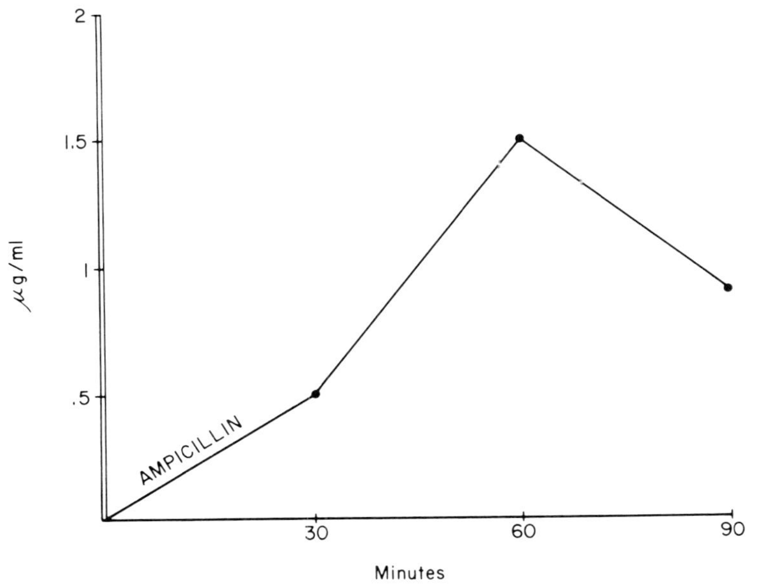


**FIG 6–11.**
Aqueous humor (rabbit) concentrations of ampicillin given intramuscularly in a dosage of 50 mg/kg. (Modified from Goldman EE, McLain JH, Smith JL: *Am J Ophthalmol* 65:717, 1968. Used by permission.)

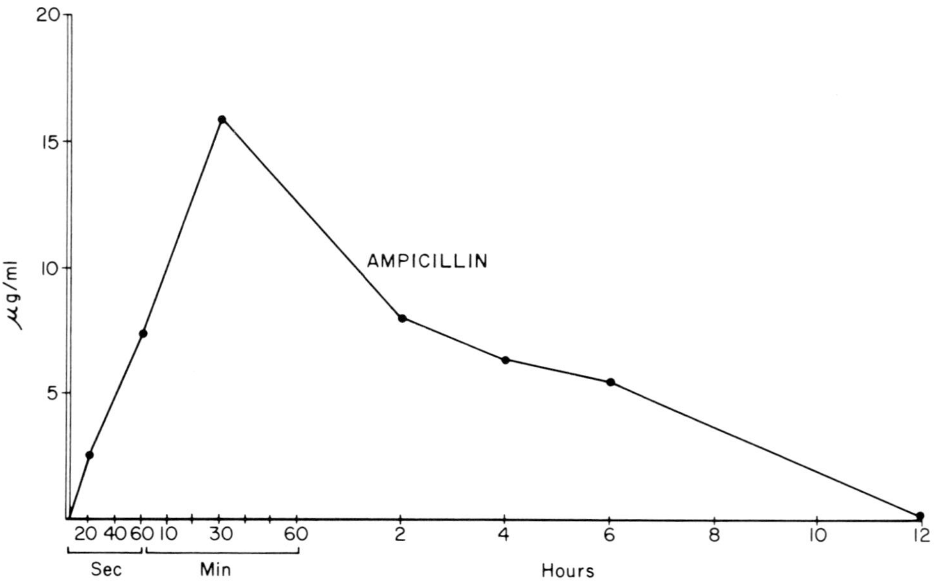


**FIG 6–12.**
Rate of entry of subconjunctivally injected ampicillin into aqueous humor (rabbit). (Modified from McPherson Jr SD, Presley GD, Crawford JR: *Am J Ophthalmol* 66:430, 1968. Used by permission.)

renders them biologically inactive and also excludes the bound portion from entry into the primary aqueous. The proportion of ampicillin bound to protein is 17%; of amoxicillin, 20%; of methicillin, 30% to 40%; of ticarcillin, 45%; of carbenicillin, 50%; of penicillin G, 35% to 60%; of penicillin V, 50% to 70%; of oxacillin, cloxacillin, and dicloxacillin, 90% or more.[120]

Similarly, a decrease in intraocular penetration follows systemic administration of these drugs.[121] There is a critical free plasma level, 21 μg/ml, below which ampicillin does not cross the blood-aqueous barrier. These authors also measured the primary aqueous levels of rabbits after subconjunctival injection of antibiotic and found the following levels of antibiotics 1

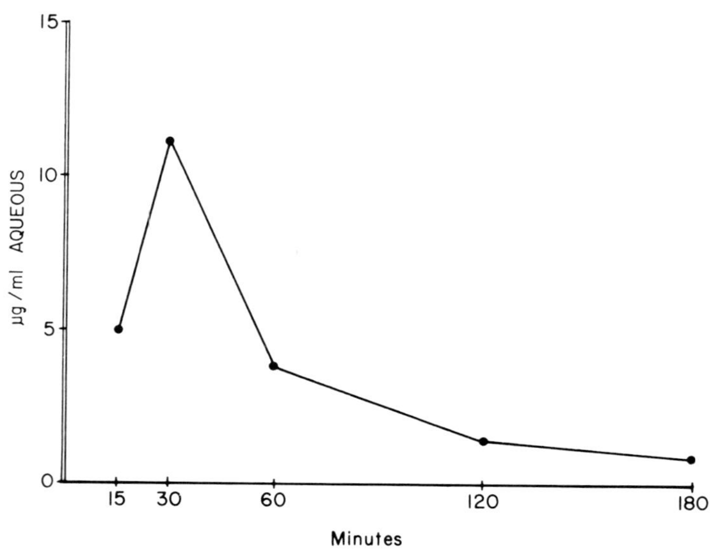


**FIG 6–13.**
Aqueous levels after topical application of 2 mg of ampicillin on rabbit cornea. (Data from Kurose Y, Leopold IH: *Arch Ophthalmol* 73:361, 1965. Used by permission.)

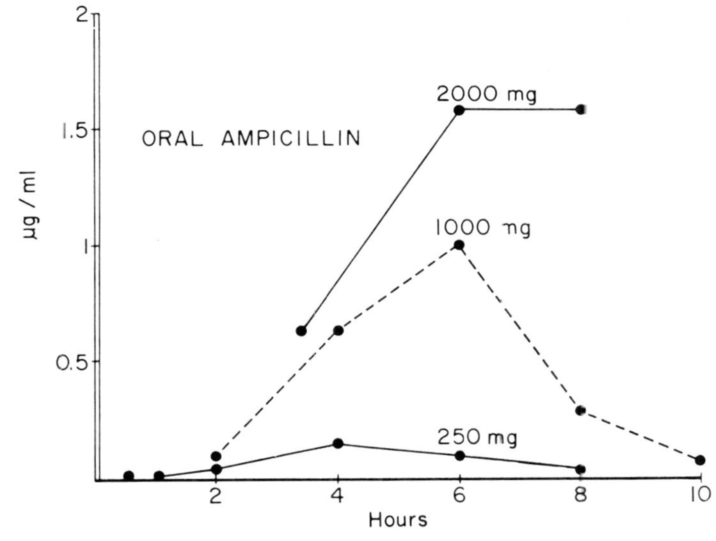


**FIG 6–14.**
Aqueous levels after a single oral dose of ampicillin. (Data from Kurose Y, Leopold IH: *Arch Ophthalmol* 73:361, 1965. Used by permission.)

hour after injection: ampicillin, 1,000 μg/ml; methicillin, 166 μg/ml; and oxacillin, 145 μg/ml. Four hours after subconjunctival injection, no detectable levels of ampicillin or methicillin were present in the aqueous.

As much as 10 mg of ampicillin has been found to be nontoxic in rabbit eyes with bacterial endophthalmitis unresponsive to other antibiotics.[122, 123]

### *Azlocillin*

Azlocillin is an acylamino penicillin similar to piperacillin and mezlocillin. It is indicated in the treatment of gram-negative infections. These drugs are synergistic but physically incompatible with aminoglycosides much like other penicillins. Tear and aqueous levels of azlocillin of 4.1 and 4.4 μg/ml, respectively, were found after intravenous injection of 4 g. These levels were in the therapeutic range for some gram-negative organisms but were marginal for *Pseudomonas.*[124]

### *Dicloxacillin*

Dicloxacillin, which is highly effective against penicillinase-producing *S. aureus,* will not penetrate into primary aqueous when given intravenously or orally but will enter secondary aqueous in concentrations as high as 12 μg/ml 2 hours after administration.[125] Subconjunctival injection of 50 mg will give aqueous concentrations as high as 181 μg/ml at 1 hour and 50 μg/ml at 4 hours. A concentration of 0.5 μg/ml will inhibit most gram-positive cocci, including penicillinase-producing *S. aureus.*

### *Carbenicillin*

Intraocular penetration of carbenicillin after intravenous administration is poor, in the same range as that of penicillin G. One hour after intravenous administration of 30 mg/kg, primary aqueous levels were 2 to 3 μg/ml. Probenecid, 200 mg, did not increase these levels significantly. In the inflamed eye, aqueous levels reached 33 μg/ml, but vitreous levels were less than 3 μg/ml. Subconjunctival injection of 100 mg gave aqueous levels averaging 172 μg/ml in normal primary aqueous and 196 μg/ml in the inflamed eye. Vitreous levels were poor, less than 4 μg/ml even in the inflamed eye. The half-life of carbenicillin in the aqueous was found to be 40 minutes.[126] Because most strains of *Pseudomonas* require more than 50 μg/ml of carbenicillin for inhibition, it is evident that vitreous concentrations of antibiotic adequate to control this microorganism were not achieved.

Twenty cataract patients received subconjunctival injections of carbenicillin varying from 50 to 500 mg. Immediate, severe, burning pain resulted, followed by a marked local chemosis that persisted for 2 to 11 days.

Aqueous levels were quite variable, but in most cases the 100-mg dosage level resulted in primary aqueous levels of about 150 μg/ml from 30 minutes to 2 hours after injection.[127]

### *Piperacillin*

Piperacillin levels exceeding the minimum inhibitory concentration (MIC) for many gram-negative and gram-positive bacteria were found in the tears and aqueous fluid of cataract patients after a single injection of 4 g of piperacillin. The mean peak tear concentration was 5.6 μg/ml, and the aqueous concentration peaked at 2.8 μg/ml.[128]

### *Therapy of Intraocular Infections*

The use of penicillin in the treatment of eye infections is limited by several factors. Most important is the susceptibility of the offending microorganism, because, of course, there will be no therapeutic response to penicillin if the organism is resistant (or if the disease is misdiagnosed and not of infectious etiology). A practical limitation is the 5% incidence of allergy after topical ocular use of penicillin. Because of this, other antibiotics and antibacterials have completely replaced penicillin in the local treatment of minor surface ocular infections. The most complex limiting factor is the resistance of the blood-aqueous barrier to the passage of penicillin. That this barrier can be bypassed is experimentally demonstrable, as shown in the following discussion.

### *Experimental Use*

Experimental intraocular infections produced by injection of 50,000 *S. aureus* organisms into the aqueous or vitreous were treated by subconjunctival injection of 1 million units of penicillin.[129] As would be expected from knowledge of the attainable intraocular concentrations, the infection was arrested with preservation of normal eyes when the penicillin was administered 4 hours after infection. If treatment was delayed for 24 hours, the anterior chamber infections cleared but left varying degrees of synechiae and corneal scarring. The 24-hour treatment of vitreous infections resulted in opaque, organized vitreous. All untreated control eyes were destroyed by panophthalmitis. These findings are compatible with those of other studies.[130]

An instructive quantitative experiment was carried out by inoculating the anterior chambers of rabbits with gonococci and then determining the least amount of penicillin required to sterilize the eye when given by various routes. Intramuscular injection required 150,000 units of penicillin, subconjunctival injection required 100,000 units, and direct inoculation into the anterior chamber required only 2.5 units. It is obvious that very effective barriers to aqueous penetration by penicillin exist, even in an infected eye.

### *Clinical Use*

Clinical use of penicillin in the treatment of corneal and anterior segment infections has shown that the human eye tolerates the subconjunctival injection of 500,000 units of crystalline penicillin in 0.5 ml of 1:1,000 concentration of epinephrine at intervals of 24 hours.[131] Injection of 0.5 ml of a 1:1,000 concentration of epinephrine is apparently safe, although some patients (with cardiac and thyrotoxic conditions) may be more sensitive to its effects than others.

A practical point is that concentrated solutions of penicillin should be made up in water rather than in normal saline solution; otherwise they will be quite hypertonic and therefore more irritating.

Very high doses of penicillin are required for the treatment or prophylaxis of eye infections.[132] One million units of crystalline penicillin administered intramuscularly or intravenously every 8 hours is recommended. Concomitant oral use of probenecid, 2 g initially and 0.5 g every 6 hours, blocks elimination of penicillin and thereby helps to maintain high concentrations within the body. After a penetrating eye injury, penicillin may be given as just described for the first 48 hours. Should no signs of infection be present at that time, penicillin may be discontinued or reduced in dosage, depending on the circumstances. Simultaneously with penicillin, an initial dose of 2 g of streptomycin, followed by 1 g every 8 hours, was recommended to give a wider antibacterial spectrum. However, the toxicity of streptomycin at this dosage level makes it unacceptable. Systemic and intraocular aminoglycosides and cephalosporins have largely supplanted penicillin in the prophylaxis of penetrating eye injuries and intraocular foreign bodies.[41]

Differences of opinion exist as to whether prophylactic antibiotics should be used after routine cataract surgery. Statistics indicate that there is as high as a 0.5% incidence of intraocular infection after cataract surgery even when performed with the best of technique. In view of this known possibility, a series of 1,202 patients were injected subconjunctivally immediately after cataract extraction with 100,000 units of penicillin G in a 0.25-ml volume, which contained 1 drop of a 1:1,000 concentration of epinephrine.[133] Intraocular infection developed in four of these eyes (0.24%), and three of the four infections were caused by penicillin-resistant organisms. Subsequently, 10 mg of streptomycin was added to the injection. Combined penicillin and streptomycin injections were then given to 3,226 patients over a 3-year period, and not one case of intraocular infection developed. A control series of 1,773 patients who were operated on in the same institution received no antibiotics and had a 0.51% incidence of infection (nine eyes). The injection caused slight postoperative conjunctival congestion, but no instance of damaging allergic or toxic reaction occurred in this large series.

Eight cases of postoperative staphylococcal endophthalmitis were reported to follow prophylactic subconjunctival injection of a solution of 100,000 units of penicillin and 10 mg of streptomycin.[134] In four of these cases there was a latent period of 21 to 40 days between surgery and infection. The long period of latency caused some clinical confusion, because the time interval was more characteristic of fungal than of bacterial infection. The incidence of infection was 3% of the operated eyes, which indicated that antibiotic prophylaxis will not reliably protect against faults in sterile operative technique.

Penicillin is effective in slowing the progress of syphilitic optic atrophy. After 8 years, only 25% of penicillin-treated patients with syphilitic optic atrophy will have lost 80% of their initial vision, whereas in the same period, 65% of untreated patients will likely become blind.[135] Combining malaria fever therapy with the penicillin treatment of syphilitic optic atrophy[135] does not alter the results obtained and is not warranted because of the risks inherent in malaria therapy.[136] Early stages of optic atrophy respond to treatment much better than do advanced stages.[137]

Treatment of syphilitic optic neuritis, a manifestation of central nervous system infection, is not easily accomplished because of the blood-brain barrier. After injection of benzathine penicillin G, 12 of 13 patients had no detectable penicillin in their cerebrospinal fluid. Even after 10,800,000 units of benzathine penicillin is given over a period of weeks, *Treponema pallidum* can be recovered from cerebrospinal fluid. Similarly, procaine penicillin G and penicillin in aluminum monostearate fail to produce treponemicidal levels (0.02 μg/ml) in cerebrospinal fluid. A reliable way of achieving treponemicidal cerebrospinal fluid levels of penicillin is to give 500,000 units of penicillin G every 6 hours together with 500 mg of probenecid by mouth every 6 hours; 27 or 31 patients so treated reached levels greater than 0.1 μg/ml, and the average exceeded 0.3 μg/ml.[138]

Official recommendations of the Centers for Disease Control for treatment of neurosyphilis advise use of 2,400,000 units of benzathine penicillin G intramuscularly given three times at weekly intervals. No controlled studies exist to confirm the validity of such advice, which is derived from extrapolation.[139] In fact, in 40% of 64 penicillin-treated neurosyphilitic patients new neurologic abnormalities developed during a 10-year follow-up period. Because only two of 33 patients using various combinations of benzathine penicillin ($\geq$4,800,000 units) and probenecid achieved a cerebrospinal fluid concentration of 0.03 μg/ml or greater (reliable treponemicidal level), long-acting penicillin regimens are of questionable efficacy. An alternate proposal is to hospitalize patients for a 14-day course of intravenous aqueous penicillin G sodium, 24 million units daily. Even with this massive level of treatment, the cerebrospinal fluid levels of penicillin should be checked after 3 days of therapy to ensure adequate penetration.[140]

Although gonorrhea is expected to cause a severe purulent conjunctivitis, appearing after a 1- to 5-day incubation period, the degree of conjunctival reaction may be quite variable. A case of culture-proven gonococcal (GC) conjunctivitis manifesting only mild bilateral hyperemia and another that was completely asymptomatic have been reported.[141] The incidence of penicillinase-producing strains of gonococcus are increasing. Initial therapy should be aqueous crystalline penicillin G, 50,000 to 100,000 U/kg/day. The therapy may be modified when susceptibility data are available. In areas with a high incidence of penicillinase-producing organisms, treatment with a penicillamine-resistant drug (nafcillin, cephalosporins) is rational.[142]

Topical therapy is 100,000 units of penicillin/ml, alternately. *Chlamydia trachomatis* neonatal conjunctivitis has been successfully treated with 25 mg of oral erythromycin ethylsuccinate/kg twice daily for 14 days.[143]

Isolation techniques should be used, because GC ophthalmia is highly contagious. The source of the infection and other potentially affected individuals should be identified and treated.

Benzathine penicillin (900,000 units intramuscularly every 2 weeks for 4 months) has been used for the treatment of trachoma[144]; 12 were completely cured, and 2 showed great improvement at the end of 4 months. Two years later, all but one of the 18 were cured. Whether penicillin acts directly on the *Chlamydia* or merely arrests secondary bacterial infection is not clear. Tetracycline is currently recommended in the treatment of trachoma and inclusion conjunctivitis in adults. Erythromycin is the alternate choice in adults and first choice in children less than 8 years of age and in pregnant women.

#### *Toxic Effects*

For practical purposes, external application of penicillin in any concentration is nontoxic to the eye. Definite toxic effects were noted in the majority of rabbit eyes receiving intravitreal injections of 2,000 to 5,000 units of the various types of crystalline penicillin.[145] These effects include ophthalmoscopically observable retinal edema (lasting up to 10 days), pigmentary migration, localized atrophic patches in the retina, irregularity and condensations in the vitreous, and blistering of the internal limiting membrane. Vacuolation of the nerve fiber layer, limited areas of neuroepithelial damage, and preretinal exudation were histologically demonstrated. Penicillin K produced neovascularization, whereas penicillin G was the least toxic. Obviously the interior of the eye will not tolerate the massive concentrations of penicillin that can be injected elsewhere in the body.

Clinically the anterior chamber will tolerate irrigation with 5,000 units of potassium penicillin G/ml. A penicillin solution of this concentration may be used for anterior chamber irrigation at the time of surgical closure of an injury or if paracentesis of a severe hypopyon is performed.

Penicillin is extremely irritating to the central nervous system and may cause serious and permanent nerve damage. Accidental injection into the sciatic nerve may cause permanent sensory and motor loss. The importance of avoiding sciatic nerve damage warrants cautioning the nurse against injecting into any portion of the buttock other than the upper outer quadrant.[146]

Penicillin not only is toxic when introduced into the central nervous system or injected into peripheral nerves but also causes severe ischemic necrosis if accidentally injected intraarterially during intended intramuscular injection. Two cases of major damage to a leg are reported, with part of the foot becoming gangrenous in one case.[147]

Five percent of the population in the United States is said to be allergic to penicillin.[148] This is presumably related to the enormous amount of penicillin used (350 tons/year, or 3 million units/inhabitant). Eighty percent of all drug eruptions are caused by penicillin. With the advent of benzathine and the other types of repository penicillin, reactions have become even more violent and prolonged.

The most common type of penicillin allergy is the delayed response that simulates serum sickness. After an incubation period, usually lasting 1 to 2 weeks, urticaria, fever, and joint pains appear. This response is a result of the development of antibodies after the injection, and therefore skin tests and the past history will not reveal penicillin sensitivity.

Sensitization may be caused by penicillin therapy, penicillin in ingested food (dairy products), or previous fungus disease of the skin. Preliminary skin or conjunctival testing may be positive or negative, even in patients who will later have severe penicillin allergy develop. These sensitized individuals will manifest allergic reactions more promptly, even after incubation periods as brief as a few minutes. Death may occur from acute serum sickness, angioedema, or anaphylaxis.[149]

The incidence of allergic reactions to penicillin in patients can be reduced by routine inquiry as to previous drug allergy. (Asthmatic patients are more likely to become sensitive to penicillin.) Juries are said to take a dim view of severe drug reactions induced in patients who know they have previously been allergic to the medication. As previously stated, however, neither the history nor skin testing will detect all patients who are allergic to penicillin. Use penicillin only when it is needed and only after ascertaining that the patient has had no previous penicillin reaction and be knowledgeable in the treatment of the allergic reactions. Subcutaneous or intravenous epinephrine is indicated for accelerated hypersensitivity. Airway management, intravenous fluid, and corticosteroids are indicated in the case of acute anaphylaxis. Desensitization may be performed to allow administration of penicillin. Cross-allergenicity may occur with other β-lactam antibiotics (cephalosporins, cephamycins, 1-oxa-β-lactams, and carbapenems).

Despite the relative infrequency of penicillin reactions, an attitude of complacency is unwarranted. Penicillin reactions are estimated to occur in 2% to 8% of patients receiving the drug. The incidence of death associated with severe reactions is from 9% to 13%.[146] Patients found to be allergic to penicillin (or any other medication, for that matter) should be cautioned against its further use and advised to inform their future medical attendants.

The local ocular use of penicillin may result in as high as a 16% incidence of allergic blepharitis.[150] For this reason, topical application for minor infections is in disrepute. Such promiscuous use of penicillin may sensitize the patient, thereby precluding later use of this valuable drug in time of need. Furthermore, the more widespread the use of an antibiotic, the more numerous will be the strains of resistant microorganisms in the community. Antibiotic-associated diarrhea also results from penicillin antibiotics.

***Summary***

Penicillin is reserved for treatment of ocular infections (excluding endophthalmitis) caused by sensitive organisms. A variety of new penicillin derivatives have quite different antimicrobic spectra; hence, laboratory sensitivity studies are essential in the management of severe infections.

Penicillin penetration into aqueous, lens, and vitreous is poor but is considerably increased by subconjunctival injection or by iontophoresis. Alternate drugs (e.g., aminoglycosides, cephalosporins, and vancomycin) are preferable for treatment of endophthalmitis.

## Cephalosporins

Cephalosporins are derivatives of cephalosporin C produced by the fungus *Cephalosporium acremonium*. The drugs are related to penicillin through their common β-lactam structure. They are also related to cephamycins and 1-oxa-β-lactams. Instead of the five-membered thiazolidine ring of penicillin, cephalosporins are composed of the β-lactam ring fused with a six-membered dihydrothiazine ring. Cleavage of the β-lactam ring at any point destroys the antibacterial activity. Once mixed in solution, cephalosporins are not stable unless frozen. They are bactericidal in action through the inhibition of mucopeptide synthesis in the bacterial cell wall. Cephalosporins are active against many gram-positive aerobic bacteria and some gram-negative aerobic bacteria, as well as some anaerobic bacteria. Cephalosporins are classified based on the spectra of their activity (Table 6–6). First-generation cephalosporins are active in vitro against gram-positive cocci, including penicillinase-producing *S. aureus* and *S. epidermidis,* group A β-hemolytic streptococci, group B streptococci, and *S. pneumoniae.* First-generation cephalosporins are not active against enterococci, methicillin-resistant *Staphylococcus, Bacteroides fragilis, Citrobacter, Enterobacter, Listeria monocytogenes, Proteus* (other than *Proteus mirabilis*), *Providencia, Pseudomonas,* and *Serratia.* Second-generation cephalosporins are noted for their increased activity against *Haemophilus influenzae* and may also show some activity against *Acinetobacter, Citrobacter, Enterobacter, E. coli, Serratia, Providencia, Proteus, Neisseria,* and *Klebsiella.* Third-generation cephalosporins show less activity against *Staphylococcus* but much greater activity against gram-negative bacteria.

Bacterial resistance may occur because of decreased permeability of the bacterial cell wall to the antibiotic or because of resistant metabolic pathways. β-Lactamase inactivates the β-lactam ring in the antibiotic neutralizing its action.

### *Aqueous Penetration of Cephalothin*

Intravenous injection of 15 mg of sodium cephalothin/kg produced no measurable primary aqueous drug concentration in rabbits.[151] In secondary aqueous, such an intravenous dosage caused a 15-minute concentration of 2 μg/ml, dropping to 0.8 μg/ml 30 minutes after injection and to 0 μg/ml at 45 minutes. Subconjunctival injection of 50 mg sodium cephalothin produced a primary aqueous concentration of 54 μg/ml at 1 hour, which persisted at a level of 35 μg/ml 4 hours after injection.

Cephalothin penetration into human aqueous was studied by aspiration of secondary aqueous at the time of cataract surgery. Fifteen minutes after an intravenous injection of 1 g of sodium cephalothin, the mean secondary aqueous concentration in 18 patients was 0.55 μg/ml, with a range from 0 to 2.50 μg/ml. After 30 minutes the mean in 18 patients was 0.48 μg/ml, with a range from 0 to 1.00 μg/ml.[152]

Intramuscular injection in rabbits of 150 mg/kg of cephalothin results in primary aqueous levels ranging from 0.2 to 1.0 μg/ml after 45 minutes (Table 6–7).[153]

### *Aqueous Penetration of Cephalexin*

Cephalexin is an orally absorbed derivative of cephalosporin. Given in an oral dose of 2 g to patients before cataract surgery, cephalexin produced primary aqueous levels of 1 to 2 μg/ml 2 to 4 hours after administration. Demonstrable aqueous levels persisted for as long as 12 hours.[154]

### *Aqueous Penetration of Cefonicid*

Patients received 1 g of intravenous cefonicid sodium before cataract surgery with removal of aqueous for measurement. Although serum concentrations were high, the aqueous levels were quite low, in the range of 0.25 and 0.27 mg/L observed at 2 and 4 hours after administration, respectively. For *S. aureus,* MICs are in the range of 3.1 μg/ml for a 50% inactivation of the bacteria.[155] Similarly, cefazolin, which also has high protein binding, delivers very low aqueous humor concentration after intravenous infection.

**TABLE 6–6.**
Classifications of Cephalosporins

| First generation | Second generation | Third generation |
|---|---|---|
| Cefadroxil | Cefaclor | Cefixime |
| Cefazolin | Cefamandole | Ceftizoxime |
| Cephalexin | Cefonicid | Ceftriaxone |
| Cephalothin | Ceforanide | Moxalactam (1-oxa-β-lactam) |
| Cephapirin | Cefotetan (cephamycin) | Cefoperazone |
| Cephradine | Cefoxitin (cephamycin) | Cefotaxime |
| | Cefuroxime | Ceftazidime |

**TABLE 6–7.**
Intraocular Cephalosporin Levels with Systemic Administration[151–163] at Peak Concentrations

| Drug | Dose* | Aqueous (μg/ml) | Dose* | Vitreous (μg/ml) |
|---|---|---|---|---|
| Cephalothin | 1 g IV | 0.55 | 2 g IV | 0.83 |
| Cephalothin | 50 mg SC | 50 | — | — |
| Cefazolin | — | — | 2 g IV | 1.19 |
| Cephaloxin | 2 g po | 1–2 | — | — |
| Cefonicid | 1 g IV | 0.27 | — | — |
| Cefoxitin | 2 g IV | 3.1 | — | — |
| Ceftriaxone | 1 g IV | 0.93 | 1–2 g IM | 11.5 |
| Ceftriaxone | 2 g IV | 2.47 | — | — |
| Ceftazidime | 2 g IV | 3.39 | — | — |
| Cefotaxime | 2 g q8h IV | 0.3–3.8 | — | — |
| Cefuroxime | 1.5 g q8h IV | 2.7–6.0 | — | — |
| Moxalactame | 2 g q8h IV | 2.4–9.5 | 2 g IV | 2.50 |
| Cefamandole | — | — | 2 g IV | 0.94 |

**IV*, Intravenously; *SC*, subcutaneously; *po*, orally; *IM*, intramuscularly.

### *Aqueous Penetration of Cefoxitin*

Intravenous administration of 2 g of cefoxitin in 10 ml of water, given over a 3-minute period before cataract extraction, produced aqueous levels averaging 1.5 μg/ml at 30 minutes, 3.1 μg/ml at 1 hour, 2.4 μg/ml at 2 hours, 1.22 μg/ml at 4 hours, and 0.8 μg/ml at 6 hours.[156] Given orally 30 minutes before the cefoxitin, 500 mg of probenecid did not increase the peak aqueous levels but did prolong these levels for 4 hours (Fig. 6–15). These peak aqueous levels would have been effective against 90% of a group of gram-positive organisms isolated from a series of eye infections but only against 30% of gram-negative organisms. The circumstances of this study of normal cataract eyes do not provide information as to drug penetration into inflamed eyes. The serum levels reported in this study (Fig. 6–16) dropped rapidly, indicating that a prophylactic intravenous antibiotic should be given within 1 hour before surgery if high levels in secondary aqueous are sought.

### *Aqueous Penetration of Ceftriaxone*

One or 2 g of intravenously administered ceftriaxone was given before cataract extraction with intraoperative sampling of aqueous for antibiotic concentration measurement. Levels of 0.93 and 0.88 μg/ml were found 2 and 12 hours after administration, respectively, with the 1-g dose. The 2-g dose increased levels to 2.47 μg/ml 2 hours after administration. These levels are in the MIC range for many gram-positive and gram-negative bacteria. Notable exceptions include *S. aureus, S. epidermidis,* and *P. aeruginosa.*[157]

### *Aqueous Penetration of Ceftazidime*

Ceftazidime, moxalactam, cefotaxime, and cefuroxime were measured in the aqueous humor after intravenous administration in the uninflamed eye during cataract extraction. Levels of each were found in the bactericidal range for most Enterobacteriaceae but not *P. aeruginosa.* Only ceftazi-

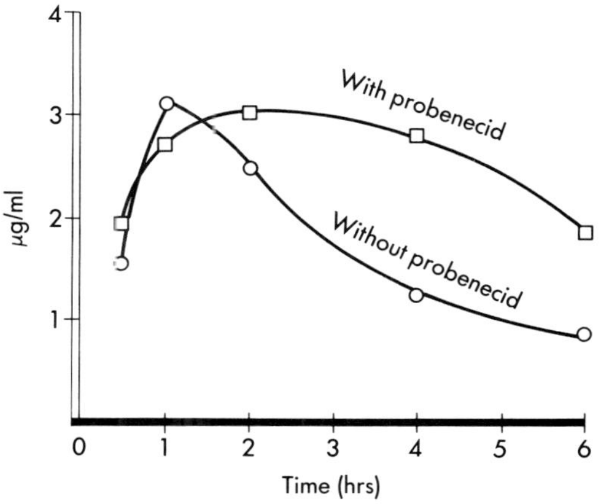


**FIG 6–15.**
Aqueous levels of cefoxitin with and without probenecid. (Modified from Axelrod JL, Kochman RS: *Am J Ophthalmol* 90:388, 1980. Used by permission.)

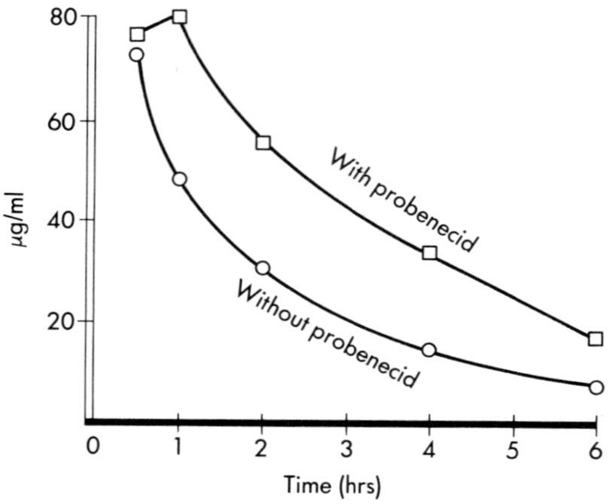


**FIG 6–16.**
Serum levels of cefoxitin with and without probenecid. (Modified from Axelrod JL, Kochman RS: *Am J Ophthalmol* 90:388, 1980. Used by permission.)

dime levels are in a range (peak 3.39 μg/ml) that inhibit a high percentage of *P. aeruginosa* strains based on a better (lower) MIC for ceftazidime for *Pseudomonas* compared with the other antibiotics.[158, 159]

### *Vitreous Penetration of Cephalosporins*

The vitreous is a much better culture medium for bacteria than aqueous humor and is therefore much more important when prophylaxis is considered in treatment of bacterial endophthalmitis. Intravitreous levels of cephalothin, cefazolin, methicillin, oxacillin, and nafcillin were compared in patients undergoing vitrectomy. Of these, only cefazolin produced vitreous concentrations (0.84 μg/ml in diabetics and 1.6 μg/ml in nondiabetics) high enough to achieve MICs for 90% of *S. epidermis* isolates. Even then, *S. aureus* strains were not covered. Patients with proliferative vitreoretinopathy and rubeosis did have higher antibiotic levels. The eyes were not otherwise inflamed, and we might expect higher intravitreous levels in the inflamed eye.[160] Intravenous cefazolin was further investigated by evaluating its intravitreal levels after repeated doses in an inflamed eye. A rabbit model was utilized, and the intraocular inflammation was created using killed *S. epidermidis* organisms. Intravitreal levels were higher in animals with inflamed eyes, as well as in animals that had undergone lensectomy and vitrectomy. The levels increased with repeated antibiotic doses and achieved concentrations well above the MICs for most organisms sensitive to cefazolin (Fig. 6–17).[161, 162]

Intravitreal levels of cefamandole and moxalactam measured in patients undergoing vitrectomy after intravenous administration were not consistently greater than the MIC (90%) for *S. aureus* and *S. epidermidis.* Levels high enough to cover Enterobacteriaceae except *P. aeruginosa* were obtained with moxalactam.[163]

Ceftriaxone may be administered intramuscularly and achieve levels that will exceed the MIC for 90% of *S. aureus,* as well as many gram-negative rods, excluding *P. aeruginosa* and *S. epidermidis.* Intravenous and intramuscular cephalosporin antibiotics play a limited role in the treatment of infectious endophthalmitis. Cefazolin may achieve MICs for important bacteria with repeated intravenous administration. These levels are improved if vitrectomy and lensectomy have been performed and if the eye is inflamed as in the case of an endophthalmitis. Prophylactic intravenous antibiotics are of minimal assistance in the case of a traumatically ruptured eye or intraocular foreign body, where higher intraocular levels can be obtained with subconjunctival or intraocular antibiotics.

### *Subconjunctival Cephalosporins*

Subconjunctival administration of 100 mg of cefsulodin was given to patients undergoing cataract surgery. Aqueous humor concentrations ranged from 32.5 to 99.3 μg/ml, with the highest concentrations present 60 to 90 minutes after subconjunctival administration. Serum levels peaked (1.1 μg/ml) at 90 to 120 minutes after subconjunctival administration. This compares with peak aqueous and serum levels of 0.45 and 9.9 μg/ml with intramuscular injection.[164] Subconjunctival injection of 100 mg of ceftriaxone in phakic and aphakic rabbit eyes achieved aqueous concentrations of 159.5 and 105.1 μg/ml at 1 hour, respectively. The vitreous levels in phakic and aphakic eyes were 25.3 μg/ml at 2 hours and 43.1 μg/ml at 1 hour, respectively. These levels were great enough to sterilize or reduce colony counts when *S. aureus* organisms were administered intravitreally.[165] Subconjunctival cephalosporins may be useful in enhancing surgical prophylaxis as an adjunct to subconjunctival aminoglycosides. Their spectrum of action is variable and in most cases would not be appropriate as a single agent.

***Intravitreal Cephalosporins***

Twenty milligrams of ceftriaxone was tolerated in the vitreous of an albino rabbit eye with only transient electroretinogram (ERG) alterations. Ceftriaxone levels greater than the MIC for *S. aureus* were present for 72 hours after injection of just 2 mg of ceftriaxone. Similar data were found for a 2-mg intravitreal dose of ceftriaxone in a monkey eye.[166] Intravitreal injection of 2.25 mg of cefazolin produced vitreous concentrations exceeding the MIC for *S. aureus* for 5 days.[167]

Intravitreal cephalosporins provide an excellent adjunct to aminoglycosides in the treatment of postoperative endophthalmitis and the prophylaxis of endophthalmitis in intraocular foreign body management. Vancomycin used in a concentration of 1 mg/0.1 ml is a good substitute for a cephalosporin intraocularly when used in combination with aminoglycosides and may provide somewhat better gram-positive coverage. Intravitreal drugs must be used with caution in all cases. A dosing error of 1,000 units may be made if the hospital formulary pharmacy, nurse, or physician confuses micrograms for milligrams. A 10-unit error can be made if there is confusion between 0.1 and 1 ml of solution. Either of these errors can result in blindness because of retinal toxicity or ineffective levels resulting in untreated endophthalmitis (see Table 6-2).

***Topical Cephalosporin***

Cephalosporins are an excellent adjunct to topical aminoglycosides in the treatment of severe infectious keratitis. Solutions should be mixed in concentrations ranging from 33 to 66 mg/ml. Cefazolin is a commonly used drug for this purpose in a dosage of 50 mg/ml alternating with an aminoglycoside every ½ hour around the clock for a severe bacterial corneal ulcer. Vancomycin may be substituted for the cephalosporin to achieve better gram-positive coverage. The vancomycin concen-

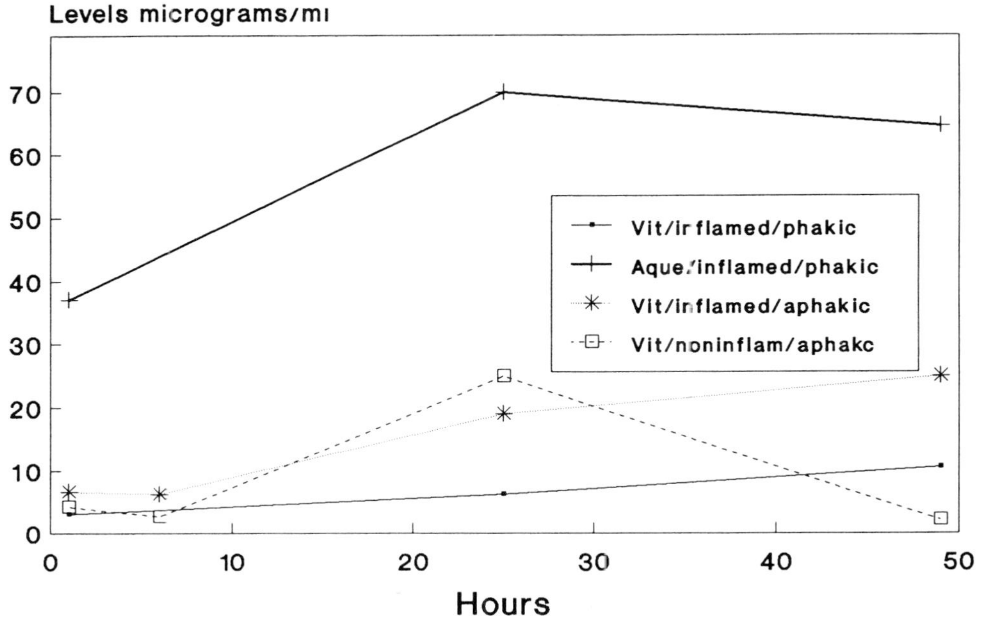


**FIG 6–17.**
Aqueous and vitreous levels in rabbits after intravenous administration of intraocular cefazolin in aphakic and phakic eyes with and without experimentally created inflammation. (Modified from Fricker L, Meredith TA, Gardner S, and others: *Invest Ophthalmol Vis Sci* 31:502, 1990. Used by permission.)

tration is also 50 mg/ml. Ciprofloxacin, with good gram-positive and gram-negative coverage, has been advocated as a single agent in the treatment of corneal ulcers. Streptococcal coverage is not as effective with ciprofloxacin compared with the cephalosporins.

#### *Toxicity*

Renal damage may result from dosages of cephaloridine in excess of 4 g/day, so its use is no longer recommended. Cephaloridine is particularly contraindicated for use with the nephrotoxic aminoglycosides.

Pseudomembranous colitis resulting from clostridial overgrowth occurs most often with clindamycin but also occurs with cephalosporins, ampicillin, chloramphenicol, and tetracyclines. A fatal case was caused by only 5 g of cephaloridine.[168] Diarrhea occurs in 20% to 30% of patients receiving cephalosporins but usually resolves spontaneously when treatment is stopped.

Clostridia were identified in all of a series of 17 patients in whom pseudomembranous colitis had developed after only cephalosporin use.[169] Oral vancomycin, 0.5 to 2.0 g daily, eradicated the clostridia in nine treated cases. Another treatment is to bind the toxin by oral administration of a cholestyramine resin.

By killing intestinal flora, cephalosporins may induce vitamin K deficiency.[170] Replacement therapy with vitamin K is effective.

Disulfiram-like (Antabuse) reactions may occur when alcohol is ingested even 2 days later because of inhibition of acetaldehyde dehydrogenase and the consequent increase in acetaldehyde concentrations. Moxalactam, cefamandole, and cefoperazone have this effect because of a specific side chain.[171]

Mild allergic reactions and rarely fatal anaphylaxis may occur with cephalosporins. Between 5% and 20% of patients with penicillin allergy may be cross-allergic to cephalosporins. Cephalosporins should be used with great caution in patients severely allergic to penicillin.

Penicillin and cephalosporin allergies may be transferred passively by blood transfusions.[172]

False positive test results for elevated creatinine levels result from cefoxitin.[173] This may lead to the erroneous conclusion that severe renal damage has occurred. Because cephalosporins are excreted in the urine, cefoxitin will be retained in the body for many hours by patients in renal failure, thereby rendering creatinine test results unreliable.

#### *Summary*

The cephalosporins are useful adjuvants to other antibiotics (aminoglycosides) in the treatment of severe ocular infections, including infectious keratitis and endophthalmitis. Their spectrum of action limits their use as a single agent for most ophthalmic purposes. Therapeutic intraocular levels have been obtained with several modes of delivery, notably subconjunctival and intravitreal injections.

### Imipenem

Imipenem is a carbapenem β-lactam antibiotic with the broadest antimicrobial spectrum of any other β-lactam antibiotic. Its action is through inhibition of mucopeptide production in the bacterial cell wall. It is bactericidal against many organisms. Imipenem is combined with cilastatin (Primaxin, MSD) for systemic use. Cilastatin inhibits in vivo metabolism of imipenem by dehydropeptidase I in the brush border of the proximal renal tubular cells, increasing urinary concentration of imipenem.

#### *Uses and Dosages*

Imipenem and cilastatin are recommended in treatment of lower respiratory tract, skin, intra-abdominal, gynecologic, bone or joints, and urinary tract infections, as well as septicemia and endocarditis caused by susceptible organisms. Mild infections are treated with 250 to 500 mg every 6 hours intravenously, and severe infections are treated with 500 mg to 1 g every 6 hours, depending on the susceptibility of the organisms. Aqueous and vitreous levels, 2.99 and 2.53 μg/ml, respectively, well above the MIC (90%) for streptococci were achieved 2 to 3 hours after a single 1-g injection of imipenem. Those levels did not exceed the

MIC (90%) of *Pseudomonas* (3.65 μg/ml) and *Proteus* (3.38 μg/ml).[174]

Imipenem's use in ophthalmology is primarily in the treatment of bacterial keratitis and endophthalmitis resistant to conventional therapy. Topical imipenem (5 mg/ml) was found to be effective in the treatment of aminoglycoside-resistant *P. aeruginosa* keratitis in rabbits. Concentrations higher than 5 mg/ml are difficult to achieve because of its solubility characteristics. Aqueous humor concentrations increased tenfold with removal of the corneal epithelium, exceeding the MIC for *P. aeruginosa*.[175]

Intravitreal infusion of imipenem in concentrations of 16 μg/ml or less was found to be nontoxic in rabbit eyes. The authors recommended imipenem infusion in the treatment of endophthalmitis in a concentration of 5 μg/ml.[176]

#### *Toxicity*

Cilastatin apparently decreases the inherent nephrotoxicity of imipenem; significant renal dysfunction is rarely reported, and transient increases in serum creatinine and BUN levels occur in only 2% of patients.

Among the most frequently reported adverse reactions include nausea, diarrhea, and vomiting in 4% of patients. Pseudomembraneous colitis *(Clostridium difficile)* has occurred in less than 0.2% of patients.

### Bacitracin

Bacitracin is a bactericidal antibiotic with a range of activity closely resembling that of penicillin. Its mechanism of action is interference with bacterial cell wall synthesis (see Table 6-5). It is active chiefly against gram-positive organisms but also affects spirochetes, gonococci, *Entamoeba histolytica,* and *Actinomyces.* Bacitracin is ineffective against gram-negative bacilli. Most gram-positive organisms are inhibited by 0.001 to 0.5 U/ml of the drug. Strains of bacteria resistant to bacitracin are much less frequently encountered than with penicillin. Of 36 strains of organisms with different resistances to penicillin and to bacitracin, 30 were more resistant to penicillin and 6 to bacitracin.[177] Bacitracin is not inactivated by blood, pus, necrotic tissue, or bacterial enzymes such as penicillinase.

#### *Clinical Use*

Concentrations of 500 to 1,000 U/g are nonirritating to the eye and other tissues and cause no undesirable systemic effects. Bacitracin does not penetrate the cornea in therapeutic amounts. It is not absorbed from the GI tract but may be given orally in treatment of intestinal infections such as *E. histolytica.* Parenteral administration may achieve effective systemic antibacterial concentrations but can damage renal tubules in doses greater than 200 to 400 U/kg. Because of this systemic toxicity, use of bacitracin is ordinarily confined to topical application. Topical bacitracin is quite effective in treatment of surface ocular infections[178] and is commonly used for this purpose.

Although bacitracin solutions are unstable, reasonable potency may be maintained for 3 weeks if the solution is refrigerated. The dry powder and ointment preparations are stable for more than 1 year at room temperature.

#### *Summary*

Although the antibacterial spectrum of bacitracin is comparable with that of penicillin for topical ocular use, bacitracin is preferable to penicillin because fewer strains of organisms are resistant, allergy is less frequent, and sensitization that prevents future use of penicillin is avoided.

### Gramicidin

Gramicidin has a spectrum of activity similar to bacitracin. It acts through altering cell wall permeability. Like bacitracin, its role is limited to topical use because of systemic toxicity. Gramicidin causes hemolytic anemia when given systemically. It is used in combination with polymixin B and neomycin in solution to treat bacterial conjunctivitis and blepharitis. Bacitracin is substituted for gramicidin in the combination ointment. These combination topical antibiotics are uniquely suited for ophthalmic use because resistance to systemic drugs will not develop as a result of their use.

## Chloramphenicol

### *Antimicrobial Spectrum*

Chloramphenicol has a broad antimicrobial spectrum, being effective against a wide variety of gram-positive and gram-negative organisms, *Chlamydia, Mycoplasma, Rickettsia,*[179] and spirochetes.[180] For example, the majority of strains of the following organisms were sensitive to less than 16 μg/ml of chloramphenicol: *Aerobacter aerogenes, Bacillus anthracis, B. subtilis, Brucella, Clostridium, Corynebacterium diphtheriae, E. coli, Haemophilus, Klebsiella, Staphylococcus* (*S. aureus,* as well as *S. albus*), *Neisseria, Pasteurella, Shigella,* and *Streptococcus.* An organism of considerable ocular significance, *P. aeruginosa,* was quite resistant, 139 of 212 strains not being destroyed by 75 μg/ml. Because great variations occur in the sensitivity of various strains of organisms, general summaries cannot be relied on. Rather, the sensitivity of the organisms responsible for a given infection must be determined, if possible.

### *Mechanism of Action*

Chloramphenicol acts by reversible binding to bacterial ribosomes and the inhibition of protein synthesis. Because of this reversibility, the drug is bacteriostatic rather than bactericidal. Chloramphenicol binding is inhibited by erythromycin, lincomycin, and clindamycin. The drug is primarily (90%) inactivated by the liver.[181]

### *Intraocular Penetration*

The ether/water partition coefficient indicates the relative solubility of a drug in lipids or water. The ether/water coefficient of penicillin is 0.0004, whereas that of chloramphenicol is 4.25. In other words, chloramphenicol is 10,000 times more fat soluble than penicillin. Its high differential solubility results in a superior intraocular penetration of chloramphenicol.[182]

The aqueous penetration of intravenously administered chloramphenicol has been studied in rabbits.[183] One hour after intravenous injection of 50 mg/kg of chloramphenicol, the serum concentration was 12 μg/ml and the aqueous concentration was 6 μg/ml. At this time no measurable concentration was detected in the vitreous. This finding suggests that aqueous penetration may be comparable to cerebrospinal fluid penetration (values approximately half of those found in the serum).

After systemic administration, chloramphenicol penetrates the eye more readily than do penicillin, streptomycin, chlortetracycline (Aureomycin), and oxytetracycline (Terramycin).[184–186] Such drugs enter the eye in much higher than normal concentration when the barriers are destroyed by surgery or paracentesis. Ideally, therefore, antibiotics should be given promptly after injury or shortly (several hours) before surgery.

Primary aqueous levels of 5 to 10 μg/ml were achieved in rabbits after subconjunctival injection of 10 mg/ml of chloramphenicol succinate.[187] These levels persisted 1 to 4 hours after injection. Intraperitoneal injection of probenecid 30 minutes before the subconjunctival chloramphenicol injection increased the chloramphenicol aqueous levels to 20 μg/ml. (Probenecid may block the active transport of antibiotics out of the eye, just as it blocks the kidney and the cerebrospinal transport system. Its mechanism of action is inhibition of organic acid transport, which is accomplished by competition for carrier systems.) Although these aqueous concentrations of antibiotic are very high, rabbits have an increased metabolic capacity to destroy chloramphenicol. Consequently, for a rabbit study to be analogous to the human situation, a rabbit must be given 20 times the human dosage of chloramphenicol. Thus, it may be inferred that a much greater intraocular penetration than reported in this experiment would be seen in humans.

Aqueous chloramphenicol levels of 3 to 6 μg/ml are present 2 hours after topical administration of 0.5% drops every 5 minutes for six doses. Demonstrable antibiotic persisted for 5 hours after drug administration. This study was performed in 18 patients undergoing cataract surgery.[188]

The superiority of an ointment vehicle has been dramatically demonstrated in both rabbit and human experiments. A single application of 0.1 ml of 1% ointment delivers 0.1 mg of drug to the ocular surface. In rabbits, the eyes were taped shut after instillation of a single dose of 1% chloramphenicol ointment. Within ½ hour, an aqueous concentration of 5 μg/ml was measured. Peak aqueous levels were reached at 2 hours, measuring 25 to 35 μg/ml. By 4 hours, the aqueous level had dropped to 5 mg/ml.[189] Aqueous levels of only 2 μg/ml were attainable by intravenous injection of 100 mg of chloramphenicol/kg. (A higher dose of 150 mg/kg caused convulsions and death within ½ hour.) Subconjunctival injection of 10 mg of chloramphenicol in polyethylene glycol gave aqueous concentrations similar to those attained by the single ointment instillation. Injection of chloramphenicol succinate was severely irritating for several days after the subconjunctival injection.

Study of 183 patients receiving chloramphenicol before cataract surgery confirmed the effectiveness of an ointment vehicle. Application of 1% chloramphenicol ointment every ½ hour for four doses resulted in human aqueous levels higher than 60 μg/ml. A single ointment application was not nearly as effective, attaining only 1 to 2 μg/ml at 2 hours. To achieve the same level as a single ointment application required 13 instillations of 0.5% chloramphenicol drops given at 15-minute intervals or 6 instillations at 5-minute intervals. A side effect to the use of chloramphenicol ointment is an intensely bitter, burning taste noted several minutes after ointment instillation.[190]

These reports uniformly confirm the effective entry of chloramphenicol into the eye. Human anterior chamber levels greater than 60 μg/ml are consistently attainable by 1% ointment instillation every ½ hour. An inference from rabbit experiments is that patching the eye will prolong the presence of the ointment by preventing the lacrimal pump action of blinking.

***Systemic Dosage***

Blood levels of chloramphenicol in excess of 15 μg/ml are easily attained in humans. The usual dosage for adults is 3 to 5 g/day, administered in divided doses every 4 hours. Chloramphenicol is readily absorbed from the GI tract, producing a peak blood level at 2 hours and declining to insignificant levels by 8 hours. Rapid renal excretion and hepatic metabolism occur.

If an immediate, high blood level is desirable, an initial dose of 3 g may be given. Oral dosage produces concentrations comparable with the intravenous route; hence, parenteral administration (intravenous or intramuscular) is indicated only if the patient cannot or should not (e.g., preceding general anesthesia) take the drug by mouth. For intravenous administration, the highly water-soluble sodium succinate derivative is recommended.

If given intramuscularly, the sodium succinate compound is painful and does not produce good antibiotic levels; therefore, the intramuscular route should not be used. The succinate form of chloramphenicol is an inactive prodrug that must be hydrolyzed to the active base.[181]

***Stability and Solubility***

Chloramphenicol is a fairly stable compound and will actually resist destruction by boiling for as long as 5 hours. In water at room temperature its solubility is only 0.25%; however, it is readily ether soluble.

***Toxicity***

The lethal dose ($LD_{50}$) for mice is 245 mg/kg. Hence, although recommended doses are well tolerated without acute side effects, the clinician must be aware that unlike penicillin, enormous doses cannot be given with impunity.

***Reaction in Infants***

In high dosage, chloramphenicol causes a typical toxic reaction in infants. This is characterized by abdominal distention, cyanosis, and vasomotor collapse. If high dosage of chloramphenicol is continued, the child may die. This peculiar reaction may be related to the inadequate amount of glucuronyl transferase produced by the immature liver. This transferase is one of the enzymes involved in the detoxification of chloramphenicol. (A genetic enzyme deficiency may be a factor in chloramphenicol-induced aplastic anemia. The only test of predictive value in selecting individuals likely to develop aplastic anemia is the determination of impaired chloramphenicol clearance 4 to 6 hours after an intravenous test dose.[191]) This reaction has not been observed in any infant given divided doses of chloramphenicol not in excess of 50 mg/kg/24 hours. Half this dose is advised for premature infants.

***Hematology***

Considerable publicity has been given to the possibility of agranulocytosis resulting from use of chloramphenicol. Although the danger of this complication is not to be underestimated, the benefits of chloramphenicol in treating eye infections (because of its excellent penetration of the blood-aqueous barrier) should not be lost.

Early recognition and proper care of drug-induced agranulocytosis demands careful observation of patients receiving drugs known to cause this condition. Of 830 cases of drug-induced agranulocytosis reported to the Council of Drugs,[192] 56 were attributed to sulfonamides and 370 to phenothiazine tranquilizers.

The mechanism of agranulocytosis may be the formation of antibodies that agglutinate leukocytes in the presence of the drug; hence, the earliest sign is leukopenia. Hematologic recovery begins when the drug is eliminated from the body, usually within 5 to 10 days after it is discontinued. The mortality rate is very low if agranulocytosis is discovered by routine white blood cell count before the development of an infection. The sudden onset of a severe prostrating infection (usually a sore throat) during treatment with chloramphenicol requires immediate evaluation of the possibility of agranulocytosis.

Aplastic anemia of delayed onset, not necessarily dose related, is the most serious complication of chloramphenicol therapy. In a survey of the Registry of Blood Dyscrasias (a series of 284 patients), the median time of onset of blood dyscrasia was found to be 38 days after discontinuation of treatment.[193] Hence, monitoring blood counts during chloramphenicol therapy is of little or no value in preventing mortality.

Unavoidable bias is present in the collection of cases of aplastic anemia with the expectation that a single given factor is responsible, thus complicating a calculation of the true incidence. Statistical studies concerning such rare problems as chloramphenicol-induced aplastic anemia are difficult to undertake and even more difficult to evaluate. For example, all aplastic anemia deaths in California during an 18-month period were studied, with the conclusion that patients receiving 4 g of chloramphenicol had a 13 times greater chance of dying from aplastic anemia than did the population as a whole.[194] Actually, only 60 patients died of aplastic anemia during this period, and only 10 had received chloramphenicol. Three of these had received the drug 8, 9, and 24 months before the onset of anemia. Perusal of the vast amount of data in this article suggests that numerous extrapolations of doubtful validity were made from uncertain data (e.g., physician questionnaires, which are notoriously inaccurate, as any physician who has filled one out will testify.) The frequency of fatal aplastic anemia subsequent to chloramphenicol treatment seems to be in the range of 1 in 50,000 patients.

For some reason, probably a statistical phenomenon, few reports incriminate the intravenous route of chloramphenicol as causing agranulocytosis. This, of course, does not seem logical from a pharmacologic standpoint. A report of prophylactic use of 1 g of intravenous chloramphenicol just before cataract extraction in 520 cases[195] describes a single case of agranulocytosis occurring 5 years after the cataract extraction. One year before the agranulocytosis the patient used phenylbutazone (Butazolidin), another drug associated with agranulocytosis. If we are to be consistent in condemning drugs that may cause agranulocytosis, not only chloramphenicol but also many analgesics and tranquilizers should be avoided, as well as sulfonamide derivatives such as tolbutamide (Orinase).

The National Registry of Drug-Induced Ocular Side Effects is aware of four cases of aplastic anemia after the topical ocular use of chloramphenicol. These have occurred during 30 years of such use. Millions of units of ophthalmic chloramphenicol were marketed during this period. The 1:50,000 risk of oral chloramphenicol-induced aplastic anemia is 13 times greater than the risk of idiopathic aplastic anemia in the general population. Statistically valid proof of a drug-related toxic effect occurring this infrequently would require accurate observation of 1.5 million cases, an impossibility for ocular usage.[196, 197]

A specific case report[196] describes fatal aplastic anemia after use of topical chloramphenicol five times daily for more than 1 month subsequent to cataract extraction. This dosage calculates to a total administration of approximately 0.5 g of chloramphenicol. The patient also took triamterene and phenacetin, both of which cause hematologic defects. Although all these statistics are meaningless with respect to causation of aplastic anemia by the ocular use of chloramphenicol, prophylactic antibiotic use five times daily for 1 month after cataract extraction must be characterized as being excessive.

#### *Optic Atrophy*

Prolonged use of chloramphenicol has been suspected to cause optic atrophy in children. More than 100 g of chloramphenicol (250 mg three times daily) was given prophylactically to two children with cystic fibrosis of the pancreas. Disabling visual loss was recognized after about 4 months of treatment. Histologic study of the optic nerves obtained at autopsy showed marked demyelination of the papillomacular bundle.[198] Such eye changes are infrequent; recognizable bilateral optic neuritis has been reported in only 6 of 200 chloramphenicol-treated patients with cystic fibrosis. Because papilledema may occur in cases of cystic fibrosis with severe pulmonary disease (presumably these patients are antibiotic treated), it is uncertain whether the optic atrophy in these cases was part of the disease or was a manifestation of chloramphenicol toxicity.[199]

In a study of 98 cystic fibrosis patients receiving long-term chloramphenicol therapy (approximately 1964–1969), visual disturbances developed in 13. Characteristically, the visual loss was sudden, bilateral, and associated with an ophthalmoscopic picture of optic neuritis. The condition was dose related, depending on the amount and duration of chloramphenicol therapy. Discontinuance of treatment resulted in a prompt improvement in vision in 11 of 13 patients. Autopsy findings in three patients who had suffered visual disturbances included bilateral optic atrophy with primary involvement of the papillomacular bundle, loss of the retinal ganglion cells, and gliosis of the nerve fiber layer.[200]

Histologic and clinical evidence of optic nerve atrophy was also reported in a case of primary infantile genetic agranulocytosis in which the patient received chloramphenicol for 4 months as treatment for serious infections associated with the primary disease. No other instance of optic neuritis is described in approximately 40 literature reports of this rare disease.[201] Attempts to produce chloramphenicol optic atrophy in rabbits with doses as high as 180 mg/kg for 35 days have been unsuccessful.

Accidental orbital injection of 2 ml of 20% chloramphenicol during intended irrigation of the upper canaliculus for a canalicular obstruction of 4 years' duration caused immediate edema of lid and orbit with limitation of eye movement, corneal edema sufficient to obstruct fundus visualization, and loss of vision to finger counting. No orbital hemorrhage was recognized. Within a few weeks the optic disc became totally atrophic. Occlusion of the central retinal artery by the toxic effect of the concentrated solution of chloramphenicol was invoked as the cause.[202]

#### *Resistant Microflora*

During prolonged therapy with chloramphenicol, as with other antibiotics, superinfection with resistant bacteria and fungi may develop in the GI tract and elsewhere.[181]

#### *Clinical Use*

Because of the potential toxicity of chloramphenicol, it should not be used systemically for trivial infections, nor should it be used for serious infections in which less toxic antibacterial drugs are equally effective. Chloramphenicol should usually be employed only after the causative organism has been isolated and determined to be sensitive to the drug. It should not be used without the precaution of frequent blood counts (every other day has been suggested if usage is prolonged, although the practicability of the recommendation may be questioned) and evaluation of the patient for acute infections, which may herald agranulocytosis.[203]

Topical application of chloramphenicol ointment (1%) or solution (0.2%) was well tolerated by human eyes in more than 200 cases with virtually no evidence of irritation or discomfort.[204] The drug was very effective against the majority of surface bacterial infections but did not alter the course of herpes simplex keratitis or epidemic keratoconjunctivitis. No instance of toxic or allergic local reaction was encountered. Comparable results were obtained with the use of 0.5% chloramphenicol solution in 46 cases of superficial ocular infection.[205]

Chloramphenicol is reported to be an effective drug against trachoma. All of a series of 19 Navajo Indians were cured by 1 g/day. An average of nine daily doses was required for cure. No topical medications were used.[206] Treatment of trachoma may be stopped when the cornea is cleared. Disappearance of the conjunctival follicular changes requires more time than does corneal clearing but will spontaneously improve without further antibiotic therapy.[207]

It is likely that antibiotics eliminate only the secondary bacterial agents that complicate trachoma. Chloramphenicol topical drops (0.25% concentration three times daily), ointment (1% concentration nightly), and oral capsules (1 g every day) used concurrently resulted in complete clearance of secondary infection in 2 to 3 days and considerably relieved all symptoms. However, in only 19 of these 60 patients did the inclusion bodies disappear and the pannus regress. Similar results were obtained after therapy with oxytetracycline, chlortetracycline, and erythromycin. A 30% solution of sulfacetamide applied four times daily was more effective, clearing inclusion bodies in 51 of 70 cases, but in this series, treatment was continued for 6 weeks.[208]

Silicone rubber is permeable to chloramphenicol. An experimental silicone implant for retinal detachment surgery was expanded by injecting into it a 25% chloramphenicol sodium succinate solution. When the animals were killed, as long as 2½ months later, inhibitory concentrations of chloramphenicol were found within the tissue specimens just external to the implant.[209]

***Summary***

Systemic and topical chloramphenicol has been supplanted by the cephalosporins, aminoglycosides, and quinolones in the treatment of severe ocular infections.

## Clindamycin

Clindamycin is a chlorinated analog of lincomycin. It is effective against both gram-positive and gram-negative microorganisms. Of particular interest to the ophthalmologist, clindamycin is effective against toxoplasmosis (and also against malaria).

Topical instillation of 1 drop of 0.2% clindamycin hydrochloride every 15 minutes resulted in average corneal concentrations of 26 μg/ml; aqueous concentrations of 6 μg/ml, and iris and ciliary body concentrations of 6 μg/ml when measured 50 minutes after the last dose. Two hours after the last dose, the average corneal concentration was still 20 μg/ml. If the 6 drops were given every 30 minutes, the drug levels were only half as high. The 0.2% clindamycin hydrochloride was well tolerated, without any toxicity.[210]

Clindamycin is available as a hydrochloride, phosphate, or palmitate. The hydrochloride form is a biologically active antibiotic. The phosphate and palmitate are prodrugs, requiring enzymatic breakdown in the body before becoming active. The hydrochloride is extremely bitter to taste and excessively irritating when given parenterally. The phosphate may be dispensed as flavored granules for oral use. Clindamycin hydrochloride is the most lipid-soluble form and therefore penetrates the cornea better than the phosphate, achieving aqueous levels twice as high. The eye possesses the enzymes required to activate the phosphate to the hydrochloride form.[211]

Fortunately for the patient with ocular toxoplasmic retinitis, clindamycin is selectively concentrated in the choroid and retina. Thirty minutes after intramuscular injection of 75 mg of clindamycin phosphate/kg in pigmented rabbits, the concentration of clindamycin in the choroid was 87 μg/g, in the retina was 23 μg/g, and in the vitreous was 1.5 μg/ml. After 1 hour these levels were 48 μg/g, 16 μg/g, and 1.2 μg/ml, respectively. After 6 hours they were 110 μg/g, 27 μg/g, and 2.2 μg/ml. Serum levels were only 19 μg/ml at 1 hour and 4.7 μg/ml at 6 hours, indicating a selective affinity for the choroid and retina. Even at 24 hours, choroidal levels were 25 μg/g and retinal levels 3.5 μg/g.[212]

Subconjunctival injection of 150 mg of clindamycin phosphate causes very severe corneal and conjunctival edema and inflammation. Subconjunctival injection of 34 mg did not cause corneal edema and at 3 hours resulted in choroidal concentrations of 152 μg/g, retinal concentrations of 16 μg/g, and vitreous concentrations of 0.9 μg/ml. At 6 hours these values were 91 μg/g, 10 μg/g, and 0.7 μg/ml; at 24 hours they were 39 μg/g, 3 μg/g, and 0.3 μg/ml.[212]

Clindamycin (7-chlorolincomycin) is effective against toxoplasmosis in rabbits. After suprachoroidal injection, active toxoplasmosis retinochoroiditis developed in the rabbits in about 4 days. Retrobulbar injection of 150 mg of clindamycin was given on the first day of recognizable activity, followed by 100 mg/kg/day intramuscularly for 8 days. Three fourths of the treated animals rapidly improved, clearing being evident by the sixth day, and retained normal retinal architecture and function. In contrast, complete disruption of the retina occurred in two thirds of the untreated eyes. No organisms could be recovered from any of the treated eyes, but *Toxoplasma* organisms were demonstrated by fluorescein antibody methods in 80% of the untreated eyes.[213]

Experimental ocular toxoplasmosis in rabbits was produced by injecting 800 organisms into Tenon's space. Retinochoroiditis appeared after 3 to 4 days and spontaneously became inactive within 12 weeks. At the time, 150 mg/kg of clindamycin phosphate was given by sub-Tenon's injection in each eye (note this is four times the intramuscular dose described just previously). On each of the next 8 days, sub-Tenon's injection of 100 mg/kg was given in each eye. Eleven rabbits were so treated; 10 received saline solution injections. Two days after completion of treatment, the rabbits were killed. In 120 histologic sections from control eyes, 46 *Toxoplasma* cysts were found compared with 14 cysts found in 132 sections from treated eyes. Injection of eye tissue into mice permitted *Toxoplasma* recovery from 18% of treated eyes and from 60% of control eyes. These results indicate susceptibility of encysted *Toxoplasma* to clindamycin.[214]

In four human patients with active toxoplasmic retinochoroiditis, 50 mg of clindamycin (form not stated) was injected subconjunctivally every other day for 4 weeks. The condition in all four eyes became inactive during the month of treatment, but in one patient it recurred at the same site 4 months later.[215] Recommended systemic dosage is 300 mg four times daily for 4 to 6 weeks.

#### *Pseudomembranous Colitis*

Most antimicrobial drugs, but especially ampicillin, cephalosporins, and clindamycin, can cause diarrhea. Endoscopic examination of the colon shows a spectrum of findings ranging from normal to pseudomembranous colitis. The responsible organism causing antibiotic-induced colitis is *C. difficile* and anaerobic gram-positive bacillus. This organism produces a specific toxin cytopathic for mucosal cells. This toxin is demonstrable in 25% of patients with antibiotic diarrhea and in most patients with pseudomembrane formation. It is rarely present in other forms of diarrheal disease. An assay for this toxin is clinically available and consists of observing a toxic reaction in cell culture, which is eliminated by specific antitoxin. No other clostridia except the *C. difficile* species produces this toxin, which is so potent that only 10 pg/ml kills cells.[216]

Of five cases of severe pseudomembranous colitis occurring before the cause and treatment were known, two patients died, indicating the serious nature of this antibiotic-induced complication.[217]

***Summary***

Subconjunctival injection of clindamycin may be effective against toxoplasmic retinochoroiditis. Systemic administration of this drug may modify intestinal microflora sufficiently to permit overgrowth of *C. difficile,* the cause of pseudomembranous colitis.

## Erythromycin

Erythromycin is quite similar to penicillin in its effect against gram-positive microorganisms. Staphylococcal resistance to erythromycin develops as readily as it does to penicillin and is related to the frequency of use.[218] Susceptible organisms are inhibited by minimal concentrations of erythromycin ranging from 0.1 to 3 μg/ml.[218, 219] Many species of *Chlamydia,* an organism of particular ocular importance, are susceptible to erythromycin. It is also effective against *Rickettsia, Treponema, Actinomyces, Mycoplasma,* and *Legionella pneumophila.* Inhibition of protein synthesis by microsomal binding is the mechanism of action.[181]

Erythromycin is well tolerated in oral dosage of 200 to 600 mg every 6 hours. The 0.5% ophthalmic ointment is nonirritating. Jaundice and abnormal liver function may occasionally occur during or after erythromycin therapy. Large doses may cause GI irritation with nausea and vomiting.

***Ocular Penetration and Tolerance***

After intravenous injection of 100 mg, erythromycin penetrates poorly into the intact rabbit eye, achieving transient aqueous concentrations of 0.7 μg/ml and vitreous concentrations of 0.1 μg/ml.

Solution concentrations of 2% or less are well tolerated as corneal baths. One hour after a 5-minute bath of the intact rabbit cornea with a 2.5% solution, erythromycin concentrations were as follows: cornea, 9 μg/ml; aqueous, 9 μg/ml; and vitreous, 0.9 μg/ml.

Subconjunctival injection of 20 mg of erythromycin causes chemosis and corneal haze lasting at least 1 week. Subconjunctival injection of 5 mg causes some conjunctival congestion lasting for 2 days but gives remarkably high drug levels: at 1 hour, cornea, 95 μg/mg; aqueous, 59 μg/ml; and vitreous 5 μg/ml; and at 4 hours, cornea, 7 μg/ml; aqueous, 9 μg/ml; and vitreous, 0.3 μg/ml.

Anterior chamber injections of 2.5 mg or more of erythromycin are quite destructive, resulting in prolonged keratitis and iritis. An anterior chamber injection of 1 mg (in 0.1-ml volumes) caused only transient mild iritis.[221]

As is true with other antibiotics, the eye does not tolerate large intravitreal injections of erythromycin. In rabbits, intravitreal injection of erythromycin gluceptate (0.1-ml volume, no preservative) resulted in total retinal atrophy and cataract formation when doses greater than 500 μg were administered.[222] After a 500-μg dose, effective antibacterial levels (24 μg/ml) were still present after 24 hours, but no antibiotic was detectable after 48 hours.

Treatment with 500 μg of intravitreal erythromycin was effective in preserving an intact retina in five of 11 rabbits infected by 1,500 *S. aureus* organisms by intravitreal injection 12 hours or less before the antibiotic was given. Even though these infected eyes showed no vitreous haze or abscess formation as late as 24 hours after infection, these eyes could not be saved by antibiotic. Severe endophthalmitis was recognizable by 48 hours after injection. The clinical implication of this study is that antibiotic therapy may be too late to be effective by the time an injured or operated eye is recognized to be infected with a highly virulent microorganism.

***Clinical Use***

Erythromycin alone has a much more limited antibacterial spectrum than most combination topical antibiotics now in common use for eye infections. It is certainly not the drug of choice for treatment of an ocular infection of unknown etiology.

Twenty-one Arizona Indian children with early trachoma (stages 1, 2, and 3) were treated with oral dosages of erythromycin, 2 to 3 mg/lb, every 4 to 6 hours. No local medication was used. At least 12 days of therapy were recommended, because recurrences were noted with shorter courses. Usually within 5 days the mononuclear cells and inclusion bodies characteristic of trachomatous exudate cleared, and the clinically evident conjunctivitis subsided. Follicles and pannus persisted for some time after the cytologic findings had become normal and the conjunctivitis had disappeared. There was no relapse among the 21 patients during an 8-month follow-up period.

Nongonococcal urethritis occurs in at least 2.5 million U.S. citizens annually, and *C. trachomatis* is recovered from two thirds of these cases. Newborn infants from these parents develop chlamydial conjunctivitis, pneumonia, and enteritis. Traditional treatment of this form of ophthalmia neonatorum has been topical erythromycin or tetracycline. Such management is inadequate to remedy the associated relatively asymptomatic but potentially serious pulmonary and enteric infections, which require systemic treatment with erythromycin or tetracycline. (Tetracyclines cause permanent discoloration of developing teeth.[223]) The pediatric oral dose of erythromycin is 30 to 50 mg/kg daily in four divided doses. The adult dose is 4 g daily in divided doses.

#### *Summary*

Erythromycin has a limited antibacterial spectrum somewhat comparable with that of penicillin. Staphylococcal resistance readily develops. The main indication for ophthalmic use is a sensitivity study that reveals it to be effective against the infecting organisms. Erythromycin is well tolerated and relatively nontoxic.

### Isoniazid

Isoniazid (isonicotinic acid hydrazide) has proved to be an effective antituberculous agent without significant toxicity. Oral dosage is 4 to 5 mg/kg/day (100 mg every 6 hours for an average adult). Peak plasma levels appear within 1½ hours after oral administration of isoniazid. Excretion is mainly renal and is fairly complete within 24 hours. Topical ocular application of a 10% solution or ointment is well tolerated, as is subconjunctival injection of 10 to 20 mg.

Isoniazid is completely ineffective against the common bacteria and viruses, but concentrations as low as 0.02 μg/ml are bacteriostatic for *Mycobacterium tuberculosis*. Corneal penetration of isoniazid is good, and aqueous concentrations are adequate for bacteriostasis by any route of administration.[224] Concentrations of 5 μg/ml are attained by oral and intramuscular administration and by hourly topical application of 10% drops. Topical application of 10% ointment and subconjunctival injection will give aqueous levels as high as 30 μg/ml. All ocular tissues, including sclera, are penetrated rapidly by isoniazid. Posterior segment concentrations obtained by systemic routes are higher than those achieved by topical administration.

#### *Clinical Use*

Isoniazid has been shown to inhibit the progress of experimental tuberculosis (human and bovine) infection of rabbit eyes.[224] Massive inoculations led to loss of the eye despite treatment, but 2½ months of isoniazid therapy cured rabbits infected with lesser doses of bacilli. It should be emphasized that in these known tuberculous infections, clinical improvement was not noted until after 3 weeks of therapy, and 2 to 3 months elapsed before clinical cure. Combination therapy with isoniazid, streptomycin, and *p*-aminosalicylic acid seemed more effective than use of any one of the drugs alone. Combination therapy with isoniazid and rifampin is said to be bactericidal instead of merely bacteriostatic.[181] Other research has confirmed the beneficial effect of isoniazid in cases of ocular tuberculosis.[224]

Clinical evaluation of the antituberculous drugs is severely handicapped by the difficulty of obtaining a definite etiologic diagnosis. The problem is compounded by the fact that spontaneous subsidence of uveitis may occur within the 1 to 3 months known to be required for an isoniazid cure of tuberculosis.

Excellent response, with less residual scarring and atrophy, is reported in the treatment of presumed tuberculous uveitis by a combination of cortisone and isoniazid.[225] Improvement was often noted in 1 week compared with 3 weeks without cortisone. This may be explained by corticosteroid inhabitation of inflammation, permitting the antituberculous medications to act more effectively. An alternative explanation is that in these cases, tuberculous infection of the eye is not actually the cause. If corticosteroids are used in the treatment of uveitis (or for other purposes), the physician should order chest x-ray examinations to rule out active pulmonary disease.

Unfortunately, resistance of tubercle bacilli to isoniazid develops rapidly. Before isoniazid therapy, 97% of the strains of tubercle bacilli were found to be susceptible to this drug. After 12 to 14 weeks of therapy, 70% to 80% had become resistant. This resistance persisted long after cessation of treatment.[226] The development of resistant strains is significantly delayed by the use of combinations of antituberculous drugs; hence, such combined use is strongly recommended (e.g., streptomycin, 1 g twice weekly; *p*-aminosalicylic acid, 12–15 g/day; and isoniazid, 4 mg/kg/day).

#### *Toxicity*

Isoniazid can cause severe hepatic damage that may result in chronic scarring of the liver or may even be fatal. In a series of 1,000 patients started on 1-year therapy for tuberculosis, monthly aspartate aminotransferase enzyme testing was performed as a measure of liver function. Enzyme elevations higher than five times normal occurred in 64 patients, 47 of whom were clinically asymptomatic. Isoniazid was discontinued in all 64 patients. With this precaution, no patient had severe liver disease develop or died from hepatic causes. In contrast, studies of patients without such monitoring of liver function report 1% to 2% incidence of severe liver disease with 10% mortality in these patients.[227]

The combination of isoniazid and ethambutol is not uncommonly used in antituberculous treatment. Both drugs interfere with enzyme functions. A case of bilateral retrobulbar neuropathy with central scotomata has been reported as a complication of such combined therapy. Improvement in vision occurred after the medications were discontinued.[228]

Isoniazid increases the excretion of pyridoxine, which is an essential coenzyme for glutamic acid decarboxylase and γ-animobutyric acid transaminase. Malfunctioning of these enzymes causes peripheral neuritis and convulsions. Such convulsions are not responsive to diazepam, phenobarbital, or phenytoin but can be stopped within 2 hours by pyridoxine treatment. The pyridoxine is given in a dosage of equal weight to the isoniazid.[229]

Peripheral neuritis occurs in 10% of patients receiving 10 mg/kg of isoniazid and may not be completely reversible. Prophylactic dosage of 50 mg of pyridoxine daily may prevent this complication.[181]

### Lincomycin

Lincomycin is the parent compound from which clindamycin is derived by chlorination. Clindamycin is better absorbed, less toxic, and more potent than lincomycin and is the preferred drug. Cross-resistance between these drugs and erythromycin can develop.[181]

Lincomycin is bactericidal against a wide range of gram-positive organisms but is ineffective against most gram-negative microorganisms. It may be given orally or parenterally in a dosage of 500 mg, which will result in effective serum levels lasting for as long as 6 hours (oral) or 20 hours (intramuscular).[230] Except for diarrhea that occurs in 10% of patients, few significant side effects have been reported.

The general term "antibiotic-associated colitis" is applicable to this type of diarrhea. It is caused by overgrowth of resistant organisms, notably *C. difficile,* and may be extremely severe. The onset of severe diarrhea is an indication for stopping the antibiotic and starting treatment with vancomycin (500 mg every 6 hours), to which *C. difficile* is highly sensitive.

#### *Aqueous Penetration*

Intramuscular injection of 600 mg of lincomycin several hours before cataract surgery results in primary aqueous levels of 1 to 2 μg/ml. These levels in uninflamed human eyes indicate that therapeutic amounts of lincomycin do enter the eye (1 mg/ml will inhibit most pneumococci and streptococci, and 2 μg/ml will inhibit 90% of staphylococci).[231, 232] Comparable levels were achieved in rabbit studies.[233]

Removal of the corneal epithelium greatly enhances penetration of topically applied lincomycin. Instillation of 1 drop of a 1% solution every 5 minutes for five doses resulted in rabbit aqueous levels of 2 to 4 μg/ml at times between 20 to 60 minutes. A similar dosage after removal of the corneal epithelium increased the aqueous levels to greater than 40 μg/ml.[234] The intravitreal half-life of lincomycin injected directly into the vitreous body was approximately 3 hours, the same as that of clindamycin.

During a cataract extraction a syringe containing α-chymotrypsin and another containing 300 mg of lincomycin in 1 ml of solution were inadvertently transposed. The lincomycin was injected into the posterior chamber, the customary site for use of α-chymotrypsin. When the error was discovered, the eye was irrigated with 2.5 ml of balanced saline solution and then with α-chymotrypsin. On the first postoperative day the patient had eyelid swelling, conjunctival chemosis, and 2+ aqueous flare and cells. After 2 weeks of corticosteroid therapy the ocular reaction subsided. The final corrected vision was 20/25.[235]

## Polymyxin B

Polymyxin B is bactericidal against most gram-negative microorganisms. For example, *E. coli, P. aeruginosa, A. aerogenes, Klebsiella pneumoniae,* and *H. influenzae* may be sensitive to polymyxin B concentrations ranging from 0.05 to 2 μg/ml. Sensitive organisms are unlikely to develop resistance. *Proteus vulgaris* is usually resistant to polymyxin B.

Polymyxin B is not absorbed from the GI tract, will not readily pass the blood-brain and blood-aqueous barriers, and does not penetrate the intact cornea after topical application. Renal tubular epithelial damage and neurotoxicity are caused by parenteral dosage in excess of 2.5 mg/kg/day. If systemic use is indicated, 1.5 to 2.5 mg/kg/day is the recommended dose. If systemic use is indicated, 1.5 to 2.5 mg/kg/day is given intramuscularly in divided doses every 8 hours. Laboratory tests subsequent to the administration of polymyxin B should include BUN and albuminuria determinations. Polymyxin B solutions are stable for at least 6 months if refrigerated.

### *Ocular Tolerance*

Concentrations of 0.25% (2.5 mg/ml) are nonirritating and may be used for topical application; hence, polymyxin B can be applied to tissues in concentrations 1,000 times greater than that required to destroy sensitive organisms. Concentrations as high as 1% cause ocular irritation. The subconjunctival injection of 10 mg of polymyxin B produced severe chemosis, localized necrosis, and bloody discharge in rabbits.[236] Subconjunctival injection of 0.5 mg was fairly well tolerated.

Currently available ophthalmic ointments contain 0 2% polymyxin B (1 mg of purified drug contains 10,000 units).

### *Ocular Penetration*

Although the intact corneal epithelium prevents penetration of polymyxin B into the corneal stroma, therapeutic concentrations do enter the stroma after epithelial damage.[237] Good stromal penetration occurs after epithelial abrasion whether drug application is by topical instillation, subconjunctival injection, or corneal bath. The greatly enhanced penetration seen after epithelial removal suggests such a step in the clinical treatment of infectious corneal ulcers. In addition, tissue obtained by curettement of the loose epithelium surrounding a corneal ulcer would be most likely to contain the infecting organisms and would therefore be ideal material for culture and staining.

No significant polymyxin B penetration into the vitreous is demonstrable after parenteral or local administration of the drug.

### *Use in Treatment of Corneal Ulcers Caused by* Pseudomonas

Corneal ulcers resulting from *Pseudomonas* infection are rapidly progressive and highly destructive. In 96 such infections reviewed in the literature, 45 eyes were lost (evisceration or enucleation), and only 10 eyes retained vision better than 6/60. Two patients treated with polymyxin B regained 6/9 vision.[237]

Treatment of experimental corneal ulcers caused by *Pseudomonas* infection with subconjunctival injections of polymyxin B gave good results, with relatively clear corneas, if therapy was started within 18 hours of infection. When therapy was delayed for 48 hours, the infection could be controlled, but dense stromal scarring resulted.[236] Comparable results are reported by other investigators.[238] Secondary bacterial contamination of ulcers resulting from *Pseudomonas* infection can readily occur.[237] The antibacterial spectrum of polymyxin B does not include many gram-positive organisms. Repeated cultures taken during the course of therapy will detect such secondary invaders and will serve as a check on the sterilization of the ulcer. The concomitant prophylactic use of other antibiotics effective against gram-positive bacteria (e.g., bacitracin and neomycin) seems logical and desirable.

Because of the great importance of early treatment, serious corneal ulcers should be treated with broad-spectrum antibiotics immediately, before culture and sensitivity results are available. The Gram stain is an unreliable predictor of the actual pathogen, and the antibiotic spectrum should not be limited based on its results.

#### *Polymyxin B and Trimethoprim Combination*

In 1989 combination polymyxin B and trimethoprim ophthalmic solution (Polytrim) was introduced for the treatment of bacterial conjunctivitis and blepharitis. Trimethoprim inhibits bacterial dihydrofolate reductase necessary for folate synthesis in bacteria. This combination covers most gram-negative organisms via polymyxin B and the gram-positive organisms are covered by trimethoprim. This alternative avoids the development of resistance that can affect the therapeutic spectrum of important systemic antibiotics such as the aminoglycosides.

#### *Summary*

Polymyxin B is effective against gram-negative organisms. Topical application achieves effective corneal stromal concentrations if the epithelium is not intact. Adequate intraocular concentrations of polymyxin B cannot be produced by topical or parenteral administration. Parenteral administration may seriously damage the kidneys and the central nervous system. Polymyxin B is best used topically in combination with an antibiotic with a good gram-positive spectrum.

### Quinolones

Quinolone anti-infective drugs exert their activity through inhibition of DNA-gyrase in susceptible organisms, preventing bacterial DNA replication. Quinolones are valuable antibiotics because of their unique antibacterial mechanism, leading to a broad spectrum of activity, including organisms that are resistant to other drugs, such as aminoglycosides and cephalosporins. The original quinolone antibiotic was nalidixic acid, synthesized in the early 1960s. Fluoroquinolones were created by the presence of fluorine at position 6 on the molecule. The fluoroquinolone antibiotics have a greater spectrum of action than nalidixic acid.

#### *Nalidixic Acid*

Nalidixic acid has a limited activity, including some *Proteus* species, *E. coli, Enterobacter, Klebsiella,* and some strains of *Salmonella* and *Shigella.* Notably nalidixic acid is not active against *Pseudomonas* or *S. aureus.* Nalidixic acid has limited clinical use, reserved mainly for urinary tract infections resistant to other standard antibiotics. Other nonfluorinated quinolones include cinoxacin and oxolinic acid. These two also have limited spectrum of antibacterial activity.

#### *Fluoroquinolones*

Fluoroquinolones have an expanded antibacterial spectrum. This group of antibiotics is characterized by a fluorine at position 6 of the four quinolone nucleus. This generally conveys both improved gram-negative and gram-positive spectrum.

#### *Ciprofloxacin*

Ciprofloxacin hydrochloride may be used either orally or topically and ciprofloxacin lactate may be used in intravenous infusion. Ciprofloxacin inhibits DNA-gyrase necessary for bacterial DNA replication and also certain aspects of transcription, repair, recombination, and transposition in susceptible bacteria. Ciprofloxacin has been approved by the FDA for use as a single agent in treatment of bacterial corneal ulcers and conjunctivitis (Ciloxan). Its spectrum of action includes most aerobic gram-negative organisms, as well as *S. aureus* and *S. epidermidis.* It has variable activity against streptococcal organisms including *S. pyogenes,* hemolytic *Streptococcus* groups B, C, F, and G, *S. pneumoniae,* and *S. faecalis.* Resistant organisms include anaerobic cocci, *Clostridium* species, and *Bacteroides* species.

Ciprofloxacin was studied for the use and treatment of bacterial conjunctivitis. Two hundred and eighty-eight cases of culture-proven bacterial conjunctivitis were randomized between 0.3% ciprofloxacin, 0.3% tobramycin, and placebo. A reduction or elimination of bacterial pathogens was found in 93.6% to 94.5% of patients using ciprofloxacin and 0.5% on the placebo and 91.9% using tobramycin. Of the nine cases of *Streptococcus* pneumonia bacterial conjunctivitis, seven showed elimination of organism after treatment, and two were unaffected by treatment. Other *Streptococcus* species also showed variable efficacy. Ciprofloxacin was 100% effective in total eradication of gram-negative organisms causing conjunctivitis. This study proved that ciprofloxacin was of similar efficacy as tobramycin in the treatment of bacterial conjunctivitis. Unfortunately, this study did not compare ciprofloxacin with other more commonly used broad-spectrum antibiotics such as sulfacetamide, erythromycin, and combination antibiotics such as polymyxin B–trimethoprim and neomycin-polymyxin B–gramicidin/bacitracin. These drugs may have the advantage of better streptococcal coverage along with lower overall cost.[239]

Ciprofloxacin may be used as single agent in the treatment of bacterial keratitis. A study of 148 cases of culture-proven bacterial keratitis showed that ciprofloxacin gave results similar to that with using combination fortified cefazolin and fortified gentamicin or tobramycin. Although less than 10% of the cases of bacterial keratitis in this study were caused by *S. pneumoniae* (13), this organism represented 25% of the clinical failures of ciprofloxacin treatment. A white precipitate in the anterior cornea developed in 16.3% of patients on topical ciprofloxacin therapy. In one case the medication was discontinued because of the severe nature of this white precipitate. In other cases, the medication was tapered after the infection cleared and the precipitates also slowly dissolved. These opacities appear to be granular or crystalline in nature and are more frequent in elderly patients. The precipitate appears to be crystallized ciprofloxacin.[240]

The benefits of substituting a commercially prepared single agent such as a fluoroquinolone for the currently used dual-fortified antibiotic regimen for the treatment of bacterial corneal ulcers include decreased chance of contamination compared with nonpreserved solutions, miscalculation of concentrations, and also increased patient compliance. The potential disadvantages include the possibility of insufficient antibacterial coverage and allergic reaction and direct toxicity to the preservative in the commercially prepared antibiotic.

Collagen shields may be used to apply ciprofloxacin, as well as other antibiotics, to the eye in the treatment of corneal ulcers. Not surprisingly, ciprofloxacin applied in a collagen shield or as drops was more effective than tobramycin similarly delivered in the treatment of experimental tobramycin-resistant *Pseudomonas* keratitis. Ciprofloxacin was somewhat more effective in reducing colony counts than its related fluoroquinolone norfloxacin. Care must be taken in the concentration used to hydrate collagen shields because epithelial damage has occurred with collagen shields soaked in high concentrations of aminoglycosides.[241, 242] Iontophoresis has also been used to deliver ciprofloxacin in an experimental model of tobramycin-resistant *Pseudomonas* corneal ulcers. The appropriate clinical role of this mode of delivery has yet to be determined.[243]

Therapeutic aqueous levels can be obtained after the intravenous administration of 200 mg of ciprofloxacin. These levels peaked at 0.21 mg/L within 1 hour after administration and dropped quickly during the subsequent 9 hours. The eyes in the study were not inflamed, and the aqueous was retrieved during routine cataract surgery. The levels obtained with inflamed eyes may be somewhat higher when the blood-eye barrier is abnormal.[244] Vitreal levels of ciprofloxacin can be measured after two 750-mg oral doses before vitrectomy surgery. These levels, 0.9 μg/ml with one dose and 0.56 μg/ml after two doses, are marginal for the treatment of gram-positive organisms such as *S. aureus, S. epidermidis,* and *Streptococcus pyogenes.* As with other antibiotics, the systemic administration of ciprofloxacin does not substitute for intravitreal antibiotic administration in the face of a bacterial endophthalmitis. It may, however, be an excellent adjuvant to intravitreal antibiotic use in selected patients.[17] Ciprofloxacin has been found to be safe when administered intravitreally in doses of 100 μg or less in phakic or aphakic rabbit eyes. Disorganization of outer rods segments was found with transmission electron microscopy after intravitreal injection with ciprofloxacin doses higher than 100 μg. Similarly, increases in corneal thickness occurred with intravitreal injections of greater than 100 μg of ciprofloxacin. The stromal edema was transient in all but one eye in which 1,000 μg of ciprofloxacin was injected. The authors recommend primate studies before recommending human use to evaluate the possibility of retinal toxicity. Because of the broad spectrum of action of ciprofloxacin, it makes an excellent empiric choice in the treatment of bacterial endophthalmitis.[245]

One case of a 65-year-old man experiencing sudden bilateral visual loss consistent with toxic optic neuropathy has been reported in association with oral ciprofloxacin use. The patient was being treated with ciprofloxacin in high doses of 1,500 mg/day over a 4-month period for osteomyelitis. Other complicating factors include the presence of alcoholic cirrhosis and diabetes mellitus. The patient had bilateral cecocentral scotomas. The ciprofloxacin was discontinued, and other medications were unchanged; the patient's vision and visual field slowly improved. The authors postulate that the quinolone group common to ciprofloxacin, quinine, chloroquine, and iodochlorhydroxyquin is responsible for the optic nerve toxicity.[246]

The systemic usage of ciprofloxacin has been criticized as being inappropriate in many cases. Of $2.4 billion spent annually on oral antibiotics, ciprofloxacin along with four other new oral antibiotics account for nearly half of this amount. More than 5 million prescriptions costing $248,000,000 were written for ciprofloxacin in 1989. Oral ciprofloxacin is not recommended for use in streptococcal infections. Its activity against *Streptococcus* is intermediate, and other antibiotics are much more effective with less cost. Ciprofloxacin is also not appropriate for the initial treatment of cellulitis. Its activity against anaerobic skin infections is poor, and its activity against streptococcal infections is variable. A more rational choice for the treatment of outpatient acquired cellulitis is either an antistaphylococcal penicillin or a first-generation cephalosporin.[247, 248]

#### *Summary*

Ciprofloxacin is a valuable systemic and topical antibiotic with a unique wide spectrum of activity against aerobic bacteria. Its role is evolving, and like many new expensive antibiotics, it is overused and misused in many incidences. Rational ophthalmic use of topical ciprofloxacin includes the treatment of bacterial conjunctivitis resistant to other less expensive broad-spectrum antibiotics and antibiotic combinations. It also includes the initial treatment of bacterial keratitis in selected patients. Because of its intermediate MICs for streptococcal organisms, a bacterial keratitis suspected to be caused by one of these organisms would be better treated with a cephalosporin or vancomycin.

### Norfloxacin

Norfloxacin has a spectrum of activity similar to that of other fluoroquinolones, including ciprofloxacin. It is active against most gram-negative aerobic bacteria and many gram-positive aerobic bacteria. Like ciprofloxacin, the MICs for streptococci are poor when compared with the other gram-positive aerobic bacteria. It is approved by the FDA for use in the treatment of bacterial conjunctivitis. Quinolones such as norfloxacin (Chibroxin) and ciprofloxacin have been shown to cause arthropathy in immature animals with systemic administration. Topical quinolones have not been shown to have any effect on weight-bearing joints. Topical norfloxacin is approved for use in children age 1 year and older. Topical ciprofloxacin hydrochloride (Ciloxan) is recommended for use in children more than 10 years of age. Norfloxacin has been used successfully in the treatment of *Pseudomonas* corneal ulceration and would seem to have similar clinical usage as ciprofloxacin.[249]

## Ofloxacin

Another fluoroquinolone, ofloxacin, is being developed for topical use. Its spectrum of activity is similar to that of norfloxacin and ciprofloxacin.[250]

***Summary***

Within a relatively short period three fluoroquinolone antibiotics will have been released for topical usage. These drugs can properly be called miracle antibiotics because of their wide spectrum of activity and slow rate of resistance. Their use will greatly add to the armamentarium against bacterial ocular surface disease. Their role in the treatment and prophylaxis of bacterial infections will slowly emerge over the next decade. The clinician must be properly aware of the economic implications of therapeutic selections in the treatment of common bacterial conjunctivitis. The use of these powerful and expensive new drugs in the treatment of routine conjunctivitis is not rational when other less expensive antibiotics can be used effectively. Fluoroquinolones will become increasingly important with the development of aminoglycoside-resistant *Pseudomonas* organisms. Clearly the advent of these broad-spectrum antibiotics for ophthalmic use do not relieve the clinician of the responsibility of performing bacterial cultures in sight-threatening ocular infections. This is demonstrated in the case of a 17-year-old girl who substituted an herbal eye drop for her prednisolone acetate in the treatment of a herpes simplex disciform keratitis. A gram-negative bacterial keratitis caused by *Pseudomonas maltophilia* developed. This organism was resistant to both aminoglycosides and ciprofloxacin. Susceptibility studies indicated that the organism was sensitive to only trimethoprim-sulfamethoxazole and responded only after trimethoprim-sulfate/polymyxin B–sulfate was initiated.[251]

## Rifampin

Although used primarily in treatment of mycobacteria, rifampin has a broad spectrum of antimicrobial activity, being effective against *Pseudomonas, Proteus, Neisseria,* and *Haemophilus,* for example. It causes cytoplasmic and ribosomal damage to cells. Rifampin concentrations ranging from 0.005 to 0.2 μg/ml inhibit *M. tuberculosis* in vitro.

Rifampin diffuses freely within body tissues and traverses the blood-brain barrier. Corneal application of 1% rifampin ointment every 15 minutes for eight doses in rabbits resulted in an aqueous concentration of 3.6 μg/ml.[252] This is well above the 0.9 μg/ml bactericidal concentration for *Mycobacterium leprae* and suggests use of topical rifampin for treatment of leprous iridocyclitis.

Rifampin and amphotericin B exhibit marked synergism (more than 100-fold enhancement of activity) against various fungi. For example, a culture of *C. albicans* containing 100,000 organisms/ml was treated with 0.5 μg of amphotericin B/ml, rifampin 50 μg/ml, and both drugs combined. After 2 days, the untreated control had increased to 20 million organisms, the amphotericin B–treated culture had increased to 2,700,000, the rifampin-treated culture had increased to 15 million, but the combined drug synergistic effect reduced the colony count to only 1,000.[253] This combination was used to treat a 14-year-old girl with *Candida* endophthalmitis contracted from prolonged intravenous feeding. Amphotericin B dosage was 0.5 mg/kg/day; rifampin, 15 mg/kg/day in a single oral dose. Within 1 week improvement was obvious, and treatment was discontinued at 10 days with dramatic recovery. The MICs of amphotericin B against the isolated *Candida* were 1 μg/ml; of rifampin, greater than 800 μg/ml. The synergistic effect just described was obtained with this isolate of *Candida*.

The synergistic effect of amphotericin B occurs because it increases cell wall permeability, thereby permitting entry of the second antibiotic. Such synergism also occurs with 5-fluorocytosine and amphotercin but is less predictable. Also, fluorocytosine is more toxic than is rifampin.

An extensive in vitro search for antifungal drug synergism used 28 isolates of 11 different fungi and yeasts and evaluated the effect of various combinations of amphotericin B, natamycin, rifampin, tetracycline, clindamycin, and gentamicin. Most combinations showed no enhancement of antifungal activity. The dramatic exception was the amphotericin B–rifampin synergism, which was effective against 75% of the organisms tested. The natamycin-rifampin combination also showed synergism but of a lesser amount.[254]

#### *Toxicity*

Rifampin commonly causes aching of muscles, joints, and abdomen and a transient jaundice. In management of tuberculosis, this drug is used for long periods and is usually tolerated well. It may cause elevation of liver enzymes and is potentially hepatotoxic. The most serious problem with rifampin is an immunologic reaction encountered with intermittent use of large doses. Hematologic, pulmonary, and renal anaphylactic reactions occur. Such reactions are uncommon despite widespread use of rifampin in tuberculotherapy.[181]

#### *Summary*

Because the synergism of rifampin with amphotericin B is so great, a tolerable combined dose can reduce the number of viable *Candida* by 20,000 times over the control. Such treatment was reported to be effective in a case of *Candida* endophthalmitis.

### Sulfonamides

The sulfonamide drugs are bacteriostatic by virtue of their ability to prevent bacterial utilization of *p*-aminobenzoic acid. Knowledge that many local anesthetics are esters of *p*-aminobenzoic acid is of practical value, because such drugs (procaine and tetracaine) will interfere with sulfonamide action. Purulent exudate also contains *p*-aminobenzoic acid and therefore interferes with the action of sulfonamides.

Generally other antibacterial drugs have replaced sulfonamides as the first choice for the treatment of major infections. However, for topical treatment of minor ocular infections, sulfacetamide in a 10% to 30% concentration is still valuable. Triple sulfonamides are used with pyrimethamine in the treatment of ocular toxoplasmosis but are not generally available.

The combination of trimethoprim and sulfamethoxazole has been found to be useful in the treatment of otherwise resistant microbial keratitis. *Nocardia* keratitis is typically a slowly progressive corneal infection resistant to intensive broad-spectrum topical antibiotic therapy. The synergistic effect of trimethoprim (16 mg/ml) and sulfamethoxazole (80 mg/ml) has been reported to allow more rapid resolution of a nocardia keratitis than would be expected with sulfacetamide alone.[255] A rare corneal ulcer–growing *Flavobacterium meningosepticum* was successfully treated with a similar dosage of topical trimethoprim-sulfamethoxazole. This aerobic, gram-negative bacillus was resistant to all other antibiotics tested, including the aminoglycosides.[256]

This combination, trimethoprim and sulfamethoxazole, has been used successfully in the treatment of *Toxoplasma gondii* posterior uveitis. All 16 reported patients had resolution of the toxoplasmosis retinochoroiditis over 4 to 6 weeks. Trimethoprim (160 mg) and sulfamethoxazole (300 mg) given orally twice daily was used with adjuvant prednisone and clindamycin in several cases. Because pyrimethamine is not used, bone marrow suppression is not encountered.[257]

Sulfonamides inhibit the growth of most gram-positive and a variety of gram-negative organisms. Microorganisms are not killed by sulfonamides, only inhibited.

Sulfacetamide is antagonistic to the inhibition of *Pseudomonas* by gentamicin.

Gentamicin alone will inhibit *Pseudomonas* growth at levels of 7 μg/ml. In the presence of sulfacetamide, gentamicin levels of 15 μg/ml are required for inhibition.[258]

### *Toxic Effects*

Sulfonamides cause a variety of undesirable reactions. Renal complications are among the most common problems and include crystalluria, hematuria, and anuria. A fluid intake sufficient to produce at least 1,000 ml of urine daily will help to avoid renal problems. Because sulfonamides are considerably more soluble in an alkaline pH, sodium bicarbonate greatly reduces the possibility of crystalluria.

Other complications include agranulocytosis, hemolytic anemia, toxic hepatitis, skin rashes and allergy, photosensitization, peripheral neuritis, drug fever, acute psychoses, and transitory myopia.[259–261]

One case of erythema multiforme major (Stevens-Johnson syndrome) has been convincingly linked to the use of topical 10% sulfacetamide solution with no history of sulfa allergy. The patient had been previously sensitized with systemic sulfa.[262] Transient myopia may occur with systemic and topical sulfonamide use. This results from ciliary body edema and concomitant zonular relaxation and anterior lens movement. This is in contrast to transient myopia associated with edema and refractive change in the crystalline lens associated with diabetes and uremia.[261] Four cases of transitory toxic amblyopia were attributed to moderate doses of sulfonamides.[263] Intravenous sulfonamide preparations are irritating and may cause local thrombophlebitis.

When sulfonamide ointments are applied in the treatment of marginal blepharitis, local photosensitization may result in circumscribed sunburning of the lid margin. The mistaken diagnosis of allergic response is commonly made.[264]

Sulfacetamide may crystallize, forming white plaques on a dry surface. White corneal plaques have been reported in a patient with severe dry-eye syndrome treated for a conjunctivitis with 10% sulfacetamide drops. The plaques were superficial, being removed with simple excision.[265] Topical use of sulfadiazine ointment for 1 year caused formation of multiple small white concretions within cysts of the palpebral conjunctiva. Spectroscopic studies identified these as being composed of sulfadiazine.[266]

The topical application of sulfanilamide powder to the abraded cornea resulted in heavily vascularized scars. Epithelial regeneration was slowed greatly, requiring more than 13 days in treated rabbits compared with 5 days for control rabbits (corneal epithelium completely removed).[267]

### *Ocular Penetration*

The intraocular penetration of topically applied sulfonamides varies considerably in different species, being 5 to 15 times greater in rabbits than in dogs. Apparently the different solubility and corneal penetrability of the various sulfonamides accounts for this variability. Topical application of sulfanilamide ointment (concentration not stated) every 30 minutes for 6 hours resulted in aqueous concentrations of 3.1 μg/ml (rabbits) and 0.6 μg/ml (dogs). Corresponding aqueous sulfapyridine concentrations were 0.23 and 0.16 μg/ml, respectively. Sulfadiazine penetration into the aqueous approximates that of sulfapyridine. A human aqueous level of 2.2 μg/ml has been reported after topical sulfanilamide application.[268]

Intraocular penetration of topically applied sulfonamides seems directly related to their solubility characteristics and inversely related to their ability to combine with protein.[268]

The intraocular penetration of sodium sulfadiazine is increased by as much as 15 times by iontophoresis compared with corneal bath. A 5-minute iontophoresis (2 mA, 45-V battery, cathode on cornea and anode on body) with a 5% solution of sodium sulfacetamide resulted in the following concentrations: cornea, 12 μg/ml; aqueous, 3.9 μg/ml; and ciliary body, 1.15 μg/ml. By contrast, a 5-minute corneal bath with the same solution achieved these concentrations: cornea, 0.9 μg/ml; aqueous, 0.25 μg/ml; and ciliary body, 0.17 μg/ml.[270] Considerably higher intraocular concentrations are attained if the corneal epithelium is absent (as high as 9.5 mg/ml in the aqueous). This iontophoretic technique was said not to cause biomicroscopically observable corneal damage.

Similarly, corneal iontophoresis greatly increased the penetration of a 5% sulfathiazole solution into both the cornea (30 μg/ml) and aqueous humor (5 μg/ml). However, vitreous penetration of sulfathiazole by iontophoresis is too small to measure reliably.[271]

Sulfathiazole penetration into the aqueous humor after oral administration is dependent on the blood levels achieved.[272] Aqueous levels in the normal eye are about one fifth of the blood levels. In contrast, sulfanilamide aqueous levels are about 80% of the blood levels.[273] Partial destruction of the blood-aqueous barrier by infection will increase the intraocular penetration of sulfathiazole in proportion to the severity of the inflammation. In the presence of an experimental vitreous abscess, the aqueous sulfathiazole levels will rise as high as 90% of the blood levels.[274] The penetration into the inflamed eye of other drugs and antibiotics, as well as the normal constituents of the blood, such as protein, is similarly enhanced.

After paracentesis the concentrations of sulfanilamide, sulfapyridine, and sulfadiazine in the secondary aqueous are approximately equal to the sulfonamide concentration in the blood. Sulfathiazole penetration of the eye is considerably less than those of the other three sulfonamides and even after paracentesis reaches aqueous concentrations of less than half the blood levels.[275]

#### Clinical Use

As soon as the sulfonamides were introduced into clinical medicine, their value in controlling ocular infections caused by susceptible microorganisms became apparent.[276, 277] However, the prognosis for salvage of eyes with serious infections (e.g., panophthalmitis after cataract extraction) remained poor despite the use of sulfonamides.[278]

Although sulfonamides have largely been replaced by other antibacterials, topical use of sulfacetamide (a 30% solution or a 10% ointment) is still a highly effective prophylaxis against corneal infection after abrasions or the entry of superficial foreign bodies and in the treatment of preexisting infections caused by susceptible organisms.[279] The sulfacetamide is instilled at the time of the first office visit and is dispensed to the patient to be used three or four times daily until epithelial healing has occurred. Although the 30% solution burns somewhat, this initial irritation is followed by an analgesic effect that is quite advantageous in the management of corneal epithelial defects. Such sulfacetamide prophylaxis was used over a 5-year period in a busy industrial practice, and not a single case progressed to corneal ulceration.[280] With the topical use of 30% sulfacetamide solution, intracorneal concentrations as high as 0.1% can be achieved within 5 minutes.

Sulfonamide therapy is an important supplement to pyrimethamine in the treatment of retinochoroiditis presumably caused by toxoplasmosis. The amount of pyrimethamine needed is greatly reduced by the synergistic effect of sulfonamides, thereby decreasing the risk of toxic effects.[281] A total of 2 g is administered daily in four divided doses. Use of triple sulfonamides (sulfadiazine, sulfamerazine, and sulfamethazine) is said to reduce the danger of crystalluria but is not readily available. Trimethoprim-sulfamethoxazole may be used without pyrimethamine.

#### Summary

The topical application of sodium sulfacetamide (30% solution and 10% ointment) is effective against minor surface ocular infections caused by a variety of microorganisms. For this purpose, sulfacetamide still compares favorably with the newer antibiotics.

Systemic administration of sulfonamides is no longer indicated in ophthalmic therapy, with the possible exception of the pyrimethamine and sulfonamide regimen for toxoplasmosis. Adequate intake of water and sodium bicarbonate will reduce the incidence of crystalluria.

### Tetracyclines

Tetracyclines are bacteriostatic through inhibition of protein synthesis through binding to the 30-S subunit of ribosomes. They may be bactericidal at high concentrations. Tetracycline absorption in the GI tract is reduced with concomitant food ingestion, particularly milk and milk products. Aluminum hydroxide, calcium, magnesium salts, and iron preparations bind to tetracycline, chelating it and decreasing absorption.

The tetracycline group includes the short-acting drugs chlortetracycline, oxytetracycline, and tetracycline, used 1 to 2 g/day with four divided doses. The intermediate-acting class includes methacycline and demeclocycline (300 mg twice daily) and the long-acting class doxycycline and minocycline (100–200 mg used once or twice daily). Doxycycline causes the least change in the intestinal flora. Minocycline achieves the highest levels in the tears. Both doxycycline and minocycline absorption are unaffected by food ingestion. The tetracyclines are termed broad-spectrum antibiotics because of their ability to inhibit the activity of a wide variety of gram-positive organisms, many gram-negative organisms (including *E. coli, Aerobacter, Klebsiella, B. subtilis,* and *Neisseria gonorrhoeae*), *Rickettsia* species, *Actinomyces, Spirochaeta* species, and *Chlamydia*. Lymphogranuloma venereum, psittacosis, molluscum contagiosum, trichomonads, organisms causing tularemia, amebas, pinworms, and anthrax bacilli also respond to tetracycline therapy. Not all strains of these organisms are susceptible; for example, one third or more of staphylococcal strains may be highly resistant. Both *P. aeruginosa* and *P. vulgaris* are rarely responsive to tetracycline.[282]

A single dose of 2.5 g of tetracycline resulted in clinical cure within 48 hours of 24 of 26 Mexican medical students with acute enteric infection. *Shigella* was isolated in stools of all of these patients. Ampicillin and cephalothin are also effective antibiotics against traveler's dysentery but require multiple doses.[283]

Concentrations of the tetracyclines ranging from 1 to 8 μg/ml are usually adequate to inhibit growth of susceptible bacteria. There is cross-resistance in therapeutic effectiveness among the tetracycline derivatives. Hence, if a patient fails to respond to one tetracycline, there is rarely any advantage in changing to another member of this same group of antibiotics.[284]

#### *Dosage*

From 1 to 4 g may be given daily in divided doses every 6 to 8 hours. Comparable amounts may be given intravenously if necessary, but therapy should be changed to the oral route as soon as practicable because of the possibility of phlebitis. For topical ocular use, 0.5% ointment is prescribed, and the frequency of application is determined by the severity of the infection.

Significant serum concentrations are reached within 1 hour after oral dosage, reach a maximum level at 4 to 6 hours, and persist to some degree for as long as 24 hours. Dosage of 1 g every 6 hours will achieve minimal, sustained serum levels as high as 5 μg/ml.

#### *Toxicity*

Nausea, vomiting, and diarrhea may complicate oral dosage. Tetracycline may cause an irritated diarrhea, which must be differentiated from the enterocolitis caused by *Staphylococcus* and the life-threatening *Pseudomonas* colitis caused by *C. difficile*. Aluminum hydroxide gels markedly reduce absorption and therefore should not be used to relieve GI symptoms. Thrombophlebitis may occur at the site of intravenous injection. Photosensitivity reactions, manifested by marked erythema after exposure to sunlight, have been reported. Overgrowth of nonsusceptible organisms (e.g., *C. albicans*) may follow tetracycline therapy.

The intravenous $LD_{50}$ of oxytetracycline in mice is 100 mg/kg. Daily oral doses of 500 mg/kg may be tolerated by dogs for as long as 2 months. Obviously there is a wide margin of safety between therapeutic and toxic doses.

In nine reported instances, death occurred late in pregnancy after prolonged intravenous use of high doses (up to 6 g/day) of tetracyclines. Autopsy revealed extensive fatty degeneration of the liver in all cases.[285]

Tetracycline that has deteriorated from aging in a moist environment may be highly nephrotoxic. Acute necrosis of the renal convoluted tubules may follow use of only a few such outdated capsules. Fortunately, such a lesion is reversible.[286, 287]

Intracranial hypertension with papilledema may follow tetracycline therapy in infants and children.[288]

Tetracycline inhibits mineralization of bone in the chick embryo. A 40% reduction of growth of the fibula results from tetracycline administration to premature children. This probably results from the strong chelation of tetracycline to cations such as calcium. Even in an adult, 3% to 11% of a dose of tetracycline becomes incorporated in bony structure and remains there cumulatively (except as 10% of the skeleton is remodeled annually). Presence of tetracycline in adult bone has no known adverse circumstances except that it causes a yellow discoloration. A 42-year-old man who had taken 500 mg of tetracycline daily for 18 years had bone as brilliantly yellow as a daffodil.[289]

### *Requiem for Tetracyclines (in Children)*

In an attempt to stop tetracycline prescribing for children less than 8 years of age, the American Academy of Pediatrics published a position paper with this section's title in 1975.[290] The reasons for this position are the unique toxicity and relative inappropriateness of tetracycline use for children. Tooth development occurs during the last half of pregnancy and continues to the age of 8 years. Tetracyclines permanently discolor developing teeth yellow and brown and also cause enamel hypoplasia. Bone growth is slowed. The "bulging fontanel syndrome" is caused by tetracycline-induced intracranial hypertension.

Tetracyclines are not only uniquely toxic to children but are also relatively inappropriate. Viruses cause 50% to 90% of respiratory tract infections in children but are not susceptible to tetracycline therapy. The usual causes of bacterial respiratory tract infections in children are *Diplococcus pneumoniae, S. pyogenes, H. influenzae,* and *S. aureus.* The tetracyclines are not the most effective antibiotics against these bacteria. For example, the really important pathogen causing tonsillitis or pharyngitis is the β-hemolytic *Streptococcus.* Twenty percent of these streptococci are resistant to tetracyclines and are better treated with penicillin or erythromycin. Penicillin is the drug of choice for pneumococci and streptococci. Ampicillin is effective against 95% of *Haemophilus.* Penicillinase-resistant semisynthetic penicillins (e.g., methicillin) are preferred for resistant staphylococci. Furthermore, an otherwise healthy child with a persistent cough and no significant physical findings will be better treated by observation than by antibiotic usage.[291]

Despite these persuasive facts, during a 2-year period, 7% of 59,000 children received tetracycline prescriptions.[290] Of 1,947 physicians attending these children, only 26 physicians wrote 54% of the tetracycline prescriptions. This leads to the obvious conclusions that most physicians already knew about these adverse facts about tetracycline usage and that identification and education of the remainder are needed.

No reports document discoloration of the teeth or any other adverse effects arising from use of topical ocular tetracycline preparations. One drop of a 1% solution contains about 0.5 mg of drug. To equal a single 250-mg capsule of tetracycline would require 500 drops, and the assumption that most of each drop would not be squeezed out by blinking as usually occurs. At 5 drops daily, 3 months would pass before the dose level reached the content of a single capsule. Even in an infant, this is not very much drug. These numbers suggest that a single drop in each eye as prophylaxis against gonococcal ophthalmia is not likely to cause complications.

### *Ocular Penetration*

When applied by corneal bath, oxytetracycline does not materially penetrate the intact rabbit cornea. If as much as one third of the corneal epithelium is abraded, a 5-minute bath with a 0.5% solution of oxytetracycline hydrochloride may produce aqueous levels of 28 μg/ml when measured 30 minutes after treatment. Similar application of chlortetracycline to the abraded cornea produced aqueous levels of 8 μg/ml.[292]

Oxytetracycline or chlortetracycline was given intravenously to rabbits in a dosage of 30 mg/kg (dosage was comparable to 2.1 g in a 70-kg man). Aqueous samples withdrawn 100 minutes later contained 3 μg of oxytetracycline/ml. No measurable concentrations of chlortetracycline were achieved.[292]

A study of human aqueous obtained at cataract surgery showed the levels of minocycline to be approximately half that in the plasma (Fig. 6–18).[293] An initial dose of 200 mg of minocycline orally, followed by two doses of 100 mg every 6 hours, produced these levels, measured at the specified time after the third dose. At 1 hour, the aqueous minocycline level was 1.15 μg/ml, which was 69% of the plasma level. The chemical structure of minocycline is more lipophilic than that of other tetracyclines, resulting in better GI absorption and greater passage across blood-brain and blood-eye barriers. Plasma protein binding of minocycline is 75%.

### *Therapy of Ocular Infections*

Surface ocular infections caused by susceptible microorganisms respond well to topical tetracycline application. The incidence of allergy and irritation is insignificant. Although intraocular penetration of tetracyclines is poor, large oral doses (6–8 g/day) produce demonstrable aqueous concentrations and may be advised for the treatment of intraocular infections.

### *Ocular Rosacea*

Tetracycline has been advocated in the treatment of acne and ocular rosacea. This is an underdiagnosed chronic skin disease affecting the forehead, cheeks, and nose, causing erythema, telangiectasia, papules, pustules, hyperemia, and enlargement of the sebaceous glands. Ocular involvement includes the entire ocular surface: lids, conjunctiva, and cornea. Associated conditions include blepharitis, chalazia, hordeolum, conjunctivitis, and keratitis. Treatment involves 1 g of tetracycline/day for 4 to 6 weeks, followed by a slow taper to 250 mg every 1 to 2 days, depending on the clinical response. This clinical improvement may, in part, result from reduced lipase production by the *Staphylococcus* organism, as well as reduction in microflora.[294]

Examination of 51 patients scheduled for chalazion surgery showed 57% of them to have signs characteristic of rosacea. In contrast, rosacea was present in only 12% of 122 patients admitted for retinal detachment or cataract surgery. Because tetracycline

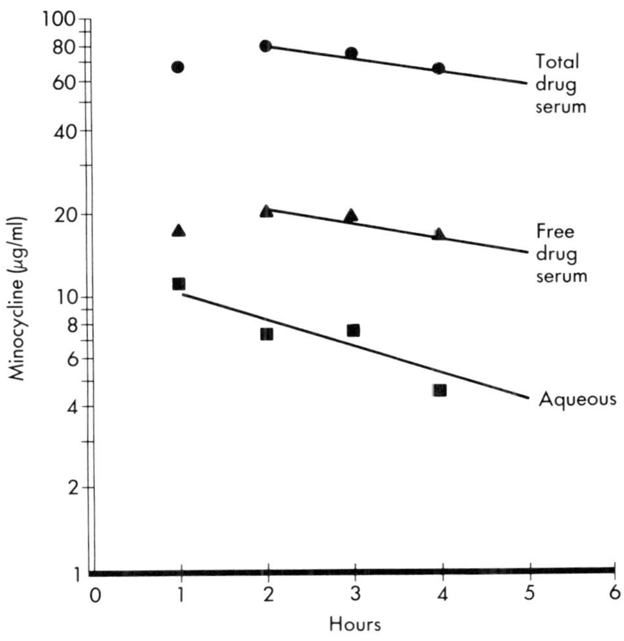


**FIG 6–18.**
Human aqueous and serum levels of minocycline at the specified time after the last of three doses of this antibiotic. (From Poirier RH, Ellison AC: *Ann Ophthalmol* 11:1859, 1979. Used by permission.)

therapy is highly effective in eliminating the findings of rosacea, such treatment would be expected to be helpful in cases of recurrent chalazia.

All 18 patients with ocular rosacea were markedly improved by 250 mg of tetracycline four times daily, reduced by one daily dose after every month of therapy until a symptom-free maintenance dose level was determined. Eleven of these patients had no previous antibiotic therapy; of these, 10 had ocular *S. aureus.* Although this finding may lead to the conclusion that rosacea is a sensitivity reaction to *S. aureus,* after successful treatment *S. aureus* was still recoverable from the eyes.[295, 296]

Gastric hypochlorhydria is characteristically associated with rosacea. A similar pH change affects the tears and may be responsible for the severe symptomatic burning and irritation of the eyes. Determination of tear pH in 44 normal patients and 20 patients with various inflammatory conditions other than rosacea showed all these to have a pH of 7.0 ± 0.20. In seven patients with rosacea, all had much more alkaline tears, measuring 8.0 ± 0.32. Five patients with inactive tetracycline-treated rosacea measured 7.0 ± 0.34.[297]

#### *Phlyctenular Keratoconjunctivitis*

Phlyctenular keratoconjunctivitis is characterized by peripheral corneal nodular lesions associated with a hypersensitivity response to *Staphylococcus.* Rosacea-like skin features occur secondary to staphylococcal hypersensitivity reaction and are improved with tetracycline.

Six children (8–14 years old) with chronic recurrent phlyctenular keratoconjunctivitis unresponsive to corticosteroid therapy all responded rapidly to oral tetracycline given 250 mg two to four times daily. After 3 weeks, when the patients were entirely asymptomatic, the dosage was reduced to a maintenance level of 250 mg/day, continued for 3 to 15 months.[298] The explanation of this response was that the phlyctenular reaction is considered to be a nonspecific hypersensitivity to bacterial proteins. Infections in skin and meibomian glands are relatively inaccessible to topical antibiotics but ideally suited to therapy with systemic tetracycline, which penetrates and accumulates within the glands of the skin and eyelids. These patients not only had the corneal phlyctenular lesion but also marginal blepharitis, nasal telangiectasia, and facial pustules, creating an appearance very similar to that of adult acne rosacea. All of these pathologic changes of skin and eye disappeared with the tetracycline therapy.

#### *Chlamydial Disease*

Adult inclusion conjunctivitis is a chronic follicular conjunctivitis acquired from genital contact. Systemic therapy is recommended for the patient and sexual partners to eliminate reinfection from untreated reservoirs of disease. A 3-week course of tetracycline or minocycline is recommended. Erythromycin is an alternative when tetracycline is not indicated (pregnancy).

Neonatal inclusion conjunctivitis is best treated with systemic and topical erythromycin or sulfa. Untreated neonatal inclusion conjunctivitis will spontaneously resolve but may leave corneal micropannis and conjunctival scarring.[299] Topical erythromycin ointment prophylaxis will prevent inclusion conjunctivitis but not pneumonitis. Prompt diagnosis and thorough systemic treatment are essential for successful resolution without sequelae.[300]

The prophylactic use of topical tetracycline antibiotics in the eyes of newborn children has been effective in several thousand patients.[301–303] The eyes of antibiotic-treated infants were open, clean, and noninflamed in contrast to the reddened, irritated, closed eyes that characteristically persist for 3 to 4 days after use of silver nitrate. Secondary bacterial conjunctivitis (75% staphylococcal) was reported in 17% to 26% of eyes treated with silver nitrate in contrast to 2.3% to 5% of the eyes treated with tetracyclines.

Credé's silver nitrate prophylaxis is not effective against *Chlamydia.* Despite such prophylaxis, conjunctival colonization occurs in half of infants born of known infected mothers. Topical 1% erythromycin ointment protected all of 24 exposed newborns against conjunctival chlamydial infection, but five of these infants contracted nasopharyngeal infection and subsequent pneumonia.[304] A large study of prophylaxis against gonococcal ophthalmia neonatorum compared more than 13,000 newborns receiving topical 1% tetracycline ointment with a similar number receiving a single intramuscular dose of penicillin G (amount unspecified).[305] Of these, 36 tetracycline-treated and 30 penicillin-treated infants developed chlamydial eye infection. (The number, if any, of gonococcal eye infections is not stated.) The number of infected mothers was unknown.

Acute trachoma may be cured by topical application of tetracyclines. An ointment vehicle is most effective. Treatment must be continued for 2 to 4 weeks.[306–309]

#### *Toxoplasmosis*

When given in intramuscular dosage of 50 mg/kg/day for 14 days, minocycline treatment of rabbits infected with toxoplasmosis retinochoroiditis was effective. *Toxoplasma* organisms could be identified from 13 of 16 control eyes but from none of 20 treated rabbits within 2 weeks. The untreated eye infections progressed to diffuse purulent infiltration of the retina and choroid. The treated eyes showed focal scarring but no persistent active inflammation. (Minocycline therapy was not started until appearance of a typical retinochoroiditis, usually present 4 to 7 days after inoculation of the suprachoroidal space with 400 to 1,200 trophozoites.) Other experiments with murine toxoplasmosis show combined therapy with minocycline and sulfadiazine to be as effective as pyrimethamine and sulfadiazine.[310]

#### *Spirochetal Infection*

Tetracycline or doxycycline is recommended for the treatment of Lyme disease caused by *Borrelia burgdorferi.* Patients 9 years of age or older are treated with 250 to 500 mg four times/day for 10 to 30 days until clinical symptoms resolve. Tetracycline is an acceptable alternative to erythromycin in the treatment of syphilis in patients with penicillin allergy. It is not recommended in the treatment of pregnant women because of fetal effects. Tetracyclines are the drugs of choice in tick-borne (epidemic) and louse-borne (epidemic) relapsing fever caused by *Borrelia.*

#### *Persistent Epithelial Defects*

Epithelial defects of the cornea may be persistent in the presence of chronic ocular or systemic inflammation or after chemical trauma. Tissue and leukocytic produced collagenase may be responsible for this as well as stromal melting and perforation. Tetracyclines have an anticollagenolytic effect independent of their antimicrobial properties. Systemic tetracyclines have been useful in healing refractory epithelial defects. Fourteen of 18 patients with persistent epithelial defects present for at least 10 days and refractory to standard therapy (lubricants, therapeutic contact lenses) showed resolution within 2 weeks after starting tetracycline therapy.[311] Tetracycline has been effective in chronic gingival disease through similar mechanisms.[312]

Tetracycline may not be as effective in the treatment of persistent epithelial defects not associated with ocular or systemic inflammation as occurs with diabetes.

#### *Identification of Neoplasms*

Oxytetracycline (Terramycin) is preferentially concentrated in rapidly growing neoplastic tissue.[313] The presence of oxytetracycline in tissue can be detected at the time of surgery by examination under ultraviolet light, which causes a brilliant yellow fluorescence. This method of tumor detection is applicable to the surgery of orbital neoplasms and may help to determine the completeness of malignant tissue removal.

Intraocular neoplasms do not selectively concentrate enough oxytetracycline to be diagnostically helpful. Possibly this is because of the inability of tetracyclines to penetrate the eye in high concentrations relative to its penetration of other tissues. Although a melanoma will not selectively fluoresce within the eye, it does so when it has extended extraocularly into the orbital tissue.

The dose of oxytetracycline required for the fluorescent detection of a neoplasm is 15 mg/kg/day for 3 days. (This is approximately 1 g/day for an adult.) No oxytetracycline is administered for at least 12 hours before surgery to permit high concentrations of the drug to leave normal structures.

#### *Summary*

The tetracycline derivatives are remarkably nontoxic antibiotics, highly effective against a wide variety of microorganisms. Unfortunately they penetrate poorly into the eye. At least 6 to 8 g/day should be given orally if these antibiotics are indicated for the treatment of an infection within the eye.

*Pseudomonas, Proteus,* and many strains of *Staphylococcus* are resistant to the tetracyclines.

### Vancomycin

Vancomycin is derived from cultures of *Nocardia orientalis.* It is a tricyclic glycopeptide. It is bactericidal through inhibition of glycopeptide polymerization in the cell wall. It is bactericidal for most gram-positive organisms. It is useful in the treatment of staphylococcal infections in patients who are allergic to or have failed to respond to the penicillins and cephalosporins. It is recommended in the treatment of methicillin-resistant streptococci. Vancomycin is used in combination with an aminoglycoside to treat *S. viridans* (or *S. bovis*) endocarditis. Vancomycin is indicated in the treatment of pseudomembranous colitis caused by *C. difficile.*[59]

#### *Ophthalmic Uses*

Vancomycin may be used topically or intraocularly to treat sight-threatening eye infections. These include infectious keratitis and endophthalmitis caused by methicillin-resistant staphylococci or streptococci.[314] It is an acceptable substitute for a cephalosporin used in combination with an aminoglycoside in the empiric treatment of infectious keratitis and endophthalmitis.[315, 316] Nearly 100% of staphylococci (coagulase positive and negative) and streptococci tested at The Ohio State University Hospitals in 1990 were susceptible (MIC $\leq 4$) to vancomycin, whereas comparable cephalosporins (cephalothin and ceftrizoxine) and ciprofloxacin had variable activity against these important pathogens.[70]

#### *Dosage*

Intravenous dosing of vancomycin in adults with normal renal function is 500 mg every 6 hours or 1 g every 12 hours. Dosing must be adjusted in children and in those with renal impairment. Dosing with renal impairment should be based on actual serum concentrations after initial empiric administration.

Topical vancomycin may be given in a concentration of 50 mg/ml in the treatment of infectious keratitis. Lower concentrations (5 mg/ml) have been used successfully in the treatment of susceptible staphylococcal blepharoconjunctivitis. Solutions mixed in sterile water have uncomfortably low pH levels. Mixing vancomycin in a buffered tear solution is better tolerated. The drug may precipitate out in solution and should be shaken before administration. Vancomycin solution remains stable up to 21 days at either 4° C or 25° C.[316]

Intravitreal vancomycin with an aminoglycoside has been recommended as initial, empiric therapy for exogenous bacterial endophthalmitis. Doses up to 2 mg were found to be nontoxic in phakic and aphakic-vitrectomized rabbit eyes by clinical histologic and electrophysiologic measures. A dose of 1 mg in 0.1 ml establishes intraocular levels significantly higher than the MIC for most gram-positive organisms.[317, 318]

#### *Adverse Reactions*

Nephrotoxicity and ototoxicity are the most important side effects of intravenous vancomycin. These occur more frequently in patients with preexisting renal insufficiency. Deafness may be preceded by tinnitus and may progress despite cessation of the drug. Serum creatinine and BUN concentrations should be monitored while the patient is on systemic vancomycin therapy. Vancomycin may cause the "red man's syndrome," with flushing or rash with hypotension.

Topical and intraocular vancomycin have not been associated with ototoxicity or nephrotoxicity. Hourly use of 50 mg of vancomycin/ml (30 μl drops) could deliver a dose of only 36 mg/day, well under the recommended systemic dose.

### Defensins

Defensins are antimicrobial peptides derived from granules of alveolar macrophages and neutrophils. This group of naturally occurring molecules appear to have activity through changes in membrane permeability or macromolecular synthesis. Rabbit defensin NP-1 had potent bactericidal activity against *Morganella morganii, P. aeruginosa, S. pneumoniae,* α-hemolytic *Streptococcus,* and *C. albicans* with a concentration of 10 μg/ml. Rabbit defensin NP-5 demonstrated minimal bacterial activity at a concentration of 50 μg/ml. These unique molecules are not yet available for clinical use but have an attractive spectrum of action that would be desirable for ophthalmic use.[319]

Defensin NP-1 has been evaluated as a macrobicide in corneal storage medium.[320] *S. aureus, S. pneumoniae,* and *P. aeruginosa* were grown in solutions of Optisol (Chiron) without antibiotics in the presence of rabbit neutrophil peptide-1 (NP-1) at concentrations of 1, 10, 100, and 200 μg/ml. Concentrations of 200 μg/ml killed the bacteria tested at temperatures of 4° C, 23° C, and 37° C. Defensins (particularly NP-1) may provide an attractive alternative to traditional agents (gentamicin) in the preservation of corneal storage solutions.

SECTION TWO

# Antiviral Drugs

For most of the past 30 years, ophthalmic antiviral therapy has consisted of the topical treatment of herpes simplex virus (HSV) infections of the cornea. Idoxuridine, vidarabine, and finally trifluoridine were available therapies (Table 6–8).[1, 2] During the past decade other ocular viral infections have appeared as opportunists in immunosuppressed patients secondary to acquired immunodeficiency syndrome (AIDS) and after organ transplantation. Of these, viral retinitis caused by cytomegalovirus (CMV), HSV, and herpes zoster virus has resulted in increased systemic and intraocular use of newer antivirals (Tables 6–9 and 6–10).[3]

## THERAPY OF ACTIVE HERPES SIMPLEX KERATITIS

Knowledge of the etiology and natural course of herpes simplex keratitis is necessary to understand appropriate therapy.[4] HSV-mediated disease is the leading cause of corneal blindness in the United States.[5] Active corneal epithelial infection may be primary or recurrent and may be caused by type 1 (usually) or type 2 HSV. Placental transfer of antibodies confers resistance to many children less than 6 months of age. Most children are asymptomatically infected with HSV through the oral route. The virus migrates to the trigeminal ganglion, where it is latent until reactivation occurs. The reactivated virus travels to the termination of a division, where active disease commences. Recurrent HSV infection may be induced through many factors (injury, heat, light, fever surgery, emotional stress, excimer laser keratectomy, epinephrine, corticosteroids, and nonsteroidal antiinflammatory agents).

Untreated HSV keratitis may persist for weeks without improvement. Most studies evaluating the natural history of HSV keratitis were performed before the advent of effective antiviral therapy[6] or were control groups in the prospective evaluation of one of the early antivirals.[7]

### Debridement

Before the development of topical antiviral drugs, the standard therapy for dendritic ulcers was debridement. This may be combined with application of iodine or phenol solutions.[6] This theoretically re-

**TABLE 6–8.**
Topical Antiviral Agents

| Agent | Dose |
|---|---|
| Trifluorothymidine | 1% solution |
| Idoxuridine | 0.1% solution |
| | 0.5% ointment |
| Vidarabine | 3% ointment |
| Acyclovir | 5% ointment for skin |
| | 3% ophthalmic ointment* |

*Available investigationally as Zovirax through Burroughs Wellcome Company, Research Triangle Park, N.C.

**TABLE 6–9.**
Systemic Antivirals

| Agent | Dose |
|---|---|
| Acyclovir | Oral: 600 mg 5 times/day<br>IV: 1,500 mg/m²/day |
| Gancyclovir | IV: Induction dose—5 mg/kg q12h for 14–21 days<br>Maintenance—5 mg/kg daily or 6 mg/kg 5 out of 7 days/wk |
| Foscarnet | IV: 20 mg/kg bolus, followed by 0.16 mg/kg/min infusion |
| Zidovidine | Oral: 500–1,500 mg/day<br>IV: 1–2 mg/kg 4 times daily |

duces the viral and antigenic load and may decrease the incidence of immunologically mediated disease (disciform keratitis).

Several studies have evaluated the role of debridement with antiviral therapy for herpes simplex keratitis. Fifty consecutive patients were randomly selected to receive either 3% acyclovir ointment after epithelial debridement or acyclovir ointment alone. The combination of debridement and topical acyclovir was associated with more rapid healing than acyclovir alone.[8]

Thirty-four patients with active herpes simplex keratitis were randomized to either trifluorodine alone (14 patients), trifluorodine and debridement (12 patients), or debridement alone (eight patients). Debridement was not associated with quicker healing when used with trifluorodine; however, the trifluorodine was not started until the day after debridement compared with immediate therapy in the trifluorodine-only group.[9]

Debridement may be best reserved for active herpes simplex keratitis with poor prognosis for improvement with antiviral treatment alone such as marginal or chronic lesions.

### Rose Bengal and Fluorescein

Active herpes simplex keratitis is frequently evaluated with rose bengal and fluorescein dyes (see Chapter 10). The antiviral effects of fluorescein and rose bengal were evaluated with a mouse herpetic keratitis model.[10] Rose bengal but not fluorescein significantly reduced the amount of replicating virus recovered from the mouse cornea. Fluorescein offers a better alternative to aid in the diagnosis of HSV if a culture is to be performed immediately after the application. As a therapeutic agent, rose bengal is surpassed by other antiviral drugs.

**TABLE 6–10.**
Intravitreal Use of Antivirals

| Agent | Dose |
|---|---|
| Gancyclovir[126,128] | 200–400 μg/0.1 ml |
| Foscarnet[134] | 1,200 μg/0.05 ml |

## IDOXURIDINE

Clinically useful selective metabolic inhibition of viruses was first achieved against herpes simplex infection of the cornea.[11] Before this was reported, no medication had ever been known to cure or improve an established virus infection without destroying the host cells.

### Mechanism of Action

Virus metabolism is closely akin to that of the nucleic acid structure within the cells. One of the fundamental building blocks of which these nucleic acids are composed is thymidine. If the 5-methyl group of thymidine is replaced by an iodine atom, the molecule becomes 5-iodo-2-deoxyuridine (IDU). IDU so closely resembles thymidine that it can substitute for thymidine in DNA synthesis. IDU-containing molecules apparently cannot function as infection-produced viruses.

An attempt to demonstrate the presence of IDU within treated virus particles was inconclusive. Microautoradiographic studies of herpes simplex treated with radioactively labeled IDU failed to show convincing superimposition of the localizing silver particles on the viral bodies.[12]

### Related Compounds

A number of antimetabolites were evaluated for their ability to inhibit virus multiplication.[13] The only antimetabolites found to be effective were those that block the final step of nucleotide (thymidine) incorporation into DNA. Blockade of earlier steps in the synthesis of DNA was ineffective, presumably because of alternate metabolic pathways. The best drug was found to be IDU. Although also effective, 5-bromo-2-deoxyuridine tends to produce chemical conjunctivitis and iritis. The chloro derivative was less effective, and the fluoro derivative was inactive. Because IDU is competitive with thymidine, addition of excess thymidine antagonizes the therapeutic effect of IDU.

### Stability

IDU is a chemically stable drug, losing only 1% to 2% of its potency per month in solution at room temperature. Solutions of IDU several months old are more variable in therapeutic effect than are fresh solutions, and the old solutions are likely to cause ocular irritation and punctate corneal staining.[14] These facts suggest that substances resulting from IDU breakdown might antagonize the therapeutic effect or cause toxicity. Iodouracil, a major breakdown product, was found to antagonize the antiviral effect of IDU in tissue culture even when present in only 0.00001% concentration. Irritation and punctate corneal staining were produced in human volunteers with 0.01% concentration of iodouracil. In experimental rabbits, a 0.01% solution of iodouracil did not inhibit the antiviral effect of a 0.1% concentration of IDU.

The practical clinical recommendation derived from these findings included storage of solution in dark bottles under refrigeration. Preparations that cause ocular burning should be considered old and should be replaced with fresh solutions. Failure of herpetic keratitis to respond as expected to IDU therapy should suggest the possibility of deterioration of the medication and may indicate a treatment trial with a fresh preparation.

### Ocular Penetration

The intraocular penetration of topically applied IDU is very poor. Radioactive iodine-labeled IDU was measured in rabbit eyes after 24 hours of instillation of a 0.1% solution of IDU every 2 hours.[15] Immediately after the last instillation of the drug, the concentration (measured as micrograms of IDU per gram of tissue) was only 6.5 in epithelium, 2.2 in corneal stroma, 0.8 in aqueous, 1 in iris, and 0.2 in vitreous; 4 hours after instillation these concentrations had decreased only slightly, to 5.3 in epithelium, 1 in corneal stroma, 0.4 in aqueous, 0.4 in iris, and 0.1 in vitreous.

### Therapeutic Concentration

In tissue culture an IDU concentration of 1 mg/ml will inhibit the growth of HSV and vaccinia virus. Concentration in excess of this MIC can be achieved in the cornea by topical application. As indicated in the preceding paragraph, the intraocular concentrations of IDU are therapeutically inadequate, a finding that probably explains the failure of herpetic iritis to respond to topical treatment.

### Adverse Reactions

Although inhibition of epithelial growth would be anticipated, IDU in a 0.1% concentration apparently is nontoxic to the corneal surface. Even if the corneal epithelium has been completely removed, healing is not inhibited by IDU. Stromal clarity is maintained, and corneal edema does not occur. No ocular abnormalities have been observed in rabbits maintained on IDU for 1 month. Even if it were absorbed systemically after topical instillation, IDU should have no toxic effect because it is rapidly metabolized. Within 4 hours after intravenous administration of radioactive iodine-labeled IDU, 75% of the labeled iodine had been excreted in the urine.

IDU may cause a severe local reaction characterized by an edematous and follicular conjunctivitis. With continuing treatment, the lacrimal puncta will become occluded and permanently stenotic.[16] This is a nonspecific reaction that may follow severe allergic response to many different drugs, including cyclopentolate, for example.

IDU has been shown to induce conjunctival cicatrization with long-term use of 1 to 3½ years in four separate patients.[17] Punctal occlusion and keratinization of the tarsal conjunctiva also occurred. Secondary corneal changes, including stromal ulceration, persistent epithelial defects, and keratinization, were found. Immunofluorescent staining of conjunctival specimens did not show the specific staining of the epithelial basement membrane that is seen in some patients with ocular cicatricial pemphigoid. The authors hypothesize that the conjunctival changes are secondary to either direct IDU cellular toxicity or from prolonged disruption of DNA synthesis.

Conjunctival cicatrization has been reported in one patient after short-term use (2 weeks) of IDU therapy.[18] Immunofluorescent examination of the conjunctiva found interepithelial staining for IgG, IgA, compliment 3, albumin, and fibrinogen. These data indicate that local autoimmunity may play a role in some patients with conjunctival cicatrization associated with IDU.

## Ocular Tolerance

Hourly instillation of IDU does not retard the healing of corneal epithelial wounds compared with the healing of control injuries treated with sterile distilled water.[19] No lens damage has been reported to follow the use of IDU. The mitotic activity of lens epithelium is unchanged after 1 month of hourly IDU treatment of an eye.

The effect of a 0.5% concentration of IDU ointment every 2 hours on the healing of corneal stromal wounds was studied by radioactive thymidine labeling of rabbit corneas that had been injured by freezing the central 6-mm portion.[20] As indicated in Fig. 6-2, at the end of 5 days the regeneration of corneal stromal cells was approximately twice as far advanced in the control eyes (treated with Neosporin ointment) as in the experimental eyes (IDU treated). Radioautograph counts indicated that the corneal stromal cell population in the injured area of the IDU-treated corneas was only half that in the control corneas.

The effect of IDU on stromal healing of the cornea was further studied by making a linear full-thickness incision across the center of rabbit corneas. A 0.1% solution of IDU was instilled into one eye every hour for 14 hours every day. The fellow eyes were treated with saline solution only. Wound strength was studied by excising a 5-mm strip of perpendicularly oriented cornea across the incision and measuring the grams of weight required to disrupt the incision. In a group of 23 rabbits sacrificed at 13 days, the average tensile strength of the IDU-treated eyes was 130 g compared with 244 g for the control eyes. Most noteworthy was the very low breaking strength of many treated eyes compared with the uniformly strong wounds in control eyes.[21] These data suggest that IDU treatment is contraindicated during the healing period of ocular surgery (e.g., after corneal transplantation for herpetic keratitis) (Table 6–11).

## Contraindications

Because of its inhibition of corneal stromal healing, use of IDU is probably not advisable during the first few weeks after

**TABLE 6–11.**
Reduction of Tensile Strength of Corneal Wounds by Treatment With IDU

| Wound Age (Days) | Tensile Strength* | |
|---|---|---|
| | IDU (g/5 mm) | Control (g/5 mm) |
| 7 | 0 | 35 |
| 9 | 10 | 510 |
| 11 | 95 | 160 |
| 12 | 45 | 120 |
| 14 | 15 | 300 |
| 15 | 200 | 205 |
| 17 | 205 | 240 |
| 19 | 50 | 250 |
| 21 | 210 | 745 |

From Payrau P, Dohlman CH: *Am J Ophthalmol* 57:999, 1964. Used by permission.
*IDU used in one eye and saline solution in control eye.

corneal transplantation or other penetrating corneal incisions. IDU is not helpful in the treatment of bacterial infections. With the possible exception of vaccinia, insufficient evidence is available to recommend use of IDU for therapy of other virus infections of the cornea.

A relevant clinical question asks whether an immunosuppressive drug that is inactive against bacteria can actually worsen infection by inhibiting host defenses. In simulation of the usual 2-week course of clinical treatment with IDU, this medication was instilled for 8 days in 1 eye of each of 20 rabbits. The other eye received bland ointment as a control.[22] On the fifth day of treatment (now termed day 0 of infection), both eyes were inoculated with *S. aureus*. On the following day (termed day 1 of infection) 15 IDU-treated eyes and 8 Lacrilube-treated eyes showed bacterial ulcers. Table 6–12 documents the marked increase in the number of infections consistently found in the IDU-treated eyes during the 4 days of observation after inoculation. This practical experiment indicates that erroneously prescribed antiviral therapy will probably worsen a bacterial keratitis and that an accurately diagnosed viral keratitis properly treated with antiviral medication is probably more vulnerable to bacterial superinfection. Other compromising host factors such as tear deficiency, chronically damaged tissue, and corticosteroid therapy should be expected to increase further the vulnerability of the diseased eye to bacterial superinfection. IDU allergy has been reported.[23]

**TABLE 6–12.**

Number of Infected Rabbit Corneas (of 20 Eyes) Treated with IDU Before and After *Staphylococcus aureus* Inoculation on Day 0 Compared with Control Fellow Eyes

| Day | IDU | Control |
|---|---|---|
| 1 | 15 | 8 |
| 2 | 20 | 15 |
| 3 | 11 | 4 |
| 4 | 14 | 6 |

Modified from Yamaguchi K: *Am J Ophthalmol* 87:202, 1979. Used by permission.

### Dosage

Because the continuing presence of IDU is required to inhibit virus growth, it is necessary that topical ocular instillation of a 0.1% concentration of IDU drops be given at least every 2 hours, *day* and *night*. It was initially recommended that drops be instilled hourly during the day and every 2 hours at night for 3 days. For the next 4 days the intervals were doubled to every 2 hours during the day and every 4 hours at night. When grossly visible staining disappears, the frequency of drops may be reduced to every 2 hours during the day. Herpetic keratitis may relapse if IDU is discontinued before microscopic staining has cleared.

When prescribed as 0.5% ointment, IDU may be used five times daily (not at night). The therapeutic response to this frequency of application of ointment is reported to equal that of drops used hourly during the day and every 2 hours at night.[15]

### Experimental Use

The effect of a 0.1% concentration of IDU every 2 hours in treatment of experimental herpetic keratitis in rabbits is unequivocal. If it is given before virus inoculation, IDU will prevent keratitis.[11] When treatment was begun 2 hours after virus inoculation, only one fourth of the eyes had dendritic keratitis develop, which appeared after 48 hours (all control eyes developed keratitis in 24 hours). The lesions in treated eyes remained small and disappeared with continuous treatment. Delay in treatment until 48 hours after virus inoculation permitted development of extensive dendritic lesions and several cases of associated herpetic iritis. After 48 hours of IDU treatment, even severely infected eyes were completely healed. Despite clinical cure, virus cultures were positive in one third of these eyes, which presumably could develop recurrences. Of 43 rabbit eyes treated after infection was established, 27 had no recurrences.

Strains of HSV isolated from three patients with severe keratitis behaved quite differently from the milder stock strain already described, producing widespread keratitis, stromal infiltration, and encephalitis, with death of most rabbits within 2 weeks. IDU was not so effective against these virulent strains, curing only seven of 17 eyes. However, in only two of the 17 treated eyes was keratitis as severe as in the 17 control eyes. Obviously these results indicate that virus resistance to metabolic antagonists will present clinical problems comparable with those encountered in antibiotic therapy of bacterial infection. Development of resistance to IDU has been demonstrated in culture propagation of HSV.[24]

HSV infections of the chicken chorioallantoic membrane can be eradicated by hourly treatment with 0.1% solution of IDU.[25] At least 6 hourly doses of IDU were required before a measurable reduction in the virus concentration was demonstrable. At least 28 hourly doses of IDU were required before the disappearance of the herpesvirus. This experimental study further confirms the need for prolonged and intensive treatment of acute herpetic keratitis.

Improving the tissue penetration of IDU, thereby permitting access of the drug to deeper sites of infection, is possible by the use of liposomes as vehicles. Liposomes are artificial microbubbles with lipid walls that can be made to enclose molecules that are not lipid soluble. Rabbit stromal HSV infections responded much better to topically applied, liposome-encapsulated IDU than to IDU alone or to saline-liposome control. On day 18 stromal infection was present in all 14 eyes of the saline-liposome control group and in none of the IDU-liposome group.[26]

## Clinical Use

### *Dendritic Ulcer*

Clinical experience with IDU has been as encouraging as the preliminary laboratory work.[27] In a series of 76 dendritic ulcers, all but one responded favorably. Subjective relief was marked within 12 to 24 hours. Conspicuous epithelial healing was already achieved within 3 days, and residual punctate staining usually disappeared within 10 days. In the single case nonresponsive to IDU, debridement and continuation of IDU therapy resulted in cure. Herpetic keratitis may relapse if IDU is discontinued before microscopic staining has cleared. However, when grossly visible staining has disappeared, the frequency of drops may be reduced to every 2 hours during the day and once during the night. Recurrence will respond to a repeat course of therapy.

During the first few weeks of healing, superficial stromal infiltrate in the pattern of a dendritic figure will persist beneath the healed epithelium. This dendritiform ghost figure is of no significance, will disappear completely, and does not in itself indicate a need for treatment to be continued.

Large and chronically active herpetic stromal ulcers with staining also respond rapidly to IDU therapy; the average healing time is 6.5 days (none more than 13 days). Herpetic iritis and deep keratitis, unassociated with surface disease, were not helped by IDU. Chronic disciform keratitis with marked corneal thickening did not respond well. Recurrent small epithelial defects overlying dense stromal scar became painful with IDU treatment, healed with the use of a bland ointment every hour as needed, and were presumed to represent some type of noninfectious recurrent erosion.

This response to IDU may be compared with the course of 53 patients.[6] (This was another series and not a control series in the same study.) The average period of staining in these cases was 21 days, and the eyes remained injected for an average of 41 days.

In three cases of ophthalmic cutaneous zoster, dendritic corneal figures were present. Virus cultures confirmed the presence of zoster virus (not simplex) in these dendritic figures. All three corneal lesions cleared promptly with corticosteroid therapy (which was combined with IDU in two cases).[28]

Because IDU is somewhat unstable, failure of a dendritic ulcer to respond promptly should arouse suspicion of faulty medication; this has been experienced, and retreatment with full-strength IDU has been shown to be effective. No IDU toxicity has appeared in 155 patients; however, allergy to the thiomersol preservative occurred three times.

### *Stromal Herpes*

The initial evaluations of IDU consisted of uncontrolled treatment in a series of cases of herpetic keratitis.[25, 29] These cases were generally divided into epithelial and stromal keratitis. About 80% of the epithelial cases and 50% of the stromal cases healed after IDU therapy. Average healing time for the epithelial cases was approximately 1 week and for the stromal cases 2 weeks. These results led to the conclusion that at last an effective treatment had been found for some cases of chronic herpetic keratitis, a condition that has been notoriously unresponsive to medical management. Unfortunately, time has not justified this conclusion.

Clinical evaluation of IDU by a group of practicing ophthalmologists showed healing of 21 of 26 dendritic ulcers in an average of 13 days.[30] Herpetic stromal involvement prolonged healing time to an average of 16 days, with good response in 14 of 21 cases.

Well-controlled double-blind studies of the effect of IDU on herpetic keratitis indicate that the spontaneous recovery rate is at least 25% and may be greater than 50%.[23, 31–33] The combined number of IDU-treated patients with acute epithelial keratitis was 57. Of these, 41 responded well to IDU; placebo treatment of 53 patients with epithelial keratitis resulted in improvement of 19. Only small numbers of patients with stromal keratitis were reported; however, a total of 34 eyes were given placebo therapy. Of these 34, 50% improved spontaneously.

Other double-blind studies agree that IDU treatment significantly improves the course of acute epithelial herpetic keratitis.[34] However, chronic stromal herpes seems to do just as well with placebo treatment as with IDU treatment. Apparently the 50% improvement of stromal herpes reported in the earlier uncontrolled studies of IDU represents merely the spontaneous recovery rate of this disease.

IDU therapy does not seem to decrease the recurrence rate of herpetic keratitis. In 23 recurrences, 12 eyes had been treated with IDU therapy and 9 with placebo therapy.

Virtually all of the original clinical studies of IDU were uncontrolled. In a series of 28 cases of acute herpetic keratitis divided into placebo and IDU groups, excellent to good results were attained in 15 IDU-treated patients and in only five placebo-treated patients. This was a statistically significant difference. In contrast, no difference could be noted between the result of IDU and placebo treatment of 43 patients presumed to have chronic herpetic keratitis.[31]

## COMBINED CORTICOSTEROID AND IDOXURIDINE THERAPY

Having available in IDU a specific antiviral drug, can the ophthalmologist simultaneously treat herpes simplex keratitis with corticosteroids?[1] Clinically, the answer seems to be yes. Cases of chronic herpetic keratitis that have stubbornly persisted for months will often become quiet and comfortable after topical corticosteroid therapy. Unfortunately, corticosteroids reactivate dendritic keratitis in some patients. Such reactivation is much less likely when antivirals and corticosteroids are simultaneously used to treat chronic herpetic keratitis.

Experimental use of hydrocortisone and IDU in the treatment of rabbit herpes simplex keratitis indicates that IDU does indeed protect the cornea against corticosteroid activation of the disease.[34] The quality of protection is directly related to the frequency of IDU application, being greater when IDU is used every 2 hours than when it is used four times daily. Increasing the frequency of hydrocortisone treatment from four times daily to every 2 hours made the IDU-treated keratitis worse in one series of rabbits. Although the clinical appearance of the rabbits receiving combined IDU and hydrocortisone treatment was good, cultures of these eyes showed persistence of virus.[2] Virus was recovered in 17 of 20 eyes receiving combined treatment but in only four of eight eyes receiving IDU only. It should further be noted that these studies lasted only 2 to 7 days and do not reveal possible late complications of corticosteroid therapy occurring thereafter. Hence, indiscriminate use of corticosteroid with IDU cannot be recommended even though the danger of enhancement of virus by corticosteroids seems to be markedly lessened by use of IDU. If a patient with a stubborn case of metaherpetic keratitis is treated with corticosteroids, simultaneous use of antivirals is clearly indicated.

The efficacy of IDU for epithelial disease drops from 85% to 90% when used alone to 70% when used in conjunction with a corticosteroid drop. Vidarabine, trifluridine, and acyclovir retain their efficacy despite corticosteroid use and are therefore indicated instead of IDU when corticosteroids are used.[35]

Although IDU is effective in the treatment of superficial corneal herpetic infection, its use is disappointing in deeper forms of infection such as disciform keratitis or herpetic iritis. This lack of effect may be because of poor penetration of the drug; however, several trials of irrigation of the anterior chamber with IDU did not enhance its effect.[36] Because these deeper infections respond to corticosteroid treatment, combined IDU and corticosteroid treatment was used for 76 patients with disciform keratitis, geographic ulcers, and diffuse keratitis with iritis.[37]

Combined therapy is guided by experimental and clinical findings that corticosteroids worsen superficial herpetic infection and facilitate its spread, whereas IDU benefits surface infections. Combinations of the two drugs give results that depend on the intensity of treatment with each medication; hence, corticosteroid dosage should be kept to the minimum amount required to benefit the deep herpetic reaction. One drop of corticosteroid three times daily was generally sufficient to suppress the deep inflammation. Concentrations of 0.1% dexamethasone, 0.12% to 1% prednisolone, and 0.5% hydrocortisone were used without obvious difference in response to the different corticosteroid compounds. IDU drops were given every 1 to 2 hours during the day.

Duration of treatment depended on the spontaneous course of the disease, which commonly lasted 1 or 2 months. When the deep infection improved, the corticosteroid drops were gradually discontinued, but the IDU dosage was maintained constant until no more corticosteroid was being used. IDU may be stopped abruptly without need to taper off when the eye is observed to remain quiet without corticosteroid treatment.

Clinically, the majority of these 76 patients responded favorably to combined treatment, which was definitely recommended for such cases of deep herpetic inflammation. Simultaneous use of corticosteroid therapy is not recommended for acute epithelial herpes, which is expected to respond to an antiviral drug.

## CYTOSINE ARABINOSIDE

Culture of HSV in media containing IDU results in development of virus strains resistant to IDU.[38] This experimental finding indicates that clinically troublesome resistant strains will emerge with continued use of this drug. In contrast, only slight resistance developed to cytosine arabinoside, an inhibitor of nucleic acid synthesis that is experimentally effective against herpetic and vaccina infections of rabbit eyes. Cytosine arabinoside has the following advantages over idoxuridine:

1. Virus resistance to cytosine arabinoside develops more slowly.
2. IDU-resistant viruses remain sensitive to cytosine arabinoside.
3. Cytosine arabinoside is quite soluble, which permits preparation of very potent concentrations.

The main *disadvantage* of cytosine arabinoside is its corneal toxicity. It causes corneal damage in doses comparable in antiviral effect to the IDU preparations now in clinical use. Beginning as punctate subepithelial opacities, cytosine arabinoside toxicity may progress to punctate staining or even corneal ulceration. Studies of tritiated thymidine uptake indicate inhibition of cellular metabolism of both corneal epithelium and stroma to a much greater degree than that caused by IDU.[39]

A fine punctate fluorescein staining of the corneal epithelium was reported to occur in human volunteers after instillation of 1% or 0.5% cytarabine six times daily for 2 days. These changes disappeared within 2 to 15 days after the drug was stopped. Similar use of 0.1% cytarabine caused no corneal changes.[40]

Corneal toxicity developed in three patients receiving 3 $g/m^2$ of cytarabine for treatment of leukemia. Corneal epithelial opacities and conjunctival redness were accompanied by eye pain, tearing, photophobia, blurred vision, and foreign body sensation. These faults were considered to be caused by inhibition of DNA synthesis in the corneal epithelium. Because of the marked sensitivity of the cornea to cytarabine toxicity, this drug has been unacceptable for clinical ocular use.[41]

A case report suggests that cytosine arabinoside therapy (1% ointment every 2 hours) combined with topical corticosteroid and a cycloplegic was responsible for curing acute vaccinial blepharitis and keratitis within several weeks.[42]

Intravenous cytarabine (100 mg/m$^2$/24 hours) caused prompt improvement (within 24 hours) of severe ophthalmic herpes zoster in three of four patients.[43]

Apparently the high doses of cytarabine routinely advocated are unnecessary for herpes zoster ophthalmic infections. In seven cases of herpes zoster, cytarabine doses varying from 10 to 40 mg/m$^2$/day were found to be effective (usual recommendation, 100 mg). Toxic effects were insignificant with these low dosage schedules.[44]

A surprising reaction has been described in patients receiving high dosages (300 mg/day for 5 days) of cytarabine for immunosuppressive treatment of leukemia. Although this antiviral agent would be expected to be particularly effective in this high dosage, at autopsy four such patients were found to have extensive herpetic visceral lesions. The postulated explanation was that in high dosage the immunosuppressive effects reduce host resistance to a greater degree than the virus is inhibited. A closely related drug, adenine arabinoside, is considerably less myelotoxic than is cytosine arabinoside and has shown more favorable clinical responses when used as an antiviral agent.[45]

## VIDARABINE (ADENINE ARABINOSIDE)

This structural analog of nucleic acid arrests the growth of the viral deoxynucleotide chain, a different mechanism from IDU, which is incorporated into the deoxynucleotide chain, creating a fraudulent DNA. It is less toxic and sometimes more effective than IDU and cytarabine and can be used effectively in treatment of patients who are allergic to IDU or who are infected with herpetic strains resistant to IDU. DNA viruses such as HSV, varicella-zoster, and vaccinia are also responsive to vidarabine treatment.[46]

Studies of the comparative penetration of vidarabine and IDU showed that a petrolatum vehicle releases nucleoside drugs slowly. In a water-soluble cream with wetting agent, release of these drugs is more rapid. Penetration is also enhanced by the wetting agent, but unfortunately this causes ocular surface irritation. Vidarabine, 3% in petrolatum (this is the commercial preparation, Vira-A) produced aqueous levels of 6 mg/ml 2 hours after topical instillation in rabbits. In cream, aqueous levels of 20 mg/ml were achieved. IDU, 0.5%, whether applied in petrolatum or cream, did not produce detectable aqueous levels.[47]

The metabolism of vidarabine produces hypoxanthine arabinoside (ara-Hx), which is also an active antiviral agent. Not only is ara-Hx 20% as active an antiviral agent as is vidarabine, but it is 10 times as soluble. Three percent ara-Hx produced aqueous levels of 12 mg/ml in petrolatum and 120 mg/ml in cream.

IDU is metabolized to uracil, which enters the eye in small quantities but has no antiviral activity. In summary, both vidarabine and its active metabolite ara-Hx enter the eye much better than does IDU. This finding is compatible with the clinical impression that herpetic uveitis may respond to vidarabine therapy.[47]

In a double-masked study of 54 herpetic corneal epithelial ulcers, the response to 3% vidarabine ointment or to 0.5% IDU ointment, instilled five times daily, were virtually identical. The mean time for complete healing was 25 days for vidarabine and 20 days for IDU. (The range of healing time was from 7 to 98 days.) Another group of 21 patients intolerant to IDU and 37 patients nonresponsive to IDU healed in a mean time of 10 days with vidarabine therapy (range up to 192 days).[48]

In a small series of patients with dendritic keratitis, six IDU-treated patients healed in an average time of 6.8 days; four vidarabine-treated patients healed in 8 days.[49]

An equivalent effect of vidarabine and IDU in treatment of epithelial herpetic keratitis was shown by a study of 29 such eyes.[50] Four patients with IDU intolerance showed no irritation by vidarabine, which is a less toxic drug.

Vidarabine was given as a 3% ointment five times daily in the treatment of 56 cases of severe herpes simplex keratitis that had been resistant to IDU therapy. Eighty percent of cases of epithelial keratitis and 52% of cases of stromal keratitis healed within 2 weeks of vidarabine therapy.[51]

In another series of 22 cases of herpes simplex keratitis uncontrolled by IDU, the administration of vidarabine resulted in healing in an average of 8 days.[52] Please note the absence of a controlled group of untreated patients in the last two cited reports. This prevents comparison with the spontaneous course of the disease.

In addition to the strain differences in herpes simplex, two distinct types are of ophthalmic interest. Type 1 causes the usual ocular or oral infection. Type 2 is the genital strain and is the most common cause of neonatal viral conjunctivitis, as well as an increasingly frequent cause of adult keratoconjunctivitis. Type 2 causes more severe clinical and experimental disease. Both types may respond almost equally well to vidarabine or IDU.[53]

Vidarabine can be given intravenously in dosage of 20 mg/kg over an 8- to 12-hour period daily for 1 week in the treatment of herpetic iridocyclitis.[54] Of 18 patients, 40% improved compared with only 10% in the placebo group. Myalgia, nausea, and leukopenia were among the reactions encountered.

An important characteristic of vidarabine is that it does not interfere with the development of host immunity as does cytosine arabinoside. For this reason, it can be used in clinical antiviral therapy without the fear that it will inactivate the patient's own defense mechanisms.[55]

Comparison of topical therapy of experimental vaccinia keratitis with 0.1% IDU or 5% vidarabine suspension resulted in a much superior response to the vidarabine. IDU is only weakly effective against the vaccinia virus. Vaccinia immune globulin may increase stromal scarring in vaccinia keratitis.[56]

Keratoconjunctivitis caused by adenovirus types 3, 7, 8, and 19 does not respond to 3.3% vidarabine ointment instilled every 4 hours.[57] The typical subepithelial infiltrates developed in 81% of the vidarabine-treated patients and in 63% of the controls.

Vidarabine adenine 5-phosphate (ara-AMP) is a nucleotide form of this antiviral drug. It has the advantage of being much more soluble than vidarabine, and it possesses equal antiviral potency. Given intravenously in a dosage of 100 mg/kg, ara-AMP will produce aqueous humor levels of 50 to 80 mg/ml lasting for 4 hours or more in rabbits. Unfortunately, topical administration of 3% ara-AMP did not result in any detectable aqueous penetration of the drug.[58] ara-AMP is metabolized to vidarabine, which, in turn, is metabolized to ara-Hx. ara-Hx has about 20% of the antiviral effect of vidarabine and is sufficiently soluble to attain aqueous levels of 2 to 8 μg/ml after topical application.[59] Iontophoresis will result in rabbit aqueous levels of 45 ng/100 mg of ara-AMP; of vidarabine, 28 ng/100 ml; of ara-Hx, 95 ng/100 ml.[60]

Punctate staining and epithelial edema occur less frequently with vidarabine than with IDU. Both drugs interfere with stromal healing to the same degree. The rupture of control corneas occurred at 41 psi. This decreased wound collagen content was demonstrated by hydroxyproline assay. The therapeutic index (highest nontoxic dose/lowest effective dose) against herpes simplex keratitis is 60 for vidarabine, 4 for IDU, and 4 for cytarabine.

Vidarabine has been used to treat herpes simplex encephalitis.[61] Mortality is reduced from 70% to 40%.[62] Brain biopsy is recommended to confirm the diagnosis, because other conditions may be otherwise indistinguishable.[63] Cytomegalovirus encephalitis is also responsive to vidarabine treatment when given 15 mg/kg/day intravenously.[64] Vidarabine treatment of zoster in a patient on chemotherapy for carcinoma resulted in death from a characteristic chromatolysis of the brain believed to be caused by synergistic DNA inhibition by the vidarabine and the chemotherapy. The neurologic toxicity of vidarabine cannot easily be distinguished from viral encephalitis because both conditions cause confusion, lethargy, tremors, ataxia, and convulsions.[65]

Retinal viral infections should theoretically be vidarabine responsive just as is encephalitis. Herpetic retinitis is rapidly destructive and will usually cause irreversible blindness before the diagnosis is established.

## TRIFLURIDINE (TRIFLUOROTHYMIDINE; VIROPTIC)

Trifluridine is a thymidine analog inhibitory against DNA viruses. In concentrations as low as 1 μg/ml, trifluridine will inhibit HSV plaque formation in culture.[66] It interferes with DNA synthesis in mammalian cells. Trifluridine is easily aqueous soluble to 1% concentrations compared with the maximum 0.1% solubility of IDU. It is also lipid soluble; this biphasic solubility accounts for good corneal penetration. Rabbit aqueous levels of 5 μg/ml are achieved 30 minutes after topical instillation of 5% trifluridine solution on intact epithelium. Epithelial disease or abrasion increases the aqueous concentration of 37 μg/ml. Kinetic study indicated that the corneal penetration of trifluridine, as well as of cytarabine and IDU, is by simple diffusion.[67]

### Adverse Reactions

No corneal toxicity was biomicroscopically evident in human volunteers receiving a 0.1% solution of trifluridine every 2 hours for 1 week or a 1% ointment five times daily for 3 weeks. Minimal epithelial damage may occur with prolonged topical use. Allergic responses to trifluridine are much less common than to IDU. The half-life of trifluridine in serum is only 12 minutes, the metabolic product being carboxydeoxyuridine, a compound with some antiviral activity. Trifluridine is quite nontoxic for this class of drug, its acute $LD_{50}$ in rats being greater than 4 g/kg.[68] Intravenous doses of 30 mg/kg/day for treatment of human cancer may produce reversible bone marrow depression. Hence, accidental ingestion of the 75 mg in an ophthalmic bottle should not be harmful, even to a child. When eight rabbits were treated with 1% trifluridine four to six times daily during pregnancy, no fetuses were anomalous, and only one was stillborn. In contrast, after similar treatment of 15 rabbits with 0.1% IDU, 42% of the fetuses were either dead or deformed.[69]

Similar to the other topical antiviral drugs IDU and adenine arabinoside, trifluridine has been found to cause conjunctival injection, superficial punctate keratopathy, occlusion of the lacrimal puncta, and conjunctival scarring. It may cause a pseudopemphigoid condition with long-term use.[70] Anterior segment ischemia has also been reported in a patient who had been treated with trifluridine for 4 months for presumed herpetic keratitis. The underlying herpetic infection cannot be ruled out as the cause of the ischemia; however, direct toxicity by trifluridine remains a possibility.[71]

### Clinical Use

In a double-blind trial of 40 patients with HSV corneal ulcers, the ulcers healed in a mean time of 6.3 days after treatment with 1.0% trifluridine was begun compared with 8.2 days after treatment with 0.1% IDU was begun. Both drugs were administered by instilling 1 drop five times daily for 2 weeks, and both were nontoxic.[72]

In another masked study, 40 patients were selected because of dendritic or geographic acute keratitis (only 30% of cultures taken were positive for virus) and treated with 0.1% idoxuridine hourly while awake and every 2 hours during the night (19 instillations/day) for 14 days or with 1% trifluridine every 2 hours while awake (9 instillations/day).[73] In both groups the ulcers healed in an average time of 5.5 days. However, the chances of successful healing by 14 days were 96% with trifluridine and only 75% with idoxuridine treatment. Also treated were 15 patients with corneal ulcers unresponsive to or intolerant of IDU or vidarabine. Of these, 75% healed completely with trifluridine. There were insufficient corticosteroid-treated patients to permit any valid conclusions, but all eight corticosteroid eyes treated with trifluridine healed and one treated with idoxuridine did not heal.

In a double-blind study of patients and treatments exactly the same as the preceding report, no statistically significant difference between the two drugs was demonstrated.[74] For your interest, the nonsignificant statistics for dendritic ulcers are 92% of 26 patients healing with trifluridine vs. 83% of 18 with IDU; healing rate was 0.79 $mm^2$/day with trifluridine and 0.57 $mm^2$/day with idoxuridine. For geographic ulcers, healing was 75% of eight with trifluridine and 33% of nine with idoxuridine; healing rate was 2.11 $mm^2$/day with trifluridine and 1.50 $mm^2$/day with idoxuridine. Of 28 dendritic ulcers unresponsive to IDU or vidarabine, all (100%) healed with trifluridine given every 2 hours while awake.[75] A recurrent dendritic ulcer developed in two of these patients at the same site 1 week after trifluridine was discontinued; these responded again to trifluridine. Two other patients had recurrences 2 to 3 months after healing of the original ulcer; these also responded to trifluridine again. These four recurrences in 10 patients suggest that trifluridine does not reduce the rate of recurrence. One patient showed an unusual toxic response after 1 month of unsupervised therapy; this was a diffuse punctate epithelial keratitis with gray areas of fine, refractile, linear, crystalline intraepithelial deposits. These changes disappeared within 10 days after therapy was stopped.

In treatment of experimental rabbit herpes simplex keratouveitis, 0.1% IDU and 1% trifluridine gave almost identical control of the conjunctivitis, keratitis, and iritis.[76]

Rabbits with experimental herpes simplex stromal keratitis respond well to 1% topical trifluridine given six times daily. Similar response was not found with substitution of the same dosage (2.5 mg) given subconjunctivally once daily. Presumably this is because tissue enzymes destroy trifluridine so rapidly that its half-life is less than 20 minutes.[77]

The virus rebound phenomenon already known for IDU also occurs with trifluridine. Treatment of experimental herpetic keratitis with trifluridine will eliminate a recoverable virus within 2 days. However, if treatment is stopped at 1 week, the virus titer reappears and rapidly rises to values higher than those of untreated control corneas. In some animals, recurrent herpetic ulcers appear during this rise in virus titer. No such herpetic relapses occurred when treatment with either IDU or trifluridine was continued for 2 weeks.[78]

Epithelial debridement used alone and in conjunction with trifluorothymidine was evaluated in 39 patients with herpes simplex dendritic keratitis.[79] Patients were randomized to either receiving debridement alone, trifluridine alone, or debridement followed by trifluridine therapy. Five of the eight cases that were randomized to debridement alone were treatment failures with new or recurrent dendrites developing or a persistent epithelial defect not healed after 2 weeks. Those patients randomized to trifluridine treatment only had an average healing time of 6.8 days with no treatment failures. Similarly, those patients randomized to debridement followed by trifluridine had an average healing time of 7.7 days, and, again, there were no treatment failures. Debridement did not improve the healing time over and above that of the use of trifluridine alone. It should be noted, however, that when the patient was given both debridement and trifluridine, the trifluridine was not started until 24 hours after the debridement.

Trifluridine is preferable to IDU and vidarabine in treatment of herpetic keratitis for a number of reasons. It requires a lesser frequency of administration, which is more convenient to the patient and leads to better compliance. It is effective against a higher proportion of cases, including those in which the other drugs have already failed. It is a solution and does not blur vision as do ointments. It is relatively nontoxic. Finally, it is not antagonized by simultaneous modest corticosteroid usage given at the same frequency.[80]

A dose of 0.5% trifluridine every 4 hours will almost eradicate experimental vaccinia keratitis within 1 week. Used in 5% concentration, trifluridine will sterilize the eye to viral culture and will clinically eradicate the ulcer. Trifluridine is much more active against vaccinia than is IDU and somewhat more active than is vidarabine.[81]

In vitro, trifluridine will reduce production of adenoviruses tenfold for type 8, 1,000-fold for type 19, and 5,000-fold for type 13. Clinically, however, IDU and vidarabine are not effective against adenoviral keratitis.[82]

### Intravitreal Use

In albino rabbits evaluated with ophthalmoscopy, electroretinopathy, and histologic examination, intravitreal injections of 200 μg/ml in 0.1 ml and infusion of an irrigating solution containing 60 μg/ml of trifluorothymidine were nontoxic to rabbit eyes.[83] Prolonged intravitreal drug levels can be obtained through the injection of liposome-encapsulated trifluorothymidine.[84] Liposome-encapsulated trifluorothymidine levels of 12.5, 24.1 and 42.9 μg were injected in 0.1 ml. Electroretinography performed 28 days after the injection was unchanged. Histopathology was also normal with light microscopy. Measurable amounts of trifluorothymidine were found in the vitreous 28 days after injection, indicating this may be a viable method of prolonged intravitreal antiviral therapy.

## ACYCLOVIR (ACYCLOGUANOSINE)

Acyclovir is the result of a truly remarkable biochemical achievement, exploiting the subtle differences of viral and cellular enzyme function in the synthesis of DNA. Viral and cellular thymidine kinase differ slightly from each other. Acyclovir is a nucleoside analog that can function as a substrate for viral thymidine kinase but not for cellular thymidine kinase. Therefore, acyclovir can enter the sequence of DNA formation only in cells infected by virus. Acyclovir is progressively transformed into acyclovir monophosphate, diphosphate, and triphosphate, from which form it enters growing chains of DNA with the aid of DNA polymerase. Once again at this step, viral DNA polymerase more effectively utilizes acyclovir triphosphate than does cellular DNA polymerase. When the acyclovir analog enters the DNA chain, its further development is stopped. Because of the selectivity of these enzyme actions, viral DNA growth is much more susceptible to acyclovir toxicity than is its cellular counterpart.[85–87]

A 50% inhibition of the in vitro cytopathic effect of HSV isolates can be achieved by acyclovir concentrations varying from 0.03% to 0.46 mg/ml.

Experimental rabbit corneal infections with HSV were treated five times daily with ointment base preparations of 0.5% IDU, 3% vidarabine, and 3% acyclovir. Within 5 days of treatment the extent of corneal epithelial loss and the severity of iritis and conjunctivitis were about half as severe in the acyclovir group as in the other two. The most impressive finding was that by day 6 of treatment only 39% of 18 acyclovir-treated eyes contained recoverable virus. In contrast, virus was cultured from 100% of control eyes, 100% of vidarabine-treated eyes, and 93% of IDU-treated eyes.[88]

Three percent acyclovir ointment or 3% vidarabine ointment were applied five times daily for 2 weeks in 41 patients with dendritic or geographic keratitis. Within 14 days, more than 90% of patients in all categories of patients had healed with no significant differences between the two drugs.[89]

More rapid healing of dendritic corneal ulcers was achieved by the combination of debridement with 3% acyclovir five times daily and 1% atropine twice daily than with the acyclovir and atropine alone. With the debridement, 75% of ulcers were healed in 2 days and without debridement in 5 days. The method used to remove the infected epithelium was gentle wiping with a cotton-tipped applicator. No cauterizing chemicals were used. Only mild discomfort from the treatment was reported.[90] Acyclovir does not interfere with the healing of corneal epithelial or stromal injuries in rabbits.[91]

With this highly selective and nontoxic antiviral drug, is it possible to eradicate the reservoirs of chronic herpetic infection, as in the trigeminal ganglion? There is reason for guarded optimism because intravenous acyclovir, 50 mg/kg twice daily, in rabbits substantially reduced the frequency of herpesvirus isolation from brain samples. However, the trigeminal ganglion could not be cleared of virus by this method.[92]

The treatment of herpes simplex keratouveitis is a difficult problem. It is frequently poorly responsive to antiviral therapy. Acyclovir ointment at 3% was compared with 2% trifluridine ointment in a rabbit model with stromal keratitis and iritis. This condition was produced by injection of a live HSV into the corneal stroma of the rabbit. Both the acyclovir and trifluridine decreased the keratouveitis when compared with the placebo ointment. Trifluridine was significantly more potent in suppressing inflammation than was the acyclovir.[93]

Patients with herpes simplex keratouveitis may be treated with systemic and topical acyclovir with good success if they have not been treated with topical corticosteroids for previous episodes. In an evaluation of 32 patients with herpetic uveitis, eight of 18 patients who had previously received corticosteroids require topical corticosteroids to clear the keratouveitis, whereas only 1 of 14 patients who had not received previous corticosteroids were unresponsive to antiviral treatment alone. The authors conclude that antiviral therapy without the use of corticosteroids was a reasonable first-line treatment for herpes simplex keratouveitis. This regimen may avoid the complications of topical corticosteroids. Unfortunately, the results were not compared with a similar control group treated with placebo. In addition, the effects of topical vs. systemic acyclovir were not ascertained.[94] An earlier study of topical and oral acyclovir in the treatment of herpetic stromal disease did not show any significant efficacy of this treatment.[95] However, patients who had previous corticosteroid treatment had a significantly worse outcome than those who had not been previously treated, confirming the apparent risks of corticosteroid treatment of herpetic keratouveitis.

In addition to the treatment of keratouveitis, oral acyclovir has been shown to reduce the incidence of herpetic keratitis after penetrating keratoplasty. In a study of rabbits with HSV type I undergoing penetrating keratoplasty and subsequent treatment with dexamethasone, those rabbits also treated with oral acyclovir did not develop any recurrent HSV infections, whereas of those not receiving prophylactic acyclovir, 82% had positive cultures for HSV. The advantages of oral acyclovir over topical antivirals is that corneal toxicity is avoided.[96, 97]

### Herpes Zoster Ophthalmicus

Oral acyclovir has been studied for the treatment of acute herpes zoster ophthalmicus. The patients were randomized to receive either oral acyclovir or placebo. Acyclovir was given 600 mg five times daily over a 10-day period. Thirty-six patients received acyclovir and 35 received placebo. Treatment with oral acyclovir resulted in quicker resolution of signs and symptoms and decreased duration of viral shedding in patients treated within 72 hours after onset of the skin rash. Treated patients were less likely to have ocular complications of herpes zoster, including episcleritis, stromal keratitis, and anterior uveitis. Pain during the acute episode of zoster was less with treatment, but postherpetic neuralgia was not affected. The oral use of acyclovir was well tolerated and does not have the same potential for systemic complications, including renal impairment, that intravenous use has. Intravenous acyclovir is currently reserved for immunocompromised patients.[98–102] Some patients are intolerant to acyclovir because of GI symptoms, including diarrhea. The addition of exogenous lactase has been found to assist in the GI tolerance of oral acyclovir because the acyclovir tablet contains lactose.[103]

### Acute Retinal Necrosis

Systemic acyclovir is useful in the treatment of the acute retinal necrosis syndrome. These patients with presumed viral cause were treated intravenously with 1,500 mg/m$^2$/day of acyclovir for 11 days. The progressive disease was halted and the retinal lesions resolved; however, 11 of 13 eyes developed retinal detachments requiring multiple operations to reattach the retina. The intravenous acyclovir was well tolerated without complications. This small group of patients indicates that acyclovir is useful in the treatment of acute retinal necrosis, but the secondary complication of retinal detachment was unaffected.[104] Another study reviewing the course of 54 patients with unilateral acute retinal necrosis indicated that the fellow eye was much more likely to remain disease free within the first 2 years after acyclovir treatment than those not treated. In the treatment group 75.3% of fellow eyes remained disease free 2 years after initial onset, whereas only 35.1% of the untreated group remained disease free.[105]

## INTERFERON

A naturally occurring species-specific defense against viruses is the intracellular manufacture of interferon, a substance that increases resistance to virus infection. Because naturally occurring interferon is difficult to obtain, synthetic analogs such as polyinosinic acid–polycytidylic acid have been used to induce patients to form their own interferon. Much interest has been expressed in this therapeutic approach. It has been shown that interferon will increase host resistance to HSV and vaccinia, but no practical clinical value has yet resulted from these studies.[106–119] Interferon has been evaluated in the treatment of adenoviral conjunctivitis. Interferon-$\alpha_2$ given topically was not found to positively effect the course of epidemic keratoconjunctivitis caused by adenovirus.[120] Interferon has been evaluated in the treatment of herpetic keratitis. Interferon-α was used in conjunction with acyclovir and compared with a placebo-acyclovir combination in 59 randomly assigned patients with superficial herpetic keratitis. Patients given the combination of interferon and acyclovir showed significantly quicker healing times than patients treated with acyclovir alone. Interferon has also been found to speed healing of an epithelial defect when used in combination with trifluridine. The dosage of interferon-α used with 30 million IU/ml was two drops per day for the first 3 days of treatment. The time for complete healing averaged 5.8 days for the combination acyclovir and interferon group vs. 9.3 days for the acyclovir-alone group. Interferon alone has little effect on the treatment of herpetic keratitis. In vitro studies of interferon in conjunction with IDU, acyclovir, and dihydroxypropoxymethylguanine assumed synergism in the inhibition of HSV replication.

Interferon-α was used to treat herpes simplex keratitis in an immunosuppressed patient with AIDS. When the infection had failed to clear with trifluridine, IDU, and vidarabine used separately, all antiviral agents were stopped and topical interferon-$\alpha_{2A}$ was given in the dosage of 12 million units/ml on a twice daily schedule. The active epithelial disease completely resolved in 3 weeks. This patient had initially been treated successfully with antiviral therapy but apparently developed resistance to the agents. Interferon seems to offer a topical adjuvant to traditional antiviral therapy in resistant herpetic keratitis.[121–124]

## GANCYCLOVIR

Gancyclovir is a nucleoside analog, 9-(12)-hydroxy-1-(hydroxymethyl)(ethoxymethyl)guanine, which is an acyclovir derivative. It has shown potency against CMV when given systemically. Its chief use in ophthalmology is in the treatment of CMV retinitis in patients with AIDS. CMV retinitis occurs in 3% to 34% of patients with AIDS and has a high incidence of retinal detachment and loss of vision. A recommended induction dose of gancyclovir in patients with normal renal function is 5 mg/kg every 12 hours for 14 to 21 days, and maintenance treatment is 5 mg/kg once daily or 6 mg/kg on 5 out of 7 days per week. The dosage should be adjusted based on clinical course and renal function.

Intravenous therapy for CMV retinitis is necessary in 18 of 109 patients with either AIDS or AIDS-related complex when evaluated prospectively over a 15-month period. All patients responded to initial gancyclovir therapy, but more than 30% of patients developed breakthrough recurrence. Thirteen percent of the patients developed neutropenia with a white blood cell count of less than 1,000 leukocytes/mm$^3$.[125]

### Intravitreal Gancyclovir

Because of the amount of suppression caused by intravenous gancyclovir therapy, intravitreal gancyclovir has been evaluated for the treatment of CMV retinitis. Use of gancyclovir will further exacerbate the myelosuppressive effect of zidovudine, and these two drugs are not used together. In patients with severe myelosuppression or when zidovudine is necessary, intravitreal gancyclovir has been found to be effective in the suppression of CMV retinitis. Intravitreal injection of 200 to 400 μg in 0.1 ml has been used. Induction therapy involves two injections per week until retinal healing followed by maintenance therapy of one injection per week until recurrence occurs. One study showed a single case of *S. epidermidis* endophthalmitis after almost 250 injections in eight patients. Another study of 44 patients showed no episodes of endophthalmitis or cataract.[126–128]

Liposome encapsulation gancyclovir and gancyclovir-trifluridine combination has shown prolonged intravitreal concentrations of gancyclovir for up to 4 weeks after a single injection. This delivery system may be valuable in the maintenance therapy of cytomegalovirus retinitis.[129, 130]

Gancyclovir has been found to be efficacious in the treatment of herpes simplex keratitis in rabbits. Its advantage over acyclovir is that it is water soluble and can be given as a drop. It would offer no particular advantage over trifluridine except in the case of a resistant herpes simplex. Its widespread use as a topical antiviral therapy could lead to development of resistant CMV decreasing the value of this drug in the treatment of important sight-threatening CMV infections.[131]

## FOSCARNET

Foscarnet (trisodium phosphonoformate hexahydrate) is a pyrophosphate analog that inhibits many viral RNA and DNA polymerases, including the reverse transcriptase of HIV. It is a virustatic drug. It is an alternative to gancyclovir in the treatment of CMV retinitis that can be used in conjunction with zidovudine because it does not induce myelosuppression. The foscarnet-gancyclovir CMV retinitis trials showed foscarnet to be preferred for most patients with the exception of those patients in renal failure with creatinine clearance less than 1.2 ml/min/kg. Dosage is initiated with a bolus of 20 mg/kg, followed by a continuous infusion of 0.16 mg/kg/min. These patients seem to do better with gancyclovir.[132, 133]

### Intravitreal Foscarnet

Intravitreal foscarnet has been reported in patients with AIDS and CMV retinitis in whom gancyclovir was contraindicated because of previous acyclovir allergy and systemic foscarnet was contraindicated because of renal failure. Foscarnet was passed through a 0.22-μg filter and then 1,200 μg (0.05 ml) was injected intravitreally. The injections were repeated every 3 days for 17 days, and then maintenance therapy was continued with one injection per week. Two vitreous samples were taken, and from these an elimination half-life of 54 hours was calculated. This treatment controlled the CMV retinitis. The authors recommended induction therapy of two injections (1,200 μg) of foscarnet per week for 3 weeks, then maintenance therapy of one injection per week.[134]

## ZIDOVUDINE

Zidovudine (formally azidothymidine [AZT]) has been shown to be beneficial in delaying the progression to AIDS in patients infected with HIV but who are asymptomatic or had very early symptoms. Zidovudine is myelosuppressive and cannot be used with systemic gancyclovir. When both zidovudine and a CMV antiviral medication are needed, foscarnet is generally recommended over gancyclovir unless severe renal insufficiency exists, in which case intraocular gancyclovir is the treatment of choice.[135–137]

Comparing the use of the combination foscarnet and zidovudine with foscarnet alone in the treatment of CMV retinitis showed a higher percentage of patients, progressing to complete resolution and a lower percentage of patients failing therapy using the combination.[132]

A patient with anterior uveitis was treated successfully with systemic zidovudine therapy after anterior chamber aspirate documented HIV presence. The patient had failed therapy with topical and systemic corticosteroids when the anterior chamber paracentesis was performed. The therapy was 100 mg of oral zidovudine four times daily for 10 days and then increased to 200 mg every 4 hours for another 14 days. Visual acuity improved to 20/20.[138]

A patient with AIDS and CMV retinitis declined treatment with gancyclovir but consented to treatment with zidovudine and had subsequent regression in the CMV retinitis, indicating some response to zidovudine treatment alone.[139]

## GERMICIDES

Inactivation of viruses is a problem common to all health care practitioners, particularly ophthalmologists with frequent contact with mucous membranes and the use of instruments from patient to patient during the day. Proper disinfection is necessary. The Centers for Disease Control recommends high-level disinfection. First, particulate matter should be removed. Usually this is not a major problem with ophthalmic devices such as tonometers. Proper hand washing and use of disposable gloves should be employed when appropriate. Disinfection solutions include 3% hydrogen peroxide, 10% dilution of household bleach (sodium hypochloride), 70% ethanol, and 70% isopropanol. After disinfection the device should be rinsed. Care must be taken not to apply the instrument to the eye immediately after disinfection because all of these solutions can damage the cornea. Rigid and soft contact lenses should be disinfected. Heat disinfection or hydrogen peroxide disinfection are both appropriate for viral inactivation, including the HIV. Ten percent povidone-iodine (Betadine) solution will completely inactivate HIV.[140]

SECTION THREE

# Antifungals

Antifungal agents may be divided into three categories: polyenes, the imidazoles, and the fluorinated pyrimidines (Tables 6–13 and 6–14).[1] Polyene antifungal agents bind preferentially to the ergosterol and the fungal plasma membrane. This alters membrane permeability and electrolyte imbalance, causing death of the fungal cell. Polyenes are fungicidal drugs.

Imidazoles act through the inhibition of ergosterol synthesis and are fungistatic at low concentrations. Direct cell membrane damage can occur at higher concentrations unrelated to the ergosterol inhibition. This fungicidal effect is not found with ketoconazole.[2]

Flucytosine is an example of a fluorinated pyrimidine. Flucytosine is enzymatically converted once inside the fungi to fluorouracil. Fluorouracil blocks fungal thymidine synthesis. Because mammalian cells cannot enzymatically change flucytosine to fluorouracil, mammalian cells are unaffected.[1]

## AMPHOTERICIN B

Amphotericin B is an antibiotic substance derived from strains of *Streptomyces nodosus*. It has a wider spectrum of activity against yeastlike fungi than any other presently available antifungal agent. Amphotericin B is the drug of choice in therapy of infections resulting from *Coccidioides immi-*

**TABLE 6–13.**
Antifungal Drugs

| Polyenes | Imidazoles | Fluorinated Pyrimidines |
|---|---|---|
| Amphotericin B | Clotrimazole | Flucytosine |
| Natamycin | Econazole | |
| Nystatin | Ketoconazole | |
| | Miconazole | |
| | Thiabendazole | |

**TABLE 6–14.**
Summary of Antifungal Dosing

| Agent | Dose |
|---|---|
| Amphotericin B | IV: Test doses of 1, 5, and 10 mg on days 1, 2, 3, respectively; then increase the dose 5 to 10 mg/day up to 1–1.5 mg/kg/day as tolerated<br>Topical: 0.15% in sterile water<br>Intravitreally: 5 μg/0.1 ml |
| Natamycin (Pimaricin)* | Topical: 5% suspension |
| Nystatin | Topical: 100,000 units/g ointment |
| Miconazole | IV: 25 mg/kg/day in 2–3 divided doses<br>Topical: 10 mg/ml<br>Subconjunctival: 10 mg<br>Intravitreal: 10–40 μg/0.1 ml |
| Ketoconazole | Orally: 300 mg/day<br>Topical: 1%–5% solution |
| Flucytosine | Orally: 50–150 mg/kg/day in divided doses<br>Topical: 1% solution |

*Natamycin 5% suspension is the only antifungal approved for by the FDA for topical ophthalmic use.

*tis, Histoplasma capsulatum, Cryptococcus neoformans, Blastomyces dermatitidis, Candida* species, and many other less common fungi. Growth of these organisms in vitro is inhibited by amphotericin B concentrations of 0.02 to 0.5 mg/ml. Isolated cases of sporotrichosis, mucormycosis, chromoblastomycosis, and aspergillosis have responded favorably to amphotericin B.[3] Viruses, protozoa, and bacteria are not affected by amphotericin B,[4] nor do actinomycosis and nocardiosis respond to this drug.

### Mechanism of Action

Amphotericin B causes increased permeability of cytoplasmic membranes, thereby permitting leakage of essential intracellular constituents. The antibiotic binds rapidly to ergosterol in susceptible cellular membranes such as those of vulnerable yeasts. The extent to which permeability is damaged is dose related. However, a more rapid death of the yeasts cannot be achieved clinically by increasing drug dosage because the same cytoplasmic membrane damage also affects human cells (the mechanism of toxicity). Synthetic derivatives with reduced toxicity also have a reduced chemotherapeutic effect, further indicating the similar mechanism of the toxic and therapeutic effects.[5]

Synergistic action may occur with the combined use of several antifungal drugs. Hypothetically, amphotericin B may damage the fungal cell membrane, increasing its permeability and thereby enhancing entry of other antibiotics such as rifampin (acts by inhibiting RNA synthesis), tetracycline (inhibits protein synthesis), or flucytosine. An increased uptake of radioactively labeled flucytosine by *Candida* occurs in the presence of amphotericin B. This synergistic activity is demonstrable in vitro.[6] Different fungi respond differently to antibiotic combinations. Antifungal action against *Candida* and *Cryptococcus* is enhanced by amphotericin B combined with flucytosine or tetracycline. Action against *Candida, Saccharomyces, Histoplasma,* and *Blastomyces* is enhanced by amphotericin B combined with rifampin. Unfortunately, combinations of these antifungal drugs also enhance toxicity against host cells, so that the therapeutic index may not be improved.

In vivo, combined treatment was evaluated against *Candida keratitis*.[7] Treatment was with drops of 0.5% amphotericin B four times daily, with subconjunctival injection once daily of 15 mg of rifampin dissolved in 0.5 ml of dimethylsulfoxide, or with a control of saline drops and DMSO (dimethylsulfoxide) injection. Evaluation was by colony count of organisms after 4 days. Combined use of amphotericin B and rifampin gave a colony count averaging 931; amphotericin B only, 4,627; control, 30,000. Whether there was a clinically observable difference in the three groups of rabbits was not reported.

Corticosteroid enhancement of fungal infections is well established. In addition to worsening the infection, the topical corticosteroid will also adversely affect the efficacy of natamycin, flucytosine, and miconazole. Topical prednisolone acetate did not adversely affect the efficacy of topical amphotericin B.[8] The institution of topical corticosteroids in the management of a suspected or proven fungal keratitis should occur only with full knowledge of the potential hazards of exacerbating the infection. Its use, if at all, should be only in the well-defined keratitis with known fungal agent while the patient is on specific antifungal therapy. Even then its use should be approached with extreme caution.

## Administration

Being relatively insoluble in water, amphotericin B is poorly absorbed from the GI tract and therefore should be administered intravenously. For intravenous infusion, a solution of 0.1 mg/ml in a 5% solution of dextrose is used. Saline solution cannot be used because the amphotericin B will precipitate. (Unused solutions should be discarded after 24 hours. Amphotericin B is both heat labile and light sensitive, and the dry powder should therefore be refrigerated and protected from light.) The rate of intravenous administration should be so adjusted that the total dose is infused over a period of 3 to 6 hours.

Because the tolerance to amphotericin B varies greatly among patients, dosage must be individually adjusted. The safest approach is to give test doses of 1, 5, and 10 mg over the first 3 days, respectively, increased by increments of 5 to 10 mg/day as tolerated. The objective is to reach a daily dosage of 1 mg/kg, which will result in blood levels of 1 to 2 μg/ml Dosage of less than 1 mg/kg may be relatively ineffective. Failure of the disease to respond necessitates a gradual increase to 1.5 mg/kg/day. This dose should not be exceeded. Many patients can never achieve maximal dose because of dose-related adverse reactions. Because renal excretion is slow and demonstrable blood levels persist for 18 hours or more after a single dose, treatment need be given only once daily or perhaps every other day. The latter schedule of alternate-day therapy is suggested when clinical improvement is noted. Relapse may occur if amphotericin B is discontinued too soon. Alternate-day therapy is advised for at least 2 months for many infections, with administration of a total dose of at least 3 g of amphotericin B. Because therapy will be prolonged for weeks or months, the clinician should not increase dosage to the highest possible level in the hope of obtaining more prompt remission. Rather, dosage should be adjusted to avoid renal damage and permit a prolonged fungistatic effect.

For topical administration, a 0.15% solution of amphotericin B may be freshly prepared with sterile water. (Amphotericin precipitates in saline solution.) The preparation must be refrigerated in a dark bottle to slow disintegration. Drops are instilled every 30 to 60 minutes for the first 3 days of treatment of a fungus keratitis. When improvement occurs, the frequency of administration may be reduced, but a level of four times daily instillation is necessary for at least 1 month.[9]

## Toxicity

Unpleasant and potentially dangerous side effects are almost inevitable when the drug is given at therapeutic levels; therefore, amphotericin B should be used only under close clinical supervision. Headaches, chills and fever, and anorexia are common with systemic use and may be minimized by the use of antipyretics and antihistaminics. Acetylsalicylic acid, 0.64 g, and promethazine (Phenergan), 25 mg, may be given orally 30 minutes before the infusion is started. Severe symptoms during the course of intravenous infusion may necessitate temporary interruption of the flow or a decrease in the dose given.

Most patients on a high dosage of amphotericin B for prolonged periods show renal damage as manifested by rising BUN levels and other indicators; kidney function tests should be done periodically during such therapy. Levels of BUN up to 30 mg/100 ml occur in the majority of patients during the second or third week of treatment. Values higher than this require interruption of treatment until the BUN level has dropped to less than 30 mg/100 ml, lest serious renal failure result. Estimations of BUN levels should be obtained every 2 to 3 days.

Moderate anemia is frequently encountered during amphotericin B therapy (75% of 30 patients).[10] The mechanism for this appears to be bone marrow depression and decreased red blood cell production. Fortunately this anemia is usually self-limited, does not progress to dangerous levels, and disappears after therapy is stopped. Complete blood cell counts should be obtained weekly and more often if values drop to borderline levels.

Nausea, vomiting, GI cramps, and diarrhea may force reduced treatment. Alternate-day dosage will often permit the patient to recover from these symptoms and to eat relatively normally on the intervening days. Hypokalemia may cause weakness or electrocardiographic changes. Supplemental potassium is curative.

Local chemical thrombophlebitis may result from the irritating nature of amphotericin B solutions. The phlebitis may be minimized by decreasing the drug concentration, reducing the rate of infusion, and avoiding reuse of the same vein.

Because of its toxicity, amphotericin B should be given in treatment of reasonably well-substantiated cases of susceptible mycotic infection. Diagnosis is preferably made by culture of the organism. Vague, undiagnosed diseases (e.g., uveitis) associated with a positive skin test result for one of the fungi do not usually justify the use of such a poisonous drug. The patient on systemic amphotericin B for ophthalmic reasons must be comanaged with an internist who will follow the patient for potential life-threatening toxicity.

### Ocular Penetration

The blood-eye barrier is highly resistant to the passage of amphotericin B. After intravenous administration of 1 mg of amphotericin B/kg, no antibiotic entered the normal rabbit aqueous, nor was any demonstrable in eyes with severe hydrochloric acid keratitis. However, in animals with an intense uveitis induced by intravitreal albumin injection, aqueous levels of 0.16 μg/ml were attained and levels of 0.13 μg/ml persisted for 24 hours.[11] In one study, trace amounts of amphotericin B, too small for reliable measurement, were found in the aqueous of normal and inflamed eyes after subconjunctival injection of 150 μg.[11]

The corneal penetration of topical antifungal medication was evaluated in a model of *Candida albicans* corneal infection. Intact corneal epithelium reduced the antifungal effect of natamycin and amphotericin B. Flucytosine was less effective in the absence of epithelium. The imidazoles were not effective topically, with or without epithelium, in this model of fungal keratitis.[12]

### Ocular Tolerance

Local application of amphotericin B is obviously much safer than the systemic use of such a toxic drug and is therefore the route of choice in treatment of corneal infection. Amphotericin B may be given topically in a concentration of 0.1% or subconjunctivally in a dose of 1 to 2 mg.[13]

Continuing topical application of 1% amphotericin B in a deoxycholate vehicle causes progressively worsening corneal epithelial defects, stromal opacities, and severe iridocyclitis.[14] Both the antibiotic and the vehicle are toxic, and the combination is worse. These toxic effects can easily be mistaken for worsening of the fungal infection, leading to a vicious cycle of more frequent antibiotic administration for an ever-increasing antibiotic toxicity. Topical application of 0.5% amphotericin B ointment causes some conjunctival irritation. An application of 5% ointment results in corneal edema and iritis so severe that it may persist for 1 week.[15]

Subconjunctival injection of 2 mg doses of amphotericin B in treatment of an *Aspergillus* corneal ulcer resulted in severe pain, marked chemosis, and localized ischemic necrosis lasting for several weeks.[16] This was followed by the development of large, raised, reddish subconjunctival nodules, permanent yellow discoloration of the conjunctiva, and a posterior subcapsular cataract. Amphotericin B was simultaneously administered as a 0.5% solution, 1 drop given hourly. After 1 week of therapy the ulcer began to improve, but less intensive therapy was continued for 2½ months, at which time all cultures and scrapings had become negative.

The effect of intraocular (anterior chamber) amphotericin B injections in rabbits has been studied.[16] A single injection of 25 μg in 0.05 ml of distilled water caused transitory and reversible iritis and slight clouding of the lens but no permanent sequelae. Increasing the injection to 50 μg considerably increased the severity of reaction, but it subsided after 4 days. Further increase to 125 μg of amphotericin B caused irreversible opacification of the cornea and interior of the eye.

A patient with metastatic coccidioidal iridocyclitis was given an anterior chamber injection of 25 μg of amphotericin B, repeated after 2 weeks.[17] The eye became phthisical and was enucleated 4 days after the second injection. Culture of the enucleated eye recovered viable organisms despite the therapy.

Treatment of a human postcataract *Volutella* fungus infection with intraocular injection of 40 μg of amphotericin B was successful in sterilizing the eye.[16] Unfortunately, there developed a corneal pannus, an updrawn pupil, a vitreous retraction, and a total funnel-shaped retinal detachment. Whether these complications were caused by the infection or by the treatment is hard to determine.

Intravitreal injection of amphotericin B can be highly destructive. Injection of 250 μg caused immediate clouding of the vitreous and retinal detachment. The vitreous remained relatively clear with injections of 100 to 250 μg, but retinal detachments occurred within 5 days. The mechanism of retinal detachment is necrosis of the retina, which can be observed as a white patch appearing almost immediately after positioning of even a small dose near the retina. Of clinical importance is the absolute necessity that an intravitreal injection of amphotericin B *must* be placed exactly in the center of the vitreous (as far as possible from the retina) and should be injected slowly to avoid streaming toward the retina. Doses as small as 5 to 10 μg, placed in the center of the vitreous, were well tolerated by rabbit eyes, resulting in no detectable clinical, microscopic, or ERG changes. Sodium deoxycholate is used as a solubilizing agent in the commercial preparation of amphotericin B. The intraocular damage described occurred with pure crystalline amphotericin B alone and did not result from sodium deoxycholate injections, indicating that the damage is caused by the antibiotic and not by the vehicle.[18]

The methyl ester of amphotericin B is said to be less toxic than is amphotericin B itself. A single 5-μg intravitreal dose of this ester caused no detectable changes in rabbit eyes yet cured experimental *Candida* endophthalmitis as long as 5 days after infection with 1,000 organisms (a dose that caused complete vitreous opacification in all untreated eyes).[19]

Focal retinal damage and vitreous band formation occurred with intravitreal doses of as low as 5 μg of amphotericin B. Up to 20 μg of amphotericin B may be given intravitreally using liposomes.[20] This liposomal-bound amphotericin B was efficacious in the treatment of fungal endophthalmitis with reduced toxicity. However, higher doses of amphotericin B are required to achieve the same efficacy level.[21]

The practical reason for intravitreal injections is that a single injection of 5 μg of amphotericin B into the center of the vitreous will cure experimental *C. albicans* endophthalmitis with retention of vision if treatment is given within 5 days of the infecting inoculation.[22] Even if the vitreous is slightly cloudy before treatment, the infection is reversible. After the retina has been destroyed by infection, it is too late for successful treatment. From the standpoint of the clinician, this allows very little time to decide whether or not a fungal endophthalmitis is present, to diagnose it by aspiration, and to institute effective treatment.

In two cases, *C. albicans* endophthalmitis was cured by a single intravitreal injection of 5 μg of amphotericin B.[23, 24] In each case a severe vitreous reaction followed the injection and lasted for several weeks. The disc was barely visible during this period of vitreous reaction, and vision dropped to counting fingers at 1 foot. One patient recovered 20/25 vision; the other, 20/200 by the last recording at 7 weeks.

Collagen shield delivery of amphotericin B offers the potential to increase compliance and has a more constant rate of drug delivery to a fungal keratitis. The anterior segment levels of amphotericin B were evaluated in rabbit eyes after application of amphotericin B with a collagen shield. The collagen shields were soaked in 0.5% amphotericin B and were compared with amphotericin B 0.15% drops. Corneal amphotericin B levels with collagen shield delivery were more than double that with drops delivery during the first 2 hours of treatment. By 3 hours the two methods were equivalent, and by 6 hours the corneal levels were higher with the drops and lower with the collagen shield. The peak levels with collagen shield delivery occurred at 1 hour, falling precipitously thereafter down to a steady state between 3 and 6 hours. The corneal levels at 6 hours with the collagen shield were still within therapeutic range. Collagen shields may make follow-up examinations difficult and, if used improperly, could cause increased toxicity. When used judiciously, however, it may aid in compliance. They achieve high corneal concentrations quickly when therapy is initiated.[25]

## Clinical Use

Clinical reports describe the use of amphotericin B in the sterilization of corneal ulcers caused by a wide variety of fungi. Topical use is quite effective. The devitalized condition of the cornea after the usual prolonged course of a fungus infection causes markedly delayed healing. Secondary bacterial infection must be prevented by routine antibacterial therapy during the period of epithelial defect. Sometimes the cornea will weaken or perforate requiring structural reinforcement with a corneal graft. The availability of an antifungal agent as effective as amphotericin B makes apparent the importance of cultures and smears (including techniques for fungus identification) in serious ocular infection. A search for fungi should be instituted early in the management of a resistant corneal infection. Persistent, slowly developing intraocular infection after trauma or surgery should arouse suspicion of fungal etiology, and, if sufficiently severe, it may warrant diagnostic surgical aspiration of material for culture.

### *Chorioretinitis*

Use of amphotericin B in the treatment of uveitis is difficult to evaluate because of the usual problems of clinical diagnosis. Nine cases of chorioretinitis were thought to be of histoplasmic etiology because skin test and complement fixation test results were positive and the chest x-ray findings were compatible with histoplasmosis.[26] Amphotericin B therapy did not seem to alter significantly the clinical course of the chorioretinitis. The amphotericin B was administered intravenously in doses of 50 mg/day to a total dosage of not more than 1 g. Because of the rather marked toxicity of this drug, it would seem best to limit its use to the treatment of patients with a most convincing diagnosis of histoplasmosis, with systemic manifestations in whom the organism can be recovered from the other tissues. Chills, fever, vomiting, abdominal and head pain, azotemia, hemorrhagic gastroenteritis, and hematologic disturbances result from amphotericin B therapy.

The effectiveness of amphotericin B in the treatment of intraocular histoplasmosis has been proved by its successful use in the therapy of rabbits infected by anterior chamber inoculation with *H. capsulatum*. Amphotericin B (0.5 mg/kg) was given intravenously once daily for 15 days. This treatment was started 2 weeks after inoculation. In eight treated rabbits, various organ cultures were negative for *Histoplasma* organisms, and six of eight inoculated eyes were sterile. In contrast, viable organisms were recovered from all untreated inoculated eyes and from the lung, liver, spleen, kidney, and blood of the untreated animals. Marked clinical improvement was grossly evident in the treated eyes in contrast to the extensive necrosis of the untreated eyes. The authors of this report emphasize that amphotericin B therapy of experimentally induced mycotic ophthalmitis is not the same as treatment of supposedly histoplasmic immunogenic eye involvement.[27]

#### *Lid Infection*

When the fungus infection to be treated is small and well localized, amphotericin B may be applied by local injection. In this way effective concentrations are achieved locally, yet systemic toxicity is avoided. For example, in treatment of a 1-cm *Aspergillus* granuloma of the lid, 1 mg of amphotericin B diluted in distilled water was injected directly into the granuloma and surrounding tissue.[28] Repeated at weekly intervals, this dosage completely cured the *Aspergillus* granuloma within 2 months. Of practical interest was the initial failure to diagnose the fungal nature of this infection, which was recognized only with special fungus stains of the second biopsy specimen.

### Summary

Amphotericin B is a moderately effective drug for combating yeastlike fungi. Unfortunately, the medication is toxic and troublesome to administer systemically. Superficial keratomycoses may respond well to topical preparations. Because its intraocular penetration with systemic administration is poor, use of amphotericin B for fungal endophthalmitis is through very careful intravitreal injection of 5 μg of amphotericin B. This may be valuable in the treatment of *Candida* endophthalmitis.

In the treatment of most superficial ocular fungus infections, natamycin (Pimaricin) is an effective alternative to amphotericin B and is available as a topical preparation.

## NATAMYCIN (PIMARICIN)

Natamycin, a semisynthetic tetraene, polyene antibiotic of the same general class as nystatin and amphotericin B, is the only antifungal drug commercially available for treatment of corneal infections. Natamycin causes a dose-related fungicidal effect by damaging fungal cell membranes. In concentrations of 1 to 25 μg/ml it will inhibit the growth of a wide variety of fungi, including species of *Aspergillus, Blastomyces, Candida, Cephalosporium, Coccidioides, Cryptococcus, Curvularia, Epidermophyton, Fusarium, Histoplasma, Microsporum, Penicillium, Sporothrix,* and *Trichomonas.* These organisms vary considerably in their susceptibility to natamycin. Viruses and bacteria are nonresponsive to natamycin treatment.

Natamycin is poorly soluble in water, does not penetrate cornea, conjunctiva, or other mucosal surfaces, and is not absorbed from the GI tract. It is stable in 5% suspension and in this form will remain in contact with the cornea for useful periods of time. Dosage is 1 drop every 1 to 2 hours initially. The frequency of use is reduced gradually, perhaps cut in half every 3 or 4 days of treatment. Effective drug levels are not attained in either cornea or aqueous after topical application; hence, it is useful only in the treatment of superficial keratomycosis.

Topical application of natamycin is well tolerated by the eye. Fifteen human volunteers used a 5% suspension of natamycin for 2 weeks, 1 drop every 2 hours while awake.[29] No ocular toxicity was observed in any of these volunteers.

### Intraocular Tolerance

Anterior chamber injection of natamycin suspension in rabbits shows the ocular structures to tolerate a dosage of 250 μg.[30] Subsequent to a dose of 500 μg, corneal decompensation and iridocyclitis developed. One hour after a 250-μg injection, iris concentrations of natamycin averaged 190 μg/g; aqueous levels averaged 62 μg/ml. The pharmacokinetics of drug clearance followed a two-compartment pattern, with an iris reservoir. At 24 hours, the iris retained

45 μg/g, whereas the aqueous had dropped to 4.8 μg/ml. The effects of intracameral natamycin treatment with 250 μg given 24 hours after intracameral injection of 5,000 spores of *Aspergillus* were difficult to evaluate because of the marked spontaneous variability in severity of the untreated infection. Of 18 eyes in each group, 12 control eyes and 8 treated eyes became infected. Blindness resulted in eight control and six treated eyes. Paradoxically, 13 of 18 eyes treated with 500 μg became blind. The combination of the infection and the drug suspension resulted in trabecular obstruction and severe glaucoma.

The intravitreal use of natamycin is apparently not practical. In rabbits 50 μg will destroy the retina. In one study a dose of 25 μg was tolerated by the eye but was not sufficient to be effective against experimental fungus infection *(Aspergillus)*.[31]

### Clinical Use

Seven patients with culture-proven fungal corneal ulcers were given 5% natamycin every 2 hours.[29] Four patients were cured of the infection within 2 to 4 weeks of therapy, whereas the other three required keratoplasty subsequent to the medical treatment. However, no viable fungus was recovered from the surgical specimens. A 1% solution of potassium iodide was also instilled at 1- to 2-hour intervals in these eyes in the belief that the potassium ion helps an injured cornea maintain its water pump system and glycolytic cycle. The iodide ion may not be helpful. Clinically, the corneal reaction to fungal infection is less with potassium iodide therapy than without it.

*Fusarium solani* is the most common cause of fungal keratitis in Florida. Natamycin in a 5% suspension applied hourly cured 16 of 18 culture-proven *Fusarium* corneal ulcers.[32] The suspension is viscous and adheres well to the cornea. It is well tolerated and causes no pain or secondary corneal damage. Improvement in the appearance of the ulcers could be recognized within 2 days. Amphotericin B had been used in the treatment of 20 previous patients with *Fusarium* ulcers, achieving a cure in only 7 cases. Also, the amphotericin B caused intense local pain and diffuse surface damage to the cornea and conjunctiva. This study stresses the differences in the antibiotic responses of different species and strains of fungi.

Three years later the same authors[33] reported a larger series of 61 cases of fungal keratomycosis. Of these, 53 were treated with natamycin, used as a 5% suspension instilled hourly during the day and every 2 hours at night, tapering the dose as a favorable response occurred. Of 36 cases of *Fusarium* keratitis, 35 were treated with natamycin, and 29 were successes. Of 10 *Monilia* corneal infections treated with natamycin, six were successful. All four yeast infections responded well to natamycin therapy. Keratoplasty was successful in saving 9 of the 13 eyes that failed to respond to medical therapy.

### Experimental Combined Therapy

In the hope that fungal inflammatory damage to the cornea could be diminished while fungal growth was inhibited by natamycin, corticosteroid therapy was also used in the treatment of *Aspergillus* corneal ulcers in rabbits.[34] Five percent natamycin and 2% potassium iodide were given every 2 to 3 hours. Also, different groups of rabbits were treated with 0.1%, 0.01%, and 0.001% dexamethasone four times daily. The eyes treated with the higher concentrations of dexamethasone showed the most improvement during the first week of treatment but subsequently showed deterioration, with larger ulcers forming and severe intraocular infection developing. The animals receiving 0.001% dexamethasone had recognizably less inflammation and did not suffer exacerbation of the fungus infection. Quite clearly, *great care* is required in the use of corticosteroids for corneal fungal infections, if they are used at all.

## NYSTATIN (MYCOSTATIN)

Nystatin is a *Streptomyces*-derived antibiotic highly active in inhibiting the growth of a wide variety of fungi, molds, and yeasts. It has little or no effect on other types of microorganisms. Nystatin is fungistatic, not fungicidal.[35]

Despite the broad antifungal spectrum of nystatin, its therapeutic effect in systemic mycoses has been disappointing because toxicity prevents administration of adequate quantities of the drug. Oral preparations are poorly absorbed, intravenous injections cause chills and fever, and intramuscular injections cause local reaction. Therefore, for ophthalmic use, nystatin is administered topically in the treatment of surface fungus infections.

The solubility and stability of nystatin are of clinical importance. As much as 200,000 units may be dissolved in 1 ml of a special commercial diluent (*N*-methyl glucamine, Tween 20, dimethyl acetamide; (E.R. Squibb and Sons, Princeton, N.J.), whereas only 300 to 600 units will dissolve in 1 ml of water. If the nystatin solution in the diluent is placed into isotonic saline solution or water, a fine suspension results. (This type of suspension was used in the rabbit tolerance experiments to be presented next.) Refrigerated aqueous suspensions retain 90% of their original activity after storage for 2 weeks.

## Experimental Therapy

### *Intraocular Infections*

The use of nystatin for experimental therapy of intraocular *Aspergillus fumigatus* infections in albino rabbits has established the therapeutic effectiveness of the drug, as well as its ocular tolerance. Nystatin is reasonably well tolerated as a topical ointment containing 100,000 units/g and as a single subconjunctival dose of 5,000 units in a 0.5-ml saline solution. Two hundred units of nystatin in a 0.1-ml solution were injected into the vitreous or aqueous chamber without causing excessive reaction. Histopathologically demonstrable hyperemia and leukocytic infiltration persisted for 48 hours after injection of the anterior chamber and for 1 week after intravitreal injection. Vitreous assays suggested that nystatin levels sufficient to inhibit *Aspergillus* growth persisted for only 24 hours after injection. A second intravitreal injection of 200 units of nystatin, 36 hours after the first, caused vitreous degeneration. Single intravitreal injection of 400 units of nystatin caused cloudiness of the vitreous that persisted for at least 1 week.

*Aspergillus* growth is inhibited by a nystatin concentration of 6 to 12 units/ml. Intravitreal injection of 1,000 *Aspergillus* spores will destroy all untreated rabbit eyes, with clinical evidence of severe infection recognizable within 3 days. Eyes infected in this manner were injected intravitreally with 200 units of nystatin at 30 minutes or 24, 48, or 72 hours after infection. Seven of the eight eyes treated 24 hours after infection showed no evidence of fungus growth during observation periods for as long as 7 weeks. Treatment 2 days or more after infection temporarily reduced the severity of infection but did not protect the eyes from destruction. Therapy 30 minutes after infection delayed but did not prevent endophthalmitis. Possibly this can be explained by the resistance of *Aspergillus* spores to nystatin before they have germinated.

The greater the number of *Aspergillus* spores injected, the more rapid is the inflammatory response. Proximity to vascular structures such as the iris or ciliary body resulted in more rapid growth than did inoculations into the central vitreous. The variable incubation period of human ocular fungus infections may be explained by differences in the size and location of the inoculum, as well as by variations in resistance and virulence.

### *Corneal Infections*

The effectiveness of nystatin against corneal infections has been evaluated in rabbits infected with *C. albicans*.[36] This study reports no toxicity after topical instillation of 100,000 units of nystatin/ml but states that subconjunctival injection of 2,000 units or more may cause localized necrosis. Subconjunctival injection of 800 units caused only transitory conjunctivitis. Bioassay failed to detect nystatin in aspirated aqueous after treatment by either topical or subconjunctival injection. (The assay method was sensitive to 80 units/ml and would therefore have failed to detect smaller amounts; *C. albicans* is inhibited by 8 units nystatin/ml.)

Treatment with 100,000 units of nystatin ointment/ml applied three times daily was begun either immediately after corneal inoculation with *Candida* or after delays of 4, 24, 48, or 72 hours. No infection developed in those eyes treated immediately.[36] Mild infections, which were controlled by treatment, occurred in one of six eyes treated 4 hours after inoculation and in six of 10 eyes treated after 24 hours. Severe infection destroyed all eyes untreated during the first 48 hours, regardless of subsequent therapy. Microscopic section of untreated eyes showed Descemet's membrane to be intact at 24 hours, but at 48 hours mycelial penetration into the anterior chamber was evident.

The ineffectiveness of topical nystatin therapy after 48 hours is compatible with the belief that the cornea blocks drug penetration. When *Candida* organisms enter the anterior chamber, they are beyond the reach of topical nystatin.

The method of inoculation was intracorneal injection of 100,000 *Candida* organisms. This invariably caused infection of prednisolone-treated corneas, with a hypopyon ulcer appearing by the fourth day and perforation usually by the seventh day. *Candida* infection of the rabbit cornea could not be produced in this way without the aid of corticosteroids. Prednisolone, 30 to 60 μg, was injected intracorneally just before fungus inoculation. The facilitation of corneal infection produced by a single prednisolone injection was found to last for at least 2 weeks.

### Clinical Use

A patient with *A. fumigatus* keratitis was cured after 1 month of treatment with nystatin.[37] Because no ophthalmic preparation of this antifungal drug is commercially available, a concentration of 50,000 units/ml was prepared by suspending sterile nystatin powder in an aqueous solution of 1.2% sodium chloride and 0.5% chlorobutanol. This nystatin suspension was instilled every 2 hours. Nystatin was also administered orally, 500,000 units every 8 hours. The effectiveness of nystatin was indicated by the facts that smears and cultures were negative by the fifth day of treatment (both smears and cultures were initially positive for *Aspergillus*) and that the hypopyon and corneal infiltrate cleared, recurred, and again cleared as nystatin was used, discontinued, and again administered. Atropine, hot compresses, and narcotics (for severe pain) were also used. Corticosteroid therapy was not used.

### Summary

Nystatin inhibits the growth of a variety of molds, yeasts, and fungi. Unfortunately, it is poorly absorbed orally and quite toxic when administered parenterally. Topical application of 100,000 units of nystatin ointment/g is of value in the treatment of external ocular infections caused by *Candida* or *Aspergillus* but is limited by topical toxicity and poor ocular penetration.

## MICONAZOLE

Miconazole is a broad-spectrum antifungal agent in the imidazole group. As 2% cream or lotion, it is effective on topical administration to skin or mucous membrane surfaces. Intravenous dosage is 25 mg/kg/day in two or three divided doses. Some examples of susceptible organisms include *Alternaria, Blastomyces, Candida, Coccidioides, Epidermophyton, Nocardia, Sporothrix,* and *Trichophyton.* Many other genera are also affected by miconazole action on the cell wall.[38] It also exhibits mild activity against gram-positive bacteria.[39]

### Ocular Penetration

In rabbits, 30 mg of miconazole/kg given intravenously over a 2-minute period produced 1-hour aqueous levels of 8 μg/ml, dropping to 2 μg/ml by 2 hours. Subconjunctival injection of 10 mg produced aqueous levels of 3 to 4 μg/ml, lasting for 10 hours. Removal of the corneal epithelium before the 10-mg subconjunctival injection increased the aqueous peak to 10 μg/ml, indicating that subconjunctival injection maintains a tear film reservoir of the drug, which then penetrates transcorneally. Drops of 1% miconazole instilled every 15 minutes for eight doses produced aqueous levels of 0.5 μg/ml with intact epithelium and 4.6 μg/ml with absent epithelium.[40]

Corneal levels were not attained by intravenous use but reached 13 μg/g after subconjunctival injection with intact epithelium and 35 μg/g with absent epithelium. Topical miconazole produced 10 μg/g corneal concentrations with intact epithelium and 93 μg/g with absent epithelium.

Vitreous levels were undetectable after intravenous or topical administration but reached 0.25 μg/ml after subconjunctival injection with absent epithelium and 1.3 μg/ml with intact epithelium (the reverse of what would be expected).

Miconazole, 1,200 mg, was given intravenously 1 hour before enucleation of a human eye for fungal endophthalmitis. No detectable levels were present in the cornea. The aqueous level was 0.6 μg/ml; the vitreous level was 2.7 μg/ml.

### Clinical Use

A *Paecilomyces* endophthalmitis after pseudophakos implantation was cured by removal of the lens, radical vitrectomy, iridectomy, and topical and systemic use of miconazole, thiabendazole, flucytosine, and amphotericin B. The surgery was performed 1½ months after cataract extraction, during which time all of these drugs had been given without apparent effect. During surgery, 25 μg of amphotericin B, 200 μg of flucytosine, and 10 μg of miconazole were given intravitreally. Exactly which component of this prolonged polypharmacologic and surgical therapy was responsible for fungal eradication is impossible to determine. Remarkably, the eye had 20/100 vision 1½ years later.[41]

Two patients with *Coccidioides* and one with *Candida* endophthalmitis were treated unsuccessfully with miconazole (400–1,000 mg three times daily intravenously). A better response was obtained with amphotericin B and flucytosine therapy, although the amphotericin B was quite toxic.[42]

## KETOCONAZOLE

Ketoconazole is similar to miconazole and the other agents in the imidazole group that are fungistatic because of inhibition of ergosterol synthesis in the fungal membrane, increasing its permeability. Ketoconazole has been used successfully to treat fungal corneal infections in humans. Orally administered ketoconazole in doses of 300 mg/day have been successful in clearing *Fusarium* corneal ulcers. It may also be given in a topical form in 1% to 5% solution.[43, 44]

### Other Imidazoles

Thiabendazole is an antiprotozoal drug that was found to have antifungal activity.[45] Subsequently, other imidazoles such as ketoconazole, miconazole, and clotrimazole were found to be more effective antifungals. Terconazole and fluconazole are examples of triazole antifungal drugs. Terconazole was found to be well tolerated in rabbit eyes with injections of 10 μg/0.1 ml. Terconazole is active against a wide spectrum of fungi. Fluconazole demonstrates unusual ocular penetrations after oral administration in the rabbit. With a single oral dose of 20 mg/kg, corneal levels were 13.3 μg/g, aqueous levels were 7.4 mg/l, vitreous levels were 9.8 mg/l, and choroid/retina levels were 5.2 μg/g. This penetration level is much higher than ketoconazole and miconazole.[46, 47]

## FLUCYTOSINE

Flucytosine is a fluorinated pyrimidine initially produced as an antimetabolite in leukemia therapy. It is enzymatically changed to fluorouracil within the fungal cell. The fluorouracil blocks fungal thymidine synthesis. Mammalian cells are not affected because they do not metabolize flucytosine.

Oral administration is 50 to 150 mg/kg/day given in divided doses. Topical therapy is a 1% solution. Fungal resistance occurs when cell membrane transport is not present. Because of induced resistance, combination treatment for keratomycosis is necessary when flucytosine is used.[1, 48–50] The efficacy of flucytosine was compared against that of amphotericin B, natamycin, and the imidazoles in a rabbit model of *C. albicans* keratitis. Epithelialized and deepithelialized corneas were compared. The polyenes (amphotericin B and natamycin) were not effective when the epithelium was intact. However, flucytosine efficacy improved with intact epithelium over what was found after the epithelium was removed. The isolate recovery rate was the lowest for amphotericin with absent epithelium (4.5 isolates at 0.15% and 5.7 isolates at 0.75%). Five percent natamycin was the next most effective antifungal. When the epithelium was absent, 11.51 isolates were recovered. Flucytosine with intact epithelium was found to have 14.53 isolates recovered from the treated cornea. The imidazoles showed no efficacy in the treatment of *Candida* keratitis in this animal model. Extrapolating these data indicates that for most *C. albicans* fungal ulcers with absent epithelium, amphotericin B and natamycin would be the treatment of choice, but flucytosine should be considered if the epithelium is intact.[12]

### Synergism

Relatively high doses of antifungal agents are ordinarily necessary to achieve fungicidal levels in the cornea. These high levels are frequently associated with clinically significant toxic effects. One study evaluated the synergistic use of low concentrations of amphotericin B, natamycin, nystatin, and clotrimazole. When all four drugs were used, the concentrations of each were decreased to approximately 1/12 of their minimum fungicidal concentrations if each were used separately. At these levels corneal endothelial changes as documented by specular microscopy were unchanged during corneal storage for potential transplantation. This synergistic activity may also be useful in the treatment of an indolent fungal ulcer with concomitant toxic drug changes.[51]

SECTION FOUR

## Antiparasitics

Fortunately, intraocular parasites are extremely rare in developed countries. They are a common cause of blindness in developing countries. The larger larvae require surgical removal, because their death induces destructive intraocular inflammation. Smaller parasites such as microfilaria may be successfully destroyed by medical treatment. Treatment of the free-living amoeba *Acanthamoeba*, an important cause of contact lens–associated keratitis, is also reviewed in this section.

### THIABENDAZOLE

Thiabendazole is an effective anthelminthic and antifungal drug. Topically applied thiabendazole is effective against experimental infections with *Trichophyton, Epidermophyton,* and *Microsporum* species. *A. fumigatus,* an organism reported as causing human keratomycosis, is highly susceptible to thiabendazole, becoming inhibited by 2 to 4 μg/ml of drug. Greater concentrations are fungicidal.[1–3]

The corneal penetration of carbon-14-labeled thiabendazole after application of a 4% suspension and maintained on the rabbit corneal for 1 hour. The peak corneal concentration of 52 μg/g far exceeds the necessary level for inhibition of *Aspergillus* (Fig. 6–19). Deeper portions of the eye attain much lower drug concentrations, for example, lens 4.0 and vitreous 0.9. Some systemic absorption followed topical application, and peak plasma levels approached 0.5 μg/ml. An average of 1,420 μg of thiabendazole was excreted via the urine in the 4-hour period.

Intraocular levels of oral administration of thiabendazole were evaluated in a 7-year-old boy undergoing pars plana vitrectomy for removal of an epiretinal membrane associated with *Toxocara canis*. A dose of 25 mg of thiabendazole/kg (total 500 mg) was administrated ½ hour before surgery. Aqueous, vitreous, and serum samples were obtained for analysis. Aqueous and vitreous levels of thiabendazole were within the therapeutic range 90 minutes after oral administration.[4]

### Toxicity

Topically applied thiabendazole is well tolerated by the eye. Repeated ocular instillation of 10% solution of 4% ointment in rabbits caused no signs of eye irritation.[5] The drug is well tolerated when given systemically, and general poisoning from absorption during ocular use seems impossible unless some type of idiosyncrasy (unreported) is present. The acute $LD_{50}$ for animals is greater than 3,000 mg/kg. Chronic dosage of 400 mg/kg interferes with weight gain and causes normochromic anemia.

An unusual toxic response to thiabendazole is of considerable ophthalmic theoretical interest. A 43-year-old woman and her 17-year-old daughter took thiabendazole for pinworm infestation. Within 2 to 3 weeks partial swelling, dryness of mouth and eyes, and jaundice developed in both. This reaction lasted for more than 1 year, finally disappearing. This was interpreted as being an autoimmune response in which the drug precipitated the formation of antibodies against the biliary, salivary, and lacrimal epithelial cells. Apparently 72% of patients with primary biliary cirrhosis (an autoimmune disease) have the sicca syndrome, and 6% of patients with sicca syndrome have hepatic disease. The only other drug known to cause a sicca syndrome is practolol, a β-adrenergic blocker.[6]

### Clinical Use

One day after administration of 2 g of thiabendazole orally, a previously visible intraretinal nematode (presumably *Toxocara*) disappeared, leaving a localized hemorrhage at its previous site.[7] Perhaps this resulted from death of the worm and body response to the dead tissue, but the possibility of escape of the worm from the eye cannot be excluded. The edematous and hemorrhagic response disappeared during the following month, leaving a permanent small scotoma.

Because of the possibility of increased reaction and retinal damage on death of the worm, a moving parasite might be permitted

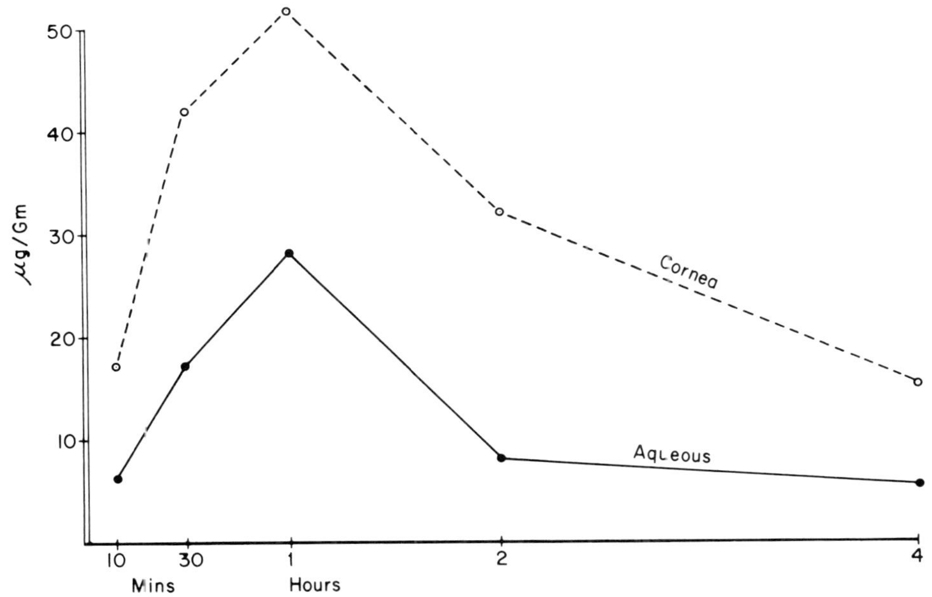


**FIG 6–19.**
Ocular concentrations of thiabendazole after topical applications for 1 hour as 4% suspension. (Data from Robinson HJ, and others: *Am J Ophthalmol* 62:710, 1966. Used by permission.)

to leave the foveal area before the thiabendazole administration. Although published photographs of two cases document presence of an actively motile parasite,[7] this condition is so rare that the effect of thiabendazole is not known with certainty.

Thiabendazole and corticosteroid therapy was of no value in treatment of two advanced cases of ocular toxocariasis, probably because the organisms were already dead. The normal fate of the parasite is to live within the tissues for several months, then to die. At the stage of disease when a leukocoria exists, the problem is usually a pure inflammatory response that cannot benefit from anthelminthic therapy.[8] Acute trichinosis infection is responsive to thiabendazole therapy, the severity and duration of symptoms being reduced.[9]

In the treatment of a patient with keratitis caused by *Phialophora verrucosa,* a 0.3% solution of thiabendazole was applied topically every 30 minutes for 1 week without improvement. The organism was again isolated in culture after this treatment. (Incidentally, covering the cornea with a thin conjunctival flap cured the patient within 2 weeks.) The low concentration of thiabendazole was selected because of poor solubility of the drug in water. However, a 12% suspension can be prepared in 1% sodium carboxymethyl cellulose, and ointment may be made in any desired concentration.[10]

Unilateral subacute neuroretinitis was found to respond to systemic thiabendazole in four patients. This condition was caused by retinal invasion by one of at least two different nematodes. The regimen used in this study was 22 mg of thiabendazole/kg twice daily orally for 2 to 4 days.[11]

## MEBENDAZOLE

Mebendazole is an anthelminthic that acts by blocking glucose uptake in nematodes but has no effect on blood glucose levels in animals or humans. A dose of 100 mg morning and evening for 3 days in children more than 2 years of age is highly effective against pinworms, whipworms, and roundworms[12] and is considered the drug of choice.

Mebendazole was used in patients with onchocerciasis-mediated posterior segment disease and found not to alter the progression of depigmentation of the chorioretinal lesions.[13] The chorioretinal disease is most likely to be a chronic inflammation rather than active parasitic disease.

## DIETHYLCARBAMAZINE

Diethylcarbamazine, the anthelminthic drug of greatest value in treatment of onchocerciasis, will destroy microfilariae within the eye. The dosage is 2 to 3 mg/kg orally three times daily. Death of the microfilariae causes localized tissue inflammation that is manifested in the eye by increased severity of uveitis and conjunctivitis. Corticosteroid therapy will reduce this undesirable inflammatory response. Unfortunately, the adult *Onchocerca* worms are not killed by diethylcarbamazine and remain as a source of new microfilariae. Repeated courses of diethylcarbamazine treatment are required over many years to control the disease.[14]

Because ocular involvement is the most commonly disabling manifestation of onchocerciasis, the ocular penetration of an ophthalmic preparation of diethylcarbamazine was studied.[15] A single topical application of 2 drops of 5% diethylcarbamazine (a nonirritating concentration) results in aqueous concentrations of 3 to 5 μg/ml, which, after oral administration, are therapeutically effective levels. These preliminary experiments suggest that some routine of topical prophylaxis might be evolved to control ocular microfilariae.

Diethylcarbamazine was evaluated as a therapy for ocular onchocerciasis in ten Liberian men with *Onchocerca volvulus* infections. These subjects had both anterior segment and posterior segment lesions. Subjects treated with oral diethylcarbamazine showed a significant increase in microfilariae found in the cornea, both living and dead after 1 week of therapy. Greater corneal inflammation, including punctate keratopathy and limbitis, were found during the first week of therapy. These responses were much higher than that found with placebo. Corneal microfilariae and ocular reaction then decreased in the eye treated with diethylcarbamazine, so that 3 months after initiation of therapy, the corneal microfilariae were not significantly different from placebo and the ocular reaction was actually somewhat less than that found with placebo. Posterior segment changes were not affected by therapy in this study.

## IVERMECTIM

Ivermectim is a semisynthetic macrocyclic lactone effective against a wide range of parasites and anthropoids. It was compared with diethylcarbamazine and placebo in the treatment of onchocerciasis and had significantly less corneal and anterior segment inflammation during the initial weeks of therapy with a similar reduction of intraocular microfilariae compared with diethylcarbamazine. In this study ivermectim was given in a dose of 200 μg/kg (12 mg), similar to diethylcarbamazine and mebendazole. As expected, ivermectim did not affect the inflammatory pigmentary chorioretinal changes found with chronic onchocerciasis.[13, 14]

## TOXOPLASMOSIS

*T. gondii* is a common cause of infectious chorioretinitis in healthy individuals. It can also occur as an opportunistic infection in patients immunocompromised by AIDS or after organ transplantation. It may appear as a multiorgan disease or as an isolated ocular infection. Indications for treatment of toxoplasmosis retinochoroiditis are reduced vision worse than 20/200; significant vitreous inflammation, giving a "headlight in the fog effect"; and lesions in the posterior pole, including the peripapillary, perifoveal, and maculopapular bundle, which can threaten the fovea. Many ophthalmologists will treat any toxoplasmosis lesions in the presence of immunosuppression. Several medical regimens have been used (Table 6–15). Most uveitis specialists surveyed indicated preference for using the combination pyrimethamine, sulfadiazine, folinic acid, and prednisone, and some preferred the addition of clindamycin. Sixteen percent used sulfadiazine, clindamycin, and prednisone without pyrimethamine, and 6% used clindamycin and prednisone alone. Sulfadiazine and clindamycin are each described in the antibacterial chapter.[16–18]

**TABLE 6–15.**
Treatment of Ocular Toxoplasmosis*

| |
|---|
| Regimen 1: Pyrimethamine, sulfadiazine, folinic acid |
| Regimen 2: Pyrimethamine, sulfadiazine, clindamycin, folinic acid |
| Regimen 3: Sulfadiazine, clindamycin |
| Regimen 4: Clindamycin |
| Regimen 5: Trimethoprim-sulfamethoxazole |

Modified from Engstrom RE, Holland GN, Nussenblatt RB, and others: *Am J Ophthalmol* 111:601, 1991. Used by permission.
*Prednisone may be added to any of the regimens.

## PYRIMETHAMINE (DARAPRIM)

Pyrimethamine (2,4-diamino-5[*p*-chlorophenyl]-6-ethylpyrimidine) is a potent folic acid antagonist that is used clinically in the treatment of toxoplasmosis and malaria.

### Pharmacology

Blood serum levels of approximately 0.2 to 0.4 mg of pyrimethamine/100 ml may be attained clinically by giving two 100-mg doses of pyrimethamine on the first day of treatment, followed by doses of 25 mg twice daily thereafter (see Fig. 6-19). If this high initial dose is not given, about 21 weeks is required for the smaller daily doses to achieve the same blood level.[19]

The concentration of pyrimethamine in the uveal tract and retina is somewhat higher than that in the serum. It is fortunate that *Toxoplasma* organisms exist within these tissues and not in the intraocular fluids, because the blood-aqueous barrier is poorly permeated by pyrimethamine. Less than 0.005 mg/100 ml was found in the aqueous of patients with serum levels of 0.1 mg/100 ml or higher. This very low aqueous concentration of pyrimethamine existed despite the presence of cells and flare in the anterior chamber of these patients with active uveitis. Because *Toxoplasma* organisms multiply only within cells and are susceptible to the action of pyrimethamine only while actively multiplying, it is the tissue concentration that determines the efficacy of the drug.

Measurement of pyrimethamine in various portions of the eye with the aid of radioactive labeling indicates a selective concentration of this drug within the retina.[20] Twelve hours after intramuscular infection of 2.5 mg/kg of labeled pyrimethamine in monkeys, the animals were killed by exsanguination (to minimize contamination of the tissues by blood radioactivity). The pyrimethamine concentrations 12 hours after this single dose were serum, 1.02 μg/ml; retina, 3.2 μg/ml; aqueous, 0.03 μg/ml; and vitreous, no measurable radioactivity. For comparison, 2.5 μg/ml may be attained in human serum with a pyrimethamine dosage of 50 mg/day. *Toxoplasma* organisms in tissue culture may be killed by exposure to 0.25 μg/ml for 4 days.[21]

There is little chance that pyrimethamine administered locally to the eye will have a therapeutic effect on the eye. Subconjunctival injection of 0.05 mg of pyrimethamine in a 0.5-ml volume produced aqueous levels of 10 μg/ml (1 mg/100 ml) within 1 hour in rabbits.[21] This aqueous level fell very rapidly (to 1 μg/ml in 2 hours). No measurable vitreous concentration was attained. Daily subconjunctival injection of 0.05 mg of pyrimethamine in rabbits was well tolerated for 2 months, causing only minimal cyclitis, which was evident on histopathologic examination. Retrobulbar injections of 0.1 mg in a 1-ml volume failed to introduce a measurable amount of pyrimethamine into the vitreous. Unfortunately, pyrimethamine concentrations in the uveal tract after local injection were not measured. Injection of 0.5 to 5 mg into the aqueous or vitreous destroyed the eyes.

### Response of *Toxoplasma* Organisms

The sensitivity of *Toxoplasma* strains to pyrimethamine varies with their rate of growth. Experimental work is usually done with rapidly multiplying strains, which may be killed by only 3.0 μg/ml of the drug. Clinical infection is usually caused by more slowly growing organisms that may be killed by 10 to 50 μg/ml in 5 days. Obviously the clinically attainable pyrimethamine concentrations are not high enough to kill resistant strains. Encysted and dormant *Toxoplasma* organisms are not affected by pyrimethamine, but, then, neither do they cause inflammation (although they may become active at some future time). Cure of a disease by an antibacterial drug does not require that their growth be slowed sufficiently to permit the body's defenses to control them. It has been demonstrated that pyrimethamine levels of 1.0 μg/ml inhibit the growth of *Toxoplasma* organisms in tissue culture.[22] This strain was killed by 10 μg/ml.

Because of considerable variations in the resistance and virulence of various strains of *Toxoplasma,* the clinical course and response to therapy will vary greatly. Because of the uncertainty of these variables, treatment should entail the highest drug dosage tolerated without toxic side effects.[23]

### Metabolic Differences Between *Toxoplasma* Organisms and Mammals

Intracellular folic acid and its subsequent active derivatives, as shown in Fig. 6–20, are derived from *p*-aminobenzoic acid by *Toxoplasma* and from folic acid by mammals. Because the folic acid molecule contains a *p*-aminobenzoic acid structure, folic acid can be utilized (although less efficiently) by *Toxoplasma* and will interfere with the therapeutic effect of pyrimethamine, as does *p*-aminobenzoic acid. Folinic acid is poorly utilized by *Toxoplasma* but is effective in mammalian metabolism. Antitoxoplasmic therapy with 25 mg of pyrimethamine and 2 g of sulfadiazine is not weakened by 5 mg of folinic acid, which is sufficient to protect the patient against toxicity. Folinic acid may be given in one fifth the amount of pyrimethamine without inhibiting its therapeutic effect.

### Combined Sulfonamide and Pyrimethamine Therapy

Remarkably, effective synergism between sulfadiazine and pyrimethamine has been demonstrated in studies of *Toxoplasma*-infected mice.[24] In these studies the median effective dose (MED) was

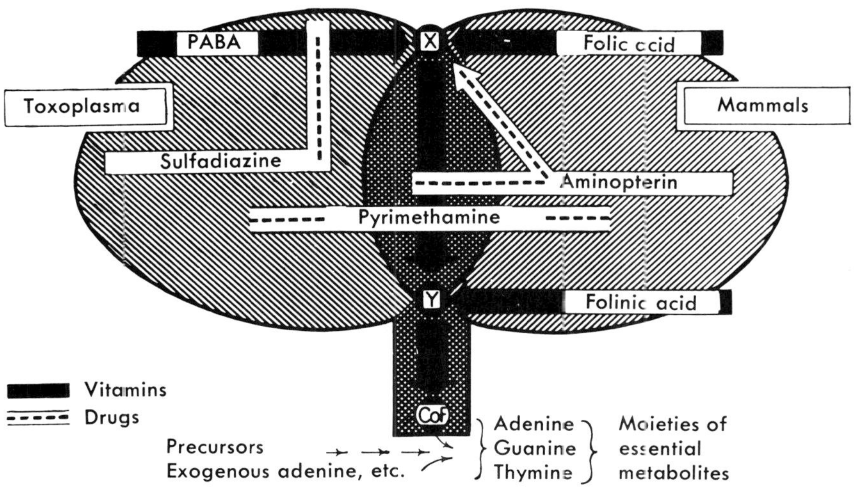


**FIG 6–20.**
Folic acid metabolism in *Toxoplasma* organisms and in mammals. Note synergistic effect of pyrimethamine and sulfadiazine, which act at two points in sequence on the same metabolic pathway. (From Frenkel JK: *Antibiot Chemother* 7:630, 1957. Used by permission.)

designated as the amount of medication permitting a 50% survival for 10 days in mice given a standard lethal inoculum (1,000 $LD_{50}$) of *Toxoplasma.* In their most efficient combination, 1/8 MED of sulfadiazine combined with 1/24 MED of pyrimethamine was the equivalent of 1 MED of either drug alone. Medication was administered via the diet and was expressed in terms of milligrams per 100 ml of diet. The MED of sulfadiazine was 40 mg% and of pyrimethamine was 9 mg%. The most efficient combination MED was 5 mg% of sulfadiazine with 0.37 mg% of pyrimethamine.

These findings clearly indicate powerful synergism between pyrimethamine and sulfadiazine when they are used in combination as therapy for toxoplasmosis. The simultaneous use of these two drugs is therefore indicated in the clinical management of patients with toxoplasmosis. Four grams of sulfapyrimidines daily is recommended.[25–27] The decreasing availability of sulfadiazine has led to use of trimethoprim-sulfamethoxazole (Bactrim) with success.

The sulfonamides vary in antitoxoplasmic potency; the most effective are the pyrimidine derivatives sulfadiazine, sulfamerazine, and sulfamethazine.[28] The MED of sulfonamide (the pyrimidines) requires a blood level of 40 mg/100 ml in contrast to 600 mg/100 ml for sulfanilamide and 450 mg/100 ml for sulfapyridine. The three sulfapyrimidines are best prescribed as a triple-sulfonamide combination, because they are independently soluble in the urine and can be administered in higher dosage with less danger of crystalluria. The therapeutic effect of such a triple mixture is additive, being equivalent to the effect of an equal amount of only one sulfonamide compound. Alkalinization with 2 g of sodium bicarbonate daily further reduces the possibility of crystalluria.

### Toxicity

The hematologic toxicity of pyrimethamine is related to the serum levels attained. Eleven patients who suffered no toxic effects had an average serum concentration of 0.25 mg/100 mg compared with an average of 0.33 mg/100 ml in eight patients who experienced bone marrow depression.[18] There are, of course, individual variations in sensitivity; one of the patients suffering from toxicity was reported to have a serum level of only 0.16 mg/100 mg. Obviously the therapeutic dose is quite close to the toxic dose, and it is therefore essential to count red blood cells, white blood cells, and platelets once or twice each week during pyrimethamine therapy. Please note that hematologic depression occurred in eight of 19 patients given 200 mg of pyrimethamine the first day and 50 mg/day thereafter.

The hematologic toxicity of pyrimethamine has been studied in 87 patients treated for at least 5 weeks (doses ranging from 25 to 100 mg/day) for uveitis caused by *Toxoplasma* infection. Although bone marrow depression caused a decrease in red blood cells, white blood cells, and platelets, thrombocytopenia was the most severe manifestation of pyrimethamine toxicity. When platelet suppression begins in a patient receiving pyrimethamine, the platelet count usually declines for 3 to 9 days after the drug is discontinued (Fig. 6–21).[29] Normal levels are regained in 1 to 2 weeks. Folinic acid did not hasten disappearance of the thrombocytopenia encountered in these patients.

Therapy should be discontinued or reduced when the platelet count drops to 80,000/mm$^3$ or less; routine counts should be made twice weekly during treatment.

Toxic manifestations of pyrimethamine also include convulsions, which have been

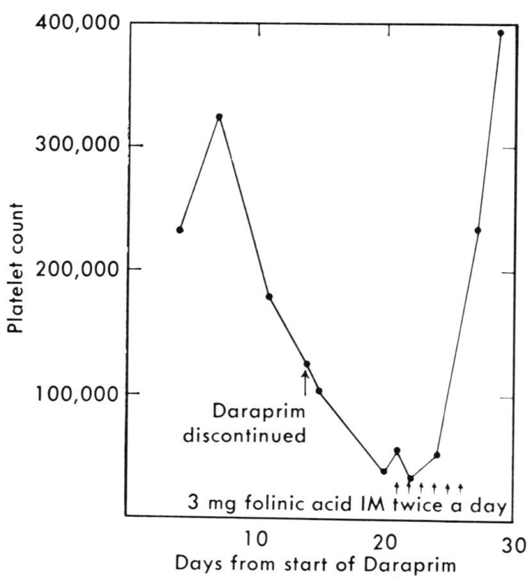


**FIG 6–21.**
Platelet counts during pyrimethamine (Daraprim) therapy. Drop in circulating platelets usually occurs after 1 week or more of therapy, continues to decline for 1 week or so after treatment is stopped, and returns to normal after another week, more or less (regardless of folinic acid). (From Kaufman HE, Geisler PH: *Arch Ophthalmol* 64:140, 1960. Used by permission.)

described in monkeys and in accidentally poisoned children.[30] Two of these children, both approximately 2 years of age, died in convulsions within 2 hours after swallowing 400 mg of pyrimethamine. (Presumably, large doses of folic acid would be indicated as emergency treatment of accidental poisoning with pyrimethamine. One is again reminded to caution patients against leaving potent medications within the reach of children.)

When administered to pregnant rhesus monkeys, pyrimethamine produces gross malformations of the fetal skull.[31] Because teratogenic drugs are particularly dangerous during early (and possibly unknown) pregnancy, the treatment of presumed toxoplasmosis uveitis in young married women should be initiated only if effective contraceptive measures are being used.

### Response of Infection to Treatment

Because of the tendency for cyst formation, it seems doubtful that a human infection can be eradicated. Clinical studies suggest that the severity of toxoplasmic chorioretinitis decreases after adequate therapy, which should be continued for at least 1 month. Typical of the published statistics is the report that 13 of 22 treated patients showed definite improvement, although only four patients were classified as being in "excellent condition."[32]

### Summary

Without doubt, *Toxoplasma*-inhibiting concentrations of pyrimethamine and sulfonamide can be attained within the retina and choroid using a clinically acceptable amount of medication. The synergism of combined therapy *greatly* enhances the therapeutic effect; combined treatment requires only ⅛ as much sulfonamide and 1/24 as much pyrimethamine as would be necessary if either were used alone.

Simultaneously administered folinic acid, *not* folic acid, results in a 100% survival rate of animals given a lethal dose of pyrimethamine and yet does not decrease the therapeutic effect of the drug. Platelet counts should be done at least once each week during the course of therapy. Counts of less than 80,000/mm$^3$ require that pyrimethamine therapy be stopped. Clindamycin may be used instead of or in addition to pyrimethamine in the treatment of toxoplasmosis. Trimethoprim-sulfamethoxazole may be used in treatment because sulfadiazine is becoming less available.

## ACANTHAMOEBA

*Acanthamoeba* keratitis is caused by a free-living amoeba that may colonize contact lenses, contact lens solutions, and contact lens cases. Clinically it may cause a corneal infiltrate, painful radial keratoneuritis, chemosis, sclerokeratitis, and dendriform epithelial lesions. Pain is usually exquisite to a degree greater than would be expected by the clinical signs. The course is complicated by delayed diagnosis and ineffective therapy.

The key to successful management is early diagnosis and aggressive and prolonged therapy. One percent propamidine isethionate (Brolene) has been shown to have activity against *Acanthamoeba*. It is not currently available in the United States but is available in Europe. Neomycin and polymyxin B both have acanthamoebal activity and are available in combination with either gramicidin (solution) or bacitracin (ointment). The antifungal drugs miconazole and clotrimazole in 1% solutions have also been shown to have acanthamoebal activity. Paromomycin sulfate is an aminoglycoside antibiotic similar to neomycin. It is a direct-acting (contact) amebicide. It has broad activity against many parasites. Concentrations of 10 μg/ml are amebicidal against *Acanthamoeba*. Paromomycin, 15 mg/ml, was more effective than neomycin and propamidine isethionate in killing *Acanthamoeba polyphaga* and *Acanthamoeba castellani* in an in vitro model. Freezing enhanced the effect of all of the antibiotics (Fig. 6–22).[33] All these antibiotics may have corneal toxicity, which may then be confused with or mask a recurring acanthamoebal infection.[34–40]

Combination treatment of neomycin-polymixin B–gramicidin, propamidine, and miconazole was used to obtain a cure in six of seven patients with *Acanthamoeba* keratitis. One of these seven patients required penetrating keratoplasty to manage the keratitis. This excellent success rate indicates that aggressive topical therapy with multiple antiamoeba drugs is indicated for

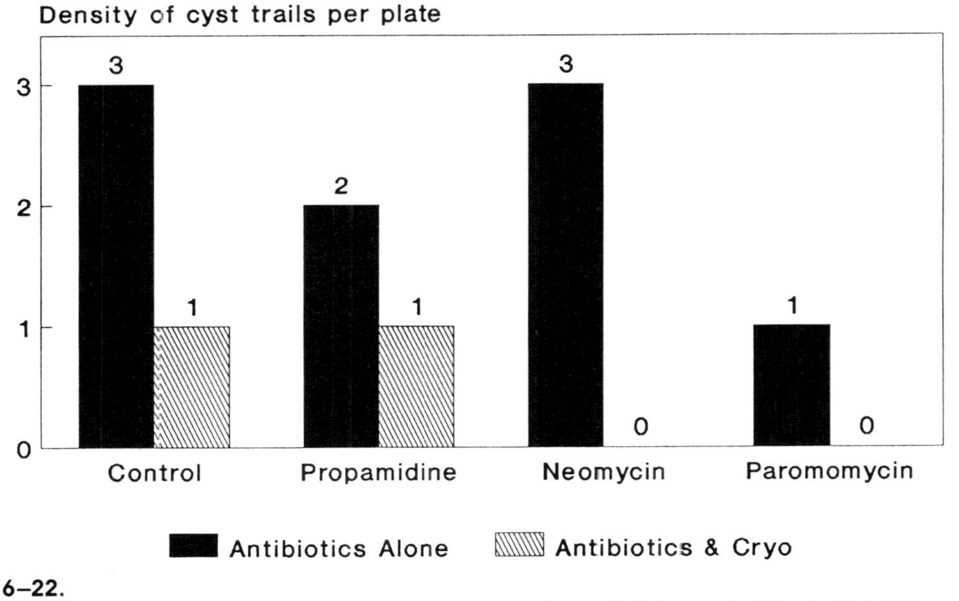


**FIG 6–22.**
Elimination of *Acanthamoeba polyphagia* cyst trails on experimental plates graded 3+ (>16 trails/plate) to 0 (no trails), with antibiotics and freezing therapy (cryo). (Modified from Matoba AY: *Arch Ophthalmol* 107:439, 1989. Used by permission.)

**TABLE 6–16.**
Agents Used in the Therapy of *Acanthamoeba* Keratitis

| |
|---|
| Propamidine isethionate |
| Neomycin sulfate |
| Paromomycin sulfate |
| Polymyxin B |
| Miconazole |
| Clotrimazole |
| Ketoconazole (systemic) |

the treatment of *Acanthamoeba* keratitis (Table 6–16). The minimum duration in treatment of this series was 4 months, with a maximum of 17 months.

Adjuvant therapy may be used in combination with antibiotics, including debridement, cryotherapy, and corneal transplant.[33, 39, 40]

## PHTHIRIUS PUBIS PALPEBRARUM

Infestation of the cilia with lice typically occurs secondary to a crab louse. It may be sexually transmitted and can spread to epidemic proportions. Therapy should include mechanical removal and shampoo of the scalp with γ-benzene hexachloride shampoo. This shampoo should not be used near the eye. Yellow mercuric oxide NF 1% ophthalmic ointment may be used on the eyelid margins twice daily. Anticholinesterase application directly to the cilia is helpful. Physostigmine will destroy the louse but leave the nits unaffected. Phospholine iodide may be applied to the cilia with a cotton swab and aid in the removal of the lice. Treatment, therefore, must be continued a full 2 weeks so that the new crab lice are treated once they are hatched from the nit. Sterilization of all clothing and bed linens must be performed, as well as examination of close personal contacts.[41, 42]

## REFERENCES

### SECTION ONE

1. Guide to choice of antibiotic therapy, 1992, Departments of Pathology and Pharmacy, Riverside Methodist Hospitals, Columbus, Ohio.
2. Fass RJ: Report of the pharmacy and therapeutic antibiotics subcommittee, 1991, Ohio State University Hospitals, Columbus, Ohio.
3. Counts GW: Review and control of antimicrobial usage in hospitalized patients, *JAMA* 238:2170, 1977.
4. Christy NE, Sommer A: Antibiotic prophylaxis of postoperative endophthalmitis, *Ann Ophthalmol* 8:1261, 1979.
5. Nagri SH, Dunkle LM, Timmerman KJ, and others: Antibiotic usage in a pediatric medical center, *JAMA* 242:1981, 1979.
6. Kagon BM, Fannin SL, Bardie F: Spotlight on antimicrobial agents, *JAMA* 226:306, 1973.
7. Truesdale R, D'Alessandri R, Manuel V, and others: Antimicrobial vs placebo prophylaxis in noncardiac thoracic surgery, *JAMA* 241:1254, 1979.
8. Jackson GG: Antibiotic policies, practices and pressures, *J Antimicrob Chemother* 5:1, 1975.
9. Shapiro M, Townsend TR, Rosner B, and others: Use of antimicrobial drugs in general hospitals. Patterns of prophylaxis, *N Engl J Med* 301:351, 1979.
10. Starr MB: Prophylactic antibiotics for ophthalmic surgery, *Surv Ophthalmol* 27:353, 1983.
11. Allensmith MR, Anderson RP, Butlerworth A: The meaning of preoperative cultures in ophthalmology, *Trans Am Acad Ophthalmol Otolaryngol* 73:683, 1969.
12. Locatcher-Khorazo D: The effect on the ocular bacterial flora of local treatment with chloramycetia (chloramphenicol), terramycin or penicillin-streptomycin ophthalmic ointment in preoperative cataract cases and miscellaneous infections, *Am J Ophthalmol* 36:475-479, 1953.
13. Dickey JB, Thompson KD, Jay WM: Anterior chamber aspirate cultures after uncomplicated cataract surgery, *Am J Ophthalmol* 112:278, 1991.
14. Yannis RA, Rissing JP, Buxton TB, and others: Multistrain comparison of three antimicrobial prophylaxis regimens in experimental postoperative pseudomonas endophthalmitis, *Am J Ophthalmol* 100:404, 1985.
15. Kolker AE, Freeman MI, Pettit TM: Prophylactic antibiotics and postoperative endophthalmitis, *Am J Ophthalmol* 63:434, 1967.
16. Sanders R, MacEwen CJ, Haining WM: A

comparison of prophylactic, topical and subconjunctival treatment in cataract surgery, *Eye* 6:105, 1992.

17. Keren G, Alhalel A, Barrov E, and others: The intravitreal penetration of orally administered ciprofloxacin in humans, *Invest Ophthalmol Vis Sci* 32:2388, 1991.
18. Peyman GA, Sathur ML, May DR: Intraocular gentamicin as intraoperative prophylaxis in South India eye camps, *Br J Ophthalmol* 61:260, 1977.
19. Stern GA, Engel HM, Driebe WT: The treatment of postoperative endophthalmitis, *Ophthalmology* 96:62, 1989.
20. Caldwell DR, Kast PR, Cook J, and others: Povidone-iodine: its efficacy as a preoperative conjunctival and periocular preparation, *Ann Ophthalmol* 16:577, 1984.
21. Grimes SR, Mein CE, Trevino S: Preoperative antibiotic and povidone-iodine preparation of the eye, *Ann Ophthalmol* 23:263, 1991.
22. Speaker MG, Menikoft JA: Prophylaxis of endophthalmitis with topical povidone-iodine, *Ophthalmology* 98:1769, 1991.
23. Buxton JN, Brownstein S: Bacterial cultures from donor eyes, *Arch Ophthalmol* 84:148, 1970.
24. Beyt BW, Waltman SR: Cryptococcal endophthalmitis after corneal transplantation, *N Engl J Med* 298:825, 1978.
25. Houff SA, and others: Human-to-human transmission of rabies virus by corneal transplant, *N Engl J Med* 300:603, 1979.
26. Keates RH, Mischler KE, Riedinger D: Bacterial contamination of donor eyes, *Am J Ophthalmol* 84:617, 1972.
27. Khudadoust AA, Franklin RM: Transfer of bacterial infection by a donor cornea in penetrating keratoplasty, *Am J Ophthalmol* 87:130, 1979.
28. Duffy P, and others: Possible person-to-person transmission of Creutzfeld-Jacob disease, *N Engl J Med* 290:692, 1974.
29. Pardos GJ, Galligher MA: Microbial contamination of donor eyes, *Arch Ophthalmol* 100:1611, 1982.
30. Sieck FA, Enzenauer RW, Cornell FM, and others: Contamination of K-sol corneal storage medium with *Propionibacterium acnes*, *Arch Ophthalmol* 107:1023, 1989.
31. Steinemann TL, Kaufman ME, Bauerman RW, and others: Vancomycin-enriched corneal storage medium, *Am J Ophthalmol* 113:555, 1992
32. Nakamura T, Popplewell J, Smith T, and others: Assessment of the antibiotic supplementation of optisol corneal storage medium, *Invest Ophthalmol Vis Sci* 33/34(suppl):927, 1992.
33. Stevens SZ, Fisher LJ, Jensen HG: Antibiotic alternatives in corneal storage media: Assessing corneal endothelial toxicity, *Invest Ophthalmol Vis Sci* 33/34(suppl):927, 1992.
34. Dohlman CH, Boruchoft A, Mobilia EF: Complications in use of soft contact lenses in corneal disease, *Arch Ophthalmol* 90:367, 1973.
35. Dart JK, Badenoch PR: Bacterial adherence to contact lenses, *CLAO J* 12:220, 1986
36. Duran JA, Refojo MF, Gipson IK, and others: *Pseudomonas* attachment to new hydrogel contact lenses, *Arch Ophthalmol* 105:106, 1987.
37. Pitts RE, Krachmer JH: Evaluation of soft contact lens disinfection in the home environment, *Arch Ophthalmol* 97:470, 1979.
38. Binder PS, Worthen DM: A continuous-wear hydrophilic lens, *Arch Ophthalmol* 94:3109, 1973.
39. Waring III GO, Flenagen JC: Pneumocephalus, *Arch Ophthalmol* 93:847, 1975.
40. Krohel GB, and others: Orbital abscess, *Arch Ophthalmol* 98:274, 1980.
41. Peyman GA, Schulman JA: Trauma: penetrating ocular injuries. In *Intravitreal surgery: principles and practice,* New York, 1986, Appleton-Century-Crofts.
42. Hahn YS, Lincoff A, Lincoff M, and others: Infection after sponge implantation for scleral buckling, *Am J Ophthalmol* 87:180, 1979.
43. Halbert SP, Locatcher-Khorazo D, Sonnkazar C, and others: Further studies on the incidence of antibiotic-producing microorganisms of the ocular flora, *Arch Ophthalmol* 58:66, 1957.
44. Pramhus C, Runyan TE, Lindberg RB: Ocular flora in the severely burned patient, *Arch Ophthalmol* 96:1421, 1978.
45. Boyce JM, White RL, Cousey WA, and others: Burn units as a source of methicillin-resistant *Staphylococcus aureus* infection, *JAMA* 249:2803, 1983.
46. Othersen MJ, Othersen MB: A history of hand washing: seven hundred years at a snail's pace, *Pharos* Spring 1987, p 23.
47. Ley AP: Experimental fungus infections of the cornea, *Am J Ophthalmol* 42:59, 1956.
48. Seligmann E: Virulence enhancing activi-

ties of aureomycin on *Candida albicans*, *Proc Soc Exp Biol Med* 79:481, 1952.
49. Rheins MS, Suie T, Van Winkle MG: Further investigation of the effects of antibiotics, *Am J Ophthalmol* 59:221, 1965.
50. Naumann G, Green WR, Zimmerman LE: Mycotic keratitis, *Am J Ophthalmol* 64:668, 1967.
51. Olson CL: Fungal contamination of conjunctiva and lid margin, *Arch Ophthalmol* 81:351, 1969.
52. Petroutsos E, Guimaraes R, Giraud J, and others: Antibiotics and corneal epithelial wound healing, *Arch Ophthalmol* 101:1775, 1983.
53. Stern GA, Schemmer GB, Farber RD, and others: Effect of topical antibiotic solutions on corneal epithelial wound healing, *Arch Ophthalmol* 101:644, 1983.
54. Mauger TF, Doctor LC, Fackler TK, and others: Aerobic and morphologic responses of the corneal epithelium to aminoglycosides, *Invest Ophthalmol Vis Sci* 33/34:997, 1992.
55. Leopold IM: The ophthalmologist and perinatal pharmacology, *Arch Ophthalmol* 77:575, 1967.
56. Visconti JA: Antimicrobial serum and urine levels, *Ohio State Univ Hosp Clin Pharm Newslett* 10:1, 1982.
57. Fedukowicz M, Wise EN, Zaret MM: Toxic conjunctivitis due to antibiotics, *Am J Ophthalmol* 40:849, 1955.
58. Paven-Longston D, Dunkel EC: Antibiotics. In *Handbook of ocular drug therapy and ocular side effects of systemic drugs*, New York, 1991, Little, Brown, p 22.
59. American hospital formulary service, drug information 92, 1992, American Society of Hospital Pharmacists, Bethesda, Md., p 52.
60. Moody MM, de Jongh CA, Schimpff SC, and others: Long-term amikacin use: effects on aminoglycosides susceptibility pattern of gram-negative bacilli, *JAMA* 248:1199, 1982.
61. Wingfield DL, McDougal RL, Roy FH, and others: Ocular penetration of amikacin following intramuscular injection, *Arch Ophthalmol* 101:117, 1983.
62. Woo FL, Johnson AP, Insler MS, and others: Gentamicin, tobramycin, amikacin, and netilmicin levels in tears following intravenous administration, *Arch Ophthalmol* 103:216, 1985.
63. Shiono T, Meyasaka S: Aminoglycoside antibiotics and lysozyme enzymes of human tears, *Arch Ophthalmol* 103:1747, 1985.
64. Yu VL, Rhame FS, Pesanti EL, and others: Amikacin therapy: use against infections caused by gentamicin-and tobramycin-resistant organisms, *JAMA* 238:943, 1977.
65. Schiffman DO: Evaluation of amikacin sulfate, *JAMA* 238:1547, 1977.
66. Talamo JM, D'Amico DJ, Kenyon KR: Intravitreal amikacin in the treatment of bacterial endophthalmitis, *Arch Ophthalmol* 104:1483, 1986.
67. D'Amico DJ, Caspers-Velu L, Libert J, and others: Comparative toxicity of intravitreal aminoglycoside antibiotics, *Am J Ophthalmol* 100:264, 1985.
68. Oum BS, D'Amico DJ, Wong KW: Intravitreal antibiotic therapy with vancomycin and aminoglycoside. An experimental study of combination and repetitive injections, *Arch Ophthalmol* 107:1055, 1989.
69. Myrdiuk RA, Snyder RW: Bacterial keratitis. In Smolin G, Thoft RA, editors: *Infectious diseases in the cornea: scientific foundations and clinical practice*, ed 2, Boston, 1987, Little, Brown, p 193.
70. Antimicrobial susceptibilities 1990, 1991, Clinical Microbiology, The Ohio State University Hospitals, Columbus, Ohio.
71. Leopold IM: Update on antibiotics in ocular infections, *Am J Ophthalmol* 100:134, 1985.
72. Debnath SC, Talukder MAS, Bartlett FW: Effect of preoperative antibiotics on bacterial colony counts of the conjunctival sac, *J Ocul Ther Surg* 4:122, 1985.
73. Burns RP: Effectiveness study of antibiotics, *Symp Ocular Ther* 5:105, 1972.
74. Fahmy JA: Bacterial flora in relation to cataract extraction. Effects of topical antibiotics on the preoperative conjunctival flora, *Acta Ophthalmol* 58:567, 1980.
75. Furgivele FP: Ocular penetration and tolerance of gentamicin, *Am J Ophthalmol* 64:421, 1967.
76. Litwack KD, Pettit T, Johnson Jr BL: Penetration of gentamicin, *Arch Ophthalmol* 82:687, 1969.
77. Golden B, Coppel SP: Ocular tissue absorption of gentamicin, *Arch Ophthalmol* 84:792, 1970.
78. Sloan S: Gentamicin penetration, *Am J Ophthalmol* 73:750, 1972.
79. Peyman GA, May DR, Homer PI, and others: Penetration of gentamicin into the aphakic eye, *Ann Ophthalmol* 9:871, 1977.
80. Furgivele FP: Penetration of gentamicin into the aqueous humor of human eyes, *Am J Ophthalmol* 73:481, 1970.
81. Abel Jr R, Mascuilli L, Boyle GL: Subconjunctival gentamicin prophylaxis against

postoperative endophthalmitis in the rabbit, *Ophthalmic Surg* 7:59, 1976.
82. May DR, Erickson ES, Peyman GA, and others: Intraocular injection of gentamicin, *Arch Ophthalmol* 91:487, 1974.
83. Cobo CM, Forster RK: The clearance of intravitreal gentamicin, *Am J Ophthalmol* 92:59, 1981.
84. Myndruk RA, Skorich DN, Davis SD, and others: Fortified antibiotic ointment in bacterial keratitis, *Am J Ophthalmol* 105:239, 1988.
85. Insler MS, Hlem CJ, George WJ: Topical vs systemic gentamicin penetration into the human cornea and aqueous humor, *Arch Ophthalmol* 105:922, 1987.
86. Waltman SR, Coffman HE: Use of hydrophilic contact lens to increase ocular penetration of topical drugs, *Invest Ophthalmol Vis Sci* 9:250, 1970.
86a. Barza M, Peckman C, Baum J: Transscleral iontophoresis of gentamicin in monkeys, *Invest Ophthalmol Vis Sci* 28:1033, 1987.
87. Awan KJ: Mydriasis and conjunctival paresthesia from local gentamicin, *Am J Ophthalmol* 99:723, 1985.
88. Leyden JJ, Kligman AM: Contact dermatitis to neomycin sulfate, *JAMA* 242:1276, 1979.
89. Peyman GA, Schulman JA: Intravitreal drug therapy, *Jpn J Ophthalmol* 33:392, 1989.
90. Woo FL, Johnson AP, Insler MS, and others: Gentamicin, tobramycin, amikacin, and netilmicin levels in tears following intravenous administration, *Arch Ophthalmol* 103:216, 1985.
91. Wilhelmus KR, Gilbert ML, Osato MS: Tobramycin in ophthalmology, *Surv Ophthalmol* 32:111, 1987.
92. Gilbert MD, Wilhelmus KR, Osato MS: Intracanalicular collagen implants enhance topical antibiotic bioavailability, *Cornea* 5:167, 1986.
93. Matoba AY, Wilhelmus KR, Robinson MM, and others: Concentration of tobramycin in preocular tear film following topical application, *Invest Ophthalmol Vis Sci* 22(suppl):215, 1982.
94. Rootman DS, Jantzen JA, Gonzalaez JR, and others: Pharmacokinetic and safety of transcorneal iontophoresis of tobramycin in the rabbit, *Invest Ophthalmol Vis Sci* 25:1397, 1988.
95. Hewitt WL: The penicillins, *JAMA* 185:264, 1963.
96. Schartz RJ, Weintzen Jr RL, Podreira F, and others: Penicillin V for group A streptococcal pharyngotonsillitis, *JAMA* 246:1790, 1981.
97. Ferrieri P: Treatment of group A streptococcal pharyngitis: reflections on glue and other things *JAMA* 246:1813, 1981.
98. Rutenburg AM, Greenberg HL: Oxacillin in staphylococcal infections, *JAMA* 187:281, 1964.
99. Anderson K, Kennedy RP, Plorde JJ: Effectiveness of ampicillin against gram-negative bacteria, *JAMA* 187:555, 1964.
100. Kurose Y, Leopold IH: Intraocular penetration of ampicillin, *Arch Ophthalmol* 73:361, 1965.
101. Rich AM, Dunlap WA, Partridge JR: The effectiveness, safety, and use of carbenicillin in ophthalmology, *Am J Ophthalmol* 75:490, 1973.
102. Antimicrobial spectrum of chloromycetin, *Ther Notes* 57:168, 1950.
103. Faris BM, Uwaydah MM: Intraocular penetration of semisynthetic penicillins, *Arch Ophthalmol* 92:501, 1974.
104. Uwaydah MM, Faris BM, Samara IN, and others: Cloxacillin penetration, *Am J Ophthalmol* 82:114, 1976.
105. Faigenbaum SJ, Boyle GL, Prywes AA, and others: Intraocular penetration of amoxicillin, *Am J Ophthalmol* 82:598, 1976.
106. Sorsby A, Ungar J: Pure penicillin in ophthalmology, *Br J Ophthalmol* 114:4480, 1946.
107. Sorsby A, Ungar J: Distribution of penicillin in the eye after injections of 1,000,000 units by the subconjunctival retrobulbar, and intramuscular routes, *Br J Ophthalmol* 32:864, 1948.
108. Weimar V: Effect of amino acid, purine, and pyrimidine analogues on activation of corneal stromal cells in take up neutral red. *Invest Ophthalmol* 1:226, 1962.
109. von Sallmann L, Meyer K: Penetration of penicillin in the eye, *Arch Ophthalmol* 31:1, 1944.
110. Boger WP, Flippin HF: Penicillin plasma concentrations, *JAMA* 139:1131, 1949.
111. Grand S: Probenecid and intraocular methicillin, *Ann Ophthalmol* 13:209, 1981.
112. Bloome MA, Golden B, McKee AP: Antibiotic concentration in ocular tissues, *Arch Ophthalmol* 83:78, 1970.
113. Green WR, Leopold IH: Intraocular penetration of methicillin, *Am J Ophthalmol* 60:800, 1965.
114. Kluge RM, Zimmerman T: The penetration of antistaphylococcal antibiotics into the aqueous humor of rabbits, *Ann Ophthalmol* 10:1248, 1978.
115. Records RE: The human intraocular pen-

etration of sodium methicillin, *Arch Ophthalmol* 76:720, 1966.
116. Records RE: Human intraocular penetration of sodium oxacillin, *Arch Ophthalmol* 77:693, 1967.
117. Goldman EE, McLain JH, Smith JL: Penicillins and aqueous humor, *Am J Ophthalmol* 65:717, 1968.
118. Goldman JN, Klein JO: Penetration of ampicillin and penicillin G into the aqueous humor, *Ann Ophthalmol* 2:35, 1970.
119. McPherson Jr SD, Presley GD, Crawford JR: Aqueous humor assays of subconjunctival antibiotics, *Am J Ophthalmol* 66:430, 1968.
120. *AMA drug evaluations,* ed. 4, Chicago, 1980, American Medical Association.
121. Records RE, Ellis PP: The intraocular penetration of ampicillin, methicillin, and oxacillin, *Am J Ophthalmol* 64:135, 1967.
122. Peyman GA, Sanders DK: *Advances in uveal surgery, vitreous surgery, and the treatment of endophthalmitis,* New York, 1978, Appleton-Century-Crofts, p 195.
123. Kleiner RE, Brucker AJ, Schweitzer JG, and others: Intraocular ampicillin in the treatment of endophthalmitis, *Am J Ophthalmol* 100:487, 1985.
124. Johnson AP, Scoper SV, Woo FL, and others: Azlocillin levels in human tears and aqueous humor, *Am J Ophthalmol* 99:469, 1985.
125. Records RE: Intraocular penetration of dicloxacillin, in experimental animals, *Invest Ophthalmol* 7:663, 1968.
126. Baraz M, Baum J, Birkby B, and others: Intraocular penetration of carbenicillin in the rabbit, *Am J Ophthalmol* 75:307, 1973.
127. Boyle GI, Gwon AE, Zinn KM, and others: Intraocular penetration of carbenicillin after subconjunctival injection in man, *Am J Ophthalmol* 73:754, 1972.
128. Woo FL, Johnson AP, Caldwell DR, and others: Piperacillin levels in human tears and aqueous humor, *Am J Ophthalmol* 98:17, 1984.
129. Sorsby A, Ungar J: The control of experimental infections of the anterior chamber and of the vitreous by subconjunctival and retrobulbar injections of crystalline penicillin in doses of 1,000,000 units, *Br J Ophthalmol* 32:873, 1948.
130. Von Sallman L, Meyer K, DiGrandi J: Experimental study on penicillin treatment of exogenous infection of vitreous, *Arch Ophthalmol* 32:179, 1944.
131. Sorsby A, Ungar J: Preliminary note on the treatment of hypopyon ulcer by crystalline penicillin in adrenalin in doses in excess of 50,000 units injected by subconjunctival or retrobulbar routes, *Br J Ophthalmol* 32:878, 1948.
132. Leopold IH: Recent advances in ocular therapy, *NY J Med* 56:2803, 1956.
133. Pearlman M: Prophylactic subconjunctival penicillin and streptomycin after cataract extraction, *Arch Ophthalmol* 55:516, 1956.
134. Aronstam RH: Pitfalls of prophylaxis, *Am J Ophthalmol* 57:312, 1964.
135. Hahn RD, Zellmann HE, Naquin H, and others: Some observations on the course of treated syphilitic primary optic atrophy, *J Chronic Dis* 1:601, 1955.
136. Kenney JA: Treatment of syphilitic optic atrophy by penicillin with and without therapy malaria, *Am J Syph* 37:449, 1953.
137. Benton CD, Harris JF: Syphilitic optic nerve atrophy treated with penicillin: observations to six years after treatment, *Arch Ophthalmol* 48:449, 1952.
138. Dunlop EMC, Al-Egaily SS, Houang ET: Penicillin levels in blood and CSF achieved by treatment of syphilis, *JAMA* 241:2538, 1979.
139. Rein MF: Treatment of neurosyphilis, *JAMA* 246:2613, 1981.
140. Ducas J, Robson HG: Cerebrospinal fluid penicillin levels during therapy for latent syphilis, *JAMA* 246:2583, 1981.
141. Podgore JK, Holmes KK: Ocular gonococcal infection with minimal or no inflammatory response, *JAMA* 246:242, 1981.
142. Raucher HS, Newton MJ: New issues in the prevention and treatment of ophthalmia neonatorum, *Ann Ophthalmol* 15:1004, 1983.
143. Sandstrom I: Treatment of neonatal conjunctivitis, *Arch Ophthalmol* 105:925, 1987.
144. Bietti GB: Repository drugs in the treatment of trachoma, *Am J Ophthalmol* 47:220, 1959.
145. Gardiner PA, Michaelson IC, Rees RJ, and others: Intravenous streptomycin: its toxicity and diffusion, *Am J Ophthalmol* 32:449, 1948.
146. Hewitt WL: The penicillins, *JAMA* 185:264, 1963.
147. Schanzer H, Gribetz I, Jacobson II JH: Accidental intra-arterial injection of penicillin G, *JAMA* 242:1289, 1979.
148. Zimmerman MC: The prophylaxis and treatment of penicillin reactions with penicillinase, *Clin Med* 5:305, 1958.

149. Waldbott GL: Anaphylactic death from penicillin, *JAMA* 139:526, 1949.
150. Noe CA: Penicillin treatment of eyelid infections, *Am J Ophthalmol* 30:477, 1947.
151. Records RE: Intraocular penetration of cephalothin: I. Animal studies, *Am J Ophthalmol* 66:441, 1968.
152. Records RE: Intraocular penetration of cephalothin: II Human studies, *Am J Ophthalmol* 66:441, 1968.
153. Uwaydah MM, Faris BM: Penetration of cephalothin in the aqueous humor of the rabbit, *Arch Ophthalmol* 83:349, 1970.
154. Boyle GL, Hein HF, Leopold IH: Intraocular penetration of cephalexin in man, *Am J Ophthalmol* 69:868, 1970.
155. Axelrod JL, Kochman RS: Cefonicid concentration in human aqueous humor, *Arch Ophthalmol* 102:435, 1984.
156. Axelrod JL, Kochman RS: Cefoxitin levels in human aqueous humor, *Am J Ophthalmol* 90:388, 1980.
157. Axelrod JL, Newton JC, Sarakhun C, and others: Ceftriaxone: A new cephalosporin with aqueous humor levels effective against Enterobacteriaceae, *Arch Ophthalmol* 103:71, 1985.
158. Criamarellou M, Kavouklis M, Petrikkos G, and others: Ceftazidine, moxalactam, cefotaxime, and cefuroxime, *J Ocular Ther Surg* 3:170, 1984.
159. Axelrod JL, Kochman RS, Horowitz MA, and others: Ceftazidine concentrations in human aqueous humor, *Arch Ophthalmol* 102:193, 1984.
160. Axelrod JL, Klein RM, Bergen RL, and others: Human vitreous levels of selected antistaphylococcal antibiotics, *Am J Ophthalmol* 100:570, 1985.
161. Fricker L, Meredith TA, Gardner S, and others: Cefazolin levels after intravitreal injection: Effects of inflammation and surgery, *Invest Ophthalmol Vis Sci* 31:502, 1990.
162. Martin DF, Ficker LA, Aguilar MA, and others: Vitreous cefazolin levels after intravenous injection, *Arch Ophthalmol* 108:411, 1990.
163. Axelrod JL, Klein RM, Bergen RL, and others: Human vitreous levels of cefamandole and moxalactam, *Am J Ophthalmol* 101:684, 1986.
164. Rubinstein E, Avni I, Tuizer M, and others: Cefsulodin levels in the human aqueous humor, *Arch Ophthalmol* 103:426, 1985.
165. Jay WM, Shockley RK, Aziz AM, and others: Ocular pharmacokinetics of ceftriaxone following subconjunctival injection in rabbits, *Arch Ophthalmol* 102:430, 1984.
166. Shockley RK, Jay WM, Friberg TR, and others: Intravitreal ceftriaxone in a rabbit model: dose and time dependent toxic effects and pharmacokinetic analysis, *Arch Ophthalmol* 102:1236, 1984.
167. Fisher JP, Civiletto SE, Forster RK: Toxicity efficacy and clearance of intravitreal injected cefazolin, *Arch Ophthalmol* 100:650, 1982.
168. Tan J, Bayne LH, McLeod PJ: Pseudomembranous colitis, a fatal case following prophylactic cephaloridine therapy, *JAMA* 242:749, 1979.
169. Bartlett JG, Willey SH, Chang TW, and others: Cephalosporin-associated pseudomembraneous colitis due to *Clostridium difficile*, *JAMA* 242:2683, 1979.
170. Henahan J: High hopes for "third generation" cephalosporins, *JAMA* 246:1398, 1981.
171. Buening MK, Wold JS, Israel KS, and others: Disulfiram-like reaction to B-lactams, *JAMA* 245:2027, 1981.
172. Branch DR, Gifford J: Allergic reaction to transfused cephalothin antibody, *JAMA* 241:495, 1979.
173. Saah AJ, Koch TR, Drusano GL: Cefoxitin falsely elevates creatinine levels, *JAMA* 247:205, 1982.
174. Axelrod JL, Newton JC, Klein RM, and others: Penetration of imipenem into human aqueous and vitreous humor, *Am J Ophthalmol* 104:649, 1987.
175. Sawusch MR, O'Brien TP, Valentine MS, and others: Topical imipenem therapy of aminoglycoside-resistant *Pseudomonas* keratitis in rabbits, *Am J Ophthalmol* 106:77, 1988.
176. Derick RJ, Paylor R, Peyman EA: Toxicity of imipenem in vitreous replacement fluid, *Ann Ophthalmol* 19:338, 1989.
177. Meleny FL: Bacitracin therapy, *Am J Ophthalmol* 133:375, 1947.
178. Bellows JG, Farmer CJ: The use of bacitracin in ocular infection. Bacitracin therapy in experimental and clinical ocular infection, *Am J Ophthalmol* 37:1211, 1948.
179. Hattwick MAW, Retailliau H, O'Brien RJ, and others: Fatal Rocky Mountain spotted fever, *JAMA* 240:1499, 1978.
180. Antimicrobial spectrum of chloromycetin, *Ther Notes* 57:168, 1950.
181. *AMA drug evaluations*, ed 4, Chicago, 1980, American Medical Association.
182. Bleeker GM, Maas EH: Penetration of

penethamate, penicillin ester, into the tissues of the eye, *Arch Ophthalmol* 60:1013, 1958.
183. Furgiuele FP, Sery TW, Leopold IH: Newer antibiotics: their intraocular penetration, *Am J Ophthalmol* 50:614, 1960.
184. Leopold IH, Nichols AC, Bogel AW: Penetration of chloramphenicol (Chloromycetin) into the eye, *Arch Ophthalmol* 44:22, 1950.
185. Leopold IH: Clinical trial with chloramphenicol in ocular infections, *Arch Ophthalmol* 45:44, 1951.
186. Leopold IH: Surgery of ocular trauma, *Arch Ophthalmol* 48:738, 1952.
187. Broughton W, Goldman JN: The intraocular penetration of chloramphenicol succinate in rabbits, *Ann Ophthalmol* 5:71, 1973.
188. Beasley H, Boltralik JJ, Baldwin HA: Chloramphenicol in aqueous humor after topical application, *Arch Ophthalmol* 93:184, 1975.
189. George FJ, Hanna C: Ocular penetration of chloramphenicol, *Arch Ophthalmol* 95:879, 1977.
190. Hanna C, Massey JY, Hendrickson RO, and others: Ocular penetration of topical chloramphenicol in humans, *Arch Ophthalmol* 96:1258, 1978.
191. Weisberger AS, Wessler S, Aviolo LV: Mechanisms of action of chloramphenicol, *JAMA* 209:97, 1969.
192. Huguley Jr CM: Drug-induced blood dyscrasias, *JAMA* 188:817, 1964.
193. Best WR: Chloramphenicol-associated blood dyscrasias, *JAMA* 201:181, 1967.
194. Wallerstein RO, Condit PK, Kasper CK, and others: Statewide study of chloramphenicol therapy and fatal aplastic anemia, *JAMA* 208:2045, 1969.
195. Snyder HP: Intravenous chloramphenicol to prevent postoperative endophthalmitis in cataract surgery—520 consecutive cases, *Ann Ophthalmol* 10:1041, 1978.
196. Fraunfelder FT, Bagby Jr GC, Kelly DJ: Fatal aplastic anemia following topical administration of ophthalmic chloramphenicol, *Am J Ophthalmol* 93:356, 1982.
197. Dutro MP: Chloramphenicol and aplastic anemia, *Am J Ophthalmol* 92:870, 1981.
198. Wong VG, Colling E: Optic atrophy in cystic fibrosis of the pancreas, *Am J Ophthalmol* 59:763, 1965.
199. Lietman PS, Di Sant'Agnese PA, Wong VG: Optic neuritis in cystic fibrosis of the pancreas, *JAMA* 189:924, 1964.
200. Harley RD, Huang NN, Macri CH, and others: Optic neuritis and optic atrophy following chloramphenicol in cystic fibrosis patients, *Trans Am Acad Ophthalmol Otolaryngol* 74:1011, 1970.
201. Cogan D: Optic neuropathy and chloramphenicol, *Invest Ophthalmol* 12:534, 1973.
202. Rothkoff L, Biedner B, Shoham K, and others: Optic atrophy after irrigation of the lacrimal ducts with chloramphenicol, *Ann Ophthalmol* 11:105, 1979.
203. Council on Drugs: *JAMA* 178:576, 1961.
204. Roberts W: Topical use of chloramphenicol in external ocular infections, *Am J Ophthalmol* 34:1081, 1951.
205. Aragones JV, Eriksen SP: Stable chloramphenicol solution for ocular infections, *Am J Ophthalmol* 66:104, 1968.
206. Chastain J: Intramuscular chloramphenicol therapy of trachoma, *Rocky Mountain Med J* 51:191, 1953.
207. Thygeson P: Criteria of cure in trachoma, with special reference to provocative tests, *Rev Int Trach* 30:450, 1953.
208. Agarwal LP, Saxena RP, Gupta BML: Antibiotic and chemotherapeutic agents in treatment of trachoma, *Am J Ophthalmol* 40:553, 1955.
209. Huamonte F, Refojo M, Banuelos A: Expandable silicone implants for scleral buckling: III Experiments in vivo, *Arch Ophthalmol* 93:354, 1975.
210. Mercer KB, De Olden JE, Leopold IH: Intraocular penetration of topical clindamycin in rabbits, *Arch Ophthalmol* 96:880, 1978.
211. Devlin JL, Mercer KB, Dea FJ, and others: Intraocular penetration of topical clindamycin in rabbits: II. Clindamycin phosphate, *Arch Ophthalmol* 96:1650, 1978.
212. Tabbara KF, O'Connor GR: Ocular tissue absorption of clindamycin phosphate, *Arch Ophthalmol* 93:1180, 1975.
213. Sugar J, Chandler JW: Experimental corneal wound strength, *Arch Ophthalmol* 92:248, 1974.
214. Tabbara KF, Ay-Liacco J, Nozik RA, and others: Clindamycin in chronic toxoplasmosis, *Arch Ophthalmol* 97:542, 1979.
215. Ferguson Jr JG: Clindamycin therapy for toxoplasmosis, *Ann Ophthalmol* 13:95, 1981.
216. Chou J: Antibiotic-associated diarrhea, *OSU Clin Lab Update* 3(6), 1981.
217. Cammerer RC, Anderson DL, Boyce Jr HW, and others: Clinical spectrum of pseudomembranous colitis, *JAMA* 235:2502, 1976.
218. Jackson GG, Lepper MH, Dowling HF: Bac-

teriophage typing of staphylococci, *J Lab Clin Med* 44:41, 1954.
219. Haight TH, Finland M: Resistance of bacteria to erythromycin, *Proc Soc Exp Biol Med* 81:183, 1952.
220. Council on Drugs: *JAMA* 173:1023, 1960.
221. Naib K, Hallet JW, Leopold IH: Observations on the ocular effects of erythromycin, *Am J Ophthalmol* 39:395, 1955.
222. Meisels HI, Peyman GA: Intravitreal erythromycin in the treatment of induced staphylococcal endophthalmitis, *Ann Ophthalmol* 8:939, 1976.
223. Gunby P: *Chlamydia trachomatis* diseases are on the rise, *JAMA* 242:2520, 1979.
224. Knapp P, von Sallmann L: Treatment of experimental ocular tuberculosis with isoniazid, *Am J Ophthalmol* 38:199, 1954.
225. Kratka WH: Isoniazid and ocular tuberculosis, *Arch Ophthalmol* 54:330, 1955.
226. Coates E: Isonicotinic acid hydrazide resistant tubercle bacilli, *N Engl J Med* 248:1081, 1953.
227. Byrd RB, Horn BR, Solomon DA, and others: Toxic effects of isoniazid in tuberculosis chemoprophylaxis, *JAMA* 241:1239, 1979.
228. Karmon G, Savir H, Zevin D, and others: Bilateral optic neuropathy due to combined ethambutol and isoniazid treatment, *Ann Ophthalmol* 11:1013, 1979.
229. Wason S, Lacouture PG, Lovejoy Jr FH: Single high-dose pyridoxine treatment for isoniazid overdose, *JAMA* 246:1102, 1981.
230. Jackson H, Cooper J, Mellinger WJ, and others: Group A, B-hemolytic streptococcal pharyngitis-results of treatment with lincomycin, *JAMA* 194:1189, 1965.
231. Becker EF: The intraocular penetration of lincomycin, *Am J Ophthalmol* 67:963, 1969.
232. Boyle G, Lichtig ML, Leopold IH: Lincomycin levels in human ocular fluids and serum following subconjunctival injection, *Am J Ophthalmol* 71:1303, 1971.
233. Coles RS, Boyle GL, Leopold IH, and others: Lincomycin levels in rabbit ocular fluids and serum, *Am J Ophthalmol* 72:464, 1971.
234. Kleinberg J, Dea FJ, Anderson JA, and others: Intraocular penetration of topically applied lincomycin hydrochloride in rabbits, *Arch Ophthalmol* 97:933, 1979.
235. Tabbara KF, Salamoun SG: Accidental intraocular injection of lincomycin, *Am J Ophthalmol* 73:596, 1972.
236. Williams RK, Hench ME, Guerry D: Pyocyaneus ulcer, *Am J Ophthalmol* 37:538, 1954.
237. Moorman LT, Harbert F: Treatment of *Pseudomonas* corneal ulcers, *Arch Ophthalmol* 53:345, 1955.
238. McNeel JW, Wood RM, Senterfit LB: Effect of polymyxin B sulfate on *Pseudomonas* corneal ulcers, *Arch Ophthalmol* 66:62, 1961.
239. Leibowitz HM: Antibacterial effectiveness of ciprofloxacin 0.3% ophthalmic solution in the treatment of bacterial conjunctivitis, *Am J Ophthalmol* 112:295, 1991.
240. Leibowitz HM: Clinical evaluation of ciprofloxacin 0.3% ophthalmic solution for treatment of bacterial keratitis, *Am J Ophthalmol* 112:345, 1991.
241. Reidy JJ, Hobden JA, Hill JM, and others: The efficacy of topical ciprofloxacin and norfloxacin in the treatment of experimental *Pseudomonas* keratitis, *Cornea* 10:25, 1991
242. Hobden JA, Reidy JJ, O'Callaghan RJ, and others: Quinolones in collagen shields to treat aminoglycoside-resistant pseudomonal keratitis, *Invest Ophthalmol Vis Sci* 31:2241, 1990.
243. Hobden JA, Reidy JJ, O'Callaghan RJ, and others: Ciprofloxacin iontophoresis for aminoglycoside-resistant pseudomonal keratitis, *Invest Ophthalmol Vis Sci* 31:1940, 1990.
244. Skoutelis AT Garfaganis SP, Chrysanthopoulos CJ, and others: Aqueous humor penetration of ciprofloxacin in the human eye, *Arch Ophthalmol* 106:404, 1988.
245. Stevens SX, Fouraker BD, Jensen JG: Intraocular safety of ciprofloxacin, *Arch Ophthalmol* 109:1737, 1991.
246. Vrabec TR, Sergott RC, Jaeger EA, and others: Reversible visual loss in a patients receiving high-dose ciprofloxacin hydrochloride (Cipro), *Ophthalmology* 97:707, 1990.
247. Frieden TR, Mangi RJ: Inappropriate use of oral ciprofloxacin, *JAMA* 264:1438, 1990.
248. U.S. pharmacy sales in 1989, *Script World Pharm News* 1500:18, 1990.
249. Vajpayee RB, Gupta SK, Angra SK, and others: Topical norfloxacin therapy in *Pseudomonas* corneal ulceration, *Cornea* 10:268, 1991.
250. Osato MS, Jensen HG, Trousdale MD, and others: The comparative in vitro activity of ofloxacin and selected ophthalmic antimicrobial agents against ocular bacterial isolates, *Am J Ophthalmol* 108:380, 1989.
251. Hufnagel TJ, Schein OD: Suppurative keratitis from herbal ocular preparation, *Am J Ophthalmol* 113:722, 1992.

252. Feldman MF, Moses RA: Corneal penetration of rifampin, *Am J Ophthalmol* 83:862, 1977.
253. Lou P, Kazdan J, Bannatyne RM, and others: Successful treatment of *Candida* endophthalmitis with a synergistic combination of amphotericin B and rifampin, *Am J Ophthalmol* 83:12, 1977.
254. Stern GA: In vitro antibiotic synergism against ocular fungal isolates, *Am J Ophthalmol* 86:359, 1978.
255. Donnenfeld ED, Cohen EJ, Barza M, and others: Treatment of *Nocardia* keratitis with topical trimethoprim-sulfamethoxazole, *Am J Ophthalmol* 111:116, 1991.
256. Bucci FA, Holland EJ: *Flavobacterium meningosepticum* keratitis successfully treated with topical trimethoprim-sulfamethoxazole, *Am J Ophthalmol* 11:116, 1991.
257. Opremcak EM, Scales DK, Sharpe MR: Trimethoprim-sulfamethoxazole therapy for ocular toxoplasmosis, *Ophthalmology* 99:920, 1992.
258. Burger LM, Sanford JP, Zweighaft BA: The effect of sulfonamides on the anti-*Pseudomonas* activity of gentamicin in vitro, *Am J Ophthalmol* 75:314, 1973.
259. Gailyey WW: Transient myopia for sulfanilamide, *Am J Ophthalmol* 22:1399, 1939.
260. Rittenhouse EA: Myopia after use of sulfanilamide, *Arch Ophthalmol* 24:1139, 1940.
261. Hook SR, Holladay JT, Prager TC, and others: Transient myopia induced by sulfonamides, *Am J Ophthalmol* 101:455, 1986.
262. Genvert GI, Cohen EJ, Donnenfeld ED, and others: Erythema multiforme after use of topical sulfacetamide, *Am J Ophthalmol* 99:465, 1985.
263. Taub RG, Hollenhorst RW: Sulfonamides as a cause of toxic amblyopia, *Am J Ophthalmol* 40:486, 1955.
264. Flach A: Photosensitivity to sulfisoxazole ointment, *Arch Ophthalmol* 99:609, 1981.
265. Tabbara KF, Veirs ER: Corneal white plaques caused by sulfacetamide eye drops, *Arch Ophthalmol* 98:378, 1984.
266. Boettner EA, Fralick FB, Wolter JR: Conjunctival concretions of sulfadiazine, *Arch Ophthalmol* 92:446, 1974.
267. Bellows FG: Chemotherapy in ophthalmology, *Arch Ophthalmol* 29:609, 1943.
268. Chinn H, Bellows JG: Corneal penetration of sulfanilamide and some of its derivatives, *Arch Ophthalmol* 27:34, 1942.
269. Gallardo E, Thompson R: Sulfonamide content of aqueous humor following conjunctival application of drug powders, *Am J Ophthalmol* 25:1210, 1942.
270. Von Sallmann L: Sulfadiazine iontophoresis in *Pyocyaneus* infection of rabbit cornea, *Am J Ophthalmol* 25:1292, 1942.
271. Boyd JL: Sodium sulfathiazole iontophoresis, *Arch Ophthalmol* 28:205, 1942.
272. Bellows JG, Chinn H: Penetration of sulfathiazole in the eye, *Arch Ophthalmol* 25:294, 1941.
273. Scheie HG, Souders B: Penetration of sulfanilamide and its derivatives into aqueous humor of eye, *Arch Ophthalmol* 25:1025, 1941.
274. Scheie HG, Leopold IH: Penetration of sulfathiazole into the eye, *Arch Ophthalmol* 27:997, 1942.
275. Liebman SD, Newman EH: Distribution of sulfanilamide and its derivatives between blood and aqueous, *Arch Ophthalmol* 26:472, 1941.
276. Guyton JS: The use of sulfanilamide compounds in ophthalmology, *Am J Ophthalmol* 22:833, 1939.
277. Thygeson P: Sulfonamide compounds in treatment of ocular infections, *Arch Ophthalmol* 29:1000, 1943.
278. Callahan A: Effect of sulfonamides and antibiotics on panophthalmitis complicating cataract extraction, *Arch Ophthalmol* 49:212, 1953.
279. Mayer LL: Sodium sulfacetamide in ophthalmology, *Arch Ophthalmol* 39:232, 1948.
280. Kuhn HS: Sodium sulfacetamide in ophthalmology, *Trans Am Acad Ophthalmol* 55:432, 1951.
281. Burnham CJ, Beuerman VA: Toxoplasmic uveitis, *Am J Ophthalmol* 42:217, 1956.
282. Salamon SM: Tetracyclines in ophthalmology, *Surv Ophthalmol* 29:265, 1985.
283. Pickering LK, Dupont HL, Olarte J: Single-dose tetracycline therapy for shigellosis in adults, *JAMA* 239:853, 1978.
284. Ory EM, Yow EM: The use and abuse of the broad-spectrum antibiotics, *JAMA* 185:273, 1963.
285. Dowling HF, Lepper MH: Hepatic reactions to tetracycline, *JAMA* 188:307, 1964.
286. Kunin CM: Nephrotoxicity of antibiotic, *JAMA* 202:204, 1967.
287. Mavromatis F: Tetracycline nephropathy, *JAMA* 193:91, 1965.
288. Giles CL, Soble AR: Intracranial hypertension and tetracycline therapy, *Am J Ophthalmol* 72:981, 1971.
289. Oklund SA, Prolo DJ, Gutierrez RV: The significance of yellow bone, *JAMA* 246:761, 1981.
290. Ray WA, Federspiel CF, Schaffner W: Prescribing of tetracycline to children less than 8 years old, *JAMA* 237:2069, 1977.

291. Yeager AS: Why now? Use of tetracycline in young children, *JAMA* 237:2101, 1977.
292. Douvas NG, Fetherstone RM, Braley AE: Role of terramycin in ophthalmology, *Arch Ophthalmol* 46:57, 1951.
293. Poirier RH, Ellison AC: Ocular penetration of orally administered minocycline, *Ann Ophthalmol* 11:1859, 1979.
294. Dougherty JM, McCulley JP, Silvany RE, and others: The role of tetracycline in chronic blepharitis: Inhibition of lipase production in staphylococci, *Invest Ophthalmol Vis Sci* 32:2970, 1991.
295. Brown SI, Shahinian Jr L: Diagnosis and treatment of ocular rosacea, *Trans Am Acad Ophthalmol Otolaryngol* 85:779, 1978.
296. Lempert SL, Jenkins MS, Brown SI: Chalazia and rosacea, *Arch Ophthalmol* 97:1652, 1979.
297. Abelson MB, Sadun AA, Udell IJ, and others: Alkaline tear pH in ocular rosacea, *Am J Ophthalmol* 90:866, 1980.
298. Zaidman GW, Brown SI: Orally administered tetracycline for phlyctenular keratoconjunctivitis, *Am J Ophthalmol* 92:178, 1981.
299. Mordhorst CH, Dawson C: Sequelae of neonatal inclusion conjunctivitis and associated disease in parents, *Am J Ophthalmol* 71:861, 1971.
300. Hammerschhlag MR, Chandler JW, Alexander FR, and others: Erythromycin ointment for ocular prophylaxis of neonatal chlamydial infection, *JAMA* 244:2291, 1980.
301. Willcockson TH, Cox CD: Bacteriological studies in newborns using Terramycin, Terramycin-polymyxin B, and silver nitrate trate, *South Dakota J Med Pharm* 6:147, 1953.
302. Clark SG, Culler AM: Aureomycin as prophylaxis against ophthalmia neonatorum, *Am J Ophthalmol* 34:840, 1951.
303. Musselman MM: *Terramycin,* New York, 1956, Medical Encyclopedia.
304. Rettig PJ: Centenary of Crede prophylaxis, *Am J Ophthalmol* 91:542, 1981.
305. Rettig PJ, Patamasucon P, Siegel JD: Postnatal prophylaxis of chlamydial conjunctivitis, *JAMA* 246:2321, 1981.
306. Thygeson P: Terramycin in ocular infections, *Trans Am Ophthalmol Soc* 49:185, 1952.
307. Mitsui Y, Tanaka C, Toya H, and others: Terramycin in the treatment of trachoma, *Arch Ophthalmol* 46:235, 1951.
308. Naggache R: Topical use of Terramycin ointment in trachoma, *Br J Ophthalmol* 37:106, 1953.
309. Bilger I: Terramycin therapy in trachoma, *JAMA* 149:1667, 1952.
310. Rollins DF, Tabbara KF, Gosheh R, and others: Minocycline in experimental ocular toxoplasmosis in the rabbit, *Am J Ophthalmol* 93:361, 1982.
311. Perry HD, Kenyon KR, Lemberts DW, and others: Systemic tetracycline hydrochloride as adjunctive therapy in the treatment of persistent epithelial defects, *Ophthalmology* 93:1320, 1986.
312. Golub LM, Ramamurthy N, McNamara TF, and others: Tetracyclines inhibit tissue collagenase activity: a new mechanism in the treatment of peridental disease, *J Periodont Res* 19:651, 1984.
313. Newell FW, Goren SB, Brizel HE, and others: The use of iodine-125 as a diagnostic agent in ophthalmology, *Trans Am Acad Ophthalmol Otolaryngol* 67:177, 1963.
314. Goodman DF, Gottsch JD: Methicillin-resistant *Staphylococcus epidermidis* keratitis treated with vancomycin, *Arch Ophthalmol* 106:1570, 1988.
315. Fleischer AE, Hoover DL, Khen JA, and others: Topical vancomycin formulation for methicillin-resistant *Staphylococcus epidermidis* blepharoconjunctivitis, *Am J Ophthalmol* 101:283, 1986.
316. Charlton JF, Kniska A, Chao GM, and others: Stability of topical fortified antibiotic solutions, *Invest Ophthalmol Vis Sci* 33/34(suppl):937, 1992.
317. Pflugfelder SC, Hernandez E, Fliesler SJ, and others: Intravitreal vancomycin: retinal toxicity, clearance, and interaction with gentamicin, *Arch Ophthalmol* 105:831, 1987.
318. Mochizuki K, Torisaki M, Wakabayashi K: Effects of vancomycin and ofloxacin on rabbit ERG in vivo, *Jpn J Ophthalmol* 35:435, 1991.
319. Cullor JS, Mannis MJ, Murphy CJ, and others: In vitro antimicrobial activity of definsins against ocular pathogens, *Arch Ophthalmol* 108:861, 1990.
320. Schwab IR, Dries D, Cullor J, and others: Corneal storage preservation with defensins, *Cornea* 11:370, 1992.

## SECTION TWO

1. Kaufman HE: Update on antiviral agent, *Ophthalmology* 92:533, 1985.
2. Donnenfeld ED, Laibson PR: Management

of epithelial herpetic keratitis, *Ophthalmic Forum* 2:195, 1984.

3. Jabs DA, Green WR, Fox R, and others: Ocular manifestations of acquired immune deficiency syndrome, *Ophthalmology* 96:1092, 1989.
4. Pavan-Langston D: Viral diseases: herpetic infections. In Sanolis G, Thoft RA, editors: *The cornea: scientific foundations and clinical practice,* Boston, 1987, Little, Brown, p 240.
5. Dawson C, Tugni B: Herpes simplex eye infections, *Surv Ophthalmol* 21:11, 1976.
6. Gunderson T: Herpes cornea, *Arch Ophthalmol* 15:225, 1986.
7. Laibson PR, Leopold IM: An evaluation of double-blind IDU therapy in 100 cases of herpetic keratitis, *Trans Am Acad Ophthalmol Otolaryngol* 68:22, 1964.
8. Wilhelmus KR, Coster DJ, Sonas BR: Acyclovir and debridement in the treatment of ulcerative herpetic keratitis, *Am J Ophthalmol* 91:323, 1981.
9. Parlato CJ, Cohen EJ, Sakauye CM, and others: Role debridement and trifluridine (trifluorothymidine) in herpes simplex dendritic keratitis, *Arch Ophthalmol* 103:673, 1985.
10. Roat MI, Romanowski E, Araullo-Cruz T, and others: The antiviral effects of rose bengal and fluorescein, *Arch Ophthalmol* 105:1415, 1987.
11. Kaufman H, Nesburn AB, Maloney ED: IDU therapy of herpes simplex, *Arch Ophthalmol* 67:583, 1962.
12. Matsumura K, Fujimoto M, Mitsui Y: Microautoradiographic studies on incorporation of 5-ido-2′-deoxyuridine into herpes simplex virus, *Jpn J Ophthalmol* 17:125, 1973.
13. Kaufman HE, Maloney ED, Nesburn A: Comparison of specific antiviral agents in herpes simplex keratitis, *Invest Ophthalmol* 1:686, 1962.
14. Maloney ED, Kaufman HE: Antagonism and toxicity of IDU by its degradation products, *Invest Ophthalmol* 2:55, 1963.
15. Kaufman HE: Chemotherapy of herpes keratitis, *Invest Ophthalmol* 2:205, 1963.
16. Cherry PMH, Falcon MG: Punctal stenosis caused by idoxuridine or acrodermatitis enteropathica? *Arch Ophthalmol* 2:205, 1963.
17. Lass JL, Thoft RD, Dohlman CP: Idoxuridine-induced congenital cicatrization, *Arch Ophthalmol* 101:742, 1983.
18. Kremer I, Rozenbaum D, Aviel E: Immunofluorescence findings in pseudopemphigoid induced by short term idoxuridine administration, *Am J Ophthalmol* 111:373, 1991.
19. Laibson PR, Sery TW, Leopold I: The treatment of herpetic keratitis and 5-iodo-2′-deoxyuridine (IDU), *Arch Ophthalmol* 70:52, 1963.
20. Polack FM, Rose J: The effect of 5-iodo-2′-deoxyuridine (IDU) in corneal healing, *Arch Ophthalmol* 71:520, 1964.
21. Payrau P, Dohlman CH: IDU in corneal wound healing, *Am J Ophthalmol* 57:999, 1964.
22. Yamaguchi K: Idoxuridine and bacterial corneal infection, *Am J Ophthalmol* 87:202, 1979.
23. Laibson PR, Leopole IH: An evaluation of double-blind IDU therapy in 100 cases of herpetic keratitis, *Trans Am Acad Ophthalmol* 68:22, 1964.
24. Kobayashi S, Nakamura T: Herpes corneae and development of IDU resistance in herpes simplex virus, *Jpn Ophthalmol* 8:14, 1964.
25. Maxwell E, Schleicher JB: Experimental and clinical experiences with IDU, *Eye Ear Nose Throat Mon* 43:39, 1964.
26. Smolin G, Okumato M, Feiler S, and others: Idoxuridine-liposome therapy for herpes simplex keratitis, *Am J Ophthalmol* 91:220, 1981.
27. Kaufman H, Martola E, Dohlman C: Use of 5-ido-2′-deoxyuridine (IDU) in treatment of herpes simplex keratitis, *Arch Ophthalmol* 68:235, 1962.
28. Pavan-Langston D, McCulley JP: Herpes zoster dendritic keratitis, *Arch Ophthalmol* 89:25, 1973.
29. Maxwell E: Treatment of herpes keratitis with 5-iodo-2′-deoxyuridine (IDU), *Am J Ophthalmol* 56:571, 1963.
30. Havener WH, Wachtel J: IDU therapy of herpetic keratitis, *Am Ophthalmol* 55:234, 1963.
31. Burns RP: A double-blind study of IDU in human herpes simplex keratitis, *Arch Ophthalmol* 70:381, 1963.
32. Jepson CN: Treatment of herpes simplex of the cornea with IDU, *Am J Ophthalmol* 57:213, 1964.
33. Hart DRL, Brightman VJF, Readsaw GG, and others: Treatment of human herpes simplex keratitis with idoxuridine, *Arch Ophthalmol* 73:623, 1965.
34. Kaufman EH, Maloney ED: IDU and hy-

drocortisone in experimental herpes simplex keratitis, *Arch Ophthalmol* 68:396, 1962.

35. Pavan-Langston D, Dunkel EL: Antivirals. In *Handbook of ocular drug therapy and ocular side effects of systemic drugs*, Boston, 1991, Little, Brown.
36. Ey RC, Hughes WF, Holmes AW, and others: Clinical and laboratory evaluation of idoxuridine (IDU) therapy in herpes simplex keratitis, *Arch Ophthalmol* 71:325, 1964.
37. Kaufman HE, Martola EL, Dohlman CH: Herpes simplex treatment with IDU and corticosteroids, *Arch Ophthalmol* 69:468, 1963.
38. Underood GE, Wisner CA, Sheldon DW: Cytosine arabinoside (CA) and other nucleosides in herpes virus infections, *Arch Ophthalmol* 72:505, 1964.
39. Kaufman HE, Capella JA, Maloney ED, and others: Corneal toxicity of cytosine arabinoside, *Arch Ophthalmol* 72:535, 1964.
40. Elliott GA, Schut AL: Studies with cytarabine HCl (CA), *Am J Ophthalmol* 60:1074, 1965.
41. Hopen G, Modino BJ, Johnson BL, and others: Corneal toxicity with systemic cytarabine, *Am J Ophthalmol* 91:500, 1981.
42. Gordon DM, Advocate S: Vaccinial blepharokeratitis: treatment with cytosine arabinoside, *Am J Ophthalmol* 59:480, 1965.
43. Pierce LE, Jenkins RB: Herpes zoster ophthalmicus treated with cytarabine, *Arch Ophthalmol* 89:21, 1973.
44. Hryniuk W, Foerster J, Shojania M, and others: Cytarabine for herpes virus infections, *JAMA* 219:715, 1972.
45. Buss DH, Scharyj M, White DR: Visceral herpesvirus infections in leukemic patients receiving cytarabine, *JAMA* 243:1903, 1980.
46. Pavan-Langston D: Use of vidarabine in ophthalmology: a review, *Ann Ophthalmol* 9:835, 1977.
47. Pavan-Langston D, Dohlman CH, Geary P, and others: Intraocular penetration of Ara A and IDU-therapeutic implications in clinical herpetic uveitis, *Trans Am Acad Ophthalmol Otolaryngol* 77:455, 1973.
48. Pavan-Langston D: Clinical evaluation of adenine arabinoside and idoxuridine in the treatment of ocular herpes simplex, *Am J Ophthalmol* 80:495, 1975.
49. Chin GN: Treatment of herpes simplex keratitis with idoxuridine and vidarabine: a double-blind study, *Ann Ophthalmol* 10:1171, 1978.
50. Pavan-Langston D, Dohlman CH: A double-blind clinical study of adenine arabinoside therapy of viral keratoconjunctivitis, *Am J Ophthalmol* 74:81, 1972.
51. O'Day DM, Poirier RH, Jones DB, and others: Vidarabine therapy of complicated herpes simplex keratitis, *Am J Ophthalmol* 81:642, 1976.
52. Hyndiuk RA, Hull DS, Schultz RO, and others: Adenine arabinoside in idoxuridine unresponsive and intolerant herpetic keratitis, *Am J Ophthalmol* 79:655, 1975.
53. North RD, Pavan-Langston D, Geary P: Herpes simplex virus types 1 and 2, *Arch Ophthalmol* 94:1019, 1976.
54. Abel RJ, Kaufman HE, Sugar J: Intravenous adenine arabinoside against herpes simplex keratouveitis in humans, *Am J Ophthalmol* 79:659, 1975.
55. Sam ZS, Centifanto YM, Kaufman HE: Failure of systemically administered adenine arabinoside to affect humoral and cell-mediated immunity, *Am J Ophthalmol* 81:502, 1976.
56. Hyndiuk RA, Okumato M, Damiano RA, and others: Treatment of vaccinial keratitis with vidarabine, *Arch Ophthalmol* 94:1363, 1976.
57. Waring III GO, Laibson PR, Satz JE, and others: Use of vidarabine in epidemic keratoconjunctivitis due to adenovirus types 3, 7, 8, and 19, *Am J Ophthalmol* 82:781, 1976.
58. Pavan-Langston D, North Jr RD, Geary PA, and others: Intraocular penetration of the soluble antiviral, Ara AMP, *Arch Ophthalmol* 94:1585, 1976.
59. Pavan-Langston D, Langston RHS, Geary PA: Prophylaxis and therapy of experimental ocular herpes simplex, *Arch Ophthalmol* 92:417, 1974.
60. Hill JM, Park NH, Gangarosa LP, and others: Iontophoresis of vidarabine monophosphate into rabbit eyes, *Invest Ophthalmol* 17:473, 1978.
61. Whitley RJ, Alford CA: Herpes simplex encephalitis: need for accurate diagnosis, *JAMA* 244:371, 1980.
62. Landry ML, Booss J, Hsiung GD: Duration of vidarabine therapy in biopsy-negative herpes simplex encephalitis, *JAMA* 247:332, 1982.
63. Bia FJ, Thornton GF, Main AJ, and others: Western equine encephalitis mimicking

herpes simplex encephalitis, *JAMA* 244:367, 1980.
64. Phillips CA, Fanning WL, Gump DW, and others: Cytomegalovirus encephalitis in immunologically normal adults, *JAMA* 238:2299, 1977.
65. Van Etta L, Brown J, Mastri A, and others: Fatal vidarabine toxicity in a patient with normal renal function, *JAMA* 246:1703, 1981.
66. Sugar J, Varnell E, Centifanto Y, and others: Trifluorothymidine treatment of herpetic iritis in rabbits and ocular penetration, *Invest Ophthalmol* 12:532, 1973.
67. O'Brien WJ, Edelhauser HF: The corneal penetration of trifluorothymidine, adenine arabinoside, and idoxuridine: a comparative study, *Invest Ophthalmol Vis Sci* 16:1093, 1977.
68. Burroughs Wellcome Co data, V-200 75M printed April 1980.
69. Itoi M, Gefter J, Kaneko N, and others: Teratogenicities of ophthalmic drugs, *Arch Ophthalmol* 93:46, 1975.
70. Udell IJ: Trifluridine-associated conjunctival cicatrization, *Am J Ophthalmol* 99:363, 1985.
71. Shearer DR, Bourne WM: Severe ocular anterior segment ischemia after long-term trifluridine treatment for presumed herpetic keratitis, *Am J Ophthalmol* 109:346, 1990.
72. Wellings PC, Awdry PN, Bors FH, and others: Clinical evaluation of trifluorothymidine in the treatment of herpes simplex corneal ulcers, *Am J Ophthalmol* 73:932, 1972.
73. Pavan-Langston D, Foster CS: Trifluorothymidine and idoxuridine therapy of ocular herpes, *Am J Ophthalmol* 84:818, 1977.
74. Sugar J, Stark W, Binder PS, and others: Trifluorothymidine treatment herpes simplex epithelial keratitis and comparison with idoxuridine, *Ann Ophthalmol* 12:611, 1980.
75. Hyndiuk RA, Charlin RE, Alpren TVP, and others: Trifluridine in resistant human herpetic keratitis, *Arch Ophthalmol* 96:1839, 1978.
76. Pavan-Langston D, Lass J, Campbell R: Antiviral drops, comparative therapy of experimental herpes simplex keratouveitis, *Arch Ophthalmol* 97:1132, 1979.
77. McNeill JI, Kaufman HE: Local antivirals in a herpes simplex stromal keratitis model, *Arch Ophthalmol* 97:727, 1979.
78. Hyndiuk RA, Kaufman HE: Newer compounds in therapy of herpes simplex keratitis, *Arch Ophthalmol* 78:600, 1967.
79. Parlato CJ, Cohen EJ, Sakauye CM, and others: Role of debridgement and trifluridine (trifluorothymidine) in herpes simplex dendritic keratitis, *Arch Ophthalmol* 103:673, 1985.
80. Kaufman HE: Antiviral update, *Trans Am Acad Ophthalmol* 86:131, 1979.
81. Hyndiuk RA, Seidman S, Leibsohn JM: Treatment of vaccinial keratitis with trifluorothymidine, *Arch Ophthalmol* 94:1785, 1976.
82. Lennetee DA, Eiferman RA: Inhibition of adenovirus replication in vitro by trifluridine, *Arch Ophthalmol* 96:1662, 1978.
83. Pang MP, Peyman GA, Nikolect J, and others: Intravitreal trifluorothymidine and retinal toxicity, *Retina* 6:260, 1986.
84. Kavan-Rong L, Peyman GA, Khoobehi B, and others: Intravitreal liposome-encapsulated trifluorothymidine in a rabbit model, *Ophthalmology* 94:1155, 1987.
85. Miller WH, Miller RL: Phosphorylation of acyclovir (acycloguanosine-monophosphate) by GMP kinase, *J Biol Chem* 255:7204, 1980.
86. Furman PA, and others: Inhibition of herpes simplex virus-induced DNA polymerase activity and viral DNA replication by 9-(2-hydroxyethoxymethyl) quanine and its triphosphate, *J Virol* 32:72, 1979.
87. Derse D, and others: Inhibition of purified human and herpes simplex virus–induced DNA polymerases by 9-(2-hydroxyethoxymethyl) guanine triphosphate, *J Biol Chem* 256:11447, 1981.
88. Pavan-Langston D, Champbel R, Lass J: Acyclic antimetabolite therapy of experimental herpes simplex keratitis, *Am J Ophthalmol* 86:618, 1978.
89. Pavan-Langston D, Lass J, Hettinger M, and others: Acyclovir and vidarabine in the treatment of ulcerative herpes simplex keratitis, *Am J Ophthalmol* 92:829, 1981.
90. Wilhelmus KR, Coster DJ, Jones BR: Acyclovir and debridement in the treatment of ulcerative herpetic keratitis, *Am J Ophthalmol* 91:323, 1981.
91. Lass JH, Pavan-Langston D, Park NH: Acyclovir and corneal wound healing, *Am J Ophthalmol* 88:102, 1979.
92. Trousdale MD, Dunkel EC, Nesburn AB: Effect of acyclovir on acute and latent herpes simplex virus infections in the rabbit, *Invest Ophthalmol* 19:1336, 1980.

93. Maudgal PC, Vrijghem JC, Molemuns M, and others: Effect of topical acyclovir therapy on experimental herpes simplex keratouveitis, *Arch Ophthalmol* 103:1389, 1985.
94. Colin J, Melet F, Chestel Z: Acyclovir in herpetic anterior uveitis, *Ann Ophthalmol* 23:28, 1991.
95. Sanitinto JJ, Asbell PA, Varnell ED, and others: Stromal disease, *Am J Ophthalmol* 98:537, 1984.
96. Schwab IR: Oral acyclovir in the management of herpes simplex ocular infections, *Ophthalmology* 95:423, 1988.
97. Beyer CF, Arens MQ, Hill GA, and others: Oral acyclovir reduces the incidence of recurrent herpes simplex keratitis in rabbits after penetrating keratoplasty, *Arch Ophthalmol* 107:1200, 1989.
98. Cobo LM, Foulks EN, Liesegang T, and others: Oral acyclovir in the treatment of acute herpes zoster ophthalmicus, *Ophthalmology* 92:1574, 1985.
99. Cobo LM, Foulks GN, Liesegang T, and others: *Ophthalmology* 93:763, 1986.
100. McGill J, MacDonald DR, Fall C, and others: Intravenous acyclovir in acute herpes zoster infection, *J Infect* 6:157, 1983.
101. Juel-Jensen BE, Khun JA, Pacvol G: High-dose intravenous acyclovir in the treatment of a double-blind, placebo-controlled trial, *J Infect* 6(suppl):31, 1983.
102. Serota FT, Starr SE, Bryan CK, and others: Acyclovir treatment of herpes zoster infections: use in children undergoing bone marrow transplantation, *JAMA* 247:2132, 1982.
103. Manka RL: Exogenous lactase in the treatment of oral acyclovir intolerance, *Am J Ophthalmol* 108:733, 1989.
104. Blumenkranz MS, Culbertson WW, Clarkson JG, and others: Treatment of the acute retinal necrosis syndrome with intravenous acyclovir, *Ophthalmology* 93:296, 1986.
105. Palay DA, Sternberg P, Davis J, and others: Decrease in the risk of bilateral acute retinal necrosis by acyclovir therapy, *Am J Ophthalmol* 112:250, 1991.
106. Weissenbacher M, Schacter N, Galin MA, and others: Intraocular production of interferon, *Arch Ophthalmol* 84:495, 1970.
107. Nesburn AB, Zinith PJ: Long-term topical poly I: C in experimental chronic ocular herpes simplex infection, *Am J Ophthalmol* 72:821, 1971.
108. Centifanto YM, Goorha RM, Kaufman HE: Interferon induction in rabbit and human tears *Am J Ophthalmol* 70:1006, 1970.
109. Kaufman HE, Ellison ED, Centifanto YM: Difference in interferon response and protection from ocular virus infection in rabbits and monkeys, *Am J Ophthalmol* 74:89, 1972.
110. Moschini GB, Oh JO: Experimental vaccinial keratoconjunctivitis, *Arch Ophthalmol* 87:211, 1972.
111. Chowchuvech E, Weissenbacher M, Schmunis G, and others: The influence of polyinosinic-polycytidylic acid complex on experimental acute toxoplasmic retinochoroiditis in rabbits, *Invest Ophthalmol* 11:182, 1972.
112. Weissenbacher M, Galin MA, Chowchuvech E, and others: Protection by polyinosinic–polycytidylic acid complex of rabbit eye tissue cultures infected with herpes simplex virus, *Invest Ophthalmol* 9:857, 1970.
113. Kaufman HE, Ellison ED, Waltman SR: Double-stranded RNA, an interferon inducer, in herpes simplex keratitis, *Am J Ophthalmol* 68:486, 1969.
114. McDonald TO, Fox LG, Timberlake GM, and others: Polyinosinic acid–polycytidylic acid in ophthalmology, *Ann Ophthalmol* 3:371, 1971.
115. Schachter N, Galin MA, Weissenbacher M, and others: Comparison of antiviral action of interferon, interferon inducers, and IDU against herpes simplex and other viruses, *Ann Ophthalmol* 2:795, 1970.
116. Chowchuvech E, Weissenbacher M, Galin M, and others: The influence of polyinosinic–polycytidylic acid complex on vaccinia keratitis in rabbits, *Invest Ophthalmol* 9:716, 1970.
117. Pollikoff R, Cannavale P, Dixon P, and others: Effect of complexed synthetic RNA analogues on herpes simplex virus infection in rabbit corneas, *Am J Ophthalmol* 69:60, 1970.
118. Interferon research report, *Ann Ophthalmol* 3:1176, 1971.
119. Baron S, Tyring SK, Fleischmann WR, and others: The interferons: mechanisms of action and clinical applications, *JAMA* 266:1375, 1991.
120. Adams CP, Cohen ES, Albrecht S, and others: Interferon treatment of adenoviral conjunctivitis, *Am J Ophthalmol* 98:425, 1984.
121. DeKoning EWJ, Van Bijsterveld OP, Cantell K: Combination therapy for dendritic

keratitis with acyclovir and alpha-interferon, *Arch Ophthalmol* 101:1866, 1983.
122. Naito T, Shiota H, Nitta K, and others: Effects on herpes simplex virus type 1 of combined use of interferon-beta and antiherpetic agents in vitro, *Jpn J Ophthalmol* 34:15, 1990.
123. McLeish W, Pflugfelder SC, Crouse C, and others: Interferon treatment of herpetic keratitis in a patient with acquired immunodeficiency syndrome, *Am J Ophthalmol* 109:93, 1990.
124. DeKoning EWJ, Van Bijsterveld OP, Cantell K: Combination therapy for dendritic keratitis with human leukocyte interferon and trifluorothymidine, *Br J Ophthalmol* 66:509, 1982.
125. Henderly DE, Fleeman WR, Causey DM, and others: Cytomegalovirus retinitis and response to therapy with gancyclovir, *Ophthalmology* 94:425, 1987.
126. Ussery FM, Gibson SR, Conklin RH, and others: Intravitreal gancyclovir in the treatment of AIDS-associated cytomegalovirus retinitis, *Ophthalmology* 95:640, 1988.
127. Cantrill HC, Henry K, Melroe NM, and others: Treatment of cytomegalovirus retinitis with intravitreal gancyclovir: Long-term results, *Ophthalmology* 96:367, 1989.
128. Cocheran-Massin I, Lehoang P, Lautier-Frau M, and others: Efficacy and tolerance of intravitreal gancyclovir in cytomegalovirus retinitis in acquired immune deficiency syndrome, *Ophthalmology* 98:1348, 1991.
129. Peyman GA, Khoobehi B, Twakol M, and others: Intravitreal injection of liposome-encapsulated gancyclovir in a rabbit model, *Retina* 7:227, 1987.
130. Peyman GA, Schulman JA, Khoobehi B: Toxicity and clearance of a combination of liposome-encapsulated gancyclovir in trifluridine, *Retina* 9:232, 1989.
131. Maudgal PC, Declerg K, Descamps J, and others: Topical treatment of experimental herpes simplex keratouveitis with 2′-0-glycylacyclovir, a water soluble ester of acyclovir, *Arch Ophthalmol* 102:140, 1984.
132. Lehoang P, Girard B, Robinet M, and others: Foscarnet in the treatment of cytomegalovirus retinitis in acquired immune deficiency syndrome, *Ophthalmology* 96:865, 1989.
133. Foscarnet-gancyclovir cytomegalovirus retinitis trial. *Clin Alert* Oct 17, 1991.
134. Diaz-Llopis M, Chipont E, Sanchez S, and others: Intravitreal foscarnet for cytomegalovirus retinitis in a patient with acquired immunodeficiency syndrome, *Am J Ophthalmol* 114:742, 1992.
135. Fischl MA, Richman DD, Grieco MH, and others: The efficacy of azidothymidine (AZT) in the treatment of patients with AIDS and AIDS-related complex, *N Engl J Med* 317:185, 1987.
136. Easterbrook PJ, Keruly JC, Creagh-Kirk T, and others: Racial and ethnic differences in outcome in zidovudine-treated patients with advanced HIV disease, *JAMA* 266:2713, 1991.
137. Lagakos S, Fischl MA, Stein DS, and others: Effect of zidovudine therapy in minority and other subpopulation with early HIV infection, *JAMA* 266:2709, 1991.
138. Farrell PL, Heinemann MH, Roberts CW, and others: Response of human immunodeficiency virus–associated uveitis to zidovudine, *Am J Ophthalmol* 106:7, 1988.
139. MMWR recommendations for preventing possible HIV-II/LAV virus from tears, *MMWR* 34, 1985.
140. Goldenheim PD: Inactivation of HIV by povidone-iodine, *JAMA* 257:2434, 1987.

## SECTION THREE

1. Johns KJ, O'Day DM: Pharmacologic management of keratomycoses, *Surv Ophthalmol* 33:178, 1988.
2. Beggs WH: Mechanisms of synergistic interactions between amphotericin B and flucytosine, *J Antimicrob Chemother* 17:402, 1986.
3. Andriole VT, Kravetz HM: The use of amphotericin B in man, *JAMA* 180:269, 1962.
4. Seabury JH, Dascomb HE: Results of the treatment of systemic mycoses, *JAMA* 188:509, 1964.
5. Butler WT: Pharmacology, toxicity, and therapeutic usefulness of amphotericin B, *JAMA* 195:371, 1966.
6. Medoff G, Kobayashi GS: Amphotericin B., old drug, new therapy, *JAMA* 232:619, 1975.
7. Stern GA, Okumoto M, Smolin G: Combined amphotericin B and rifampin treatment of experimental *Candida albicans* keratitis, *Arch Ophthalmol* 97:721, 1979.
8. O'Day DM, Ray WA, Robinson RD, and others: Efficacy of antifungal agents in the cornea: II. Influence of corticosteroids, *Invest Ophthalmol Vis Sci* 25:331, 1984.

9. Wood TO, Williford W: Treatment of keratomycosis with amphotericin B 0.15%, *Am J Ophthalmol* 81:847, 1976.
10. Brandriss MW, Solff SM, Moores R, and others: Anemia induced by amphotericin B, *JAMA* 189:663, 1964.
11. Green WR, Bennett JE, Goos RD: Ocular penetration of amphotericin B, *Arch Ophthalmol* 73:769, 1965.
12. O'Day DM, Ray WA, Herd S, and others: Influence of the corneal epithelium of the efficacy of topical antifungal agents, *Invest Ophthalmol Vis Sci* 25:855, 1984.
13. *AMA drug evaluations*, ed 4, Chicago, 1980, American Medical Association, p 386.
14. Leopold IH: Antibiotics and antifungal agents, *Invest Ophthalmol* 3:504, 1964.
15. Foster JBT, Almeda E, Littman ML, and others: Some intraocular and conjunctival effects of amphotericin B in man and in rabbits, *Arch Ophthalmol* 60:555, 1958.
16. Bell RW, Ritchey JP: Subconjunctival nodules after amphotericin B injection, *Arch Ophthalmol* 90:402, 1973.
17. Cutler JE, Binder PS, Paul TO, and others: Metastatic coccidioidal endophthalmitis, *Arch Ophthalmol* 96:689, 1978.
18. Axelrod AJ, Peyman GA, Apple DJ: Toxicity of intravitreal injection of amphotericin B, *Am J Ophthalmol* 76:578, 1973.
19. McGetrick JJ, Peyman GA, Nyberg MA: Amphotericin B methyl ester: evaluation for intravitreous use in experimental fungal endophthalmitis, *Ophthalmic Surg* 10:25, 1979.
20. Tremblay C, Baraz M, Szoka F, and others: Reduced toxicity of liposomal-associated amphotericin B injection intravitreally in rabbits, *Invest Ophthalmol Vis Sci* 26:711, 1985.
21. Liv K, Peyman GA, Khoobehi B: Efficacy of liposomal-bound amphotericin B for the treatment of experimental fungal endophthalmitis in rabbits, *Invest Ophthalmol Vis Sci* 30:1527, 1989.
22. Axelrod AJ, Peyman GA: Intravitreal amphotericin B treatment of experimental fungal endophthalmitis, *Am J Ophthalmol* 76:584, 1973.
23. Stern GA, Fetkenhour CL, O'Grady RB: Intravital amphotericin B treatment of *Candida* endophthalmitis, *Arch Ophthalmol* 95:89, 1977.
24. Perraut Jr LE, Perraur LE, Bleiman B, and others: Successful treatment of *Candida albicans* endophthalmitis with intravitreal amphotericin B, *Arch Ophthalmol* 99:1565, 1981.
25. Schwartz SD, Harrison SA, Engstrom RE, and others: Collagen shield delivery of amphotericin B, *Am J Ophthalmol* 109:701, 1990.
26. Falls H, Giles C: The use of amphotericin B in selected cases of chorioretinitis, *Am J Ophthalmol* 49:1288, 1960.
27. Sethi KK, Schwartz J: Amphotericin B in ocular histoplasmosis of rabbits, *Arch Ophthalmol* 75:818, 1966.
28. Harrell ER, Wolter JR, Gutow RF: Localized aspergilloma of the eyelid, *Arch Ophthalmol* 76:322, 1966.
29. Newmark E, Ellison AC, Kaufman HE: Pimaricin therapy of *Cephalosporium* and *Fusarium* keratitis, *Am J Ophthalmol* 69:458, 1970.
30. Ellison AC, Newmark E: Intraocular effects of pimaricin, *Ann Ophthalmol* 8:897, 1976.
31. Ellison AC: Intravitreal effects of pimaricin in experimental fungal endophthalmitis, *Am J Ophthalmol* 81:157, 1976.
32. Jones DB, Forster RK, Rebell G: Fusarium solani keratitis treatment with natamycin (Pimaricin), *Arch Ophthalmol* 88:147, 1972.
33. Forster RK, Rebell G: The diagnosis and management of keratomycoses, *Arch Ophthalmol* 93:1134, 1975.
34. Newmark E, Ellison AC, Kaufman HE: Combined Pimaricin and dexamethasone therapy of keratomycoses, *Arch Ophthalmol* 93:1134, 1975.
35. Bailey JC, Fulmer J: Asperigillosis of orbit, *Am J Ophthalmol* 51:671, 1961.
36. Montana JA, Sery TW: Effect of fungistatic agents on corneal infections with *Candida albicans*, *Arch Ophthalmol* 60:1, 1958.
37. Mangiaracine A, Liebman S: Fungus keratitis *(Aspergillus fumigatus)*, *Arch Ophthalmol* 58:695, 1957.
38. *AMA drug evaluations*, ed 4, Chicago, 1980, American Medical Association.
39. Van Cutsem JM, Thienpont D: Miconazole, a broad spectrum antimycotic with antibacterial activity, *Chemotherapy* 17:392, 1972.
40. Foster CS, Stefanyszyn M: Intraocular penetration of miconazole in rabbits, *Arch Ophthalmol* 97:1703, 1979.
41. Miller GR, Rebell G, Magoon RC, and others: Intravitreal antimycotic therapy and the cure of mycotic endophthalmitis caused by a *Paecilomyces lilacinus* contaminated pseudophakos, *Ophthalmic Surg* 9:54, 1978.
42. Blumenkranz MS, Stevens DA: Therapy of endogenous fungal endophthalmitis, *Arch Ophthalmol* 98:1216, 1980.
43. Torres MA, Mohemed J, Cavezos-Adine H,

and others: Topical ketoconazole for fungal keratitis, *Am J Ophthalmol* 100:293, 1985.
44. Komadina TG, Wilkes TKI, Shock JP, and others: Treatment of *Aspergillus fumigatus* keratitis in rabbits with oral and topical ketoconazole, *Am J Ophthalmol* 99:476, 1988.
45. Robinson HJ, Phares HF, Graessle OE: Antimycotic properties of thiabendazole, *J Invest Dermatol* 42:479, 1964.
46. Schulman JA, Peyman GA, Dietlein J, and others: Ocular toxicity after intravitreal injection of terconazole, *Ann Ophthalmol* 21:345, 1989.
47. O'Day DM, Foulds G, Williams JE: Ocular uptake of fluconazole following oral administration, *Arch Ophthalmol* 108:1006, 1990.
48. Drouhet E, Dupont B: Evolution of antifungal agents: past, present, future, *Rev Infect Dis* 9(suppl I):S4-SM, 1987.
49. Richards AB, Jones BR, Whitwell J, and others: Corneal and intraocular injection by *Candida albicans* treated with 5-fluorocytosine, *Trans Ophthalmol Soc UK* 89:862, 1969.
50. Hoeprich MR, Ingraham JL, Klecker E: Development of resistance to 5-fluorocytosine in *Candida parapsilosis* during therapy, *J Infect Dis* 130:112, 1974.
51. Kowalski RP, Raj CVS, Stuart JC, and others: Antifungal synergism: a proposed dosage for corneal storage medium, *Arch Ophthalmol* 103:250, 1985.

## SECTION FOUR

1. Robinson HJ, Graessle OE, Lehman EG, and others: Ocular absorption of thiabendazole-$^{14}$C by the rabbit, *Am J Ophthalmol* 62:710, 1966.
2. Robinson HJ, Phares HF, Graessle OE: Antimycotic properties of thiabendazole, *J Invest Dermatol* 42:479, 1964.
3. Blank H, Rebell G: Thiabendazole activity against the fungi of dermatophytosis mycetomas and chromomycosis, *J Invest Dermatol* 44:219, 1965.
4. Maguire AM, Zarbin MA, Connor TB: Ocular penetration of thiabendazole, *Arch Ophthalmol* 108:1675, 1990.
5. Robinson HJ, Stoerk HC, Graessle OE: Studies on the toxicologic and pharmacologic properties of thiabendazole, *Toxicol Appl Pharmacol* 7:53, 1965.
6. Fink AI, MacKay CJ, Cutler SS: Sicca complex and cholangiostatic jaundice in two members of a family probably caused by thiabendazole, *Trans Am Acad Ophthalmol Otolaryngol* 86:1892, 1979.
7. Rubin ML, Kaufman HE, Tierney JP, and others: An intraretinal nematode (a case report), *Trans Am Acad Ophthalmol Otolaryngol* 72:855, 1968.
8. Schimek RA, Perez WA, Carrera GM: Ophthalmic manifestations of visceral larva migrans, *Ann Ophthalmol* 11:1387, 1979.
9. *AMA drug evaluations,* ed 4, Chicago, 1980, American Medical Association.
10. Wilson LA, Sexton RR, Ahearn D: Keratochromomycosis, *Arch Ophthalmol* 76:811, 1966.
11. Gass JDM, Callahan DG, Bowmen B: Oral therapy in diffuse unilateral subacute neuroretinitis, *Arch Ophthalmol* 110:678, 1992.
12. Wolfe MS, Wershing JM: Mebendazole: treatment of trichuriasis and ascariasis in Bavarian children, *JAMA* 230:1408, 1974.
13. Semba RD, Murphy RP, Newland HS, and others: Longitudinal study of lesions of the posterior segment in onchocerciasis, *Ophthalmology* 97:1334, 1990.
14. Taylor HR, Murphy RP, Newland HS, and others: Treatment of onchocerciasis: the ocular effects of ivermectin and diethylcarbamazine, *Arch Ophthalmol* 104:863, 1986.
15. Lazar M, Lieberman TW, Furman M, and others: Ocular penetration of Hetazan in rabbits, *Am J Ophthalmol* 66:215, 1968.
16. Engstrom RE, Holland GN, Nussenblatt RB, and others: Current practices in the management of ocular toxoplasmosis, *Am J Ophthalmol* 11:601, 1991.
17. Hollarn GN, Engstrom RE, Glasgow RS, and others: Ocular toxoplasmosis in patients with acquired immunodeficiency syndrome, *Am J Ophthalmol* 106:653, 1988.
18. Lakhanpal V, Schockel SS, Nirankari VS: Clindamycin in the treatment of toxoplasmic retinochoroiditis, *Am J Ophthalmol* 95:605, 1983.
19. Kaufman HE, Caldwell LA: Pharmacological studies of pyrimethamine (Daraprim) in man, *Arch Ophthalmol* 61:885, 1959.
20. Kaufman HE: The penetration of Daraprim (pyrimethamine) into the monkey, *Am J Ophthalmol* 52:402, 1961.
21. Chang SC: Penetration of pyrimethamine (Daraprim) into ocular tissues of rabbits, *Arch Ophthalmol* 60:603, 1958.
22. Cook MK, Jacobs L: The effect of pyrimethamine and sulfadiazine on *Toxoplasma* in tissue culture, *Am J Trop Med* 5:376, 1956.

23. Kaufman HE, Remington J, Melton M, and others: Relative resistance of slow-growing strains of *Toxoplasma gondii* to pyrimethamine (Daraprim), *Arch Ophthalmol* 62:611, 1959.
24. Eyles DE, Coleman N: Synergistic effect of sulfadiazine and Daraprim against experimental toxoplasmosis in the mouse, *Antibiot Chemother* 3:483, 1953.
25. Frenkel JK, Jacobs L: Ocular toxoplasmosis, *Arch Ophthalmol* 59:260, 1959.
26. Hogan MJ: Ocular toxoplasmosis, *Arch Ophthalmol* 55:333, 1956.
27. Eyles DE: Newer knowledge of the chemotherapy of toxoplasmosis, *Ann NY Acad Sci* 64:252, 1956.
28. Eyles DE: The relative activity of the common sulfonamides against experimental toxoplasmosis in the mouse, *Am J Trop Med* 2:54, 1953.
29. Kaufman HE, Geisler PH: The hematologic toxicity of pyrimethamine (Daraprim) in man, *Arch Ophthalmol* 64:140, 1960.
30. McGowan JB, Lupovitch A, Katase RY: Daraprim: a folic acid antagonist, *Am J Ophthalmol* 58:608, 1964.
31. Grisham RSC: Central nervous system toxicity of pyrimethamine (Daraprim) in man, *Am J Ophthalmol* 54:1119, 1962.
32. Jacobs L, Naquin H, Hoover R, and others: Comparison of the toxoplasmic skin tests, the Sabin-Feldman dye tests, and complement fixation tests for toxoplasmosis in various forms of uveitis, *Trans Am Acad Ophthalmol* 60:655, 1956.
33. Matoba AY, Pare PD, Le TE, and others: The effect of freezing and antibiotics on the viability of *Acanthamoeba* cysts, *Arch Ophthalmol* 107:439, 1989.
34. Hirst CW, Green WR, Merz W, and others: Management of *Acanthamoeba* keratitis, *Ophthalmology* 91:1105, 1984.
35. Lindquist TD, Sher NA, Doughman DJ: Clinical signs and medical therapy of early *Acanthamoeba* keratitis, *Arch Ophthalmol* 106:73, 1988.
36. Driebl WT, Stern GA, Epstein RS, and others: *Acanthamoeba* keratitis: potential role for topical clotrimazole in combination chemotherapy, *Arch Ophthalmol* 106:1196, 1988.
37. Johns KJ, Head S, O'Day DM: Corneal toxicity of propamidine, *Arch Ophthalmol* 106:68, 1988.
38. John T, Lin J, Sahm DF: *Acanthamoeba* keratitis successfully treated with prolonged propamidine isethionate and neomycin-polymyxin-gramicidin, *Ann Ophthalmol* 22:20, 1990.
39. Ishibashi Y, Matsumoto Y, Kabato T, and others: Oral triconazole and topical miconazole with debridement for *Acanthamoeba* keratitis, *Am J Ophthalmol* 109:121, 1990.
40. Berger ST, Mondino BJ, Holt RJ: Successful medical management of *Acanthamoeba* keratitis, *Am J Ophthalmol* 110:393, 1990.
41. Couch JM, Green WR, Hirst LW, and others: Diagnosing and treating phthirius pubis palpebrarum, *Surv Ophthalmol* 26:219, 1982.
42. Cogan DG, Grant WM: Treatment of pedulogis cilaris with anticholinesterase agents, *Arch Ophthalmol* 41:627, 1949.

CHAPTER 7

# Antiinflammatory Agents

SECTION ONE

## NONSTEROIDAL ANTIINFLAMMATORY DRUGS

E. MITCHEL OPREMCAK

Nonsteroidal antiinflammatory drugs (NSAIDs) have been widely used in general medicine as a result of their analgesic, antipyretic, antiplatelet, and antiinflammatory actions. In the United States approximately 14% of the population is on an oral NSAID therapy, and more than 100 million prescriptions are dispensed each year.[1–3] Historically the role for NSAIDs in ophthalmology has been less well defined. Recently this class of drugs has been used in several clinical trials, and indications for the use of NSAIDs in ocular disease are expanding.

Nonsteroidal antiinflammatory drugs inhibit prostaglandin (PG) and thromboxane formation from arachidonic acid through the inhibition of the enzyme cyclo-oxygenase.[4] Another newer class of NSAIDs blocks the enzyme lipoxygenase. Lipoxygenase products are also generated from arachidonic acid and include leukotrienes and hydroperoxyeicosatetraenoic acids (HPETEs).[5] The metabolites from both enzymatic pathways have a wide range of biologic activities. The PGs are a large group of 20-carbon, unsaturated fatty acid derivatives that promote a nonspecific inflammatory response.[6] They are synthesized de novo after tissue injury. In the eye, PGs increase vascular permeability, produce miosis, and result in the breakdown of the blood-eye barrier.[7–9] Inhibition of cyclo-oxygenase in platelets blocks thromboxane formation and the ability of platelets to induce clotting. Lipoxygenase products and leukotrienes also have a potent effect on the immune response and similarly to PGs promote inflammation after tissue injury.[2] The widespread use and clinical effectiveness of NSAIDs result largely from their inhibitory action on these two enzymes.

There are several classes of NSAIDs that differ in their chemical structure, serum half-lives, and pharmacokinetics (Table 7–1),[3] but all NSAIDs are absorbed rapidly from the gastrointestinal (GI) tract and have high protein-binding to albumin in the bloodstream.[10] Drug distribution depends in part on the lipid solubility of the individual drug. Agents such as naproxen and ketoprofen with higher lipid solubility exhibit greater ocular and central nervous system (CNS) penetration, action, and side effects.[11, 12] Certain NSAIDs have longer half-lives and are thereby more convenient for patient compliance (Table 7–1). These agents, however, including naproxen, diflunisal, phenylbutazone, and sulindac, require a loading dose to achieve an earlier therapeutic blood level. Several NSAIDs are available as topical preparations for ophthalmology, as discussed later on (Table 7–2).

Clinical trials comparing the various NSAIDs have shown very little difference in antiinflammatory efficacy.[13–15] Individual patient preferences, however, do vary significantly. It is not uncommon for a patient to respond poorly to one agent or group of

NSAIDs but to benefit from a trial with a second drug or class of NSAID. In certain disorders, one drug may appear to have better antiinflammatory effect than other NSAIDs. For example, rheumatoid scleritis and HLA-B27 associated diseases (ankylosing spondylitis, Reiter's syndrome, etc.) appear to respond to indomethacin better than to other drugs.[16, 17]

As a group, oral NSAIDs are associated with several potentially serious side effects. The most commonly reported adverse symptoms are gastrointestinal. PGs increase gastric blood flow, increase mucin production, and decrease acid production. $PGE_2$ has 2,000 times more potency than cimetidine as an inhibitor of gastric acid secretion. NSAIDs block these protective actions of PG through inhibition of cyclo-oxygenase in the mucosal cell lining of the stomach. Gastric erosion, dyspepsia, ulceration, perforation, and hemorrhage all are associated with the use of NSAIDs.[2, 18, 19] Relative risks for peptic ulcer disease are estimated between two and four times greater in patients taking NSAIDs compared with case-controlled subjects not taking these drugs.[20, 21] Elderly patients or those with a history of peptic ulcer disease have a higher risk for these systemic side effects. As well, patients taking anticoagulants should avoid NSAIDs to avoid potentially serious gastrointestinal hemorrhage. Patients at higher risk for gastrointestinal complications may benefit from the use of histamine $H_2$ antagonists. Misoprostol, cimetidine, and ranitidine are potent $H_2$ inhibitors that have been shown to reduce endoscopically diagnosed gastric and duodenal ulceration.[22, 23]

**TABLE 7–1.**
Nonsteroidal Antiinflammatory Drug Classification and Serum Half-Lives of Common Agents

|  |
|---|
| Carboxylic acids |
| Acetylated, aspirin (0.25 hr) |
| Nonacetylated, diflunisal (Dolobid) (13 hr) |
| Acetic acids |
| Tolmetin (Tolectin), 1 hr |
| Diclofenac (Voltaren), 1 hr |
| Etodolac (Lodine), 3 hr |
| Indomethacin (Indocin), 5 hr |
| Sulindac (Clinoril), 14 hr |
| Propionic acids |
| Ketoprofen (Orudis), 2 hr |
| Ibuprofen (Advil, Motrin, Nuprin), 2 hr |
| Suprofen (Profenal), 2 hr |
| Fenoprofen (Nalfon), 3 hr |
| Flurbiprofen (Ansaid, Ocufen), 4 hr |
| Naproxen (Anaprox, Naprosyn), 14 hr |
| Fenamic acids |
| Meclofenamic acid (Meclomen), 2 hr |
| Metafenamic acid (Ponstel), 2 hr |
| Fenolic acids |
| Phenylbutazone (Butazolidin), 77 hr |
| Piroxicam (Feldene), 57 hr |
| Pyrrole-pyrrole |
| Ketorolac (Toradol), 5 hr |

**TABLE 7–2.**
Nonsteroidal Antiinflammatory Drug Topical Ocular Preparations

|  |
|---|
| 0.1% Diclofenac (Voltaren) |
| 1.0% Indomethacin (Indocin) |
| 1% Suprofen (Profenal) |
| 0.03% Flurbiprofen (Ocufen) |
| 0.5% Ketorolac (Toradol) |

Long-term use of NSAIDs have other potentially serious side effects. Renal failure, hyperkalemia, and interstitial renal necrosis have been reported with oral NSAID administration.[1, 24, 25] All classes of NSAIDs have these potential side effects, and renal function should be monitored accordingly. Potentially serious drug-drug interactions may also be noted with the use of NSAIDs. These interactions include reduced clearance of digoxin, methotrexate, lithium, and aminoglycosides and can result in elevated blood levels of these medications.[3]

## PREVENTIVE OPHTHALMIC INDICATIONS

The Early Treatment Diabetic Retinopathy Study (ETDRS) was a multicenter, randomized controlled study designed to address the role of both laser treatment and aspirin therapy in diabetes mellitus.[26] Aspirin was given at a dose of 650 mg/day to reduce PG formation and platelet aggregation, postulated to play an important role in diabetic retinal ischemia. Aspirin was found to be safe and did not complicate intraocular diabetic hemorrhages. It was not found to be effective, however, in preventing high-risk proliferative diabetic retinopathy or visual loss in this collaborative national study.[26]

A randomized trial of low-dose (325-mg), alternate-day aspirin therapy in 22,071 male physicians was used to determine whether NSAIDs could slow down or prevent cataract formation.[27] Several earlier studies suggested a protective effect of aspirin in cataract formation via acetylation of lens proteins.[28–30] There was no difference noted in the prevalence of cataract formation with this intervention; the aspirin-treated group had 173 cataracts develop, and the placebo-treated group formed 180 cataracts. This randomized study excluded any large benefit of aspirin therapy in the prevention of cataract formation.

Several topical NSAID preparations have been formulated and used to prevent miosis that often develops during intraocular surgical procedures (see Table 7–2). Pupillary reduction to 4 mm or less has been reported to occur in 28% to 56% of cataract extractions.[30, 31] Intraoperative miosis significantly increases the difficulty and risks of cataract surgery.[32, 33] Flurbiprofen (0.03%) has been shown in controlled clinical trials to reduce intraoperative miosis by 36%.[34, 35] Other topical agents, including 1% suprofen and 1% indomethacin, have been shown to be effective in preventing intraoperative miosis as well.[36, 37] These preparations do not appear to have as much beneficial effect in preventing miosis in vitreoretinal surgery,[38] probably because of the longer duration and more traumatic nature of these procedures.

## THERAPEUTIC OPHTHALMIC INDICATIONS

### Conjunctiva

Vernal keratoconjunctivitis (VKC) is a bilateral, seasonal allergic disorder of the ocular surface. Mast cell degranulation and PG formation is thought to play a mediating role in this disorder. One of the important products synthesized by activated mast cells is $PGD_2$.[39, 40] In both animals and humans, this PG, when applied topically, can produce conjunctival vasodilation, chemosis, and discharge.[39, 40] In one small series, three patients with refractory VKC were treated with 325 mg of aspirin (3–12 times daily) to inhibit $PGD_2$ formation.[41] Ocular symptoms and signs improved in all patients. Inhibition of $PGD_2$ through the use of aspirin was the postulated mechanism of action. The authors conclude that patients with recalcitrant VKC may benefit from adjunctive systemic aspirin. Topical NSAID therapy for patients with VKC has not been reported.

### Cornea

Topical corticosteroids are often employed to treat inflammation after surgical or traumatic corneal injuries. Corneal wound healing and tensile strength, however, are diminished with the use of topical corticosteroids.[42] NSAIDs may provide anti-inflammatory effects without compromising wound strength. Most animal models have shown that topical NSAIDs do not inhibit corneal burst strength. In one study, 1% suprofen, when applied hourly, did not reduce tensile strength compared with 1% dexamethasone.[43] In two additional studies, topical indomethacin, phenylbutazone, and flurbiprofen were found to delay corneal epithelialization but did not inhibit wound strength.[44, 45] Only one study reported decreased burst strength with topical 0.03% flurbiprofen comparable with 1% prednisolone acetate.[46] From these studies it would appear that topical NSAIDs delay epithelial growth but do not significantly reduce tensile wound strength.

The role for topical NSAIDs in treating inflammatory corneal disorders is not well established and is controversial. Animal models employing an intrastromal clove oil model of keratitis showed clinical and histologic benefit from the use of topical 1% suprofen only if applied 48 hours before challenge.[47] Treatment with suprofen immediately with onset of keratitis was ineffective in controlling ongoing inflammation. In one clinical study, patients with ocular discomfort from a variety of noninfectious corneal disorders (corneal scars, edema, erosions, infiltrates, etc.) were found to have a reduction in symptoms with the use of topical 1% indomethacin compared with placebo control.[48] The authors proposed clinical application for this drug in certain noninfectious forms of keratitis.

NSAIDs should be used with caution in certain infectious forms of keratitis. Investigators have shown that topical NSAIDs do not appear to worsen viral keratitis but may complicate bacterial corneal infections. Topical 0.03% flurbiprofen and 0.1% diclofenac given four times daily in both murine and rabbit models of herpesvirus-mediated keratitis did not worsen clinical disease course.[49, 50] This is in contrast to the augmented keratitis noted in control animals treated with topical corticosteroids. In both animal models, the topical application of NSAIDs was noted to have a beneficial effect on reducing the severity of both clinical and histologic corneal inflammation and did not prolong viral shedding compared with control and corticosteroid treatment groups.[49, 50]

The clinical course of bacterial keratitis appears to be complicated by the use of topical NSAIDs. In two rabbit models of *Pseudomonas* and pneumococcal keratitis, clinical disease was aggravated by the use of topical 0.03% flurbiprofen.[51, 52] Corneal ulceration was accelerated in all animals compared with controls and was worse in rabbits treated with corticosteroids alone. The authors postulated that topical corticosteroids block both cyclo-oxygenase and lipoxygenase activity, thereby controlling the corneal inflammation. Shunting of the metabolites into the lipoxygenase pathway occurred as a result of the use of a cyclo-oxygenase inhibitor, allowing the generation of leukotrienes.[52] Lipoxygenase by-products accumulated in the cornea and aggravated the keratitis. A similar observation and hypothesis have been forwarded in an animal model of granulomatous lens–induced uveitis.[53] Topical NSAIDs should be used with caution in bacterial keratitis until effective control with antibacterial agents has been achieved.

### Sclera

Scleritis is a painful and potentially destructive ocular disease.[54–56] The scleral coat of the eye can be inflamed as an idiopathic condition or as a result of several infectious or autoimmune systemic diseases. In several series, rheumatoid arthritis is the most common cause for this disorder. Topical therapy employing corticosteroids is commonly ineffective in controlling disease progression. Several clinical studies have suggested that oral indomethacin (75–150 mg/day) is the drug of choice for the treatment of scleritis.[54] Adjunctive oral corticosteroids may be needed for recalcitrant cases.[55] Patients with necrotizing rheumatoid scleritis may even require second-generation immunosuppressive agents such as cyclophosphamide to control both ocular and systemic manifestations of the disease.[56]

### Glaucoma

PGs have a complex and variable effect on aqueous humor production and intraocular pressure (IOP). Arachidonic acid and certain prostaglandins (PGE and PGF) can produce an acute rise in IOP.[57, 58] Other prostaglandins ($PGD_2$) and chronic administration of PGs appear to lower IOP in animals when applied topically.[59, 60] Intraperitoneal indomethacin can abrogate the acute rise in IOP noted after topical delivery of PGE or arachidonic acid.[61] In one rabbit study, 14 topical NSAIDs were compared for efficacy in preventing arachidonic acid–mediated pressure rise.[62] NSAIDs were given 30 minutes before challenge with topical 5% arachidonic acid, and 0.03% flurbiprofen was shown to be the most effective topical agent in preventing a rise in IOP.

Topical epinephrine is commonly used to lower IOP in patients with glaucoma. It is interesting to note that the pressure-lowering effect of epinephrine is abrogated by the use of oral indomethacin.[63] This observation not only suggests a possible mechanism of action for epinephrine but may be important clinically in glaucoma patients who require both types of medication. Epinephrine is an adrenergic agonist and stimulates both α- and β-receptors. The beta-agonist activity is unlikely to play a role in the reduced IOP because β-blocking agents are potent antiglaucomatous drugs. The α-adrenergic effect may be mediated in part by epinephrine-induced disruption of the blood-eye barrier. Epinephrine appears to stimulate PG synthesis via release of arachidonic acid from tissues and may act as a cofactor for cyclo-oxygenase.[64–66] This would result in a low-grade inflammation, a breakdown of the blood-eye barrier, and a lower IOP. These actions may also explain the increased incidence of macular edema with the use of topical epinephrine.

PGs have been postulated to play a role in a unique form of glaucoma, Posner-Schlossman syndrome. Patients with Posner-Schlossman syndrome develop a low-grade iritis and an acute rise of their IOP. In one report, topical and oral NSAIDs were used to inhibit the formation of intraocular PGs in this syndrome.[67] Sixteen of 21 patients were controlled with topical 0.5% indomethacin four times daily, oral indomethacin (200 mg/day), and 0.5% timolol maleate. The other patients in this series were not controlled and required surgical procedures to reduce the IOP.

Postoperative inflammation and an acute rise in IOP are frequently observed after argon laser trabeculoplasty (ALT).[68] In one trial, 1% indomethacin and 0.03% flurbiprofen were given before ALT in 70 glaucomatous eyes.[69] These agents were not noted to reduce postoperative inflammation. Long-term pressure reduction was not affected and was similar for both placebo and indomethacin groups. Topical 0.03% flurbiprofen pretreatment, however, appeared to have a detrimental effect on IOP. A significantly smaller number of patients were noted to have lower IOP both at 1 day and 5 weeks after ALT when compared with indomethacin- or placebo-treated eyes. In another study, topical indomethacin was ineffective in reducing the acute IOP rise noted after ALT.[70] It appears that topical NSAIDs do not significantly inhibit intraocular inflammation or the acute IOP rise noted after ALT and may have an adverse effect on lowering IOP.

### Postoperative and Traumatic Inflammation

Topical NSAIDs are often employed before cataract surgery to prevent PG-mediated intraoperative miosis.[33–35] They have also been used to prevent and treat postoperative inflammation. Several investigators have demonstrated that topical NSAIDs reduce the disruption of the blood-eye barrier and lessen postoperative inflammation after cataract surgery.[71–75] In these studies, blood-eye barrier integrity was assessed by clinical evaluation of cell and flare and by fluorophotometry. After intracapsular or extracapsular cataract extractions with intraocular lens implantation, postoperative inflammation was lessened with the topical application of 0.03% flurbiprofen, 1% indomethacin, and 0.5% ketrolac.[75–79] The antiinflammatory effect was equal or superior to the use of topical corticosteroid.[76, 77] Topical NSAIDs were not found to have significant adverse side effects or produce an elevation in IOP. Both topical 0.03% flurbiprofen and 0.1% dexamethasone phosphate were found to be ineffective in preventing postoperative inflammation after more aggressive and destructive surgical procedures such as cyclocryablation.[80] It would appear that topical NSAIDs are safe and effective in controlling postoperative inflammation after routine cataract surgery.

### Cystoid Macular Edema

Cystoid macular edema (CME) is a common complication after uncomplicated cataract surgery.[81–83] Postoperative inflammation and PG release have been postulated to play a role in this condition.[84, 85] Several studies have shown that topical indomethacin in combination with corticosteroids can prevent the development of angiographic proven CME after both intracapsular and extracapsular cataract surgery.[86–88] These three studies looked at a total of 948 eyes and demonstrated an overall 50% reduction in incidence of postoperative CME with the use of topical NSAIDs. In another study of 98 eyes, a 70% reduction in fluorescein angiographic CME was noted with the use of topical 0.03% flurbiprofen alone. This study showed that flurbiprofen may be more effective than indomethacin and that corticosteroids may have an antagonistic action when used with NSAIDs. Topical indomethacin has also been used to prevent CME after retinal detachment surgery.[89] Postoperative CME was reduced from 33% (placebo-treated group) to 13% (indomethacin-treated group) in 63 eyes after scleral buckle procedure.

The treatment of clinically significant CME has been more challenging. Burnett et al.[90] treated 14 patients with aphakic CME with topical 1% fenoprofen and found no significant effect when compared with placebo alone. Another randomized study found no significant visual improvement using oral indomethacin compared with placebo in patients with severe CME.[85] More recently, Yunnuzzi[85] reported two trials using topical indomethacin alone or in combination with topical corticosteroids. Treatment with topical 1% indomethacin alone neared significance with respect to benefit in this small pilot study. When topical indomethacin was combined with corticosteroid drops in 40 consecutive patients with chronic CME, 80% were noted to have improved visual acuity by 6 weeks. More recently, a larger, randomized trial was performed comparing topical 0.5% ketorolac four times daily to placebo therapy in 120 patients with chronic pseudophakic CME.[91] A statistically significant improvement in visual acuity was noted in the ketorolac-treated group after 30, 60, and 90 days of therapy.

### Uveitis

Surprisingly, very few studies have been reported investigating the role of NSAIDs in uveitis. Granulomatous inflammation was better controlled in a rat model of lens-induced uveitis with lipoxygenase inhibitors than cyclo-oxygenase inhibitors.[53] The authors postulated that lipoxygenase inhibitors better interfere with macrophage functions that play an important role in this model of granulomatous uveitis. In a rabbit model of an endotoxin-induced iridocyclitis, both parenteral indomethacin and aspirin were found to be effective in reducing uveitis.[92] Only one clinical trial has employed oral NSAIDs in patients with uveitis. Olson et al.[93] reported a beneficial effect from adjunctive use of oral NSAIDs in chronic childhood iridocyclitis. In a crossover study of 14 patients, intraocular inflammation was significantly improved in all eyes when patients took oral agents. A corticosteroid-sparing effect was noted in patients when using NSAIDs.

### Summary

NSAIDs have a wide potential for use in ophthalmology. The analgesic, antiplatelet, and antiinflammatory actions of this group of drugs can be exploited to treat a wide variety of disorders. Patients appear to have a variable response to individual agents with regard to efficacy and side effects. Gastrointestinal and renal complications of oral NSAIDs are of concern, and patients should be monitored for side effects while using these drugs. The benefits and risks of NSAIDs should be compared with alternative therapies, including topical and parenteral corticosteroids.

SECTION TWO

## IMMUNOMODULATORY AGENTS

DAVID K. SCALES

Immunosuppressive drugs have played an increasingly important role in the practice of ophthalmology during the last 30 years. For patients and ophthalmologists alike, these cytotoxic, antimitotic, or antimetabolite agents offer new therapeutic options (Table 7–3), frequently where none previously existed. This has been particularly true within the fields of glaucoma surgery, cornea, and uveitis. Before using these powerful and potentially toxic medications, the ophthalmologist must possess a complete understanding of the indications, risks, and benefits and accept the commitment to follow the patient closely.

Fortunately, the number of ophthalmologists with training in the use of specific immunosuppressive and antimetabolite drugs is increasing. However, for those ophthalmologists who do not have special expertise with these drugs, consultation with an internist, rheumatologist, or hematologist will provide assistance in following

**TABLE 7–3.**
Currently Used Ophthalmic Immunosuppressive and Antimitotic Agents*

| Drug Class | Indications | Dosages | Toxic Reaction |
|---|---|---|---|
| Alkylating agent | | | |
| Cyclophosphamide | Behçet's, Wegener's, cicatricial pemphigoid, Mooren's, rheumatoid, sympathetic ophthalmia | 1–2 mg/kg/day po IV | Hemorrhagic cystitis, mylosuppression, secondary malignancies, alopecia, infections |
| Chlorambucil | Behçet's, sympathetic ophthalmia | 2–12 mg/day po | Same as for cyclophosphamide, gonadal atrophy |
| Antimetabolite agents | | | |
| Azathioprine | Behçet's, cicatricial pemphigoid, SLE, Wegener's, rheumatoid, scleritis | 1–2.5 mg/kg/day po | Mylosuppression, secondary infections, nausea |
| Methotrexate | Rheumatoid, scleritis, HLA-B27 (Reiter's) sympathetic ophthalmia | 10–25 mg/wk in divided doses, po, IV, IM | Hepatotoxicity, mucosal ulcerations, myelosuppression |
| 5-Fluorouracil | High-risk glaucoma at surgery | 5–7.5 mg SC (7–14 days) | Wound leaks, hypotony, corneal epitheliopathy |
| Anti-inflammatory agent | | | |
| Colchicine | Behçet's | 0.5–0.6 g/day bid po | Myelosuppression, nausea, diarrhea |
| Ergot alkaloid agent | | | |
| Bromocriptine | Adjunct with cyclosporine, anterior uveitis (idiopathic) | 2.5 mg/day qid po | Postural hypotension, nausea, vomiting |
| Antibiotics | | | |
| Cyclosporin A | Behçet's, sympathetic ophthalmia, birdshot, VKH, corneal graft rejection | 5–7 mg/kg/day po; 2% topical | Nephrotoxicity, hypertension, hyperuricemia, neurotoxicity (mild) |
| Mitomycin C | High-risk glaucoma surgery, pterygium removal | 0.5 mg/ml; 0.4% topical | Wound leak, hypotony, scleral melting |
| Dapsone | Cicatricial pemphigoid | 25–50 mg bid/tid, po | Hemolytic anemia, nausea, neuropathy |
| Doxyrubicin | Essential and hemifacial spasm (experimental) | N/A, IM | Skin ulceration, local scarring |

**po*, Orally; *IV*, intravenously; *SLE*, systemic lupus erythematosus; *IM*, intramuscularly; *SC*, subcutaneously; *bid*, twice daily; *qid*, four times daily; *VKH*, Vogt-Koyanagi-Harada syndrome; *tid*, three times daily; *N/A*, not available.

the systemic parameters of drug treatment as the ophthalmologist follows the clinical response to treatment.

The available information regarding these medications is quite extensive and beyond the scope of this chapter. The intent of this chapter is not to provide a comprehensive algorithm for immunosuppressive therapy but to provide a useful introduction for the general ophthalmologist. Emphasis here is on ocular responses rather than biochemical mechanisms or action sites.

## IMMUNOSUPPRESSIVE AGENTS

### Alkylating Agents

Alkylating agents were developed after the observation that exposure and systemic absorption of nitrogen mustards lead to widespread bone marrow depression with leukopenia and degeneration of lymphoid tissue. After World War II these compounds and their derivatives were investigated and found to have antimitotic effects beneficial in the treatment of neoplasia. The basic mechanism of alkylating agents is the ability to interfere with cell division in rapidly dividing tissue principally by cross-linking DNA. In the bone marrow the lymphocytic cells appear to be more sensitive to these effects, hence their use in immunosuppression. Lymphocytopenia may be seen within several days, and depression of platelets and erythrocytes may be seen within several weeks.

*Cyclophosphamide* is a derivative of nitrogen mustard that is converted by liver enzymes to active compounds. These active metabolites form covalent bonds with 7-nitrogen guanine and cross-link DNA, producing significant cytotoxic effects. Dosages for cyclophosphamide are about 1 to 2 mg/kg/day orally or intravenously for adults, which is a somewhat lower dose than those used in treating neoplasms. The drug is carefully tailored to the patient's clinical response with careful monitoring of the white blood cell and platelet count. Metabolites are excreted in the feces and urine. Complications of therapy include hemorrhagic cystitis, alopecia, sterility, anemia, leukocytopenia, thrombocytopenia, and decreased resistance to infection. Of particular note is the predisposition of patients treated with alkylating agents to have secondary malignancies develop (urinary bladder, myeloproliferative, and lymphoproliferative neoplasms). This must be considered in the decision to treat nonfatal ocular inflammatory or autoimmune syndromes with alkylating agents and should be discussed in detail with the patient.

*Chlorambucil* is a derivative of nitrogen mustard and has similar attributes and toxicities. Dosage for adults is in the range of 2 mg/day orally, increased to a maximum of 6 to 12 mg/day. The toxicity profile is similar to cyclophosphamide, including reports of irreversible gonadal atrophy, late secondary neoplasms (leukemias), and myelosuppression.

## Antimetabolites

### *Purine Analogs*

Purine analogs have many important uses in human disease, including immunosuppressive (azathioprine), antiviral (vidarabine), and antigout (allopurinol) medications. Their principal immunosuppressive mechanisms of activity have not been clearly established, but they appear to interfere with induction of enzymes required for DNA, as well as RNA synthesis, resulting in cell death. Lymphocytes seem to be particularly susceptible to several of these enzymatic deficiencies after mercaptopurine administration, resulting in immunosuppression.

*Azathioprine* is a prodrug of 6-mercaptopurine, which is activated in the liver and interferes with purine bases incorporated in DNA and RNA, thereby generating errors in the genetic code. Oral dosage in adults is 1 to 2.5 mg/kg/day, and the drug is commonly used in conjunction with low-dose corticosteroids to allow lower dosages of both drugs with lower side effects. The primary toxicity of azathioprine involves reversible myelosuppression and epithelial injury, resulting in esophagitis and mild GI complaints. Close monitoring of the complete blood cell count is essential.

### *Antifolates*

The enzyme dihydrofolate reductase is the principal site of action for this class of drugs. Immunosuppression results from inhibition of cellular metabolism by interruption of folate coenzymatic activity. Because cells in the logarithmic phase of growth are more affected by these medications (methotrexate), lymphoid tissues are rapidly inhibited, resulting in immunosuppression.

*Methotrexate* is a folate analog that appears to act through inhibition of cellular dihydrofolate reductase activity. It can be given orally, intravenously, or intramuscularly in several timetables. Generally a weekly dose of 10 to 25 mg is given as a single or divided dose over 36 to 48 hours. Toxicity and side effects are relatively common with methotrexate and seem to be dose related. Common complaints are gastric discomfort characterized by mucosal ulceration and diarrhea. More severe complications of therapy are hepatic fibrosis (hepatic toxicity related to total dose), cirrhosis, bone marrow suppression with leukopenia and thrombocytopenia, and pulmonary fibrosis. Close follow-up of the patient's hepatic function with consideration of pretreatment and intratreatment liver biopsies and complete blood cell counts are required. Use of methotrexate in patients with liver disease or associated hepatic compromise should be avoided.

#### *Pyrimidine Analogs*

These drugs contain several important properties, including antineoplastic (fluorouracil, cytarabine), antiviral (idoxuridine), and antifungal (flucytosine) actions. Pyrimidine analogs produce immunosuppression by blocking the biosynthesis of pyrimidine nucleotides.

*5-Fluorouracil* is a pyrimidine analog that blocks the enzyme thymidylase synthetase and ultimately inhibits RNA, as well as DNA synthesis, leading to cell death. It is particularly active against rapidly dividing cells such as fibroblasts. Used as an adjunctive medication in glaucoma surgery, it is injected subconjunctivally to lessen scarring and surgical failure. Complications of therapy are wound leaks, hypotony, flat anterior chamber, and corneal epitheliopathy.

### Antibiotics

The actions of antibiotics in producing immunosuppression are varied and are covered within the individual discussions of each drug. Varying levels of leukopenia are known to be associated with certain routinely used antibiotics and for the most part are considered undesirable side effects of therapy. The drugs reviewed here have relatively weak antibiotic properties compared with their immunosuppressive properties.

*Cyclosporine* (cyclosporin A) was discovered as a natural product of several fungal species. Originally investigated for antibiotic properties, it was found to have special immunosuppressive properties, particularly inhibiting T-helper cell responses to antigen presentation. Cyclosporine is water insoluble and must be prepared in either olive or corn oil (100 mg/ml orally or 2% topically) or as an ointment (0.2%–0.5%). An oral capsule (100 mg) is available as well. Doses for adults are initially 5 mg/kg/day and range from 5 to 7 mg/kg/day. Cyclosporine may be used alone or as a corticosteroid-sparing agent. Cyclosporine has been associated with significant dose-related (10 mg/kg/day) nephrotoxicity, and the serum creatinine level must be carefully followed for elevation. Patients are at risk for the development or exacerbation of hypertension during treatment. Other complications of therapy include mild neurotoxicity, hypertrichosis, gingival hyperplasia, and elevation of serum cholesterol levels. Patients with underlying renal disease, poor renal function (decreased creatinine clearance), or poorly controlled hypertension or older patients should be carefully screened and evaluated before use.

*Mitomycin C* is a compound isolated from the fungus *Streptomyces caespitosus*. After enzymatic alteration within the cell, the parent compound becomes a bifunctional or trifunctional alkylating agent that inhibits DNA synthesis and cross-links DNA. Mitomycin's immunosuppressive properties are fairly weak; however, it is a potent inhibitor of fibroblast proliferation. It is used as a single topical application during glaucoma filtering operations to impede scarring and prevent surgical failure. Complications of therapy are wound leaks, hypotony, and localized scleral melting.

*Dapsone* is a sulfone antibiotic related to the sulfonamides used to treat leprosy. Its mechanism of immunomodulation is not fully understood. Dosage in adults is 25 to 50 mg in divided doses two or three times per day adjusted to clinical response. Dapsone is completely absorbed in the GI tract. It is metabolized in the liver, and 70% to 80% is excreted in the urine. A severe hemolytic anemia may develop in individuals who are glucose-6-phosphate dehydrogenase deficient, and this level must be measured before treatment is initiated. Other side effects include dose-dependent hemolytic anemia, GI complaints, peripheral neuropathy, and methemoglobinemia.

### Antiinflammatory Agents

Immunosuppressive properties are not a prominent feature of most antiinflammatory (nonsteroidals, gold, salicylates) drugs.

Colchicine is a specific antiinflammatory agent for gouty arthritis primarily because of its effect on granulocytes and inhibition of microtubule formation. It is not active as an analgesic or found to be effective in most other forms of arthritis.

*Colchicine* has antimitotic effects by virtue of its ability to inhibit microtubule formation. This effect leads to interruption of mitotic spindle formation and inhibition of granulocyte migration and other motile cells. Adult dosages are 500 to 600 mg two to three times/day. It is rapidly absorbed from the GI tract and excreted primarily in the feces. Common toxicity reactions involve GI symptoms. Acute toxicity results in hemorrhagic gastroenteritis, nephrotoxicity, neurotoxicity with ascending CNS paralysis, and extensive vascular injury. Administration on a chronic basis can lead to profound bone marrow depression.

### Ergot Alkaloid

Ergot compounds are products of fungal infection of grain. The effects of ergot compounds are myriad and have been documented for more than 2,000 years. They are highly toxic and have been a source of significant morbidity and mortality since 600 B.C., usually as a result of ingestion of infected grain. Principal uses today are in obstetrics, migraine therapy, Parkinson's disease, and secretion of prolactinomas.

*Bromocriptine* is a dopamine agonist whose precise immunomodulatory effects are not well understood. It decreases secretion of prolactin, which is an immunopotentiator, as well as a competitive inhibitor of cyclosporine, for receptors on T cells (increasing the effect of a given dose of cyclosporine). Adult dosage is 2.5 mg three to four times/day orally. It is rapidly absorbed and excreted largely in feces. Toxicity reactions are commonly GI, but postural hypotension and keratitis sicca are also reported.

## UVEITIS

Together with our increased understanding of the immune system, particularly T-cell interactions, our ability to use immunosuppressive agents has expanded in the field of uveitis. In certain disease states, such as Behçet's disease, sympathetic ophthalmia, and Wegener's granulomatosis, immunosuppressives have become the treatment of choice. Other diseases with relative indications are Vogt-Koyanagi-Harada syndrome, severe juvenile rheumatoid arthritis, pars planitis, and chronic and diffuse uveitis. Immunosuppressive agents have not been found to be useful in Eales' disease, uveal effusion syndrome, tuberculosis, toxoplasmosis, or the presumed ocular histoplasmosis syndrome.

For most uveitic entities general indications for using these drugs remain (1) corticosteroid-resistant or intolerant uveitis, (2) severe or bilateral sight-threatening disease, and (3) the presence of unacceptable corticosteroid-related side effects. One important requirement is a well-informed, reliable patient. General contraindications are (1) infectious uveitis (fungal endophthalmitis, toxoplasmosis, etc.), (2) end-stage prephthisical uveitis without reasonable hope of some visual recovery, and (3) renal or hepatic disease. Pregnancy and childhood should be considered relative contraindications because of possible teratogenicity and long-term side effects.

Properly used and monitored, these drugs appear to have a lower level of adverse consequences or complications than corticosteroids alone. In many cases the role for systemic antimitotic or immunosuppressive agents is that of a "corticosteroid-sparing" agent to allow a lower dose of systemic corticosteroids. This allows systemic corticosteroids to be used to control acute exacerbations of disease activity and then tapered as the dose of immunosuppressive agent is adjusted to appropriate levels and to the clinical response. In some instances (particularly with alkylating drugs), remissions and occasionally cures of the underlying uveitis have been achieved.

### Clinical Use

Behçet's disease is a chronic disease with systemic manifestations and severe intraocular inflammation that leads to blindness in approximately three fourths of eyes in 6 to 10 years.[1] Although initially responsive to corticosteroids, the disease eventually becomes corticosteroid resistant and requires the use of immunosuppressives for effective control of intraocular inflammation. Chlorambucil (Leukeran) has been found to be an effective agent in the control of ocular inflammation[2]; however, other reports have stressed that significant side effects (azoospermia, gonadal atrophy) can accompany its use.[3] Despite use of chlorambucil, 75% of treated eyes had vision worse than 20/200 after treatment. Colchicine has been used with success primarily in Japan.[4] Colchicine seems to be of limited benefit in white patients in controlling active inflammation and may be more useful as prophylaxis against recurring ocular attacks.[5] Most recently cyclosporine has been noted to have excellent activity in controlling Behçet's disease.[6, 7] Nephrotoxicity appears to be dose related and is less frequent with lower dosages of 5 to 7 mg/kg/day.

*Sympathetic ophthalmia* is a rare, bilateral, but often asymmetric, diffuse granulomatous uveitis that is associated with penetrating trauma to the eye. An autoimmune basis has been suggested.[8] Initial therapy with systemic corticosteroids is the treatment of choice. For severe disease resistant or intolerant to corticosteroids, cyclosporine is a reasonable second-line drug showing stabilization of the disease process and improvement of vision in 80% of patients.[5] Rarely other cytotoxic drugs will be required to control the progression of disease.

*Wegener's granulomatosis* is a potentially lethal, multisystem disease with prominent ocular complications that may comprise the presenting symptoms. Although systemic corticosteroids may minimally prolong the survival time, they do not significantly improve the long-term prognosis.[9] Cytotoxic agents, primarily cyclophosphamide, are most effective at controlling the complications of this disease and may provide lasting improvement or cure.[10, 11] Other respiratory vasculitides with significant ocular sequelae such as polyarteritis nodosa, Churg-Strauss syndrome, and Cogan's syndrome have been noted to respond to cytotoxic drugs, particularly the alkylating agents.[9–13]

*Vogt-Koyanogi-Harada disease* and *birdshot chorioretinopathy* are distinct clinical entities that have demonstrated elevated immunologic cellular responsiveness to retinal S antigen. This seems to be mediated by T (helper) cells.[14, 15] Both diseases may respond initially to systemic corticosteroids. For cases that become resistant or intolerant to corticosteroids, the use of oral cyclosporine has proved an effective alternative or corticosteroid-sparing agent.[16, 17]

The indications for systemic immunosuppressives in the treatment of *idiopathic uveitis* are somewhat more difficult to define. It should be noted that many older studies, although commendably important in the progression and dissemination of information regarding potentially successful drug therapy in diseases commonly associated with loss of all useful vision, were uncontrolled, generally anecdotal, with imprecise endpoints for success or failure, and limited by contemporary diagnostic abilities and knowledge of immunology. The large numbers of patients diagnosed with chronic cyclitis, diffuse uveitis, and panuveitis would undoubtedly have more specific categorizations with current knowledge. These issues do not lessen the importance of these early reports but do tend to make application to specific diagnoses in modern uveitic therapy difficult. It should not be inferred that immunomodulatory treatment based on a diagnosis of idiopathic uveitis is acceptable without having exhausted every reasonable avenue to arrive at a more specific underlying diagnosis. Most patients with uveitis today can be specifically diagnosed, with only approximately 10% remaining "idiopathic" after 2 years of close observation with rigorous, repeated medical and surgical immunologic investigations.[18] It is essential that patients have as specific a diagnosis as possible before use of these potentially dangerous medications to more fully justify the risks and allow the patient the best possible hope of therapeutic success.

## CORNEA

The use of cyclosporine immunosuppression for *corneal graft survival* was first explored in animal models.[19, 20] Investigations in high-risk human corneal transplantation rejection using topical 2% cyclosporine revealed that 91% of transplanted corneas were clear, with an average follow-up of 16 months.[21] There was no evidence of systemic absorption. Side effects other than transient punctate epitheliopathy were not reported. Systemic cyclosporine has also been evaluated in high-risk corneal transplants.[22] Compared with topical corticosteroids alone, combination topical and systemic corticosteroids, systemic cyclosporine added to the combination of topical and systemic corticosteroids improved graft survival from 10.5% and 5% to 88.9%, respectively. Side effects of systemic cyclosporine in this group were mild, with one case of creatinine elevation and one complaint of hirsutism, both of which responded to lowering or stopping therapy.

Topical cyclosporine has been evaluated in the treatment of both ligneous conjunctivitis, keratoconjunctivitis sicca, and vernal keratoconjunctivitis. Three reported cases of *ligneous conjunctivitis* responded to treatment with 2% topical cyclosporine.[23, 24] Immunohistologic analysis showed decrease in both T and B cells, with loss of interleukin-2 receptors after treatment.[23] One case responded to topical therapy after reactivation following 4 years of remission.[24] A double-masked placebo-controlled study[25] of 2% topical cyclosporine in *vernal keratoconjunctivitis* confirmed other reports[26, 27] that showed there was a statistically significant decrease in conjunctival hyperemia, papillary hypertrophy, punctate corneal epitheliopathy, and Trantas' dots after treatment with 2% cyclosporine.

Multiple drug regimens have been tried to control the progression of *ocular cicatricial pemphigoid*. One early report noted that therapy with cyclophosphamide and prednisone halted conjunctival shrinkage, but severe side effects were encountered.[28] Other investigators reported success with several agents—dapsone, prednisone, cyclophosphamide, and azathioprine alone or in combination—but stressed that relapses (22%) necessitated continued follow-up after therapy.[29–31] A stepwise, tiered approach to the use of immunosuppressive agents was suggested, with dapsone employed as the most effective initial agent for mild and moderate inflammation, cyclophosphamide useful for more severe disease, and azathioprine most effective when added to other regimens.[32]

The use of systemic immunosuppressives for autoimmune *peripheral ulcerative keratitis* associated with vasculitis or bilateral and progressive disease was evaluated. Vision was stabilized, and 94% of patients showed no progression of disease.[33] A nonrandomized clinical trial of systemic cytotoxic immunosuppression with nonsteroidal and corticosteroidal antiinflammatory agents in the treatment of rheumatoid arthritis–related peripheral ulcerative keratitis strongly suggested that in addition to improvement in ocular disease, the systemic manifestations benefited from immunosuppression. Mortality decreased from 53% over 10 years in conventionally treated patients to 6% when systemic immunosuppressives were used.[34] Similarly, disease progression was arrested with preservation of visual function in patients with bilaterally progressive *Mooren's ulceration* who received adequate immunosuppression with systemic corticosteroids and cyclophosphamide.[35] In that series no patients discontinued therapy because of systemic effects, but it should be stressed that these patients were followed closely by a physician trained in the specific use of these agents.

Topical mitomycin C has been recommended for use in the prevention of recurrence after pterygium excision. Recommended dosage is 0.02% to 0.04% used four times daily for 1 to 2 weeks after surgery. The recurrence rate with such therapy has been reported as low as 0% to 11%.[36–38] Unfortunately, a recent report identifies sight-threatening complications in ten patients receiving topical mitomycin, including corneal edema, corneal perforation, corectopia, iritis, cataract, and intractable pain.[39] A primary conjunctival graft after pterygium removal may offer similar low recurrence rates without these serious complications.[40]

## GLAUCOMA

The primary goal of glaucoma filtering procedures is to interfere with the normal wound-healing mechanisms of the eye, producing a stable fistula to allow aqueous flow into the subconjunctival space. Pharmacologic adjunctive treatments have been developed to assist this goal. Numerous antimitotic agents have been evaluated, such as bleomycin,[41] D-penicillamine,[42] β-aminopropionitrile,[43] 5-fluorouracil,[44] and mitomycin C.[45, 46] The majority of clinical interest in human filtration surgery has centered around the use of subconjunctival 5-fluorouracil and topical mitomycin C.

Postoperative 5-fluorouracil injections have been recommended for use in eyes with uncontrolled glaucoma and poor prognosis, especially after previous cataract surgery or prior failed filtering surgery.[47] Other investigators have described success in using 5-fluorouracil in primary filtering in young patients,[48] as well as adjunctive therapy in other high-risk groups such as aphakia, neovascular glaucoma,[49, 50] and inflammatory glaucoma.[51] Toxicity seen with this agent is related primarily to the effect on dividing cells (corneal epithelial defects, wound leaks, corneal perforation), which are more severe in patients with preexisting corneal abnormalities.[52] Prolonged postoperative hypotony and associated complications (choroidal detachment, flat anterior chamber, maculopathy) are also seen.[53] Efforts to minimize the numbers and seriousness of these complications have led to reductions in the dose of 5-fluorouracil.[51]

Topical mitomycin C has recently been used in filtering surgery with the advantage of its ability to be used as a single intraoperative application rather than the repeated postoperative injections required with 5-fluorouracil.[54, 55] Randomized comparative studies of mitomycin C with 5-fluorouracil in high-risk patients show lower average pressures with less corneal surface and hypotony related complications in the mitomycin C–treated groups.[53, 56] Severe toxicity has been reported in an animal model of intraocular instillation of mitomycin C, resulting in irreversible progressive bullous keratopathy in three of four rabbits so studied.[57] Complete irrigation of the episclera after application should be accomplished to avoid this potential complication in humans.

## OCULOPLASTICS AND NEUROPHTHALMOLOGY

Response to systemic cyclosporine in *granulomatous optic neuropathy* and orbitopathy in one patient with orbital pseudotumor and three with sarcoidosis has been reported.[58] All patients were corticosteroid resistant or intolerant. Cyclosporine (2–5 mg/kg/day) therapy over 2 years was associated with marked visual recovery in two patients, visual stabilization in two, and substantial regression of intracranial lesions in one patient with neurosarcoid. Side effects were reversible hypercholesterolemia and hirsutism. Renal toxicity was not noted.

A single-blind randomized trial of cyclosporine vs. oral prednisone in *Graves' orbitopathy* showed a 66% response for the cyclosporine-treated group compared with 22% for those who had received prednisone alone.[59] Response was measured by improvement in the visual acuity, ocular muscle enlargement and proptosis, objective (NOSPECS), and subjective eye scores. Further improvement was noted when both agents were used additively. Major and moderate side effects were less common with the cyclosporine treatment group and were limited to diverticulitis, rise in serum creatinine level, hypertension, and hirsutism.

Three patients with *orbital vasculitis* were treated with intravenous and oral cyclophosphamide after failure to respond to systemic corticosteroids and loss of vision in one eye.[60] Vision was maintained in each remaining eye, and disease progression was halted. Side effects of therapy were not mentioned.

Doxyrubicin, a cytotoxic anthracycline antibiotic, binds with DNA and inhibits synthesis of DNA, RNA, and protein. Clinical use in cancer chemotherapy revealed skeletal muscle toxicity. This observation led to its experimental use in humans as a chemomyectomy agent in the treatment of *benign essential* and *hemifacial spasm*.[61] This pilot investigation suggests that this technique, although requiring more study before clinical use, may have promise as an adjunctive treatment in facial spastic disorders. No systemic toxicity was encountered; however, some significant local toxicity reactions were seen after local infiltration such as recurrent herpes simplex eruptions, eyelid ulceration, and consecutive lower lid entropion.

Optic neuropathy resulting from sarcoid and Wegener's granulomatosis have been commented on earlier.[58] A report of improved optic neuropathy related to multiple sclerosis (measured by significant reduction of latency in the P-100 peak of the visual evoked potential) after systemic cyclosporine is of interest.[62]

## RETINA

Employment of various antimitotic agents in animal models of *proliferative vitreoretinopathy* after complicated retinal detachment has been investigated and reviewed.[63] The intraocular use of 5-fluorouracil revealed that doses of up to 1.0 mg were tolerated in a rabbit model[64] with no evidence of functional or histologic toxicity. Subsequent studies by the same authors used periocular and intravitreal injections of 5-fluorouracil in human detachments with advanced proliferative retinopathy as an adjunctive treatment to surgical repair.[63] Six months after retinal repair, 60% of patients still had attachment. No serious systemic or ocular toxicity was noted, but mild delay in corneal epithelial defect healing and subepithelial scarring was observed.

Other agents have been investigated as well and found to have potential for inhibiting fibroblastic activity in vitro. In a comparative study of eight neoplastic drugs and dexamethasone, doxyrubicin was found to be superior at nontoxic concentrations in inhibiting proliferation of retinal epithelial cells and fibroblasts than combination drug therapy or dexamethasone alone.[65] In vivo toxicity studies of intraocular infusions with antineoplastic agents during vitrectomy have demonstrated that these agents can be well tolerated in an animal model.[66, 67] Further studies will be required and should be encouraged to determine if these agents will be of use in the treatment of human proliferative vitreoretinopathy.

## COMPLICATIONS OF SYSTEMIC IMMUNOSUPPRESSIVE AGENTS

Antineoplastic and immunosuppressive agents used in the treatment of extraocular malignancies and inflammations may cause intraocular morbidity, and the ophthalmologist should be aware of this. Systemic use of immunosuppressives in the treatment of collagen vascular disease or malignancy may result in systemic immune depression and intraocular hemorrhage because of thrombocytopenia, anemia, or bleeding diathesis as a result of hepatic injury. As well, immune cell inhibition may allow the emergence of opportunistic infections such as cytomegalovirus or severe manifestations of toxoplasmic retinitis, herpetic retinitis, and endogenous fungal infection.

Intracarotid administration of carmustine (BCNU) has been associated with ipsilateral significant visual loss, secondary glaucoma, and internal ophthalmoplegia.[68] Intracarotid administration of cisplatin has been noted to cause pigmentary retinopathy and cavernous sinus syndrome.[68] The incidence of visual loss with BCNU occurs in approximately 70% of patients treated with intracarotid injection and can be avoided if the infusing catheter is advanced beyond the origin of the ophthalmic artery before infusion.[69] This avoids high concentrations of drug reaching the ophthalmic circulation.

## SUMMARY

The use of immunosuppressives has become an important tool both in surgical and medical ophthalmology. Its role is certain to increase and become more commonplace in the future. For several systemic diseases with primary ophthalmic manifestations (Wegener's, Behçet's, polyarteritis nodosa, relapsing polychondritis, etc.), these agents are now specifically indicated and may be considered for first-line treatment in preserving vision and life. As the use of these drugs becomes more widespread, it is incumbent on the ophthalmic physician to be aware of the changing indications and use of these powerful medications. Although use of these medications should be specifically reserved for those with expertise in their usage and prepared to follow any potential complications, the pivotal role of the ophthalmologist in the management of ocular inflammation and observation of ocular complications after use of these agents cannot be disputed. The ophthalmologist is constituted with the knowledge of human response to systemic medication and human pathophysiology, together with ophthalmic examination skills that are unique and not found in those not equally trained. Hence, the integral requirement for an ophthalmologist's active participation in the care and management of these patients is without question.

SECTION THREE

# CORTICOSTEROID DRUGS

KARL S. PAPPA

Before the advent of corticosteroids, their synthetic derivatives, and adrenocorticotropic hormone (ACTH), ophthalmologists achieved similar, although less intense, effects by means of foreign protein injection or anterior chamber paracentesis.[1] Fever therapy induced by foreign protein injection is believed to stimulate pituitary production of ACTH.[2, 3] Discovery of ACTH made it possible to obtain the desirable effects of fever therapy without the accompanying unpleasant and sometimes dangerous fever, aching, and generalized illness. ACTH provided the desired antiinflammatory effects, as well as undesired metabolic effects. ACTH itself has no antiinflammatory or metabolic effects but achieves these effects through stimulation of the adrenal cortex to produce corticosteroids. Topical application of ACTH to an inflamed eye is therefore irrational and valueless. Oral administration of ACTH is also ineffective, because it is destroyed in the GI tract.

Cholesterol is the required intermediate compound in the biosynthesis of corticosteroids. The 27-carbon cholesterol is metabolized enzymatically to a 21-carbon compound in the adrenal cortex.[4] The chemical structures of hydrocortisone and other synthetic corticosteroids that are in current clinical use are illustrated in Fig. 7–1. Certain structural characteristics are required for all biologically active corticosteroids. A double bond between C4,5 and the C3 ketone is necessary for adrenal cortical activity. The presence of an oxygen function at C11 appears essential for significant antiinflammatory activity. Also, the complete expression of antiinflammatory activity requires the presence of the 17-hydroxyl group, which is present in nearly all antiinflammatory corticosteroids in clinical use with the exception of medrysone. Methylation at C6 increases antiinflammatory activity, whereas fluorination in the 9-$\alpha$-position enhances both glucocorticoid and antiinflammatory effects.[4]

Cortisol (hydrocortisone) is synthesized by the cells of the zona fasciculata and zona reticularis and released into the circulation under the influence of ACTH.[5] Normal daily output is 15 to 25 mg of cortisol and 5 mg of corticosterone.[6] The normal plasma concentration of 11-hydroxycorticoids averages approximately 20 μg/100 ml. The rate of secretion changes with diurnal fluctuations.[5] Plasma concentrations usually peak near 8 A.M. and drop to their nadir at about midnight (Fig. 7–2).

In plasma, cortisol is bound to plasma proteins. Corticosteroid-binding globulin (CBG) is an $\alpha_2$-globulin synthesized by the liver and binds 95% of the circulating hormone at any given time. The remaining 5% is free or loosely bound to albumin and is considered biologically active. This free form appears to be involved in the regulation of corticosteroid blood levels through the hypothalamic-pituitary axis.[4]

The half-life of cortisol in the circulation is normally about 90 to 100 minutes.[5] Cortisol is metabolized by the liver, where it is reduced and conjugated to form water-soluble compounds that are excreted in the urine. Plasma levels of free corticosteroid are determined by the degree of plasma

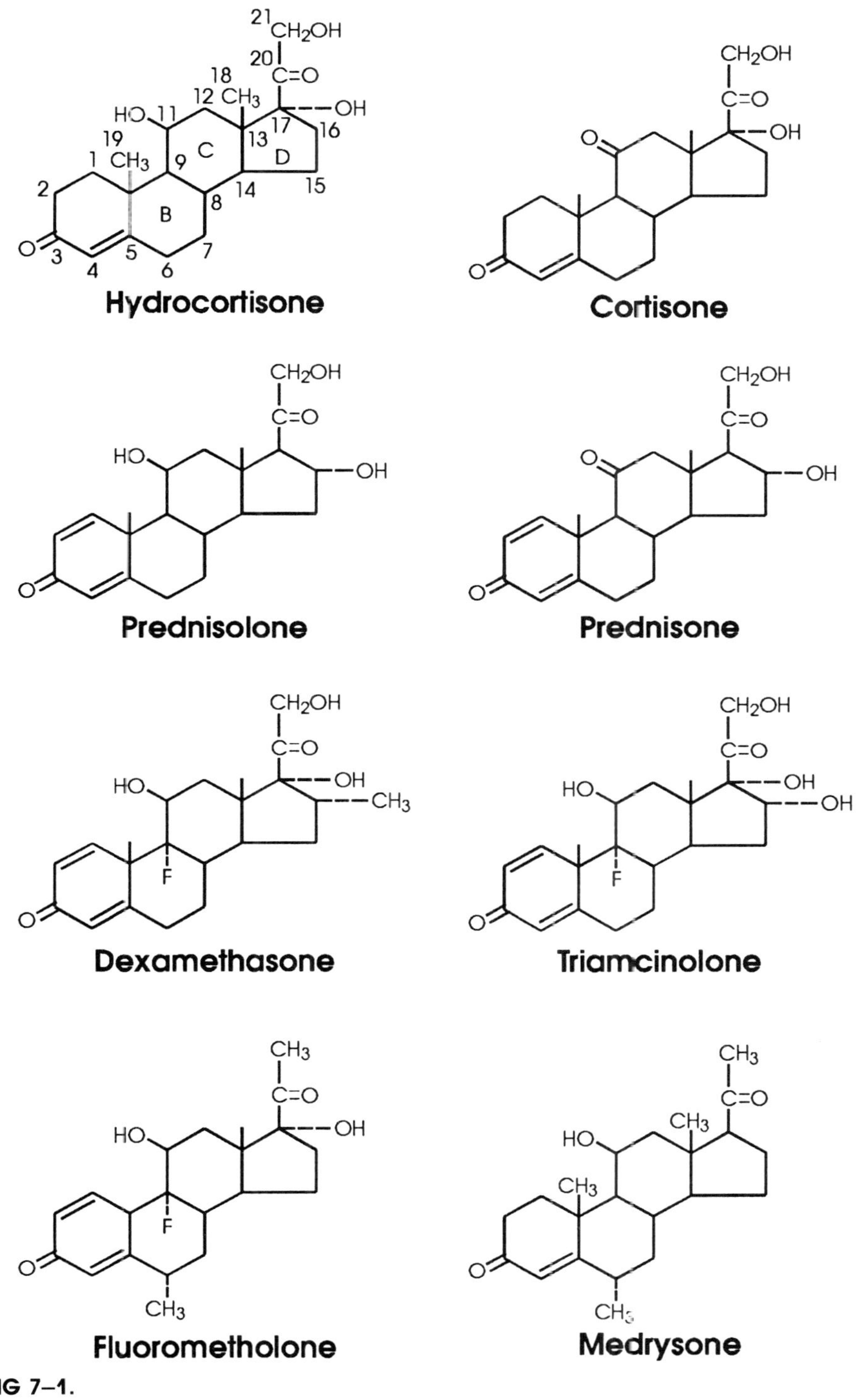


**FIG 7–1.**
Chemical structures of hydrocortisone and the more commonly used corticosteroid derivatives.

protein binding, the metabolic activity of the liver, and the secretion of ACTH.[4]

The advantages of tablet and topical therapy were achieved with cortisone. Almost immediately hydrocortisone was found to be biologically more active and more potent and has been demonstrated to be more clinically effective than cortisone. A significant disadvantage of cortisone compared with ACTH is the marked ad-

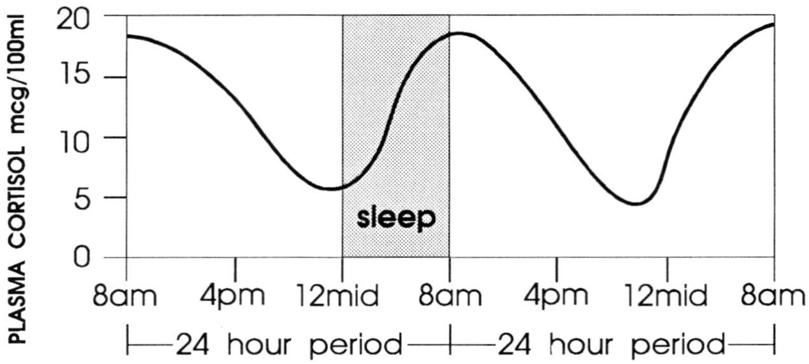


**FIG 7–2.**
The diurnal rhythm of plasma cortisol (free and protein bound). (Adapted from Goldfien A: Adrenocortical steroids and adrenocortical antagonists. In Katzung BG, editor: *Basic and clinical pharmacology,* Los Altos, Calif, 1984, Lange Medical Publications. Used by permission.)

renal atrophy that results from prolonged therapy.

A further advance in the field of corticosteroid therapy was the synthesis of prednisone and prednisolone. Not only are these drugs five to 10 times as potent as cortisone, but, more important, their antiinflammatory effect is relatively greater than their metabolic side effects. This should not be interpreted to mean that prednisone will be effective in cases where cortisone is not, but simply that prednisone requires a smaller (one-fifth) dose. The results of treatment of experimental horse serum uveitis in rabbits with different corticosteroids is illustrated in Fig. 7–3.[7] The amounts used in this program of experimental therapy are listed in Table 7–4. Note that prednisone therapy was only one-fifth the amount of cortisone or hydrocortisone.

One of the most potent synthetic corticosteroid derivatives is dexamethasone, which has an antiinflammatory effect 30 to 50 times that of cortisone (measured in activity by weight). Clinical administration of dexamethasone employs dosages of 4 to 10 mg/day; 10 mg of dexamethasone is the antiinflammatory equivalent of 100 mg of prednisolone. Most ocular diseases responsive to corticosteroids may be treated successfully with 4 mg dexamethasone/day. Dexamethasone has a tissue half-life of 3

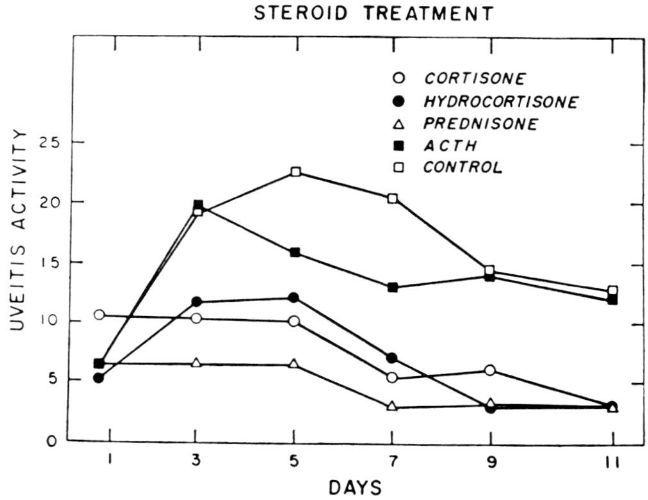


**FIG 7–3.**
Effect of various corticosteroids in therapy of horse serum uveitis in rabbits. Note the latent period before adrenocorticotropic hormone (ACTH) effect. Prednisone was given in one-fifth the dose of cortisone or hydrocortisone. (From O'Rourke JF, Iser G, Ryan T: *Arch Ophthalmol* 55:323, 1956. Used by permission.)

**TABLE 7–4.**
Dosage Schedule of Different Corticosteroids Used in Treatment of Experimental Horse Serum Uveitis in Rabbits*

| Drug | Daily Intramuscular Dose |
|---|---|
| Cortisone | 25 mg/kg |
| Hydrocortisone | 25 mg/kg |
| Prednisone | 5 mg/kg |
| Corticotropin | 10 units/kg |
| Saline solution | 1 ml/kg |

From O'Rourke JF, Iser G, Ryan R: *Arch Ophthalmol* 55:323, 1956. Used by permission.
*Data presented in Fig. 7–3 based on this dosage schedule. Note that only one-fifth as much prednisone was used.

days compared with 9 hours for hydrocortisone and therefore requires only a single daily dose. As is true for all other corticosteroids, higher doses are required for treatment of exceptionally severe cases of uveitis. The most important characteristic of dexamethasone is not its extraordinary potency but its improved therapeutic ratio. Effective antiinflammatory doses of dexamethasone are less likely to produce systemic side effects than are equivalent amounts of other corticosteroids. Sodium and water retention, potassium loss, and abnormal sugar metabolism are minimal with use of dexamethasone. Negative nitrogen, phosphorus, and calcium balances are produced, however. Gastrointestinal ulceration, tuberculosis, psychosis, and dendritic keratitis are all contraindications to its use.[8, 9]

Reference to Table 7–5 indicates that all corticosteroid derivatives have some undesirable side effects, although they vary considerably in intensity.[10] The newer corticosteroids only change the proportionate risk of such side effects but do not eliminate them.[11] Interestingly, therapeutic response to locally applied corticosteroid seems to require approximately the same amount or concentration no matter which corticosteroid is used. This seems to confirm the hypothesis that at least one reason for the increased potency of newer derivatives is their slower metabolism within the body.

Medrysone and fluorometholone are claimed to be much less likely to cause an elevation of IOP. Medrysone does not penetrate into the eye and is recommended only for treatment of surface disorders. Fluorometholone is poorly soluble in both lipid and water vehicles and is dispensed as a microsuspension. As expected, it does not penetrate as well as the more soluble corticosteroids. Thirty minutes after instillation of 0.1% fluorometholone, corneal concentrations are only 1.45 μg/g, and aqueous

**TABLE 7–5.**
Comparative Effects of Corticosteroids

| | Cortisone | Hydrocortisone | Prednisone | Prednisolone | Methylprednisolone | Triamcinolone | Dexamethasone |
|---|---|---|---|---|---|---|---|
| Equivalent daily dose (mg) | 25 | 20 | 5 | 5 | 4 | 4 | 0.75 |
| Edema, sodium retention | + + + + | + + + | + | + + | + | 0 | + |
| Weakness or potassium depletion | + + + | + + | + | + | + | + + | + |
| Hypertension | + + | + | + | + + | + | + | + |
| Mental stimulation | + + + | + | + + | + + | + | 0 to − | + + + + |
| Increased appetite and weight gain | + + | + + | + + | + + | + | − | + + + + |
| Peptic ulcer | + + | + | + + + | + + + | + + | + + + | + + |
| Purpura | + | + | + + + | + + + | + + | + + + | + + |
| Moon face | + + + | + + | + + | + + | + + | + + + | + + |
| Hirsutism | + + | + + | + + | + + | + + | + + + + | + |
| Skin effects | + | + | + | + | + | + + + + | + |
| Osteoporosis | + + + | + + | + + + | + + + | + + + | + + + | + + |
| Diabetes | + + | + + | + + + | + + + + | + + + | + + | + |
| Infections | + + | + + | + + | + + | − + | + + | + + |
| Topical effect | + | + + + | + | + + + | − + | + + + | + + |
| Adrenal atrophy | + + + | + + + | + + + | + + + | + + + | + + + | + + + |

From Hollander JL: *JAMA* 172:306, 1960. Used by permission.

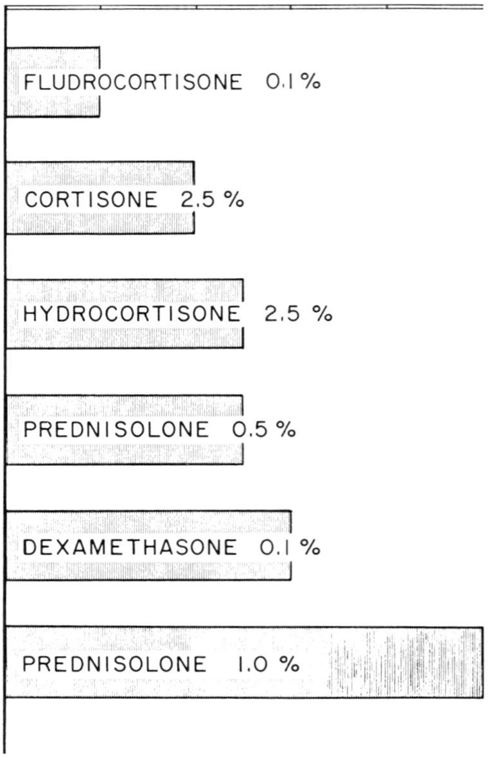


**FIG 7–4.**
Relative antiinflammatory action of various corticosteroid preparations. (Modified from a commercial by Allergan Pharmaceuticals.)

levels are 0.137. Remarkably, these concentrations do not increase with removal of the corneal epithelium or when the eye is inflamed, presumably because the drug remains relatively insoluble under all circumstances.[12] Not only does fluorometholone achieve low tissue concentrations, it is also eliminated more rapidly than prednisolone and dexamethasone.[13] Hence, the reduced tendency to cause glaucoma appears to be related more to concentration and potency differences than to dissociation of therapeutic and toxic effects.

Widespread clinical use has kept pace with the evolution of all these new drugs, and their behavior, indications, and contraindications can be stated precisely.[14–17] The relative potencies of commercially available corticosteroid ophthalmic preparations can be compared graphically (Fig. 7–4).[18] Such comparison emphasizes the fact that concentration of a preparation, as well as the absolute strength of a drug, affects its potency. Table 7–6 shows relative antiinflammatory potency of corticosteroids expressed in equivalent dosages.[19]

## ANTIINFLAMMATORY EFFECTS

Corticosteroids decrease cellular and fibrinous exudation and tissue infiltration, inhibit fibroblastic and collagen-forming activity, retard epithelial and endothelial regeneration, diminish postinflammatory neovascularization, and restore toward normal the excessive permeability of inflamed capillaries.[20] Failure of cortisone to inhibit epithelial or fibroblastic proliferation in vitro suggests the probability of an indirect action such as suppression of the substances that induce tissue activity in response to inflammation or trauma. The antiinflammatory effects of corticosteroids are nonspecific, occurring whether the con-

**TABLE 7–6.**
Relative Potency and Equivalent Dosage of Corticosteroids

| Corticosteroid | Antiinflammatory Potency | Sodium Retention | Equivalent Dose (mg) |
|---|---|---|---|
| Cortisone | 0.8 | 0.8 | 25.0 |
| Hydrocortisone | 1 | 1.0 | 20.0 |
| Prednisone | 4 | 0.8 | 5.0 |
| Prednisolone | 4 | 0.8 | 5.0 |
| Methylprednisolone | 5 | 0.5 | 4.0 |
| Triamcinolone | 5 | 0.0 | 4.0 |
| Paramethasone | 10 | 0.0 | 2.0 |
| Fluprednisolone | 13.5 | 0.0 | 1.5 |
| Fludrocortisone | 10 | 125.0 | 0.1 |
| Betamethasone | 25 | 0.0 | 0.75 |
| Dexamethasone | 25 | 0.0 | 0.75 |

Adapted from Kreines K, Weinberg IC: *Ohio State Med J* 71:698, 1975. Used by permission.

dition being treated is allergic, traumatic, or infectious. The degree of response is related to dosage, and therefore corticosteroid therapy must be titrated against the severity of the individual disease. Subject to the limitations of toxic side effects, enough corticosteroid is given to obtain a therapeutic response. It must be emphasized that an infectious or allergic cause of inflammation is not eliminated by corticosteroid therapy but continues to be present even though the inflammatory response of the body is inhibited. The clinical implication is that treatment must be continued after apparent cure, and dosage must be tapered off gradually to avoid relapse.

The antiinflammatory effects of corticosteroids have been most useful to ophthalmologists because the delicate and transparent ocular structures are particularly susceptible to functional damage by inflammation and scarring. Properly used, corticosteroids will markedly reduce the amount of permanent scarring and may make the difference between useful vision and its loss. In general, therapeutic responses are obtained in clinically nonpyogenic inflammations such as uveitis and scleritis and in all forms of ocular allergy. Although pyogenic inflammations are initially reduced in severity, the ultimate tissue destruction will be more extensive because of the loss of bodily defense mechanisms. Corticosteroids reduce resistance to many types of invading microorganisms—bacteria, viruses, fungi, and the like—and should not be used in the presence of such infections except simultaneously with an *effective* antibiotic or other antibacterial medication. Degenerative diseases are completely refractory to corticosteroids. These facts indicate the great practical significance of accurate differential diagnosis. As an illustration, the similar-appearing lesions of idiopathic paramacular chorioretinitis, tuberculous choroiditis, and age-related macular degeneration will, respectively, be greatly improved, be made considerably worse, and be unaffected at great expense to the patient through corticosteroid therapy.

Additional details of the antiinflammatory effects of corticosteroids are as follows. Normally the intraocular capillaries are relatively impermeable, and for this reason the transfer of fluorescein across the blood-aqueous barrier measures primarily capillary permeability rather than rate of blood flow. By this measure, corticosteroids do not alter the permeability of normal intraocular capillaries. Inflammation breaks down the normal blood-aqueous barrier, permitting leakage into the aqueous of protein and cells, a fact easily demonstrated biomicroscopically. Both clinically and experimentally, cortisone will reduce toward normal the increased capillary permeability characteristic of inflammation. The therapeutic benefit of stopping this abnormal cellular and protein leakage into the aqueous is evident.

The tissue infiltration and surface exudation of polymorphonuclear leukocytes,

A

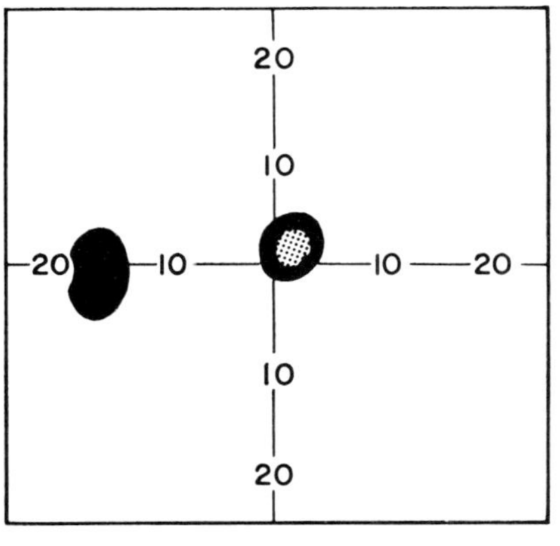


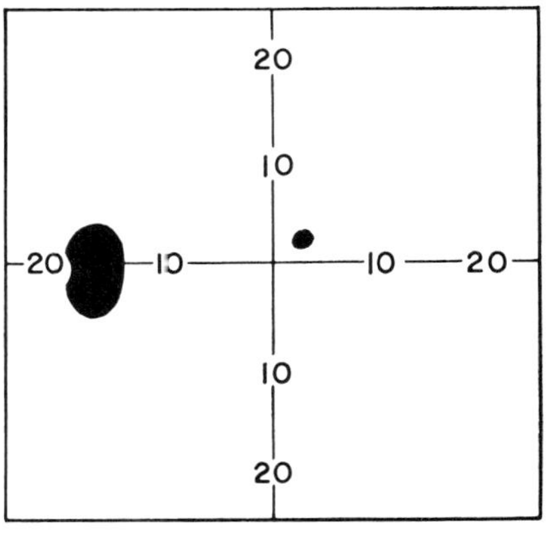


B

**FIG 7–5.**
**A,** Scotoma of acute chorioretinitis in a 33-year-old woman whose other macula had been destroyed by old inflammation. **B,** Greatly reduced scotoma in same eye after 4 days of intensive corticosteroid therapy (20 mg of dexamethasone/day) given in hospital under supervision of endocrinologist. Vision has been restored to 20/20.

lymphocytes, and mononuclear cells are markedly inhibited by corticosteroids. Edema is also reduced. The dramatic corticosteroid-induced decrease in size and intensity of a scotoma caused by chorioretinitis is shown in Fig. 7–5. Such an improvement of function is accompanied by an ophthalmoscopically observable decrease in the activity of the lesion.

## FIBROBLAST-COLLAGEN EFFECTS

Wound healing and the maintenance of normal tissue structure are dependent on the interrelationships of collagen and the cells (fibroblasts) that form it. Because of its avascular and isolated anatomy, the cornea is a unique example of a keratocyte-collagen fiber functional unit. Probably normally and certainly after injury, collagen is both removed (by collagenase) and renewed (by keratocytes). A unique type of injury, the corneal burn, destroys the keratocytes and renders the remaining collagen vulnerable to collagenolysis without the capacity for renewal. Corticosteroids may be both helpful and harmful in this process.

Corticosteroids impair fibroblastic and keratocytic activity.[21] This effect slows the replacement of collagen, which constitutes wound healing. It also slows the repopulation of the cornea with keratocytes. Although such corticosteroid action may slow scar formation, it also slows corneal healing, maintenance, and replacement. Although this is desirable in the prevention of corneal scarring, it is disadvantageous during the healing of surgical wounds. That scarring from corneal burns may be minimized by cortisone therapy is clearly indicated by experimental studies.[22] Standard corneal alkali, acid, and thermal burns were produced in 90 rabbits (30 for each type of burn). Cortisone therapy was administered by drops, subconjunctival injection, or intramuscular injection, and adequate controls were left untreated. The data given in Table 7–7 leave no doubt that the final densities of the corneal scars were significantly less in the eyes treated with cortisone. It can be inferred from these data that the topical instillation of cortisone drops is an effective route for the treatment of corneal burns and that subconjunctival or systemic administration will not produce added benefits. Incidentally, not one of these eyes developed a secondary infection even though no antibiotics were used. This fact should be interpreted in light of the knowledge that rabbit corneas have an inherent resistance to infection that is far greater than that of human eyes. Certainly antibiotics are indicated in the management of human corneal burns.

In contrast, chemical burns of rat eyes are reported not to respond to corticosteroid therapy.[23] Topical and subconjunctival routes were used; however, in most of their experiments, corticosteroid treatment was given only once daily.

**TABLE 7–7.**

Severity of Corneal Scarring Resulting from Standardized Acid, Thermal, and Alkali Burns in Cortisone-Treated and Control Rabbit Eyes

| | Density of Corneal Scar | | | |
|---|---|---|---|---|
| Eyes | 1 | 2 | 3 | 4 |
| Acid burns | | | | |
| Cortisone treated | 31 | 8 | 1 | |
| Control | | 13 | 7 | |
| Thermal burns | | | | |
| Cortisone treated | 29 | 11 | | |
| Control | | 20 | | |
| Alkali burns | | | | |
| Cortisone treated | | | 35 | 50 |
| Control | | | 4 | 16 |

Data from Leopold IH, Maylath F: *Am J Ophthalmol* 35:1125, 1952. Used by permission.

## COLLAGENASE AUGMENTATION

Keratocytes apparently form a collagenase precursor that can be activated by polymorphonuclear leukocyte lysosome enzymes (which themselves have collagenolytic activity) and by dexamethasone. Corticosteroids also stabilize lysosomal membranes and inhibit the release of leukocytic lysosomes. Hence, corticosteroids may have the opposing effects of both activating and inhibiting collagenase formation. Collagenase is irreversibly inhibited by molecular binding with cysteine and British antilewisite and reversibly inhibited by calcium chelation with edetate sodium (*not* by edetate calcium). Calcium is essential to collagenase activity. Collagenase is also produced by injured corneal epithelial cells. The exact circumstances under which corticosteroids are beneficial or harmful to burned corneas are not precisely defined.[24, 25]

Although corneal scarring can be reduced by corticosteroid therapy, in some cases of corneal alkali burn or infection, the use of corticosteroids results in a rapid destruction of the corneal stroma so dramatic that it has been referred to as "melting." The destruction of the corneal stroma is a result of the enzyme collagenase, which may be produced by damaged corneal epithelial cells.

In vitro demonstration of the effect of hydrocortisone on collagenase used a substrate of collagen gel lysed by collagenase obtained from alkali-burned corneas. The area of collagen lysis was 42% greater in diameter in the presence of $10^{-2}$M hydrocortisone than without it.[26] In the presence of $10^{-5}$M dexamethasone the diameter of the area of lysis was 13% greater than without it. Both 0.01M cysteine and ethylenediamine tetraacetic acid 0.01M were able to inhibit completely the lytic effect of collagenase, with or without corticosteroids.

### Inhibition of Wound Healing

Inhibition of fibroblastic activity by corticosteroids significantly interferes with the healing of corneal incisions. The amount of inhibition is related to the dosage. Although

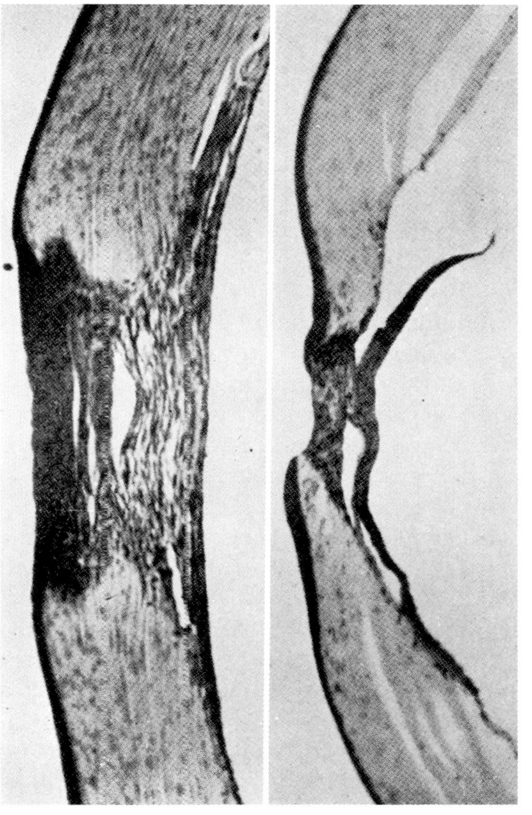

**FIG 7–6.**
*Left,* Normal healing of corneal incision 10 days postoperatively in control rabbit. Epithelial healing is complete, normal corneal thickness is restored, and the wound is bridged by a mass of fibrocytes. *Right,* Impaired healing of corneal incision 10 days postoperatively. This rabbit received 15 mg of cortisone subconjunctivally daily, beginning 2 days preoperatively. Note thinness of fibrous union and failure of epithelium and endothelium to regenerate. (From Ashton N, Cook C: *Br J Ophthalmol* 35:708, 1951. Used by permission.)

small doses alter the histologic course of healing, the final wound closure is adequate. Large doses may greatly impair corneal healing (Fig. 7–6).[27] Corneal wound healing normally proceeds as follows:

1. *First day:* Sealing of wound with fibrinous coagulum; epithelial regeneration rapid.
2. *Second day:* Considerable polymorphonuclear and macrophage infiltration of wound edges.
3. *Third day:* Conversion of keratocytes to fibroblasts.
4. *Fifth day:* Evident fibroblastic

activity; endothelial proliferation visible.

5. *Seventh day:* Fibroblastic closure of outer half of wound, with displacement of the previously inverted epithelium.
6. *Tenth day:* Normal corneal thickness restored by fibroblastic bridge.

Cortisone therapy, even in small amounts, inhibits all of the reparative activity just described.[27]

Study of the traction force required to disrupt rabbit corneal wounds of less than 2 weeks' duration indicated a high incidence of decreased tensile strength secondary to use of topical cortisone.[28] The strength of cortisone-treated wounds was, in some cases, less than half that of the untreated controls. Great individual variation existed, however, and several cortisone-treated wounds were stronger than their controls. Administration of cortisone was identical with accepted clinical usage, 0.5% suspension six times daily or subconjunctival injection of 0.15 mg.

The impairment of wound healing resulting from corticosteroid treatment is dose related. Weak concentrations of corticosteroids and infrequent drug application cause little or no impairment of healing of experimental corneal wounds. For example, 0.1% dexamethasone used four times daily or 0.01% 12 times daily did not impair corneal wound strength. However, 0.1% dexamethasone applied topically 12 times daily reduced wound strength to approximately half the normal.[29]

After experimental rabbit corneal incisions, 0.05% dexamethasone ointment applied twice daily for 21 days did not alter the tensile strength of the wound when tested 21 days postoperatively.[30]

Not only the type and concentration of corticosteroid but also its molecular form may substantially alter clinical effectiveness. For example, equal molar concentrations of dexamethasone in the form of 0.1% alcohol, 21-acetate, or 21-phosphate were applied in dosages of 2 drops five times daily to rabbit eyes with 180-degree limbal incisions. The eyes were subsequently ruptured with oxygen under increasing pressures. Fig. 7–7 shows that dexamethasone alcohol completely inhibited the fibroblastic component of healing between 3 and 6 days.[31] Even 2 weeks later the average bursting strength of the treated eyes was 18 psi compared with 24 psi for the control. Although inhibition of wound healing was also demonstrated for

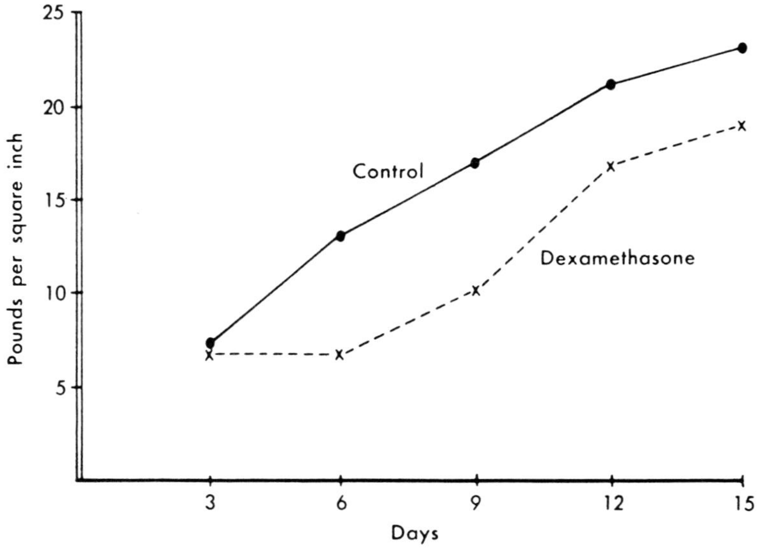


**FIG 7–7.**
Effect of 0.1% dexamethasone alcohol, 2 drops five times daily, on bursting strength of 180-degree limbal incision in rabbit eyes. (Modified from McDonald TO, and others: *Invest Ophthalmol* 9:703, 1970. Used by permission.)

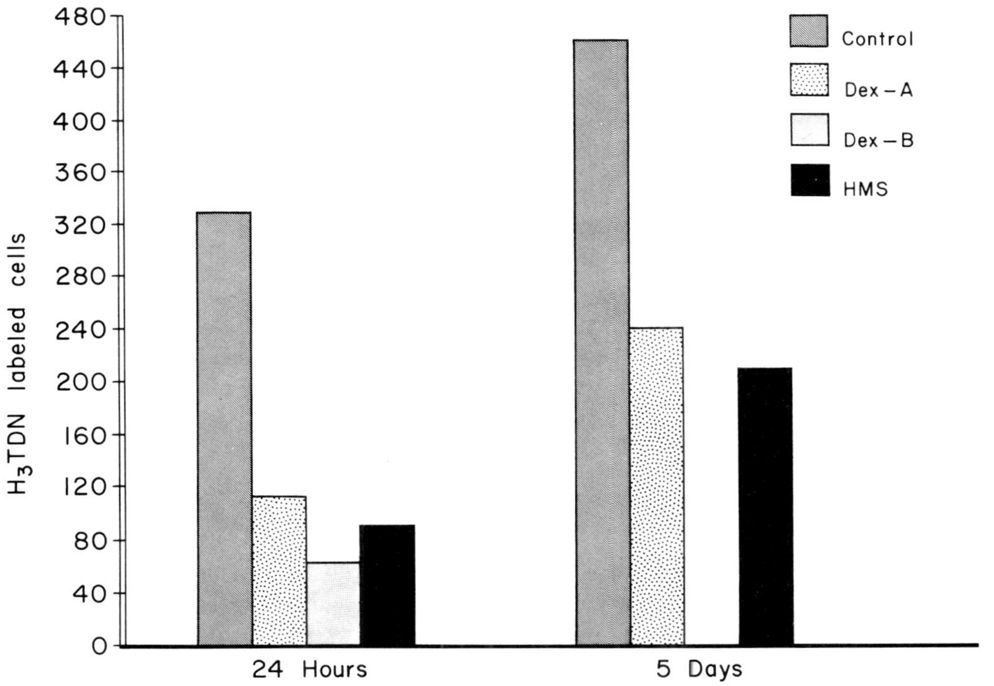


**FIG 7–8.**
Tritium-labeled keratocyte inhibition by corticosteroid therapy. *Dex-A,* 0.05% dexamethasone ointment three times daily after freezing; *Dex-B,* dexamethasone three times daily 1 day before and 1 day after freezing; *HMS,* 1% medrysone solution three times daily. (From Polack FM, Rosen PN: *Arch Ophthalmol* 77:400, 1967. Used by permission.)

the acetate and phosphate forms of dexamethasone, the amount of inhibition was only half as great as for the alcohol form. Even in 0.001% concentrations, dexamethasone alcohol reduced the 6-day wound strength by 3 psi. Sufficient systemic absorption occurred in the animals receiving 2 drops of 0.1% dexamethasone alcohol to reduce the 6-day bursting strength of the untreated opposite control eye by 4 psi.[31] In comparable experiments, 0.5% indomethacin and 1% phenylbutazone did not impair wound healing.

A particularly sensitive experimental measure of the effect of corticosteroids on wound healing is the cellular uptake of tritiated thymidine after a freezing injury. Tritiated thymidine selectively enters cellular deoxyribonucleic acid (DNA) before mitosis and remains there during the life of the cell. Hence, this method will demonstrate the number of cells undergoing active multiplication. The number of labeled keratocytes 1 and 5 days after a 1-minute freezing injury is shown in Fig. 7–8.[32] Obvious and marked inhibition of cellular multiplication by corticosteroid therapy is apparent.

Despite the general agreement that corticosteroids tend to inhibit experimental wound healing, clinical experience indicates that ocular surgery can be performed with impunity during corticosteroid therapy in moderate dosage. The ophthalmologist may encounter, however, occasional cases that seem to incriminate corticosteroid therapy as the cause of serious wound disruptions.

In fairness to the opposite point of view, it should be stated that the tensile strength of healing corneal incisions has been reported as completely unaffected by 15 mg of cortisone/kg in rabbits.[33] Similarly, topical and subconjunctival application of corticosteroids are reported to cause no alteration in the healing of thermal corneal burns.[34]

### Glucocorticoid Receptors

The actions of corticosteroids are mediated by the binding of corticosteroid molecules to receptor molecules located within cells sensitive to corticosteroid influence. Sensitive cells can be detected and measured with the use of radioactive corticosteroids. The complexity of the interaction is revealed by the discovery that a typical sensitive cell will contain approximately 60,000 receptor molecules. Radiolabeling techniques applied to a uniform cell population derived from tissue culture can study as few as 500,000 cells and can identify the affinities and the location of the receptors. Dexamethasone has twice the receptor affinity of hydrocortisone and four times the affinity of progesterone. Of the corticosteroid receptors, 60% are found in the cell nucleus and 40% in the cytoplasm. Within 30 minutes after corticosteroid injection, two thirds of the labeled cytoplasmic receptors have migrated to the nucleus. Within 2½ hours, the amount of cytoplasmic receptor has returned to normal, although it cannot be determined whether this is return migration of the molecules or synthesis of new receptor protein. The hormonal response occurs when the corticosteroid-receptor complex associates with the nuclear chromatin and transmits the functional message that initiates appropriate synthesis of effector molecules (Fig. 7–9).

Corticosteroid receptors are present in human trabecular meshwork cells and in rabbit iris–ciliary body tissue; hence, these cells can be expected to have cortisone-sensitive functions.[35–37]

Radioautographic localization of labeled dexamethasone applied topically was used to identify its binding to the nuclei of corneal epithelial cells and keratocytes and to conjunctival epithelial cells and the endothelial cells of blood vessels. Prior incubation with an excess of unlabeled hormone suppressed in this localization indicates that these cells are corticosteroid-receptor cells. No corneal endothelial localization occurred.[38]

Receptor cells for intravenously administered radioactive dexamethasone include stromal and endothelial cells of the trabecular meshwork, conjunctiva, iris muscle, choroid, retina, and sclera. Presumably these tissues can exhibit physiologic responses to corticosteroids.[39]

### Lysosome Stabilization

Ciliary body lysosomes are stabilized by corticosteroids. Because these lysosomes contain enzymes capable of breaking down mucopolysaccharide structure,

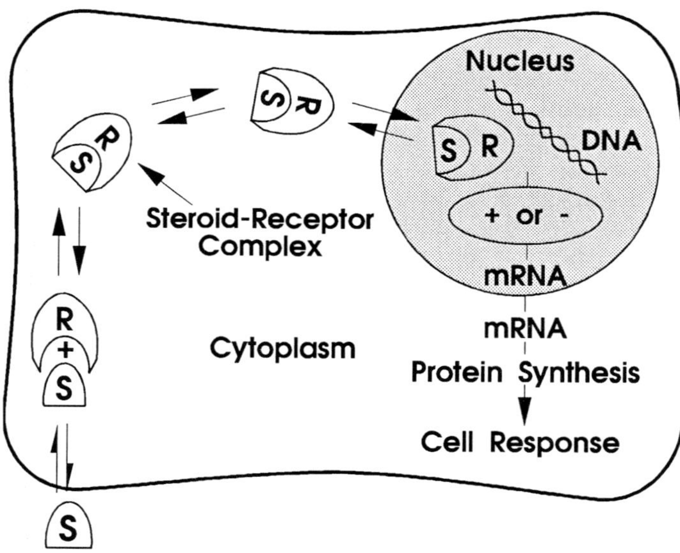


**FIG 7–9.**
Proposed mechanism of action for corticosteroid hormones. The steroid enters the cell after binding with a specific cytoplasmic receptor. This complex then migrates to the cell nucleus, where it alters DNA transcription, resulting in changes in protein synthesis that affect cell function.

corticosteroid-induced increase in mucopolysaccharides may occur and may be related to the mechanism of corticosteroid-induced glaucoma.[40]

The hypothesis that corticosteroid-induced glaucoma is caused by clones of susceptible goniocytes stipulates that the inherited original goniocytes will produce populations of cells that form part of the trabecular meshwork. If a sufficient number of these cells are corticosteroid sensitive, their lysosomes will be stabilized by corticosteroids, and the mucopolysaccharides of the trabecula will increase, thereby reducing outflow facility. The gradation of the pressure response will depend on the number of clones of genetically determined goniocytes, which can vary independently of inheritance. This explanation is compatible with the fact that only 62% of monozygotic twins are concordant in their pressure response to corticosteroids.[41]

Corticosteroid stabilization of lymphocyte lysosomes correlates with open-angle glaucoma and susceptibility to the corticosteroid ocular hypertensive response. Lymphocytes may be activated (sensitized; transformed) to function by exposure to various immunologic substances formed within the body or by plant extracts called phytohemagglutinins. This activation is decreased by corticosteroids, and the amount of corticosteroid inhibition is greater in glaucoma-susceptible individuals. Glaucoma-susceptible lymphocytes are also stabilized to a greater degree than normal lymphocytes by theophylline. Theophylline preserves cyclic adenosine monophosphate (cAMP) from destruction by cAMP phosphodiesterase. cAMP is the energy molecule that transmits messages into a cell. This similar response suggests that corticosteroids stabilize lysozymes via the cAMP pathway. This same cAMP pathway may be involved in the ciliary body regulation of aqueous humor formation.[42] This is apparently the biochemical explanation of why coffee and tea can cause elevated IOP in some glaucoma patients.[43]

A recent double-masked crossover study of caffeine vs. placebo was performed in normal patients. This study showed no clinically significant effect on aqueous humor formation and IOP.[44] However, the authors also point out that any small change in IOP produced by caffeine in normal patients could possibly be amplified in glaucomatous eyes.

Of more general applicability, corticosteroid stabilization of leukocytic lysosomal vacuoles prevents enzymatic destruction of inflamed host tissues by the immunologic and cellular defense mechanisms of the body. This response is desirable in the eye, because it preserves structure and function. On the other hand, the stabilized leukocyte cannot manifest its defensive capabilities, which renders the host vulnerable to invasion by alien microorganisms.

For example, herpes simplex activation does not result from an enhancement of virus growth but from corticosteroid inhibition of antibody-dependent, cell-mediated cytotoxicity against viral growth.[45]

Just to confuse the matter, the existence of increased glaucomatous lymphocyte sensitivity to corticosteroids has been affirmed by some laboratories and denied by others.[46]

### Leukocytic Response

Not only the activation of leukocytes but also their migration is affected by corticosteroids. Partial removal of corneal epithelium stimulates the appearance of polymorphonuclear leukocytes in the tear fluid within 2 to 5 hours. This appearance of leukocytes is greatly reduced by 1% prednisolone (cell count reduced from 2,400/ml to 400/ml), 0.5% indomethacin (reduced to 50/ml), 0.01% flurbiprofen (reduced to 50/ml), and 0.5% aspirin (reduced to 100/ml). Topical use of 0.1% flurbiprofen was less effective, because an irritant response to the stronger concentration slightly increased the polymorphonuclear mobilization. The reason antiprostaglandin drugs were more effective than corticosteroids is that they act further down the sequence of PG synthesis. This sequence is phospholipid → phospholipase $A_2$ → arachidonic acid → PG. Corticosteroids inhibit phospholipase $A_2$. PG inhibitors block arachidonic acid transformation.[47] Corticosteroids actually lyse and destroy lymphocytes.

When experimental rabbit corneal infections with *Staphylococcus aureus* or *Pseudomonas aeruginosa* were treated with adequate amounts of bactericidal antibiotics (e.g., gentamicin, polymyxin B, and neomycin) to which the organisms are demonstrably sensitive, the eradication of the infection proceeded equally well whether or not 1.0% prednisolone was also used. Both antibiotic and corticosteroid were instilled hourly.[48] This result is to be expected, inasmuch as corticosteroids do not enhance microbial growth or interfere with the mechanisms of antibiotic killing. Corticosteroids do impair mobilization of phagocytes and their defensive capabilities. Simultaneous use of corticosteroid and bactericidal antibiotic will reduce lytic damage to the host.

This concept must be restated to be clearly understood. If clinically you treat an unknown microorganism with a bacteriostatic or ineffective antibiotic and also with corticosteroid, you will reduce host defenses and enhance the amount of microbial damage to the host. Because the clinician initially does not know the type of organism and its sensitivity, corticosteroid therapy started before culture and sensitivity reports are complete may be dangerous. "Corticosteroids have no place in the therapy of bacterial keratitis in the absence of concurrent administration of appropriate antibiotics."[48]

If polymorphonuclear leukocytes are radiolabeled, the relative ability of corticosteroids to reduce their mobilization to an inflamed cornea is easily measured. Table 7–8 shows the efficacy of various corticosteroids in reducing leukocyte mobilization.[49] These data suggest that 1% prednisolone acetate is the most effective of the products tested in this study for suppressing corneal inflammation.

**TABLE 7–8.**

Percentage of Decrease in Polymorphonuclear Leukocyte Mobilization to an Inflamed Cornea by the Designated Corticosteroid

| Corticosteroid | Reduction (%) |
|---|---|
| 1% prednisolone acetate (Econopred Plus; Pred Forte) | 51 |
| 0.1% dexamethasone alcohol (Maxidex) | 40 |
| 0.1% fluorometholone (FML Liquifilm) | 31 |
| 1% prednisolone phosphate (Inflamase Forte) | 28 |
| 1% dexamethasone phosphate (Decadron Phosphate) | 19 |

Data from Leibowitz HM: *Ophthalmology* 87:753, 1980. Used by permission.

It appears from Table 7–8 that the particular corticosteroid derivative used is crucial in determining the antiinflammatory activity of the drug. Thus, in rabbit corneas with an intact epithelium, prednisolone acetate demonstrates greater antiinflammatory activity than prednisolone phosphate.[49] A human clinical trial comparing equal concentrations of the acetate and alcohol derivatives of fluorometholone showed a significantly greater antiinflammatory effect with the acetate derivative.[50] Fluorometholone concentrations of 0.1% and 0.25% were recently compared in rabbit corneas, and there was no significant difference in their antiinflammatory effects.[51] Fluorometholone acetate, 0.1%, was significantly more effective in inhibiting corneal inflammation when compared with either 0.1% or 0.25% fluorometholone (Table 7–9). However, when it was directly compared with 1% prednisolone acetate, there was no significant difference shown in their ability to suppress external ocular inflammation.[51]

Topical application of corticosteroids to the cornea provides enormously greater concentrations than can be achieved by systemic administration. Clinically we can control the dosage of ocular topical corticosteroids by changing both the concentration and frequency of application. The frequency of administration correlates directly with

**TABLE 7–9.**

Effect of Topical Corticosteroids on Leukocyte Mobilization into an Inflamed Cornea

| Drug | Reduction (%) |
|---|---|
| Fluorometholone | |
| 0.1% | 31.3 |
| 0.25% | 34.7 |
| Fluorometholone acetate, 0.1% | 47.9 |
| Prednisolone acetate | |
| 0.125% | 33.8 |
| 1.0% | 51.7 |

Data from Leibowitz HM, Ryan WJ, Kupferman A: *Arch Ophthalmol* 110:119, 1992. Used by permission.

**TABLE 7–10.**
Percentage of Decrease in Polymorphonuclear Leukocyte Mobilization to an Inflamed Cornea by 1% Prednisolone Given at the Designated Frequency

| Frequency | Total Drops | Reduction (%) |
|---|---|---|
| 1 drop q4h | 6 | 11 |
| 1 drop q2h | 10 | 30 |
| 1 drop qh | 18 | 51 |
| 1 drop every 30 min | 34 | 61 |
| 1 drop every 15 min | 66 | 68 |
| 1 drop each min for 5 min qh | 90 | 72 |

Data from Leibowitz HM: *Ophthalmology* 87:753, 1980. Used by permission.

the effectiveness. Table 7–10 shows the effectiveness of various doses over an 18-hour period.

In practice, bacterial keratitis is treated with antibiotic alone for the first 24 hours. At that time, if the appearance of the eye is clinically stable and the culture report provides evidence that the antibiotic regimen should be effective, topical corticosteroid treatment may be started. Suddenly discontinuing corticosteroid therapy in the management of a severe keratitis may induce a massive necrotizing rebound invasion of leukocytes.[49]

### Membrane Permeability

In general terms, corticosteroids preserve or restore toward normal the permeability of cell membranes or layers of cells. This may be demonstrated in rabbit corneas stored in McCarey-Kaufman medium, commonly used in eye banks. Under such circumstances a bicarbonate leak occurs from the aqueous side to the stromal side, and the cornea becomes hydrated. This leak can be decreased by $10^{-8}$M hydrocortisone, resulting in better preservation.[52]

The physiologic basis for this situation is that the normal rabbit cornea maintains its dehydration by means of an active transport of bicarbonate ion and water across the endothelium into the aqueous. This flow is great enough to account for all water removal from the cornea.

### Neural Response

After 40 mg of prednisone/day for 3 weeks, retinal sensitivity increases, causing a supernormal electroretinogram (ERG) that may be up to 300% greater than normal. Patients with adrenocortical hyperplasia also show supernormal ERGs. The mechanism of this effect is unknown but is not related to variations in sodium or potassium concentration, as established by ERG measurement of renal dialysis patients.[53–55] Excitability of the cerebral cortex is also increased by corticosteroids.[56]

### Inhibition of Neovascularization

Another useful therapeutic action of cortisone is inhibition of neovascularization. This effect is readily reproduced experimentally, provided that minimal lesions are studied. Naturally a sufficiently severe injury will heal with neovascularization despite use of corticosteroids. The rate of development of alloxan-induced corneal vascularization in cortisone-treated and control rabbits is shown in Fig. 7–10.[57] Cortisone has a nonspecific vasoconstrictor effect that may contribute to this inhibition of neovascularization and that may induce regression of existing vessels.[58]

### Vascular Proliferation

Growth of rat retinal blood vessel endothelial cells is reduced 50% by 0.2 mg of dexamethasone/kg/day but not by 10 mg of indomethacin/kg/day (PG antagonist).[59, 60]

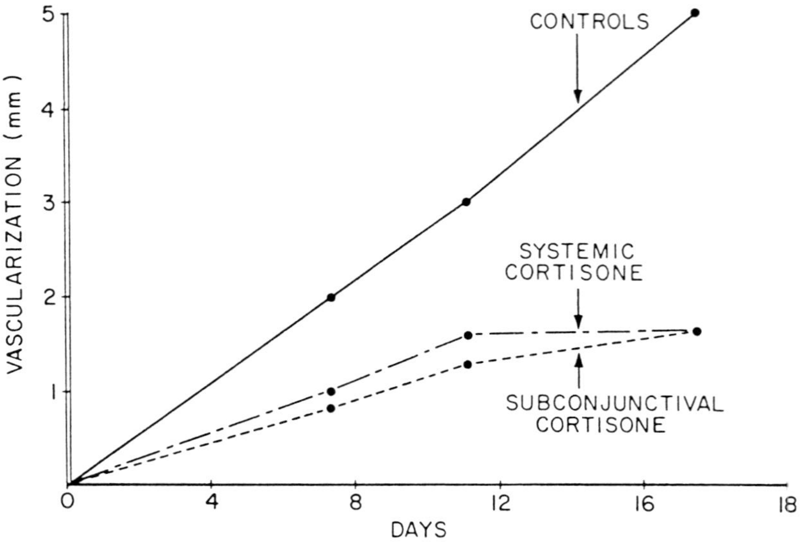


**FIG 7–10.**
Rate of development of alloxan-induced corneal neovascularization in control and cortisone-treated rabbits. (From Ashton N, Cook C, Langham M: *Br J Ophthalmol* 35:718, 1951. Used by permission.)

### Inhibition of Epithelial Regeneration

A relatively minor disadvantage of corticosteroids is the inhibition of epithelial and endothelial regeneration. The data given in Table 7–11 indicate that epithelial regeneration after standard thermal corneal burns occurred in 3 days in control animals but was delayed until the fourth day in three fifths of the cortisone-treated rabbits. This was not only an effect of topical administration but also occurred with intramuscular injection of cortisone. Similar slight retardation of epithelial regeneration is reported in experimental wound healing and is observed clinically as persistent fluorescein staining.

Scanning electron microscopy shows loss of corneal microvilli subsequent to topical prednisolone therapy. Continuing therapy destroys the cytoplasmic membrane of the epithelial cells, eroding downward layer after layer into the corneal epithelium.[61]

## INTRAOCULAR PENETRATION

Radioactive carbon–labeled cortisone acetate has been used to study the penetration of this substance into the eye.[62] One milliliter of a 0.25% suspension of radioactive cortisone acetate was applied to rabbit

**TABLE 7–11.**
Retardation of Epithelial Regeneration by Cortisone in Standard Corneal Thermal Burns in Rabbits

| | Days Required for Epithelization | | | |
|---|---|---|---|---|
| Eyes | 1 | 2 | 3 | 4 |
| Cortisone treated | | | 16 | 24 |
| Control | | | 19 | 1 |

Data from Leopold IH, Maylath F: *Am J Ophthalmol* 35:1125, 1952. Used by permission.

corneas with a special stirring applicator. After 20 minutes, the eyes were thoroughly washed, enucleated, divided into their various portions, and subjected to chromatography and radioactivity counting. Cortisone acetate concentrations were extremely minute, being measured in millimicrograms (Table 7–12). Although only cortisone acetate was used, measurable quantities of radioactive cortisone and hydrocortisone were found in the tissues, indicating rapid metabolic transformation of these substances. Highest concentrations were found in the cornea and aqueous, considerably lower concentrations in the iris, and no measurable quantity in the lens, vitreous, and retina. Considerable activity in the sclera and choroid might have been caused by posterior venous drainage or possibly by contamination, although the latter was believed unlikely. Because it is known that clinical response occurs to applications of corticosteroids of this concentration, it is apparent that these substances are biologically effective in extraordinarily dilute concentrations (e.g., 5 billionths of 1 g in the entire iris).

Radioactive labeling permits identification of the distribution of cortisone after topical ocular instillation. An astonishing amount of corticosteroid is rapidly distributed throughout the body. Thirty minutes after instillation into rabbit eyes, only 1.6% of the radioactive corticosteroid was present within eye tissue.[63] Twenty-nine percent was still present in the conjunctival sac and was recovered by surface washing. The unusually long persistence of medication in the conjunctival sac resulted from the method of application, namely, pooling of 0.25 ml of solution between the lids that were held open by sutures. Nasal washings contained only 0.5%, suggesting that relatively little absorption occurred by this route (or that it was rapidly absorbed into the general circulation and therefore did not accumulate within the nose). Liver, kidneys, adrenal glands, and gallbladder contained 21.4% of the radioactivity. The remaining 47.5% was presumably distributed throughout the other body tissues.

All parts of the eye contained radioactivity 30 minutes after cortisone application; however, the highest counts were obtained from cornea and conjunctiva. Counts per minute values for various eye tissues were cornea, 70; iris and ciliary body, 30; sclera and choroid, 20; retina, 16; aqueous, 8; lens, 4; vitreous, 1. (The total dose instilled on the eye was 10,000 counts/min of radioactivity.)

The corticosteroids present in the normal primary aqueous humor of rabbits have been analyzed by chromatography.[64] No cortisone was found by a method capable of detecting as little as 60 mμg/ml. The only corticosteroid present had characteristics identical to those of crystalline hydrocortisone and was found in a concentration of 0.17 mμg/ml.

The aqueous concentrations of prednisolone alcohol after topical ocular instillation of a drop of 1% prednisolone (labeled with radioactive tritium) are shown in Fig. 7–11.[65]

As is true of all medications applied to the cornea, penetration of hydrocortisone compounds is also determined by differential solubility characteristics. It is pointed out in Table 7–13 that the water-soluble succinate and phosphate compounds of hydrocortisone did not penetrate the normal cornea enough to elevate the aqueous corticosteroid concentration significantly above the normal control level.[66] In contrast, the lipid-soluble acetate compound penetrated in effective concentration. Obviously the fact that a given corticosteroid prepara-

**TABLE 7–12.**

Range of Concentration (mμg) of Some Corticosteroid Derivatives in Specific Tissues After 20-minute Application of 0.25% Solution of Cortisone Acetate to Rabbit Corneas

| Derivative | Cornea | Aqueous | Iris and Ciliary Body | Choroid and Sclera |
|---|---|---|---|---|
| Cortisone acetate | 70–99 | 28–90 | 6–10 | 13 |
| Cortisone | 29–69 | 5–6 | 5–12 | 66 |
| Hydrocortisone | 14–26 | 6–30 | — | 8 |

Data from Hamashige S, Potts A: *Am J Ophthalmol* 40:211, 1955. Used by permission.

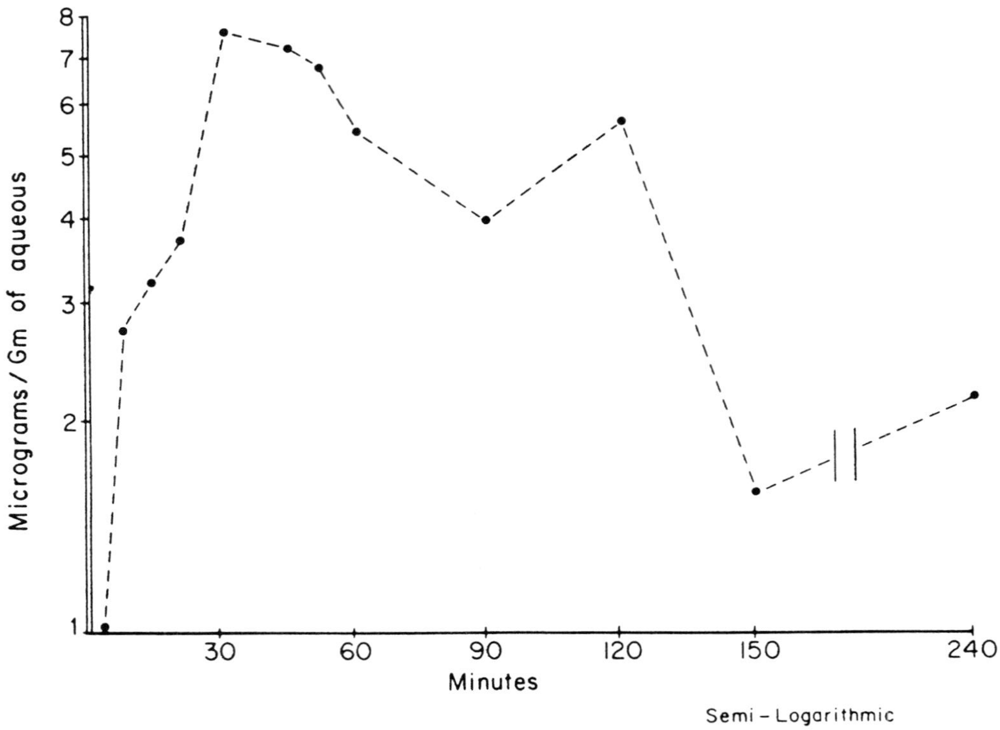


**FIG 7–11.**
Aqueous concentrations of prednisolone at specified intervals after ocular instillation of a drop of 1% suspension. (From Murdick PW, and others: *Arch Ophthalmol* 76:602, 1966. Used by permission.)

tion is a clear solution rather than a suspension does not necessarily indicate that it will penetrate to the interior of the eye.

Ocular penetration studies have been performed comparing topical and subconjunctival cortisone or hydrocortisone (Table 7–14).[67] Aqueous levels of cortisone were much higher than hydrocortisone and were higher for both in the presence of corneal damage. Cortisone entered the aqueous readily via both topical and subconjunctival administration.

Repeated topical applications of cortisone acetate will produce progressively higher aqueous cortisone levels, reaching a plateau after 3 days of therapy. Aqueous concentrations of 50 mμg/ml may be attained by topical application of cortisone acetate suspension nine times daily (Fig. 7–12).[22] A similar concentration was attained (but within 1 rather than 3 days) by subconjunctival injection of 1.25 mg every 12 hours and by intramuscular injection of 100 mg every 8 hours. Twenty-five milligrams of cortisone acetate by retrobulbar injection every day reached a peak of 35 mμg/ml. (This was a relatively early study, and the absolute values may be a little high.) By all

**TABLE 7–13.**
Hydrocortisone (mμg/ml) Recovered From Rabbit Aqueous After Topical Application Every 5 Minutes for Six Times of 0.5% Solutions of Some Hydrocortisone Compounds

| Hydrocortisone Compound | Test Eye | Control Eye |
|---|---|---|
| Acetate | 6.0 | 0.52 |
| Succinate | 0.48 | 0.65 |
| Phosphate | 0.9 | 0.70 |

Data from Fleming TC, Merrill DL: *Research report no. 5*, Alcon Laboratories. Used by permission.

**TABLE 7–14.**

Aqueous Levels of Corticosteroid (μg/ml) After Subconjunctival Injection or Topical Use of Drops of Cortisone or Hydrocortisone in Normal and Alkali-Burned Rabbit Eyes

| Corticosteroid | Normal Eye | Burned Eye |
|---|---|---|
| Subconjunctival injection of cortisone (50 mg) | 5–10 | 15–17 |
| Topical use of 2.5% cortisone (6 mg) | 5–8 | 13–22 |
| Subconjunctival injection of hydrocortisone (50 mg) | Not measurable | 2–5 |
| Topical use of 2.5% hydrocortisone (6 mg) | 2 | 3–5 |

Data from Leopold IH: *Arch Ophthalmol* 52:769, 1954. Used by permission.

routes, cortisone penetrated in appreciable quantity to the vitreous, although never quite attaining the aqueous concentrations. Topical applications gave the smallest vitreous concentrations. Cortisone was rapidly cleared from the aqueous, being virtually gone within 24 hours after the last of the series of applications by any route. From these penetration studies it would seem that anterior segment lesions could be treated equally well by topical, subconjunctival, or systemic routes, and the posterior lesions would be reached by systemic administration or subconjunctival injections.

Considerable variance exists in the intraocular penetration of prednisone and prednisolone, depending on whether free alcohol or acetate forms are employed and whether the cornea is normal or abraded. Fig. 7–13 shows aqueous concentrations of prednisone and prednisolone, in alcohol or acetate form, attained by topical instillation

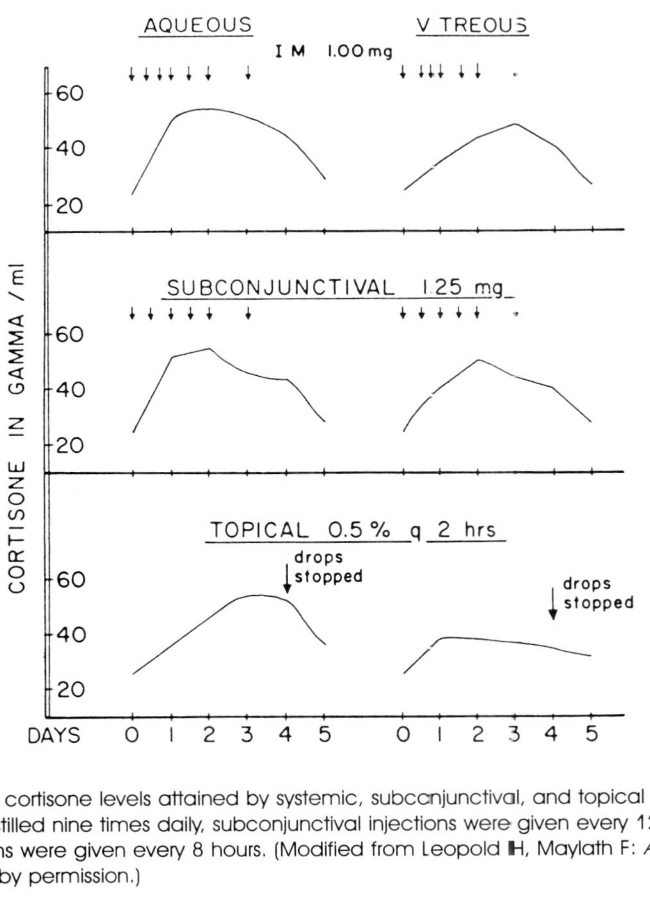


**FIG 7–12.**

Aqueous and vitreous cortisone levels attained by systemic, subconjunctival, and topical routes of administration. Drops were instilled nine times daily, subconjunctival injections were given every 12 hours, and intramuscular injections were given every 8 hours. (Modified from Leopold IH, Maylath F: *Am J Ophthalmol* 35:1125, 1952. Used by permission.)

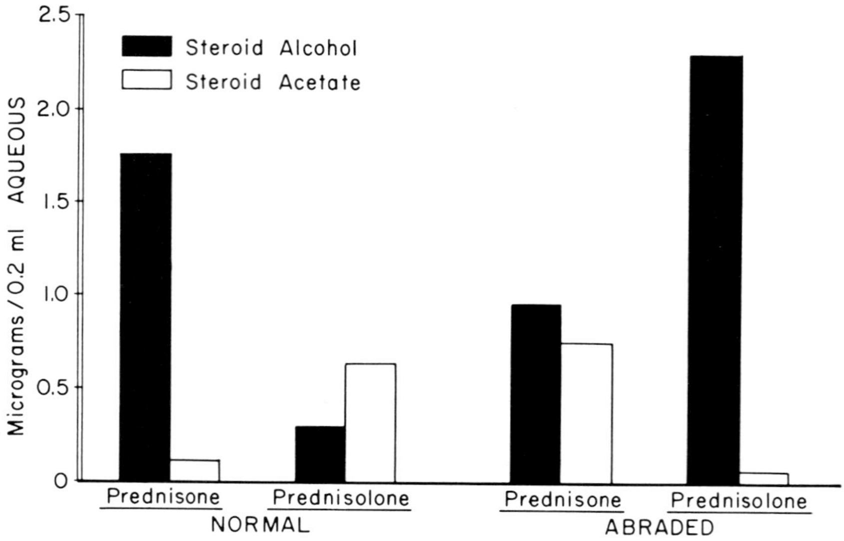


**FIG 7–13.**
Penetration of topically applied corticosteroids, 0.5% suspension, given four times at 15-minute intervals. (Data from Leopold IH, Kroman H, Green H: *Trans Am Acad Ophthalmol* 59:771, 1955. Used by permission.)

in rabbit eyes of 0.5% suspension every 15 minutes for 1 hour; aspiration of aqueous was done 15 minutes after the last drop.[68]

Prednisolone sodium phosphate is a highly water-soluble compound and is almost lipid insoluble. Theoretically it should not penetrate the intact corneal epithelium. Nevertheless, 30 minutes after instillation of 1 drop of 1% drug, corneal concentrations of 10 μg/g and aqueous levels of 0.5 μg/g are attained. If the epithelium is removed, corneal concentrations reach 235 μg/g and aqueous levels 17 μg/g.[69]

The intraocular penetration of topically applied prednisolone derivatives varies considerably. The aqueous concentration of corticosteroids attained by placing 1 drop of 0.5% suspension into a rabbit cul-de-sac every 15 minutes for 1 hour is shown in Fig. 7–14; the sample was drawn 15 minutes after the last drop.[70] It is apparent that triamcinolone is present in far lower aque-

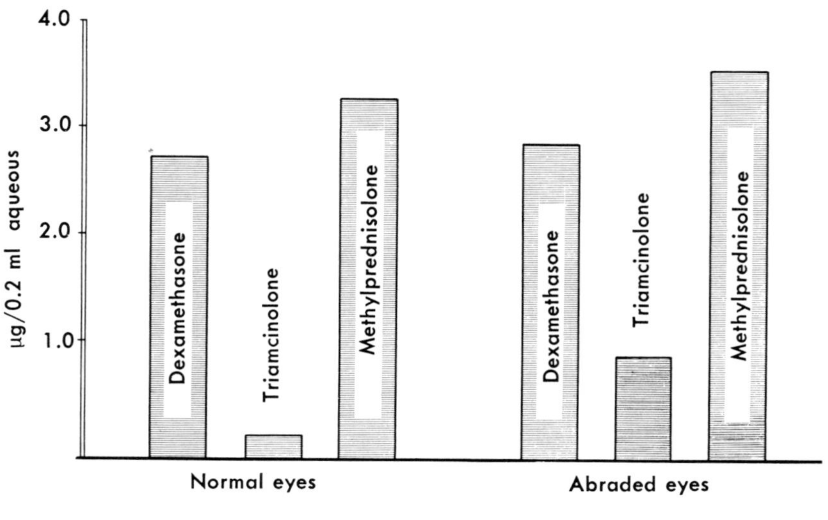


**FIG 7–14.**
Aqueous concentrations of corticosteroids 15 minutes after topical application of 0.5% suspension for times at 15-minute intervals. (Modified from Leopold IH, Kroman HS: *Arch Ophthalmol* 63:943, 1960. Used by permission.)

ous concentrations than are dexamethasone and methylprednisolone.

The blood-aqueous barrier definitely limits the intraocular penetration of intravenously administered corticosteroids. After intravenous administration of 25 mg of dexamethasone (Fig. 7–15), no corticosteroid is demonstrable in the aqueous humor during the first 30 minutes. By 1 hour, a peak level is reached that is only slightly higher than that attained by topical application. Within 2 hours, the aqueous level of dexamethasone has fallen to half its peak value. (Triamcinolone given intravenously was found to penetrate much less well than dexamethasone, just as happened via the topical route.)

It was concluded from these studies (blue tetrazolium technique for determining corticosteroids) that triamcinolone penetrates poorly into the aqueous humor of rabbits compared with dexamethasone and methylprednisolone.

The following year the same investigators, using a paper chromatography technique (stated to be more sensitive than the blue tetrazolium method), concluded that the prednisolone derivatives (dexamethasone [methylfluoroprednisolone], triamcinolone [fluorohydroxyprednisolone], and methylprednisolone) appeared to have equal ability to penetrate into the aqueous humor. Concentrations between 1 and 1.5 μg/1.5 ml of aqueous could be attained in 18- to 27-kg rabbits by intravenous injection of 25 mg of corticosteroid 1 hour before sampling or by topical instillation of 0.5% suspension of corticosteroid every 15 minutes for 1 hour. Slightly higher concentrations were attained by the topical route of administration in these experiments.[71]

Dexamethasone acetate penetrates into the cornea more poorly than does the alcohol or phosphate forms. The antiinflammatory activity of these dexamethasone derivatives is not directly related to their concentration at the site of action. For example, the acetate form produces the lowest concentrations in the cornea but the largest antiinflammatory effect (Table 7–15).[72] At the same time it is least likely to cause a rise in IOP, again presumably because of its failure to penetrate beyond the cornea.[72]

Obviously these corticosteroid derivatives have different abilities to penetrate the eye. Their variable penetration appears to be

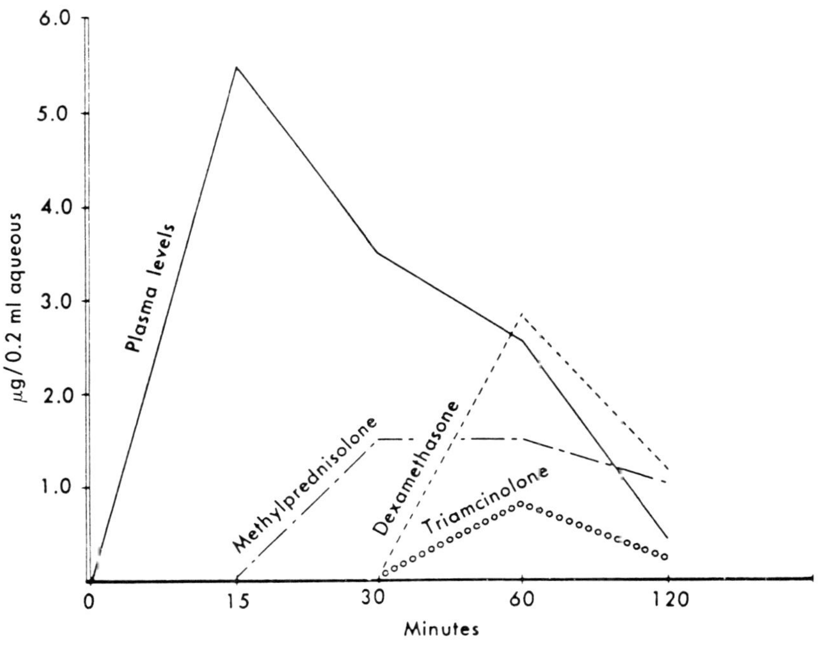


**FIG 7–15.**
Aqueous concentrations of corticosteroids after intravenous administration of 25 mg in rabbits. (Modified from Leopold IH, Kroman HS: *Arch Ophthalmol* 63:943, 1960. Used by permission.)

**TABLE 7–15.**
Corneal Inflammatory Suppression and Bioavailability of Dexamethasone Derivatives

| Corticosteroid | Corneal Inflammatory Suppression (%) | Corneal Bioavailability (μg/min/g) |
|---|---|---|
| Epithelium intact | | |
| Dexamethasone acetate, 0.1% | 55 | 111 |
| Dexamethasone alcohol, 0.1% | 40 | 543 |
| Dexamethasone sodium phosphate, 0.1% | 19 | 1,068 |
| Epithelium absent | | |
| Dexamethasone acetate, 0.1% | 60 | 118 |
| Dexamethasone alcohol, 0.1% | 42 | 1,316 |
| Dexamethasone sodium phosphate, 0.1% | 22 | 4,642 |

Data from Leibowitz HM, Kupferman A, Stewart RH, and others: *Am J Ophthalmol* 86:418, 1978. Used by permission.

related to the lipophilic barrier formed by the corneal epithelium. When the epithelium is removed, there is a marked increase in corneal penetration of the hydrophilic dexamethasone derivatives but little change in penetration with the lipophilic dexamethasone acetate derivative (see Table 7–14). Very lipophilic drugs will be absorbed readily into the corneal epithelium and usually saturate this layer before entering the hydrophilic stromal layer. These drugs usually will achieve low concentrations in the aqueous even when the epithelium is removed. Fluorometholone is an example of this; it penetrates the corneal epithelium poorly but produces moderate corneal antiinflammatory activity.[73] It does not penetrate well into the aqueous even when the corneal epithelium has been removed. Perhaps for this reason it is less likely to elevate IOP than other corticosteroids.

Depending on their solubility, topical corticosteroid derivatives can be formulated as solutions, suspensions, ointments, or gels. The rate of release of drug particles from the vehicle and their solubility in the precorneal tear film can greatly affect intraocular penetration. For example, the ointment form of dexamethasone phosphate does not penetrate the cornea as well as the solution, even with its increased viscosity and contact time.[74] In this case dexamethasone phosphate has a greater affinity for the ointment vehicle itself. It is poorly released into the precorneal tear film, and thus there is little drug available for corneal absorption.

High-viscosity gel corticosteroid preparations have been designed to improve ocular penetration and therapeutic efficacy. A gel preparation used in rabbit corneas enhanced the antiinflammatory activity of prednisolone acetate.[75]

After reading about the endless variations of ocular penetration and therapeutic effect resulting from these different corticosteroid derivatives and vehicles, I find it reassuring that reputable manufacturers produce consistently effective products. For example, comparison of two brands (Pred Mild Suspension and Econopred, both 0.125% prednisolone acetate) showed no differences in concentration of drug in cornea and anterior chamber or in their antiinflammatory effect against experimental clove oil keratitis.[76]

## PRINCIPLES OF CORTICOSTEROID THERAPY

The route of administration of corticosteroids depends primarily on the site of involvement and type of inflammation. Topical therapy is effective in anterior segment disease, including disorders of lids, conjunctiva, cornea, iris, and ciliary body. Severe anterior segment disease may sometimes require supplementary systemic or periocular corticosteroids if drops alone fail to control the inflammation.

The course of posterior segment disease (i.e., optic neuritis and posterior scleritis) is not appreciably affected by topical corticosteroids and requires systemic corticosteroids, periocular corticosteroids, or both. Patients obviously prefer oral administration of corticosteroids to injections. Because the peak concentration of plasma corticosteroids occurs within 1 hour after oral administration, it is unnecessary to resort to intravenous injections for faster results. Four to 8 hours after an oral dose of cortisone, plasma corticosteroid levels have returned to normal; therefore, one dosage regimen is to divide the total daily dose into equal amounts to be taken every 4 to 6 hours.

A careful medical history should be performed before beginning any type of corticosteroid therapy, especially for systemic treatment. The dosage should be individualized for each patient and the specific disease. Each patient should be frequently monitored and the dosage reassessed during therapy for both desired and undesired corticosteroid effects. Generally, low-dose topical therapy over a short term can be discontinued without a tapered regimen. However, any high-dose, long-term therapy should be gradually tapered and never abruptly discontinued.

The basic pharmacologic principle that drugs have dose-response relationships is, of course, of great practical importance. Not only therapeutic efficacy but also toxicity follows dose-response relationships. However, the amount of a clinically useful drug required for a therapeutic response will usually not induce a toxic response. From a practical standpoint, therefore, the smallest amount of drug that will achieve the desired therapeutic response for the shortest time necessary should always be used.

As a specific example, 0.001% dexamethasone drops five times daily will reliably prevent experimental corneal graft reactions, whereas smaller doses fail to do so. Tensile strength of healing corneal wounds is impaired by 0.1% dexamethasone drops 12 times daily but not by smaller doses. If delayed until the seventh postoperative day, corticosteroid therapy does not impair corneal wound healing. The clinical implications of these dose relationships are obvious insofar as they relate to avoidance of toxicity.[77] A less apparent implication is that corticosteroid overtreatment is probably the clinical rule rather than the exception to the detriment of the patient. "More is not necessarily better" applies not only to vitamins but also to corticosteroids.

As a reminder, topical ocular medications are absorbed systemically. The only difference between topical and systemic routes of administration is the lesser amount of drug usually given topically. For example, adrenal gland atrophy occurs in rabbits given 1 drop of dexamethasone five times daily for 21 days. (Of course, a rabbit is smaller than a human, and this is a proportionately much higher dose.[78])

The typical dose-response curve describing the effect of corticosteroid therapy of keratitis would show an increasing response to greater concentrations of drug. This response is not limitless, however, because increments of response to further increases of dosage become smaller as a maximum value is reached. Theoretically, such a curve is somewhat S shaped. There will also be a toxic response curve, which will be located somewhere to the right of the therapeutic curve, depending on the therapeutic index of the given drug. Ideally, a dose C (Fig. 7–16) would give a substantial therapeutic response yet almost no toxic response. Unfortunately, variations in disease and host do not permit exact choice of this ideal dose C.

Dose D gives the maximal response possible; knowledge of this level is useful, because there is no benefit from further dosage increase.

Can a maximal corticosteroid response dose be established? Measurement of the

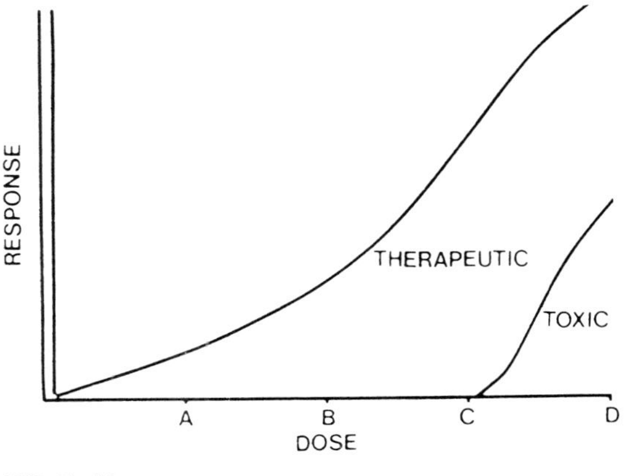


**FIG 7–16.**
Theoretical dose-response curve, indicating both therapeutic and toxic responses.

**TABLE 7–16.**
Current Topical Ocular Corticosteroids

| Corticosteroid | Derivative | Dosage Form | Concentration (%) | Brand Name |
|---|---|---|---|---|
| Prednisolone | Acetate | Suspension | 0.125 | Econopred |
| | | | | Pred Mild |
| | | | 1.0 | Econopred Plus |
| | | | | Pred Forte |
| | | | | AK-Tate |
| Prednisolone | Sodium phosphate | Solution | 0.125 | Inflamase Mild |
| | | | | AK-Pred |
| | | | 0.5 | Metreton |
| | | | 1.0 | Inflamase Forte |
| | | | | AK-Pred |
| Dexamethasone | Alcohol | Suspension | 0.1 | Maxidex |
| Dexamethasone | Sodium phosphate | Solution | 0.1 | Decadron phosphate |
| | | Ointment | 0.05 | Decadron phosphate |
| Fluorometholone | Alcohol | Ointment | 0.1 | FML |
| | | Suspension | 0.1 | FML |
| | | | 0.25 | FML Forte |
| | Acetate | Suspension | 0.1 | Flarex |
| Medrysone | Alcohol | Suspension | 1.0 | HMS |

radioactively labeled polymorphonuclear leukocyte response to the intracorneal injection of clove oil permits exact measurements that may be used to formulate a dose-response curve applicable to this specific toxic keratitis (not necessarily applicable to any given disease, though). Using this experimental technique, the maximal attainable therapeutic response was reduction of the leukocytes invading the cornea to 40% of their untreated number. This was achieved with 1% prednisolone acetate, topically applied (rabbits). Increasing the strength of the prednisolone to 3% did not significantly further decrease the number of leukocytes. The use of 0.125% prednisolone reduced the leukocytes to only 70% of their untreated number.[79]

## ROUTES OF ADMINISTRATION AND DOSAGE

### Topical Therapy

Topical therapy is generally preferred when it is clinically effective because of the ease of application, moderately low cost, and relative absence of systemic complications. Table 7–16 shows the current topical corticosteroid products available. These corticosteroids have been shown to be both clinically effective and safe when used topically at these standard concentrations. Dosage will vary with the severity of disease. Increased frequency of application is usually equal to or more effective than use of a stronger concentration of either solution or suspension. In unusually severe cases, 1 drop each minute for 5 minutes every hour may be employed the first 24 to 48 hours; frequency may then be reduced gradually to two to four times daily to control inflammation.[49, 80] The possibility of relapse exists, especially with high dosages if therapy is prematurely stopped in a disease such as iritis. Therefore, topical usage should be tapered off over several days to weeks, depending on the response of a given eye.

Experimentally 1% prednisolone acetate is reported to be the most effective agent against corneal inflammation.[49] Usually little difference is noted clinically between these derivatives of prednisolone, dexamethasone, and fluorometholone acetate (see Table 7–16). Should a disappointing result be obtained from one of these medications, change to another is sometimes suggested. Fluorometholone produces moderate suppression of corneal inflammation when compared with prednisolone acetate and dexamethasone alcohol.[49] It appears to be useful for chronic inflammatory diseases that required extended periods of therapy. Medrysone is a very weak antiinflammatory agent that should be used only for relatively minor conjunctival inflammation. Both medrysone and, to a lesser degree, fluorometholone penetrate the cornea poorly and have low potential for elevating IOP.[49, 50] As mentioned earlier, recent in vitro and clinical studies suggest that modification of fluorometholone from its alcohol base to its acetate derivative changes the drug from a moderately effective to a highly effective antiinflammatory agent. These studies showed no significant difference in ability to suppress extraocular inflammation when directly compared with prednisolone acetate 1%.[50, 51]

### Systemic Therapy

Systemic corticosteroids remain the treatment of choice for severe bilateral posterior segment inflammation. Defined treatment goals should be established by the ophthalmologist and carefully explained to each patient before therapy is initiated. Also, the patient should be aware of the planned length of treatment and potential adverse effects. Because of the greater risk for systemic side effects, the ophthalmologist should use the lowest effective dose for the shortest time period needed to control inflammation. Concurrent use of antacids, cimetidine, or ranitidine may be beneficial in preventing GI ulceration.

The choice of the available corticosteroid agents and dosage remains somewhat empirical and should be individualized (see Table 7–6). Most ophthalmologists prefer using short- to intermediate-acting agents with minimal mineralocorticoid activity and a favorable side effect profile (see Tables 7–5 and 7–6). Prednisone has become the corticosteroid of choice because it is inexpensive, short acting, and relatively free from sodium retention. It may be used in divided doses, a single daily dose, or a single alternate-day dose. For mild to moderate inflammation, daily doses of 20 to 40 mg are usually recommended. For patients with severe sight-threatening inflammation, an initial daily dose of 1 to 1.5 mg/kg daily is recommended.[80] This dosage should be maintained for a reasonable time period until one sees a clinical effect.

Once clinical improvement is noted, the corticosteroid dosage should be reduced in a gradual stepwise fashion. This should occur over days to weeks, depending on the duration of treatment and the course of the disease. The daily dosage can be reduced in 10-mg increments from high doses and 2- to 5-mg increments from low doses. A daily dosage of 15 to 20 mg appears to be a reasonable adult maintenance dose. This should be continued for at least 1 to 2 weeks before the drug is discontinued to prevent recurrence of disease.[80]

If a given reduction is followed by exacerbation of the inflammation, therapy must immediately be raised to the initial high doses (Fig. 7–17).[81] Such escape of the disease from therapeutic control is a serious complication and should be avoided if at all possible by slow and gradual reduction of dosage. As long as any evidence of active inflammation persists, it is hazardous to discontinue therapy. A few patients will require months of treatment at fairly high dosage levels.

Although it is to be expected that some patients with uveitis will not respond to corticosteroid therapy, many such patients are found to have received inadequate treatment and will respond to increased dosage. Uveitis made worse by properly intensive and continued corticosteroid treatment is uncommon.

Although there is no doubt that frequent massive doses of corticosteroid achieve the greatest effect, this is not always necessary and may, in fact, be undesirable. Such intensive usage will give the greatest systemic toxicity and pituitary-adrenal suppression. As little as 5 mg of prednisone given twice daily can cause adrenal suppression.

### Single Daily Dose

For long-term low-dosage maintenance as for chronic uveitis, a single morning, daily dose of prednisone may be optimal. If this daily dose does not exceed 7.5 mg of prednisone, the adrenal response to ACTH is

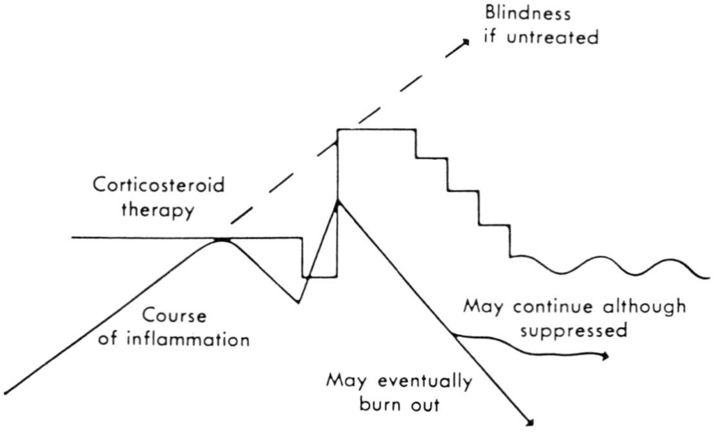


**FIG 7–17.**
Modification of course of chronic intraocular inflammation by corticosteroid therapy. Diagram is designed to illustrate the prevention of blindness by treatment, relapse with reduction of treatment, control by higher level treatment, and final quiescence. (From Gordon D: *Arch Ophthalmol* 62:400, 1959. Used by permission.)

unchanged. At a daily dose of 15 mg, 50% of patients have a reduced ACTH response. At a daily dose of 20 mg, 50% of patients are completely suppressed. If desired, an evening time can be substituted for morning without changing this effect on the pituitary axis. Nocturnal doses of longer-acting corticosteroids will suppress the ACTH response.

As mentioned previously, the normal circadian rhythm for corticosteroids is lower at night (see Fig. 7–2). The average daily adrenal secretion of cortisol (hydrocortisone) is 15 to 25 mg; of cortisone, 1.5 to 4 mg; of aldosterone, 30 to 150 μg. The plasma half-life of hydrocortisone is 90 to 100 minutes; its tissue half-life is 8 to 12 hours.[5, 82, 83]

Single daily dose or alternate-day dose therapy with dexamethasone does not prevent pituitary-adrenal suppression, because its tissue half-life is 3 days. This long duration of action does permit single daily dosage for the purpose of achieving a therapeutic effect. In fact, there is no reason for giving the long-acting corticosteroids (dexamethasone, betamethasone, triamcinolone) in divided daily doses, which simply is a bother to the patient and reduces compliance.

Any patient on prolonged systemic corticosteroid therapy should receive supplemental corticosteroid if a major operation, accident, or illness occurs. Without this precaution, severe hypotension or hypoglycemia may occur.

### Alternate-day Therapy

The undesirable side effects of systemic corticosteroid therapy can be substantially reduced by using alternate-day therapy rather than divided dosage. Briefly stated, the entire total dose of corticosteroid that would have been given during a 2-day period is administered as a single dose every other morning. Such alternate-day dosage causes less suppression of the adrenal glands and other endocrine glands, minimizes growth alterations, and does not completely suppress cell-medicated immune responses, for example, those measured by skin testing with histoplasmosis antigen.

How effective is this alternate-day regimen in the control of disease? Apparently in the control of systemic diseases (e.g., asthma and arthritis) this therapeutic ratio of 2 : 1 (double dose on alternate days) is effective. Evaluation of a corneal graft rejection model in rabbits indicated that the therapeutically equivalent ratio was 2.6 : 1 (2.5 times the daily dose given every other morning).[84] Inasmuch as we do not know in the individual case how large a corticosteroid dosage will be required on a daily basis, we then do not know how large a dose is 2 to 2.6 times as great. This corneal graft rejection model does demonstrate, however, that if the appropriate level of alternate-day corticosteroid dosage is empirically determined, it should control ocular inflammation (or at least corneal rejection), as well as the more toxic method of multiple daily dosage.

Alternate-day corticosteroid therapy with corticosteroids having a short or intermediate tissue half-life may not provide a maximal immunosuppressive effect. In a study of 53 renal transplant patients, 80% maintained a stable transplant glomerular filtration rate while receiving 16 mg of methylprednisolone every other day, but 20% did not and required a daily dosage.[85] Methylprednisolone has a 2-day half-life.

Alternate-day systemic corticosteroid therapy in children will minimize growth suppression and seems to be a worthwhile method. In adults there may also be a lesser adrenal suppression.[86]

Alternate-day therapy is considered to be a strongly preferable method of systemic corticosteroid administration if prolonged therapy is necessary.

Study of the circadian plasma cortisol rhythm can be used as a measure of stress. Of 19 cataract extractions with the patient under local anesthesia, two thirds showed no interruption of circadian rhythm. In contrast, this rhythm was disrupted by increased cortisol production in 90% of 11 cataract patients receiving general anesthesia.[87]

## Periocular Therapy

Periocular (repository) corticosteroids may be given by injection in the subconjunctival, sub-Tenon's, or retrobulbar space as a long-acting preparation. They are ideal for uniocular disease. They can be used as a supplement to topical therapy for severe anterior segment inflammation or for posterior segment disease such as CME.[80] Periocular therapy rapidly places a relatively high concentration of corticosteroid near the actual sight of inflammation. At the same time it avoids most of the adverse effects of systemic therapy. It also provides a nice alternative when a poorly compliant patient is treated and is a valuable adjunct when surgery is performed on a uveitic eye.[80]

In severe inflammation a synergistic therapeutic effect does occur with simultaneous use of topical and periocular corticosteroids. However, use of periocular injection alone does not offer any significant advantage over topical therapy when anterior segment disease is treated. When equal doses of topical and periocular corticosteroids were compared, there was a greater reduction in corneal inflammation with topical therapy.[88] This suggests that topical corticosteroids should be the primary treatment for anterior segment inflammation.

Sub-Tenon's injection with the long-term depot vehicle of methylprednisolone acetate (Depo-Medrol) has been successfully used for a variety of ocular inflammatory diseases.[89] This suspension form of methylprednisolone provides a constant source of corticosteroid that lasts for 2 to 4 weeks. Sub-Tenon's injection of the long-acting preparation of triamcinolone acetonide (Kenalog) has also been reported to benefit a variety of chronic inflammatory ocular diseases.[90] These two commercial products appear clinically to be equally effective. However, anecdotally the residual vehicle left after injections with methylprednisolone acetate is not as well tolerated by some patients and can cause an allergic response.

Does retrobulbar injection of a depot-type corticosteroid result in prolonged effective concentrations in the intraocular tissues? This question was answered by a study using radiolabeled methylprednisolone acetate. The results indicate that retrobulbar injection can deliver high concentrations of corticosteroid to the optic nerve, sclera, choroid, and retina for 1 week or longer (Fig. 7–18).[91] This was demonstrated to be clinically significant in a rabbit model of herpetic chorioretinitis.[92]

Before periocular injection is performed, there should be liberal use of topical anesthetic. This includes direct contact of the area to be injected with a cotton swab soaked in topical anesthetic. The usual technique is to inject 0.5 ml (20–40 mg) of the repository corticosteroid beneath Tenon's capsule near the equator in the superior temporal quadrant.

Even with liberal topical anesthesia these injections are somewhat uncomfortable for the patient. Mixing the corticosteroid preparation with a local anesthetic

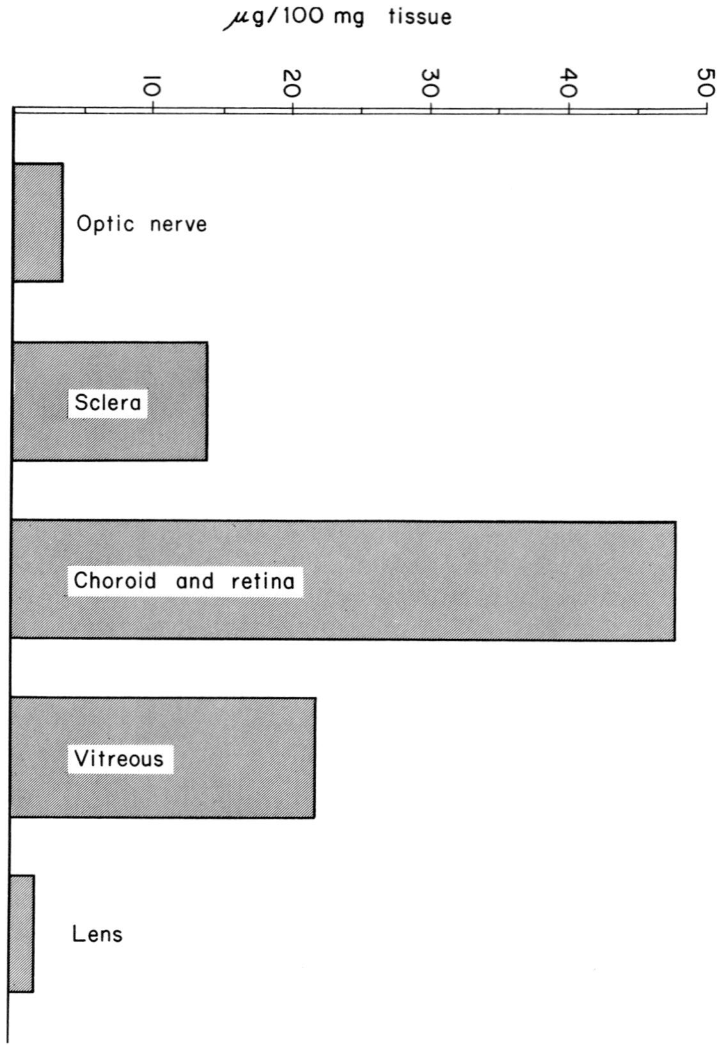


**FIG 7–18.**
Concentration gradient of methylprednisolone in ocular tissues 2 days after retrobulbar injection. (Modified from Hyndiuk RA, Reagan MG: *Arch Ophthalmol* 80:499, 1968. Used by permission.)

only increases the volume of the injection and the pain of the procedure. After injection, pain and tenderness can persist for 6 to 12 hours. The patient should be given a mild analgesic or ice pack to relieve this initial pain. The eye should be patched to improve comfort.

The physician using corticosteroid injections in the area of the eye should always be aware of the possibility of scleral perforation. The small, sharp needles used to permit comfortable injection will also enter the eye with minimal resistance. Of a series of six cases of accidental intraocular injection of depot corticosteroids, irreparable organized retinal detachment developed in three.[93]

In the treatment of pars planitis, 0.4 ml of methylprednisolone was injected into the choroid. The whitish material was seen in the choroidal vessels and dissected forward into the anterior chamber, where it appeared as white flocculent debris. This disappeared uneventfully after 2 months. The pars planitis did not improve.[94]

Permanent paralysis of the superior rectus muscle, found to be thin and atrophic on surgical exploration, followed injection of

1 ml of methylprednisolone into the sub-Tenon's space superiorly.[95]

After six subconjunctival injections of corticosteroid for persistent uveitis, atrophy of subcutaneous tissue over the inferior orbital rim resulted. A depression of the lower lid was cosmetically visible, but no enophthalmos was present.[96]

The injection of repository corticosteroid may cause a susceptible eye to develop intractable glaucoma. In such cases, surgical removal of the depot corticosteroid may be needed to control the glaucoma, and sometimes this can be difficult.[97]

Periocular corticosteroid injections are contraindicated in cases of ocular toxoplasmosis and scleritis.[80] A rapidly high intraocular corticosteroid dose may block the patient's normal local defense mechanisms against toxoplasmosis and cause an exacerbation of the ocular disease. Corticosteroid injections in the presence of scleritis may inhibit new collagen production and predispose the sclera to perforation.

A considerable amount of scarring and fibrosis of Tenon's capsule is evident on surgical exploration of an injected area.[98] Some of these effects may be caused by the vehicle itself rather than the actual corticosteroid drug. One study has demonstrated no ocular toxicity in rabbits when triamcinolone acetonide is injected intravitreally without its vehicle.[99]

Local intralesionally injected corticosteroids offer a reasonable alternative or adjunct to incision and curettage in the treatment of chalazia.[100–102] Complications of chalazion injection include local hypopigmentation, increased IOP, orbital fat atrophy, and yellow discoloration of epibulbar tissue.[103]

Permanent unilateral vision loss has been reported in an 8-year-old child who received a 0.5-ml injection of a repository corticosteroid.[104] A recurrent, previously excised chalazion was injected, and 2 days later vision on the injected side decreased to light perception with no subsequent improvement. Fundus examination and fluorescein angiography revealed both retinal and choroidal microemboli causing vascular occlusion.

The local injection of repository corticosteroids has also been reported to successfully treat eyelid and periocular hemangiomas.[105] Obviously there may be an increased risk of intraarterial injection when a vascular tumor is treated. Extreme caution should be taken both during and immediately after any periocular corticosteroid injection. A thorough postinjection assessment of visual acuity, ocular motility, and fundus vasculature in all patients is highly recommended.

### Intravitreal Therapy

Previous studies suggest that intravitreal dexamethasone exerts a protective effect on the blood-ocular barrier and decreases intraocular inflammation.[106, 107] A significant reduction in intraocular inflammation was described in a rabbit model of *Pseudomonas* endophthalmitis when a combination of intravitreal antibiotic and dexamethasone was used compared with intravitreal antibiotic alone.[107] No improvement in either group was seen when treatment was delayed beyond 5 hours. This result was most likely related to the virulence of the *Pseudomonas* pathogen studied.

A more recent study created a rabbit model for endophthalmitis using *Staphylococcus epidermidis,* a less virulent bacteria. In this study the histologic findings of four different treatments for endophthalmitis were evaluated (Table 7–17). Both groups treated with dexamethasone, with or without vitrectomy (groups 3 and 4), showed fewer histologic signs of inflammation.[108] This study suggests that intravitreal dexamethasone used in the presence of severe intraocular inflammation (i.e., endophthalmitis) can preserve retinal architecture, which potentially could improve retinal function.

### Controlled-release Vehicles

Ocusert devices delivering 10 μg of hydrocortisone acetate/hr were used to treat allergic conjunctivitis (to bovine albumin) in rabbits. The response to the continuous low-level drug delivery was as good as or better than that obtained by five times daily

**TABLE 7–17.**
Summary of Histologic Findings in Endophthalmitis Treatment Groups*

| Histologic finding | 1 (TPPV) | 2 (TPPV + ATB) | 3 (TPPV + ATB/ Corticosteroid) | 4 (ATB/Corticosteroid Without TPPV) |
|---|---|---|---|---|
| Anterior chamber angle leukocytes (avg. no.) | 60 | 60 | 15 | 10 |
| Retina | | | | |
| Photoreceptor Loss | Severe | Moderate | None | Mild |
| Intraretinal edema | Severe | Moderate | Minimal | Mild |
| Choroid | | | | |
| Leukocytic Infiltration | Moderate | Moderate | Minimal | Mild |

Data from Maxwell DP, Brent BD, Diamond JG, and others: *Ophthalmology* 98:1373, 1991. Used by permission.
**TPPV*, Trans pars plana vitrectomy; *ATB*, intravitreal gentamicin, 400 μg; *corticosteroid*, intravitreal dexamethasone, 800 μg.

instillation of eye drops. This response establishes that the very high level of medication briefly attained with an eye drop is not necessary for successful treatment of allergic conjunctivitis.[109]

## OCULAR INDICATIONS

Corticosteroids can be useful in treating a vast array of ocular inflammatory diseases, including various allergic and hypersensitivity responses, as well as uveitic, traumatic, and immunologic disease processes. Table 7–18 lists ocular indications in which corticosteroids have been beneficial by anatomic location of the disease process. Some have only recently been added to this growing list. For example, large randomized clinical trials have suggested that corticosteroids can be of benefit to certain patients with traumatic hyphema and optic neuri-

**TABLE 7–18.**
Ocular Indications for Corticosteroid Treatment

| | |
|---|---|
| Eyelids | Uvea |
| Allergic blepharitis | Iritis, iridocyclitis |
| Contact dermatitis | Postoperative iritis |
| Chalazion | Intermediate uveitis/pars planitis |
| Hemangioma | Posterior uveitis |
| Chemical burns | Sympathetic ophthalmia |
| Herpes zoster | Vogt-Koyanagi-Harada syndrome |
| | Phacoanaphylactic endophthalmitis |
| Conjunctiva | |
| Allergic conjunctivitis | Retina |
| Vernal conjunctivitis | Cystoid macular edema |
| Chemical burns | Retinal vasculitis |
| Herpes zoster | |
| Mucocutaneous lesions | Optic nerve |
| | Optic neuritis |
| Sclera | Giant cell arteritis |
| Episcleritis | Pseudotumor cerebri |
| Scleritis | Traumatic optic neuropathy |
| | Radiation optic neuropathy |
| Cornea | |
| Epithelial punctate keratitis | Orbit/extraocular muscle |
| Herpes simplex disciform | Graves' disease |
| Keratitis | Pseudotumor |
| Herpes zoster keratitis | Tolosa-Hunt |
| Immune graft rejection | Myasthenia gravis |
| Marginal ulcers | |
| Interstitial keratitis | Globe |
| Acne rosacea keratitis | Traumatic hyphema |
| Chemical burns | Endophthalmitis |

tis.[110, 111] The appropriate discussion that is warranted for this exhausting topic is subject matter for a separate book and beyond the scope of this chapter. Thus, further reading in an outside source is recommended.

## CONTRAINDICATIONS AND COMPLICATIONS

Undesirable effects of corticosteroids are most conveniently discussed when they are divided into systemic and local manifestations. The greatest contraindication to corticosteroid therapy, however, holds for both systemic and topical routes of administration; it is the *lack of a specific indication for corticosteroid use.*

### Systemic Complications

Undesirable systemic side effects of corticosteroids do not ordinarily occur from topical use, even of long duration. Frequent topical use of concentrated preparations of potent corticosteroids can cause measurable systemic effects, however. Study of four volunteers receiving 1 drop of 0.01% dexamethasone in both eyes every 2 hours (24-hour 0.75-mg dexamethasone dosage) for 4 days showed a reduction of urinary excretion of 17-hydroxycorticosteroids to a range of 19% to 72% of normal. Endogenous cortisol production rate was decreased to 11% to 43% of normal.[112] Because of this not inconsiderable physiologic effect, the same precautions should be observed in patients receiving frequent topical corticosteroids as in patients receiving small doses of systemic corticosteroids. The relative vulnerability of patients with some types of disease will be reviewed subsequently. Also, the ophthalmologist should realize that as little as 10 mg of prednisone or the equivalent daily for 4 weeks may suppress normal growth in children.

One drop of 0.1% dexamethasone sodium phosphate in each eye four times daily is a systemic dosage of 0.25 mg/day. Six weeks of such medication resulted in a lowering of plasma cortisol level from 22 to 17 μg/100 ml. However, testing showed the hypothalamic-pituitary-adrenal function to be normal (metyrapone test).[113]

Daily orbital injections of 4 mg of dexamethasone for 6 days reduced plasma cortisol levels from an average of 19 to 6.0 μg/100 ml, indicating that prolonged injection therapy can have systemic side effects.[114]

With systemic administration, the following complications may arise[115]:

1. Mental changes, ranging from euphoria to psychosis
2. Activation of infection, notably serious in tuberculosis
3. Temporary increase in severity of diabetes and hypertension
4. GI ulceration
5. Osteoporotic changes, sometimes leading to pathologic fracture
6. Electrolyte imbalance, causing edema and the like
7. Delay in wound healing, infrequently noted with high dosage
8. Moon face and other manifestations of Cushing's syndrome

Relative contraindications to corticosteroid therapy, therefore, are present in patients with preexisting disease of the types just mentioned. Low-level dosage (e.g., 5 mg of prednisolone four times daily) in the average healthy patient can be safely carried out with minimum supervision, including weekly weight and blood pressure readings, urinalysis, and a brief history to detect GI disorders and early evidence of psychotic manifestations. A chest x-ray film should be obtained at the onset of therapy and should be repeated monthly in long-term treatment. If high dosage is required, it is well to enlist the aid of a primary care physician in the supervision of the patient.

### Gastrointestinal Ulceration

The physician must know that the newer corticosteroids such as prednisone and prednisolone, although they produce less electrolytic imbalance, still may cause other serious systemic complications. In a series of 18 patients with rheumatoid arthritis treated for as long as 7 months with prednisone or prednisolone, three patients had radiologic evidence of GI ulcer develop and 1 had severe depression psychosis develop.[116] The ulcers were asymptomatic, and it is emphasized that perforation or severe hemorrhage may occur without previous warning in patients on corticosteroid therapy. Routine administration of antacids or oral histamine antagonists may minimize GI ulceration in corticosteroid-treated patients.

Cortisone not only enhances the formation of GI ulcers but also increases the severity of ulceration. Experimental surgical anastomosis of stomach to colon greatly predisposes dogs to peptic ulceration. In a control group of 13 such dogs, 31% had ulcers develop and 15% had perforations develop. Of 10 dogs similarly operated on and treated with cortisone (200-mg daily injections), all developed ulcers, and perforation occurred in 80%.[117]

Drug-induced hypokalemia may result from use of thiazide diuretics or from corticosteroid therapy. Administration of potassium chloride in enteric-coated potassium chloride has been responsible for a definite increase in ulcerative lesions and stenosis of the small intestine (300 reported cases). These lesions are not the result of surface irritation but seem to result from rapid release of potassium chloride and its absorption over a short segment of intestine. This high concentration causes vasospasm and subsequent infarction. A typical, virtually pathognomonic circumferential ulceration and stenosis result.[118, 119] To prevent potassium chloride intestinal lesions, one should attempt to supply potassium by dietary means (e.g., orange juice), or, if absolutely necessary, supplemental potassium should be given with meals rather than on an empty stomach. Potassium administration should immediately be discontinued if any unusual GI symptoms develop during treatment.[120]

### Osteoporosis

Pathologic vertebral fractures may spontaneously develop as a result of osteoporosis induced by prolonged systemic corticosteroid therapy.[121]

### Femoral Head Ischemic Necrosis

Ischemic necrosis of the femoral head occurs because the vascular supply of the femoral head is easily compromised in conditions such as fracture, sickle cell disease, nitrogen emboli, and chronic alcoholism. Prolonged corticosteroid therapy may cause vasculitis and capillary fragility and is implicated as a cause of ischemic femoral head necrosis. This condition occurs in more than one third of renal transplant patients treated by corticosteroids. The onset is with vague, continuous hip pain that may occur months after the corticosteroid therapy has been stopped. Another 6 months may elapse before faint areas of radiologic discontinuity appear in the femoral head. The nutrition of the bone is already irreparably compromised by the time the diagnosis can be made.[122]

Although other bones may also be involved by corticosteroid-induced avascular necrosis, the head of the femur is by far the most common site, being found in 91 of 95 patients.[123] Experimental corticosteroid administration to rabbits and pathologic study of human femoral heads indicate the probable mechanism of bone involvement is corticosteroid mobilization of fat with resultant hyperlipidemia and fatty degeneration of the liver. Fatty emboli result, and intravascular fat deposits can be found in the femoral heads of both rabbits and humans. These emboli lodge preferentially in the subchondral region because of the terminal vessels anatomically located there. The osteocytes die, and a line of subchondral resorption of bone can be seen by x-ray examination. Microfractures and sequestration of dead bone cause gradually progressive loss of the femoral head.[124]

The fatty emboli incriminated are of microscopic size, perhaps 40 by 80 μm. A single milliliter of fat would represent 10 million such emboli. Emboli of this soft character are capable of distending and traversing terminal arterioles in soft tissue but become trapped in the terminal arterioles in the haversian systems of bone. Over long periods, masses of these emboli accumulate and cause retrograde occlusion of the intraosseous circulation. A dosage of methylprednisolone equivalent to 1.5 mg/kg/

day of cortisone in rabbits caused an increase of serum lipids by 3 to 100 times. Interestingly, chronic administration of alcohol, as well as of cortisone, causes such fatty changes.[125]

Serum lipids were abnormal in the majority of 77 cases of corticosteroid-associated ischemic necrosis of the femoral head.[126]

A study of 72 cases of femoral head necrosis unassociated with injury or local disease elicited in every case a history of prolonged administration of some unusual substance, specifically, corticosteroids (32 cases), alcohol (10 cases), iron overload from home brew (16 cases), and nonsteroidal antiinflammatory drugs (14 cases). The duration of corticosteroid injection varied between 6 months to 3 years. Only seven of the 32 had received more than the equivalent of 10 mg of prednisone/day. Many patients were being treated for rheumatoid arthritis; the hip pains of aseptic necrosis resulted in continuing corticosteroid treatment for supposed arthritic hip. The facts that iron overload does not cause fat emboli and that large amounts of fat may be found in normal femoral heads cast some doubt on the fat embolus theory and suggest osteoporosis as an alternate cause.[127]

Vasculitis was proposed as the mechanism of ischemic necrosis, because 87% (20 of 23 patients) of systemic lupus erythematosus patients with ischemic necrosis showed such vascular changes. Of these 23 patients, all had received corticosteroids. The onset of symptoms occurred from 7 to 132 months after starting corticosteroid therapy. Twenty patients received 10 mg or more of prednisone daily. One patient had discontinued corticosteroid treatment 13 years before the onset of the ischemic necrosis.[128]

A mechanism of bleeding or clotting defect was proposed in a study of 50 patients with nontraumatic femoral head necrosis. Of these patients, 37 were alcoholic. Coagulation studies showed defects in 30 patients. Blood sludging, thrombosis, or hemorrhage were postulated as causes of the necrosis.[129]

A relationship exists between the corticosteroid dosage and the incidence of aseptic necrosis. Of 68 renal transplant patients receiving 120 to 200 mg of prednisone/day for 2 to 3 weeks, 16 patients developed femoral head necrosis. Of 136 transplant patients receiving 120 to 200 mg/day for only 2 to 4 days, only two had necrosis develop. (In both groups a maintenance dose of 30 mg/day was continued.[130])

The relative frequency of corticosteroid therapy as a cause of ischemic necrosis of the femoral head is difficult for an ophthalmologist to determine from the literature. Trauma must be by far the most common cause. Nitrogen emboli in divers can cause femoral head necrosis, as can sickle cell anemia (six of 38 patients). Of 52 patients seen between 1935 and 1960, 17% had a history of alcoholism and 10% had a history of corticosteroid therapy.[131] Reports of patients selected because of corticosteroid therapy do not permit estimates of incidence.[132, 133]

Treatment of idiopathic femoral head ischemic necrosis is unsatisfactory, requiring limitation of use for long periods. Less severe cases may stabilize with time; more severe ones require hip prostheses and apparently do well.

The purpose of such prolonged manifestation is to emphasize that prolonged corticosteroid use has dangers with which ophthalmologists are relatively unfamiliar. Long-term use of corticosteroids without sound medical indications seems unwarranted.

### Pediatric Problems

Being infrequently confronted with uveitis in growing children, the ophthalmologist is relatively unfamiliar with the response of persons in this age group to prolonged corticosteroid therapy. In general, the response of the disease and the side effects in the patient are comparable to what would be expected in adults. In addition, growth may be retarded. Rather serious changes in the appearance of the child that adversely affect the child's entire future life may be produced, as seen in Fig. 7–19.[134] This series of pictures documents the development of a most unsightly moon face and buffalo hump during the course of 1½ years' treatment with prednisone. The pa-

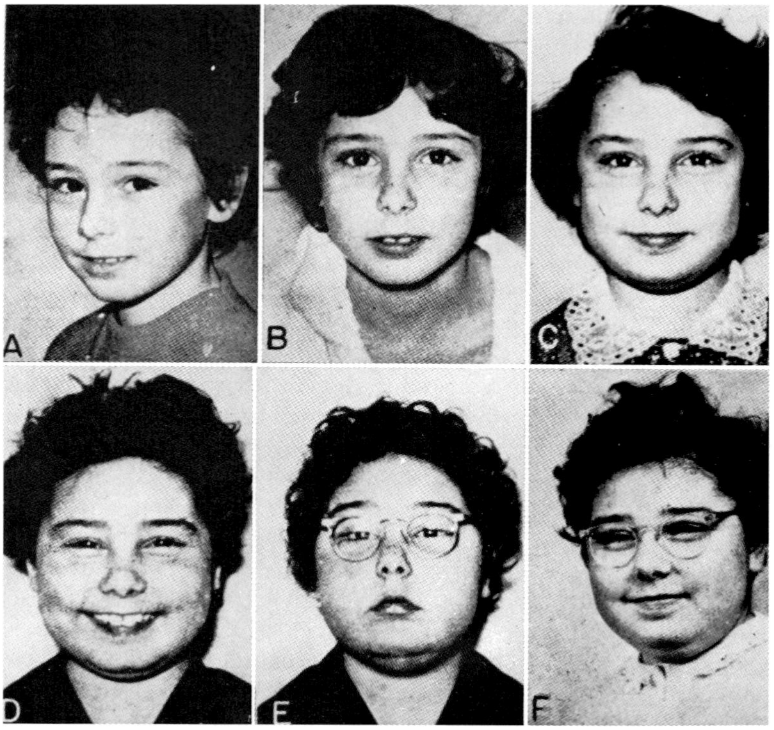

**FIG 7–19.**
Serial photographs made during prolonged prednisolone therapy. **A,** Patient at 7 years of age. **B,** Patient at 8½ years of age. **C,** Patient after 1 month of prednisolone therapy, 30 to 75 mg/day. **D,** Patient after 2 months of prednisolone therapy (20 mg/day was given during the second month). **E,** Patient after 6 months of prednisolone therapy. **F,** Patient after 1½ years of prednisolone therapy (still takes 20 mg/day). (From Sudarsky RD: *Arch Ophthalmol* 1959, 62:5. Used by permission.)

tient suffered from a severe case of Harada's syndrome of exudative retinal detachment and, through this therapy, achieved a final vision of 20/50. Clearly, the necessity for preservation of vision will warrant prolonged prednisone therapy with its associated side effects. Obviously such treatment can be justified only by the existence of serious disease known to be responsive to corticosteroids and is not to be undertaken lightly.

An 11-month-old child died from Cushing's syndrome induced by postkeratoplasty periocular injections of triamcinolone (total of 120 mg over 8 weeks).[135] Partial adrenal suppression occurred in adults receiving 8 drops daily of 0.1% dexamethasone for 6 weeks.

### *Pseudotumor Cerebri*

The syndrome of pseudotumor cerebri may develop rather suddenly if long-term corticosteroid therapy in children is abruptly discontinued or reduced. Twenty-eight such cases of corticosteroid-associated pseudotumor cerebri have been reviewed and reported.[136] Bilateral papilledema, headache, and vomiting were present in almost all patients. There was generalized abnormality of the electroencephalograms and increased pressure of the cerebrospinal fluid. Eight of the 28 patients had paresis of the sixth cranial nerve.

Treatment of this type of pseudotumor cerebri is fairly simple. An increase in the corticosteroid dosage will alleviate the symptoms. Dosage should then be reduced gradually. If the condition does not improve within a few weeks, a more thorough neurosurgical evaluation is in order.

Although pseudotumor cerebri after abrupt cessation of prolonged corticosteroid therapy has been thought to be peculiar to children only, several comparable cases have been cited in adults. Withdrawal of corticosteroid in such patients must be very gradual, requiring as long as several months.[137]

***Skin Damage***

Permanent depigmentation of the lower eyelid of a black child followed injection of a chalazion with 3 mg of triamcinolone preserved with 0.9% benzyl alcohol. Such injections are not advised for facial use. The mechanism of this depigmentation may be corticosteroid inhibition of melanosomes or benzyl alcohol toxicity.[138]

Prolonged corticosteroid therapy causes marked skin thinning and predisposes to easy bruising. In extreme cases, even minor trauma can cause large tears of the skin.[139]

### Exophthalmos

Exophthalmos as great as 25 mm may be caused by long-term corticosteroid therapy in patients with no demonstrable thyroid disease. This will subside only slowly and incompletely when the medication is discontinued.[140]

### Possible Teratogenic Effect

Although no clinical evidence indicates that corticosteroids are teratogenic when administered to pregnant women, caution should be observed in administration of all potent drugs during pregnancy. Maternal treatment with cortisone did cause adverse effects in hybrid mice; the offspring of parents with recessive albinism were mated to those with dominant pigmentation. No such control hybrids were albino, but 62 of 520 (12%) hybrid offspring were albino after maternal treatment with cortisone (12.5% solution, 3 minims of which were injected subcutaneously on the seventh, eighth, and ninth days of gestation). In this experiment, maternal treatment with cortisone uncovered a normally recessive trait, albinism.[141]

Intramuscular injection of 10 mg of triamcinolone/kg of body weight on days 21, 23, and 25 of pregnancy will cause hydrocephalus in 90% of rhesus monkey fetuses.[142, 143]

Triamcinolone given during any trimester of pregnancy causes hypoplastic thymus glands and generalized defects of the lymphatic system in infant baboons.[144]

## LOCAL CONTRAINDICATIONS AND COMPLICATIONS

### Corticosteroid Activation of Infections

Because corticosteroids reduce the resistance of the body to most types of infection, their use should be avoided in ocular infections. Exceptions to this rule may arise if the infection is controlled by antibiotics and the physician wishes to reduce the ocular inflammatory reaction and in herpes zoster, which seems to be benefited by corticosteroid therapy.

### Adverse Effects in Viral Infection

General agreement exists that corticosteroid treatment of the typical dendritic keratitis caused by herpes simplex infection leads to more severe corneal scarring than would otherwise be expected. That such observations are not merely clinical impressions of doubtful validity is established by controlled experimentation. Forty-eight rabbits were inoculated with herpes simplex virus by corneal scratch or sub-Tenon's capsule injection.[145] Half were treated by subconjunctival injection of 20 to 50 mg (quite a large dose) of hydrocortisone or prednisolone every third day. Unequivocally, corticosteroid therapy caused the virus infection to become much worse. All 25 control rabbits recovered within 14 days, with corneal scarring so faint as to be visible only with magnification. Thirteen treated rabbits died of encephalitis, five were killed when signs of encephalitis were recognized (herpes simplex virus was recovered from the brains of four of these rabbits), three survived but corneal perforation developed, and the remaining two showed marked corneal scarring. The appearance of treated and untreated eyes 8 days after inoculation is shown in Fig. 7–20. Such experimental results are reproducible.[146]

The literature contains many such experiments indicating that corticosteroids potentiate herpes simplex infections. Another study, including clinical, pathologic,

A

B

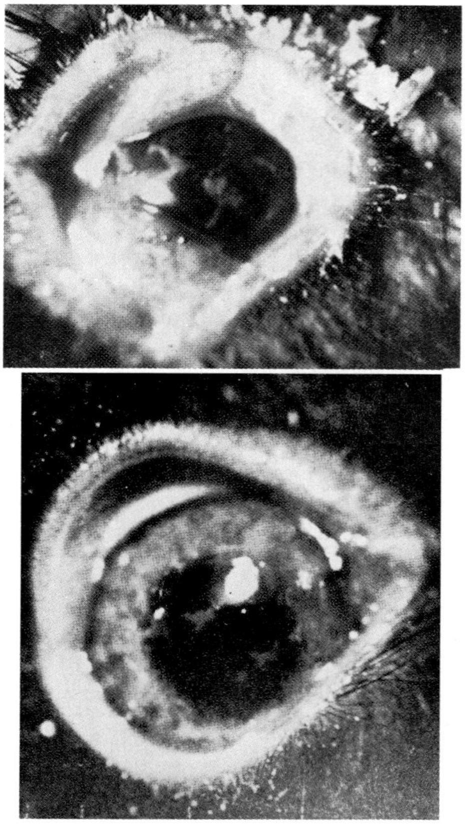

**FIG 7–20.**
**A,** Prednisolone-treated experimental herpes simplex infection 8 days after inoculation of sub-Tenon's space with virus. **B,** Untreated control rabbit eye 8 days after inoculation of sub-Tenon's space with herpes simplex virus in the same manner as in **A.** The severe exacerbation produced by corticosteroid therapy is shown in **A.** (From Kimura SJ, Okumoto M: *Am J Ophthalmol* 43:131, 1957. Used by permission.)

and histochemical evaluation, reported the effect of 5 mg of prednisolone injected subconjunctivally every other day in rabbits.[147] Herpes simplex inoculation was by injection beneath Tenon's capsule. In all rabbits, treated and control, keratoconjunctivitis developed; however, it was of earlier onset, greater severity, and longer duration in the prednisolone-treated groups. The incidence of uveitis was twice as great in the treated animals. Half the treated rabbits but no control rabbits had disciform keratitis develop. Inclusion bodies could be found for 19 days in the prednisolone-treated rabbits and for 12 days in the control rabbits. Pathologic sections showed more severe damage, including stromal necrosis, in the treated rabbits.

The virus-enhancing effect is also a property of the newer corticosteroid derivatives. Triamcinolone, methylprednisolone, and dexamethasone in 1% solutions were instilled three times daily topically on rabbit corneas inoculated with herpes simplex virus.[148] As illustrated in Fig. 7–21, the healing time of control corneas varied from 10 to 13 days; of triamcinolone-treated corneas, from 12 to 17 days; of methylprednisolone-treated corneas, from 14 to 24 days; and of dexamethasone-treated corneas, from 17 to 25 days.

Because the initial stages of herpetic keratoconjunctivitis may not be recognized without slit-lamp examination, the prudent physician will not prescribe corticosteroids indiscriminately for red eyes. Unfortunately shotgun therapy of red eyes with the commercially available and advertised antibiotic-corticosteroid mixtures is relatively common and has produced many cases of serious metaherpetic keratitis.

Although presented in a pro and con format, a discussion of corticosteroid therapy of acute herpes simplex keratitis produced no controversy. Both sides agreed that corticosteroid therapy was contraindicated in acute epithelial herpes. It may be helpful in advanced stromal disease if used together with antiviral drugs.[149, 150]

Diffuse, exudative bilateral retinal detachment caused by cytomegalovirus followed corticosteroid therapy in a previously healthy 30-year-old patient.[151] Cytomegalovirus optic neuritis developed in an immunosuppressed lymphocytic lymphoma patient.[152]

### Fungus-promoting Effect

Many ophthalmologists are in agreement that the topical use of corticosteroids increases ocular susceptibility to fungus infection. Clinical reports of cases of fungus keratitis typically describe minor injuries treated with corticosteroid or corticosteroid-antibiotic medications.[153] Gradually progressive, gray-white corneal infiltrates develop and result in extensive corneal scarring or total loss of the eye.

Because virtually all chronic corneal inflammations at some time receive a trial of corticosteroid therapy, it is doubtful that such reports alone establish a relationship between corticosteroids and fungus growth.

Fungi have been cultured from the eyes of 67% of patients receiving topical corticosteroids for 3 weeks or more compared with 18% of untreated control subjects.[154] Of 18 patients with negative cultures for fungus, 9 became positive for fungi after 3 weeks of topical use of corticosteroids. It is relevant to note that another author[155] was able to culture fungi from 25% of normal eyes and 35% of diseased eyes.

A report from India states that 71 fungus-free eyes were treated with topical 1% hydrocortisone three times daily for 1 month; at the end of this period, repeat cultures were positive for fungi in 41% of cases.[156]

Experimental fungus keratitis was produced in 80% of corticosteroid-treated rabbit eyes but in only 20% of untreated control eyes.[157]

*Candida albicans* inoculation of abraded rabbit corneas resulted in keratitis in 37% of untreated eyes and in 75% of eyes treated with 1% hydrocortisone, 1 drop every 6 hours.[158]

The combined weight of clinical and experimental evidence strongly indicates that corticosteroid therapy decreases human resistance to ocular fungus infections. Fortunately, the incidence of major infections is low. In material from the Armed Forces Institute of Pathology, fungus infection was found in 1 of every 727 cases of perforated ulcers or posttraumatic vitreous abscesses. However, before the advent of corticosteroids, fungi were found in only 1 of every 11,329 such eyes. Review of Birge's excellent 30-page article will convince one that fungus infection is frequent (e.g., *C. albicans* in 20% of women) and must be considered in the differential diagnosis of persistent eye inflammations.[159] Consideration of the foregoing facts suggests that corticosteroid therapy of minor corneal abrasions is unwise.

## Response of Bacterial Infection

Not only viral and fungal but also bacterial corneal infections may be made worse by cortisone. Experimental *Pseudomonas*

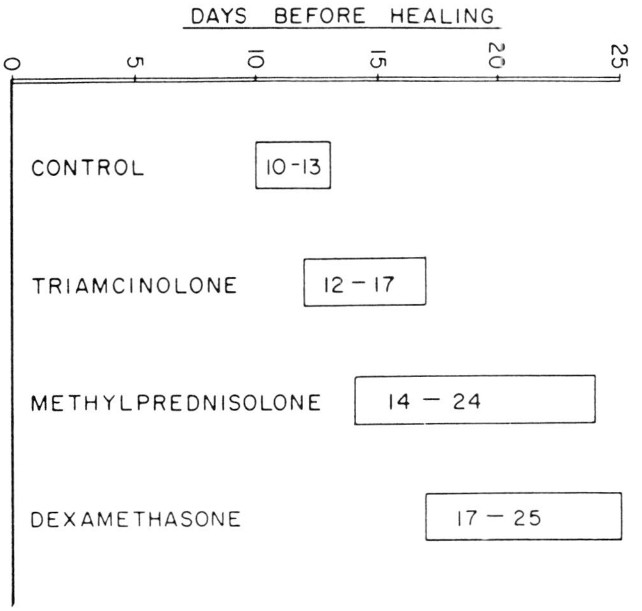


**FIG 7–21.**
Retardation of healing of experimental herpes simplex corneal infections by corticosteroids. Bars represent time span between minimum and maximum times required for healing. (Data from McCoy GA, Leopold IH: *Am J Ophthalmol* 49:1355, 1960. Used by permission.)

A

B

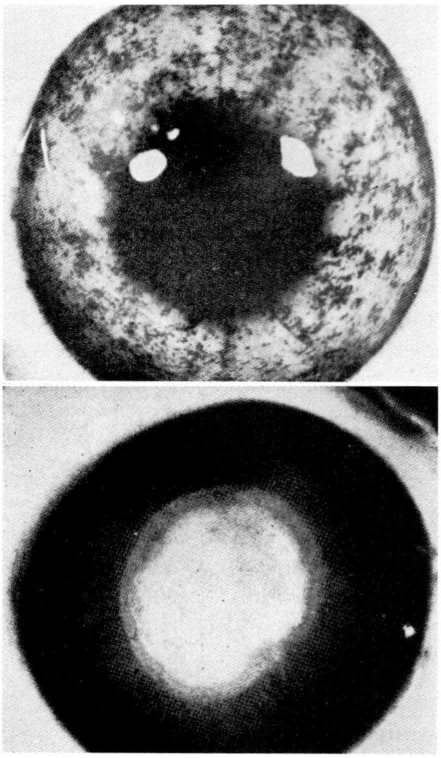

**FIG 7–22.**
**A,** Minimal superficial corneal involvement in control rabbit inoculated with *Pseudomonas* organisms in the same manner as shown in **B.** No cortisone therapy was given. **B,** Typical *Pseudomonas* corneal ulcer in cortisone-treated rabbit. (From Suie T, Taylor FW: *Arch Ophthalmol* 56:53, 1956. Used by permission.)

corneal ulcers were demonstrated to produce much more extensive ulcerations and scarring when treated with cortisone (Fig. 7–22).[160] Fifty-four percent of cortisone-treated corneas and only 9% of control corneas showed extensive and deep ulceration and scarring. Simultaneous treatment with polymyxin B, however, prevented extension of corneal involvement whether or not cortisone was used.

Numerous isolated reports document ocular infections with organisms of low virulence that have apparently succeeded in invading tissues because of corticosteroid-reduced resistance.[161–163]

### Activation of Tuberculosis

Clinicians are quite familiar with the hazard of activating tuberculous infections with corticosteroid therapy. Presence of such infection is generally considered to be a strong contraindication to corticosteroid use. If corticosteroids are essential for the treatment of another condition, coexisting tuberculosis can ordinarily be controlled by simultaneous rifampin and isoniazid therapy. Studies of experimental ocular tuberculosis indicate that the apparent initial cortisone-induced improvement of inflammatory signs is transient and is followed by severe caseating disease that destroys a high proportion of cortisone-treated eyes.[164] The long-term results of various types of therapy are illustrated in Fig. 7–23. This study concludes that cortisone therapy of ocular tuberculosis is specifically contraindicated even when accompanied by antituberculous medications. It is only fair to point out that treatment of these rabbits was for just 1 month, during which period no real difference existed between those streptomycin-treated rabbits that received cortisone and those that did not. Clinically, treatment would not have been stopped arbitrarily while activity of the uveitis persisted. This study does not permit conclusions as to the ultimate outcome had therapy continued. As seen in Table 7–19, treatment was insufficient to sterilize these eyes in the majority of any group of rabbits. Expert opinion on tuberculosis therapy recommends at least 3 to 6 months of continuing treatment because of the characteristic slow growth and susceptibility of these organisms.

Because it is impossible to prove the etiology of many cases of human uveitis, and because ultimate intraocular scarring can unquestionably be reduced by corticosteroid therapy, corticosteroids should be used in the management of endogenous uveitis. If tuberculosis is suspected, simultaneous specific therapy is prudent.

Prolonged corticosteroid administration may activate latent systemic tuberculous infection and adversely affect the course of active tuberculosis. These facts have been established by animal experimentation[165] and by clinical observation.[166] To prevent such exacerbation of tuberculosis, all patients requiring corticosteroid treatment for 2 weeks or more should first be examined for tuberculosis (history of past

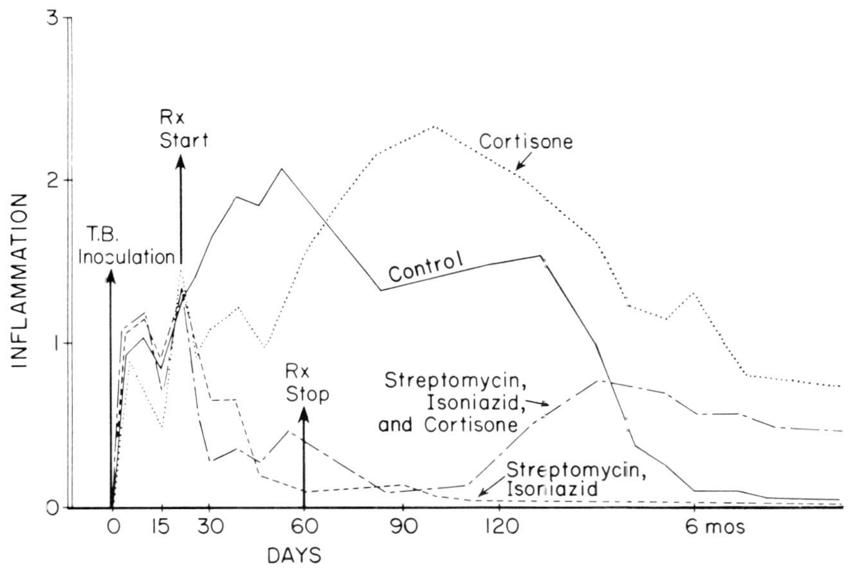


**FIG 7–23.**
Degree of activity of experimental ocular tuberculosis during a 6-month period. Note that cortisone treatment causes an initial favorable response, but at the cost of much more severe disease later. Even when simultaneous streptomycin and isoniazid treatment was given, cortisone caused late exacerbation. Note, however, that all therapy was discontinued after 1 month. (Data from Woods AC: *Arch Ophthalmol* 59:559, 1958. Used by permission.)

symptoms or treatment, chest x-ray films, and tuberculin skin test). Prophylactic isoniazid (300 mg/day for adults; 8 mg/kg for children) should be prescribed during corticosteroid treatment of all patients with evidence of previous tuberculosis. A chest x-ray film at the close of therapy is advised to be sure that reactivation of infection has not occurred.

### Uveitis

Mild anterior uveitis of 2 to 3 weeks' duration developed in two patients after provocative testing for responsiveness to topical corticosteroids. The uveitis responded promptly to dexamethasone (the same drug used for the provocative testing). Whether this was a coincidental finding in a series of 2,000 patients or related in some way to a corticosteroid reduction of ocular resistance was impossible to determine.[167]

Subsequently, 17 more patients (15 of whom were black) had severe anterior nongranulomatous uveitis develop during or subsequent to corticosteroid testing for glaucoma. A positive fluorescent treponemal antibody, absorbed (FTA-ABS) serologic test result was found in 82% of these patients (14), although only 4 had positive Venereal

**TABLE 7–19.**
Demonstration of Tuberculosis Bacilli by Culture and by Acid-Fast Stain at End of 6-Month Experimental Period*

| | Culture Positive for Tuberculosis Bacilli (%) | Acid-fast Stains Positive for Tuberculosis Bacilli (%) |
|---|---|---|
| Untreated controls | 100 | 38 |
| Cortisone treated only | 100 | 50 |
| Streptomycin and isoniazid therapy | 60 | 0 |
| Streptomycin, isoniazid, and cortisone therapy | 57 | 30 |

Data from Woods AC: *Arch Ophthalmol* 59:559, 1958. Used by permission.
*It is obvious that bacteria persisted within all groups of eyes despite treatment

Disease Research Laboratory (VDRL) test results. This suggests the possibility that corticosteroids may activate latent spirochetal ocular infection.[168]

In summary, the physician must be aware that the intensive use of local corticosteroids will render the eye immunologically incompetent and hence unable to resist normally the invasion of microorganisms of all types.

### Corticosteroid-induced Glaucoma

A decade elapsed between the introduction of corticosteroids into ophthalmology and the recognition and acceptance of the fact that these drugs can produce the clinical picture of primary open-angle glaucoma and that they do so with a frequency of undeniable clinical importance. A chronologic outline of these discoveries may be more interesting than a simple presentation of the facts.

Originally it was believed that ACTH and cortisone did not elevate IOP or cause positive glaucoma provocative test results in normal persons. In occasional patients with severe uveitis treated with corticosteroids a hypertensive response was noted.[169] This secondary type of glaucoma occurred only in eyes damaged so extensively as to hinder the normal aqueous outflow. Two explanations of this phenomenon were suggested:

1. Aqueous production is greatly reduced by the cyclitis and is permitted to return to normal levels by the corticosteroid therapy.
2. Increased permeability of inflamed iris vessels destroys the blood-aqueous barrier, thereby eliminating the osmotic differential responsible for maintaining IOP. Corticosteroid-induced return to normal permeability blocks this abnormal leakage, thereby producing the hypertensive response.

Prolonged use of topical corticosteroids was subsequently incriminated as a cause of chronic glaucoma.[170] This form of glaucoma is characterized by painless increased pressure in a white eye. Optic atrophy and visual field loss occur, but glaucomatous cupping is absent, and the field defects are said to be "uncharacteristic" of glaucoma. The published fields showed irregular constriction. Outflow facility is severely decreased. Despite discontinuance of corticosteroid therapy, surgery and antiglaucoma medications were necessary in treatment of these eyes. The five cases reported included one patient with myopic degeneration with retinal detachment and corneal infiltrates of unstated etiology, one patient with recurrent iritis and severe diabetes with neuropathy, a 57-year-old woman whose visual field appeared to have a typical nasal step, one patient with recurrent uveitis of such severity as to cause extensive synechiae, iris atrophy, and band keratopathy, and a 34-year-old woman whose mother had glaucoma. The descriptions of these cases certainly suggested that the patients were predisposed to glaucoma whether or not corticosteroid therapy was employed. If anyone but Goldmann had presented these cases, they would have been dismissed as pure coincidence. However, there could be no quarrel with his recommendation for periodic tonometry in eyes sufficiently diseased to require prolonged corticosteroid therapy.

Whether long-term systemic corticosteroid therapy might induce glaucomatous change was studied in 48 patients under treatment for rheumatoid arthritis and skin and collagen diseases.[171] The mean applanation pressure of the treated group was found to be statistically significantly increased and the facility of outflow to be decreased. Mean applanation pressure was higher (18.8 mm Hg) in patients receiving corticosteroid therapy for more than 4 years than in patients treated less than 1 year (15.9 mm Hg). The authors concluded that corticosteroid therapy was responsible for these changes. Although this conclusion may be justified, it must be recognized that the normal control group did not suffer from severe arthritis or collagen disease, although the group was matched for age, sex, race, and refractive error. Furthermore, examination of the data suggests that the control and corticosteroid-treated patients were very similar, with the exception of about six

**TABLE 7–20.**
Reversible Glaucoma Produced in Normal Human Eyes by Topical Use Three Times Daily of 0.1% Solution of Dexamethasone in Left Eye

| | Right Eye | | Left Eye | |
|---|---|---|---|---|
| | Ocular Pressure | Outflow Facility | Ocular Pressure | Outflow Facility |
| 3 mo with drug | 16 | 0.28 | 29 | 0.10 |
| 3 mo without drug | 17 | 0.26 | 16 | 0.28 |
| 3 wk with drug | 17 | 0.24 | 33 | 0.08 |
| 3 wk without drug | 15 | 0.30 | 17 | 0.25 |
| 4 wk with drug | 16 | 0.26 | 36 | 0.06 |
| 2 wk without drug | 17 | 0.26 | 17 | 0.27 |

From Armaly MF: *Arch Ophthalmol* 70:482, 1963. Used by permission.

individuals in the corticosteroid-treated group who appeared predisposed to glaucoma.

The concept of corticosteroid-induced glaucoma was further substantiated by sporadic case reports. In two such cases of structurally normal eyes, pressures of 40 to 60 mm Hg developed after daily use of dexamethasone drops for 4 to 6 months.[172] The glaucoma disappeared in each case within a few days after the dexamethasone was discontinued.

Systemic or topical corticosteroid therapy was found to cause a decrease in facility of outflow and a corresponding increase of IOP.[173] This glaucomatous change may affect one eye alone in the case of topical therapy. The corticosteroid effect may be completely reversible within 1 month's time.

Conclusive proof of the glaucoma-producing effect of corticosteroids was provided by patients in whom IOP could be reversibly elevated again and again by topical use of corticosteroids. The data in Table 7–20 illustrate the magnitude of changes in coefficient of outflow and IOP resulting from instillation three times daily of a 0.1% solution of dexamethasone in the left eye. (The right eye was an untreated control.) This 42-year-old patient developed glaucoma during treatment of uveitis of the left eye. He had no family history of glaucoma, and for 29 months of follow-up care after the last use of dexamethasone his IOPs remained normal.

In a group of 19 patients with untreated primary open-angle glaucoma, administration three times daily of a 1.0% solution of dexamethasone for 2 to 3 weeks caused pressure elevations of 11 mm Hg or more in 18 of these patients.[174] These pressures returned to their original levels within 1 to 3 weeks after corticosteroid instillations were discontinued. The pressure and outflow facility values in a representative patient are shown in Fig. 7–24.

Dexamethasone-induced hypertension is markedly greater in a glaucomatous eye than in a normal eye. Fig. 7–25 gives the pressure increases resulting from topical use of dexamethasone three times daily in the right eye in four groups of patients (young normal patients, old normal patients, patients with known low-tension glaucoma, and patients with untreated primary open-angle glaucoma). The lines represent the ratio of IOP in the right eye (treated) to that in the left eye (untreated). Note that pressure increased even in normal young eyes, but the increase was much greater and more rapid in the glaucomatous eyes.

Dexamethasone glaucoma is only partly reversed by miotic, epinephrine, and carbonic anhydrase inhibitor therapy. Because corticosteroids are commonly used medications, inquiry should be made as to their use in all patients found to have glaucoma.

Further confirmation of the hypertensive effect of topical use of corticosteroids was provided by a study of 44 glaucoma patients (average rise in pressure 15.2 mm Hg), 32 persons suspected of having glaucoma (average rise in pressure 11.2 mm Hg), and 30 normal persons (average rise in pressure 4.6 mm Hg).[175] This hypertensive response resulted after 3 to 8 weeks of treatment with betamethasone, prednisolone, dexamethasone, hydrocortisone, or triamcinolone. The outflow and pressure changes were completely reversible when treatment was discontinued.

Use of 1% prednisolone sodium phosphate (Inflamase Forte), 1% prednisolone acetate (Econopred Plus), 0.1% dexamethasone sodium phosphate (Maxidex), and 0.1% dexamethasone phosphate (Decadron Phosphate) four times daily for 3 to 6 weeks all gave comparable ocular hypertensive responses.[176]

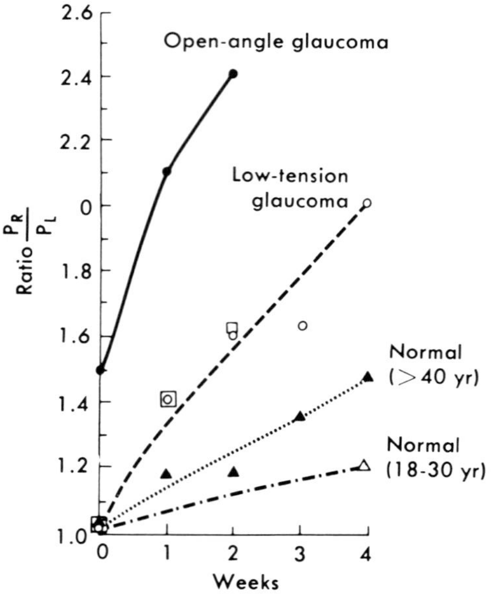


**FIG 7–25.**
Increase of IOP in dexamethasone-treated right eyes compared with untreated left eyes. (From Armaly MF: *Arch Ophthalmol* 70:482, 1963. Used by permission.)

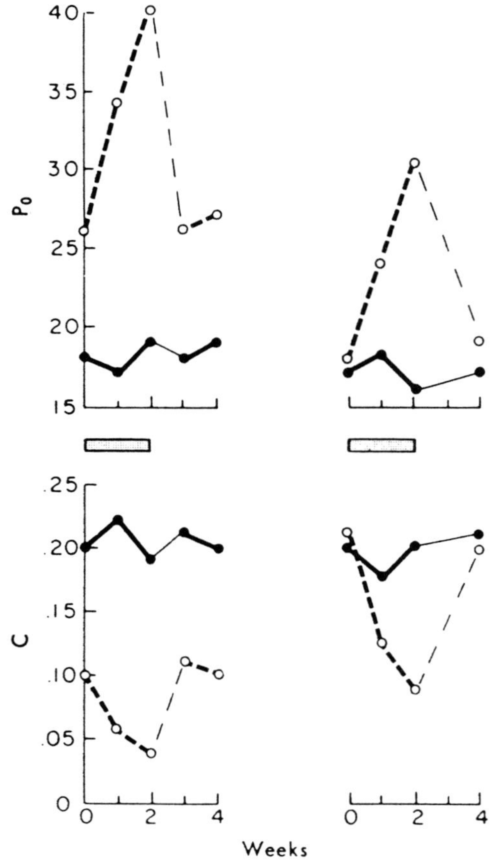


**FIG 7–24.**
Response of primary open-angle glaucoma to a 0.1% suspension of dexamethasone three times daily. *Solid line,* pilocarpine-treated left eye. *Broken lines,* cortisone-treated right eye. *Heavy bars,* dexamethasone treatment for 2 weeks in right eye. Left-hand response was obtained without miotic treatment of right eye and right-hand response with a 2% solution of pilocarpine four times daily in right eye. Note that pilocarpine decreases but does not abolish the hypertensive effect of dexamethasone. $P_o$, Intraocular pressure (IOP); *C,* coefficient of aqueous outflow. (From Armaly MF: *Arch Ophthalmol* 70:482, 1963. Used by permission.)

The relative effectiveness of the corticosteroid pressure response induced by 1% medrysone (hydroxymethylprogesterone), 0.1% fluorometholone, and 0.1% dexamethasone phosphate was 1, 4, and 7.6, respectively. That is, the pressure response of a given eye to fluorometholone would be four times as great as to medrysone and half as great as to dexamethasone.[177]

The potency of various corticosteroids to inhibit lymphocyte activation is generally comparable with their pressure-elevating potency. An exception is fluorometholone, which has relatively much less hypertensive effect. This may be related to poor intraocular penetration.[178]

One clinical study reports that 0.1% fluorometholone acetate exhibits a lower propensity to elevate IOP when compared with dexamethasone.[179] This effect, along with its increased potency, would certainly be advantageous over the currently available drugs. The authors also suggest that the pressure-elevating effects of fluorometholone acetate and fluorometholone are very similar when compared with dexamethasone. This supports a previous study suggesting that the specific ester fluorometholone has little effect on IOP.[176] However, direct comparison in a double-masked crossover study is needed.

Corticosteroid provocative testing for glaucoma is a safe research tool. Of 645 tested patients, none showed permanent changes attributable to the test.[180]

Dexamethasone-induced glaucoma will cause visual field defects measurable with a $1/_{1,000}$ white stimulus.[181] These field defects are similar to those typical of primary open-angle glaucoma and include an enlarged blind spot, arcuate scotomas, and peripheral constriction. The field defects are not related to the duration of corticosteroid therapy but to the elevation of IOP. Although these field defects may be slowly reversible when dexamethasone therapy is discontinued, as long as 2 months is required for disappearance of the field defect. Dexamethasone-induced pressure rise in eyes with primary open-angle glaucoma will cause an increase in size of preexisting field defects (Fig. 7–26).

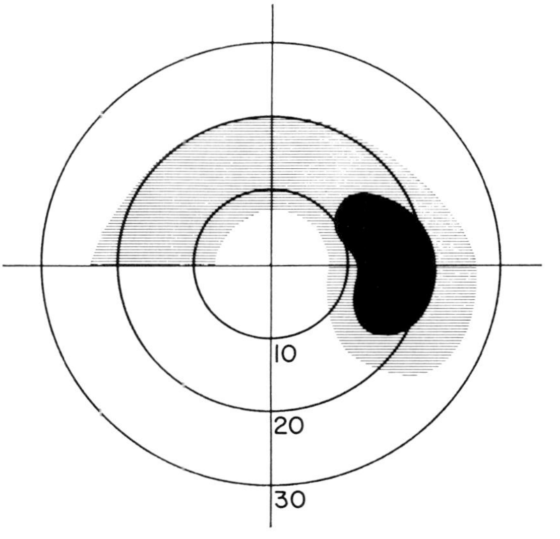


**FIG 7–26.**
Dexamethasone-induced increase in field defect. Black area indicates pretreatment scotoma in well-controlled glaucoma (IOP, 14 mm Hg). After 4 weeks of dexamethasone, 0.1% solution three times daily, the arcuate scotoma increased as represented by the stippled area (IOP, 29 mm Hg). (From Armaly MF: *Arch Ophthalmol* 71:636, 1964. Used by permission.)

The clinical importance of corticosteroid-induced glaucoma is emphasized by a report of 26 patients seen during a 6-month period.[182] All were threatened by a progressive loss of visual fields, and several had been subjected to glaucoma surgery. All 26 were using corticosteroid topically, sometimes without the knowledge of their ophthalmologist. In some instances the corticosteroid had been prescribed to counteract the redness caused by irritation from miotics. When the corticosteroid drops were discontinued, control of the glaucoma was easily achieved in all cases; indeed, a few eyes required no glaucoma therapy at all. Without doubt, these cases of glaucoma had been induced or made worse by the topical use of corticosteroids.[183]

Statistical analysis of the corticosteroid hypertensive response indicates the existence of three separate groups of individuals within the general population. The largest group, 66.2% of the study, responded with an average rise in pressure of 1.6 mm Hg after 4 weeks of 0.1% dexamethasone three times daily.[184] The second group, 28.8%, responded with an average rise of 10 mm Hg. A pressure rise greater than 16 mm Hg occurred only in the third group (5% of sample). Although these three groups were differentiated on the basis of the magnitude of pressure rise, the time of pressure rise was also different and is of clinical significance. Fig. 7–27 shows that group 1 patients (66%) responded with only a slight pressure

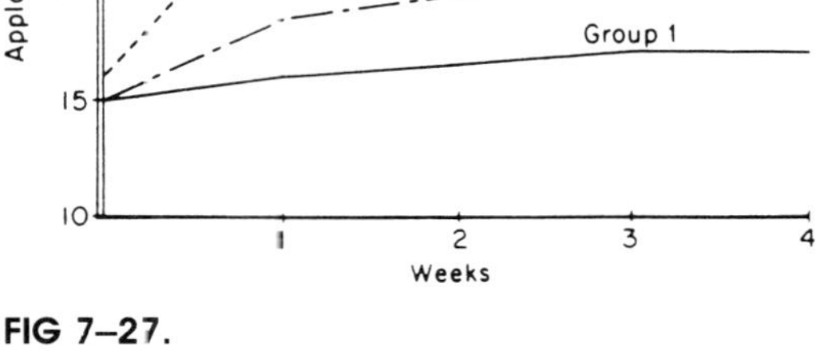


**FIG 7–27.**
Mean weekly applanation pressures after dexamethasone administration, three times daily, showing different rates of rise for the three groups previously separated by magnitude of corticosteroid response. (Modified from Armaly MF: *Invest Ophthalmol* 4:187, 1965. Used by permission.)

rise at the end of several weeks and that the pressure did not continue to rise. In contrast, during the month of study, the group 2 and 3 pressures continued to rise at a steady rate that presumably would continue with further treatment. The clinical implication is that a patient who has received corticosteroid treatment for 1 month but still has pressure less than 21 mm Hg is unlikely to have glaucomatous complications from such treatment. Should the pressure be greater than 21 mm Hg at the end of 1 month, subsequent corticosteroid therapy should include careful supervision of IOP.

The genotypic basis for these three groups of corticosteroid responsiveness was confirmed by a study of parents of individuals who were or were not corticosteroid responsive. The expected proportion of parental and offspring genotypes was found in this study of 109 families.[185]

The glaucomatous response to corticosteroids is a recessive trait found in one third of the population.[186] The homozygous state (double dose) of this gene causes primary open-angle glaucoma. Hence, the glaucomatous response to corticosteroids will be found in all patients with primary open-angle glaucoma, in both their parents, and in all offspring. Eyes with angle-closure or secondary glaucoma will not respond to corticosteroids with increased pressure (unless the patient happens to carry this genetic trait, which occurs in one third of cases). A positive correlation has been noted between the presumably genetic traits of corticosteroid-induced glaucoma, inability to taste phenylthiocarbamide,[187] plasma cortisol suppression by oral dexamethasone,[188] absence of proliferative retinopathy in diabetic patients, and corticosteroid inhibition of lymphocyte activation.[189, 190]

Patients with increased IOP have significantly higher plasma hydrocortisone levels than do those with normal IOP.[191–193] Thyroid parameters do not differ between corticosteroid pressure responders and nonresponders. This indicates that dexamethasone suppression of thyroid-stimulating hormone secretion does not share the enhanced corticosteroid sensitivity found to be associated with glaucoma in the eye, the lymphocyte, and hypothalamic control of the level of plasma hydrocortisone.[194]

To confirm this theory of recessive inheritance of glaucoma, both parents of a glaucoma patient and all the children of a glaucoma patient should show a positive corticosteroid provocative test result. Betamethasone, 0.1%, three times daily for 3 to 6 weeks, caused a positive response in only one of six parents and only 29 of 87 children of glaucoma patients.[195] The authors concluded that a positive corticosteroid test result indicates a predisposition to develop the disease but that these data did not confirm the theory of recessive inheritance. Of considerable interest is the fact that six of 210 positive reactors to the corticosteroid test continued to have glaucoma (previously absent) after betamethasone was discontinued. Prolonged miotic therapy was required in these patients, who developed early perimetric defects. That these patients would have developed glaucoma anyway could be proposed as an explanation.

In a study of 63 twins it was found that the pressure response to topical dexamethasone was more consistent between dizygotic twins than monozygotic twins. The significance of this unexpected finding is unclear.[196]

Although 100% of monozygotic twins would be expected to show the same corticosteroid pressure response, this actually occurs in only 65%.[197, 198] A possible explanation for this discrepancy is that the pressure response is not consistently reproducible in the same individual; it is, in fact, only 73% reproducible.[199]

Should eyes with secondary glaucoma be treated with corticosteroid? Will this control inflammation and reduce pressure, or is this group of patients genetically predisposed to corticosteroid glaucoma as is true in the case of contusion-angle glaucoma?

Corticosteroid provocative testing caused a glaucomatous response in approximately one third of 28 eyes with secondary glaucoma. This incidence is the same as in the general population of nonglaucomatous patients; therefore, it indicates the response is a result of a genetic trait rather than a characteristic of eyes with damaged outflow channels.[200]

What is the relationship between retinal detachment and open-angle glaucoma? Of 20 patients with nontraumatic rhegmatogenous retinal detachment, 20% were high corticosteroid responders (5% expected) and 53% had a cup/disc ratio greater than 0.3 (18% expected). Patients with recognizable open-angle glaucoma were excluded from the study group.[201] The practical application of this genetic relationship is that postoperative use of corticosteroid can be expected to increase pressure in one of every five detachment patients.

Pigmentary glaucoma apparently has a different etiology than does primary open-angle glaucoma, because it does not show the same corticosteroid response.[202]

Of 17 patients who had early postoperative cataract IOP increases, none showed a positive dexamethasone pressure response. This indicates the postoperative pressure rise results from surgical factors rather than genetic predisposition.[203]

When digital pressure comparable with that used before cataract surgery was performed on 10 ocular hypertensive patients, the pressure dropped by an average of 7 mm Hg but rebounded to 1.7 mm Hg higher than baseline by 30 minutes later. If pretreated with 600 mg of aspirin, the pressure overshoot did not occur; in fact, the pressure was still subnormal at 60 minutes. Aqueous flare appeared at the time of pressure elevation but did not develop in the aspirin-treated patients. Indomethacin treatment of rabbits also blocked the postcompression aqueous flare and pressure rise. These findings suggest that a PG mechanism is responsible for the secondary pressure rise and that digital massage released PGs.[204] The corticosteroid effect on digital pressure rebound was not evaluated.

One should not conclude that the eyes respond uniquely to corticosteroids. Genetically determined differences in corticosteroid responsiveness occur in many tissues, including circulating lymphocytes and skin fibroblasts.[205]

Corticosteroid provocative testing for glaucoma is a more sensitive examination than is the water-drinking tonography test. Evaluation of offspring of glaucomatous patients by the latter test showed 47% to be positive in contrast to 97% positive to the betamethasone test.[186] This provocative test requires instillation four times daily of a 0.1% solution of betamethasone for 3 weeks. The tonographic and pressure criteria for a positive test result are comparable with those for a positive test result for positive water-drinking tonography. Corticosteroid provocative testing is impractical for diagnosis of glaucoma; it takes too long and is too much of a nuisance. Furthermore, it is positive for 30% of the population, diagnosing this genetic trait, as well as cases of glaucoma.

A recent large retrospective review of patients provocatively tested with dexamethasone reinforces this point. In this study, the high corticosteroid responders (IOP greater than 31 mm Hg during treatment) had a significantly elevated false-positive rate of 87%. A much better predictive power was demonstrated when a multivariate model that included patient age, race, baseline IOP, baseline outflow facility, baseline cup/disc ratio, and systemic hypertension was used.[206]

As would be expected, glaucoma may also be induced by subconjunctival injection of corticosteroids in susceptible individuals. One of the particular hazards of this route of administration is that the depot will continue to release corticosteroid for some months, during which time pressure elevation will continue. The clinician should exercise appropriate judgment before giving such an injection. Was it indicated, for example, to give subconjunctival corticosteroids to four patients reported to have glaucoma develop from this treatment?[207] Their diagnoses were macular degeneration, vascularized corneal scar (all conditions nonresponsive to corticosteroids), and episcleritis (easily controlled by corticosteroid drops).

Surgical excision of the subconjunctival corticosteroid depot may be necessary before the glaucoma can be controlled.[97] Such a dissection is not a minor matter such as is removal of a pterygium, because the repository mass diffuses within the tissues and requires painstaking dissection, with concern to avoid vital structural damage.

The potential seriousness of corticosteroid-induced glaucoma is illustrated by the tragedy of a 15-year-old boy who used prednisolone drops several times daily for hay fever. When first seen by the ophthalmologist, this boy had advanced glaucomatous cupping, 20/70 vision, a pressure of 50 mm Hg, and field loss to within 5 degrees of fixation.[208] This irreversible damage apparently occurred within a 6-month period.

The mineralocorticoids are much less likely to cause increased IOP than are the glucocorticoids. Of 17 glaucomatous patients receiving parenteral desoxycorticosterone (30 mg intramuscularly every day for 3 to 6 days) or aldosterone D (2 mg intravenously), only two patients showed elevation of IOP.[209] A pressure rise occurred despite unchanged coefficient of outflow, indicating that increased aqueous production (presumably on the basis of electrolyte alteration) was the mechanism of action.

The intensity of the glaucomatous response in a given individual depends on the potency of the corticosteroid compound used and the frequency and duration of administration. For instance, use four times daily of suspensions of 0.1% prednisolone will elevate IOP about as much as use once daily of 0.1% solutions of dexamethasone. The less effective corticosteroids also require a much longer period of use before they cause pressure elevation.

Attempts have been made to develop antiinflammatory corticosteroids without the property of increasing IOP.[210] As mentioned earlier, medrysone is a very weak antiinflammatory agent compared with prednisolone. Topical instillation of 1% medrysone three times daily for 1 month in 23 patients caused no increase of IOP. These patients were chosen because they had previously shown an average increase of 6.7 mm Hg after use of 0.1% dexamethasone.[211]

Medrysone was used in a variety of eye conditions in 61 patients.[212] No increased IOP was noted. Furthermore, no reactivation of herpetic ulcers occurred.

The relative pressure-elevating potency and antiinflammatory effect of medrysone and dexamethasone have been determined. In a selected group of 28 high responders, the pressure elevations caused by 1% medrysone and by 0.001% dexamethasone were found to be virtually identical. In a rabbit corneal graft rejection model, the protection resulting from 1% medrysone and 0.001% dexamethasone was comparable for both drugs. The clear implication from these data is not that medrysone has a better therapeutic index with respect to causing glaucoma but that medrysone is simply 1,000-fold less strong than dexamethasone in its capability both to cause glaucoma and suppress inflammation.[213]

This concept of dose-related pressure response to corticosteroid is, of course, of practical clinical significance. Use the least amount of corticosteroid necessary to achieve the therapeutic goal. Fig. 7–28 shows clearly this dose-response relationship as measured in 24 eyes known to be high responders to corticosteroid.[214]

#### *Other Hormonal Responses*

An extensive review of the possible influence of a large variety of hormones other than corticosteroids on IOP concluded that certainly such influences did exist, but their relationship to physiologic maintenance of IOP and to open-angle glaucoma was not evident.[215]

#### *Summary*

The implications of this information are clear. Topical administration of corticosteroids should be used only for limited periods and under adequate tonometric supervision in patients with primary open-angle glaucoma and in their relatives. The possibility of pressure elevation should be considered in all patients receiving long-term corticosteroid therapy.

### Corticosteroid-induced Cataract

Posterior subcapsular cataract formation has been reported as a complication of long-term high-dosage systemic corticosteroid therapy.[216] This report evaluated 72 patients receiving long-term corticosteroid therapy and 23 control patients with rheumatoid arthritis not treated by corticosteroids. Posterior subcapsular cataracts were found in no patients receiving corticosteroids for less than 1 year, in 42% of those treated for 1 to 3 years, and in 58% treated for 4 years or more. As shown in Fig. 7–29,

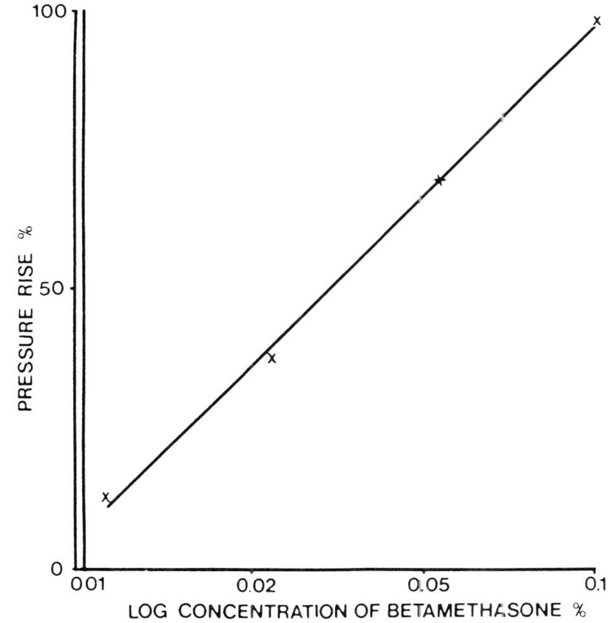


**FIG 7–28.**
Dose-response relationship between betamethasone and increased IOP in known high responders. (Data from Kitazawa Y: *Am J Ophthalmol* 82:492, 1976. Used by permission.)

cataract incidence was also closely related to corticosteroid dosage. Only 11% of patients receiving less than 10 mg daily of prednisone (or the equivalents) had cataracts develop compared with 30% receiving 10 to 15 mg and 80% receiving more than 15 mg/day. Most cataracts were clinically insignificant because they did not interfere with vision.

The dosage and duration of systemic corticosteroid administration appeared to be the primary determining factor in the production of posterior subcapsular cataract in a series of 38 patients with rheuma-

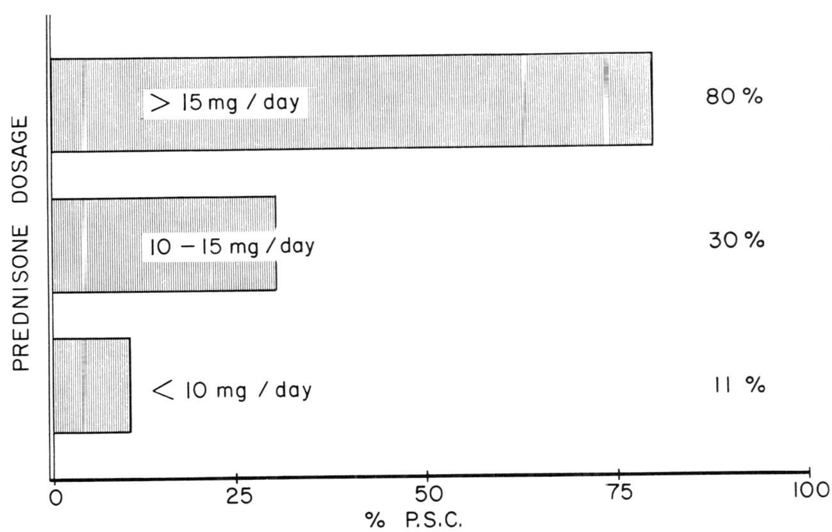


**FIG 7–29.**
Incidence of posterior subcapsular cataract in patients receiving corticosteroid therapy. (Data from Oglesby R, and others: *Arch Ophthalmol* 66:625, 1961. Used by permission.)

toid arthritis.[217] Fourteen (37%) of these patients receiving long-term corticosteroid therapy had such cataracts; these patients had no history of previous eye disease, injury, or radiation exposure. A control group of 24 arthritic patients had no cataracts. The duration and severity of the arthritis were comparable in the two groups. In addition, two of 12 asthmatic patients receiving corticosteroid therapy had characteristic posterior subcapsular cataracts.

In 86 eyes that had undergone keratoplasty for keratoconus, a correlation was found between amount and duration of corticosteroid dosage and posterior subcapsular cataract formation.[218] The cataract formation$_{50}$ (required to produce cataract in half the patients) dose was 765 drops of 0.1% dexamethasone (8 bottles of 5 ml) given over 10½ months. However, a substantial difference in susceptibility exists, with one patient developing a cataract after only 220 drops in 2½ months.

The relationship between corticosteroid therapy and posterior subcapsular cataract was evaluated in 106 patients from a hematology-oncology clinic. Of these, 39 had received corticosteroid therapy. Of the corticosteroid-treated patients, 51% had posterior subcapsular cataract compared with only 15% of the 67 noncorticosteroid-treated patients. No correlation could be found between the severity of cataract and total dose of corticosteroid or age of patient. Scatter-graph plotting did not seem to show any difference in severity whether the dosage had been only several hundred milligrams or 11,000 mg of prednisone. These data were interpreted to mean that patients with posterior subcapsular cataract may be more sensitive to the effects of corticosteroids.[219] The postulate that some patients are predisposed to corticosteroid cataract seems undeniable; not everyone gets it.

No cataracts were found in 20 patients with renal failure or immediately after renal transplant. Of 78 posttransplant patients, 53% had posterior subcapsular cataracts. No cataracts were found during the first 5 months of immunosuppressive therapy. In patients treated for more than 1 year, 92% had cataracts. Age and duration of pretransplant hemodialysis did not influence cataract formation. The total dose of prednisone was the only variable directly correlated with cataract formation.[220]

With the hope that corticosteroid-induced increased IOP would benefit diabetic retinopathy, 11 diabetic patients were given 2 to 4 drops of 0.1% dexamethasone in one eye two to four times daily, as necessary to maintain their pressures between 24 and 33 mm Hg. Over treatment periods from 14 to 36 months, nine of the 11 treated eyes developed cataract (five required surgery), but only one untreated eye did. Apparently diabetic eyes are highly susceptible to corticosteroid-induced cataract.[221] The article did not mention what happened to the retinopathy. The frequency of posterior subcapsular cataract was determined in 159 control patients, in 65 patients with rheumatoid arthritis who were not corticosteroid treated, and in 76 patients with corticosteroid-treated rheumatoid arthritis. In the patients less than 55 years of age in these groups, the frequency of cataract was 2%, 4.5%, and 16.6%, respectively.[222]

The appearance of the presumably corticosteroid-induced cataract is shown in Fig. 7–30.[223] This cataract cannot be differentiated biomicroscopically from early complicated cataract, radiation cataract, cataract associated with ocular disease, and senile posterior subcapsular cataract.

Histologically, these cataracts consist of multiple vacuoles resulting from liquefactive necrosis and aberrant migration of nucleated epithelial cells to the posterior pole of the lens.[224, 225]

Progression of these cataracts occurred in three of five patients whose corticosteroid dosage was reduced. In one patient the cataract worsened 2 months after therapy was discontinued.[223]

Complete disappearance of posterior subcapsular cataract happened in nine of 14 corticosteroid-treated children with nephrosis. In three of these, the cataract disappearance happened despite continued corticosteroid therapy. Only one of the cataracts was severe enough to reduce vision to less than 20/30. The least amount of prednisone taken by any cataract patient was 6.0 g and

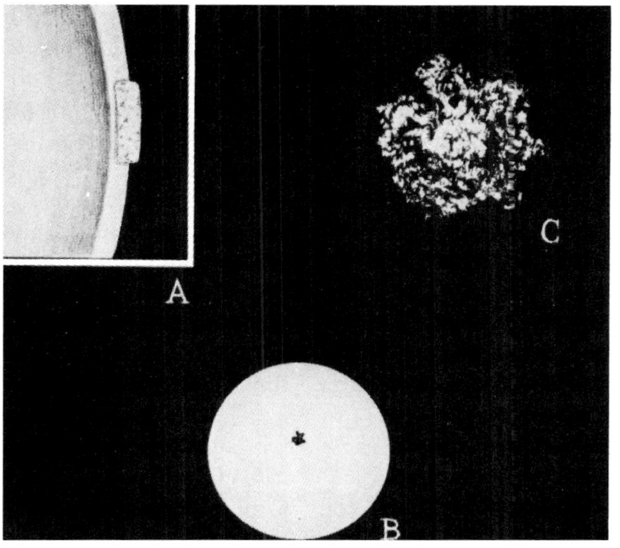


**FIG 7–30.**
Corticosteroid-induced posterior subcapsular cataract. (Modified from Oglesby R, and others: *Arch Ophthalmol* 66:97, 1961. Used by permission.)

the shortest duration of therapy was at least 1 year. Cushing's syndrome was more fre quent in the children with cataracts, although the total corticosteroid dosage was higher in children without cataracts. The study included 39 children with nephrosis. The reversibility of these cataracts was believed to represent a changed metabolic response to corticosteroid.[226] Perhaps the mechanism of corticosteroid cataract is interference with an easily reversible biochemical reaction.

It should be recognized that patients with rheumatoid arthritis not receiving corticosteroid treatment have an unusually high incidence of posterior subcapsular cataract. In a series of 43 patients with rheumatoid arthritis (not treated with corticosteroids) who had posterior subcapsular cataract requiring surgery, 19 were less than 50 years of age at the time of operation. The youngest was only 27 years old.[227]

No posterior subcapsular cataracts were found in a group of 48 asthmatic patients who had been receiving corticosteroid therapy for many years.[228] Nineteen of these patients had used 16 mg or more of methylprednisolone equivalent for 2 to 7 years. In a control group of 148 patients without corticosteroid therapy, 9 patients had cataracts, two of these being posterior subcapsular.

In another series of 40 patients with rheumatoid arthritis receiving corticosteroid therapy, only 2 cases of posterior subcapsular cataract were found.[229] Both of these patients had a family history of cataracts, a fact with obvious implications. Ten of these patients had received the equivalent of 15 to 20 mg of prednisone for 1 to 4 years. One of the cataract patients had been treated for less than 1 year and the other for more than 4 years.

Three of 14 children on long-term corticosteroid therapy (>1 year) were found to have bilateral asymptomatic posterior subcapsular cataracts.[230] The corticosteroid dosage was sufficiently high to cause typical cushingoid obesity.

Further documentation of the cataractogenic potential of prolonged systemic corticosteroid therapy appears in a report of 15 children so treated for 2 years or more.[231] Eight of these 15 children had posterior subcapsular cataracts. Three months after corticosteroid therapy was discontinued in three children, no regression of the cataracts was recognizable.

Of 109 children on long-term (>6 months) corticosteroid therapy, 22% had posterior subcapsular cataracts develop.[232]

A single case has been reported in which a posterior subcapsular cataract developed unilaterally in a 20-year-old man after 1 year's treatment of chronic herpetic keratitis with idoxuridine (IDU) and topical use of corticosteroids.[233]

Two other cases of cataracts after topical use of corticosteroids seem especially tragic. These young girls, aged 17 and 20 years, used corticosteroid drops for the redness resulting from contact lens wearing. One used prednisolone daily for almost 2 years. The other used dexamethasone or prednisolone twice daily for 4 years. Both girls had posterior subcapsular cataracts and glaucoma so resistant to medical therapy that sclerectomy was required for control. Both had also lost approximately half of their visual fields.[234] Millions of patients wear contact lenses and may gain access to corticosteroid drops to alleviate ocular irritation. Characteristically, these drops will be used for long periods without medical supervision. *Do not grant contact lens wearers access to corticosteroids!*

A possible mechanism of cataract formation might be biochemical changes in the aqueous humor resulting from corticosteroid exposure. Prolonged topical use of methylprednisolone in rabbits causes marked chemical changes in the aqueous to occur. For example, the ascorbic acid level is lowered from 36 to 25 mg/100 ml; the potassium level is lowered from 6 to 4 mEq/L, and pH increases from 7.6 to 7.8.[235]

Phospholipid and adenosine triphosphate levels decrease in the lens with corticosteroid-induced posterior subcapsular cataracts. Adenosine triphosphate is important in the transport systems that maintain lens transparency.[236]

Both clinical and experimental data strongly suggest a relationship between prolonged corticosteroid therapy and cataracts. The risk increases proportionally to the duration and amount of therapy. In most cases the cataract causes minimal, if any, visual complaints.[236] Clinical perspective will identify situations where the risk of withholding beneficial treatment is a consideration at least as important as the possibility of cataract formation.

### "Corticosteroid" Mydriasis

Experimental use of topical corticosteroids to provoke a glaucomatous response has disclosed another effect, dilatation of the pupil. For instance, all of 39 volunteers receiving 0.1% dexamethasone four to five times daily in one eye showed dilatation of the treated pupil. Dilatation occurred as early as the first week of treatment, averaged 1 mm, and disappeared in all cases promptly after dexamethasone was stopped. The amount of dilatation bears no relationship to the ocular hypertensive response.[237]

The mydriatic effect of corticosteroids was studied on isolated monkey intraocular muscle preparations.[238] As expected, the tonus of the dilator muscle was increased and that of the sphincter was decreased. More careful analysis, however, revealed that the specific corticosteroid components of these medications did not alter the muscle status. Rather, the response was caused by some effect of the vehicle (preservatives or surface tension-reducing agents).

Also in living monkeys, ptosis and mydriasis resulted from instillation of dexamethasone in its commercial vehicle and from use of the vehicle alone but not from dexamethasone in saline solution. The vehicle contains various preservatives, antioxidants, and surface-active agents. The combination of surface-active agents (polysorbate 80, phenylmethanol, and disodium edetate) appeared to be responsible for a direct myopathic effect.[239]

Exposure of the dilator, sphincter, and ciliary muscle preparations to the vehicles of corticosteroid eye drops (no corticosteroid) inhibited muscle responses to both acetylcholine and epinephrine, as well as to potassium chloride. (Potassium chloride bypasses specific receptor sites and induces muscle contractions by direct depolarization of cell membranes.) Apparently these vehicles disturb the selective semipermeability of the cell membrane, thereby altering the ability of the muscle to respond.

Inasmuch as altered response of intraocular smooth muscle might be responsible for such clinically observed side effects as mydriasis, difficulty of accommodation, and increased resistance to aqueous outflow (glaucomatous response), the demonstration that such smooth muscle changes are a result of the eye drop vehicle rather than of the corticosteroid may be of great significance. Possibly other of our existing concepts as to "corticosteroid-induced complications" will need to be changed to "vehicle-induced" changes. Such speculation is presently premature.

## Corneal Perforation

Patients with rheumatoid arthritis and Sjögren's syndrome are vulnerable to development of spontaneous sterile corneal ulcers that may perforate. Topical corticosteroids, possibly by activating collagenase, can accelerate corneal melting, and their use is contraindicated in such patients. Of 18 such eyes, seven corneas perforated (four perforations had received corticosteroids). Treatment is by protection with a soft contact lens and artificial tears.[240]

In a series of nine rheumatoid patients with peripheral corneal furrows, two had peripheral corneal perforations develop after corticosteroid use.[241] None of these nine patients with rheumatoid corneal disease was helped by corticosteroid therapy. Five additional cases of central corneal perforation after corticosteroid therapy were reported in the paper.

A possible explanation for this untoward effect of corticosteroid therapy is reduction of corneal fibroblast metabolism by these drugs. The combined effect of a disease and a drug, both damaging the corneal stroma, may account for corneal thinning and perforation. A relevant fact is that the skin of a rheumatoid patient (but not of a normal patient) thins when corticosteroids are applied topically.[242]

In general, corticosteroid therapy of corneal or scleral disease in patients with rheumatoid arthritis is more likely to be harmful than to be beneficial.

A report from the Wills Eye Hospital indicates that even in this huge patient population, corneal perforation does not occur from untreated keratoconjunctivitis sicca.[243] However, over a 2-year period four patients were seen who had suffered corneal perforation after corticosteroid treatment of keratoconjunctivitis sicca. There is no rational reason to treat keratoconjunctivitis sicca with corticosteroids, and it is evident that some type of collagenase activation or fibroblastic repair inhibition may result in corneal melting from corticosteroids in such cases.

### *Scleromalacia Perforans*

Another collagen disease that is at least partially helped by corticosteroid is scleromalacia perforans. Histologic study of a single such cortisone-treated eye has been compared with the findings in six untreated eyes.[244] It is pertinent to state that this eye was treated when supplies of cortisone were limited and received what would now be considered relatively light treatment, namely, 100 mg of cortisone every day for several weeks. Thereafter, cortisone drops were administered every 4 hours for some months. Clinically, reduction in redness, nodule formation, and photophobia were attributed to the cortisone. Histologically, the treated eye showed a much less severe inflammatory reaction and had almost no polymorphonuclear cells and eosinophils in contrast to the large number of these cells found in the six untreated eyes. Surprisingly, fibroblastic regeneration over the ulcerated areas of sclera and uniformly palisaded arrangement of the new fibroblasts were much more definite in the cortisone-treated eye. Apparently corticosteroids prevent further inflammatory activity in scleromalacia perforans, thereby creating suitable conditions for fibrous regeneration. Excessive corticosteroid therapy may, however, inhibit the regenerative process, and in some cases scleral thinning seems to be accelerated by such treatment.

In another case the clinical response of scleromalacia perforans to ACTH therapy was not significant.[245] This patient suffered onset and progression of scleromalacia during a 13-month course of corticosteroid therapy for rheumatoid arthritis. Dosage was 100 mg of cortisone every day for 4 months and then 400 mg of ACTH twice weekly. This patient also had retinitis pigmentosa and suffered progressive loss of field and acuity during the 13 months of cortisone therapy.

### Corneal Thickness

After 4 weeks of treatment with topical dexamethasone, 35% of patients developed a 3% increase in corneal thickness. This may be related to the effects of increased IOP.[246]

### Corticosteroid Retinopathy

Dexamethasone, 1.0 mg/kg/day for 10 days, will produce fan-shaped neovascularization and vascular tortuosity in young rabbit and rat retinas that are vascularized to the approximate stage of the 6-month-old human fetus. This is somewhat similar to oxygen-induced retinopathy.[247]

### Hypersensitivity

Allergy to corticosteroid preparations must be extremely rare, and the probability of reaction to vehicle or impurities should be suspected. After repeated retrobulbar injections of methylprednisolone suspension for 5 years of chronic cyclitis, severe inflammatory reaction believed to be allergic developed in a patient. Repeated patch testing with the methylprednisolone was negative, but intradermal injection caused a 1-cm erythematous response with eosinophils.[248]

### Mechanical Trauma

Inadvertent intraarterial injection of corticosteroid in treatment of nose, scalp, lip, and tonsillar regions can result in retinal emboli and permanent visual field defects.[249] The combination of epinephrine and corticosteroid reproducibly resulted in experimental retinal emboli. Experimentally, unilateral injection of a dog carotid artery will consistently result in embolization of both retinas.[250, 251]

## SUMMARY

Corticosteroid therapy is here to stay—for use *when indicated.* It is a two-edged sword, however, and can cause serious complications and side effects if it is used unwisely.[252]

## REFERENCES

## SECTION ONE

1. Clive DM, Stoff JS: Renal syndromes associated with nonsteroidal antiinflammatory drugs, *N Engl J Med* 1984, 310:563–572.
2. Langman MJS: Ulcer complications and nonsteroidal antiinflammatory drugs, *Am J Med* 1988, 84(suppl 2A):15–19.
3. Brooks PM, Day RO: Nonsteroidal antiinflammatory drugs—differences and similarities, *N Engl J Med* 1991, 324: 1716–1725.
4. Hamberg M, Svenson J, Samuelsson B: Thromboxanes: new group of biologically active compounds derived from prostaglandin endoperoxides, *Proc Natl Acad Sci USA* 1975, 72:2994–2998.
5. Samuelsson B, Borgeat P, Hammarstrom S, and others: Leukotrienes: a new group of biologically active compounds. In Samuelsson B, Ramwell PW, Paoletti R, editors: *Leukotrienes and other lipoxygenase products,* New York, 1980, Raven Press, pp 1–18.
6. Kass MA, Holmberg NJ: Prostaglandin and thromboxane synthesis by microsomes of rabbit ocular tissues, *Invest Ophthalmol Vis Sci* 18:166, 1979.
7. Bhattacherjee P, Eakins KE: A comparison of the inhibitory activity of compounds on ocular prostaglandin biosynthesis, *Invest Ophthalmol Vis Sci* 1974, 13:967–972.
8. Van Haeringen NJ, Oosterhuis JA, van Delft JL, and others: A comparison of the effects of nonsteroidal compounds on the disruption of the blood-aqueous barrier, *Exp Eye Res* 1982, 35:271–277.
9. Araie M, Sawa M, Takase M: Topical flurbiprofen and diclofenac suppress blood-aqueous barrier breakdown in cataract surgery: a fluorometric study, *Jpn J Ophthalmol* 1983, 27:535–542.
10. Van den Ouweland FA, Gribnau FWJ, van Ginneken, and others: Naproxen kinetics and disease activity in rheumatoid arthritis:

a within patient study, *Clin Pharmacol Ther* 1988, 43:79–85.
11. Goodwin JS, Regan M: Cognitive dysfunction associated with naproxen and ibuprofen in the elderly, *Arthritis Rheum* 1982, 25:1013–1015.
12. Netter P, Lapicque F, Bannwarth B, and others: Diffusion of intramuscular ketoprofen into the cerebrospinal fluid, *Eur J Clin Pharmacol* 1985, 29:319–321.
13. Orme M, Baber N, Keenan J, and others: Pharmacokinetics and biochemical effects in responders and non-responders to nonsteroidal antiinflammatory drugs, *Scand J Rheum* 1981, 39(suppl):19–27.
14. Huskisson EC, Woolf DL, Balme HW, and others: Four new antiinflammatory drugs: responses and variations, *BMJ* 1976, 1:1048–1049.
15. Gall EP, Caperton JF, McComb JE, and others: Clinical comparison of ibuprofen, fenoprofen calcium, naproxen, tolmectin sodium in rheumatoid arthritis, *J Rheumatol* 1982, 9:402–407.
16. Heller CA, Ingelfinger JA, Goldman P: Nonsteroidal antiinflammatory drugs and aspirin—analyzing the scores, *Pharmacotherapy* 1985, 5:30–38.
17. Watson PG, Hayreh SS: Scleritis and episcleritis, *Br J Ophthalmol* 1976, 60:163–191.
18. Bjarnason I, Zanelli G, Prowse P, and others: Blood and protein loss via small intestinal inflammation induced by nonsteroidal antiinflammatory drugs, *Lancet* 1987, 2:711–714.
19. Henry DA: Side effects of nonsteroidal antiinflammatory drugs, *Baillieres Clin Rheumatol* 1988, 2:425–454.
20. Beard K, Walker AM, Perera DR, and others: Nonsteroidal antiinflammatory drugs and hospitalization for gastroesophageal bleeding in the elderly, *Arch Intern Med* 1987, 147:1621–1623.
21. Sommerville K, Faulkner G, Langman M: Non-steroidal antiinflammatory drugs and bleeding peptic ulcer, *Lancet* 1986, 1:462–464.
22. Hawkey CJ: Non-steroidal antiinflammatory drugs and peptic ulcers, *BMJ* 1990, 300:278–284.
23. Soll AH: Pathogenesis of peptic ulcer and implication for therapy, *N Engl J Med* 1990, 322:909–916.
24. Garella S, Matarese RA: Renal effects of prostaglandins and clinical adverse effects of nonsteroidal antiinflammatory agents, *Medicine (Baltimore)* 1984, 64:165–181.
25. Lifschitz MD: Prostaglandins and renal blood flow: in vivo studies, *Kidney Int* 1981, 19:802–815.
26. Early Treatment Diabetic Retinopathy Study Research Group: Effects of aspirin treatment on diabetic retinopathy: ETDRS report number 8, *Ophthalmology* 1991, 98:757–765.
27. Seddon JM, Christen WG, Manson JE, and others: Low-dose aspirin and risks of cataract in a randomized trial of US physicians, *Arch Ophthalmol* 1991, 109:252–255.
28. Kremer M, Baikoff G, Charbonnel B: ProstaglandinE2 inside effects of ocular surgery in man: preventative action of indomethacin. In Samuelsson R, Paoletti R, Ramwell P, editors: *Advances in prostaglandins, thromboxane and leukotriene research*, vol 12, New York, 1983, Raven Press, pp 121–126.
29. Kulkarni PS, Eakins HM, Saber WL, and others: Microsomal preparations of normal bovine iris ciliary body generate prostacyline like but not thromboxane-A2-activity, *Prostaglandins* 1977, 14:689–700.
30. Kulen-de Vos HCJ, van Rij G, de Lavalette JCGR, and others: Effect of indomethacin in preventing surgically induced miosis, *Br J Ophthalmol* 1983, 67:94–96.
31. Sawa M, Masuda K: Topical indomethacin in soft cataract aspiration, *Jpn J Ophthalmol* 1976, 20:514–519.
32. Clayman HM: Pupillary, iris and other complications. In *The surgeon's guide to intraocular lens implantation*, Thorofare, NJ, 1985, Slack, pp 107–137.
33. Thrasher B, Keller DA: Extracapsular cataract extraction, phacoemulsification and posterior chamber intraocular lens implantation. In Ginsberg S, editors: *Cataract and intraocular lens surgery*, Amsterdam, 1984, Kugler Publications, pp 255–278.
34. Keates RH, McGowan KA: Clinical trial of flurbiprofen to maintain pupillary dilation during cataract surgery, *Ann Ophthalmol* 1984, 16 919–921.
35. Flurbiprofen—an ophthalmic NSAID, *Med Lett Ther* 1987, 29:58–59.
36. Stark WJ, Fagadau WR, Stewart RH, and others: Reduction of pupillary constriction during cataract surgery using suprofen, *Arch Ophthalmol* 1986, 104:364–366.
37. Gimbel HV: The effect of treatment with topical nonsteroidal antiinflammatory drugs with and without intraoperative epinephrine on the maintenance of mydriasis during cataract surgery, *Ophthalmology* 1989, 96:585–588.

38. Vander JF, Greven CM, Maquire JI, and others: Flurbiprofen sodium to prevent intraoperative miosis during vitreoretinal surgery, *Am J Ophthalmol* 1989, 108:288–291.
39. Roberts LJ, Lewis RA, Oates JA, and others: Prostaglandin, thromboxane and 12-hydroxy-5,8,10,14-eicosatraenoic acid production by iontopho-stimulated rat serosal mast cells, *Biochem Biophys Act* 1979, 575:185–188.
40. Lewis RA, Roberts LJ, Holgate ST, and others: Immunologic generation of mast cell prostaglandins and their effects on mast cell cyclic nucleotides, *J Allergy Clin Immunol* 1980, 65:235–237.
41. Abelson MB, Butrus SI, Weston JH: Aspirin therapy in vernal conjunctivitis, *Am J Ophthalmol* 1983, 95:502–505.
42. Gasset AR, Lorenzetti DWC, Ellison EM, and others: Quantitative corticosteroid effect on corneal wound healing, *Arch Ophthalmol* 1969, 81:589–591.
43. Lee BP, Kupferman A, Leibowitz: Effect of suprofen on corneal wound healing, *Arch Ophthalmol* 1985, 103:95–97.
44. Hersh PS, Rice BA, Bear JC, and others: Topical nonsteroidal agents and corneal wound healing, *Arch Ophthalmol* 1990, 108:577–583.
45. McDonald TO, Borgmann AR, Roberts MD, and others: Corneal wound healing: I. Inhibition of stromal healing by three dexamethasone derivatives, *Invest Ophthalmol Vis Sci* 1970, 9:703–709.
46. Miller D, Greunberg P, Miller R, and others: Topical flurbiprofen or prednisone: effect on corneal wound healing in rabbits, *Arch Ophthalmol* 1981, 99:681–682.
47. Frucht-Pery J, Levinger S, Zauberman H: The effect of topical administration of indomethacin on symptoms in corneal scars and edema, *Am J Ophthalmol* 1991, 112:186–190.
48. Leibowitz HM, Ryan WJ, Kupferman A, and others: Effect of concurrent topical corticosteroid and NSAID therapy of experimental keratitis, *Invest Ophthalmol Vis Sci* 1986, 27:126–129.
49. Trousdale MD, Barlow WE, McGuigan LJ: Assessment of diclofen on herpes keratitis in rabbit eyes, *Arch Ophthalmol* 1989, 107:1664–1666.
50. Hendrick RL, Barfknecht CF, Schoenwald RD, and others: The effect of flurbiprofen on herpes simplex virus type 1 stromal keratitis in mice, *Invest Ophthalmol Vis Sci* 1990, 31:1503–1511.
51. Moreira H, McDonnell PJ, Fasano AP, and others: Treatment of experimental pseudomonas keratitis with cyclo-oxygenase and lipoxygenase inhibitors, *Ophthalmology* 1991, 98:1693–1697.
52. Gritzz DG, Lee TY, Kwitko S, and others: Topical antiinflammatory agents in an animal model of microbial keratitis, *Arch Ophthalmol* 1990, 108:1001–1005.
53. Rao NA, Patchett R, Fernandez MA, and others: Treatment of experimental granulomatous uveitis by lipoxygenase and cyclo-oxygenase inhibitors, *Arch Ophthalmol* 1987, 105:413–415.
54. Watson PG: The diagnosis and management of scleritis, *Ophthalmology* 1980, 87:716–720.
55. Foster CS: Immunosuppressive therapy for external ocular inflammatory disease, *Ophthalmology* 1980, 87:140–150.
56. Mondino BJ, Phinney RB: Treatment of scleritis with combined oral prednisone and indomethacin therapy, *Am J Ophthalmol* 1988, 106:473–479.
57. Beitch BR, Eakins KE: The effect of prostaglandins on the intraocular pressure of the rabbit, *Br J Pharmacol* 1969, 37:158–167.
58. Bito LZ: Comparison of the ocular hypotensive efficacy of eicosanoids and related compounds, *Exp Eye Res* 1984, 38:181–194.
59. Battacherjee P, Kulkarni PS, Eakins KE: Metabolism of arachidonic acid in the rabbit ocular tissues, *Invest Ophthalmol Vis Sci* 1979, 18:172–178.
60. Goh Y, Nakajima M, Azuma I, and others: Effects of prostaglandin D2 and its analogues on the intraocular pressure in rabbits, *Jpn J Ophthalmol* 1988, 32:471–480.
61. Bhattacherjee P, Eakins KE: A comparison of the inhibitory activity of compounds on ocular prostaglandin biosynthesis, *Invest Ophthalmol* 1974, 13:967–970.
62. Podos SM, Becker B: Comparison of ocular prostaglandin synthesis inhibitors, *Invest Ophthalmol* 1976, 15:841–844.
63. Camras CB, Feldman SG, Podos SM, and others: Inhibition of the epinephrine-induced reduction of intraocular pressure by systemic indomethacin in humans, *Am J Ophthalmol* 1985, 100:169–175.
64. Yousufzai SYK, Abdel-Latif AA: Effect of Norepinephrine and other pharmacological agents on prostaglandin E release by rabbit and bovine irides, *Exp Eye Res* 1983, 37:279–281.
65. Miyaki K, Kayazawa F, Manabe R, and others: Indomethacin and epinephrine induced breakdown of the blood-ocular

barrier in rabbits, *Invest Ophthalmol Vis Sci* 1987, 28:482–486.
66. Engstrom P, Dunham EW: Alpha-adrenergic stimulation of prostaglandin release from rabbit iris–ciliary body in vitro, *Invest Ophthalmol Vis Sci* 1982, 22:557–560.
67. Reibaldi A, Avitabile T: Topical indomethacin in Posner Schlossman's syndrome, *Ann Ophthalmol* 1983, 4:28–29.
68. Thomas JV, Simmons RJ, Belcher CD: Argon laser trabeculoplasty in the presurgical glaucoma patient, *Ophthalmology* 1982, 89:187–197.
69. Hotchkiss ML, Robin AL, Pollack Quigley HA: Nonsteroidal antiinflammatory agents after argon laser trabeculoplasty, *Ophthalmology* 1984, 91:969–976.
70. Pappas HR, Berry DP, Partamain L, and others: Topical indomethacin therapy before argon laser trabeculoplasty, *Am J Ophthalmol* 1985, 99:571–575.
71. Araie M, Sawa M, Takase M: Topical flurbiprofen and diclofenac suppress blood-aqueous barrier breakdown in cataract surgery: a fluorophotometric study, *Jpn J Ophthalmol* 1983, 27:535–542.
72. Araie M, Sawa M, Takase M: Effect of topical indomethacin on the blood-aqueous barrier after intracapsular extraction of a senile cataract—a fluorophotometric study, *Jpn J Ophthalmol* 1981, 25:237–247.
73. Eguchi K, Ohara K, Tobari I, and others: Effects of topical indomethacin on suppression of inflammation after ocular surgeries—double mask study of antiinflammatory effects on the intracapsular lens extraction, *Acta Soc Ophthalmol Jpn* 1982, 86:2198–2212.
74. Mochizuki M, Sawa M, Masuda K: Topical indomethacin in intracapsular extraction of a senile cataract, *Jpn J Ophthalmol* 1977, 21:215–226.
75. Sanders DR, Kraff MC, Leiberman HL, and others: Breakdown and re-establishment of blood-aqueous barrier with implant surgery, *Arch Ophthalmol* 1982, 100:588–590.
76. Flach AJ, Kraff MC, Sanders DR, and others: The quantitative effect of 0.5% ketorolac tromethamine solution and 0.1% dexamethasone sodium phosphate solution on post-surgical blood-aqueous barrier, *Arch Ophthalmol* 1988, 106:480–483.
77. Flach AJ, Jaffe NS, Akers WA: The effect of ketorolac tromethamine in reducing post-operative inflammation: double mask parallel comparison with dexamethasone, *Ann Ophthalmol* 1989, 21:407–411.
78. Sabiiston D, Tessler H, Sumers K, and others: Reduction of inflammation following cataract surgery by the nonsteroidal antiinflammatory drug flurbiprofen, *Ophthalmic Surg* 1987, 18:873–877.
79. Flach AJ, Lavelle CJ, Olander KW, and others: The effect of ketorolac tomethamine solution 0.5% in reducing postoperative inflammation after cataract extraction and intraocular lens implantation, *Ophthalmology* 1988, 95:1279–1284.
80. Hurvitz LM, Spaeth GL, Zakhour I, and others: A comparison of the effect of flurbiprofen dexamethasone and placebo on cyclocryotherapy-induced inflammation, *Ophthalmic Surg* 1984, 15:394–399.
81. Stark WJ, Worthen DM, Halladay JT: The FDA report on intraocular lenses, *Ophthalmology* 1983, 90:311–317.
82. Irvine AR: Cystoid macular edema, *Surv Ophthalmol* 1976, 21:1–17.
83. Miami Study Group: Cystoid macular edema in aphakic and pseudophakic eyes, *Am J Ophthalmol* 1979, 88:45–48.
84. Jampol LM: Pharmacologic therapy of aphakic and pseudophakic cystoid maculae edema, *Ophthalmology* 1985, 92:807–810.
85. Yannuzzi LA: A perspective on the treatment of aphakic cystoid macular edema, *Surv Ophthalmol* 1984, 28:540–551.
86. Miyake K, Sakamura S, Miura H: Long-term follow-up study on prevention of aphakic cystoid macular edema by topical indomethacin, *Br J Ophthalmol* 1980, 64:324–328.
87. Yannuzzi LA, Landau AN, Turtz AI: Incidence of aphakic cystoid macular edema with the use of topical indomethacin, *Ophthalmology* 1981, 88:947–954.
88. Kraff MC, Sanders DR, Jampol LM, and others: Prophylaxis of pseudophakic cystoid macular edema with topical indomethacin, *Ophthalmology* 1982, 89:885–890.
89. Miyake K: Indomethacin in the treatment of postoperative cystoid macular edema, *Surv Ophthalmol* 1984, 28:554–568.
90. Burnett J, Tessler H, Isenberg S, and others: Double-masked trial of fenoprofen sodium: treatment of chronic aphakic cystoid macular edema, *Ophthalmic Surg* 1983, 14:150–152.
91. Flach AJ, Jampol LM, Weinberg D, and others: Improvement in visual acuity in chronic aphakic and pseudophakic cystoid macular edema after treatment with topical 0.5% ketorolac tromethamine, *Am J Ophthalmol* 1991, 112:514–519.
92. Howes EL, McKay DG: The effect of aspirin and indomethacin on the ocular response

to circulating bacterial endotoxin in the rabbit, *Invest Ophthalmol* 1976, 15:648–651.

93. Olson NY, Lindsley CB, Godfrey WA: Nonsteroidal antiinflammatory drug therapy in chronic childhood iridocyclitis, *Am J Dis Child* 1988, 142:1289–1292.

## SECTION TWO

1. BenEzra D, Cohen E: Treatment and visual prognosis in Behçet's disease, *Br J Ophthalmol* 1986, 70:589.
2. Abdalla MI, Bahgat N: Long-lasting remission of Behçet's disease after chlorambucil therapy, *Br J Ophthalmol* 1973, 57:706.
3. Tabbara KF: Chlorambucil in Behçet's disease. A reprisal, *Ophthalmology* 1983, 90:906.
4. Hijikata K, Matsuda K: Visual prognosis in Behçet's disease: effects of cyclophosphamide and colchicine, *Jpn J Ophthalmol* 1978, 22:506.
5. Nussenblatt RB, Palestine AG: *Uveitis: fundamentals and practice,* Chicago, 1989, Mosby.
6. Nussenblatt RB, Palestine AG, Chan CC, and others: Effectiveness of cyclosporin therapy for Behçet's disease, *Arthritis Rheum* 1985, 28:671.
7. BenEzra D, Brodsky M, Peer J, and others: Cyclosporin (CyA) versus conventional therapy in Behçet's disease. Preliminary observations of a masked study. In Shindler R, editor: *Cyclosporin in autoimmune diseases,* New York, 1985, Springer-Verlag New York, pp 158–161.
8. Chan CC, BenEzra D, Su-Ming H, and others: Granulomas in sympathetic ophthalmia: immunohistochemical study, *Arch Ophthalmol* 1985, 103:198.
9. Robin JB, Schanzlin DJ, Meisler DM, and others: Ocular involvement in the respiratory vasculitides, *Surv Ophthalmol* 1985, 30:127.
10. Fauci AS, Wolf SM: Wegener's granulomatosis: studies in eighteen patients and a review of the literature, *Medicine (Baltimore)* 1973, 52:535.
11. Bullen CL, Liesegang TJ, McDonald TJ, and others: Ocular complications of Wegener's granulomatosis, *Ophthalmology* 1983, 90:279.
12. Issak BL, Liesang TJ, Michet Jr CJ: Ocular and systemic findings in relapsing polychondritis, *Ophthalmology* 1986, 93:681.
13. Cheson BD, Bluming AZ, Alroy JA: Cogan's syndrome: a systemic vasculitis, *Am J Med* 1976, 60:549.
14. Nussenblatt RB, Gery I, Ballintine EJ, and others: Cellular immune responsiveness of uveitis patients to retinal S-antigen, *Am J Ophthalmol* 1980, 89:173–179.
15. Nussenblatt RB, Mittal KK, Ryan S, and others: Birdshot retinochoroidopathy associated with HLA-29 antigen and immune responsiveness to retinal S-antigen, *Am J Ophthalmol* 1982, 94:147.
16. Nussenblatt RB, Palestine AG, Chan CC: Cyclosporin A therapy in the treatment of intraocular inflammatory disease resistant to systemic corticosteroids and cytotoxic agents, *Am J Ophthalmol* 1983, 96:275.
17. Nussenblatt RB, Palestine AG, Chan CC, and others: Randomized, double masked study of cyclosporine compared to prednisolone in the treatment of endogenous uveitis, *Am J Ophthalmol* 1991, 112:138.
18. Opremcak EM: Personal communication, 1992.
19. Coster DJ, Shepherd WFI, Dhim Fook T, and others: Prolonged survival of corneal allografts in rabbits treated with cyclosporin A, *Lancet* 1979, 2:688.
20. Salisbury JD, Gebhardt BM: Suppression of corneal allograft rejection by cyclosporin A, *Arch Ophthalmol* 1981, 99:1640.
21. Belin MW, Bouchard CS, Frantz S, and others: Topical cyclosporine in high risk corneal transplants, *Ophthalmology* 1989, 96:1144.
22. Hill JC: The use of cyclosporine in high risk keratoplasty, *Am J Ophthalmol* 1989, 107:506.
23. Holland EJ, Chan CC, Kuwabara T, and others: Immunohistologic findings and results of treatment with cyclosporine in ligneous conjunctivitis, *Am J Ophthalmol* 1989, 107:160.
24. Rubin BI, Holland EJ, de Smet MD, and others: Response of reactivated ligneous conjunctivitis to topical cyclosporine, *Am J Ophthalmol* 1991, 112:95.
25. Bleik JH, Tabbara KF: Topical cyclosporine in vernal keratoconjunctivitis, *Ophthalmology* 1991, 98:1679.
26. BenEzra D, Pe'er J, Brodsky M, and others: Cyclosporine eye drops for the treatment of severe vernal keratoconjunctivitis, *Am J Ophthalmol* 1986, 101:178.
27. Secchi AG, Tognon MS, Leonardi A: Topical use of cyclosporine in the treatment of vernal keratoconjunctivitis, *Am J Ophthalmol* 1990, 110:641.

28. Mondino BJ, Brown SI: Immunosuppressive therapy in ocular cicatricial pemphigoid, *Am J Ophthalmol* 1983, 96:453.
29. Foster CS: Cicatricial pemphigoid, *Trans Am Ophthalmol Soc* 1986, 84:527.
30. Foster CS, Wilson LA, Ekins MB: Immunosuppressive therapy for progressive ocular cicatricial pemphigoid, *Ophthalmology* 1982, 89:340.
31. Neumann R, Tauber J, Foster CS: Remission and recurrence after withdrawal of therapy for ocular cicatricial pemphigoid, *Ophthalmology* 1991, 98:858.
32. Tauber J, de la Maza MS, Foster CS: Systemic chemotherapy for ocular cicatricial pemphigoid, *Cornea* 1991, 10(3):185.
33. Tauber J, de la Maza MS, Hoang-Xuan T, and others: An analysis of the therapeutic decision making regarding immunosuppressive chemotherapy for peripheral ulcerative keratitis, *Cornea* 1990, 9(1):66.
34. Foster CS, Forstot SL, Wilson LA: Mortality rate in rheumatoid arthritis patients developing necrotizing scleritis or peripheral ulcerative keratitis: effects of systemic immunosuppression, *Ophthalmology* 1984, 91:1253.
35. Foster CS: Systemic therapy for progressive bilateral Mooren's ulcer, *Ophthalmology* 1985, 92:1436.
36. Singh G, Wilson MR, Foster CS: Mitomycin eye drops as treatment for pterygium, *Ophthalmology* 1988, 95:813.
37. Hayasaka S, Noda S, Yamamoto Y, and others: Postoperative instillation of low-dose mitomycin-C in the treatment of primary pterygium, *Am J Ophthalmol* 1988, 106:715.
38. Hayasaka S, Noda S, Yamamoto Y, and others: Postoperative instillation of mitomycin-C in the treatment of recurrent pterygium, *Ophthalmic Surg* 1989, 20:580.
39. Rubinfeld RS, Pfister RR, Stein RM, and others: Serious complications of topical mitomycin-C after pterygium surgery, *Ophthalmology* 1992, 99:1647.
40. Shaw EL: A modified technique for conjunctival transplant, *CLAOJ* 1992, 18:112.
41. Kay JS, Litin BS, Jones MA, and others: Delivery of antifibroblastic agents as adjuncts to filtration surgery, part II. Delivery of 5-fluorouracil and bleomycin in a collagen implant: Pilot study in a rabbit, *Ophthalmic Surg* 1986, 17:796.
42. McGuigan LJ, Cook DH, Yablonski ME, and others: Dexamethasone, D-penicillamine, and glaucoma filtration surgery in rabbits, *Invest Ophthalmol Vis Sci* 1986, 27:1755.
43. McGuigan JB, Mason RP, Sanchez R, and others: D-penicillamine and beta-aminoproprionitrile effects on experimental filtering surgery, *Invest Ophthalmol Vis Sci* 1987, 28:1625.
44. Gressel MG, Parrish II RK, Folberg R: 5-fluorouracil and glaucoma filtering surgery: I. An animal model, *Ophthalmology* 1984, 91:378.
45. Bergstrom TJ, Wilkinson WS, Skuta GL, and others The effects of subconjunctival mitomycin-C on glaucoma filtration surgery in rabbits, *Arch Ophthalmol* 1991, 109:1725.
46. Pasquale LR, Thibault D, Dorman-Pease MW, and others: Effect of topical mitomycin-C on glaucoma filtration surgery in monkeys, *Ophthalmology* 1992, 99:14.
47. Fluorouracil Filtering Surgery Study Group: Fluorouracil filtering surgery one-year follow-up, *Am J Ophthalmol* 1989, 108:625.
48. Heuer DK, Parrish II RK, Gressel MG, and others: 5-fluorouracil and glaucoma filtering surgery: II. A pilot study, *Ophthalmology* 1984, 91:384.
49. Heuer DK, Parrish II RK, Gressel MG, and others: 5-fluorouracil and glaucoma surgery: III. Intermediate follow-up of a pilot study, *Ophthalmology* 1986, 93:1537.
50. Ruderman JM, Welch DB, Smith MF, and others: A randomized study of 5-fluorouracil and filtration surgery, *Am J Ophthalmol* 1987, 104 218.
51. Weinreb RN: Adjusting the dose of 5-fluorouracil after filtration surgery to minimize side effects, *Ophthalmology* 1987, 94:564.
52. Knapp A, Heuer DK, Stern GA, and others: Serious corneal complications of glaucoma surgery with postoperative 5-fluorouracil, *Am J Ophthalmol* 1987, 103:183.
53. Skuta GL, Beeson CC, Higginbotham EJ, and others: Intraoperative mitomycin-c versus 5-fluorouracil in high-risk glaucoma filtering surgery, *Ophthalmology* 1992, 99:438.
54. Chen CW: Enhanced intraocular pressure controlling effectiveness of trabeculectomy by local application of mitomycin-C, *Trans Asia Pacific Acad Ophthalmol* 1983, 9:172.
55. Palmer SS: Mitomycin as adjunct chemotherapy with trabeculectomy, *Ophthalmology* 1991, 98:317.
56. Kitazawa Y, Kawase K, Matsushita H, and others: Trabeculectomy with mitomycin: a comparative study with fluorouracil, *Arch Ophthalmol* 1991, 109:1693.
57. Derick RJ, Pasquale L, Quigley HA, and

others: Potential toxicity of mitomycin-C, *Arch Ophthalmol* 1991, 109:1635.
58. Bielory L, Frohman LP: Low-dose cyclosporine therapy of granulomatous optic neuropathy and orbitopathy, *Ophthalmology* 1991, 98:1732.
59. Prummel MF, Mourits MP, Berghout AB, and others: Prednisone and cyclosporine in the treatment of severe graves ophthalmopathy, *N Engl J Med* 1989, 321:1353.
60. Garrity JA, Kennerdall JS, Johnson BJ, and others: Cyclophosphamide in the treatment of orbital vasculitis, *Am J Ophthalmol* 1986, 102:97.
61. Wirtschaffter JD: Clinical doxyrubicin chemomyectomy: an experimental treatment for benign essential blepharospasm and hemifacial spasm, *Ophthalmology* 1991, 98:357.
62. Nussenblatt RB, Palestine AG, Chan CC: Improvement of uveitis and optic nerve disease by cyclosporine in a patient with multiple sclerosis, *Am J Ophthalmol* 1984, 96:790.
63. Peyman GA, Schulman J: Proliferative vitreoretinopathy and chemotherapeutic agents, *Surv Ophthalmol* 1985, 29:434.
64. Blumenkranz M, Hernandez E, Ophir A, and others: 5-Fluorouracil: new applications in complicated retinal detachments for an established antimetabolite, *Ophthalmology* 1984, 91:122.
65. Fiscella RR, Elvart J, Peyman GA, and others: In vivo evaluation of cellular inhibitory potential of various antineoplastic drugs and dexamethasone, *Ophthalmic Surg* 1985, 16:247.
66. Barrada A, Peyman GA, Greenburg D, and others: Toxicity of antineoplastic drugs in vitrectomy infusion fluids, *Ophthalmic Surg* 1983, 14:845.
67. Peyman GA, Stelmack T, Barrada A, and others: Toxicity of antineoplastic drug concentrations in vitrectomy infusion fluid, *Ophthalmic Surg* 1984, 15:844.
68. Miller DF, Bay JW, Lederman RJ, and others: Ocular and orbital toxicity following intracarotid injection of BCNU (carmustine) and cisplatinum for malignant gliomas, *Ophthalmology* 1985, 92:402.
69. Chrousos AK, Oldfield EH, Doppman JL, and others: Prevention of ocular toxicity of carmustine (BCNU) with supraophthalmic intracarotid infusion, *Ophthalmology* 1986, 93:1471.

## SECTION THREE

1. Leopold I: Corticosteroids in aqueous, *Am J Ophthalmol* 1954, 38:101.
2. Arendshorst W, Falls H: Role of the adrenal cortex in treatment of ocular diseases with pyrogenic substances, *Arch Ophthalmol* 1950, 44:635.
3. Makley TA, Opremcak EM: Foreign protein shock therapy in ophthalmology, *J Toxicol Cutan Ocular Toxicol* 1991, 10:27.
4. Haynes RC, Muroll F: Adrenocorticotropic hormone. Adrenocortical steroids and their synthetic analogs. In Gilman AG, Goodman LS, Rall TW, and others, editors: *The pharmacologic basis of therapeutics,* ed 7. New York, 1985, Macmillan, p 1459.
5. Goldfien A: Adrenocorticosteroids and adrenocortical antagonists. In Katzung BG, editor: *Basic and clinical pharmacology,* Los Altos, Calif, 1984, Lange Medical Publications, p 453.
6. Leopold IH: The steroid shield in ophthalmology, *Trans Am Acad Ophthalmol Otolaryngol* 1967, 71:273.
7. O'Rourke JF, Iser G, Ryan R: An initial evaluation of prednisone therapy in ocular inflammation, *Arch Ophthalmol* 1956, 55:323.
8. Neilson RH: The use of dexamethasone in ophthalmologic steroid therapy, *Arch Ophthalmol* 1959, 62:438.
9. Gordon D: Dexamethasone in ophthalmology, *Am J Ophthalmol* 1959, 48:656.
10. Hollander JL: Clinical use of dexamethasone, *JAMA* 1960, 172:306.
11. Boland EW: Chemically modified adrenocortical steroid, *JAMA* 1960, 174:835.
12. Kupferman A, Leibowitz HM: Penetration of fluorometholone into the cornea and aqueous humor, *Arch Ophthalmol* 1975, 93:425.
13. Yamauchi H, Kito H, Uda K: Studies on intraocular penetration and metabolism of fluorometholone in rabbits: a comparison between dexamethasone and prednisolone acetate, *Jpn J Ophthalmol* 1975, 19:339.
14. Hogan MJ, Thygeson P, Kimura S: Effects of prednisone and prednisolone in ocular inflammation, *Trans Am Acad Ophthalmol* 1955, 59:779.
15. Gordon D: Prednisone and prednisolone in ocular disease, *Am J Ophthalmol* 1956, 41:593.
16. King Jr JH, Passmore JW, Skeehan Jr RA, and others: Prednisone and prednisolone

in ophthalmology, *Trans Am Acad Ophthalmol* 1955, 59:759.
17. Woods A: The present status of ACTH and cortisone in clinical ophthalmology, *Am J Ophthalmol* 1951, 34:945.
18. Commercial, Allergan Pharmaceuticals, Santa Ana, Calif.
19. Kreines K, Weinberg IC: The selection of adrenocorticosteroid preparations, *Ohio State Med J* 1975, 71:698.
20. Duke-Elder S, Ashton N: Action of cortisone on tissue reactions of inflammation and repair with special reference to the eye, *Br J Ophthalmol* 1951, 35:695.
21. Francois J, Feher J: Studies with the polarization microscope of the fibroblastic activity of the regenerating rabbit's cornea under the influence of corticosteroids, *Exp Eye Res* 1973, 15:201.
22. Leopold IH, Maylath F: Intraocular penetration of cortisone and its effectiveness against experimental corneal burns, *Am J Ophthalmol* 1952, 35:1125.
23. Bahn GC, Sonnier E, Allen JH: Therapeutic studies in experimental chemical injury of the cornea, *Am J Ophthalmol* 1959, 48:253.
24. Hook RM, Hook CW, Brown SI: Fibroblast collagenase partial purification and characterization, *Invest Ophthalmol* 1973, 12:771.
25. Brown SI: Collagenase and corneal ulcers, *Invest Ophthalmol* 1971, 10:203.
26. Brown SI, Weller CA, Vidrich A: Effect of corticosteroids on corneal collagenase of rabbits, *Am J Ophthalmol* 1970, 70:744.
27. Ashton N, Cock C: Effect of cortisone on healing of corneal wounds, *Br J Ophthalmol* 1951, 35:708.
28. Palmerton ES: The effect of local cortisone on wound healing in rabbit corneas, *Am J Ophthalmol* 1951, 35:708.
29. Gasset AR, Lorenzetti DWC, Ellison EM, and others: Quantitative corticosteroid effect on corneal wound healing, *Arch Ophthalmol* 1969, 81:589.
30. Beams R, Linabery L, Grayson M: Effect of topical corticosteroids on corneal wound strength, *Am J Ophthalmol* 1968, 66:1131.
31. McDonald TO, Borgmann AR, Roberts MD, and others: Corneal wound healing, *Invest Ophthalmol* 1970, 9:703.
32. Polack FM, Rosen PN: Topical steroids and tritiated thymidine uptake, *Arch Ophthalmol* 1967, 77:400.
33. Fink A, Baras I: Effect of steroids on tensile strength of corneal wound, *Am J Ophthalmol* 1956, 42:759.
34. Basu PK: Effect of different steroids on the healing of nonperforating corneal wounds in rabbits, *Arch Ophthalmol* 1958, 59:657.
35. Weinstein BI, Altman K, Gordon GG, and others: Specific glucocorticoid receptor in the iris-ciliary body of the rabbit, *Invest Ophthalmol* 1977, 16:973.
36. Southren AL, Gordon GG, Yeh HS, and others: Nuclear translocation of the cytoplasmic glucocorticoid receptor in the iris–ciliary body of the rabbit, *Invest Ophthalmol* 1979, 18:517.
37. Weinreb RN, Bloom E, Baxter JD, and others: Detection of glucocorticoid receptors in cultured human trabecular cells, *Invest Ophthalmol* 1981, 21:403.
38. Hernandez MR, Wenk EJ, Weinstein BI, and others: Corneal-conjunctival uptake of topical $^3$H-dexamethasone in the rabbit eye, *Invest Ophthalmol* 1981, 20:120.
39. Tchernitchin A, Wenk EJ, Hernandez MR, and others: Glucocorticoid localization by radio-autography in the rabbit eye following systemic administration of $^3$H-dexamethasone, *Invest Ophthalmol* 1980, 19:1231.
40. Kasavina BS Chesnokova NB: Lysosomal hydrolases of the eye tissues and the effect of corticosteroids on their activity, *Exp Eye Res* 1973, 16:227.
41. Francois J: Corticosteroid glaucoma, *Ann Ophthalmol* 1977, 9:1075.
42. Nathanson JA: Adrenergic regulation of intraocular pressure: Identification of $B_2$-adrenergic-stimulated adenylate cyclase in ciliary process epithelium, *Proc Natl Acad Sci USA* 1980, 77:7420.
43. Zink HA, Palmberg PF, Bigger JF: Increased sensitivity to theophylline associated with primary open-angle glaucoma, *Invest Ophthalmol* 1973, 12:603.
44. Adams BA, Brubaker RF: Caffeine has no clinically significant effect on aqueous humor flow in normal eyes, *Ophthalmology* 1990, 97:1030.
45. Cooper JAD, Daniels CA, Trofatter KF: The effect of prednisolone on antibody-dependent cell-medicated cytotoxicity and the growth of type I herpes simplex virus in human cells, *Invest Ophthalmol* 1978, 17:381.
46. McCarty G, Schwartz B, Miller K: Absence of lymphocyte glucocorticoid hypersensitivity in primary open-angle glaucoma, *Arch Ophthalmol* 1981, 99:1258.
47. Srinivasan BD, Kulkarni PS: Polymorpho-

nuclear leukocyte response, *Arch Ophthalmol* 1981, 99:1085.
48. Leibowitz HM, Kupferman A: Topically administered corticosteroids, *Arch Ophthalmol* 1980, 98:1287.
49. Leibowitz HM: Management of inflammation in the cornea and conjunctiva, *Ophthalmology* 1980, 87:753.
50. Leibowitz HM, Hyndiuk RA, Lindsey C, and others: Fluorometholone acetate: clinical evaluation in the treatment of external ocular inflammation, *Ann Ophthalmol* 1984, 16:1110.
51. Leibowitz HM, Ryan WJ, Kupferman AK: Comparative antiinflammatory efficacy of topical corticosteroids with low glaucoma-inducing potential, *Arch Ophthalmol* 1992, 110:118.
52. Hull DS, Green K, Buyer J: Cornea endothelial bicarbonate fluxes following storage in moist chamber, MK medium, and MK medium with added hydrocortisone, *Invest Ophthalmol Vis Sci* 1979, 18:484.
53. Zimmerman TJ, Dawson WW, Fitzgerald CR: Part I. Electroretinographic changes in normal eyes during administration of prednisone, *Ann Ophthalmol* 1973, 5:757.
54. Zimmerman TJ, Dawson WW, Cade JR: Part II. Electroretinographic changes, *Ann Ophthalmol* 1973, 5:769.
55. Zimmerman TJ, Dawson WW, Fitzgerald CR: ERG in human eyes following oral adrenocorticoids, *Invest Ophthalmol* 1973, 12:777.
56. Streeten DHP: Corticosteroid therapy: I. Pharmacological properties and principles of corticosteroid use, *JAMA* 1975, 232:944.
57. Ashton N, Cook C, Langham M: Effect of cortisone on vascularization and opacification of the cornea induced by alloxan, *Br J Ophthalmol* 1951, 35:718.
58. Ashton N, Cook C: In vivo observations of the effects of cortisone upon the blood vessels in the rabbit ear chambers, *Br J Exp Pathol* 1952, 33:32.
59. Heffernan JT, Futterman S, Kalina RE: Dexamethasone inhibition of experimental endothelial cell proliferation in retinal venules, *Invest Ophthalmol* 1978, 17:565.
60. BenEzra D: Dexamethasone inhibition of cell proliferation, *Invest Ophthalmol* 1979, 18:220.
61. Takashima R: Corticosteroid effects on the corneal surface of rabbits studied by scanning electron microscopy, *Jpn J Ophthalmol* 1975, 19:393.
62. Hamashige S, Potts A: The penetration of cortisone and hydrocortisone into the ocular structures, *Am J Ophthalmol* 1955, 40:211.
63. Janes RG, Stiles JF: The penetration of cortisol into normal and pathologic rabbit eyes, *Am J Ophthalmol* 1963, 56:84.
64. Green H, Kroman H, Leopold IH: Corticosteroids in the aqueous humor of the rabbit, *Arch Ophthalmol* 1955, 54:853.
65. Murdick PW, Keates RH, Donovan EF, and others: Ocular penetration studies, *Arch Ophthalmol* 1966, 76:602.
66. Fleming TC, Merrill DL: Water soluble and non-water soluble hydrocortisone, Research report no 5, Alcon Laboratories, Fort Worth, Tex.
67. Leopold IH: Intraocular penetration of local hydrocortisone and cortisone, *Arch Ophthalmol* 1954, 52:769.
68. Leopold IH, Kroman H, Green H: Intraocular penetration of prednisone and prednisolone, *Trans Am Acad Ophthalmol* 1955, 59:771.
69. Kupferman A, Leibowitz HM: Topically applied steroids in corneal disease, *Arch Ophthalmol* 1974, 92:331.
70. Leopold IH, Kroman HS: Methyl and fluoro-substituted prednisolones in the blood and aqueous humor of the rabbit, *Arch Ophthalmol* 1960, 63:943.
71. Kroman HS, Leopold IH: Studies upon methyl- and fluoro-substituted prednisolones in the aqueous humor of the rabbit, *Am J Ophthalmol* 1961, 52:77.
72. Leibowitz HM, Kupferman A, Stewart RH, and others: Evaluation of dexamethasone acetate as a topical ophthalmic formulation, *Am J Ophthalmol* 1978, 86:418.
73. Kupferman A, Leibowitz HM: Penetration of fluorometholone into the cornea and aqueous humor, *Arch Ophthalmol* 1975, 93:425.
74. Cox WV, Kupferman A, Leibowitz HM: Topically applied steroids in corneal disease: II. The role of the drug vehicle in stromal absorption of dexamethasone, *Arch Ophthalmol* 1972, 88:549.
75. Kupferman A, Ryan WJ, Leibowitz HM: Prolongation of antiinflammatory effect of prednisolone acetate. Influence of formulation in high viscosity gel, *Arch Ophthalmol* 1981, 99:2028.
76. Kupferman A, Leibowitz HM: Biological equivalence of ophthalmic prednisolone acetate suspensions, *Am J Ophthalmol* 1976, 82:109.

77. Kaufman HE: *Ocular antiinflammatory therapy,* Springfield, Ill, 1970, Charles C Thomas, Publisher.
78. McDonald TO, Kasten K, Hervey R, and others: Comparative toxicity of dexamethasone and its tertiary butyl acetate ester after topical ocular instillation in rabbits, *Am J Ophthalmol* 1973, 76:117.
79. Leibowitz HM, Kupferman A: Kinetics of topically administered prednisolone acetate, *Arch Ophthalmol* 1976, 94:1387.
80. Nussenblatt RB, Palestine AG: Philosophy, goals and approaches to medical therapy. In *Uveitis, fundamentals and clinical practice,* Chicago, 1989, Mosby, p 115.
81. Gordon D: The treatment of chronic uveitis, *Arch Ophthalmol* 1959, 62:400.
82. Klinefelter HF, Winkenwerder WL, Bledsoe T: Single daily dose prednisone therapy, *JAMA* 1979, 241:2721.
83. *AMA drug evaluations,* ed 4, Chicago, 1980, American Medical Association.
84. Sugar A, Benson W, Burder RM, and others: Alternate-day versus daily systemic corticosteroids in corneal homograft rejection, *Am J Ophthalmol* 1973, 75:486.
85. Breitenfield RV, Hebert LA, Lemann J, and others: Stability of renal transplant function with alternate-day corticosteroid therapy, *JAMA* 1980, 244:151.
86. Kaufman HE: Practical considerations in the selection of antiinflammatory agents, *Trans Am Acad Ophthalmol Otolaryngol* 1975, 79:80.
87. Krupin T, Johnson MF, Haimann MH, and others: Plasma cortisol and elective cataract surgery, *Am J Ophthalmol* 1978, 85:475.
88. Leibowitz HM, Kupferman A: Periocular injection of corticosteroids, *Arch Ophthalmol* 1977, 95:311.
89. Cloes RS, Krohn DL, Breslin H, and others: Depo-Medrol in treatment of inflammatory diseases, *Am J Ophthalmol* 1962, 54:407.
90. Sturman RM, Laval J, Sturman MF: Subconjunctival triamcinolone acetonide, *Am J Ophthalmol* 1966, 61:155.
91. Hyndiuk RA, Reagan MG: Radioactive depot-corticosteroid penetration into monkey ocular tissue, *Arch Ophthalmol* 1968, 80:499.
92. Bohigian G, Dawson C, Coleman V: Retrobulbar administration of steroids in herpes simplex uveitis, *Arch Ophthalmol* 1971, 85:320.
93. Schlaegel Jr TF, Wilson FM: Accidental intraocular injection of depot corticosteroids, *Trans Am Acad Ophthalmol Otolaryngol* 1974, 78:847.
94. McLean EB: Inadvertent injection of corticosteroid into the choroidal vasculature, *Am J Ophthalmol* 1976, 81:835.
95. Raab EL: Limitation of motility after periocular corticosteroid injection, *Am J Ophthalmol* 1974, 78:996.
96. Nozik RA: Orbital rim fat atrophy after repository periocular corticosteroid injection, *Am J Ophthalmol* 1976, 82:928.
97. Herschler J: Increased intraocular pressure induced by repository corticosteroids, *Am J Ophthalmol* 1976, 82:90.
98. O'Connor GR: Periocular corticosteroid injections: uses and abuses, *Eye Ear Nose Throat Mon* 1976, 55:83.
99. McCuen BW, Bressler M, Tano Y, and others: The lack of toxicity of intravitreally administered triamcinolone acetonide, *Am J Ophthalmol* 1981, 91:785.
100. King RA, Ellis PP: Treatment of chalazia with corticosteroid injections, *Ophthalmol Surg* 1986, 17:351.
101. Epstein GA, Putterman AM: Combined excision and drainage with intralesional corticosteroid injection in the treatment of chronic chalazia, *Arch Ophthalmol* 1988, 106:514.
102. Garrett GW, Gillespie ME, Mannix BC: Adrenocorticoid injection vs. conservative therapy in the treatment of chalazia, *Ann Ophthalmol* 1988, 20:196.
103. Pizzarella LD, Jakobiec FA, Hofeldt AJ, and others: Intralesional corticosteroid therapy of chalazia, *Am J Ophthalmol* 1979, 87:582.
104. Thomas EL, Laborde RP: Retinal and choroidal vascular occlusion following intralesional corticosteroid injection of a chalazion, *Ophthalmology* 1986, 93:405.
105. Kushner BJ: Local steroid therapy in adnexal hemangioma, *Ann Ophthalmol* 1979, 11:1005.
106. Raichand M, Peyman GA, Schwartz H, and others: Antiinflammatory action of dexamethasone in vitrectomy infusion fluid, *Ophthalmol Surg* 1982, 13:493.
107. Graham RO, Peyman GA: Intravitreal injection of dexamethasone, *Arch Ophthalmol* 1974, 92:149.
108. Maxwell DP, Brent BD, Diamond JG, and others: Effect of intravitreal dexamethasone on ocular histopathology in a rabbit model of endophthalmitis, *Ophthalmology* 1991, 98:1370.
109. Keller N, Longwell AM, Birss SA: Intermit-

tent vs. continuous steroid administration, *Arch Ophthalmol* 1976, 94:644.
110. Farber MD, Fiscella R, Goldberg M: Aminocaproic Acid versus prednisone for treatment of traumatic hyphema. *Ophthalmology* 1991, 98:279.
111. Beck RW, Cleary PA, Anderson MA, and others: A randomized controlled trial of corticosteroids in the treatment of acute optic neuritis, *N Engl J Med* 1968, 278:911.
112. Burch PG, Migeon CJ: Systemic absorption of topical steroids, *Arch Ophthalmol* 1968, 79:174.
113. Krupin T, Mandell AI, Podos SM, and others: Topical corticosteroid therapy and pituitary-adrenal function, *Arch Ophthalmol* 1976, 94:919.
114. O'Day DM, McKenna TJ, Elliott JH: Ocular corticosteroid therapy: systemic hormonal effects, *Trans Am Acad Ophthalmol Otolaryngol* 1975, 79:71.
115. Hogan M, Thygeson P, Kimura S: Uses and abuses of adrenal steroids and corticotropin, *Arch Ophthalmol* 1955, 53:165.
116. Ballet AJ, Black R, Bunim J: Major undesirable side effects from prednisolone and prednisone, *JAMA* 1955, 158:459.
117. Nicoloff DM, Soisin H, Peter ET, and others: The effect of cortisone on peptic ulcer formation, *JAMA* 1963, 183:1019.
118. Boley SJ, Allen AC, Schultz L, and others: Potassium-induced lesions of the small bowel, *JAMA* 1965, 193:997.
119. Allen AC, Boley SJ, Schultz L, and others: Potassium-induced lesions of the small bowel, *JAMA* 1965, 193:1001.
120. Lawrason FD, Albert E, Mohr FL, and others: Ulcerative-obstructive lesions of the small intestine, *JAMA* 1965, 191:641.
121. Curtiss PH, Clark WS, Herndon C: Vertebral fractures resulting from prolonged cortisone and corticotropin therapy, *JAMA* 1954, 156:467.
122. Griffiths HJ: Etiology, pathogenesis, and early diagnosis of ischemic necrosis of the hip, *JAMA* 1981, 246:2615.
123. Cruess RL: Steroid-induces avascular necrosis of the head of the humerus, *J Bone Joint Surg* 1976, 58B:313.
124. Cruess RL, Ross D, Crawshaw E: The etiology of steroid-induced avascular necrosis of bone, *Clin Orthop* 1975, 113:178.
125. Fisher DE, Bickel WH, Holley KE, and others: Corticosteroid-induced aseptic necrosis: II. Experimental study, *Clin Orthop* 1972, 84:200.
126. Fisher DE, Bickel WH: Corticosteroid-induced avascular necrosis, *J Bone Joint Surg* 1971, 53A:859.
127. Solomon L: Drug-induced arthropathy and necrosis of the femoral head, *J Bone Joint Surg* 1973, 55B:246.
128. Klipper AR, Stevens MB, Zizic TM, and others: Ischemic necrosis of bone in systemic lupus erythematosus, *Medicine (Baltimore)* 1976, 55:251.
129. Boettcher WG, Bonfiglio M, Hamilton HH, and others: Nontraumatic necrosis of the femoral head, *J Bone Joint Surg* 1970, 52A:312.
130. Harrington KD, Murray WR, Kountz SL, and others: Avascular necrosis of bone after renal transplantation, *J Bone Joint Surg* 1971, 53A:203.
131. Patterson RJ, Bickel WH, Dahlin DC: Idiopathic avascular necrosis of the head of the femur, *J Bone Joint Surg* 1964, 46A:267.
132. Velayos EE, Leidholt JD, Smyth CJ, and others: Arthropathy associated with steroid therapy, *Ann Intern Med* 1966, 64:759.
133. Heimann WG, Freiberger RH: Avascular necrosis of the femoral and humeral heads after high-dosage corticosteroid therapy, *N Engl J Med* 1960, 263:672.
134. Sudarsky RD: Exudative type of retinal separation, *Arch Ophthalmol* 1959, 62:5.
135. Romano PE, Traisman HS, Green OC: Fluorinated corticosteroid toxicity in infants, *Am J Ophthalmol* 1977, 84:287.
136. Walker AE, Adamkiewicz JJ: Pseudotumor cerebri associated with prolonged corticosteroid therapy, *JAMA* 1964, 188:779.
137. Ivey KJ, DenBesten L: Pseudotumor cerebri associated with corticosteroid therapy in an adult, *JAMA* 1969, 208:1698.
138. Cohen BZ, Tripathi RC: Eyelid depigmentation after intralesional injection of a fluorinated corticosteroid for chalazion, *Am J Ophthalmol* 1979, 88:269.
139. Gottlieb NL, Penneys NS: Spontaneous skin tearing during systemic corticosteroid treatment, *JAMA* 1980, 243:1260.
140. Slansky HH, Kolbert G, Gartner S: Exophthalmos induced by steroids, *Arch Ophthalmol* 1967, 77:579.
141. Barber AN, Afeman C, Willis J: Inheritance of congenital anophthalmia in mice, *Am J Ophthalmol* 1959, 48:763.
142. Michejda M, Hodgen GD: In utero diagnosis and treatment of non-human primate fetal skeletal anomalies, *JAMA* 1981, 246:1093.
143. Hodgen GD: Antenatal diagnosis and treat-

ment of fetal skeletal malformations, *JAMA* 1981, 246:1079.

144. There's no "safe trimester" with teratogenic drugs, *JAMA* 1975, 234:264.
145. Kimura SJ, Okumoto M: The effect of corticosteroids on experimental herpes simplex keratoconjunctivitis in the rabbit, *Am J Ophthalmol* 1957, 43:131.
146. Thygeson P, Geller HO, Schwartz A: Effect of cortisone on experimental herpes simplex keratitis of the rabbit, *Am J Ophthalmol* 1951, 34:885.
147. Kumura SJ, Bonnet V, Okumoto M, and others: The effect of corticosteroid hormones on experimental herpes simplex keratitis, *Am J Ophthalmol* 1961, 51:945.
148. McCoy G, Leopold IH: Simplex infections of the cornea, *Am J Ophthalmol* 1960, 49:1355.
149. Ostler HB: Glucocorticoid therapy in ocular herpes simplex: I. Limitations, *Surv Ophthalmol* 1978, 23:35.
150. Pavan-Langston D, Abelson MB: Glucocorticoid therapy in ocular herpes simplex: II. Advantages, *Surv Ophthalmol* 1978, 23:35.
151. Berger BB, Weinberg RS, Tessler HH, and others: Bilateral cytomegalovirus panuveitis after high-dose corticosteroid therapy, *Am J Ophthalmol* 1979, 88:1020.
152. Marmor MF, Egbert PR, Egbert BM, and others: Optic nerve head involvement with cytomegalovirus in an adult with lymphoma, *Arch Ophthalmol* 1978, 96:1252.
153. Anderson B, Shaler SR, Cesar G: Mycotic ulcerative keratitis, *Arch Ophthalmol* 1959, 62:169.
154. Mitsui Y: Corneal infections after cortisone therapy, *Br J Ophthalmol* 1955, 39:244.
155. Fazakas: Magyar Orvosi A. 35:325, 1934, K.M. Aug. 96:227, 1936. Cited in Duke-Elder S: *Textbook of ophthalmology,* vol 5, St Louis, 1952, Mosby, p 5299.
156. Nema HV, Ahuja OP, Bal A, and others: Effects of topical corticosteroids and antibiotics on mycotic flora of conjunctiva, *Am J Ophthalmol* 1968, 65:747.
157. Ley AP: Fungus keratitis, *Arch Ophthalmol* 1956, 56:877.
158. Berson EL, Kobayashi GS, Becker B, and others: Topical corticosteroids and fungal keratitis, *Invest Ophthalmol* 1967, 6:512.
159. Birge HL: Ocular aspects of mycotic infections, *Arch Ophthalmol* 1952, 47:354.
160. Suie T, Taylor FW: The effect of cortisone on experimental *Pseudomonas* corneal ulcers, *Arch Ophthalmol* 1956, 56:53.
161. Elliott ID, Halde C, Shapiro J: Keratitis and endophthalmitis caused by *Petriellidium boydii, Am J Ophthalmol* 1977, 83:16.
162. Ballen PH, Loffredo FR, Painter B: *Listeria* endophthalmitis, *Arch Ophthalmol* 1979, 97:101.
163. Schwartz LK, Loignon LM, Webster RG: Post traumatic phycomycosis of the anterior segment, *Arch Ophthalmol* 1978, 96:860.
164. Woods AC: Studies in experimental ocular tuberculosis, *Arch Ophthalmol* 1958, 59:559.
165. Laboratory Subcommittee of the Committee on Medical Research: The effect of cortisone and/or corticotropin on experimental tuberculosis infection in animals [statement prepared by the subcommittee], *Am Rev Tuberc* 1952, 66:257.
166. Committee on Therapy: The effect of cortisone and/or corticotropin on tuberculosis infection in man [statement prepared by the committee], *Am Rev Tuberc* 1952, 66:254.
167. Krupin T, LeBlanc RP, Becker B, and others: Uveitis in association with topically administered corticosteroid, *Am J Ophthalmol* 1970, 70:883.
168. Shin DH, Kass MS, Kolker AE, and others: Positive FTA-ABS tests in subjects with corticosteroid-induced uveitis, *Am J Ophthalmol* 1976, 82:259.
169. Laval J, Collier R: Elevation of intraocular pressure due to hormonal steroid therapy in uveitis, *Am J Ophthalmol* 1955, 39:175.
170. Goldman H: Cortisone glaucoma, *Arch Ophthalmol* 1962, 68:621.
171. Bernstein HN, Schwartz B: Effects on long-term systemic steroids on ocular pressure and tonographic values, *Arch Ophthalmol* 1962, 68:742.
172. Briggs HH: Glaucoma associated with the use of topical corticosteroid, *Arch Ophthalmol* 1963, 70:312.
173. Bernstein HN, Mills DW, Becker B: Steroid-induced elevation of intraocular pressure, *Arch Ophthalmol* 1963, 70:15.
174. Armaly MF Effect of corticosteroids on intraocular pressure and fluid dynamics, *Arch Ophthalmol* 1963, 70:482.
175. Becker B, Mills DW: Corticosteroids and intraocular pressure, *Arch Ophthalmol* 1963, 70:500.
176. Mindel JS, Goldberg J, Tavitian HO: Similarity of the intraocular pressure response to different corticosteroid esters when compliance is controlled, *Trans Am Acad Ophthalmol* 1979, 86:99.

177. Mindel JS, Tavitian HO, Smith H, and others: Comparative ocular pressure elevation by medrysone, fluorometholone, and dexamethasone phosphate, *Arch Ophthalmol* 1980, 98:1577.
178. Cantrill HL, Palmberg PF, Zink HA, and others: Comparison of in vitro potency of corticosteroids with ability to raise intraocular pressure, *Am J Ophthalmol* 1975, 79:1012.
179. Stewart RH, Smith JP, Rosenthal AL: Ocular response to fluorometholone acetate and dexamethasone sodium phosphate, *Curr Eye Res* 1984, 3:835.
180. LeBlanc RP, Stewart RH, Becker B: Corticosteroid provocative testing, *Invest Ophthalmol* 1970, 9:946.
181. Armaly MF: Effect of corticosteroids on intraocular pressure and fluid dynamics, *Arch Ophthalmol* 1964, 71:636.
182. Becker B, Mills DW: Corticosteroid eye drops and intraocular pressure, *Sight Sav Rev* 1963, 33:130.
183. Becker B, Mills DW: Elevated intraocular pressure following corticosteroid eye drops, *JAMA* 1963, 185:170.
184. Armaly MF: Statistical attributes of the steroid hypertensive response in the clinically normal eye, *Invest Ophthalmol* 1965, 4:187.
185. Armaly MF: The heritable nature of dexamethasone-induced ocular hypertension, *Arch Ophthalmol* 1966, 75:32.
186. Becker B, Hahn KA: Topical corticosteroids and heredity in primary open-angle glaucoma, *Am J Ophthalmol* 1964, 57:543.
187. Becker B, Ballin N: Glaucoma and corticosteroid provocative testing, *Arch Ophthalmol* 1965, 74:621.
188. Rosenbaum LJ, Alton E, Becker B: Dexamethasone testing in Southwestern Indians, *Invest Ophthalmol* 1970, 9:325.
189. Foon KA, Yuen K, Ballintine EJ, and others: Analysis of the systemic corticosteroid sensitivity of patients with primary open-angle glaucoma, *Am J Ophthalmol* 1977, 83:167.
190. Becker B, Bresnick G, Chevrette L, and others: Intraocular pressure and its response to topical corticosteroids in diabetes, *Arch Ophthalmol* 1966, 76:477.
191. Schwartz B, Seddon JM: Increased plasma cortisol levels in ocular hypertension, *Arch Ophthalmol* 1981, 99:1791.
192. Schwartz B, Golden MA, Wiznia RA, and others: Differences of adrenal stress control mechanisms in subjects with glaucoma and normal subjects, *Arch Ophthalmol* 1981, 99:1770.
193. Ray S, Mehra KS, Misra S, and others: Plasma cortisol in glaucoma, *Ann Ophthalmol* 1977, 9:1151.
194. Krupin T, Jacobs LS, Podos SM, and others: Thyroid function and the intraocular pressure response to topical corticosteroids, *Am J Ophthalmol* 1977, 83:643.
195. Francois J, Heintz-DeBree C, Tripathi RC: The cortisone test and the heredity of primary open-angle glaucoma, *Am J Ophthalmol* 1966, 62:844.
196. Schwartz JT, Reuling Jr FH, Feinleib M, and others: Twin heritability study of the corticosteroid response, *Trans Am Acad Ophthalmol Otolaryngol* 1973, 77:126.
197. Schwartz JT, Reuling FH, Feinleib M, and others: Twin study on ocular pressure following topically applied dexamethasone: II. Inheritance of variation in pressure response, *Arch Ophthalmol* 1973, 90:281.
198. Schwartz JT, Reuling FH, Feinleib M, and others: Twin study on ocular pressure after topical dexamethasone: I. Frequency distribution of pressure response, *Am J Ophthalmol* 1973, 76:126.
199. Palmberg PF, Mandell A, Wilensky JT, and others: The reproducibility of the intraocular pressure response to dexamethasone, *Am J Ophthalmol* 1975, 80:844.
200. Becker B: The effect of topical corticosteroid in secondary glaucomas, *Arch Ophthalmol* 1964, 72:769.
201. Shammas HF, Halasa AH, Faris BM: Intraocular pressure, cup-disc ratio, and steroid responsiveness in retinal detachment, *Arch Ophthalmol* 1976, 94:1108.
202. Zink HA, Palmberg PF, Sugar A, and others: Comparison of in vitro corticosteroid response in pigmentary glaucoma and primary open-angle glaucoma, *Am J Ophthalmol* 1975, 80:478.
203. Rothkoff L, Biedner B: Response to corticosteroid testing in patients with early increased intraocular pressure after cataract, *Glaucoma* 1980, 1:257.
204. Obstbaum SA, Podos SM: Ocular compression and noncorticosteroidal antiinflammatory agents, *Am J Ophthalmol* 1975, 79:1008.
205. Bigger JF, Palmberg PF, Zink HA: In vitro corticosteroid: correlation response with primary open-angle glaucoma and ocular corticosteroid sensitivity, *Am J Ophthalmol* 1975, 72:92.
206. Lewis JM, Priddy T, Judd J, and others:

Intraocular pressure response to topical dexamethasone as a predictor for the development of primary open-angle glaucoma, *Am J Ophthalmol* 1988, 106:607.
207. Kalina RE: Increased intraocular pressure following subconjunctival corticosteroid administration, *Arch Ophthalmol* 1969, 81:788.
208. Roberts W: Rapid progression of cupping in glaucoma, *Am J Ophthalmol* 1968, 66:520.
209. Frenkel M, Krill AE: Effects of two mineralocorticoids on ocular tension, *Arch Ophthalmol* 1964, 72:315.
210. Dorsch W, Thygeson P: The clinical efficacy of medrysone, a new ophthalmic steroid, *Am J Ophthalmol* 1968, 65:74.
211. Spaeth GL: Hydroxymethylprogesterone, *Arch Ophthalmol* 1966, 75:783.
212. Bedrossian RH, Eriksen SP: The treatment of ocular inflammation with medrysone, *Arch Ophthalmol* 1969, 81:184.
213. Podos SM, Krupin T, Asseff C, and others: Topically administered corticosteroid preparations, *Arch Ophthalmol* 1971, 86:251.
214. Kitazawa Y: Increased intraocular pressure induced by corticosteroids, *Am J Ophthalmol* 1976, 82:492.
215. Kass MA, Sears ML: Hormonal regulation of intraocular pressure, *Surv Ophthalmol* 1977, 22:153.
216. Oglesby R, Black R, von Sallmann L, and others: Cataracts in patients with rheumatic disease treated with corticosteroids, *Arch Ophthalmol* 1961, 66:625.
217. Giles CL, Mason GL, Duff IF, and others: The association of cataract formation and systemic corticosteroid therapy, *JAMA* 1962, 182:719.
218. Donshik PC, Cavanaugh HD, Boruchoff SA, and others: Posterior subcapsular cataracts induced by topical corticosteroids following keratoplasty for keratoconus, *Ann Ophthalmol* 1981, 13:29.
219. Skalka HW, Prchal JT: Effect of corticosteroids on cataract formation, *Arch Ophthalmol* 1980, 98:1773.
220. Pfefferman R, Gombos GM, Kountz SL: Ocular complications after renal transplantation, *Ann Ophthalmol* 1977, 9:467.
221. Yablonski ME, Burde RM, Kolker AE, and others: Cataracts induced by topical dexamethasone in diabetics, *Arch Ophthalmol* 1978, 96:474.
222. Wiesinger H, Irby R: Posterior subcapsular cataract (PSC) in patients with rheumatoid arthritis treated with corticosteroids, *Invest Ophthalmol* 1963, 2:294.
223. Oglesby RB, Black RL, von Sallmann L, and others: Cataracts in rheumatoid arthritis patients treated with corticosteroids, *Arch Ophthalmol* 1961, 66:97.
224. Greiner JV, Chylack LT: Posterior subcapsular cataracts, *Arch Ophthalmol* 1979, 97:135.
225. Eshagian J, Rafferty NS, Goossens W: Human cataracts complicata, clinicopathologic correlation, *Ophthalmology* 1981, 88:155.
226. Forman AR, Loreto JA, Tina LU: Reversibility of corticosteroid-associated cataracts in children with the nephrotic syndrome, *Am J Ophthalmol* 1977, 84:75.
227. Gordon DM, Kammerer WH, Freyberg RH: Examination for posterior subcapsular cataracts, *JAMA* 1961, 175:127.
228. Leibold JE, Itkin IH: Cataracts in asthmatics treated with corticosteroids, *JAMA* 1963, 185:448.
229. Pfahl SB, Makley TA, Rothermich N, and others: The relationship of steroid therapy and cataracts in patients with rheumatoid arthritis, *Am J Ophthalmol* 1961, 52:831.
230. Havre DC: Cataracts in children on long-term corticosteroid therapy, *Arch Ophthalmol* 1965, 73:818.
231. Braver DA, Richards RD, Good TA: Posterior subcapsular cataracts in steroid treated children, *Arch Ophthalmol* 1967, 77:161.
232. Ohguchi M, Ohno S, Shiono H, and others: Posterior subcapsular cataracts in children in long-term corticosteroid therapy, *Jpn J Ophthalmol* 1975, 19:254–260.
233. Cronin TP: Cataract with topical use of corticosteroid and idoxuridine, *Arch Ophthalmol* 1964, 72:198.
234. Burde RM, Becker B: Corticosteroid-induced glaucoma and cataracts in contact lens wearers, *JAMA* 1970, 213:2075.
235. Virno M, Schirru A, Percori-Giraldi J, and others: Aqueous humor alkalosis and marked reduction in ocular ascorbic acid content following long-term topical cortisone (9a-fluoro-16a-methylprednisolone), *Ann Ophthalmol* 1974, 6:983.
236. Sundmark E: The cataract-inducing effect of systemic corticosteroid therapy, *Acta Ophthalmol* 1966, 44:291.
237. Spaeth GL: Effects of topical dexamethasone on intraocular pressure and the water drinking test, *Arch Ophthalmol* 1966, 76:772.

238. Kern R, Macri FJ: Steroid eye drops and effect on isolated intraocular muscles of monkeys, *Arch Ophthalmol* 1967, 78:794.
239. Newsome DA, Wong VG, Cameron TP, and others: "Steroid-induced" mydriasis and ptosis, *Invest Ophthalmol* 1971, 10:424.
240. Pfister RR, Murphy GE: Corneal ulceration and perforation associated with Sjögren's syndrome, *Arch Ophthalmol* 1980, 98:89.
241. Brown SI, Grayson J: Marginal furrows, *Arch Ophthalmol* 1968, 79:563.
242. Greenwood BM: Capillary resistance and skin-fold thickness in patients with rheumatoid arthritis: effect of corticosteroid therapy, *Ann Rheum Dis* 1966, 25:272.
243. Krachmer JH, Laibson PR: Corneal thinning and perforation in Sjögren's syndrome, *Am J Ophthalmol* 1974, 78:917.
244. Ashton N, Hobbs HE: Effect of cortisone on rheumatoid nodules of the sclera, *Br J Ophthalmol* 1952, 36:373.
245. Mathias D: Scleromalacia perforans, *Am J Ophthalmol* 1955, 39:161.
246. Baum JL, Levene RZ: Corneal thickness after topical corticosteroid therapy, *Arch Ophthalmol* 1968, 79:366.
247. Aihara Y: A study of fluorescein angiography on steroid-induced retinopathy in rabbits, *Jpn J Ophthalmol* 1980, 24:196.
248. Mathias CGT, Maibach HI, Ostler HB, and others: Delayed hypersensitivity to retrobulbar injections of methylprednisolone acetate, *Am J Ophthalmol* 1978, 86:816.
249. Byers B: Blindness secondary to steroid injections into the nasal turbinates, *Arch Ophthalmol* 1979, 97:79.
250. Wilson RS, Havener WH, McGrew RN: Bilateral retinal artery and choriocapillaris occlusion following the injection of long-acting steroid suspensions in combination with other drugs: I. Clinical studies, *Trans Am Acad Ophthalmol* 1978, 85:967.
251. Wilson RS, McGrew RB, White HJ: Bilateral retinal artery and choriocapillaris occlusion following the injection of long-acting steroid suspensions in combination with other drugs: II. Animal experimental studies, *Trans Am Acad Ophthalmol* 1978, 85:975.
252. Havener WH: Corticosteroid misuse. In Leopold I, Burns R, editors: *Symposium on ocular therapy,* vol 8, New York, 1975, John Wiley & Sons.

CHAPTER 8

# Biologic Drugs

Kenneth V. Cahill

Mary Lou Kachmer McGregor

## TETANUS

Wounds about the eye, just as those elsewhere in the body, may be the site of entry of *Clostridium tetani*. The management of each ocular wound therefore requires consideration of specific prophylactic measures against tetanus. The physician's task in the management of these cases is considerably more involved than making a decision between use of antitoxin and toxoid booster on the basis of prior immunization. Proper judgment of the management of potential cases of tetanus (every patient with an unsterile wound has a potential case of tetanus) requires knowledge of the following facts.[1–4]

The tetanus organism is widespread, developing in the gastrointestinal tracts of humans and animals and existing in spore form in soil and dust. Development of the spores requires anaerobic conditions such as exist in wounds that are contaminated by foreign material or contain devitalized tissue. The symptoms of tetanus result from toxemia and not from spread of infection through the body. Tetanus produces one of the most potent neurotoxins known. A lethal amount of tetanus toxin is too small to induce immunity, which accounts for the well-established fact that a patient who has survived a tetanus infection has no resistance against reinfection and must be immunized just as anyone else. Once the toxin has reached the nerve fibers, it cannot be removed by antitoxins.

A wound contaminated with tetanus does not suppurate unless there is associated infection with other bacteria. An apparently trivial or already well-healed wound may contain viable tetanus organisms. The incubation period varies from 2 to 30 days, depending on the nature of the wound and the severity of contamination, and may be prolonged if antitoxin has been given. Signs of local tetanus about the wound precede systemic manifestations in the majority of patients. Dirty wounds, extensive wounds, or wounds for which treatment has been delayed should be considered more dangerous potential sources of tetanus. Thorough cleaning with soap and water, careful removal of foreign material, and debridement of severely injured tissue that may be sacrificed without functional or cosmetic loss are of importance in minimizing the possibility of tetanus infection of such a wound. Because of routine immunization of infants for tetanus, the incidence of tetanus in Europe and North America is very low. About 70 cases in the United States are reported to the Centers for Disease Control each year, which probably represents 50% of the actual occurrence. The incidence is much higher in Asia and Africa where immunization is not administered as widely.

### Passive Immunization

Tetanus antitoxin (tetanus immune globulin) is a biologic product obtained from humans or horses that have been immunized against tetanus toxin. Human tetanus immune globulin (HTIG) is preferable to horse tetanus immune globulin and is now used routinely when temporary passive immunization is indicated. It is virtually free of the risk of inducing hypersensitivity, which may be seen in patients receiving horse tetanus immune globulin. The half-life of HTIG in the patient is 3 to 4 weeks, whereas the half-life of horse tetanus immune globulin may be only a few days. The dosage of HTIG is 4 units/kg of body weight given intramuscularly, or for adults, a dose of 250 units is usually administered.[5]

Horse tetanus immune globulin is administered only in rare situations when HTIG is not available. Much higher intramuscular doses of horse tetanus immune globulin have been given (up to 10,000 units) because of the body's destruction of this foreign (heterologous) immune globulin.

Determination of sensitivity to horse serum is through intradermal injection of 0.1 ml of a 1:10 dilution of antitoxin. Before this injection, the patient should be questioned carefully about previous allergic conditions, especially asthma, urticaria, known sensitivity to horses, and reactions to past injections of sera. Epinephrine should be available for instant injection should it be needed. If the antitoxin test dose is placed peripherally on an extremity, a tourniquet may be applied in the event of a reaction, temporarily arresting further absorption. If no reaction appears within 30 minutes, the test is repeated with 0.1 ml of undiluted antitoxin. If this test result is also negative, the antitoxin may be given intramuscularly or subcutaneously. A positive skin reaction consists of a wheal, which is supposed to be larger in more sensitive individuals. A wheal less than 5 mm in diameter may represent a nonspecific reaction to injury, which may be determined by a control test with normal saline solution (use a different syringe and needle). If an equal reaction occurs to the saline solution, the tetanus antitoxin reaction is considered negative. Negative skin test results do not exclude the possibility of later severe serum sickness.

The value of administration of horse tetanus immune globulin to a patient sensitive to horse serum is doubtful. Such a sensitized patient has antibodies that will destroy the antitoxin, thereby decreasing or completely nullifying the desired therapeutic effect of passive immunity. Furthermore, the risk of acute anaphylactic reaction, delayed serum sickness, damage to the central nervous system, and similar allergic complications may far outweigh the possible benefit to be obtained from prophylactic use of horse antitoxin.

### Active Immunization

Because of the transient and possibly inadequate protection attained by passive immunization, active immunization is far preferable and is advised for all persons beginning in infancy. Inoculation with tetanus toxoid is virtually free of significant side effects and is highly effective. During World War II only 12 cases of tetanus occurred among members of the U.S. Armed Forces (only one case was fatal), and six of these were in patients who had not yet been properly immunized. Hospital admissions for service injuries numbered 2,735,000 during this period. In contrast to this military record, 500 to 600 civilians die of tetanus in the United States each year.

Active immunity is attained by giving three intramuscular injections of 0.5 ml of alum-precipitated tetanus toxoid. During the first month of immunization the antitoxin titer is very low, and the patient cannot be considered protected (Fig. 8–1). Very soon after the second injection, satisfactory titers are attained and last for about 1 year but not reliably longer. The third injection is a vital part of the basic immunization and should not be considered an optional booster. After the third injection, a rapid and prolonged elevation of antitoxin titer occurs, averaging 10 units/ml 1 month after injection. Once this basic level of immunization has been attained, subsequent booster doses will stimulate an adequate and prompt antibody response for as long as 15 years and possibly for a lifetime. In fact, the immunity attained from booster doses is so effective that a repeat booster is not recommended for a wound incurred less than 10 years after the last booster injection unless the wound is exceptionally contaminated.

The duration of effective tetanus immunization is usually much longer than generally realized.[6] Approximately 90% of indi-

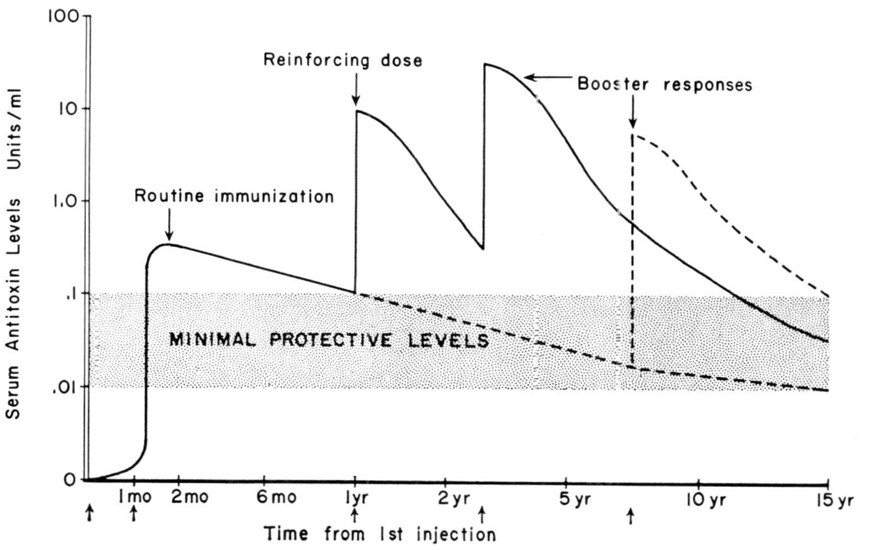


**FIG 8–1.**
Average response to tetanus toxoid injections. Arrows indicate times of injection of 0.5 ml of toxoid. *Solid line:* rise in circulating antitoxin levels attained by initial, 1-month, 1-year, and booster injections. *Broken line:* drop in titer in patients who did not receive subsequent injections (Modified from Filler RM, Ellerbeck WJ: *JAMA* 174:1, 1960. Used by permission.)

viduals immunized to tetanus during World War II still had protective levels of antibody 20 years later. Twelve years after immunization in infancy, only 4% of 190 children had antibody levels less than the threshold of protection. Of 45 immunized children encountered in routine pediatric practice for the purpose of receiving a booster shot (for summer camp, a wound, etc.), all were found to have tetanus antibody levels from 40 to 2,500 times higher than the minimum protective level. Exaggerated local reactions to tetanus toxoid may develop in some hyperimmunized individuals.

At the time of an injury all patients who have not previously been immunized should begin active immunization. Tetanus antitoxin should be considered a medication to be administered only once in a lifetime. If it is used, simultaneous or subsequent active immunization should be mandatory and is the responsibility of the physician giving the antitoxin. Active and passive immunization may be initiated simultaneously, provided that the injections are made into different extremities with separate syringes. Alum-precipitated (not fluid) toxoid must be used if antitoxin is to be given simultaneously. (It is not definitely established that fluid toxoid is superior to alum-precipitated toxoid for any purpose, including attaining a more rapid effect from a booster dose.) The second and third toxoid injections should subsequently be given at the usual intervals of 1 month and 1 year.[7]

Infants receive combined diphtheria-pertussis-tetanus (DPT) immunizations at 2, 4, and 6 months of age, a fourth at 18 months of age, and a fifth at 5 years of age.

Past adverse reactions to tetanus toxoid were reported by 740 Air Force recruits. Of these, 730 had negative skin test results and were uneventfully immunized. Ten had positive skin test results; of these, one fainted and one had a fever 4 days later. Three patients showed a local allergy to the thimerosal preservative.[8] Apparently historic reports of reactions to tetanus toxoid are not valid and certainly do not contraindicate booster immunization when indicated, with prophylactic medications at hand should an unexpected reaction occur. This risk of immunization is weighed against the fact that even trivial puncture wounds can cause tetanus in a nonimmunized individual.[9]

## Antibiotic Prophylaxis

The vegetative form of *C. tetani* (not the spores) is very sensitive to metronidazole, penicillins, cephalosporins, imipenem, erythromycin, the macrolides, and tetracycline. These antibiotics may be employed to kill the organisms before toxin is produced. Antitoxin neutralizes toxin but has no effect on the organisms in the local wound.

Antibiotics should not be used as a substitute for active immunization or for clearly indicated passive immunization. If antibiotic prophylaxis for tetanus is employed in addition to immunization, blood levels should be maintained for 3 weeks to protect against late-germinating spores. This prolonged antibiotic therapy is usually reserved for large contaminated wounds.

### Summary

The principles of tetanus prophylaxis may be summarized as follows:

1. Tetanus-prone wounds are those contaminated with dirt, feces, or saliva; punctures (including the use of unsterile needles and injections through unprepared skin); missile wounds; burns; frostbite; avulsions; and crush injuries.
2. All wounds should receive accepted local surgical care.
3. Immunized patients should receive tetanus toxoid at the time of injury if:
   a. It has been at least 10 years since they last received tetanus toxoid.
   b. They have a tetanus-prone wound and it has been at least 5 years since they received tetanus toxoid.
4. Nonimmunized patients should begin active immunization with tetanus toxoid at the time of injury. If they have sustained a tetanus-prone wound, they should receive 250 units of HTIG intramuscularly.
5. Patients with an uncertain history of immunization should be treated as nonimmunized patients until their immunization status can be determined.
6. Patients with humoral immunodeficiencies, including human immunodeficiency virus (HIV) infection, should receive HTIG for any tetanus-prone wound in addition to the previously listed guidelines.
7. Patients with symptoms of tetanus from a prior injury require emergent intensive medical care.

## *CLOSTRIDIUM PERFRINGENS*

*Clostridium perfringens* is an anaerobic bacillus closely related to tetanus and particularly destructive to tissue. It can cause gas gangrene panophthalmitis, which typically results in rapid purulent ocular destruction, usually with loss of vision within 12 hours after injury. A review of 53 cases indicates that the eye has invariably been lost despite treatment with penicillin or gas gangrene antitoxin.[10] The characteristics of intraocular *Clostridium* infection include unusually severe pain, early rise in intraocular pressure, coffee-colored discharge (hemolysis), gas bubbles in the anterior chamber, and loss of vision. Unfortunately, destruction of the eye is so rapid that cultural diagnosis of the organism is of no value in guiding antibiotic selection.

## RUBELLA

The congenital rubella syndrome, with its severe damage to eyes, heart, and brain, came dramatically to our attention during the 1964–1965 pandemic. The United States suffered 20,000 malformed infants and 30,000 stillbirths at an estimated cost of $1.5 billion. Introduction of the clinical use of rubella vaccine in 1969 permitted an effective attack on the problem. In the decade between 1967 and 1977, the incidence of rubella in schoolchildren decreased by 90%. Vigorous enforcement of school laws requiring rubella vaccination for entry should continue. Efforts to vaccinate susceptible women are still recommended, because there remains a proportion of these women who are vulnerable to the risk of a malformed infant.[11–14] Adult female rubella screening can be implemented at various opportunities, including enrollment in higher education, application for marriage licenses, abortion and family planning clinics, and even in obstetric wards to protect the children of subsequent pregnancies.[15]

A 1978 California study of 450 women between the ages of 14 and 35 years showed 33% to have low serum titers, indicating susceptibility to rubella. The patient's history of having had a clinical attack of German measles was worthless. Of women who believed they had sustained such an infection, only 74% actually had serum titer–proved immunity. Of women who denied having had rubella, 65% were immune. Serologic testing is the only way to establish immune status.

An outbreak of rubella in Chicago in 1978 resulted in at least 31 infants with congenital rubella syndrome (incidence of 49/100,000 live births).[14] None of these mothers had been immunized, 74% were unmarried, and 64% were primigravidas.[14] Another outbreak of 23 infants born with congenital rubella syndrome occurred in 1990 in southern California.[15] Of the 21 mothers, nine were born in other countries. Of the 12 mothers educated in California, only four were subject to the 1982 California law requiring rubella vaccination for enrollment in ninth grade. These episodes prove that our communities are still vulnerable to rubella-induced tragedies.

After vaccination, seroconversion to an immune status occurs in 98% of patients and persists for at least 10 years.[16] These data support the policy of vaccinating schoolchildren and indicate that protection should extend to the childbearing years without revaccination.

The fetal risk of inadvertent rubella immunization during early pregnancy was studied in 215 cases. Elective abortion was chosen by half of these women in preference to the risk of fetal abnormality. Rubella virus was isolated from placental or fetal specimens in seven of these cases. However, the other half of the pregnancies that were not interrupted resulted in not a single infant with evidence of rubella infection or damage.[17, 18]

Of another 94 women inadvertently vaccinated during pregnancy, all gave birth to healthy infants.[19] The practice of recommending abortion under such circumstances is not endorsed. Only four children born with congenital rubella syndrome after first trimester vaccination have been reported, and in each instance historic information suggested the probable cause to be a concomitant infection with wild rubella.[20]

Although the purpose of rubella immunization is not the protection of the vaccinated individual but of a potentially exposed and as yet nonexistent fetus, immunization of hospital employees has been suggested.[21] Securing the cooperation of the target population is apparently not easy. Of 11 obstetrics-gynecology specialists known to be nonimmune and vulnerable to infection that could spread to their patients, only one consented to vaccination. The presumed reason for failure to cooperate was knowledge that 50% of vaccinated persons have reactions consisting of fever and joint pain lasting from 1 to 6 days, with onset 8 to 12 days after vaccination.[22] Some hospitals now require proof of immunity to rubella for employment and for physician staff privileges.

Passive protection against rubella is conferred by intravenous injection of 30 ml of human serum obtained from volunteers approximately 3 weeks after disappearance of their rubella rash. To be effective, this serum must be injected within 5 days after exposure to rubella infection.[23]

Such passive rubella prophylaxis may be indicated for women during the first trimester of pregnancy because the incidence of serious congenital malformations caused by rubella in the first trimester is about 17%.[24, 25] Unfortunately, the results of passive rubella prophylaxis in protecting an unborn fetus are equivocal.

## Summary

After first-trimester rubella, perhaps 20% of infants will suffer from the congenital rubella syndrome. Rubella vaccine was introduced in 1969, and compulsory school entry vaccination occurred subsequently. Many women of childbearing age have not been vaccinated and are not immune as a result of naturally occurring infection. This pool of potential mothers would benefit from immunization, which is strongly recommended. Ophthalmologists should encourage this effective preventive measure against congenital cataract, glaucoma, and even worse eye conditions.

## RUBEOLA

The dramatic potential of an immunization program is illustrated by the fact that between 1962 (the year of licensure of measles [rubeola] vaccine) and 1982, the incidence of measles in the United States decreased by 99.4%. This disease is on the verge of elimination.[26]

## HEPATITIS B

The hepatitis B carrier rate in the United States is 0.3%, and 200,000 new infections occur annually. In addition to causing a severe acute illness, hepatitis B may cause death from cirrhosis, hepatic carcinoma, or immune complex diseases such as polyarteritis nodosa. As high as 20% of surgeons show serologic evidence of past hepatitis B infection.[27]

In 1982, a plasma-derived hepatitis B vaccine (Heptavax-B) was approved. In 1986, hepatitis B vaccines derived from hepatitis B surface antigen (HBsAg) using recombination DNA technology in yeast cultures became available (Engerix-B, Heptavax-B). This newer form of vaccine has no known possibility of transmitting the acquired immunodeficiency syndrome (AIDS) virus. It is contraindicated in people who are hypersensitive to yeast. The vaccination regimen consists of three doses, with one given initially, one at 1 month, and one 6 months after the initial dose. Each dose should be 2.5 μg for children from birth through 10 years of age, 5 μg for patients aged 11 through 19 years, and 10 μg for patients 20 years and older. A dialysis formulation containing 40 μg is recommended for adult dialysis patients. The injections should be given in the anterolateral thigh for young children and in the deltoid muscle of older children and adults. Protective levels of antibody are induced in 96% of children and adults. The duration of the protective effect is unknown at present, and the need for booster doses has not been defined. Adverse effects of hepatitis B vaccination have been reported at the site of the injection in 17% of injections and systemically in 15% of the injections. Injection site reactions include pain, tenderness, pruritus, erythema, ecchymosis, swelling, warmth, and nodule formation. The most frequent systemic complaints are fatigue, weakness, headache, fever, and malaise. The Occupational Safety and Health Administration (OSHA) requires that all health care workers who are at risk for hepatitis B exposure be educated about this risk and be given the opportunity to be vaccinated at no cost.

Infants born to HBsAg-positive mothers should receive 0.5 ml of human hepatitis B immune globulin intramuscularly in the anterolateral thigh. Active immunization with the HBsAg vaccine should be initiated within 7 days. The first vaccine dose may be given at the same time as the immune globulin but should be injected into the contralateral thigh.

Human hepatitis B globulin is also advised for individuals exposed to hepatitis B virus through (1) needlestick, ocular, or mucous membrane exposure to blood known or presumed to contain HBsAg; (2) human bites that penetrate the skin by known or presumed HBsAg carriers; or (3) intimate sexual contact with known or presumed HBsAg carriers. Human hepatitis B immune globulin (0.06 ml/kg) should be administered intramuscularly as soon as possible after exposure. Active immunization should be initiated with intramuscular HBsAg vaccine at a separate site within 7 days. The worldwide use of hepatitis B vaccination has been hampered by the cost of the three vaccination doses, which exceeds $100 per person.[28]

## HERPES SIMPLEX

γ-Globulin obtained from human blood has been studied for treatment or prophylaxis of ocular virus infections, including herpes simplex, herpes zoster, rubella, and vaccinia. The improvement of vaccinia ocular lesions seems to be well established. The response of herpetic infections is uncertain.

Human γ-globulin has been used topically and parenterally in the treatment of herpetic keratitis, generally with disappointing results. Such failures have been attributed to the inability of the antibody proteins to penetrate the avascular cornea and the inaccessibility of the intracellular virus. To determine whether immunoglobulin could penetrate to the iris and ciliary body, the severity of herpetic iridocyclitis was studied in control rabbits and in rabbits preinoculated with 5 ml of γ-globulin.[29] During the first 4 days after virus inoculation and after 8 days, the iridocyclitis was equal in treated and control groups. No treated animals were protected against infection. From the fifth through the seventh day, the eyes of treated animals were less inflamed than those of control animals.

In the treatment of experimental rabbit herpes simplex keratitis, γ-globulin with a specific antibody titer of 1:512 was not of value during the acute epithelial stage of infection.[30] However, γ-globulin seemed to reduce the severity of inflammation during the chronic stromal stage of the disease.

Active and passive immunization of rabbits, even when very high titers of serum antibodies were achieved, did not protect the animals against herpes simplex keratitis, nor was the course of the disease modified.[31] Treatment with topical application of serum antibody to the infected corneas was of absolutely no benefit. However, the immunized rabbits were protected against an intravenous dose of virus sufficient to cause death from encephalomyelitis in three of four rabbits. Presumably this indicates that circulating or locally applied antibodies cannot penetrate the cornea in therapeutic amounts.

Rabbits immunized by limbal injection of killed herpes simplex virus have a less severe keratitis develop than do control animals inoculated intracorneally with live virus.[32]

The available evidence seems to indicate that immune globulin treatment of herpes simplex ocular infections is ineffective. Acyclovir offers a systemic therapy for herpes simplex in addition to the topical ocular antiviral medications available.

## HERPES ZOSTER

Administration of 250 ml of serum obtained from patients previously infected with herpes zoster was reported to improve the course of ocular herpes zoster.[33] Of 22 treated patients, 83% retained vision better than 6/18. In comparison, 60% of 39 untreated patients maintained 6/18 or better vision. These series of patients were uncontrolled and subject to some variables in selection; hence, the value of herpes zoster immunotherapy is difficult to assess.

In a double-blind study of zoster immune plasma, this treatment did not alter the course of cutaneous herpes zoster. Furthermore, the untreated patients actually had higher antibody titers develop than did those treated.[34]

Herpes zoster occurs with selective frequency in patients with blood dyscrasia.[35] One might speculate that this indicates reduced immunologic resistance, possibly replaceable by administration of immune serum.

Systemic acyclovir has been approved for the treatment of herpes zoster and appears to lessen the intensity and duration of infection.

## INTERFERONS

The interferons are proteins produced by the body in response to foreign antigens, such as those found on viruses, bacteria, and tumor cells.[36, 37] Interferons can induce the synthesis of RNA and protein, inhibit cellular proliferation, and produce other immunomodulary effects. Three major classes of interferons have been designated based on the cell type found to produce them They are interferon-α (leukocyte interferon), interferon-β (fibroblast interferon), and interferon-γ (immune interferon). Interferons can now be produced by recombinant DNA techniques, making their clinical use possible.

Interferon therapy has been approved by the U.S. Food and Drug Administration for five clinical indications. Interferon-α is approved for hairy-cell leukemia, condyloma acuminatum, Kaposi's sarcoma in AIDS, and type C viral hepatitis. Interferon-γ is approved as an immunomodulatory treatment for chronic granulomatous disease. Interferons have also shown some promise in the treatment of basal cell carcinoma, chronic myelogenous leukemia, cutaneous squamous cell carcinoma, early HIV infection, hepatitis B, and laryngeal papillomatosis caused by the human papillomavirus.

Interferons have shown some benefit in treating ophthalmic diseases.[38–41] Topical interferon has shown some activity in the treatment of herpes simplex keratitis and has a potentiating effect with acyclovir or trifluorothymidine. Topical interferon may have some effect on adenoviral keratoconjunctivitis and enteroviral acute hemorrhagic conjunctivitis. Interferons have also been studied for Behçet's disease, Sjögren's syndrome, Graves' disease, retinoblastoma, cytomegalovirus retinitis, subretinal neovascularization, and recurrent conjunctival papillomas, but their therapeutic role is uncertain. The side effects of systemic interferon therapy limit their usefulness, because they often cause an influenza-like syndrome and other systemic problems.

## FIBRINOLYTIC AGENTS

The body contains both clotting and anticlotting mechanisms. Plasminogen, the precursor of plasmin, may be activated by streptokinase (from streptococci), urokinase (from urine), and tissue plasminogen activator (tPA). Plasmin dissolves fibrin and thereby hastens absorption of blood clots not more than a few days old. The use of tPA is reviewed in Chapter 16.

## BOTULINUM TOXIN

### Strabismus

Dr. Alan B. Scott began his research on the effect of botulinum A toxin in the 1970s, and in 1977 the first injection into human extraocular muscles was performed.[42, 43] Since then many thousands of patients have been treated around the world using this technique. The idea of using botulinum A toxin was sparked by the observation that blurred vision, double vision, or both are observed in approximately 90% of patients with systemic botulism. Dr. Scott believed that the effects of this potent toxin could be harnessed in a therapeutic fashion. Once the mechanism of action and the clinical efficacy in strabismus were determined, it became apparent that there were many other important uses for this toxin. Botulinum A toxin is now used in the treatment of strabismus,[44-48] blepharospasm,[49-56] lateral rectus palsy, hemifacial spasm, Meige syndrome, facial synkinesis after facial nerve palsy, and spasmodic torticollis (Table 8–1).[44]

Before clinical trials could be established, it was important to understand the pharmacology and the physiology of botulinum toxin. Botulinum toxin is produced by the bacteria *Clostridium botulinum*. There are at least six antigenically separate toxins: A, B, C, D, E, and F. Clinical work has focused on type A toxin. The reason for this is that type A toxin retains its toxigenicity very well during the isolation process and is highly potent in a variety of media. The toxin can also be easily crystallized to obtain a stable form that maintains its potency for several years.[57]

Botulinum toxin is a very potent neuroparalytic agent. It acts primarily on peripheral cholinergic synapses. Here it inhibits the release of the neurotransmitter acetylcholine. Without acetylcholine, widespread muscular paralysis is generated. The gradual overwhelming paralysis that ensues after botulism poisoning can be fatal.

**TABLE 8–1.**
Uses of Botulinum A Toxin

| |
|---|
| Strabismus |
| Lateral rectus palsy |
| Essential blepharospasm |
| Hemifacial spasm |
| Meige syndrome |
| Facial synkinesis after facial nerve palsy |
| Spasmodic torticollis |
| Creation of temporary ptosis to protect the cornea |

Botulinum toxin type A is a large molecular weight neurotoxin that has a high affinity for skeletal muscle. Once it binds to the membrane receptors at the presynaptic neuromuscular junction, it inhibits muscle contraction. The exact mechanism by which it inhibits muscle contraction can be divided into several stages.[58]

The first stage is the binding to the membrane. Next there is translocation of the toxin across the cell membrane. The last stage is the actual step responsible for long-term paralysis. The neurotoxin prevents the release of acetylcholine into the synaptic junction. This is the result of an enzymatic action on calcium ion channels. Paralysis ensues over the next several days. Histologic changes can be identified after paralysis has been present for several weeks. It is noted that terminal and preterminal motor nerve fibers develop new sprouts and new muscle receptors develop. Because of this rearborization of motor nerve fibers, paralysis is a temporary phenomenon. The length of paralysis varies extensively, however.

Once the pharmacologic effect of toxin causes paralysis of the muscle, a mechanical effect occurs. This mechanical effect must occur for long-term effects to be seen after injection of botulinum toxin for strabismus. The belief is that after paralysis there is an alteration in the muscle length-tension relationship. The classic example is in a cranial nerve VI palsy where the lateral rectus muscle is paralyzed. The ipsilateral medial rectus contracts against the paralyzed lateral rectus muscle. It is believed that this contracture increases with time and that there is an eventual shortening of the muscle. Once this occurs, the medial rectus then exerts an increased passive tension on the paretic lateral rectus muscle. As a lateral rectus muscle is pulled, it elongates as if it is being stretched. This results in the inability of abduction or persistent esotropia even if there is full recovery of the sixth nerve palsy.

Dr. Scott believes that botulinum toxin can "balance the forces" and prevent the change in the length-tension relationship. Therefore, as the lateral rectus regains function, it is able to fully assume its mechanical action without having been affected by a change in its length. The same change in mechanical action is postulated to occur in other forms of strabismus. The treated muscle becomes paralyzed and allows its antagonistic muscle to "take up the slack." After the pharmacologic effect of the toxin has worn off, it is hoped that the antagonistic muscle has recoiled in a manner that makes it stronger. If this occurs, one would see long-term stability in the new alignment.[60]

When the treatment of strabismus is discussed, it is important to remember that fusion is sometimes a driving force in the maintenance of good alignment. Botulinum toxin may also work through a sensory modality. Temporary realignment provides the opportunity for single binocular vision. Fusion may be regained and then maintained because of sensory status.[61] If alignment can be achieved in an infant, there is an opportunity for stimulation of binocular cortical cells. This may prevent their atrophy and improve their function if the patient is young enough. This is the reasoning of many of the ophthalmologists who treat infantile esotropia with botulinum toxin injection into the medial rectus muscle.[62]

## Method of Injection for Strabismus

Botulinum A toxin is strictly controlled and distributed by Allergan Pharmaceuticals (Irvine, Calif.) under the trade name Botox at this time. Directions for reconstitution are enclosed with each vial of toxin. It is very important to remember that one must use saline solution without any preservatives when the toxin is reconstituted. The material rapidly loses potency when left open. Twenty-six-gauge needles attached to an electromyogram (EMG) signal are necessary for inserting the toxin into the desired extraocular muscle. Currently there are multiple injection electrodes available. Some institutions fashion their own and maintain their desired sharpness. A standard bipolar concentric electrode technique is preferable, but a monopolar needle technique is also possible. Monopolar signals can be sufficiently strong when one is injecting into a previously uninjected, unoperated muscle. However, the signal becomes very weak and difficult to find when the muscle has been previously injected or there is significant scar tissue because of previous surgery. When the EMG signal is weak, the bipolar electrode method is helpful. A battery-driven differential amplifier has been developed that allows for easier detection of the muscle signal. The patient is placed in a comfortable position either flat on their back or in a chair that reclines. The eye to be injected is anesthetized with 5 topical anesthetic drops over 5 minutes before the procedure. Next it is helpful to put 1 drop of epinephrine into the eye to constrict the blood vessels and help prevent unnecessary bleeding of conjunctival vessels. The appropriate ground wires are placed. The syringe is filled with toxin. The needle is then placed on the syringe and the toxin injected until it comes through the tip of the syringe. This is to ensure that there is no dead space within the needle. These small details are very important because only a very small amount of toxin is to be injected. Next the attachment electrodes and ground wire are checked. The patient is asked to look away from the muscle to be injected. For example, if the right lateral rectus muscle is to be injected, the patient is asked to look into left gaze. An experienced ophthalmic surgeon can usually detect where the muscle lies. The needle is inserted tangentially through the conjunctiva at the level of the muscle. Once the conjunctiva has been entered, the patient is now asked to look in primary position to allow minimal contact of the extraocular muscle with the globe. The needle is then gradually pushed into the orbit to follow the line of the muscle for 10 to 20 mm. You can be certain you are in the muscle by having the patient look right and left. You can hear the EMG recording rise as the muscle contracts and fall as it relaxes. Once the EMG signal is strong, the appropriate unit dose is given. One should then hold the needle in position for approximately one minute to help prevent the seeping of the toxin from the injection site. The needle is then removed and the ground wire is removed from the patient. It is best to patch the patient because the eye is anesthetized. The patient is usually told to remove the patch several hours later.

### Therapeutic Information

When the initial study of botulinum toxin for use in strabismus was performed, all forms of strabismus were involved in the study. Only patients who had a stable deviation for 6 months or more before injection were enrolled. The goal of the study was to determine the appropriate dose of toxin. It was determined that the threshold effect for any amount of paralysis lies between $1.25 \times 10^{-5}$ and $6.25 \times 10^{-5}$ μg.[63] Once the dose was determined, there were several other important factors that required investigation. There was a concern that some people might show increasing tolerance through development of an antibody to botulinum toxin. It was noted that no patient has shown any tolerance to botulinum. It is believed that the small dose used is not recognized by the immune system, and therefore no antibody is formed. It was also noted in these initial studies that there was quite a significant variability between patients who were injected with the same dose. Because of this variable response to recommended doses, a percentage of patients will require a second injection at a later time.

Complications after injection of the toxin include:

1. Corneal irritation.
2. Discomfort at the time of the injection.
3. Prolonged discomfort of the eye after injection. This complication usually occurs if the needle tip touches orbital periosteum or there is significant scar tissue from previous surgeries. There is no way to prevent it, and analgesic medication is recommended after the procedure.
4. Subconjunctival hemorrhage from needle insertion. Vertical rectus muscles are more prone to hemorrhage. Pressure can be applied to the eye if the hemorrhage continues to enlarge once the needle is removed.
5. Effect of the drug on adjacent muscles. This complication is usually a temporary side effect.
6. No effect of the toxin injection. This usually occurs because the dose was inadequate or the injection was not into the muscle itself.

7. Diplopia. This complication can be caused when the new alignment does not involve a suppression scotoma.

8. Penetration of the sclera. Such penetration has occurred, and there was no effect on the final vision of the patient.[64]

9. Retrobulbar hemorrhage. Retrobulbar hemorrhage is possible if one enters the muscle cone.

In most causes of strabismus, extraocular muscle surgery still produces a more stable and predictable result than botulinum A toxin injections.[65] Botulinum A toxin is helpful in weakening the antagonist muscle and decreasing chances for contracture in cases of acute paralytic strabismus, especially cranial nerve VI palsy.[66] Injections are also useful in the treatment of small deviations and sensory deviations and as a trial in adults to see if intractable diplopia might occur after surgical correction.

### Essential Blepharospasm

Botulinum A toxin has become the most commonly used treatment for patients with benign essential blepharospasm, idiopathic orofacial dystonia (Meige's syndrome), idiopathic oromandibular dystonia (Breughel's syndrome), and hemifacial spasm. Subcutaneous injections in the areas of abnormal muscle contraction result in a temporary weakening of these muscles. The effect gradually increases during the first 2 weeks after injection and gradually decreases thereafter. The muscular weakening usually provides patients with adequate symptomatic relief to perform normal activities for 2 to 6 months, with 3 months being average. Patients typically can be managed with three or four sets of injections per year. The injections do not eliminate the involuntary orbicularis muscle spasms but weaken them so that they can be overcome by the voluntary action of the levator muscle.

The placement of the injections can be adjusted for the characteristics of the spasms in each patient. The central upper lid is usually avoided to minimize chances of levator muscle weakening with subsequent ptosis. The central and medial lower lid is typically not treated to minimize chances of ectropion and diplopia. A typical dosage and distribution of the botulinum A toxin for a patient with benign essential blepharospasm is shown (Fig. 8–2). This type of figure can be reproduced in the patient's chart to facilitate efficient and accurate record keeping. Some practitioners advise that the first treatment for a patient should be half of the usual dose. The patient can be rechecked in 3 weeks when the maximum effect should already have been achieved. If adequate muscle weakening has not occurred, additional toxin can be injected. Alcohol should not be used to clean off injection vials or to prep the skin because it can inactivate the botulinum A toxin.

Regardless of whether half or full doses are injected, patients must be prepared to cope with the side effects of botulinum A toxin.[67–69] Incomplete spontaneous blinks and lagophthalmos during sleep are nearly inevitable. Frequent instillation of artificial teardrops during the day and petrolatum ophthalmic ointment at bedtime usually provides adequate relief. Most patients with blepharospasm already have decreased tear production with dry eye symptoms and should increase their use of ocular lubricants when the injections are given.

Other ocular side effects of injections for eyelid spasms include ptosis from diffusion into the levator muscle, diplopia from

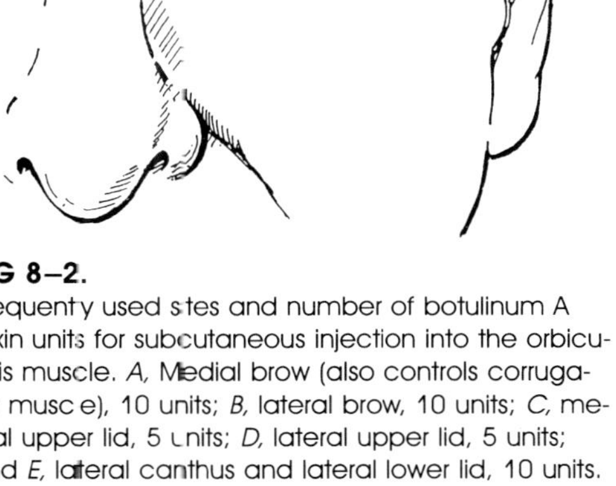


**FIG 8–2.**
Frequently used sites and number of botulinum A toxin units for subcutaneous injection into the orbicularis muscle. *A,* Medial brow (also controls corrugator muscle), 10 units; *B,* lateral brow, 10 units; *C,* medial upper lid, 5 units; *D,* lateral upper lid, 5 units; and *E,* lateral canthus and lateral lower lid, 10 units.

diffusion into extraocular muscles, and ectropion from excessive lower lid paresis. These side effects usually reach their greatest magnitude when the effect of the botulinum A toxin peaks 2 weeks after injection. Fortunately, the side effects usually resolve more quickly than does the desired weakening of the orbicularis oculi muscles. These side effects of botulinum A toxin may be used to advantage in select patients.[70–72] Central upper lid subcutaneous injections can be used to create a temporary ptosis that lasts 1 to 2 months in patients who need prolonged occlusion and corneal protection. Central lower lid injections can provide temporary relief from spastic entropion.

Once an effective dose and distribution of botulinum A injections have been achieved, this same schedule should remain effective for subsequent treatments. Antibody formation has not been noted in patients receiving treatment of facial spasms, and resistance to the medicine is not usually seen.[73, 74] Muscle degeneration is not evident either, even after 5 or more years of botulinum A treatment.[75] Some injections seem to be more or less effective, presumably because of variations in the injection technique or biologic activity of different toxin batches.

## GROWTH FACTORS

Growth factors are naturally occurring mitogenic proteins involved in tissue repair and maintenance. Epidermal growth factor (EGF) is the most widely studied growth factor in ophthalmic applications. On binding to cell membrane receptors, EGF can stimulate RNA, DNA, and protein synthesis, as well as cell division of epidermal and many other cells. It appears to be produced naturally in many tissues and is found in very high concentration in mouse submaxillary glands. It is also present in human urine. These have been the most common sources of EGF used in research. Recently EGF has been produced through recombinant DNA technology.

EGF has been studied extensively in corneal disorders[76]: epithelial wound healing, stromal wound healing, stromal collagen reformation, and endothelial regeneration. The concentration and frequency of EGF application appear to be important.[77] It has also been studied in conjunction with fibronectin[78] and corticosteroids. Fibronectin is a naturally occurring glycoprotein involved with the formation of cell attachments. Corticosteroids may be helpful to decrease inflammation during the healing process, as in the case of alkali burns. Other growth factors exist in the body and may prove to be effective in modifying the healing of various ophthalmic disorders and injuries.[79]

## REFERENCES


1. Edsall G: Specific prophylaxis of tetanus, *JAMA* 171:417, 1959.
2. Hampton OP, Altemeier WA, Edsall G, and others: Principles of prophylaxis against tetanus, *Ohio Med J* 57:164, 1061.
3. Stafford ES: Active and passive antitetanus immunization, *JAMA* 173:539, 1960.
4. Filler RM, Ellerbeck W: Tetanus prophylaxis, *JAMA* 174:1, 1960.
5. Council on Drugs: A new agent for prophylaxis of tetanus, *JAMA* 192:471, 1965.
6. Edsall G, Elliott WM, Peebles TC, and others: Excessive use of tetanus toxoid boosters, *JAMA* 202:17, 1967.
7. Recommendation of the Immunization Practices Advisor Committee (ACIP): Diphtheria, tetanus, and pertusis: guidelines for vaccine prophylaxis and other preventive measures, *MMWR* 1985; 34:405–426.
8. Jacobs RL, Lowe RS, and Lanier BQ: Adverse reactions to tetanus toxoid, *JAMA* 247:40, 1982.
9. Rothstein RJ, Baker FJ: Tetanus prevention and treatment, *JAMA* 240:675, 1978.
10. Leavelle RB: Gas gangrene panophthalmitis, *Arch Ophthalmol* 53:634, 1955.
11. Orenstein WA, Greaves WL: Congenital rubella syndrome: a continuing problem, *JAMA* 247:1174, 1982.
12. Rubella and congenital rubella syndrome, *Ohio Dep Health Commun Dis Newslett* vol 4, no 4, April 1980.
13. Shlian DM: Screening and immunization of rubella-susceptible women, *JAMA* 240:662, 1978.
14. Lamprecht C, Schauf V, Warren D, and others: An outbreak of congenital rubella in Chicago, *JAMA* 247:1129, 1982.
15. Lee SH, Ewert DP, Frederick PD, and

others: Resurgence of congenital rubella syndrome in the 1990's: report on missed opportunities and failed prevention policies among women of childbearing age, *JAMA* 267:2616, 1992.

16. Herrmann KL, Halstea SB, Wiebenga NH: Rubella antibody persistance after immunization, *JAMA* 247:193, 1982.
17. Wyll SA, Herrmann KL: Inadvertent rubella vaccination of pregnant women, *JAMA* 225:1472, 1973.
18. Sabin AB: Immunization, evaluation of some currently available and prospective vaccines, *JAMA* 246:236, 1981.
19. Preblud SR, Stetler HC, Frank JA, and others: Fetal risk associated with rubella vaccine, *JAMA* 246:1413, 1981.
20. Fox JP: Fetal perspective of rubella vaccine efficacy and safety, *JAMA* 246:1444, 1981.
21. Orenstein WA, Heseltine PNR, LeGagnoux SJ, and others: Rubella vaccine and susceptible hospital employees, *JAMA* 245:711, 1981.
22. Preblud SR, Hinman AR: Rubella vaccination of hospital employees, *JAMA* 245:736, 1981.
23. Ward H, Parker G: Passive protection against rubella, *Med J Aust* 1:81, 1956.
24. Rauh LW: Rubella and pregnancy, *Ohio Med J* 51:875, 1955.
25. Cotlier E: Effective vaccines for rubella, *Am J Ophthalmol* 67:424, 1969.
26. Hinman AR, Eddins DL, Kirby CD, and others: Progress in measles elimination, *JAMA* 247:1592, 1982.
27. Recommendations of the Immunization Practices Advisory Committee (ACIP): Update on hepatitis B prevention, *MMWR* 36:353, 1987.
28. Bryan JP, Sjögren M, Iqbal M, and others: Comparative trial of low-dose, intradermal, recombinant and plasma-derived hepatitis B vaccines, *J Infect Dis* 162:789, 1990.
29. Howard J, Allen HF: Treatment of experimental herpes simplex iridocyclitis with human serum gamma globulin, *Arch Ophthalmol* 59:68, 1958.
30. Hudnell AB, Osterhout S: The effect of gamma globulin on experimental herpes simplex keratitis, *Invest Ophthalmol* 2:295, 1963.
31. Gispen R: Immunization against herpes keratitis in rabbits, *Am J Ophthalmol* 44:88, 1957.
32. Metcalf JF: Protection from experimental ocular herpetic keratitis by a heat-killed virus vaccine, *Arch Ophthalmol* 98:893, 1980.
33. Gundersen T: Convalescent blood for treatment of herpes zoster ophthalmicus, *Arch Ophthalmol* 24:132, 1940.
34. Groth KE, McCullough J, Marker SC, and others: Evaluation of zoster immune plasma, *JAMA* 239:1877, 1978.
35. Wechsler HF, Wolf JJ: Agammaglobulinemia, *JAMA* 161:526, 1956.
36. Baron S, Tyring SK, Fleischmann WR, and others: The interferons. Mechanisms of action and clinical applications, *JAMA* 266:1375, 1991.
37. Teich SA, Cheung TW, Friedman AH: Systemic antiviral drugs used in ophthalmology, *Surv Ophthalmol* 37:19, 1992.
38. Arvin AM: Interferon as an antiviral and anti-tumor therapeutic agent, *Ophthalmology* 87:1236, 1980.
39. Negoro Y, Imanishi J, Matsuo A, and others: Treatment of epidemic keratoconjunctivitis by human leukocyte interferon, *Jpn J Ophthalmol* 24:125, 1980.
40. Pollikoff R, Jankauskas P, DiPuppo A, and others: Studies on the effect of bacterial endotoxin on primary herpetic keratitis, *Invest Ophthalmol* 7:397, 1968.
41. Fung WE: Interferon alpha 2A for treatment of age-related muscular degeneration, *Am J Ophthalmol* 112:349, 1991.
42. Scott AB, Rosenbaum A, Collins CC: Pharmacologic weakening of extraocular muscles, *Invest Ophthalmol* 12:924, 1973.
43. Scott AB: Botulinum toxin injection into extraocular muscles as an alternative to strabismus surgery, *Ophthalmology* 87:1044, 1980.
44. Carruthers JD: Ophthalmologic use of botulinum A exotoxin, *Can J Ophthalmol* 20:135, 1985.
45. Elston JS: The use of botulinum toxin A in the treatment of strabismus, *Trans Ophthalmol Soc UK* 104:208, 1985.
46. Elston JS: Botulinum A toxin for ocular muscle disorders, *Lancet* 1:265, 1986.
47. Gammon JA, Gemmill M, Tigges J, and others: Botulinum chemodenervation treatment of strabismus, *J Ophthalmic Nurs Tech* 5:51, 1986.
48. Osako M, Keltner JL: Botulinum A toxin (Oculinum) in ophthalmology, *Surv Ophthalmol* 36:28, 1991.
49. Freuh BR, Felt DP, Wojno TH, and others: Treatment of blepharospasm with botulinum toxin. A preliminary report, *Arch Ophthalmol* 102:1464, 1984.
50. Scott AB, Kennedy PA, Stubbs HA: Botulinum A toxin injection as a treatment for

blepharospasm, *Arch Ophthalmol* 103:347–350, 1985.
51. Shorr N, Seiff SR, Kopelman J: The use of botulinum toxin in blepharospasm, *Am J Ophthalmol* 99:542, 1985.
52. Tsoy EA, Buckley DG, Dutton JJ: Treatment of blepharospasm with botulinum toxin, *Am J Ophthalmol* 99:176, 1985.
53. Savine PJ, Sergott RC, Bosley TM, and others: Hemifacial spasm treated with botu linum A toxin injection, *Arch Ophthalmol* 103:1305, 1985.
54. Perman KI, Baylis HI, Rosenbaum AL, and others: The use of botulinum toxin in the medical management of benign essential blepharospasm, *Ophthalmology* 93:1, 1986.
55. Shore JW, Leone CR, O'Connor PS, and others: Botulinum toxin for the treatment of essential blepharospasm, *Ophthalmic Surg* 17:747, 1986.
56. Engstrom PF, Arnoult JB, Mazow ML, and others: Effectiveness of botulinum toxin therapy for essential blepharospasm, *Ophthalmology* 94:971, 1987.
57. Dunlop D, Pittar G, Dunlop C: Botulinum toxin in ophthalmology, *Aust NZ J Ophthalmol* 16:15, 1988.
58. Melling J, Hambleton P, Shone CC: *Clostridium* botulinum toxins: nature and preparation for clinical eye, *Eye* 2:16, 1988.
59. Hoffman RO, Helveston EM: Botulinum in the treatment of adult motility disorders, *Int Ophthalmol Clin* 26:241, 1986.
60. Jampolsky A: Botulinum toxin injections in strabismus. In Crawford JS, Flynn JT, Haik BG, and others, editors: Transaction of the New Orleans Academy of Ophthalmology: pediatric ophthalmology and strabismus, New York, 1986, Raven Press, p 526.
61. Elston JS, Lee JP, Powell CM, and others: Treatment of strabismus in adults with botulinum toxin A, *Br J Ophthalmol* 69:718, 1985.
62. Dunlop C: Botulinum toxin—the rationale of its use, *Aust NZ J Ophthalmol* 16:15, 1988.
63. Scott AB: Botulinum toxin injection of eye muscles to correct strabismus, *Trans Am Ophthalmol Soc* 79:734–770, 1981.
64. Fells P: Sausages and squints. *Br J Ophthalmol* 69:717, 1985 (editorial).
65. Flanders M, Tischler A, Wise J, and others: Injection of type A botulinum toxin into extraocular muscles for correction of strabismus, *Can J Ophthalmol* 22:212, 1987.
66. Elston JS, Lee, JP: Paralytic strabismus: the role of botulinum toxin, *Br J Ophthalmol* 69:891, 1985.
67. Freuh BR, Nelson CC, Kapustiak JF, and others: The effect of omitting botulinum toxin from the lower eyelid in blepharospasm treatment, *Am J Ophthalmol* 106:45, 1988.
68. Dutton JJ, Buckley EG: Long-term results and complications of botulinum A toxin in the treatment of blepharospasm, *Ophthalmology* 95:1529, 1988.
69. Lingua RW: Sequelae of botulinum toxin injection, *Am J Ophthalmol* 100:305, 1985.
70. Magoon EH: Botulinum injection for treatment of blepharospasm, corneal exposure, and entropion, *J Ocular Ther Surg* 4:133, 1985.
71. Burns CL, Gammon JA, Gemmill MC: Ptosis associated with botulinum toxin treatment of strabismus and blepharospasm, *Ophthalmology* 93:1621, 1986.
72. Kirkness CM, Adams GGW, Dilly PN, and others: Botulinum toxin A induced protective ptosis in corneal disease, *Ophthalmology* 95:473, 1988.
73. Gonnering RS: Negative antibody response to long-term treatment of facial spasm with botulinum toxin, *Am J Ophthalmol* 105:313, 1988.
74. Tsui JK, Wong NLM, Wong G, and others: Production of circulating antibodies to botulinum A toxin in patients receiving repeated injections for dystonia, *Ann Neurol* 23:181, 1988.
75. Harris CP, Alderson K, Nebeker J, and others: Histologic features of human orbicularis oculi treated with botulinum A toxin, *Arch Ophthalmol* 109:393, 1991.
76. Tripathi RC, Raja SC, Tripathi BJ: Prospects for epidermal growth factor in the management of corneal disorders, *Surv Ophthalmol* 34:457, 1990.
77. Leibowitz HM, Morellos, Stern M, and others: Effect of topically administered epidermal growth factor on corneal wound strength, *Arch Ophthalmol* 108:734, 1990.
78. Smiddy WE, Glaser BM, Green WR, and others: Transforming growth factor beta. A biologic chorioretinal glue, *Arch Ophthalmol* 107:577, 1989.
79. Soong HK, Hassan T, Varani J, and others: Fibronectic does not enhance epidermal growth factor–mediated acceleration of corneal epithelial wound closure, *Arch Ophthalmol* 107:1052, 1989.

# CHAPTER 9

# Alcohol

Elson L. Craig

The consumption of alcohol in this country creates an enormous number of societal and economic problems. Consider that one third of the U.S. population consumes four or more alcoholic drinks per week, 10% of the population chronically abuses alcohol, and more than 10 million people are chronic alcoholics. The medical cost attributable to the use of alcohol in the United States alone has been estimated to be in excess of $50 billion, which is nearly 7.5% of the total dollars spent on health care in the United States in 1990 ($666 billion[1]). Manning et al.[2] in their book on the cost of poor health habits estimate the external cost of each ounce of alcohol consumed in the United States to be $0.48.

Medical complications caused by drinking alcohol can be divided into acute and chronic forms. The term ethyl alcohol poisoning should be used only when referring to acute alcohol ingestion with its associated direct tissue damage. The many systemic conditions that are associated with chronic alcoholism are probably not caused directly by toxicity to the alcohol but are related to the concomitant imbalances in nutrition and metabolism. Suter et al.,[3] in their review of the effects of drinking alcohol on dietary intake, pointed out that alcohol accounts for 5.6% of the energy in the average American diet, 10% of the energy in persons who consume moderate amounts of alcohol, and as much as 50% in chronic alcoholics. The substitution of alcohol for other dietary foods leads to nutritional imbalances. Clearly the most significant complication of alcohol use is its role in causing automobile accidents. It was estimated by the U.S. Department of Transportation that of the 39,500 motor vehicle fatalities that occurred in the United States in 1992, 17,700 (45%) involved the use of alcohol.

Ethyl alcohol has value as a therapeutic agent in a number of conditions. In ophthalmology the most widely known of these is in the treatment of acute methanol poisoning.

## ETHYL ALCOHOL

Ethyl alcohol is absorbed unaltered from the stomach and small intestines and is detectable in the blood within minutes after ingestion. Peak levels are reached within 1 to 2 hours. From the blood, alcohol enters the tissues of the body and is found primarily in the cerebrospinal fluid, urine, and pulmonary alveoli. Alcohol is metabolized in the liver to acetaldehyde by the enzyme alcohol dehydrogenase. The rate of metabolism of pure ethyl alcohol is fairly constant in healthy adults, occurring at about 10 ml/hr. Increased intake beyond this level will result only in increased blood levels. In the adult, blood levels of approximately 0.2% produce intoxication, and levels between 0.5% and 0.8% may be fatal. Alcohol acts as a central nervous system (CNS) depressant, affecting the cortical inhibitory control centers first, but with increased blood levels the more critical centers in the medullary region are depressed and respiratory arrest may occur. Morphologic changes occurring with acute alcohol ingestion are nonspecific but can include congestion and edema of the viscera with superficial and deep hemorrhages in the stomach wall and cerebral edema with congestion of the meningeal and superficial cortical vessels.[4]

Acute alcohol poisoning has been found to produce a number of ocular side effects (Table 9–1). Some of these alterations in normal function may be attributed to the vascular congestion and acute edema occurring in the CNS. Ethyl alcohol increases the serum osmotic pressure, creating an osmotic gradient. In experimental animals alcohol enters the aqueous humor more rapidly than the vitreous. At equilibrium the vitreous concentration is approximately half that of blood. The osmotic effect created causes the vitreous volume to decrease, lowering intraocular pressure. Sturner and Coumbis[5] have suggested that the alcohol content of the brain is about the same as that in the vitreous. A more potent osmotic mechanism caused by ethyl alcohol is the suppression of endogenous antidiuretic hormone formation. The decrease in this hormone permits water loss and consequent increase of serum osmotic pressure. The net result of these effects is to produce acute circulatory changes in the CNS, leading to intracellular fluid retention and CNS edema. Other possible causes for CNS dysfunction produced by alcohol may be anoxia, depression of nerve conduction, or loss of cortical inhibitions. Whatever mechanism is involved, the effects are for the most part transient in acute alcohol poisoning.

Complications associated with chronic alcohol use are thought to be unrelated to the direct effects of the alcohol but more likely are related to inadequate diet and resultant deficiencies of vitamins, protein, and lipotrophic factors. Chronic alcoholism produces psychomotor dysfunction, psychoses, polyneuritis, and liver disease and is probably the most frequent cause of cortical atrophy in the adult age 40 to 50 years.[6]

### Fetal Alcohol Syndrome

Chronic alcohol use by pregnant women causes a particular pattern of malformations in their offspring, which was first reported from a study of French children by Lamache in 1967[7] and Lemoine et al.[8] in 1968 and in the United States by Jones et al.[9] in 1973. Jones et al.[10] later named the condition the fetal alcohol syndrome (FAS).[10] Children with the FAS display a triad of symptoms consisting of growth retardation, CNS dysfunction, and congenital anomalies. The incidence of the FAS in the United States was reported by Hanson et al.[11] to be 1:750 births. The amount of alcohol intake necessary to cause the FAS is approximately 89 ml/day, or six average drinks.[12] Lesser amounts are believed to increase the risk of fetal anomalies.

Streissguth et al.[13] listed the primary findings in the FAS as growth deficiency of prenatal origin, including both height and weight; a pattern of specific anomalies that includes characteristic facies defined by short palpebral fissures, midface hypoplasia, smooth and long philtrum, and thin upper lip; and CNS manifestations, including microcephaly, delayed development, attention deficits, learning disabilities, intellectual deficits, and seizures.[13] The FAS is recognized as the leading known cause of mental retardation in the United States.[14] Stromland[15] reviewed the ocular involve-

**TABLE 9–1.**
Ocular Side Effects of Acute Alcohol Poisoning

| |
|---|
| Lowering of ocular pressure |
| Range of fusion decreased; exophoria for near, esophoria for distance; produces tropias |
| Accommodation reduced; lowering of accommodative convergence/accommodation ratio |
| Diplopia; impairment of binocular fusion mechanism |
| Nystagmus (posttraumatic see-saw nystagmus may be abolished by ethanol) |
| Decreased color vision (80% of chronic alcoholics have red-green defects) |
| Reduced flicker fusion frequency |
| Slowed dark adaptation |
| Prolonged recovery time from glare |
| Reduced visual-evoked potential |
| Transient blindness |

ment of the eye in the FAS and reported that the most frequent findings in the outer eye region consist of short horizontal palpebral fissures and ptosis. These facial features seem to be more marked in early childhood (about 1 year of age) and become less apparent as the child grows. This finding was confirmed in the study of the FAS in adolescents and adults conducted by Streissguth et al.[13] Vision was reduced in nearly half of children with FAS, and they had a higher incidence of myopia than the general population. Esotropia was found in 50% to 65% of all children evaluated in separate studies. Corneal opacities, anterior chamber angle abnormalities, iris defects, and combinations of these were the most frequently encountered anterior segment malformations. Optic nerve hypoplasia and pallor and tortuosity of retinal vessels (arteries) were obvious changes in the posterior pole. The mechanism of the teratogenic effects of alcohol is unknown. Stromland[15] pointed out that women who are alcoholics usually use narcotics, sedatives, and other neurotrophic drugs, all of which may be teratogenic as well. He also suggested the possibility that the ocular abnormalities may be secondary to the overall developmental retardation. For example, the tortuosity of the retinal vessels could be caused by microphthalmia, making the fundus too small for the normal growth of the vascular tree. Mennella and Beauchamp[16] found that alcohol could be transferred to the infant through breast milk if present in the mother's blood during feeding. They stated that this had an effect on the flavor of the mother's milk and the infant's behavior.

### Tobacco-alcohol Amblyopia

Tobacco-alcohol amblyopia is a condition that many investigators consider to be a nutritional amblyopia that can cause bilateral progressive optic neuropathy. Most cases occur in men who are smokers, drink alcohol, and have poor nutrition. This combination most likely has a synergistic effect on the optic nerve because the toxic effect of alcohol or tobacco alone in a person with normal nutrition seems to be much less. Vitamin $B_{12}$ (cyanocobalamin) and vitamin $B_1$ (thiamine) deficiency may play an important role in the optic nerve damage. Normally vitamin $B_{12}$ in food is liberated by peptic enzymes and hydrochloric acid in the stomach and is then bound to protein and absorbed into the blood from the small intestines. In pernicious anemia vitamin $B_{12}$ deficiency occurs because of decreased intrinsic factor secretion by the stomach. Optic neuropathy with central and cecocentral scotomas and decreased vision has been reported to occur in this condition.[17]

Elevated thiocyanate levels in healthy smokers suggest that cyanide released into the blood may accumulate in body tissue and act as a toxin. Cyanide is normally detoxified in tissues by conversion to thiocyanate, which is then complexed with sulfur. The hydroxyl group of natural vitamin $B_{12}$ (hydroxycobalamin) can also exchange with excessive tissue levels of cyanide. Diets deficient in vitamin $B_{12}$, in coenzymes folate and pyridoxine needed to synthesize homocysteine and cysteine, and in sulfur-containing amino acids decrease the tissues' ability to convert cyanide to thiocyanate. This in turn allows for the accumulation of high levels of cyanide. The exact role of cyanide toxicity in causing optic nerve damage in tobacco-alcohol amblyopia is uncertain. Equally as unclear is the role that vitamin $B_{12}$ plays in tobacco-alcohol amblyopia, particularly because serum levels may frequently be normal in affected patients. Vitamin $B_{12}$ may not play a major role in this condition. Treatment of tobacco-alcohol amblyopia with hydroxycobalamin is beneficial in some cases; cyanocobalamin (a form of vitamin $B_{12}$ found in most multivitamins) is not effective. Hydroxycobalamin can be given only by intramuscular injection and should be given two times weekly for at least 1 month and then weekly for several months.

## METHANOL POISONING

Methyl alcohol (wood alcohol) is sometimes ingested by accident or intentionally. When less than a minimum lethal dose of methanol (3 g/kg) is swallowed, mild intoxication will occur during the first 24 hours, and the patient usually recovers completely. When double the minimal lethal dose is ingested, semicoma may develop. By the second day the patient seems to have recovered and appears normal for a brief period. This is followed by progressive weakness, respiratory failure, and death. Before death pupillary dilatation and horizontal nystagmus are common. Severe acidosis develops, with carbon dioxide–combining powers as low as 15 vol% (normal 40–55 vol%). In eight monkeys given twice the minimum lethal dose of methanol, acidosis was treated by giving adequate doses of sodium bicarbonate (dosage determined by carbon dioxide–combining power). Four of the eight monkeys survived. The others died as a result of CNS damage. Retinal edema occurred in all animals despite adequate treatment of the acidosis.[18]

Methanol poisoning of humans and experimentally in monkeys can be divided into three components.[19] The first component is the narcotic action that methanol manifests, as do other alcohols and organic solvents. The lethal dosage required for narcotic death is approximately 10 g/kg, which may be all methanol, all ethanol, or a combination of the two. The second component is characterized by a latent period and is a metabolic acidosis probably caused indirectly by the toxic metabolic products of methanol and directly by tissue damage from formaldehyde. The minimal lethal dose of methanol is 2 to 3 g/kg. Death usually occurs about 1 day after an untreated fatal dose. The third component of methanol poisoning occurs only if the patient survives for 30 hours or more. It is characterized by ocular and CNS necrosis, including death of retinal ganglion cells and the basal ganglia.

Methanol is metabolized by alcohol dehydrogenase, which is also used for ethanol metabolism. The two alcohols compete for this enzyme. Ethanol is markedly selective to the extent that inhibition of methanol metabolism is already demonstrable when the ethanol concentration is only 1⁄16 that of methanol. Repeated administration of ethanol is capable of blocking completely the methanol breakdown. Evidence of this is the increased amount of methanol in the urine and the absence of formate (methanol metabolite) when ethanol is given. Urinary and pulmonary excretion of unchanged methanol will occur if sufficient ethanol is given for a long enough period. If ethanol treatment is begun early, acidosis, CNS damage, and eye damage may be completely prevented. The initial dose of ethanol should be 0.75 g/kg; another 0.50 g/kg is given every 4 hours for 2 to 3 days. For a 68-kg man this would be an initial dose of 4.5 ounces (135 ml of 100-proof [50%] whiskey), followed by 3 ounces (90 ml) every 4 hours.

Prompt treatment with ethanol is essential if the toxic effects of methanol are to be minimized. In a series of nine monkeys receiving 6 g of methanol/kg, the poisoning was reversible if ethanol treatment was begun within 8 to 12 hours. After a 16-hour delay in the start of ethanol treatment, death was postponed but not prevented.[20] Because methanol is demonstrable in the plasma for as long as 4 days, ethanol treatment of human poisoning seems rational even if the treatment is not started for several days after methanol ingestion. At least the damage resulting from the metabolism of the remaining methanol could be prevented. Because the outcome varies with the dosage, the previously mentioned 16-hour time should not be considered an absolute contraindication for subsequent therapy.

## ETHYLENE GLYCOL POISONING

Poisoning from antifreeze (ethylene glycol) ingestion closely parallels methanol poisoning. Ethylene glycol is not itself poisonous, but 100 ml is a lethal dose for an adult. Death comes as a result of renal occlusion caused by the crystallization of calcium oxalate in renal tubules and parenchyma. Alcohol dehydrogenase blockade by the administration of ethyl alcohol prevents metabolism of ethylene glycol. The unchanged ethylene glycol is then excreted in 3 to 5 days. During this period the patient should be given repeated doses of ethyl alcohol and maintained in a state of mild intoxication.

## ETHANOL EFFECT ON INTRAOCULAR PRESSURE

The intraocular pressure was decreased in 32 of 33 eyes of normal and glaucomatous subjects studied by Peczon and Grant.[21] The intraocular pressure drop was observed to occur during the first hour, and the pressure returned to normal in 4 to 5 hours. In general, the patient with the higher pressure experienced the greatest pressure drop, which averaged 9 mm Hg in the glaucoma patients. Facility of outflow was not increased. As discussed previously, ethyl alcohol causes a transitory increase in serum osmotic pressure by a direct osmolar effect but, more important, by the suppression of endogenous antidiuretic hormone. Support for the latter mechanism of lowering intraocular pressure is derived from the experimental finding that the administration of vasopressin (the antidiuretic hormone) will partially or completely block the reduction of intraocular pressure by ethanol.[22]

## ALCOHOL USES

Alcohol has a number of uses in patient care. The use of alcohol scrubs to sterilize the skin before an injection is given is commonplace. Gram-negative and gram-positive organisms, particularly *Staphylococcus aureus,* as well as most viruses, have been shown by many investigators to be effectively eliminated from the skin after the skin is swabbed with alcohol.[23–25] Unfortunately, this effect is very transient because the alcohol evaporates rapidly and does not leave any germicidal residue.

A major concern to the ophthalmologist is the sterilization of the applanation tonometer tip. Fear of spreading such conditions as epidemic keratoconjunctivitis, herpes simplex virus, or human immunodeficiency virus is a real concern and has prompted the American Academy of Ophthalmologists to make specific recommendations for the sterilization of applanation tonometer tips.[26] Effective sterilization is thought to occur if the tonometer head is soaked in 70% isopropyl alcohol, 3% hydrogen peroxide, or 0.5% sodium hypochlorite (diluted household bleach).

Craven et al.[27] surveyed 89 ophthalmologists in the Dallas–Fort Worth area to determine the method used to sterilize the applanation tonometer tip. From the 89 who responded, 16 methods were being used. The most common was alcohol wipes (26%), followed by 0.5% sodium hypochlorite soaks (23%). These authors reported their findings on the applanation sterilization techniques and the recoverability of adenovirus type 8 (epidemic keratoconjunctivitis). All techniques, including plain tissue wiping, were effective in removing inoculates of adenovirus except air drying. These authors suggested that wiping the tonometer tip with an alcohol sponge was a convenient and effective technique for removing most contaminates. Ventura and Dix[28] have shown that herpes simplex virus type 1 was not removed by tissue wiping but was effectively removed by wiping with 70% isopropyl alcohol; they also recommend this as a routine procedure. Key and Whitman[29] reported that soaking the applanation tonometer tip in 70% isopropyl alcohol for only 10 to 15 minutes caused damage to the prism of the tonometer head and that soaking the tip overnight produced unavoidable severe damage. Soukiasian et al.[30] found corneal complications from the use of alcohol sterilization of the applanation tonometer tip. A 38-year-old patient had severe corneal epithelial damage develop from the residual alcohol on the tip of the tonometer. This healed in 18 hours with patching. They suggested that at least 1 minute be allowed to elapse before the instrument is applied to the patient's cornea. This allows adequate time for the alcohol to evaporate. Similar corneal damage has occurred from the use of tips soaked in hydrogen peroxide.[31, 32] Swabbing the applanation tonometer tip with 70% isopropyl alcohol is convenient, practical, and effective in removing common contaminants, but care should be taken to allow the alcohol to evaporate before the tip is applied to the corneal surface.

Bacteriologic studies using a platinum spatula for scraping of the cornea require effective sterilization, which can be easily

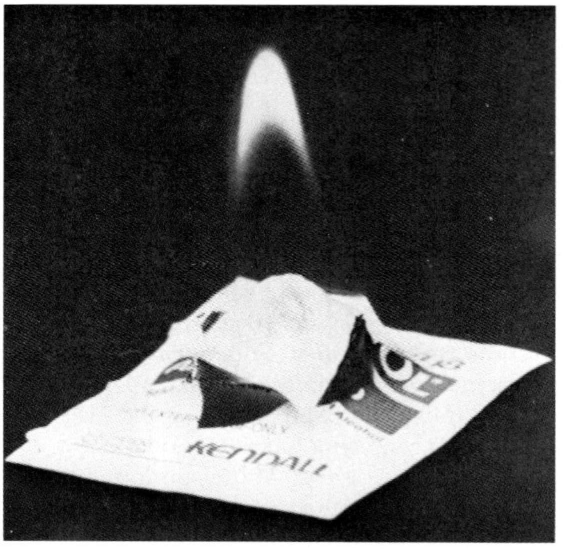


**FIG 9–1.**
Disposable alcohol flame sterilizer. (From Salisbury JA, Cobo LM, Brown JL: *Am J Ophthalmol* 91:261, 1981. Used by permission.)

accomplished with an alcohol lamp. A convenient substitute for the lamp is a commercially packaged alcohol wipe such as that used for skin sterilization. Simply split the middle of the package cover, pull out the alcohol-saturated wipe as a wick, and light it. The flame will last for 2 to 3 minutes (Fig. 9–1).

## ALCOHOL RETROBULBAR INJECTION

Prolonged local anesthesia is sometimes desirable in the treatment of painful, blind eyes and offers a good alternative to enucleation. Retrobulbar injection of absolute or 95% alcohol has been commonly used for such treatment. Alcohol injections can be very painful and must be preceded by an injection of a short-acting anesthetic, such as lidocaine or procaine. After the anesthetic is injected into the muscle cone, 0.5 to 1 ml of alcohol is injected through the same needle, which is left in position while the syringes are changed. To decrease or completely eliminate any discomfort from the alcohol injection, May and May[33] recommended that separate injections be used. Once the anesthetic is given, the needle is removed, and the second injection, which is the alcohol, is not given for 15 minutes. They believe that this allows ample time for complete retrobulbar anesthesia, and there is little chance that the patient will feel the second needle entrance or the alcohol injection.

The retrobulbar needle should be inserted with caution to be certain that the tip is within the muscle cone and as far anterior as possible. Although destruction of the sensory nerves may be accomplished by injection anywhere within the muscle cone, undesirable paralysis of the extraocular muscles occurs only if their motor nerves are damaged by infiltration of the posterior orbit. Because of the thickness of the protective sheath of the optic nerve, it is less likely to be damaged than are the smaller ciliary nerves. The patient will usually experience no further decrease in light perception when retrobulbar alcohol injection is employed for pain control in eyes with severely impaired vision. However, the risk of severe and permanent damage to the optic nerve or its blood supply is too great to permit this treatment of eyes with useful vision. Breakdown of corneal epithelium as seen in neuroparalytic keratitis is not a common complication of retrobulbar alcohol injection. For several days after injection, however, disturbing orbital edema and conjunctival chemosis with moderate discomfort may develop in some patients. More commonly, the patient will experience minimal symptoms and be pain free shortly after the injection. Apparently the sensory fibers of the ciliary nerves are capable of regeneration, because months after the injection the pain may recur, requiring reinjection.

Discomfort and conjunctival chemosis immediately after the injection of alcohol can be reduced or avoided completely by preventing the anterior diffusion of the alcohol into the subconjunctival tissues. This can best be accomplished by being certain that the needle tip is within the muscle cone during injection. Flushing the needle out with anesthetic solution as the needle is being withdrawn prevents escape of residual alcohol from the syringe and needle into the anterior tissues.

## SUMMARY

Alcohol is uniquely valuable in ophthalmology and has a number of uses. Its use to sterilize skin areas before injections are given and before minor surgical procedures are performed, and to sterilize instruments such as the applanation tonometer tip is not only convenient but also effective. Ethyl alcohol is specifically valuable in the treatment of methanol or ethylene glycol poisoning and may be lifesaving. On the other hand, the abuse of alcohol creates a number of major problems in our society. A review article by Eckardt[34] summarizes the multiple destructive effects of alcohol on brain tissue, the peripheral nervous system, liver, pancreas, gastrointestinal tract, cardiovascular system, endocrine organs, fetal development, and general and psychosocial adaptation. The many benefits of alcohol use in medicine are obvious; equally as obvious are the complex problems created by its abuse.

## REFERENCES


1. Sullivan LW: The Bush Administration Health Care Plan, sounding board, *N Engl J Med* 327:801, 1992.
2. Manning WG, Keeler EB, Davis SR, and others: The cost of poor health habits, Cambridge, Mass, 1991, Harvard University Press.
3. Suter PM, Schutz Y, Jequier E: The effect of ethanol on fat storage in healthy subjects, *N Engl J Med* 326:983, 1992.
4. Robbins SL: *Textbook of pathology with clinical application,* Philadelphia, 1962, WB Saunders Co.
5. Sturner WQ, Coumbis RS: The quantitation of ethyl alcohol in vitreous humor and blood by gas chromatography, *Am J Clin Pathol* 49:349, 1966.
6. Walsh FB, Hoyt WF: Clinical neuroophthalmology, vol 3, Baltimore, 1969, Williams & Wilkins Co.
7. Lamache MA: Reflections sur la déscendance des alcooliques, *Bull Acad Natl Med* (Paris) 151:517, 1967.
8. Lemoine P, Harousseau H, Borteyru JR, and others: Lés enfants de parents alcooliques. Anomalies observées. A propos de 127 cas, *Quest Med* 21:476, 1968.
9. Jones KL, Smith DW, Ulleland CN, and others: Patterns of malformation in offspring of chronic alcoholic mothers, *Lancet* 1:1267, 1973.
10. Jones KL, Smith DW: Recognition of the fetal alcohol syndrome in early infancy, *Lancet* 2:999, 1973.
11. Hanson JW, Streissguth AD, Smith DW: The effects of moderate alcohol consumption during pregnancy and fetal growth and morphogenesis, *J Pediatr* 92:457, 1978.
12. Clarren SK, Smith DW: The fetal alcohol syndrome, *N Engl J Med* 298:1063, 1978.
13. Streissguth AP, Aase JM, Clarren SK, and others: Fetal alcohol syndrome in adolescents and adults, *JAMA* 265:1961, 1991.
14. Abel EL, Sokol RJ: Incidence of fetal alcohol syndrome and economic impact of FAS-related anomalies, *Drug Alcohol Depend* 19:51, 1987.
15. Stromland K: Ocular involvement in the fetal alcohol syndrome, *Surv Ophthalmol* 31:277, 1987.
16. Mennella JA, Beauchamp GK: The transfer of alcohol to human milk—effect on flavor and the infant's behavior, *N Engl J Med* 326:981, 1991.
17. Foulds WS, Chisholm FA, Steward JB, and others: The optic neuropathy of pernicious anemia, *Arch Ophthalmol* 82:427, 1969.
18. Potts AM: Visual toxicity of methanol; clinical aspects of experimental methanol poisoning treated with base, *Am J Ophthalmol* 39:86, 1955.
19. Gigler AP, Potts AM, Farkas IS: Studies on visual toxicity of methanol; effect of ethanol on methanol poisoning in rhesus monkey, *Am J Ophthalmol* 42:244, 1956.
20. Gilger AP, Farkas IS, Potts AM: Studies on visual toxicity of methanol, *Am J Ophthalmol* 48:152, 1959.
21. Peczon JD, Grant WM: Glaucoma, alcohol, and intraocular pressure, *Arch Ophthalmol* 6:145, 1967.
22. Houle Re, Grant WM: Alcohol, vasopressin, and intraocular pressure, *Invest Ophthalmol* 6:145, 1967.
23. Lilly HA, Lowbury EJ: Transient skin flora: their removal by cleansing or disinfection in relation to their mode of deposition, *J Clin Pathol* 31 919, 1978.
24. Evans CA, Mattern KL: The bacterial flora of the anticubital fossa: the efficacy of alcohol disinfection of this site, the palm of the hand, and the forehead, *J Invest Dermatol* 75:140, 1980.
25. Ojajarvi J: Effectiveness of hand washing and disinfection methods in removing

transient bacteria after patient nursing, *J Hyg (Lond)* 85:193, 1980.
26. Recommendations for preventing possible transmission of human T-lymphotropic virus type III/lymphadenopathy–associated virus from tears, *MMWR* 34:533, 1985.
27. Craven ER, Butler BS, McCulley JP, and others: Applanation tonometer tip sterilization for adenovirus type 8, *Ophthalmology* 94:1538, 1987.
28. Ventura LM, Dix RD: Viability of herpes simplex virus type 1 on the applanation tonometer, *Am J Ophthalmol* 103:48, 1987.
29. Key CB, Whitman J: Alcohol soaking damages applanation tonometer heads, *Arch Ophthalmol* 104:800, 1986 (letter to the editor).
30. Soukiasian SH, Asdourian GK, and others: A complication from alcohol-swabbed tonometer tips, *Arch Ophthalmol* 105:424, 1988 (letter to the editor).
31. Levenson JE: Corneal damage from improperly cleaned tonometer tips, *Arch Ophthalmol* 107:1117, 1982 (letter to the editor).
32. Pogrebniak AE, Sugar A: Corneal toxicity from hydrogen peroxide–soaked tonometer tips, *Arch Ophthalmol* 106:1505, 1988.
33. May DR, May WN: Decreasing discomfort caused by retrobulbar alcohol injection, *Am J Ophthalmol* 95:262, 1983.
34. Eckardt M: Health hazards associated with alcohol consumption, *JAMA* 246:648, 1981.

CHAPTER **10**

# Fluorescein and Other Dyes

Elson L. Craig

## FLUORESCEIN

Sodium fluorescein is a water-soluble hydroxyxanthene dye with a molecular weight of 376 daltons. It produces a green fluorescent color in alkaline solution (pH > 5.0), and this color is detectable in concentrations as dilute as 1 ppm. Fluorescein dye is nontoxic and nonirritating to the eye even when it is injured. Fluorescein dye is useful in evaluating both normal physiology and diseases of the anterior and posterior segments of the eye. Clearly, the improvement in the quality of fluorescein dye and the great improvements in imaging equipment that have occurred in recent years have been instrumental in advancing our understanding of the pathophysiology and treatment of diseases of the choroid and retina. More recently developed procedures for iris and corneal angiography and improved techniques for fluorophotometry have also been useful in understanding disease processes in these tissues and in detecting leakage of dye into the aqueous and vitreous as an indicator of blood-ocular disruption in various conditions.

### Mechanism of Color Effect from Sodium Fluorescein

Fluorescein, as viewed by the usual methods, does not appear to actually stain tissues, but it is useful as an indicator dye by virtue of its visibility in very dilute solutions. The normal precorneal tear film is slightly acid, and when a fluorescein solution is applied, the tear film appears yellow or slightly orange. When a very dilute solution is applied, the fluorescein turns greenish. The intact corneal epithelium, having a high lipid content, resists penetration of the water-soluble fluorescein dye and is not colored by it. Any break in the epithelial barrier permits rapid penetration of fluorescein into Bowman's membrane and into the corneal stroma. If the epithelial loss is extensive, topically applied fluorescein can penetrate into the anterior chamber, mix with aqueous, and become visible biomicroscopically as a green flare. When the epithelial surface has regenerated, it will no longer color regardless of the persistence of damage to the underlying corneal stroma.

Fluorescence is an important property of fluorescein dye that makes it possible to selectively visualize fluorescein-colored solutions. Fluorescence occurs when a substance absorbs light of one wavelength and reemits a portion of that light at a longer wavelength. In ophthalmic usage a blue light (wavelength approximately 465–490 nm) is used to illuminate the dye, and it is reflected back as a yellow-green light (wavelength approximately 520–530 nm). Because most instruments used to perform angiography on the eye employ white light for illumination, optical filters must be used. A blue light transmitting filter is placed in front of the exciting light, and the ocular fundus is examined or photographed through a yellow-green passing filter. For best results both filters must be matched so that no blue light escapes back to the observer or the camera.

### Topical Use

Fluorescein may be applied as 1 drop of 0.5% to 2.0% solution or by the use of a strip of fluorescein-impregnated filter paper placed in the conjunctival cul-de-sac until it becomes moistened by the patient's tears. If the purpose of the fluorescein use is to detect an epithelial defect, excessive dye should be irrigated from the surface of the eye with a sterile saline solution. Because inadequate irrigation lessens the contrast between stained pathologic lesions and adjacent normal areas, irrigation should be continued until the tear film is entirely colorless. Blinking between irrigations helps to remove excess fluorescein beneath the lids. Fluorescein coloring of the eye is transient, disappearing within 30 minutes.

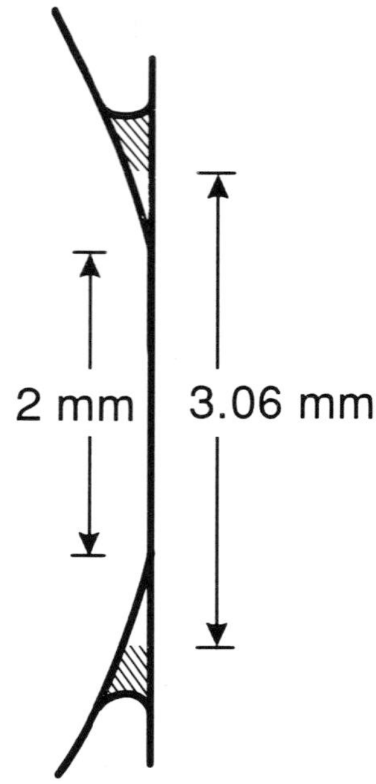


**FIG 10–1.**
Cornea partially flattened by applanation tonometer. Above and below flattened area are wedges of fluorescein-stained solution, the apices of which are too dilute and therefore invisible. The 3.06 mm endpoint of applanation appears to have been reached but in reality is composed of an erroneously small flattened area surrounded by the invisible apex of inadequately stained fluid. (From Moses RA: *Am J Ophthalmol* 49:1149, 1960. Used by permission.)

### Uses

#### *Fitting of Contact Lenses*

Fluorescein dye is used as an aid in the fitting of rigid contact lenses. Fluorescein in the tear layer beneath the contact lens is used to determine areas of lens-cornea contact and the overall fit of the lens. Fluorescein cannot be used in the fitting of soft contact lenses because the dye enters the pore structure of the hydrogel and remains within the lens for many hours. If fluorescein has been placed on the eye, soft contact lenses should not be inserted for at least 1 hour. Fluorexon has staining properties similar to fluorescein, but because it has a larger molecular structure, it will not readily enter the pores of a soft lens and can therefore be safely used with hydrogel lenses.[1]

#### *Applanation Tonometry*

During applanation tonometry fluorescein is used to delineate the margins of the applanated area. The dye can be viewed with white light but more appropriately with blue light to produce fluorescence. On cross section the fluorescein pool between the cornea and the applanation tonometer will be triangular, with its apex directed toward the applanated area (Fig. 10–1).[2] This fluid pool may be invisible if the fluorescein concentration is too low or if the fluorescein has been destroyed by an anesthetic solution. Because unstained fluid cannot be differentiated from applanated cornea, the applanation endpoint will be made up of these two factors rather than the applanated corneal surface alone, causing an underestimation of intraocular pressure (IOP). The extent of this error has been estimated to be as much as 5 to 6 mm Hg.[2] As previously discussed, fluorescence is helpful in identifying fluorescein dye in the tear pool. Certain anesthetic agents markedly reduce the fluorescent property of fluorescein. For example, fluorescence is least impaired by a 0.1% solution of benoxinate, whereas 0.5% proparacaine causes a marked reduction. Potential errors of underestimation of IOP with applanation tonometry may be avoided by using adequate fluorescein dye and a minimum of anesthetic solution. Applanation tonometry is best performed with a 0.25% solution of fluorescein dye, which produces distinct lines, whereas more concentrated solutions tend to do just the opposite. Using no fluorescein during applanation tonometry resulted in an underestimation of pressure of 5 mm Hg (a range between 3 and 10 mm Hg), which is similar to the error caused by using a very dilute solution.[3, 4] A fluorescein-anesthetic combination Fluress, specifically prepared for use in applanation tonometry, was introduced in 1966. This solution combines 0.25% fluorescein sodium with 0.4% benoxinate hydrochloride and 1% chlorobutanol. Benoxinate hydrochloride was chosen because of its effectiveness, stability, and patient comfort.[5] A single drop of this solution provides adequate anesthesia for applanation tonometry with an onset within 15 seconds and a duration of 15 minutes. Benoxinate does not cause significant reduction in fluorescence and does not induce tearing to dilute the fluorescein dye. A wetting and stabilizing agent, povidone, is incorporated into the solution to prevent precipitation of the relatively insoluble benoxinate-fluorescein combination and to permit incorporation of 1% chlorobutanol in the preparation. Povidone also increases the duration of fluorescein-corneal contact. Unlike methylcellulose and polyvinyl alcohol, povidone does not blur the definition of the margins of fluorescence at the applanation edge.

The propensity for fluorescein solutions used in ophthalmology to become contaminated with bacteria, particularly *Pseudomonas aeruginosa,* has been known since 1955.[6] This very significant clinical problem was essentially eliminated by the introduction of Fluress. Deliberate heavy contamination of Fluress with many types of organisms (including *Escherichia coli, Staphylococcus aureus,* and *Candida albicans*) was self-sterilized within 14 to 180 minutes.[5] In other studies, open bottles of Fluress were found to remain sterile in the clinical area for periods of 1 month or more. The solution was self-sterilizing even when deliberately contaminated with *Pseudomonas.*[7] When compared with other available fluorescein-anesthetic combinations in a laboratory experiment chosen to simulate the clinical setting, Fluress proved to be superior in self-sterilization after deliberate contamination with *P. aeruginosa* and *S. aureus.* All other solutions tested remained contaminated for up to 2 hours after inoculation.[8]

In Fluress, a 0.25% concentration of fluorescein was selected because it provides adequate fluorescence to avoid applanation reading errors, yet it does not cause objectionable residual lid staining. The pH adjustment to 5.0 was selected to provide stability for benoxinate. Fluress is a carefully designed, stable, bacteriostatic, nontoxic, and nonirritating solution useful in applanation tonometry. Fluress can be used for simultaneous staining and anesthetization of the cornea but should not be used in the evaluation of a possible keratitis or corneal ulcer because of its antimicrobial properties. A sterile fluorescein strip is more appropriate for these cases.

***Corneal Surgery***

Dilute solutions of fluorescein dye can be very useful during anterior segment surgery. For instance, the raw and the epithelial surface of a free conjunctival graft look very much alike and may become accidentally reversed. Fluorescein may be used to identify the raw surface, because only this side will color. The green color change of previously instilled fluorescein indicates immediately the presence of aqueous when the corneal transplant trephine enters the anterior chamber. This is particularly helpful in cases where the surrounding cornea is too opaque to permit the surgeon to see the iris.

Should a persistent postoperative flat anterior chamber require surgical reformation, fluorescein solution may be injected into the anterior chamber at the time of surgery. A stream of fluorescein-colored solution will identify the site of a wound leak if it is present.

The rare condition of extensive stripping of Descemet's membrane from the corneal stroma during a surgical procedure is difficult to evaluate because of the transparency of the membrane lying against the iris and the haziness of the overlying cornea. Intravenous fluorescein will appear in the anterior chamber, and the color difference on the two sides of the detached membrane aids in the evaluation of this condition. Placement of a large bubble of air behind the membrane is one method that can be used to reappose it to the stroma, with possible return of corneal transparency.[9]

### Detection of Aqueous Leaks

An aqueous leak that may occur after anterior segment surgery or after trauma may be easily detected with a solution of fluorescein. In this examination several drops of fluorescein are instilled, and the excess is not irrigated out. The eyelids are held widely apart, the surface of the eye is observed under good illumination, and the property of fluorescence is not used. The normal appearance of such an application is a uniform tear film that is somewhat yellowish. If there is an aqueous leak of any magnitude, a tiny rivulet of green or clear aqueous will be seen flowing downward from the perforation site. If this is not evident at first, gentle pressure on the globe may cause sufficient leakage from the site to produce a visible rivulet. In those cases where the aqueous leak is diffuse, as in a large wound, no rivulet will form, and instead there will be an immediate bright green color change of the instilled fluorescein as contrasted with the yellow-orange color. This color change usually is first evident above the margin of the lower lid, but if the leak is under a conjunctival flap, the color change may first be seen at the conjunctival edge.

### Lacrimal Drainage System Patency

Although the mechanical flow of irrigating solution usually proves to the physician and the patient whether the nasolacrimal drainage system is open or not, the addition of fluorescein to the irrigating solution provides visible evidence that the solution has indeed entered the throat. The patient may be asked to spit out this green material as a convincing demonstration of the success of the procedure. Fluorescein testing of the patency of the lacrimal drainage system does not necessarily require mechanical irrigation. The primary dye test was evaluated in 25 normal subjects by three physicians of differing levels of experience in performing the test.[10] The difference between obtaining a 100% positive primary test result or a lower 80% was the technique employed. The 100% positive results occurred when four moistened fluorescein strips were placed consecutively in the area of the punctum. The patient was instructed to blink normally, and the examiner waited for at least 10 minutes before the subject was instructed to blow out of the nostril into white tissue paper while the opposite nostril was occluded. The paper was examined for fluorescein, and, if found, the test result was considered to be positive. If the paper did not show fluorescein after two attempts, a cotton-tipped curved nasal wire moistened with a topical anesthetic was inserted into the nose using a nasal speculum. The cotton-covered tip of the wire was placed beneath the inferior turbinate near the nasolacrimal duct opening. If fluorescein was detected, the test result was considered to be positive. In those subjects with negative results, only two consecutive fluorescein strips were used, and the strips were applied in the center of the cul-de-sac and dragged to the area of the punctum. The high percentage of positive results was attributed to the higher concentration of dye used, the placement of the dye over the punctum, and the longer period before attempting to identify fluorescein stain in the nose. From this study and others it is evident that the use of fluorescein to demonstrate the patency of the nasolacrimal duct is a highly reliable test, and the likelihood of a negative result in a normal patient is small. The test is made more sensitive with the aid of ultraviolet light or a blue light. This test has the advantage of simplicity, comfort, and safety and is a more physiologic measure of lacrimal function than are probing and irrigation; however, it permits study of only one nasolacrimal system per examination.

## Intravenous Fluorescein

### Fluorescein Angiography

Intravenous fluorescein is an extremely valuable aid in the study of ocular physiology and in the diagnosis of diseases of the choroid and retina. Fluorescein angiography was first described in 1960 by McClean and Maumenee[11] in their report of a hemangioma of the choroid. Since that time its use in research and clinical practice has become routine. The techniques for the performance of fluorescein angioscopy and angiography have been the subject of a number of articles and books.[12–17] A monograph published by the American Academy of Ophthalmology provides a current review of this subject.[16]

For fluorescein angiography, a dose of 5 ml of a 10% fluorescein solution or 3 ml of a 25% solution is rapidly injected into a vein large enough for a 21-gauge needle. To increase the speed of the bolus to the eye, a 5-ml flush of sterile saline solution may be used immediately after the fluorescein injection. Normally the dilution of the dye between the arm and the eye is approximately 600 times for a 5-ml bolus.[18] Despite this significant dilution, in the normal person, the dye can be readily seen in the ocular circulation in about 13 seconds after injection, and it persists for about 20 seconds. Fluorescein may also be administered orally. One gram of the dye is mixed with 200 ml of a liquid drink that has a taste and color adequate to mask that of the fluorescein. Peak blood concentration is reached within 30 minutes. Oral fluorescein is almost totally absorbed within a few hours and is excreted in the urine, usually within 48 hours. This route of administration produces a slow rise in serum concentration and is therefore effective only in evaluating conditions that retain dye in the late venous and recirculation phases of the angiogram, as occurs in cystoid maculopathy.

Nearly 80% of the intravenous fluorescein binds to the albumin in the plasma and to erythrocytes. Fig. 10–2 shows the concentration of unbound fluorescein in blood subsequent to oral and intravenous administration.[19] Presumably only the unbound portion of fluorescein leaves the ocular vessels unless the blood-eye barrier is so damaged as to admit plasma proteins. In contrast to the belief that 80% of fluorescein is plasma bound, Ianacone et al.[20] showed

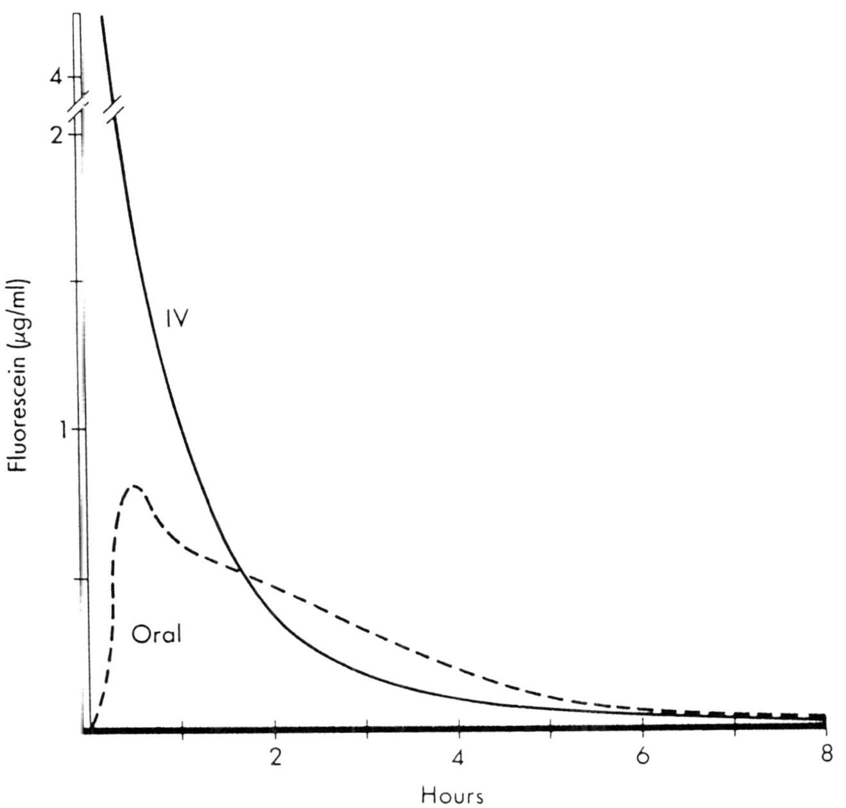


**FIG 10–2.**
Unbound fluorescein concentration in blood after oral or intravenous routes of administration. (Modified from Palestine AG, Brubaker RF: *Invest Ophthalmol* 21:542, 1981. Used by permission.)

by electrophoresis of human plasma sampled 10 minutes after intravenous injection of fluorescein that no detectable amounts of bound fluorescein could be found. From these results these investigators assumed that the fluorescence observed in the angiogram was produced by 100% of the injected dye.[20]

Fluorescein is metabolized by the liver to a glucuronide molecule that is only ⅓ to 1/30 as fluorescent as is fluorescein, depending on the wavelength of the excitation light. After either oral or intravenous administration of fluorescein, fluorescein glucuronide reaches concentrations many times greater than fluorescein. Within 3 hours after systemic administration, 95% of the fluorescein has been glucuronidated. McLaren and Brubaker[21] reported that by 6 hours fluorescein glucuronide concentration in the anterior chamber of living human eyes was 10 to 30 times more concentrated than fluorescein after oral administration and three to 10 times more concentrated after intravenous administration. Abnormal levels of background protein, as well as variable production of metabolites of fluorescein, may influence ocular fluorophotometry and must be taken into account in the interpretation of physiologic studies performed with systemically administered fluorescein.[22, 23]

Although we assume that fluorescein simply diffuses in and out of tissues, this may not be true for ocular tissues. Isolated rabbit iris and ciliary body have been shown to accumulate fluorescein by means of an active transport system that can act against a concentration gradient, is saturable by excess fluorescein, and is inhibited by cyanide, dinitrophenol (both inhibitors of oxidative metabolism), and anoxia. Transport systems for organic anions such as penicillin, probenecid, *p*-aminohippuric acid, and prostaglandins are known to exist in ocular tissues. Fluorescein effectively competes with *p*-aminohippuric acid for its transport mechanism.[24] Fluorescein is therefore actively transported out of the eye much as is penicillin.

Abnormalities of the fundus demonstrated by fluorescence may be explained by three general mechanisms:

1. The normal fluorescence of the choriocapillaris may become more apparent as a result of thinning of the retinal pigment epithelium.
2. Neovascularization may produce new vascular channels that contain the circulating fluorescein.
3. Any abnormality that increases capillary permeability may permit fluorescein to leak into the lesion.

These three mechanisms may be differentiated by the time of onset of the fluorescence. Choriocapillaris fluorescence appears as early as the arterial phase. Neovascularization fluorescence coincides with the arteriolar or venous phase, depending on the origin of the new vessels, and also shows characteristic irregular configurations. Fluorescence resulting from abnormal capillary permeability appears later and slowly increases as the injected fluorescein recirculates and further infiltrates the affected tissue. Hypofluorescence results from reduced circulation flow or from concealment by overlying material such as pigment or hemorrhage. A thorough review of the various patterns of fluorescence seen in ocular lesions is beyond the scope of this chapter but should be carefully reviewed by any ophthalmologist who treats lesions of the posterior portion of the eye.

#### *Fluorophotometry*

The technique for fluorophotometry to detect fluorescein in the anterior chamber and vitreous has been known for nearly as long as that for fluorescein angiography.[25] This procedure is one of the most accurate methods of measuring aqueous flow in human eyes and has contributed greatly to our understanding of aqueous formation and response to autonomic drugs. Briefly, fluorophotometric measurement of the rate of disappearance of fluorescein from the anterior chamber permits calculation of the rate of aqueous flow.[26] Cannulation of the anterior chamber with the introduction of fluorescein permits estimation of its volume.[27]

Ocular fluorophotometry is probably the best available method to evaluate changes in the blood-ocular barrier and is a more sensitive measure than fluorescein angiography. Oral or intravenously administered fluorescein can be measured in the aqueous or the vitreous by commercially available fluorophotometric equipment. By careful quantification of the concentration of fluorescein in these areas, conclusions can be made about breakdown in the blood-ocular barrier. Numerous investigators have used this technique to study normal and pathologic conditions, as well as the effect of various medications on ocular vascular tissues.[28–33]

### *Iris Examination*

Anterior segment fluorescein angiography, first introduced in 1968,[34] is useful in evaluating the vasculature of the iris, conjunctiva, and episclera and in the diagnosis of iris lesions. The procedure is performed using a photo slit lamp modified to give increased light output in a short period, usually 1.0 to 2.5 seconds. A blue filter (420–495 nm) is placed in front of the excitation light, and a barrier filter (515 nm) is placed in front of the film. For iris angiography fluorescein dye is injected in the usual manner, and photographs are taken using high-speed film. Watson[35] reported that when performing angiography on conjunctival and episcleral vessels, he obtained different information injecting 5 ml of 10% fluorescein compared with 0.6 ml of 20% solution. The lower-dose angiography is valuable when fine capillaries and fine details are important, and the higher dose, especially when viewed or photographed at low magnification, is best when the identification of gross, generalized changes are important.

Normally, in iris fluorescein angiography the iris vessels are straight in configuration and leak fluorescein only slightly. Iris vessels fill about 19 seconds after the injection of fluorescein dye into an antecubital vein; simultaneously the anterior ciliary arteries at the limbus fill from inside out and flow posteriorly on the sclera.[36] Iris neoplasms tend to show dilated and tortuous vessels with early hyperfluorescence and late leakage of fluorescein. In rubeosis iridis the new vessels are usually on the iris surface, are irregular in distribution, and leak fluorescein readily.

## Complications of Fluorescein Injection

About 10% to 15% of all patients receiving intravenous fluorescein complain of moderate nausea and headache, usually for a few minutes. Vomiting occurs in 2% to 3% of patients, and when it does, it lasts for only a few minutes. Of 547 patients, 10% had minor reactions to intravenous fluorescein, nausea being the most common problem. Male patients were affected more often; 12.8% had a reaction compared with 7.3% of females.[37] The concentration of the fluorescein is the most significant factor related to postinjection nausea. After intravenous injection of 25% fluorescein, nausea occurred in 23% of patients. Only 11% were nauseated with 10% fluorescein, and only 2% were nauseated with 5% fluorescein.[38] Kwiterovich et al.[39] conducted a prospective study to determine the frequency of adverse reactions in fluorescein angiography. They reported that reactions occurred 12 times more frequently when the dye was injected slowly, premedication was associated with more reactions, and patients who had a previous reaction to fluorescein had a 48.6% chance of another adverse reaction. Unlike other dyes, fluorescein does not cause photosensitization.[40]

True allergic reactions to fluorescein may be minor and are characterized by itching and hives. More serious reactions include laryngeal edema, convulsive seizure, anaphylactic shock, myocardial infarction, and even death. Halperin[41] reported that rapid sneezing in a 15-year-old was the first sign of a severe allergic reaction to intravenous fluorescein that led to dyspnea and shock.

Histamine plasma levels were measured in blood drawn from the arm opposite to the one receiving fluorescein.[42] In all subjects the level of histamine rose within 3 minutes of fluorescein injection and returned to baseline by 30 minutes. The amount of histamine was greater in those patients with adverse reactions (Fig. 10–3). The known histamine-induced symptoms of nausea and

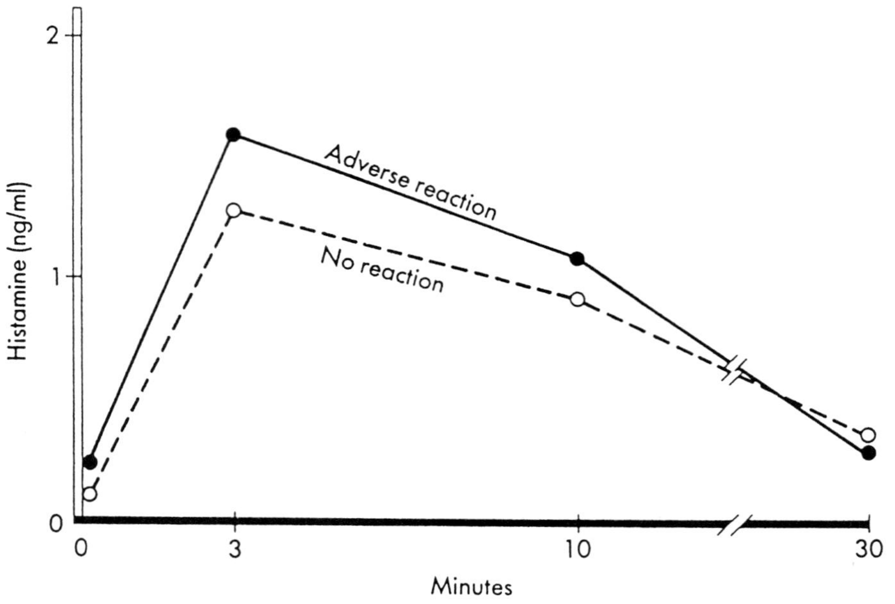


**FIG 10–3.**
Mean plasma histamine levels after intravenous fluorescein. (Modified from Arroyave CM: *Am J Ophthalmol* 87:474, 1979. Used by permission.)

vomiting, itching, paresthesias, dizziness, and fainting are very similar to the allergic reactions that can occur after fluorescein injection.

Yannuzzi et al.[43] reported on the results of a national survey designed to study the nature and frequency of moderate and severe complications of fluorescein angiography. In this survey, 2,434 responding ophthalmologists reported on 221,781 fluorescein angiograms performed in 1984. From this large pool of data the estimated frequency of mild adverse reactions was 5% or less, of moderate adverse reactions was 1:63, of severe adverse reactions was 1:1,900, and for death was 1:222,000. When fluorescein is injected, appropriate precautions should be taken, and resuscitative drugs, equipment, and trained personnel should be immediately available.

Concerns as to fluorescein teratogenicity arose from abortions and birth defects noted in experimental animals given intravenous fluorescein during pregnancy. Subsequent evaluations failed to reproduce the findings of these earlier studies, but the recommendation to avoid fluorescein use whenever possible in pregnant women is still observed.[44] Fluorescein crosses the placenta in humans, as shown by the finding of fluorescein in the amniotic fluid obtained from amniocentesis in a patient 33 weeks pregnant 2 days after an angiogram.[45]

Halperin et al.[46] surveyed 424 retina specialists to obtain information on patients who had fluorescein angiography during pregnancy. Of the 399 who responded, 77% had never performed fluorescein angiography on a pregnant woman, and 23% had performed at least one fluorescein angiogram on a pregnant woman. Side effects included nausea and vomiting in a few patients. Birth defects were rare, and only one stillbirth was reported. Because the majority of the pregnancies were complicated by major health problems such as diabetes, hypertension, or toxemia, the risk for fetal abnormalities and mortality was not thought to be increased. The authors concluded that fluorescein angiography does not increase the risk of birth anomalies when performed on a pregnant patient and that it is reasonable to perform a fluorescein angiogram on such a patient when it is necessary to direct treatment to a serious, sight-threatening lesion.

The decision to perform fluorescein angiography on any patient should be based on a need to obtain data for treatment not available by any other means. In many cases a careful examination with a clear determination of treatment objectives will be adequate. The use of routine fluorescein studies are not in the best interest of the patient, and the risk of the examination should be considered. Wilkinson[47] provided a good overview of the use of fluorescein angiography in retinal lesions most frequently examined by this technique. His conclusions were that most cases of age-related macular degeneration and diabetic retinopathy could be effectively treated without angiography.

### Fluorescein-Conjugated Compounds

The ability to conjugate fluorescent material to other substances and use the resultant fluorescent property as a specific marker to identify the conjugated compound is an important adjunct in pathologic diagnosis and was first introduced in 1941 by Coons. Immunofluorescence has become an indispensable diagnostic tool in autoimmune diseases, and the application of immunohistology and immunopathology has helped to expand diagnostic techniques in other areas. For instance, the rapid identification of suspected organisms is important for the effective treatment of corneal infections. In cases of infection with fungi or acanthamoebae, the culture is slow to grow, and routine Gram's and Giemsa stains may not be specific enough to identify the offending organisms from other cellular elements in the smear. For these reasons, rapid, more specific staining techniques are highly desirable. Robin et al.[48] reported their results using fluorescein-conjugated lectins for the rapid visualization of fungi and acanthamoebae in 18 cases of infectious keratitis. Specimens obtained from corneal scraping and paraffin embedded tissue with documented mycotic and acanthamoebic keratitis were studied with two fluorescein-conjugated lectins, concanavalin A and wheat germ agglutinin. After binding of the conjugated compounds with the organisms, examination with fluorescent microscopy was reported to readily reveal hyphae, yeast, and sporulating forms. The most positive staining was confined to the mycotic cell wall and acanthamoebic cysts and trophozoites. In similar experiments these same authors demonstrated that fluorescein-conjugated lectins can bind to several species of aerobic and anaerobic bacteria, fungi, atypical mycobacteria, and acanthamoebae.[49, 50] They suggest that this procedure may eventually become an effective first-line stain for the rapid identification of microorganisms in ocular infections. Similarly, the use of fluorescein-conjugated monoclonal antibodies has widespread application in identifying specific infectious agents and has been applied in infections such as chlamydial conjunctivitis.[51]

Calcofluor white is a laundry brightener that binds to polysaccharides such as cellulose and chitin. Cellulose is a major component of the cell wall of acanthamoebic cysts, and when bound by calcofluor white, the substance then acts as a biologic stain. Calcofluor white powder is dissolved in distilled water to form a 0.1% solution, and Evans blue dye (0.1%) is used as a counterstain. Tissues are stained for 1 minute, after which slides are examined with a fluorescein microscope. The cell walls of the mycotic organisms stain an intense bright green-white fluorescence against a reddish orange background produced by the Evans blue dye counterstain.[52] Calcofluor white is highly effective in staining the cell wall of the acanthamoebic endocyst but is not useful in identifying the trophozoite stage.[53] Cellufluor is a yellow fluorescent dye similar to calcofluor white. Sutphin et al.[54] used induced fluorescence from cell wall–bound Cellufluor to detect microorganisms in 109 ocular specimens from corneal, aqueous, vitreous, orbital, lacrimal gland, and lacrimal sac drainage.[54] These investigators reported that 50% of smears previously thought to be negative for organisms showed typical fungal elements with fluorochrome staining. This technique enhanced the detection of fungal elements and amoebic cysts and was considered to be an important adjunct to the standard Gram, Giemsa, and methenamine-silver stains.

## Antidote to Poisoning by Aniline Dyes

An unusual use of fluorescein dye is in the detoxification of aniline dyes such as those used for indelible pencils.[55] Indelible pencils consist of 30% methylrosaniline chloride (methyl violet) in a graphite and gum tragacanth base. These compounds are highly dissociated salts, and the cations are protoplasmic poisons. These salts will readily combine with the anion of sodium fluorescein to produce a slightly dissociated salt, methylrosaniline fluorescein. Precipitation of this insoluble compound effectively removes the toxic cation from tissues.

Methyl violet is very toxic, spreads rapidly through ocular tissues and the lids, produces intense purple staining, and causes severe edema and rapid necrosis (within several hours). Because of these, ocular injuries by indelible pencils, if significant dye is retained, may lead to loss of an eye after only relatively minor trauma. Treatment requires prompt surgical removal of the pencil point and as much dye as possible, after which the eye is irrigated with a 2% sodium fluorescein solution every 10 minutes until a blue-black precipitation no longer forms. Thereafter, fluorescein irrigation should be repeated every 30 minutes for 12 to 24 hours, at which time the eye may be completely free of purple staining. Healing will be slower than normal after such a chemical injury. A 2% fluorescein solution must be used because the commonly available 0.5% ophthalmic preparation is not strong enough. Gentian violet (hexamethylrosaniline chloride) is another cationic dye that binds to protein, causing tissue necrosis. Instillation of a 2% solution into rabbit eyes is known to cause severe damage.

## Experimental Studies

Because fluorescein is visible, it is an excellent tracer substance for physiologic studies of the penetration of water-soluble molecules into the eye. For example, in a study of iontophoresis, an electric current was found to drive fluorescein rapidly into the aqueous. After a 4-minute period of iontophoresis, 20 times as much fluorescein had entered the eye as when no current was used.[56] Breakdown of the blood-eye barrier with the resultant leakage of injected fluorescein into the vitreous is detectable even before the angiogram becomes abnormal. This provides a valuable method of studying the vasculopathy that occurs in such conditions as diabetic retinopathy. The pharmacokinetics of fluorescein in the vitreous are complex, however, and include blood-eye barrier permeability, active transport out of the eye, entry from both retinal and ciliary body sources, and intravitreal mixing, all of which are subject to a variety of measurement errors.[57]

## Other Dyes for Angiography

Sodium fluorescein given by intravenous injection is currently the standard method of performing angiography. Other dyes such as calcein and carboxyfluorescein have been investigated in animal experiments,[58] and indocyanine green has been investigated in humans.[59] Angiography using carboxyfluorescein encapsulated in heat-sensitive liposomes has been performed in animal studies. Liposomes are phospholipids that can be made to encapsulate water-soluble molecules such as carboxyfluorescein within their inner aqueous phase. These liposomes, when injected into the blood, isolate the dye from the serum, but with a small rise in temperature (approximately 4° C greater than body temperature), the liposomes are lysed, releasing the encapsulated dye. Because carboxyfluorescein, once released from the liposome, fluoresces intensely when exposed to blue light, its presence can be detected by fluorophotometry or photography.[60] Such a delivery system offers several advantages. If, for instance, the blue light of the laser is used, laser-triggered repetitive fluorescein angiography can be performed. Single or multiple pulses of laser light energy can be used to create the rise in temperature necessary to lyse the liposomes, but, in addition, the blue light of the laser allows fluorescence to be observed in individual vessels or to measure blood flow rates.[61–64] Because not all dye is released by a single exposure to the laser light, repeated angiograms can be performed rapidly over an extended period. Although these techniques may prove to be superior to conventional fluorescein angiography, toxicity of liposomes in humans has not been fully determined.

Indocyanine green is well tolerated intravenously and can be used in humans for infrared angiography as a clinical procedure.[65–68] Indocyanine green is used for determining cardiac output, liver blood flow, and liver function, as well as for angiography in ophthalmology. It is largely protein bound and has a peak absorption at 805 nm and peak fluorescence at 835 nm in the infrared spectrum. Indocyanine angiography is more effective in revealing choroidal neovascular membranes than are comparable studies with fluorescein. Apparently, because of the longer wavelength of indocyanine green, it is more easily detected through pigment, blood, and lipid and produces overall enhanced image resolution.[69] With the use of infrared videoangiography, choroidal neovascular membranes obscured by subretinal hemorrhage can be more clearly identified with this technique compared with fluorescein angiography.[70, 71] Clinical research using the diode light source (Candela Laser Corp., Wayland, Mass.) has been shown to be more efficient than conventional light sources, resulting in lower light levels on the retina but still producing clear, sharp angiograms.

Yannuzzi et al.[72] reported the results of their study of a consecutive series of 129 patients with exudative age-related macular degeneration and ill-defined or occult choroidal neovascularization (CNV) using a new system for digital indocyanine green videoangiography. In this study 39% of the patients with occult CNV were reclassified as having a well-delineated CNV. This technique was reported to be particularly useful in identifying occult CNV in eyes with serous pigment epithelial detachments and in eyes that had undergone previous laser photocoagulation. The improved visualization of the occult CNV allowed for more effective laser treatment that would not have been possible with standard fluorescein angiography.

Adverse reactions to indocyanine green have been reported. Wolf et al.[73] reported that nausea and vomiting, sometimes occurring with fluorescein angiography, were almost never seen with the use of indocyanine green dye. However, these same authors reported a case of severe anaphylactic reaction in a 62-year-old woman after intravenous injection of indocyanine green. The anaphylactic reaction was thought to be caused by the iodine additive. Other studies have found that fatal reactions can occur in 1:10,000 to 1:100,000 procedures after intravenous injection of iodine-containing contrast media

Indocyanine green in a 1% solution is nontoxic to living corneal endothelial cells and stains diseased or dead endothelial cells. It may be used for evaluation of donor corneal viability.[74]

## Rose Bengal

It has been generally accepted that rose bengal (dichloro-tetra-iodofluorescein) selectively stains devitalized corneal and conjunctival cells and does not stain normal, healthy cells. Rose bengal is thought to actually stain cells and their nuclei a visible red without causing damage to the cells; thus, the dye has been referred to as a vital dye. Feenstra et al.[75, 76] in two extensive reviews of the mechanisms of action of rose bengal and fluorescein have challenged this notion. These investigators showed that both commercial additive-containing rose bengal and additive-free rose bengal stain healthy rabbit corneas and culture cells whenever they are not covered by albumin, mucin, or tear substitutes such as carboxycellulose. This staining was described as rapid, predominantly nuclear, and visible with the unaided eye in concentrations as low as 0.025% for the additive-free solution. With the fluorescence microscope the stain could be detected at levels of 0.001% solution. They also demonstrated that rose bengal at concentrations as low as 0.01% was cytotoxic to culture cells and that cell death occurred even at concentrations of 0.001% when the cells were exposed to room light. Fluorescein was also found to stain healthy culture cells but could be observed only with the aid of the fluorescence microscope and appropriate excitation and emission filters. The conclusions were that both dyes stain healthy living cells, rose bengal stains more strongly than fluorescein, rose bengal does not stain the normal ocular surface because of the blocking effect of the precorneal tear film, and rose bengal but not fluorescein is cytotoxic. Fluorescein staining is enhanced over rose bengal because of its ability to pass through intercellular spaces and its rapid diffusion through the corneal stroma.

The main clinical use of rose bengal is the identification of tear deficiencies in such conditions as keratoconjunctivitis sicca and Sjögren's syndrome. In keratoconjunctivitis sicca the lesions cause interpalpebral limbus-based triangles of staining associated with relatively minor corneal staining. Typically rose bengal staining is a somewhat more sensitive and reliable test for keratoconjunctivitis sicca than is the Schirmer filter paper test for tear secretion. However, the diagnosis should not be made on the basis of insignificant punctate corneal staining.

Rose bengal is instilled as a 1% aqueous solution. Irritation and discomfort are more marked with rose bengal than with fluorescein, but it usually does not require preliminary use of a local anesthetic. Excess rose bengal is removed as in fluorescein staining. Discoloration of the skin of the patient's lid and the examiner's fingers, as well as the ocular staining, is more persistent than is fluorescein coloring. Application of rose bengal staining via a filter paper strip is much less irritating.[77]

Photosensitization with rose bengal and subsequent exposure to light causes erythrocyte hemolysis. Perfusion of the anterior chamber of enucleated rabbit eyes with $5 \times 10^{-6}$M rose bengal and subsequent exposure for 30 seconds to 5 minutes of light from a 24-W bulb at 5 cm (intervening water barrier to absorb heat) caused sufficient endothelial photodynamic damage to increase the rate of corneal swelling up to six times baseline. Catalase (200 μg/ml) eliminated the light-induced swelling, indicating that the photodynamic endothelial damage resulted from hydrogen peroxide produced by superoxide-free radicals. Whether rose bengal photosensitization of the corneal surface is clinically significant was not specified, but this seems possible.[78]

A newly developed technique for photothrombosis of corneal vessels in rabbits has been reported.[79] In corneal experiments, corneal neovascularization in well-healed surface wounds were occluded with argon laser irradiation after a single intravenous injection of 40 mg of rose bengal/kg of body weight. A dose of 8 mg/kg was determined to be adequate for photothrombotic occlusion of the corneal vessels. The authors concluded that this technique produces thrombosis with much less laser energy and therefore less tissue damage than photocoagulation because photothrombosis is mediated by electron-state transition between the photosensitizing dye and molecular oxygen, which generates oxygen singlets. Thermal damage to endothelial cells is therefore not required as in photocoagulation. The thrombus produced by photothrombosis has been shown to be composed entirely of aggregated platelets with little or no fibrin. The occluded vessels remained blocked for at least 16 weeks and apparently resist thrombolysis. Huang et al.[80] used this same technique to induce corneal transdifferentiation in previously injured rabbit corneas. They concluded that because transdifferentiation is inhibited by corneal vascularization, occluding these vessels would be beneficial to healing. The treated vessels remained occluded for the duration of the 18-week study, and corneal clarity and epithelial integrity improved.

Similar photochemical initiated thrombosis of preretinal and choroidal vessels has been studied.[81] Fluorescein angiography and electron microscopy were used to document the resultant pathologic changes in the vessels over time. After an intravenous injection of 10 mg of rose bengal/kg the selected retinal area was exposed to a 330-W xenon arc lamp light beam filtered to 550 nm. After treatment the eyes were studied with fluorescein angiography, then removed for histopathologic evaluation. Endothelial cells in both preretinal and choroidal vessels were damaged, with platelet adhesion and aggregation producing thrombosis. In this study the occlusion was only temporary, and endothelial cell regeneration began at 7 days and was complete by 28 days. Both of these studies demonstrate a technique that has the potential to be a new modality for treating neovascularization in human ocular tissues.

Photoradiation therapy to treat solid malignant tumors in humans using a pigment, an acid-extracted form of hematoporphyrin called hematoporphyrin derivative, was first reported in 1976.[82] After intravenous administration the dye appears to have an affinity for tissue with a rapid turnover such as a neoplasm and remains in this tissue long after it has been cleared from normal tissue. When the malignant cells containing the hematoporphyrin derivative are exposed to an exciting light, a sequence of photochemical reactions occurs, leading to the intracellular formation of singlet oxygen. This potent oxidizing agent causes changes in cellular amino acids and unsaturated fatty acids, leading to other intracellular changes that ultimately cause death of the tumor cells. Hematoporphyrin derivative can be photoactivated by several wavelengths of visible light, but 630 nm is usually used for treatment because the red light has greater tissue penetration.[83] This technique has been used to treat cutaneous,[84] intraocular, and orbital neoplasms.[85, 86] Disadvantages of the procedure are inability to determine tissue margins; side effects of cutaneous photosensitization, which may be severe and last for as long as 30 days; possible necessity for multiple injections; and possible occurrence of ocular complications such as transient glaucoma and tissue necrosis. Before this treatment modality can be recommended for the treatment of ocular neoplasms, a significant amount of additional study is needed.

## Methylene Blue

Vital staining of nerve tissue may be achieved with a 0.5% solution of methylene blue, which stains the corneal nerves as delicate blue filaments. Methylene blue is more irritating than rose bengal, and topical anesthetic is recommended before its use. Vital staining of corneal nerves requires at least three instillations of dye at 5-minute intervals. Bluish ocular discoloration may persist for as long as 1 day after methylene blue staining.

Methylene blue irrigation of the lacrimal sac before dacryocystorhinostomy will stain the mucosal lining a readily identifiable blue. The dye should remain in the sac for several minutes. Before starting the operation, the surgeon should wash the sac free of excess methylene blue, because this solution would otherwise spill out on incision of the sac and stain the surrounding tissues.

## Alcian Blue

Counterstaining with Alcian blue may be used to differentiate mucous deposits from diseased cells. A 1% solution of Alcian blue is employed. With this dye, mucus and connective tissue stain blue, but diseased epithelial cells do not stain. Rose bengal stains both diseased epithelial cells and mucus.

## Lissamine Green

A 1% solution of this dye will stain dry or devitalized corneal and conjunctival cells, and this has been suggested as a simple screening method for the detection of vitamin A deficiency xerophthalmia.[87] Unfortunately, the test has an unacceptable high incidence of false-negative results. The eyes of 57% of vitamin A–deficient night-blind children did not stain with lissamine green dye, 29% with vitamin A–responsive Bitot's spots did not stain, and 26% with vitamin A deficiency corneal involvement also did not stain. A good history of visual symptoms appears to be equally as effective as staining with this dye.

## Argyrol

Instillation of Argyrol (10% or 20% silver protein solution) into the conjunctival sac before the surgical scrub of the eye serves as an excellent indicator of the adequacy of the preparation. Mucus strands and debris on the lid margins and the skin surface appear discolored by the dark stain produced by the Argyrol. The tissues themselves are not stained, and the Argyrol easily washes off;

when no stain is seen, the preparation is complete. Because of the great importance of a thorough and complete washing of the field before intraocular surgery, such use of Argyrol or a comparable marker is highly advisable. Argyrol has no antimicrobial activity.

## SUMMARY

Techniques for fluorescein angiography and angioscopy have improved greatly since first introduced more than 30 years ago. The use of dyes other than sodium fluorescein such as indocyanine green and potentially calcein and carboxyfluorescein may prove to be superior in certain circumstances. Indocyanine green has already been used to detect choroidal neovascular membranes that are obscured by hemorrhage, lipid, or pigment and not easily visible by standard fluorescein angiography. Laser-stimulated fluorescence from dyes contained in heat-sensitive liposomes allows select angiography at specific sites in the retina in experimental animals. Such a delivery system may, in the future, provide another means of investigating both normal and abnormal retinal and choroidal circulation.

Yet another experimental method that could lead to a new treatment modality for producing occlusions of retinal and choroidal vessels in humans is photochemical activation of intravenously injected rose bengal.

Dyes used in the evaluation of anterior segment conditions have not changed greatly, but newer instrumentation for fluorophotometry and anterior segment angiography provides important clinical tools for the evaluation of blood-ocular barrier disruptions such as occur in diabetes or uveitis. The use of various dyes continues to be important in the evaluation and treatment of anterior and posterior segment ocular diseases.

## REFERENCES


1. Refojo MF, Miller D, Fiore AS: A new fluorescent for soft hydrophilic lens fitting, *Arch Ophthalmol* 87:275, 1972.
2. Moses RA: Fluorescein in applanation tonometry, *Am J Ophthalmol* 49:1149, 1960.
3. Roper DL: Applanation tonometry with and without fluorescein, *Am J Ophthalmol* 90:668, 1980.
4. Rumelt MB: Applanation tonometry without fluorescein, *Am J Ophthalmol* 89:309, 1980.
5. Quickert MH: A fluorescein-anesthetic solution for applanation tonometry, *Arch Ophthalmol* 77:734, 1967.
6. Valghan DG: The contamination of fluorescein solutions, *Am J Ophthalmol* 39:55, 1955.
7. Stewart HL: Prolonged antibacterial activity of a fluorescein-anesthetic solution, *Arch Ophthalmol* 88:385, 1972.
8. Duffner LR, Pflugfelder SC, Mandelbaum S, and others: Potential bacterial contamination in fluorescein-anesthetic solutions, *Am J Ophthalmol* 110:199, 1990.
9. Hecht SD: The use of intravenous fluorescein to estimate the extent of planar Decemet's membrane detachment, *Eye Ear Nose Throat Mon* 54:375, 1975.
10. Wright MM, Bersani TA, Frueh BR, and others: Efficacy of the primary dye test, *Ophthalmology* 96:481, 1989.
11. McClean AL, Maumenee AE: Hemangioma of the choroid, *Am J Ophthalmol* 50:3, 1960.
12. Schatz H, Burton TC, and others: *Interpretation of fundus fluorescein angiography,* St Louis, 1978, Mosby.
13. Ernest JT: Recent correlates of ocular physiology and fluorescein angioscopy, angiography, and fluorophotometry—CME credit article, *J C E Ophthalmol* July: 5, 1979.
14. Robert G, Sobrance G, Lieb W: *Fluorescein angiography,* New York, 1990, Thieme Medical Publishers (translated by Blodi FC).
15. Nanjiani M: Fluorescein angiography. *Technique, interpretation, and application,* New York, 1992, Oxford University Press.
16. Berkow JW, Orth DH, Kelley JS: *Fluorescein angiography-technique and interpretation,* Ophthalmology Monogr No 5, 1991, American Academy of Ophthalmology.
17. Jalkh AE, Celorio JM: *Atlas of fluorescein angiography,* Philadelphia, 1993, WB Saunders Co.
18. Flower RW: Injection technique for indocyanine green and sodium fluorescein dye angiography of the eye, *Invest Ophthalmol* 12:881, 1973.
19. Palestine AG, Brubaker RF: Pharmacokinetics of fluorescein in the vitreous, *Invest Ophthalmol* 21:542, 1981.

20. Ianacone DC, Felberg NT, Federman JL: Tritiated fluorescein binding to normal human plasma proteins, *Arch Ophthalmol* 98:1643, 1980.
21. McLaren JW, Brubaker RF: Measurement of fluorescein and fluorescein monoglucuronide in the living human eye, *Invest Ophthalmol Vis Sci* 27:966, 1986.
22. Arie M, Sawa M, Mishima S: Aqueous humor dynamics in man as studied by oral fluorescein, *Jpn J Ophthalmol* 24:346, 1980.
23. Barsotti MF, Bartels SP, Kamm RD, and others: Background-protein effects on fluorophotometric data, *Invest Ophthalmol Vis Sci* 31:2046, 1990.
24. Stone RA, Wilson CM: Fluorescein transport in the anterior uvea, *Invest Ophthalmol* 22:303, 1982.
25. Maurice DM: A new objective fluorophotometer, *Exp Eye Res* 2:82, 1963.
26. Coakes RL, Brubaker RF: Method of measuring aqueous humor flow and corneal endothelial permeability using a fluorophotometry nomogram, *Invest Ophthalmol* 18:288, 1979.
27. Johnson SB, Passmore JA, Brubaker RF: The fluorescein distribution volume of the anterior chamber, *Invest Ophthalmol* 16:633, 1977.
28. Zeimer RC, Cunha-Vas JG, Johnson ME: Studies on the technique of vitreous fluorophotometry, *Invest Ophthalmol Vis Sci* 22:668, 1982.
29. Zeimer RC, Blair NP, Cunha-Vas JG: Vitreous fluorophotometry for clinical research: I. Description and evaluation of a new fluorophotometer, *Arch Ophthalmol* 101:1753, 1983.
30. Zeimer RC, Blair NP, Cunha-Vaz JG: Vitreous fluorophotometry for clinical research: II. Method of data acquisition and processing, *Arch Ophthalmol* 101:1757, 1983.
31. McLaren JW, Brubaker RF: A two-dimensional scanning ocular fluorophotometer, *Invest Ophthalmol Vis Sci* 26:144, 1985.
32. Ruy MS, Bonner RF, Bungay PM, and others: Posterior vitreous fluorophotometry in normal subjects, *Arch Ophthalmol* 104:1004, 1986.
33. Jackson WE, Chase HP, Garg SK, and others: Vitreous fluorophotometry in insulin-dependent diabetes mellitus, *Arch Ophthalmol* 108:1733, 1990.
34. Jensen VA, Lundbaek K: Fluorescein angiography of the iris in recent and long-term diabetes, preliminary communication, *Acta Ophthalmol* 46:584, 1968.
35. Watson PG: Anterior segment fluorescein angiography in the surgery of immunologically induced corneal and scleral destructive disorders, *Ophthalmology* 94:1452, 1987.
36. Talusan ED, Schwartz B: Fluorescein angiography, *Arch Ophthalmol* 99:1074, 1981.
37. Greene GS, Bell LW, Hitching DR, and others: Adverse reactions to intravenous fluorescein: evidence for sex difference, *Ann Ophthalmol* 8:533, 1976.
38. Willerson D, Tate GW, Baldwin HA, and others: Clinical evaluation of fluorescein 25%, *Ann Ophthalmol* 8:833, 1976.
39. Kwiterovich KA, Maguire MG, Murphy RP, and others: Frequency of adverse systemic reactions after fluorescein angiography, *Ophthalmology* 98:1139, 1991.
40. Valenzeno DP, Pooler JP: Phototoxicity, the neglected factor, *JAMA* 242:453, 1979.
41. Halperin LS: Sneezing as an early indicator of allergy to fluorescein dye, *Am J Ophthalmol* 112:601, 1991 (letter).
42. Weiter JJ: Intravenous fluorescein effects, *Am J Ophthalmol* 71:771, 1971.
43. Yannuzzi LA, Rohrer KT, Tindel LJ, and others: Fluorescein angiography complication survey *Ophthalmology* 93:611, 1986.
44. McEnerney JK, Wong WP, Peyman GA: Evaluation of the teratogenicity of fluorescein sodium, *Am J Ophthalmol* 84:847, 1977.
45. Shekleton P, Fidler J, Grimwade JA: A case of benign intracranial hypertension in pregnancy, *Br J Obstet Gynecol* 87:345, 1980.
46. Halperin LS, Olk RJ, Soubraine G, and others: Safety of fluorescein angiography during pregnancy, *Am J Ophthalmol* 109:563, 1990.
47. Wilkinson CF: The clinical examination: Limitation and over-utilization of angiographic services, *Ophthalmology* 93:401, 1986.
48. Robin JB, Chan R, Narsing RA, and others: Fluorescein-conjugated lectin visualization of fungi and acanthamoebae in infectious keratitis, *Ophthalmology* 96:1198, 1989.
49. Robin JB, Arffa RC, Avni I, and others: Rapid visualization of three common fungi using fluorescein-conjugated lectins, *Invest Ophthalmol Vis Sci* 27:500, 1986.
50. Robin JB, Chan R, Andersen BR: Rapid visualization of *Acanthamoeba* using fluorescein-conjugated lectins, *Arch Ophthalmol* 106:1273, 1988.
51. Vrabec MP, McCanna PJ: The effect of topically applied fluorescein on fluorescein

monoclonal antibodies in the diagnosis of chlamydial conjunctivitis, *Ann Ophthalmol* 20:424, 1988.
52. Marines HM, Osato MS, Font RA: The value of calcofluor white in the diagnosis of mycotic and *Acanthamoeba* infections of the eye and ocular adenexa, *Ophthalmology* 94:23, 1987.
53. Wilhelmus KR, Osato MS, Font RL, and others: Rapid diagnosis of *Acanthamoeba* keratitis using calcofluor white, *Arch Ophthalmol* 104:1309, 1986.
54. Sutphin JE, Robinson NM, Wilhelmus KR, and others: Improved detection of oculomycoses using induced fluorescence with Cellufluor, *Ophthalmology* 93:416, 1986.
55. Hosford G: Treatment of ocular methylrosaniline poisoning with fluorescein, *JAMA* 150:1482, 1952.
56. Tonjum AM, Green K: Quantitative study of fluorescein iontophoresis through the cornea, *Am J Ophthalmol* 71:1328, 1971.
57. Palestine AG, Brubaker RF: Pharmacokinetics of fluorescein in the vitreous, *Invest Ophthalmol* 21:542, 1981.
58. Fang T, Naguib KS, and others: Comparative study of three fluorescein dyes for angiography; sodium fluorescein, carboxyfluorescein, and calcein, *Ophthalmic Surg* 21:250, 1990.
59. Hyvarinen L, Flower RW: Indocyanine green fluorescein angiography, *Acta Ophthalmol* 58:528, 1980.
60. Zeimer RC, Khoobehi B, Niesman MR, and others: A potential method for local drug and dye delivery in the ocular vasculature, *Invest Ophthalmol* 29:1179, 1988.
61. Khoobehi B, Niesman MR, Peyman GA, and others: Repetitive, selective angiography of individual vessels of the retina, *Retina* 9:87, 1989.
62. Khoobehi B, Peyman GA, Niesman MR, and others: Measurement of retinal blood velocity and flow rate in primates using a liposome-dye system, *Ophthalmology* 96:905, 1989.
63. Zeimer RC, Khoobehi B, Peyman GA, and others: Feasibility of blood flow measurement by externally controlled dye delivery, *Invest Ophthalmol Vis Sci* 30:660, 1989.
64. Zeimer RC, Guran T, Shahidi M, and others: Visualization of the retinal microvasculature by targeted dye delivery, *Invest Ophthalmol Vis Sci* 31:1459, 1990.
65. Hochheimer BF: Angiography of the retina with indocyanine green, *Arch Ophthalmol* 86:564, 1971.
66. Flower RW: Choroidal angiography today and tomorrow, *Retina* 12:189, 1992 (guest editorial).
67. Flower RW: Injection technique for indocyanine green and sodium fluorescein dye angiography of the eye, *Invest Ophthalmol* 12:881, 1973.
68. Orth DH, Patz A, Flower RW: Potential clinical applications of indocyanine green choroidal angiography: preliminary report, *Eye Ear Nose Throat Mon* 55:15, 1976.
69. Guyer DR, Puliafito CA, Monés JM, and others: Digital indocyanine-green angiography in chorioretinal disorders, *Ophthalmology* 99:287, 1992.
70. Destro M, Puliafito CA: Indocyanine green videoangiography of choroidal neovascularization, *Ophthalmology* 96:846, 1989.
71. Hayashi K, Hasegawa Y, Tokor T, and others: Value of indocyanine green angiography in the diagnosis of occult choroidal neovascular membrane, *Jpn J Clin Ophthalmol* 42:827, 1988.
72. Yannuzzi LA, Slakter JS, Sorenson JA, and others: Digital indocyanine green videoangiography and choroidal neovascularization, *Retina* 12:191, 1992.
73. Wolf S, Arend O, Shulte K, and others: Severe anaphylactic reaction after indocyanine green fluorescence angiography, *Am J Ophthalmol* 114:638, 1992.
74. McEnerney JK, Payman GA: Indocyanine green, *Arch Ophthalmol* 96:1445, 1978.
75. Feenstra RP, Scheffer CG, Tseng CG: What is actually stained by rose bengal? *Arch Ophthalmol* 110:984, 1992.
76. Feenstra RP, Scheffer CG, Tseng CG: Comparison of fluorescein and rose bengal staining, *Ophthalmology* 99:605, 1992.
77. Scott PM: Rose bengal strips, *Am J Ophthalmol* 87:572, 1979.
78. Hull DS, Strickland EC, Green K: Photodynamically induced alteration of corneal endothelial cell function, *Invest Ophthalmol* 18:1226, 1979.
79. Huang AJW, Watson BD, Hernandez E, and others: Photothrombosis of corneal neovascularization by intravenous rose bengal and argon laser irradiation, *Arch Ophthalmol* 106:680, 1988.
80. Huang AJW, Watson BD, Hernandez E, and others: Induction of conjunctival transdifferentiation on vascularized corneas by photothrombotic occlusion of corneal neovascularization, *Ophthalmology* 95:228, 1988.
81. Royster AJ, Nanda SK, Hatchell DL, and

others: Photochemical initiation of thrombosis, *Arch Ophthalmol* 106:1608, 1988.

82. Kelly JF, Snell ME: Hematoporphyrin derivative: a possible aid in the diagnosis and treatment of carcinoma of the bladder, *J Urol* 115:150, 1976.
83. Dougherty TJ, Kaufman JE, Goldfarb A, and others: Photoradiation therapy for the treatment of malignant tumors, *Cancer Res* 38:2628, 1978.
84. Tse DT, Kersten RC, Anderson RL: Hematoporphyrin photoradiation therapy in managing nevoid basal-cell carcinoma syndrome: a preliminary report, *Arch Ophthalmol* 102:990, 1984.
85. Liu LHS, Ni C: Hematoporphyrin phototherapy for experimental intraocular malignant melanoma, *Arch Ophthalmol* 101:901, 1983
86. Tse DT, Dutton JJ, Weingeist TA, and others: Hematoporphyrin photoradiation therapy for intraocular and orbital malignant melanoma, *Arch Ophthalmol* 102:833, 1984
87. Norn MS: Vitamin A–responsive keratopathy in xerophthalmia, *Am J Ophthalmol* 88:955, 1979.

# CHAPTER 11

# Oxygen

Elson L. Craig

Recent data from many investigators have shown that oxygen plays a major role in ocular tissue damage beyond that previously attributed to excess concentrations or oxygen deprivation (hypoxia). High concentrations of oxygen have been known for some time to damage the eyes of both infants and adults, although the adult retina is much more resistant. Mild to severe hypoxia causes disturbances in tissue function that may lead to a number of serious eye diseases such as retinopathy in diabetics or vascular occlusive disease, intraocular neovascularization, age-related macular degeneration, and optic nerve ischemia. The effects of mild hypoxia on the retina/retinal pigment epithelium/choriocapillaris complex have been extensively reviewed by Steinberg.[1] The conversion of tissue oxygen to the superoxide molecule is now known to produce damage to tissues with high concentrations of polyunsaturated fatty acids such as exist in retinal photoreceptors and the retinal pigment epithelium. Superoxide may prove to be important in the development of age-related macular degeneration, as well as in the formation of cataracts. The therapeutic use of oxygen has both toxic and beneficial effects; however, both normobaric and hyperbaric oxygen is useful in treating a number of conditions.

## EFFECT OF OXYGEN ON PREMATURE INFANTS

Terry[2] in 1942 was the first to observe a correlation between extreme prematurity and the overgrowth of fibrovascular tissue behind the lens. Keeping the premature infant in an oxygen atmosphere until the retina became more vascularized was suggested as a prophylaxis for this condition.[3] Patz et al.[4] in 1952, Gordon et al.[5] and Lenman et al.[6] in 1954, and Kinsey[7] in 1956 suggested a causal relationship between oxygen therapy in premature infants and retrolental fibroplasia. This led to a reduction in the use of oxygen to support premature infants, with a concomitant decrease in the incidence of retrolental fibroplasia. Withholding oxygen therapy, however, was thought to have contributed to an increased death rate from respiratory problems. Because this condition is found almost exclusively in premature infants who receive supplemental oxygen therapy, the term retinopathy of prematurity was used to distinguish it from other forms of retrolental fibroplasia. From studies performed in the early 1980s and from more recent studies, it is thought that retinopathy of prematurity is a multifactorial disease and includes not only supplemental oxygen therapy but also low birth weight ($<$ 1,300 g), low Apgar score ($<$ 5), possibly a genetic predisposition, light-induced oxygen-free radical formation causing membrane damage by lipid peroxidation,[8] secondary factors such as vitamin E,[9, 10] and prostaglandins.[11]

The level of oxygen required to cause retinopathy of prematurity has not been clearly established even when continuous transcutaneous oxygen monitoring was used.[12] In the early studies by Patz,[13] premature infants were maintained in incubators in 60% to 70% oxygen for 4 to 7 weeks. After 3 weeks infants showed extreme attenuation of retinal vessels. In experimental animals and in humans the effect of oxygen was shown to occur in two phases. The primary phase was a vasotoxic and vasoconstrictive phase, and the secondary phase was a phase of abnormal vascular proliferation.[13] From this and other studies it became apparent that oxygen in high concentrations has the capability of selectively causing constriction and obliteration of growing vessels in immature animals. That constriction of mature retinal vessels can be produced in adults has been demonstrated by Riva et al.[14] Using the laser Doppler velocimetry technique, they were able to show in normal adult volunteers that after 5 minutes of breathing 100% oxygen retinal vessel diameter decreased by 12%, red blood cell velocity by 53%, and blood flow by 60%.

Vasoproliferation and subsequent cicatrical changes at the junction of vascularized and nonvascularized retina lead to the complications associated with retinopathy of prematurity. In 1984 the International Classification of Retinopathy of Prematurity was published.[15] This classification was developed to provide the examining ophthalmologist with a more reproducible method of characterizing the location and extent of the disease clinically. The diagnosis, severity, and natural history of retinopathy of prematurity were further reviewed by Flynn et al.[16]

There is no concentration of oxygen in excess of that in air that is not associated with some risk of developing some degree of retinopathy of prematurity.[17, 18] In addition, the increased affinity of fetal hemoglobin for oxygen may make even low concentrations of oxygen (as low as 20%) hazardous.[19] The length of time the infant is in an oxygen-enriched atmosphere is an important factor in causing retinal damage. As short an exposure as 11 hours was found to cause some degree of retinal scarring. When the use of oxygen has been necessary, it should be terminated as soon as possible without tapering off. Transcutaneous monitoring either continuously or during the more acute stage of the infant's illness did not significantly reduce the incidence of retinopathy of prematurity in 296 infants studied.[12]

Johnson and Ahdab-Barmada[20] examined the retinas of 132 premature neonates and provided histologic evidence of a form of retinal neuronal necrosis occurring in the central portion of the retina and affecting primarily ganglion cell nuclei. Common among those demonstrating this form of neuronal necrosis was low birth weight (of the 30 affected histologically all weighed less than 2,000 g, and 80% of those weighed less than 1,500 g) and the use of supplemental oxygen. In most cases arterial oxygen pressure was reported to be greater than 150 mm Hg for more than 2 hours. Neuronal necrosis was characterized by karyorrhexis primarily of ganglion cells in the macula region, although neurons in the inner and outer nuclear layers were also involved in a few cases. These authors reported this as a distinctive type of acute hyperoxemic retinal necrosis occurring in premature infants and further suggested that certain developing neuronal cells show increased sensitivity to the toxic effects of oxygen. They also suggested that this represents a second toxic effect of hyperoxemia that can occur in some premature infants. Similar findings in brain tissue have been reported by other investigators.[21]

The benefits of cryotherapy for retinopathy of prematurity studied by a multicenter trial started in 1985 and, more recently, laser therapy have provided a direction for treating the complications of this disease.[22, 23] Tasman[24] points out that this is a lifetime disease and that even infants who never require treatment during the active stages of their disease may later develop myopia, exudative or rhegmatogenous retinal detachment, cataracts, angle-closure glaucoma, or visual loss from retinal pigment epithelial changes or cystoid macular edema.

## EFFECT OF OXYGEN ON ADULTS

Severe ocular and general toxic effects result from prolonged exposure to 90% to 100% oxygen at atmospheric pressure. Bilateral retinal detachment developed in more than half of adult dogs maintained at such oxygen levels within 2 to 3 days. Removal from the oxygen caused spontaneous reattachment of the retina. Other changes included ciliary cysts, iritis with hyphema, and edema of the cornea and conjunctiva. Continuous oxygen exposure for 3 days was fatal to all 10 adult dogs so exposed and to 6 of 9 dogs removed to normal atmospheric oxygen for 1 to 2 hours daily.[25]

During these experiments, promazine was used as a tranquilizer to facilitate handling the dogs. Subsequent experiments revealed this sedative to have significant retinal toxicity in combination with oxygen.[26] The toxic effect of oxygen on the retina was greatly increased by the simultaneous administration of phenothiazine or chloroquine. Concurrent exposure to 98% oxygen and daily intramuscular injections of 50 mg of promazine caused extensive retinal detachments in 27 of 37 dogs within 4 days, whereas oxygen alone caused only localized detachments in two of 10 dogs. The mechanism of this oxygen-induced retinal detachment has not been established; however, the probability of choriocapillaris damage has been suggested.[27] Contrary to the tissue damage that occurs in high oxygen concentrations, barbiturates were found to protect retinal cells from hypoxia in cell culture. Tissue culture cells from rat retinas were used to screen certain glutamate antagonists, anesthetics, calcium blockers, and thiopental sodium for their protective effect. Thiopental was shown to significantly reduce hypoxia-induced damage to retinal cells in these cultures.[28]

The rods and cones of rabbits selectively degenerate when exposed to high concentrations of oxygen. In rabbits, death of the visual cells occurred after 5 days in 60% oxygen and after 2 days in 90% to 100% oxygen.[29] Such levels should not be administered to humans for prolonged periods.

A 32-year-old man was unable to breathe because of myasthenia gravis. Respiration was maintained with an iron lung, and 80% oxygen was administered for about 150 days. At the end of this period the patient complained of rapid, almost complete loss of vision occurring within a 2-day span. The retinal arterioles were severely sheathed. The visual loss was permanent, with one eye reduced to hand movement and the other to total blindness.[30]

## HYPERBARIC OXYGEN

Hyperbaric medicine is now a recognized subspecialty, and in most major medical centers hyperbaric oxygen treatment is available as standard therapeutic modality. Most chambers used today are capable of providing compressed oxygen to at least 3 atm. The therapeutic effects are usually based on inhaled oxygen under pressure; consequently, the patient must be enclosed in the chamber during the treatment period. All monitoring systems, including transcutaneous oxygen pressure ($Po_2$) and carbon dioxide pressure ($Pco_2$), can be maintained during treatment. Conditions in which hyperbaric oxygen may be of benefit are listed in Table 11–1.

Under hyperbaric conditions, oxygen is even more toxic to retinal tissues. Electroretinograms recorded during exposure of rabbits to 100% oxygen under pressure as high as 7 atm showed a more rapid loss of retinal function with progressive increases in pressure.[31] The B wave was extinguished after less than 1 hour of exposure to 100% oxygen at less than 6 atm. Breathing pure oxygen at less than 3 atm caused a 10% decrease in the diameter of retinal arterioles in healthy young men,[32] which is similar to that shown by Riva et al.[14] when individuals

**TABLE 11–1.**
Conditions Where Hyperbaric Oxygen May Be Indicated

| |
|---|
| Actinomycosis/mucormycosis infections |
| Anaerobic soft tissue infections |
| Air embolism |
| Arterial insufficiency |
| Burns |
| Carbon monoxide poisoning |
| Crush injuries |
| Compromised skin grafts and flaps |
| Cyanide poisoning |
| Decompression sickness |
| Gas gangrene |
| Optic neuropathy |
| Osteomyelitis, chronic or refractory |
| Osteoradionecrosis |
| Ischemic wounds that are refractory (e.g., diabetes) |

are breathing 100% oxygen. During this oxygen exposure the blood $P_{CO_2}$ level was not significantly altered; hence, the vasoconstriction was thought to be oxygen induced and unrelated to carbon dioxide changes.

Hyperbaric oxygen has been used in scleral buckling procedures to protect the anterior segment in patients with sickling hemoglobinopathies. Experimental studies in rabbits have shown that hyperbaric oxygen may be beneficial in raising the anterior chamber $P_{O_2}$ level in traumatic hyphemas in sickle cell patients and in so doing decrease the sickling of erythrocytes.[33]

As might be expected, the toxic effects of hyperbaric oxygen are manifested earlier in diseased eyes. For example, a patient with old inactive retrobulbar neuritis exposed to 100% oxygen at 2 atm had an almost complete loss of visual field of the affected eye develop within 2 hours. The normal eye was unaffected. It required 2 weeks for the field loss to recover.[34] Because a diseased eye may have reduced oxygen tolerance, hyperbaric oxygen therapy should not be used indiscriminately in the management of various circulatory disorders. Prolonged hyperbaric oxygen treatment has been shown to cause a reversible myopia and nuclear sclerotic cataracts in some patients.[35]

Several investigators have studied the effects of hyperoxia and hyperbaric oxygen on neovascularization induced by corneal trauma in rabbits, guinea pigs, and rats. In each of these studies there was little effect on the neovascular response.[36–38]

## OXYGEN DEFICIENCY

Hypoxia caused by reduced blood flow to vital ocular tissues produces a number of complex problems that cannot be adequately addressed in this chapter. Several acute conditions treatable by oxygen therapy are important to consider, however.

Carbon monoxide poisoning acts by blocking access of oxygen to hemoglobin, thereby causing tissue anoxia. This results in headache, nausea, vomiting, loss of dexterity, memory loss, irritability, confusion, and death. These symptoms may give the false impression that the person has some obscure psychiatric or organic brain syndrome. The problem is most common during wintertime when heaters and gasoline engines may be operated within closed environments. Definitive treatment is identification and removal of the pollutant source. In acute carbon monoxide poisoning, supplemental oxygen and avoidance of exertion is required. The half-life of carboxyhemoglobin is substantially reduced by 100% oxygen, which competes more effectively for binding sites. Hyperbaric administration of oxygen is even more effective.

Corneal damage caused by the overwear of contact lenses is a local manifestation of inadequate oxygen. The critical oxygen tension beneath a contact lens is 10 mm Hg; values less than this will result in corneal swelling.[39, 40] Holden and Mertz[41] found the critical oxygen transmissibility of daily and extended wear contact lenses to be 12.1%, which reduced overnight corneal swelling to approximately 8%.

## RETINAL ARTERIOLAR OCCLUSION

Oxygen is used for the emergency treatment of central retinal artery occlusion. A mixture of 95% oxygen and 5% carbon dioxide (Carbogen) given by mask should be initiated as soon as possible, preferably within 5 to 10 minutes. Usually retinal edema secondary to ischemia becomes visible within 15 to 20 minutes after the occlusion. The purpose of the carbon dioxide is to induce vasodilation; the oxygen is to help maintain the viability of retinal tissue.

Alder et al.,[42] using oxygen-sensitive microelectrodes to measure intraretinal $P_{O_2}$ levels in cats, found that occluding the retinal circulation caused the intraretinal $P_{O_2}$ level to fall to zero within 60% of the retina measured from the choriocapillaris to the internal limiting membrane. If the animal was then allowed to breathe 100% oxygen, the $P_{O_2}$ level rose throughout the retina so that the values within the inner retina were as high as that for air breathing with an intact retinal circulation. Similar results were reported using monkeys.[43, 44] From these and other studies it has been concluded that in animals who breathe 100% oxygen, the choroid can adequately supply the whole retina with oxygen if the retinal circulation is lost. Because the ocular circulation and oxygen consumption may be different in human eyes, these findings may not apply. Inhalation of 100% oxygen at 3 atm was not of benefit in the management of two cases of branch retinal arteriolar occlusion and one case of central retinal artery occlusion.[45] The distance from the choriocapillaris to the inner retinal layers was thought to be too far for effective oxygen diffusion. The accumulation of toxic metabolites and the lack of essential nutrients may also contribute to the inability of the retina to survive. It should be noted that the reduction of oxygen consumption by the outer layers of the retina and increased oxygen diffusion from the choroid into the inner retinal layers are thought to be two of the major beneficial effects of retinal photocoagulation.[46–51]

The toxicity of 95% oxygen will of necessity limit treatment of an artery occlusion to short periods. Experimental studies in monkeys have shown that irreversible loss of retinal function occurs within 105 minutes after occlusion.[52] If improvement does not occur promptly, the oxygen/carbon dioxide mixture should be discontinued.

## ACTIVATED OXYGEN RADICALS

Increased awareness of the ability of the superoxide molecule to cause damage to tissues with high concentrations of polyunsaturated fatty acid has led to a number of speculations as to its role in causing injury to retinal and other ocular tissues. The use of oxygen and glucose to form activated oxygen radicals is an important function of phagocytic cells, which include retinal pigment epithelial cells. Lipid peroxide formation from polyunsaturated fatty acids contributes to the breakdown of biologic membranes. The molecules that form the retinal photoreceptors have many double bonds, which makes them highly susceptible to breakdown by these free radicals. Dorey et al.[53] pointed out that lipid peroxidation has been implicated in causing retinal degeneration, age-related accumulation of lipofuscin in the retinal pigment epithelium, and photooxidative damage to the retina. The latter is thought to occur because of the production of singlet oxygen in the retina by ultraviolet light. Several metalloenzymes, some of which contain zinc and copper, are involved in the early stages of superoxide degradation and are protective to tissues. Interestingly, the highest concentration of zinc in the body is found in the eye, particularly in the retina, retinal pigment epithelium, and choroid.[54] The elderly are thought to be at risk for zinc deficiency,[55, 56] and oral zinc has been suggested as a preventive measure and treatment for age-related macular degeneration. The beneficial effects of such treatment are yet to be established, although some positive results have been reported.[57]

Because the lens is exposed to ultraviolet light, it is thought that oxidative mechanisms may contribute to cataract formation. The human lens has protection from this type of insult because it contains enzymes such as glutathione peroxidase, superoxide dismutase, and catalase. Jacques et al.[58] studied the status of antioxidants in the lenses of 112 subjects with and without cataracts. Although the sample size was small, they concluded that antioxidant levels did not appear to differ between the two groups.

## SUMMARY

Normal oxygen levels are essential for the routine function of tissues. The retina, in particular, has a very high metabolic rate and is vulnerable to alteration in oxygen levels. Acute hypoxia can cause rapid loss of function, and in situations such as arterial occlusion, breathing high concentrations of oxygen for short periods may be of benefit. Laser therapy, which is widely used to treat chronic hypoxia in diabetic retinopathy, decreases oxygen requirements in the outer retina and improves the perfusion of oxygen from the choroid to the inner layers of the retina. Excessive concentrations of oxygen, however, are toxic to the eyes of both infants and adults and, in the case of premature infants, contribute to the development of retinopathy of prematurity. The use of hyperbaric oxygen has yet to be shown to have significant benefit in treating ocular diseases, except possibly in patients with sickle cell disease. Tissue toxicity from the formation of singlet oxygen may play a role in the development of age-related macular degeneration and has stimulated the use of trace metals such as zinc to increase the concentration of metalloenzymes needed to deactivate this oxidant. The role of activated oxygen radicals in producing cataracts has not been fully established.

## REFERENCES


1. Steinberg RH: Monitoring communications between photoreceptors and pigment epithelium cells: effect of "mild" systemic hypoxia, Friendenwald Lecture, *Invest Ophthalmol Vis Sci* 28:1888, 1987.
2. Terry TL: Extreme prematurity and fibroblastic overgrowth of persistent vascular sheath behind each crystalline lens: 1. Preliminary report, *Am J Ophthalmol* 25:203, 1942.
3. Szewezyk MX, Parsa CF, Hudak ML: Retrolental fibroplasia: etiology prophylaxis: a preliminary report, *Am J Ophthalmol* 34:1649, 1951.
4. Patz A, Hoeck LE, De La Cruz E: Studies on the effects of high oxygen administration in retrolental: 1. Nursery observation, *Am J Ophthalmol* 35:1248, 1952.
5. Gordon HH, Lubchenco L, Hix I: Observations on the etiology of retrolental fibroplasia, *Bull John Hopkins Hosp* 94:34, 1954.
6. Lanman JT, Guy LP, Dancis J: Retrolental fibroplasia and oxygen therapy, *JAMA* 155:223, 1954.
7. Kinsey VE: Retrolental fibroplasia: a cooperative study of retrolental fibroplasia and the use of oxygen, *Arch Ophthalmol* 56:481, 1956.
8. Ahdab-Barmada M, Moossy J, and others: Hyperoxia produces neuronal necrosis in the rat, *J Neuropathol Exp Neurol* 45:233, 1986.
9. Hittner HM, Godio LB, and others: Retrolental fibroplasia. Efficacy of vitamin E in a double-blind clinical study of premature infants, *N Engl J Med* 305:1365, 1981.
10. Schaffer DB, Johnson L, and others: Vitamin E and retinopathy of prematurity. Follow-up of one year, *Ophthalmology* 92:1005, 1985.
11. Flower RW, Blake DA, and others: Retrolental fibroplasia: evidence of a role of the prostaglandin cascade in the pathogenesis of oxygen-induced retinopathy in the newborn beagle, *Pediatr Res* 15:1293, 1981.
12. Flynn JT, Bancalari E, and others: Retinopathy of prematurity. A randomized, prospective trial of transcutaneous oxygen monitoring, *Ophthalmology* 94:630, 1987.
13. Patz A: The effect of oxygen on immature retinal vessels. In Bettman JW, chairman: *Vascular disorders of the eye,* St Louis, 1966. Mosby, p 16.
14. Riva CE, Grunwald JE, Sinclair SH: Laser Doppler velocimetry study on the effect of pure oxygen breathing on retinal blood flow, *Invest Ophthalmol Vis Sci* 24:47, 1983.
15. Committee on the Classification of Retinopathy of Prematurity: An international classification of retinopathy of prematurity, *Arch Ophthalmol* 102:1130, 1984.
16. Flynn JT, Eduardo B, and others: Retinopathy of prematurity: diagnosis, severity, and natural history, *Ophthalmology* 94:620, 1987.
17. Kinsey VE, Arnold HJ, Kalina RE, and others: $PaO_2$ levels and retrolental fibroplasia: a report of the cooperative study, *Pediatrics* 60:655, 1977.
18. Yu VYH, Hookham DM, Nave JRM: Retrolental fibroplasia—a controlled study of 4 years' experience in a normal intensive care unit, *Arch Dis Child* 57:247, 1982.
19. Naiman J, Green WR, Patz A: Retrolental fibroplasia in hypoxic newborns, *Am J Ophthalmol* 88:55, 1979.
20. Johnson BL, Ahdab-Barmada M: Hyperoxemic retinal neuronal necrosis in the premature neonate, *Am J Ophthalmol* 102:423, 1986.
21. Ahdab-Barmada M, Moossy J, Painter M: Pontosubicular necrosis and hyperoxemia, *Pediatrics* 66 840, 1980.
22. Cryotherapy for Retinopathy of Prematurity Cooperative Group: Multicenter trial of cryotherapy for retinopathy of prematurity. Preliminary results, *Arch Ophthalmol* 106:471, 1988.
23. Sternberg Jr P, Lopez PF, Lambert HM, and others: Controversies in the management of retinopathy of prematurity, *Am J Ophthalmol* 113:198, 1992 (perspectives).
24. Tasman W: Threshold retinopathy of prematurity revisited, *Arch Ophthalmol* 110:623, 1992 (editorial).
25. Beehler CC, Newton NL, Tredici TJ: Retinal detachment in adult dogs resulting from oxygen toxicity, *Arch Ophthalmol* 71:665, 1964.
26. Beechler CC, Roberts W: Experimental retinal detachments, *Arch Ophthalmol* 79:759, 1968.
27. Yanoff M, Miller WW, Waldhausen JA: Oxygen poisoning of the eye, *Arch Ophthalmol* 84:627, 1980.
28. Pulido JS, Masakatsu F, Howe CA, and

others: Barbiturates protect retinal cells from hypoxia in cell culture, *Arch Ophthalmol* 107:1809, 1989.
29. Noell WK: Metabolic injuries of visual cells, *Am J Ophthalmol* 40:60, 1955.
30. Kobayashi T, Murakami S: Blindness of an adult caused by oxygen, *JAMA* 219:741, 1972.
31. Bridges WZ: Electroretinographic manifestations of hyperbaric oxygen, *Arch Ophthalmol* 75:812, 1966.
32. Anderson Jr B, Salzman H, Frayser R: Changes in arterial $pCO_2$ and retinal vessel size with oxygen breathing, *Invest Ophthalmol* 6:416, 1967.
33. Wallyn CR, Jampol LM, Goldberg MF, and others: The use of hyperbaric oxygen therapy in the treatment of sickle cell hyphema, *Invest Ophthalmol Vis Sci* 26:1155, 1985.
34. Nichols CW, Lambertsen CJ, Clark JM: Transient unilateral loss of vision associated with oxygen at high pressure, *Arch Ophthalmol* 81:548, 1969.
35. Palmquist BM, Philipson B, Barr PO: Nuclear cataract and myopia during hyperbaric oxygen therapy, *Br J Ophthalmol* 68:113, 1984.
36. Henkind P: Hyperbaric oxygen and corneal neovascularization, *Lancet* 2:836, 1964.
37. Kaiser RJ, Klopp DW: Hyperbaric air and corneal vascularization, *Ann Ophthalmol* 5:44, 1973.
38. Culton MC, Chandler AD, Proia AD, and others: The effect of oxygen on corneal neovascularization, *Invest Ophthalmol Vis Sci* 31:1277, 1990.
39. Polse KA, Decker M: Oxygen tension under a contact lens, *Invest Ophthalmol Vis Sci* 18:188, 1079.
40. Binder PS: The physiologic effects of extended wear soft contact lenses, *Ophthalmology* 87:745, 1980.
41. Holden BA, Mertz GW: Critical oxygen levels to avoid corneal edema for daily and extended wear contact lenses, *Invest Ophthalmol Vis Sci* 25:1161, 1984.
42. Alder VA, Ben-Nun J, Cringle SJ: $PO_2$ profiles and oxygen concentration in cat retina with an occluded retinal circulation, *Invest Ophthalmol Vis Sci* 31:1029, 1990.
43. Landers MB: Retinal oxygenation via the choroidal circulation, *Trans Am Ophthalmol Soc* 76:528, 1978.
44. Wolbarsht ML, Stefansson E, Landers MB: Retinal oxygenation from the choroid in hypoxia, *Exp Biol* 47:49, 1987.
45. Anderson Jr B, Saltxaman HA, Heyman A: The effects of hyperbaric oxygenation on retinal arterial occlusion, *Arch Ophthalmol* 73:315, 1965.
46. Diabetic Retinopathy Study Research Group: Preliminary report on effects of photocoagulation therapy, *Am J Ophthalmol* 81:383, 1976.
47. Diabetic Retinopathy Study Research Group: Preliminary report on effects of proliferative diabetic retinopathy: the second report of diabetic retinopathy study findings, *Trans Am Acad Ophthalmol Otolaryngol* 85:82, 1978.
48. Diddie KR, Ernest JT: The effect of photocoagulation on the choroidal vasculature and retinal oxygen tension, *Am J Ophthalmol* 84:62, 1977.
49. Landers MB, Stefansson E, Wolbarsht ML: Panretinal photocoagulation and retinal oxygenation, *Retina* 2:167, 1982.
50. Molnar VA, Poitry S, Tsacopoulos M, and others: Effect of laser photocoagulation on oxygenation of the retina in miniature pigs, *Invest Ophthalmol Vis Sci* 26:1410, 1985.
51. Alder VA, Cringle SJ, Brown M: The effect of retinal photocoagulation on vitreal oxygen tension, *Invest Ophthalmol Vis Sci* 28:1078, 1987.
52. Hayreh SS, Weingeist TA: Experimental occlusion of the central artery of the retina: IV. Retinal tolerance time to acute ischaemia, *Br J Ophthalmol* 64:818, 1980.
53. Dorey KC, Khouri GG, Syniuta LA, and others: Superoxide production by porcine retinal pigment epithelium in vitro, *Invest Ophthalmol Vis Sci* 30:1047, 1989.
54. Galin MA, Nano HD, Hall T: Ocular zinc concentration, *Invest Ophthalmol Vis Sci* 1:142, 1962.
55. Wagner PA: Zinc nutriture in the elderly, *Geriatrics* 40:111, 1985.
56. Turnland J, Costa F, Fargen S: Zinc, copper, and iron balance in elderly men, *Am J Clin Nutr* 34:2641, 1981.
57. Newsome DA, Swartz M, Leone NC, and others: Oral zinc in macular degeneration, *Arch Ophthalmol* 106:192, 1988.
58. Jacques PF, Chylack LT, McGandy RB, and others: Antioxidant status in persons with and without senile cataract, *Arch Ophthalmol* 106:337, 1988.

CHAPTER 12

# Germicides

Thomas F. Mauger

The choice of chemical antiseptics used to disinfect living tissue (e.g., the conjunctiva) is based on a number of factors. Of primary importance is the *toxicity* of the antiseptic, which determines the concentration that may be applied to the tissue.

The highest nonirritating concentrations of a number of antiseptic compounds are given in Table 12–1. This nonirritating concentration is the highest concentration that will produce not more than a slight inflammation of a rabbit eye 1 hour after the last of six instillations of 2 drops each, 5 minutes apart. These concentrations would probably be safe for a single application to a healthy human eye.

The *rate of destruction* of bacteria by a germicide depends on the kind of organism, the degree of dispersion of the organism (presence or absence of clumps), the amount of other organic matter present, the temperature, and the pH. Complete sterilization of a living tissue such as the conjunctiva is impossible from the practical standpoint; however, the number of microorganisms present can be greatly reduced by chemical germicides. The bactericidal effectiveness of the highest nonirritating concentration of a number of antiseptics is shown in Table 12–1. This germicidal activity was determined against a strain of *Staphylococcus aureus* suspended in a mixture of 10% serum in physiologic saline solution (intended to approximate tear fluid).[1]

**TABLE 12–1.**
Bactericidal Effect of Nonirritating Concentrations of Antiseptics

| Antiseptic | Maximum Nonirritating Concentration (%) | Original No. of Organisms Surviving (%) | |
|---|---|---|---|
| | | After 1 Min | After 10 Min |
| Merthiolate | 0.1 | 84.7 | 70.9 |
| Argyrol | 50 + (12.5 used) | 55.2 | 19.8 |
| Phenyl mercuric nitrate | 0.01 | 53.2 | 2.9 |
| Gentian violet | 0.01 | 45.4 | 0.01 |
| Chlorazene | 0.1 | 22.8 | 2.3 |
| Acriflavine | 0.05 | 19.8 | 0.46 |
| Mercurochrome | 2.0 | 5.5 | 0.25 |
| Silver nitrate | 0.25 | 5.5 | 5.5 |
| Iodine | 0.025 | 1.0 | 0.39 |
| Alba* | 0.04 | 0.0 | |

From Thompson R, Isaacs ML, Khorazo D: *Am J Ophthalmol* 20:1087, 1937. Used by permission.
*Proprietary quaternary ammonium surface-active germicide.

Experimental increase of the organic matter by use of 20% serum reduces the rate of destruction of staphylococci by these germicides. This inactivation of the germicide is a variable characteristic of different chemicals, as tabulated in Table 12–2. Presence of conjunctival discharge would cause such inactivation.

Another pertinent characteristic (Table 12–2) of germicides is the effect of dilution on disinfectant action. Progressive dilution by tears of the antiseptics introduced into the conjunctival sac may rapidly destroy germicidal activity. The tabulated dilution effect is a 1:1 dilution from the highest nonirritating concentration.

Injurious effects on the natural defense factors may occur from germicide concentrations too dilute to affect bacteria. Phagocytosis by leukocytes and lysozyme activity is affected in such dilution (see Table 12-2).

Obviously the circumstances under which a germicide is to be used will determine the "best" agent. For instance, leukocytic damage (relatively little with iodine) would be of little consequence if the chemical were used once for preoperative cleaning but might impair resistance if the chemical were used repeatedly in treatment of an infection. Other properties might be of value, such as the coloring effect of Argyrol that is used to stain and identify mucous debris during the preoperative cleaning of an eye. Note that Argyrol is one of the poorest germicides. The rapid killing effect and the surface-active cleaning properties of the quaternary ammonium compounds suggest their use to flush the conjunctival sac before surgery. Unfortunately, they are rapidly adsorbed to fabric surfaces (e.g., cotton balls) or organic material, thereby being rendered useless. It is interesting that silver nitrate, historically valuable in prophylaxis of ophthalmia neonatorum, is rapidly inactivated by organic matter (e.g., the vernix caseosa on an infant's skin). Gentian violet kills bacteria slowly but has a much more persistent germicidal effect that is only slightly diminished by organic matter. No doubt this accounts for its usefulness in treatment of chronic marginal blepharitis during the preantibiotic era.

The evaluation of the effectiveness of an antiseptic is not simply a matter of determining a phenol coefficient or some com-

**TABLE 12–2.**
Summary of Characteristics of Chemical Germicides

| Antiseptic | Relative Disinfection Action | Persistency of Action | Drop in Action With 1:1 Dilution (%) | Drop in Action by Increase of Organic Matter | Bacteriostatic Concentration (Leukocytic Injury Concentration) | Usable Concentration (Leukocytic Injury Concentration) | Usable Concentration (Lysozyme Injury Concentration) |
|---|---|---|---|---|---|---|---|
| Alba | Best | Good | 50 | Slow, but marked | 10 | 40.0 | 10.0 |
| Iodine | Very good | Poor | 75 | Marked | 4 | 0.4 | 50.0 |
| Silver nitrate | Good | Least persistent | | Very marked | | | |
| Mercurochrome | Good | Very good | 75 | Slight | 8 | 33.0 | 1,000.0 |
| Acriflavine | Moderate | Very good | 50 | Marked | No injury | | 12.5 |
| Chlorazene | Moderate | Good | 75 | Slight | 2 | 0.4 | 100.0 |
| Gentian violet | Fair | Best | 75 | Very slight | 4 | 166.0 | 1.6 |
| Phenyl mercuric nitrate | Fair | Very good | 10 | Slight | No bacteriostasis | 1.4 | 8.3 |
| Argyrol | Fair | Good | 0 | Slight | 4 | 40.0 | 1,040.0 |
| Merthiolate | Poor | Good | 0 | | 4 | 3.3 | 0.16 |

From Thompson R, Isaacs ML, Khorazo D: *Am J Ophthalmol* 20:1087, 1937. Used by permission.

parable measurement. A given in vitro measurement may be entirely different from the clinical in vivo effect. The factors responsible for such differences include (1) drug absorption, (2) tissue affinities for the drug, (3) ability of the drug to diffuse or spread on surfaces and through tissues, (4) concentrations that are safe and practicable, (5) stability under adverse conditions, (6) rate of destruction or elimination of the drug, (7) difference of effect of the pH of tissues compared with experimental conditions, (8) binding of the drug to proteins or to the other constituents of body fluids and discharges, (9) presence of drug inhibitors, and (10) the factors of resistance and metabolism of the microorganism.[2]

## SURFACE-ACTIVE GERMICIDES

Surface-active agents are substances that alter the relationship of interfaces. These chemicals may be anionic (possess a negatively charged structure, e.g., sulfonate), cationic (possess a positively charged structure, e.g., quaternary ammonium), or nonionic (possess no ionized groups, e.g., alcoholic esters). Such chemicals are useful as wetting agents, detergents, and emulsifying agents; however, their bactericidal properties are of most value in ophthalmology.

The mechanism of the bactericidal action of surface-active chemicals is not positively established but may result from partial disruption of the cellular membranes. The consequent increase in permeability may permit loss of vital intracellular constituents. A direct toxic effect against enzymes and other proteins is also possible.

The germicidal activity of a representative surface-active agent, cetyl pyridinium chloride aqueous solution (Ceepryn), is shown in Table 12–3. The critical killing dilution is defined as the highest dilution of germicide that kills in 10 minutes but not in 5 minutes.[3] It is evident that many common pathogenic microorganisms are destroyed by concentrations far more dilute than are employed for the usual germicidal purposes. However, some *Pseudomonas* strains may be very resistant. Spores may be highly resistant. Fungi and viruses vary in susceptibility; some, such as the psittacosis virus, are extremely resistant.

Surface-active germicides such as the quaternary ammonium compounds are valuable in disinfecting tissue surfaces (or such instruments as the tonometer that will contact the corneal surface) because their toxicity index (ratio of bacterial toxicity to tissue toxicity) is more favorable than that of germicides containing chlorine, alcohol, and other irritant chemicals. The quaternary ammonium compounds have low toxicity on oral administration, are relatively nonirritating to skin, and are virtually odorless and tasteless. As chemical compounds, they are stable, noncorrosive, and neutral.

Disadvantages of quaternary ammonium compounds include their incompatibilities. They are inactivated by soap, anionic surface-active compounds, proteins, fats, and other organic matter. Although these compounds penetrate and wet surfaces by virtue of their surface activity, clumping of organisms and their adherence to instrument surfaces reduce germicidal effectiveness. Also, bacteria contained within clotted blood adherent to an instrument may be protected against destruction.

### Benzalkonium (Zephiran)

One of the most popular cationic detergents is benzalkonium chloride. This drug may be used in ophthalmology for the preservation of eye drops, for instrument sterilization, for cleaning of skin and mucous membranes, and to enhance corneal penetration of drugs.

#### *Preservative Action*

Benzalkonium is well suited to use as a preservative for eye drops, because a 1:5,000 solution is well tolerated by the eye. No irritation or sensitization results from use of this concentration. Solutions as strong as 1:750 begin to irritate the eye. Accidental use of the 12.8% concentrated stock solution for tonometer sterilization has resulted in almost immediate complete desquamation of the corneal epithelium. Fortunately, in several cases where this misfortune occurred, healing was rapid with no residual stromal scarring (personal observation).

**TABLE 12–3.**
Germicidal Activity of Cetyl Pyridinium Chloride Aqueous Solution*

| Organism | No. of Strains Tested | No Serum | 10% Bovine Serum |
|---|---|---|---|
| *Staphylococcus aureus* | 5 | 1:83,000 | 1:12,500 |
| *Staphylococcus albus* | 1 | 1:73,000 | 1:12,000 |
| *Streptococcus viridans* | 1 | 1:42,500 | 1:12,000 |
| *Streptococcus haemolyticus* | 2 | 1:127,500 | 1:17,000 |
| *Neisseria catarrhalis* | 2 | 1:84,000 | 1:13,000 |
| *Diplococcus pneumoniae I* | 1 | 1:95,000 | 1:14,000 |
| *Diplococcus pneumoniae III* | 1 | | 1:20,000 |
| *Pseudomonas aeruginosa* | 2 | 1:5800 | < 1:1,000 |
| *Klebsiella pneumoniae* | 2 | 1:49,000 | 1:5,500 |
| *Corynebacterium diphtheriae* | 1 | 1:64,000 | 1:14,000 |
| *Mycobacterium phlei* | 1 | 1:1,500 | 1,:1,000 |
| *Eberthella typhosa* | 5 | 1:48,000 | 1:3,000 |
| *Escherichia coli* | 2 | 1:66,000 | < 1:1,000 |
| *Proteus vulgaris* | 2 | 1:34,000 | 1:2,000 |
| *Shigella dysenteriae* | 1 | 1:60,000 | 1:5,000 |
| *Shigella paradysenteriae* | 2 | 1:52,000 | 1:3,500 |
| *Shigella paradysenteriae* | 1 | 1:49,000 | 1:2,000 |
| *Shigella sonnei* | 2 | 1:68,000 | 1:6,500 |
| *Lactobacillus acidophilus* | 1 | | 1:16,500 |
| *Brucella abortus* | 1 | | 1:19,500 |
| *Trichomonas vaginalis* | 1 | | 1:3,000† |
| *Candida albicans* | 1 | 1:37,000 | 1:3,500 |
| *Cryptococcus neoformans* | 1 | 1:61,000 | 1:6,000 |
| *Trichophyton mentagrophytes* | 1 | 1:36,000 | 1:3,000 |
| *Microsporum canis* | 1 | 1:34,000 | 1:5,000 |

From Glassman HN: *Bacteriol Rev* 12:105, 1948. Used by permission.
*The critical killing dilution is defined as the highest dilution of germicide that will kill in 10 min but not in 5 min.
†Twenty-five percent human serum.

The ophthalmologist should be aware that eye medications formulated with antiseptic "preservatives" contain bacteriostatic rather than bactericidal concentrations of these drugs. Hence, appropriate precautions against contamination of the solution during use are still necessary. When evaluated by in vitro cultures without proper neutralization, benzalkonium chloride appears to sterilize a solution contaminated with *Pseudomonas* after 5 minutes of contact. However, injection of these supposedly sterilized solutions into a rabbit cornea almost invariably results in *Pseudomonas* ulceration. The actual sterilizing time for *Pseudomonas* is 3 days for a 1:5,000 concentration of benzalkonium chloride (1 day for a 0.5% chlorobutanol solution and 30 minutes for polymyxin B, 1,000 units/ml).[4] The reason for the difference between in vivo and in vitro testing is persistence of the antiseptic in the culture medium.

Benzalkonium is incompatible with some anions, including nitrate, salicylate, fluorescein, and sulfonamides. Although pilocarpine nitrate and physostigmine salicylate cannot be preserved with benzalkonium, the hydrochloride salts of these alkaloids are entirely compatible with benzalkonium.

Wetting agents such as benzalkonium enhance the transcorneal penetration of drugs. This enhanced penetration is necessary for some medications to be effective. A notable example is carbachol, which is a rather unreliable miotic in aqueous solution because of its poor penetration.

### *Instrument Disinfection*

Equipment that would be damaged by heat may be disinfected by immersion in a 1:750 aqueous solution of benzalkonium chloride. Thirty minutes of exposure to the 1:750 solution is advised. Inactivators of cationic detergents (soap, blood clots, etc.) must be completely removed from the equipment before immersion by mechanical scrubbing or wiping and thorough rinsing in water. The common practice of placing cotton gauze in the bottom of the sterilizing tray to protect delicate instruments from mechanical injury actually destroys the germicidal effect of benzalkonium through adsorption of the chemical on the cotton fibers. Similarly, the soaking of cotton balls in benzalkonium solution is useless, because the germicidal effect is rapidly inactivated. Because benzalkonium does not reliably kill spores, fungi, and viruses, soaking of instruments in this solution is not a dependable means of sterilization.

A popular method of tonometer sterilization was suspension of the footplate assembly in a solution of 1:5,000 benzalkonium between uses. The efficacy of this procedure was studied by contamination of the footplate with *Pseudomonas* organisms and culture of the footplate on trypticase soy agar at intervals.[5] In only 25% of the trials was the footplate sterilized within 1 minute of immersion in the 1:5,000 benzalkonium solution. After 5 minutes, 56% of the footplate cultures still showed contamination with viable organisms. Obviously this is less than a foolproof method of sterilization. The ophthalmologist must avoid gross contamination of the instrument, which should never be used on a recognizably infected eye.

Ultrasonic energy has been used to enhance the benzalkonium effect by achieving more effective cleaning and contact.[5] The device used was a 500-W ultrasound generator specifically devised to support the tonometer. This machine produces sufficient energy to cause visible dispersion of the water surface into a fine mist. Ultrasonic agitation of the 1:5,000 benzalkonium solution sterilized 75% of the *Pseudomonas*-contaminated tonometers within 1 minute and 100% within 3 minutes. Ultrasonic vibration in distilled water does not destroy *Pseudomonas* organisms.

When used for instrument sterilization, benzalkonium solutions contain 0.5% sodium nitrate as a rust inhibitor. This solution should not be applied to skin or mucous membranes. Methemoglobinemia may result from nitrate absorption if a sufficiently large body area is treated with this instrument solution. Sodium nitrate may damage aluminum instruments.

Optical instruments with lenses fastened by cement may be damaged by the solvent action by benzalkonium.

### *Skin Preparation*

The germicidal and detergent properties of benzalkonium are useful in cleaning skin and mucous membranes. Normal skin will tolerate a 1:750 solution without irritation. Mechanical rubbing is essential in skin preparation with any solution to remove dirt, desquamating epithelium, skin fats, and superficial bacteria.

Anionic detergents such as soap or pHisoHex must be removed thoroughly with water and alcohol before use of benzalkonium, which is inactivated by these substances. Skin preparation techniques using such a combination of anionic and cationic detergents are irrational and ineffective and should be discontinued.

In a 1:5,000 concentration, quaternary ammonium compounds comparable to benzalkonium may be used as germicidal detergents for eye irrigation before surgery.[6] Prior to the antibiotic era, irrigations with a 1:5,000 benzalkonium solution were advised for the treatment of acute catarrhal conjunctivitis and acute blepharoconjunctivitis.[7]

Unfortunately, despite all the literature describing the effectiveness of quaternary ammonium compounds, they do not work very well clinically. For example, after routine preoperative eye preparation with benzalkonium chloride, 40% of skin cultures were still positive (compared with 12% prepared with povidone-iodine).[8]

Fifty-four cases of *Pseudomonas* infection followed inadequate disinfection of cystoscopes and bronchoscopes with 1:750 benzalkonium chloride. The epidemic strain was isolated from the basin used to "disinfect" the instruments.[9] An outbreak of *Pseudomonas* septicemia affected nine patients whose intravenous skin and equipment sterilization was performed with 1:750 benzalkonium chloride from a contaminated stock bottle.[10] *Pseudomonas* contaminated blood cultures from 79 patients, again because of infected benzalkonium solutions.[11] These three articles describing not only the failure of benzalkonium to sterilize but its being the source of infection were published in the same edition of the *Journal of the American Medical Association* with the intent of attracting the attention of physicians.[12]

### *Toxicity*

Benzalkonium chloride cannot be used in any solutions intended for intraocular use. The threshold concentration that produced recognizable irritation or increase of corneal thickness after a single intraocular instillation of 0.25 ml was 0.03% in physiologic salt solution. Although the next-tested concentration, 0.01%, did not show toxicity, a safety factor of 10× was believed to be necessary, thereby making 0.001% the safe dose for intraocular benzalkonium chloride. In this dilution, the drug is valueless as a preservative.[13]

Irrigating rabbit anterior chambers for 10 seconds with 0.05% benzalkonium chloride in distilled water and then rinsing them out with saline solution uniformly resulted in total and permanent endothelial destruction.[14]

Oxygen uptake of rabbit corneas was unchanged by exposure to 0.01% benzalkonium chloride but was reduced by a concentration of 0.025%.[15] The thimerosal threshold was 1.0%.

A more sensitive study method, scanning electron microscopy, was used to evaluate the response of cat corneal epithelium to single instillations of benzalkonium chloride in saline solution. At concentrations of 0.0025%, cells showed loss of microvilli and elevated margins. At 0.0075% the surface cells peeled off.[16] Chlorhexidine caused damage at 0.005%.

Electrophysiologic functions such as ion transport were damaged by only 0.001% benzalkonium chloride, 0.0004% thimerosal, 0.05% chlorobutanol, and 0.00025% amphotericin B.[17]

A soft contact lens wearer changed from her usual irrigating solution to one containing 0.01% benzalkonium chloride. After 3 days a red, painful, ulcerated cornea developed that required about 1 week to heal, after which she was again able to wear a contact lens without benzalkonium preservative.[18] No cause could be determined unless the preservative was blamed.

Since the introduction of carbachol in benzalkonium chloride in 1942, these "wetting agents" are known to increase corneal penetration of drugs. This was considered to be a desirable effect that enhanced therapy and was therefore to be sought. The reason for enhanced penetration must be damage to the epithelial cells. Fortunately, they grow back so rapidly as to be completely replaced every 3 days, so damage to them is relatively inconsequential or at least transitory. The irreplaceable endothelial cells do not enjoy this margin of safety, and it has been well established clinically that the practice of instilling preserved medications, such as epinephrine, intraocularly causes prompt corneal clouding.

## Thimerosal

An epidemic is said to have occurred in 3% to 50% of soft contact lens wearers in the United States.[19] The condition causes red, irritated eyes with epithelial changes ranging from faint barely visible irregularities to a coarse, punctate keratopathy. Photophobia and lacrimation may be present. Vision may be reduced by several lines or more. Bilaterality is the rule. This syndrome is not self-limited but progressively worsens. Of 38 such patients reported, 31 demonstrated ocular sensitivity to thimerosal, and 27 showed positive patch test results.[19] The symptoms disappeared when the patients stopped using thimerosal-preserved solutions. This article briefly states the historical origin of the problem, which developed when preservative use in eye drops was required because of an anecdotal series of corneal infections. Thimerosal is surpassed by benzalkonium, chlorhexidine, and chlorobutanol as a germicide.[20] Thimerosal required more than 24 hours to kill *S. aureus* and more than 4 hours to kill *Pseudomonas* in contrast to less than 15 minutes for benzalkonium. Additional reports of this syndrome of thimerosal allergy may be found in the literature.[21–23] The rapid deposition of calcium superficially in the cornea in a distribution somewhat reminiscent of band keratopathy has been attributed to mercurial preservatives.[24]

## Chlorobutanol

One of the most popular preservatives for eye drops is 0.5% chlorobutanol solution. Although primarily bacteriostatic, chlorobutanol is often bactericidal when exposure is prolonged for 24 hours or more. Growth of *Pseudomonas* and *S. aureus* in nutrient broth was invariably prevented by 0.5% chlorobutanol solution.[25] Both gram-positive and gram-negative bacteria, as well as many species of fungi, are inhibited by chlorobutanol.

Chlorobutanol is stable and resists destruction by autoclaving at pH of 6.0 or less, but more alkaline solutions are rapidly hydrolyzed by heat. Because sodium fluorescein solutions are more alkaline than this, heat sterilization of chlorobutanol-preserved fluorescein completely destroys the preservative.

Although eye drops containing 0.5% chlorobutanol as a preservative have been instilled several times daily for years without ill effect, such solutions may not be tolerated as a continuous bath. Diffuse epithelial damage of the cornea results from bathing the eyes for as long as 20 minutes with 0.4% chlorobutanol in isotonic saline solution. Use of chlorobutanol-preserved solutions for gonioscopy is inadvisable, because epithelial damage lasting for several hours may ensue after this prolonged chemical contact. Biochemical studies indicate that chlorobutanol inhibits oxygen utilization by the cornea and loosens epithelial adhesion.[26]

In practice, a 0.5% solution of chlorobutanol is an effective and nonirritating preservative. No instance of sensitization has been recognized during these many years of extensive use. In a study of 576 bottles of eye medications containing chlorobutanol as a preservative, only a single instance of contamination (the organisms were *Pseudomonas*) was detected. The pharmacologic activity of ophthalmic medications is not reduced by chlorobutanol.

## Chlorhexidine

Chlorhexidine is very similar to chlorobutanol and benzalkonium in its efficacy and toxicity when used as an ophthalmic preservative.[27] It may be used in combination with detergent such as the preoperative disinfectant Hibiclens. Two patients were reported to have severe keratitis develop, which was associated with Hibiclens preoperative preparation. One patient was a 9-month-old girl who underwent a craniotomy for craniofacial asymmetry. The preoperative preparation was Hibiclens. The eyes were then covered with conformers during the surgery. Total epithelial defect with diffuse corneal haze developed in one eye. The epithelial defect healed, but the cornea became opaque. The second patient reported was an elderly woman who was given Hibiclens preoperative preparation before cataract surgery and had epithelial defect and dense opacity of the cornea develop.[28] Five additional patients have been reported with postoperative corneal opacity and edema associated with accidental Hibiclens exposure during preoperative preparation.[29] Hibiclens should not be used near the eye or even on the face because of the severe ocular reaction.

## pHisoHex

A proprietary germicidal cleaning agent, pHisoHex was widely used for preoperative skin preparation around the eye. It contains 80% sodium octylphenoxyethoxyethyl ether sulfonate, 3% hexachlorophene, and lanolin esters. Ophthalmologists should be aware that the first ingredient is extremely toxic to the cornea.

Two near tragedies have been reported after use of pHisoHex.[30] In each case the operated eye was being removed with the patient under general anesthesia, and the normal remaining eye was unknowingly contaminated with the cleaning solution, which remained on the eye during surgery. At the close of surgery the good eye was noted to be red with a hazy cornea despite the fact it had been covered to prevent exposure damage. Inflammation was severe by the first postoperative day, most of the corneal epithelium was absent, the cornea was diffusely hazy, and striate keratopathy was marked. Two weeks postoperatively the eye showed marked superficial punctate staining, heavy folds of Descemet's membrane, pigment keratic precipitates, and aqueous flare. Folds in Descemet's membrane and photophobia were still present 6 weeks postoperatively. By 8 months, healing was complete, with only minor residual scarring, and the patient was asymptomatic. Both cases had a very similar course.

Experimental exposure of a rabbit eye for as short a time as 30 seconds causes superficial punctate staining that lasts for 24 hours.[30] Exposures of 1 or 2 minutes cause damage lasting for 2 weeks. Histologic examination shows changes in all layers of the cornea, including sloughing of the endothelium.

Clearly, prevention is the preferred treatment of pHisoHex keratitis. This germicide should not be allowed to enter the eye even briefly. Particularly if the patient is under general anesthesia, ocular contamination with pHisoHex must be avoided, because the unconscious patient cannot complain. No local anesthetic should be placed in the fellow eye of a conscious patient, because the burning sensation of accidentally instilled germicide is of protective importance. Thorough irrigation of the eye should follow cleansing of the skin with pHisoHex.

During surgery for retinal detachment, which requires a clear cornea, accidental contamination of the eye with even slight amounts of pHisoHex is immediately evident. The cornea dries rapidly, losing its luster and transparency. pHisoHex is a good germicide, but it is quite destructive to the cornea; hence, it represents a tragedy ready to happen in a careless moment.

Hexachlorophene is a potent neurotoxic agent and causes brain damage after ingestion or with use to clean areas of broken skin. Its topical use in preventing staphylococcal skin injection in infants has caused diffuse central and peripheral nerve damage. As little as 3 tablespoons of pHisoHex was fatal to a 7-year-old boy. A 31-year-old woman had gradual progressive loss of superior visual fields and bilateral optic atrophy with 20/400 vision caused by daily ingestion of 1 teaspoon of hexachlorophene for treatment of facial acne.[31]

### Povidone-iodine

Presently we use povidone-iodine for our ophthalmic preoperative preparations. It will kill all bacteria in less than 1 minute and spores more slowly. It does not burn the skin even though left on underneath the bandages. The stained skin is virtually impossible to reinfect for at least 1 hour. The stain is water soluble and washes off easily, unlike the stain of tincture of iodine. In routine preparation before eye surgery, when half-strength povidone-iodine was used, bacteria could be recovered in only 12% of cases after the preparation.[8] The effectiveness of a preoperative preparation is related not only to the germicide chosen but also to the thoroughness of the scrub. The importance of a meticulous prep cannot be exaggerated. Povidone-iodine may be diluted and used to clean the conjunctival cul-de-sac before surgery.

In a study of 56 eye surgery patients, 100% were positive for bacterial growth before scrub, but only 9.3% were positive after iodophor scrub.[32] Skin cultures are reported to be sterile twice as often after scrub with an iodophor than with the hexachlorophene-benzalkonium combination.

Povidone-iodine (0.1%, 1%, 5%; 1 minute exposure) was found to sterilize isolates of herpes simplex virus type II and *Neisseria gonorrhoeae* in the laboratory. *Chlamydia trachomatis* titers were reduced with 5% and 1% solutions. The authors of this report suggest a clinical trial of povidone-iodine as a potential prophylactic agent for ophthalmia neonatorum.[33]

Povidone-iodine is so nontoxic that it can actually be used intraperitoneally in one-fourth strength.[34] This antiseptic can also be used to scrub lacerations without devitalizing the raw tissue surfaces.[35] Repeated irrigation of a large abdominal wound with povidone-iodine, maintained in the wound with a gauze pack, caused an iododerma that cleared uneventfully.[36]

### Iodide

A wide variety of inflammatory and degenerative diseases, including those of the eye, were once empirically treated with this drug.[37] Of a series of 115 eyes with age-related macular degeneration treated with oral administration of iodides (0.015 mg protiodide of mercury three times daily), 56 were reported to show improved visual acuity. However, 29 of these subsequently lost vision,[38] and these results probably represent the expected spontaneous course of age-related macular degeneration.

The physician prescribing systemic iodide should be aware that this drug can cause fever (with temperatures as high as 40° C after 5 days of treatment with 3 ml of a saturated solution of potassium iodide in a daily dose). Skin eruptions, conjunctivitis, and coryza are other manifestations of iodide sensitivity.[39]

#### *Treatment of Herpetic Keratitis*

A strong solution of iodine (containing 7% iodine and 5% potassium iodide in alcoholic solution) was originally used in treatment of acute herpetic keratitis.[40] In the untreated control series (53 eyes), the average duration of conjunctival redness was 41 days, and the shortest period of corneal staining encountered in any eye was 10 days. In 97 eyes treated with iodine cautery, the average duration of redness was 15 days, and in 85% corneal staining had disappeared by 10 days. Metaherpetic complications developed in 11 of the 53 control eyes and in 25 of the 97 treated eyes, a virtually equal incidence.

Topical instillation of a 5% potassium iodide solution alone was not helpful in treatment of dendritic ulcers. By contrast, epithelial curettement without chemical cautery definitely shortens the course of dendritic keratitis. Neither iodine cautery nor curettement benefits metaherpetic keratitis.

Because of the danger of permanent stromal scarring, the generous use of a strong solution of iodide has been abandoned in favor of the sparing use of a mild solution of iodine. The physician should avoid discoloration of Bowman's membrane, because such treatment causes irreversible, although superficial, corneal damage. Specific antiviral therapy with topical trifluorodine, idoxuridine, and vidarabine has displaced chemical cauterization for herpetic keratitis.

One percent potassium iodide used every 1 to 2 hours reduces the corneal reaction to fungal ulcers.[41] This benefit is believed to be a result of the potassium ion, which helps an injured cornea maintain its water pump system and glycolytic cycle. The iodide ion may not be helpful.

## STERILIZING AGENTS

### Cresol

An apparently effective solution (Post's solution No. 4) for chemical sterilization of sharp instruments contains the following constituents:

| | |
|---|---|
| Liquor cresolis compound | 8 ml |
| Oil of lavender | 2 ml |
| Thymol crystals | 2 g |
| Ethyl alcohol | 88 ml |

The thymol and oil of lavender are used primarily to disguise the unpleasant odor of the cresol. This solution is not corrosive to metal instruments and does not dull sharp edges. Surgical instruments experimentally contaminated by bacteria are invariably sterilized within 2 minutes of immersion in this solution and usually within 60 seconds. Even when the solution has been contaminated by 5% whole blood and when spore-forming organisms such as *Bacillus subtilis* were used, materials difficult to sterilize, such as gauze or string, become sterile within 4 minutes.[42]

More recent evaluation of such chemical sterilizing solutions indicates that they are completely unreliable against spores.[43] The differences in method of evaluation include use of *B. subtilis* strains with a high spore count, selection of culture media particularly adapted to growth of spores, saving of all solutions to identify presence of spores washed but not killed, and drying of a proteinaceous film of spores on the instruments before use of the sterilizing solution. With these more rigid methods, all instruments were found to remain contaminated after 30 minutes of soaking in Post's solution No. 4. In most instances, Post's solution itself contained viable spores after 30 minutes. The current belief is that no chemical method will effectively sterilize instruments contaminated with spores, with the exception of ethylene oxide.

### Ethylene Oxide

The sharp instruments used in eye surgery tend to be dulled by autoclaving, which was the reason for the past extensive use of sterilizing solutions (which inadequately sterilize spores). Ethylene oxide sterilization has been shown to be efficacious for autoclaving and yet not to damage sharp edges, glass, or plastic. This gas, in a concentration of 10 g/L of space, will sterilize even resistant organisms and spores within a 2-hour period. The explosive properties of pure ethylene oxide are eliminated by mixing it with hydrocarbon gases. The gas is toxic and should be handled with reasonable care. Three cases of leukemia have been reported in workers exposed to ethylene oxide.[44] The ethylene oxide gas sterilizer is standard equipment in many hospitals. A small portable sterilizer has been developed and is practicable for private ophthalmic use.[45] Ethylene oxide sterilization of intraocular lenses has been suspected of causing postoperative inflammation.[46]

## DETERGENT-INDUCED CORNEAL EDEMA

A report of 18 patients with corneal decompensation after intraocular surgery at the same institution implicated an increase of detergent (a nonionic ethoxylated fatty alcohol) concentration from 0.4% to 4.0%. When the detergent was discarded and cannulas were replaced, the epidemic of corneal edema subsided. Interestingly, the 4% concentration was within the detergent manufacturer's guidelines for medical use. Obviously the manufacturer did not expect direct intraocular instillation. The other problem was inadequate flushing of the cannulas after disinfection. Even after the problem was identified and the cannulas were flushed with 0.4% solution, three additional cases occurred indicating that residual 4% solution remained despite aggressive irrigation. The use of disposable cannulas will eliminate this complication, but other ophthalmic instruments (irrigation-aspiration tips) may also be susceptible.[47, 48]

Intraocular lens sterilization may also leave toxic residues. Sodium hydroxide was found to be less endothelial toxic (cultured bovine corneas) than ethylene oxide, formaldehyde, and $\gamma$-radiation.[49] Fungal endophthalmitis related to sodium hydroxide sterilization was related to contaminated sodium bicarbonate used for neutralization.[50]

## METALLIC GERMICIDES

Preantibiotic treatment of surface infections has included application of a variety of metallic salts, dyes, and so forth. Most of these medications do, indeed, have bacteriostatic or bactericidal activity, but their use on the eye is limited by ocular tolerance. Topical use of most of these medications is now obsolete.

Not only are the antiseptic solutions used in ophthalmology before the introduction of antibiotics relatively ineffective germicides, but they actually greatly delay healing of corneal epithelial defects and in most instances may cause permanent corneal opacity.[51] Such drugs include 10% (mild) silver protein, 2% merbromin (Mercurochrome), 0.5% zinc sulfate, 1:3,000 benzalkonium chloride (Zephiran), 1:1,000 acriflavine (Neutroflavin), 1:2,500 nitromersol (Metaphen), 1:2,500 thimerosal (Merthiolate), and 1:5,000 mercuric oxycyanide.

Mercury is not an infrequent allergen.[52] The typical reaction is delayed, reaching a peak 1 to 2 days after application of the thimerosal. The area of skin around the eye exposed to mercury (e.g., by skin preparation or preserved drops) is locally affected with a weeping, swollen, reddened allergic dermatitis of very typical appearance. It hurts more than it itches. Perhaps 1 week is required for the reaction to subside.

## Copper

Copper has been used to destroy bacteria, fungi, viruses, and algae. Copper sulfate has been shown to inhibit fungus *(Cephalosporium)* grown in vitro in concentrations as dilute as 0.06%. Topical application every hour of 0.12% copper sulfate solution was tolerated by the human eye and was believed to be helpful in treatment of two patients with developed keratitis resulting from *Cephalosporium;* however, 8 weeks of therapy was necessary for one of the patients.[53] Increased penetration of copper may be attained by iontophoresis.

Copper sulfate iontophoresis has been reported to be an effective treatment for herpes simplex keratitis, whether epithelial or stromal. The rationale for this treatment is that the copper ion, with its known antimicrobial effect, may be forced into cell membranes by an electromotive force. A 5% solution of cocaine was instilled at 2-minute intervals over a 10-minute period to render cell membranes more permeable and for its anesthetic effect. An aqueous solution of 0.125% copper sulfate was placed in a corneal bath electrode and connected to the anode of a 45-V B battery. One milliampere of current was passed for 2 minutes. After treatment, 0.25% scopolamine solution was instilled and an eye pad applied.

All 20 patients had a burning sensation in the eye immediately after the treatment, which lasted for 4 to 5 hours. Because this was anticipated, codeine was given before treatment. The treatment caused conjunctival hyperemia, loss of epithelium surrounding the ulcer, stromal edema, and slight anterior chamber flare. The eye may appear slightly worse the day after iontophoresis. On the average, corneal staining disappeared 4 to 5 days after iontophoresis. All 20 eyes (nine with dendritic ulcers, 10 with stromal keratitis, and one with disciform keratitis) healed after iontophoresis, although one patient required three treatments during a 2-week period. No case recurred during the 21 months between the first treatment and publication of the paper.[54] This treatment should not be substituted for accepted antiviral therapy (trifluridine) in the treatment of herpes simplex keratitis.

Copper is selectively stored in the liver and in the central nervous system. Presumably this selective storage explains the damage to these two organs in Wilson's hepatolenticular degeneration.[55] Certainly systemic toxic effects will not follow any ocular use of copper.

## Silver

The ability of silver ions, even in dilution of $10^{-5}$M, to kill microorganisms is the basis for their ophthalmic use. This lethal action is not selective for microorganisms but is a protein denaturation that indiscriminately destroys conjunctiva and corneal epithelium, as well as bacteria. Silver nitrate is well suited to destroy surface organisms. For this reason, it is an effective eye prophylactic against gonorrhea if it is used immediately after birth. However, the antiinfectious potency of silver nitrate is not lasting, and it is too toxic for repeated instillation. Furthermore, the chemical burn of corneal epithelium temporarily reduces ocular resistance and predisposes the eye to pyogenic infections.

Tissue chlorides precipitate insoluble (and therefore inactivated) silver chloride. This precipitation prevents deep tissue penetration and protein destruction by silver (provided the solution is not too concentrated). Simultaneously it shields subsurface infection from cure. Presumably this is the reason why bacteria that cause surface conjunctival infection (e.g., gonococci) are destroyed and why deeper infections (e.g., the virus of inclusion blennorrhea and established gonococcal infections) are not cured.

### *Ocular Tolerance*

A 1% silver nitrate solution is extremely irritating (as anyone brave enough to try 1 drop in his or her own eye will testify). However, it is not extremely destructive, and usually within several days after silver prophylaxis the average newborn eye has stopped discharging. If 2% silver nitrate solution is used, prompt irrigation with saline solution is advised to prevent excessive eye irritation. A 6% silver nitrate solution causes extensive scar formation, and 12% may cause total blindness in rabbits.[56] Tragic results may follow confusion of 10% silver protein solutions (Argyrol) with 10% silver nitrate solutions, which may blind a child. A survey of 85 ophthalmologists in 1952 disclosed 17 who had encountered blindness that had resulted from use of excessively strong solutions of silver nitrate.[57] This is largely of historic interest in the 1990s when silver nitrate solution is limited largely to use in some cases of superior limbic keratoconjunctivitis.

Silver nitrate applicator sticks have been used as tissue-cauterizing devices. For example, exuberant granulation tissue in an exenteration socket can be eradicated by application of a silver nitrate stick. A 35-year-old woman had the base of an incised chalazion cauterized with a silver nitrate stick. The eye was then patched. When next seen, the cornea was densely opaque, concealing all detail of the underlying iris. Corneal transplantation and cataract extraction were required. The corneal button was heavily infiltrated with silver granules.[58] Use of silver nitrate stick within the eyelids does not seem prudent. Not only dense scarring but also extensive neovascularization results from silver nitrate stick applications to the cornea.[59] A nurse used a silver nitrate stick for ocular prophylaxis of a newborn.[60] Despite a perfectly dreadful initial reaction of extensive surface necrosis, only slight corneal scarring remained after 1 year.

### *Credé Prophylaxis*

In 1881 the incidence of gonorrheal ophthalmia was reduced from 10% to 0.5% simply by the instillation of a 2% silver nitrate solution into each conjunctival sac of newborns immediately after the delivery.[61]

Gonorrhea is still sufficiently prevalent (and actually may be increasing) that some type of eye prophylaxis continues to be desirable. The various antibiotics and sulfonamide drugs, systemically or topically instilled, have repeatedly been proved to be effective in gonorrheal prophylaxis, more than silver nitrate.[57, 62, 63] These new drugs are far less irritating and also protect against eye infections from common pyogenic organisms that are prevalent after the use of silver. Erythromycin ointment is used in many states for prophylaxis and has the advantage of some effect against *Chlamydia*-induced conjunctivitis.

### *Antiviral Effect*

Silver nitrate (as well as a large number of other chemicals) was evaluated in treatment of experimental herpes simplex keratitis.[64] Silver nitrate, mercuric chloride, benzoquinone, and chloranil all inactivated herpes virus when used in vitro in concentrations as dilute as $10^{-5}$M. A rather surprising finding in this study was virus inactivation by prednisolone in a $10^{-2}$M concentration. Iodine is effective in a $10^{-3}$M concentration.

Unfortunately, none of the large number of chemicals studied was found to be therapeutically effective when applied topically to the infected cornea in the form of drops. Presumably this limitation exists because the virus lies within the epithelial cells, and a virucidal chemical concentration is destructive to the cornea. Use of 0.17% silver nitrate solution was said to reduce the number of dendritic figures in 10 to 21 rabbit eyes but did not shorten their duration. These results were interpreted as being equivocal.

### *Antibacterial Effect*

Silver nitrate is extremely toxic to microorganisms. For example, a concentration of 1 μg of silver nitrate/ml of solution killed 98.3% of *Pseudomonas* in 5 minutes and 99.997% in 15 minutes.[65] The presence of chloride ions in tissue fluids greatly reduces the antibacterial effectiveness of silver because of precipitation of insoluble silver chloride. Nevertheless, the minimal inhibitory concentrations for *Pseudomonas* are in the range of 20 to 40 μg/ml of silver nitrate, even in the presence of 7 mg of sodium chloride/ml. The antibacterial activity of the medium seems to be related to the total concentration of silver and not only to the silver ions present.

Tissue toxicity of silver ions may be estimated by the measurement of respiration of skin cells in tissue cultures. One milligram per milliliter (0.1%) of silver nitrate caused a 22% inhibition of respiration; 2.5 mg/ml caused 39% inhibition; 5 mg/ml caused 61% inhibition; and 10 mg/ml caused 76% inhibition. The minimal amount of silver nitrate causing inhibition of respiration of skin in tissue culture was 25 times greater than the minimal concentration of silver nitrate that inhibited growth of *Pseudomonas aeruginosa.* Obviously there is a favorable therapeutic index for the topical use of silver as an antibacterial agent. The author has advocated the use of 0.5% silver nitrate solution applied as a moist compress to prevent infection in burns of the skin.

### *Argyrosis*

Argyrosis is the well-known bluish gray discoloration caused by tissue deposits of silver.[66] Because tissue chlorides are almost exclusively confined to the intercellular areas, silver staining of tissue is selectively deposited outside the cells.[67] This discoloration is permanent; however, superficial skin, conjunctival, and corneal silver deposits can be removed by subcutaneous or subconjunctival injection of a freshly prepared solution of sodium thiosulfate and potassium ferricyanide. Solutions of 12% sodium thiosulfate and 0.5% potassium ferricyanide are more stable than is the mixture. When mixed in equal proportions, a solution of 6% sodium thiosulfate and 0.25% potassium ferricyanide results, which must be used within 30 minutes. Topical ocular instillation is said to be effective but acts much more slowly. Deeper silver deposits (e.g., on Descemet's membrane) cannot be removed in this way.[68]

## CONTACT LENS STERILIZATION

Having smooth surfaces, the traditional "hard" methyl methacrylate contact lens is rather easily sterilized, cleaned, and washed. Almost any detergent or germicide can be used, provided that it is thoroughly rinsed off before insertion into the eye.

The hydrophilic "soft" lenses are porous and retain microorganisms, as well as chemicals. Heat sterilization is the accepted method; however, 3% hydrogen peroxide will sterilize soft lenses within 5 minutes, destroying *Pseudomonas, Candida,* and all other common microorganisms. Hydrogen peroxide is painful to the eye but does not cause any significant damage. Soaking the soft lens in 2.5% sodium thiosulfate solution (harmless to the eye) for 15 minutes will inactivate the hydrogen peroxide, after which the lens may be rinsed and inserted.[69] Contact lens fitting sets should be disinfected between uses. Hydrogen peroxide solutions will kill *Acanthamoeba castellani* and *Acanthamoeba polyphaga.*

A substantial mythology has arisen that soft contact lenses may concentrate the preservatives from eye drops and thereby damage the eye. This, of course, cannot happen. To the extent that the lens binds the preservative, it is not released to affect the eye. Dire consequences do not result from preservative binding.[70]

Not only may contact lenses become contaminated with microbes, but the contact lens case may also serve as a reservoir. One hundred and thirty-two contact lens cases out of 247 tested positive for microbial agents. A higher percentage of cases were contaminated with preservative-free solution use. A group of patients who had contact lens care instructions reinforced had a much lower rate of microbial contamination. Hydrogen peroxide solutions were associated with only a one out of 12 rate of contamination in the asymptomatic users and one out of 78 in those who had special care instruction reinforced. A glycocalyx biofilm was found in the contact lens cases that contributed to the contamination. This biofilm protected the microbes from chemical inactivation. This study reinforces the importance of regular mechanical contact lens case cleaning to remove biofilm and also contact lens case exchange. The cases may also get small cracks or fissures that can harbor organisms such as *Acanthamoeba*.[71]

## ULTRAVIOLET LIGHT

The germicidal properties of ultraviolet light are well known and widely used for sterilization. Before the discovery of antibiotics, ultraviolet radiation was successfully employed in treatment of corneal ulcers caused by microorganisms. Resistance of viruses, fungi, and many bacteria to antibiotics and the development of new ultraviolet radiation sources suggest reevaluation of this old method of therapy.

Peak germicidal activity occurs at a wavelength of about 2,650 Å (most effective wavelength against viruses and fungi, as well as against bacteria). Nucleoprotein absorption of ultraviolet light has a similar peak, which suggests that the germicidal effect is a result of nucleoprotein destruction. For some unexplained reason, actinic keratitis is produced most effectively at a wavelength of 2,880 Å.[72] Superimposition of the germicidal and keratitis producing spectral curves (Fig. 12-1) indicates that at 2,537 Å the germicidal effect is 85% of maximum, whereas the keratitis effect is only 20% of maximum.[73] The 2,537-Å wavelength was chosen because it is the wavelength emitted by a low-pressure mercury vapor lamp.

Experimental studies with 2,537-Å ultraviolet light indicate that a dosage of as much as 1,250 μW sec/cm$^2$ can be tolerated by the human cornea in a single dose without causing permanent scarring. Rabbit experiments indicate that stromal vascularization and scarring occur after 5 million μW sec/cm$^2$. Corneal epithelial damage is moderately severe after 800,000 μW sec/cm$^2$, but by 5 to 7 days after treatment, the cornea has returned to normal. In remarkable contrast to corneal resistance is bacterial susceptibility to this wavelength. Complete in vitro bacterial destruction requires only 2,500 to 26,400 μW sec/cm$^2$. Fungus destruction requires 6,600 to 330,000 μW sec/cm$^2$. Virus susceptibility is assumed to be in the same range as bacterial susceptibility. The human eye can tolerate without sequelae more than three times the dose required to kill in vitro the most resistant microorganism tested.

Treatment appears to be quite simple, requiring only an accurately timed exposure of the cornea to the calibrated lamp positioned 5 mm away. Apparently the energy output of these bulbs varies considerably (600–3,000 μW cm$^2$ at 5 minutes); hence, each bulb requires individual calibration. Because the radiation intensity varies with the inverse square of the distance, accurate dosage requires precise positioning.

The discomfort of radiation keratitis can be minimized by cycloplegics and patching and is said to be less severe than that of chemical cautery. Topical anesthesia is used before treatment. Mechanical removal of diseased epithelium or discharge presumably permits better ultraviolet penetration.

Hudnell and Chick[73] report treatment of seven patients having acute dendritic ulcers. One ulcer recurred but was successfully treated by repeat ultraviolet therapy. Unlike x-ray therapy, the ultraviolet effect is not cumulative. This presentation of ultraviolet

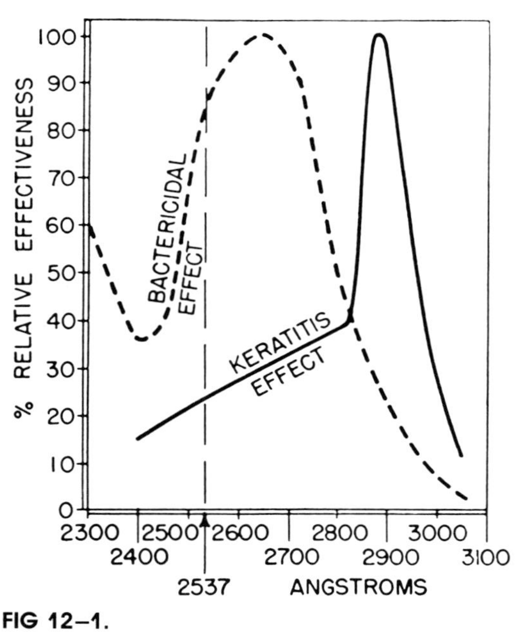


**FIG 12–1.**
Relative action spectra of bactericidal and keratitis-producing effects of ultraviolet light. (From Hudnell AB, Chick EW: *Arch Ophthalmol* 68:304, 1962. Used by permission.)

treatment is most interesting, although it is not yet pragmatically established.

Exposure of a tonometer footplate to ultraviolet light within a special sterilizer holder destroyed all organisms within 15 minutes.[74] The microbial challenge was by swabbing the footplate. This is not exactly the same as the in-use moist contact with the plunger, which moves up and down in the central cavity, shielded from ultraviolet light. Fortunately, the applanation tonometer prism is an easily cleaned smooth surface.

## TONOMETER TIP DISINFECTION

In the ophthalmologist's office preventing transmittal of infectious disease is critical because of our repeated contact to patients' eyes with instruments. The chief mode of transferral of viral conjunctivitis is tonometer tip use. Equally important is the transmittal of disease through improper hand washing. With the advent of human immunodeficiency virus (HIV), tonometer disinfection has become paramount. Goldmann tonometer tips were inoculated with HIV type I and then cleaned with either a disposable tissue or gauze or disinfected with 3% hydrogen peroxide or a 70% isopropyl alcohol swab. Both the hydrogen peroxide and alcohol were found to completely disinfect the tonometer tips. The simple wiping with a tissue or gauze still showed active virus present.[75] Alcohol soaking of tonometer tip heads for 5 to 10 minutes at a time will eventually destroy a tonometer tip. Simple wiping of the tip with isopropyl alcohol and then allowing it to air dry seems to be effective at disinfection without destroying the tip. Other methods of disinfection such as a 10% dilution of household bleach (sodium hypochlorite) and hydrogen peroxide 3% were not found to functionally destroy the tonometer.[76] Seventy percent isopropyl alcohol will totally denude the epithelium with a 10-second application. Hydrogen peroxide that has been left in a Petri dish overnight will concentrate to a level that will cause gas formation in the anterior chamber if applied to the cornea using a tonometer tip. Sodium hypochlorite will cause severe epithelial damage but not quite as extreme as that found with isopropyl alcohol. The message is that none of these solutions is compatible with normal corneal health; therefore, the tonometer tip should be allowed to thoroughly dry after disinfection or be thoroughly rinsed before use.[77]

## WHY GERMICIDES?

Just as examples of why we cannot disregard microorganisms, consider the following: Hepatitis B surface antigen is found in the tears of 44% of 25 patients known to be carriers. Chimpanzee experiments show that the infecting dose of hepatitis B is actually smaller than a detectable amount. You can spread hepatitis with your tonometer. One in every 300 patients walking into your office is a carrier.[78]

Do you reuse the leftover eye drops from the hospital? Of 218 such recycled bottles, 44% were found to be contaminated. Of 45 used ointment tubes (antibiotic), 36% were contaminated.[79]

## REFERENCES


1. Thompson R, Isaacs ML, Khorazo D: A laboratory study of some antiseptics with reference to ocular application, *Am J Ophthalmol* 20:1037, 1937.
2. Theodore FH: Newer concepts in treating external eye disease, *Am J Ophthalmol* 40:744, 1955.
3. Glassman HN: Surface-active agents and their application in bacteriology, *Bacteriol Rev* 12:105, 1948.
4. Reigelman S, Vaughan DG, Okumoto M: Rate of sterilization as a factor in the selection of ophthalmic solutions, *Arch Ophthalmol* 54:725, 1955.
5. Hok R, Wachtel J, Havener WH: Ultrasonic tonometer sterilization, *Am J Ophthalmol* 58:676, 1964.
6. Bell RP, Johnson LV: Cetydimethylbenzylammonium chloride—a new ophthalmic irrigation solution, *Ohio State Med J* 47:231, 1951.
7. Lawrence CA: Chemical preservatives for ophthalmic solutions, *Am J Ophthalmol* 39:385, 1955.
8. Hale LM: Povidone-iodine in ophthalmic surgery, *Ophthalmic Surg* 1:9, 1970.
9. Dixon RE, Kaslow RA, Mackel DC, and others: Aqueous quaternary ammonium an-

tiseptics and disinfectants, *JAMA* 236:2415, 1976.
10. Frank MJ, Schaffner W: Contaminated aqueous benzalkonium chloride, *JAMA* 236:2418, 1976.
11. Kaslow RA, Mackel DC, Mallison GF: Nosocomial pseudobacteremia, *JAMA* 236:2407, 1976.
12. Hussey HH: Benzalkonium chloride: failures as an antiseptic, *JAMA* 236:2433, 1976.
13. Britton B, Hervey R, Kasten K, and others: Intraocular irritation evaluation of benzalkonium chloride in rabbits, *Ophthalmic Surg* 7:46, 1976.
14. Maurice D, Perlman M: Permanent destruction of the corneal endothelium in rabbits, *Invest Ophthalmol* 16:646, 1977.
15. Burton GD, Hill RM: Aerobic responses of the cornea to ophthalmic preservatives, measured in vivo, *Invest Ophthalmol* 21:842, 1981.
16. Burstein NL: Preservative cytotoxic threshold for benzalkonium chloride and chlorhexidine digluconate in cat and rabbit corneas, *Invest Ophthalmol* 19:308, 1980.
17. Burstein NL, Klyce SD: Electrophysiologic and morphologic effects of ophthalmic preparations on rabbit cornea epithelium, *Invest Ophthalmol* 16:899, 1977.
18. Gasset AR: Benzalkonium chloride toxicity to the human cornea, *Am J Ophthalmol* 84:169, 1977.
19. Wilson LA, McNatt J, Reitschel R: Delayed hypersensitivity to thimerosal in soft contact lens wearers, *Ophthalmology* 88:804, 1981.
20. Norton DA, Davies DJG, Richardson NE, and others: The antimicrobial efficiencies of contact lens solutions, *J Pharm Pharmacol* 26:841, 1974.
21. Binder PS, Rasmussen DM, Gordon M: Keratoconjunctivitis and soft contact lens solutions, *Arch Ophthalmol* 99:87, 1981.
22. Mondino BJ, Gordon LR: Conjunctival hyperemia and corneal infiltrates with chemically disinfected soft contact lenses, *Arch Ophthalmol* 98:1767, 1980.
23. Spizziri LJ: Stromal corneal changes due to preserved saline solution used in soft contact lens wear, *Ann Ophthalmol* 13:1277, 1981.
24. Lemp MA, Ralph RA: Rapid development of band keratopathy in dry eyes, *Am J Ophthalmol* 83:657, 1977.
25. Murphy JT, Allen HF, Mangiaracine AB: Preparation, sterilization, and preservation of ophthalmic solution, *Arch Ophthalmol* 53:63, 1955.
26. Grant WM: *Toxicology of the eye,* Springfield, Ill, 1962, Charles C Thomas.
27. Green K, Livingston V, Bowman K, and others: Chlorhexidine effects on corneal epithelium and endothelium, *Arch Ophthalmol* 98:1273, 1980.
28. Hamed LM, Ellis FD, Boudreault G, and others: Hibiclens keratitis, *Am J Ophthalmol* 104:50, 1987.
29. Phinney RB, Mondino BJ, Hofbauer JD, and others: Corneal edema related to accidental Hibiclens exposure, *Am J Ophthalmol* 106:210, 1988.
30. Browning C, Lippas J: pHisoHex keratitis, *Arch Ophthalmol* 53:817, 1955.
31. Slamovits TL, Burde RM, Klingele TG: Bilateral optic atrophy caused by chronic oral ingestion and topical application of hexachlorophene, *Am J Ophthalmol* 89:676, 1980.
32. Chase RC, Ellis PP: Iodophors and skin asepsis, *Am Ophthalmol* 2:312, 1970.
33. Benevento WJ, Murray P, Reed ID, and others: The sensitivity of Neisseria gonorrhea, chlamydic trachomatous, and herpes simplex type II disinfection with povidone-iodine, *Am J Ophthalmol* 109:329, 1990.
34. Kiernan PD, Hubert JP, Beahrs OH: Intraperitoneal povidone-iodine lavage, *JAMA* 243:863, 1981.
35. Nelson RH: Reattaching the severed auricle, *JAMA* 242:2833, 1979.
36. Bishop ME, Garcia RL: Iododerma from wound irrigation with povidone-iodine, *JAMA* 240:249, 1978.
37. Goodman L, Gilman A: *The pharmacologic basis of therapeutics,* ed 4, New York, 1970, Macmillan.
38. Laird RG: Iodine therapy for senile macular degeneration, *Am J Ophthalmol* 28:287, 1945.
39. Steffen GE: Iodine fever, *JAMA* 192:571, 1965.
40. Gundersen R: Herpes cornea, *Arch Ophthalmol* 15:225, 1936.
41. Newmark E, Ellison AC, Kaufman HE: Pimaricin therapy of *Cephalosporium* and *Fusarium* keratitis, *Am J Ophthalmol* 69:458, 1970.
42. Post MH, Moor W: The sterilization of sharp instruments by chemical solutions, *Am J Ophthalmol* 25:579, 1942.
43. Reigelman S, Vaughan Jr DG, Okumato M: Evaluation of the sporicidal activity of Post's sterilizing solution, *Arch Ophthalmol* 53:847, 1955.
44. Hogstedt C, Malmqvist N, Wadman B: Leu-

kemia in workers exposed to ethylene oxide, *JAMA* 241:1132, 1979.

45. Linn JG: Use of gas sterilization for ophthalmic surgery. *Arch Ophthalmol* 62:619, 1959.
46. Stark WJ, Rosenblum P, Maumenee AE, and others: Postoperative inflammatory reactions to intraocular lenses sterilized with ethylene oxide, *Ophthalmology* 87:385, 1980.
47. Breebaart AC, Nuyts RMMA, Pels E, and others: Toxic endothelial cell destruction of the cornea after routine extracapsular cataract surgery, *Arch Ophthalmol* 108:1121, 1990.
48. Nuyts RMMA, Edelhauser HF, Pels E, and others: Toxic effects of detergent on the corneal epithelium, *Arch Ophthalmol* 108:1158, 1990.
49. Singh G, Bohnke M, vonDomarus D, and others: Toxicity of methods of implant material sterilization on corneal endothelium, *Ann Ophthalmol* 17:727, 1985.
50. Pettit TM: Fungal endophthalmitis following intraocular lens implantation, *Arch Ophthalmol* 98:105, 1980.
51. Bellows JG: Influence of local antiseptics on regeneration of corneal epithelium of rabbits, *Arch Ophthalmol* 36:70, 1946.
52. Taub SJ: Delayed hypersensitivity to Merthiolate preservative, *Eye Ear Nose Throat Mon* 49:235, 1970.
53. Byers JL, Holland MG, Allen JH: *Cephalosporium* keratitis, *Am J Ophthalmol* 49:267, 1960.
54. Brown SI, Holland MG, Allen JH: Treatment of herpes simplex keratitis with copper sulfate iontophoresis, *Arch Ophthalmol* 67:453, 1962.
55. Gubler CJ: Copper metabolism in man, *JAMA* 161:530, 1956.
56. Calvery HO, Lightbody HD, Rones B: Effects of some silver salts on the eye, *Arch Ophthalmol* 25:839, 1941.
57. Wachter HE, Pennoyer MM: Prophylaxis in the eyes of newborn infants, *Mo Med* 53:187, 1956.
58. Grayson M, Pieroni D: Severe silver nitrate injury to the eye, *Am J Ophthalmol* 70:227, 1970.
59. Goren SB, Eisenstein R, Choromokos E: The inhibition of corneal vascularization in rabbits, *Am J Ophthalmol* 84:305, 1977.
60. Horblass A: Silver nitrate ocular damage in newborns, *JAMA* 231:245, 1975.
61. Newell FW: Centenary Crede prophylaxis, *Am J Ophthalmol* 90:874, 1980.
62. Ormsby HL: Ophthalmia neonatorum, *Am J Ophthalmol* 39:90, 1955.
63. Chapman KJ: A comparable study of Neo-Silvol and teramycin as prophylactic treatments in the eyes of the newborn, *Ohio Med J* 52:591, 1956.
64. Sery TW, Furgiuele FP: The inactivation of herpes simplex virus by chemical agents, *Am J Ophthalmol* 51:42, 1961.
65. Ricketts CR: Mechanism of prophylaxis by silver compounds against infection of burns, *BMJ* 1 444, 1970.
66. Gutman FA, Crosswell Jr HH: Argyrosis of the cornea without clinical conjunctival involvement, *Am J Ophthalmol* 65:183, 1968.
67. Collin HB: Endothelial cell lined lymphatics in the vascularized rabbit cornea, *Invest Ophthalmol* 5:337, 1966.
68. Moss AP, Sugar A, Hargett NW, and others: The ocular manifestations and functional effects of occupational argyrosis, *Arch Ophthalmol* 97:906, 1979.
69. Gassett AR, Ramer RM, Katzin D: Hydrogen peroxide sterilization with hydrophilic contact lenses, *Arch Ophthalmol* 93:412, 1975.
70. Mackeen DL: The safety and efficacy of chemical disinfection with hydrophilic gel contact lenses, *Contact Lens J* 8:17, 1974.
71. Wilson LA, Sawart AD, Simmons RB, and others: Microbial contamination of contact lens storage cases and solutions, *Am J Ophthalmol* 110:193, 1990.
72. Cogan DG, Kinsey VE: Action spectrum of keratitis produced by ultraviolet radiation, *Arch Ophthalmol* 35:670, 1946.
73. Hudnell AB, Chick EW: Corneal ultraviolet phototherapy, *Arch Ophthalmol* 68:304, 1962.
74. Sherman SE: Evaluation of an improved ultraviolet tonometer sterilizer, *Am J Ophthalmol* 78:329, 1974.
75. Pepose JS, Linette E, Lee SF, and others: Disinfection of Goldmann tonometers against human immunodeficiency virus type I, *Arch Ophthalmol* 107:983, 1989.
76. Key CB, Whitman J: Alcohol soaking damage applanation tonometer heads, *Arch Ophthalmol* 104:800, 1986.
77. Mauger TF, Laxson LC: Effect of hydrogen peroxide and sodium hypochlorite on the corneal oxygen uptake note, *J Toxicol Cut Ocular Toxicol* 11:369, 1992.
78. Moniz E, Feldman F, Newkirk M, and others: Removal of hepatitis B surface antigen from a contaminated applanation tonometer, *Am J Ophthalmol* 91:522, 1981.
79. Jarte VJ, O'Hanrahan MT, Timoney RF: Microbial contamination in residues of ophthalmic preparations, *Surv Ophthalmol* 24:257, 1980.

CHAPTER **13**

# Wetting Agents and Tear Substitutes

Thomas F. Mauger

The tear film is a multilayered structure with a mucin base adherent to the corneal epithelium, a lipid surface to prevent evaporation, and a watery middle zone. The function of this tear film is governed by complex forces of surface tension and interfacial tensions that are the properties of the individual components and their interactions. The wettability of surfaces and adsorbed polymers is an important component of the stability of thin films.[1]

## SURFACE TENSION

Surface tension is the property of a surface to maintain its integrity, to resist rupture by the attraction of its molecules to each other. We most readily understand this with respect to liquids, where it is apparent this property is not the hardness associated with solids. However, solids also have a surface tension, which is important because the relationship of solid and liquid surface tensions determines whether the solid can be wetted by the liquid. Water has an exceptionally high surface tension (70 dynes/cm at 37° C). (A dyne is the amount of force that will, when acting continuously on a mass of 1 g, impart to it an acceleration of 1 cm/sec$^2$.) Surface tension forces are powerful. The tear film may be as thin as 7 μm, which would result in a weight [exclusive of tear meniscus] of 0.000,02 g. A force of 70 dynes would accelerate this weight by about 35 km/sec. This calculation explains why the eyelids cannot open so rapidly as to leave behind a dry corneal surface uncovered by the tear film. This force causes the surface of the water droplet to attempt to shrink to its smallest possible area and also to maintain its integrity.

## SURFACTANTS

A surfactant is a molecule that has an affinity for surfaces and the ability to act there to reduce surface tension. Large molecules of biologic or synthetic origin perform surfactant functions in natural and artificial tears. Soaps and detergents are smaller molecules with comparable surfactant activity, but they are toxic to the lipoidal surfaces of the cornea and cell membranes. Dissolved molecules with surfactant capability have a high affinity for the water surface and adsorb to this surface, reducing its surface tension. The amount of surface tension reduction caused by the surfactant is called its *film pressure.* The surface tension of the solution equals the algebraic sum of the surface tension of the water (or any solvent) and the film pressure of the surfactant. If multiple surfactants are present, the strongest one has theoretically the greatest affinity for the surface and will displace the weaker ones. Usually interactions occur so that the combined film pressure of multiple surfactants is usually less than that of the strongest single one. In some instances, a weaker surfactant will strongly adsorb at an interface, thereby resisting displacement by stronger surfactants.

The glycoproteins secreted by the conjunctival goblet cells are collectively called *mucin*. Mucin is a surfactant and in physiologic concentrations will lower the surface tension of pure water by 35 dynes/cm. Physiologically, the tears are covered by the surface lipid film, and there is no free aqueous-air interface. The surface tension of tear fluid is 40 dynes/cm. This is the surface tension of the lipid combined with the mucin. With respect to water, mucin has a twofold surface-stabilizing action. It is a surfactant and in addition is capable of forming hydrogen bonds with water. Mucin holds the water to the surface lipid film, as well as to the lipoidal corneal epithelium.

## INTERFACIAL TENSIONS

Water cannot wet a lipid surface whether it is solid or liquid. Only when the interfacial tension is lower than the surface tension of both the water and the lipid surfaces will the surfaces adhere to each other. The firmer this adherence, the more secure will be a film of one substance on the other. The film may be of oil on water (surface lipid layer on tears) or of water on lipid (aqueous tear component on corneal epithelium). In each instance, mucin or a substitute surfactant must be present to reduce the interfacial surface tension to a lower level than the surface-free energy of the solid or the surface tension of the liquid.

In the case of a solid, a surfactant is not dissolved within it but is absorbed to the solid surface. The liquid film does not then adhere to the solid directly but to the surfactant molecules. The wettability of an adsorbed surfactant is the important property of a tear substitute; this is the mucomimetic behavior that is sought to restore the tear film. (A dry eye may be caused by diminished tear production or may exist despite profuse tearing. Instability of the tear film occurs when the corneal epithelial surface is poorly wetted because of inadequate mucin.)

The wetting characteristics of various materials can be studied by measuring the contact angle of 1 drop of saline solution on the experimental surface. This measurement indicates the effectiveness of the preparation in causing wettability of the cornea or of a contact lens. This wetting angle measurement changes considerably with various additives, whether they are viscous agents, wetting agents, polymers, preservatives, stabilizers, or other chemicals. Hence, the final properties of a preparation may be modified greatly by its formulation. The contact angle measurements of 12 popular ocular contact lens solutions varied from 51 to 20 degrees.[2] For reference, bovine salivary mucin has a contact angle of 24 degrees.[3]

Fig. 13–1[1] illustrates 1 drop of solution

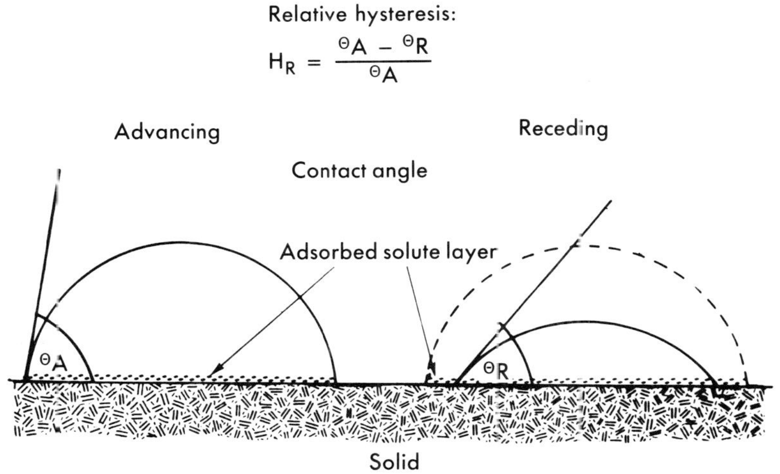


**FIG 13–1.**
Contact angle hysteresis caused by solute adsorption. (From Holly FJ: *Med J* 4:14, 1978. Used by permission.)

on a solid surface. The angle between the base of the drop and the solid is the contact angle. This angle is constant for any pure fluid and solid interface at a given temperature. The figure is more complex because it depicts a property of surfactant-containing liquids termed *hysteresis.* Hysteresis is the failure of coincidence of two related phenomena, in this case the advancing and receding contact angles. Because both normal tears and artificial tears contain surfactants, this behavior is highly relevant, as will shortly be explained.

## CORNEAL CHARACTERISTICS

The wettability of the cornea is significantly influenced by its surface microvilli, which secure the mucin layer (Fig. 13–2). Disruption and loss of the microvilli are demonstrable by scanning electron microscopy of rabbit corneas permitted to dry for as short as 5 minutes. Dried cells apparently sustain irreversible damage to their membranes and slough off, leaving unwetted spots that absorb fluorescein.[4]

Overt drying is not necessary to cause corneal damage. Hyperosmolarity occurs with evaporation when only small amounts of fluid are available. The average osmolarity of tears from normal eyes was 302 mOsm/L compared with 343 mOsm/L from keratoconjunctivitis sicca eyes. This explains the damage occurring in the lower portion of the cornea even though the tear breakup time is longer than the blink interval. Based on this finding, perhaps artificial tear solutions should be hypotonic rather than isotonic.[5]

Under other circumstances, hypertonicity is a desirable attribute of tear fluid and favors epithelial adherence to the cornea. This is the basis for treatment of recurrent epithelial erosion with hypertonic medications, such as 2% sodium chloride. Technically, the adhesion tension of a liquid to a solid equals the product of the liquid surface tension and the cosine of the contact angle. This affinity of water for various surfaces is relevant to the healing of injured cornea because of the great differences in wetting angles, depending on the extent of an injury. As shown in Fig. 13–3,[6] the water contact angle for the normal mucin-covered corneal surface is 20 degrees, for the hydrophobic

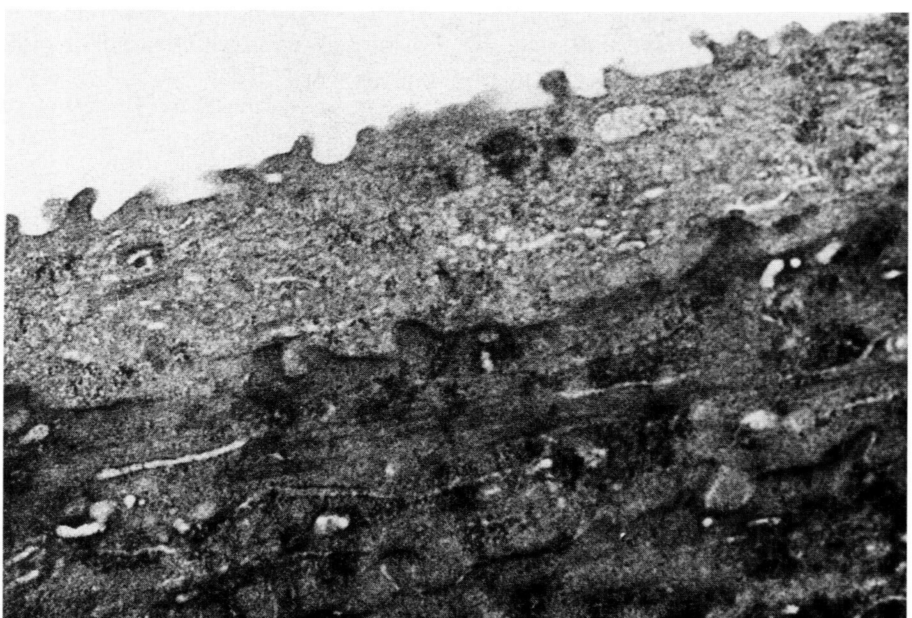

**FIG 13–2.**
Corneal microvilli by transmission electron microscopy (magnification ×47,000).

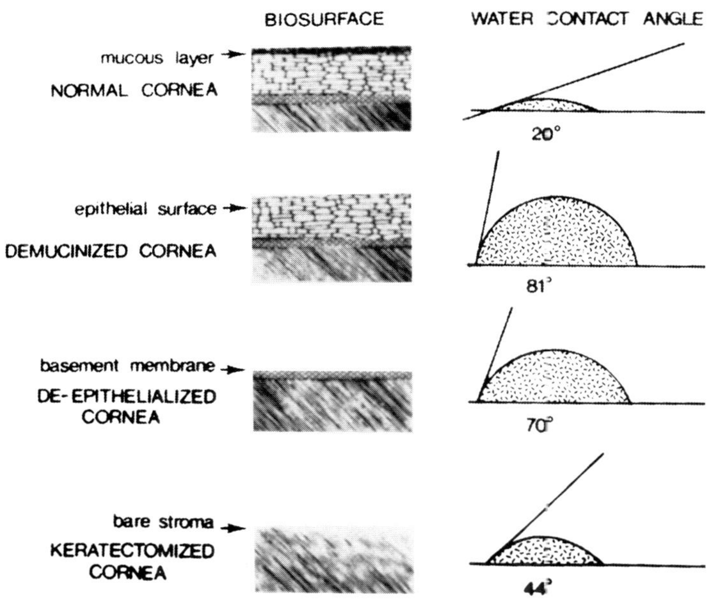


**FIG 13–3.**
Water wettability of various cornea surfaces. (From Holly FJ: *Invest Ophthalmol Vis Sci* 17:552, 1978. Used by permission.)

corneal epithelium it is 81 degrees, for Bowman's membrane it is 70 degrees, and for stroma it is 44 degrees. Adhesion between various liquids and surfaces decreases with greater water content (hypotonicity).[6]

## SUPERFICIAL LIPID LAYER

The superficial lipid layer of the tear film is derived from meibomian gland secretion, a tiny amount of which is expressed from the glands by each blink. The composition of meibomian secretion is very different from that of the sebaceous glands of the skin and contains mainly long-chain waxy esters. This meibomian secretion has a number of very unique properties. It has a high interfacial tension with water (at least 28 dynes/cm). It can form films on water that are monolayers or multiple layers (duplex films) and therefore can be as thin as 0.1 μm in the wide open eye or as thick as 100 μm when the lids are completely closed. The speed of movement of the lipid film is faster than the movement of the eyelid, leaving no uncovered aqueous portion of the tear film. Mucin also enters into the superficial lipid layer, causing the lipid film to become more resilient and thicker and therefore better able to compress and expand with each blink.[7]

The integrity of this very important lipid layer can be compromised by many artificial tear preparations. The component causing the lipid layer damage is the surface-active preservative benzalkonium chloride. In its usual 0.01% concentration, benzalkonium chloride causes almost instantaneous disruption and solubilization of the tear film. Even a 0.004% concentration causes such disruption. Chlorobutanol, thimerosal, methylparaben, and propylparaben are preservatives that do not disrupt the lipid layer. Of the various polymeric ingredients found in artificial tears, none disrupted the lipid film except polysorbate 80, which reduced the durability of the lipid film to about 9 minutes (under the experimental conditions of measurement, the usual duration of the lipid film was at least 15 minutes). Because of these various factors, the most stable lipid films obtained with 12 of the popular tear substitutes occurred with Liquifilm Tears and Adsorbotear.[7] The composition of vari-

**TABLE 13–1.**
Tear Substitutes*

| Name | Manufacturer | Polymer | Preservative/ EDTA |
|---|---|---|---|
| Murocel | Bausch & Lomb | MC 1% | MP |
| TearGard | Bio Products Ophthalmic | HEC | SA, EDTA |
| Neo Tears | Barnes-Hind | HEC, PVA | Thim, EDTA |
| Adsorbotear | Alcon | HEC, POV | Thim, EDTA |
| Tearisol | IOLAB | HPMC 0.5% | BAK, EDTA |
| Tears Naturale II | Alcon | HPMC, DEX | PQ |
| Lacril | Allergan | HPMC, GEL | CB, PS |
| Liquifilm Tears | Allergan | PVA 1.4% | CB |
| Liquifilm Tears Forte | Allergan | PVA 3.0% | Thim, EDTA |
| HypoTears | IOLAB | PVA, PEG-400, and dextrose | BAK, EDTA |
| Murine | Ross | PVA 1.4% POV 0.6% | BAK, EDTA |
| Tears Plus | Allergan | PVA 1.4% POV 0.6% | CB |
| Cellufresh | Allergan | CMC 0.5% | |
| Celluvisc | Allergan | CMC 1.0% | |
| Refresh | Allergan | PVA 1.4% POV 0.6% | |
| Tears Naturale Free | Alcon | HPMC, DEX | EDTA |
| HypoTears PF | IOLAB | PVA, PEG-400, and dextrose | |

**MC*, Methylcellulose; *MP*, methylparaben and propylparaben; *HEC*, hydroxy ethylcellulose; *SA*, sorbic acid; *EDTA*, edetate disodium; *PVA*, polyvinyl alcohol; *Thim*, thimerosal; *POV*, povidone; *HPMC*, hydroxypropyl methylcellulose; *BAK*, benzalkonium chloride; *DEX*, dextran 70; *PQ*, polyquad; *GEL*, gelatin A; *CB*, chlorobutanol; *PS*, polysorbate 80; *CMC*, carboxymethylcellulose.

ous commercial artificial tears is of practical interest and is reported in Table 13–1.

## SURFACTANT AFFINITY TO CORNEA

Affinity of a macromolecular compound for the corneal surface is another characteristic of importance in an artificial tear. Most studies evaluating the retention time of such a substance utilize visible markers such as Argyrol or nickel chloride and show retention times of 3 to 10 minutes. Such methods show the duration of the traced substance but not necessarily of the portion of the vehicle adsorbed to the corneal surface. Almost all artificial tear preparations substantially prolong the tear breakup time, increasing it from the normal 25 seconds to 30 to 50 seconds. Tear breakup time was measured every 15 minutes on 12 normal subjects. This report states that the prolongation of tear breakup time produced by a given instillation remains constant on repeated measurements and then drops abruptly to baseline values, thereby permitting an accurate estimate of duration.[8]

## EYELIDS

The constant blinking motion of the eyelids results in spreading and renewal of the tear film and mixing of its components. A detailed cinematographic study of the eyelids determined that the average duration of the closing phase of a blink was 80 msec; the opening phase was 175 msec. The total duration of a blink was 260 msec. The maximum closing velocity was 18 cm/sec; opening velocity was 10 cm/sec. The tear film mixing efficiency of the lids is so great that a 1-ml drop of fluorescein placed in the temporal corner of the conjunctiva is well mixed after only a single blink. The dye runs along the lid and then is lifted up across the entire exposed surface of the eye.[9]

## OSMOLARITY, OSMOLALITY, pH, AND BUFFERING

The terms osmolarity and osmolality are frequently confused. Osmolality refers to the total number of dissolved particles in solution expressed as moles per kilogram of solvent. Osmolarity refers to the moles per liter of solution. Colloid osmotic pressure is caused by the effect of large molecules that do not easily pass through cellular membranes.[10] Crystalloids are of smaller molecular weight and can usually permeate vascular membranes easily. An example of a colloid would be dextran, whereas an example of a crystalloid would be the electrolytes.

Patients with keratitis sicca often complain of burning induced by artificial tear instillation, which results from pH or osmolarity of the solutions rather than from irritation by the polymers used. Allergy to the preservative, especially thimerosal, is another common reason for intolerance of eye drops. A study of the preference of 15 patients with keratitis sicca for various osmolarities showed that 6 selected a 260-mOsm solution, 4 selected a 200-mOsm solution, and 4 preferred a 150-mOsm solution. (One patient could not decide.) Isotonicity is 300 mOsm. The hypotonic solutions are apparently preferred because the tear film in a dry eye is already too hypertonic for comfort The patients also preferred an alkaline (pH 8.5) solution to isotonic (pH 7.0) or acid solutions.[11]

Although lower osmolarity is generally preferred, it seems that higher colloidal osmolality is more beneficial to the cornea. The corneal stroma may be dehydrated during cornea transplant preservation even in the absence of intact epithelium if the colloidal osmotic pressure is high enough. Interestingly, one of the lowest osmolality artificial tears, HypoTears (Iolab, Claremont, Calif.), has the highest colloidal osmolality.[10]

The range of pH tolerance of the rabbit endothelium extends from 6.5 to 8.5. Outside this range the cells and their barrier function break down. Eyes from human eye banks behave similarly. Presumably this physiologic range would be comparable for the surface of the eye.[12, 13]

The buffering capacity of tears is not great but is sufficient to maintain a reasonable pH in the face of the significant environmental stress it receives on the surface of

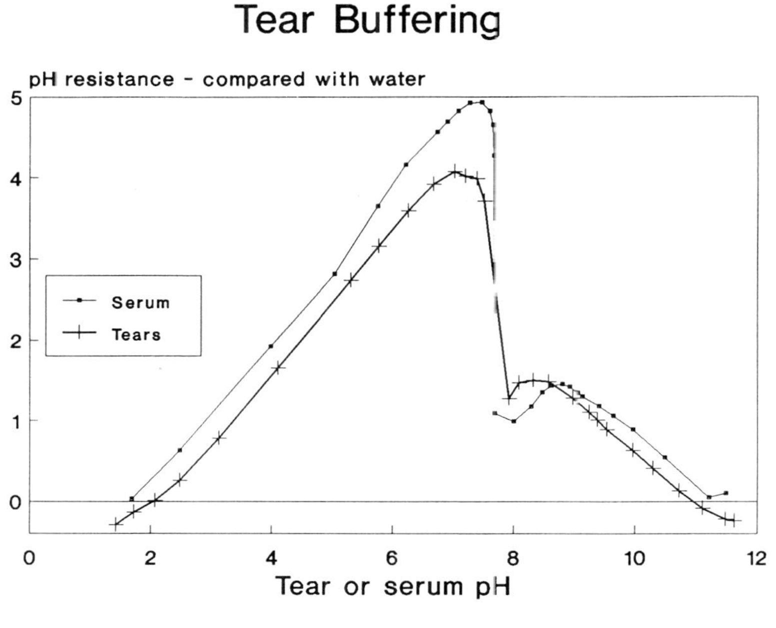


**FIG 13–4.**
Buffering characteristics of tears and serum titrated with HCl and NaOH. The Y-axis shows the pH difference from water undergoing an identical titration. Note greater buffering in the acid range because of bicarbonate present. (Modified from Carney LE, and others: *Invest Ophthalmol Vis Sci* 30:747, 1989. Used by permission.)

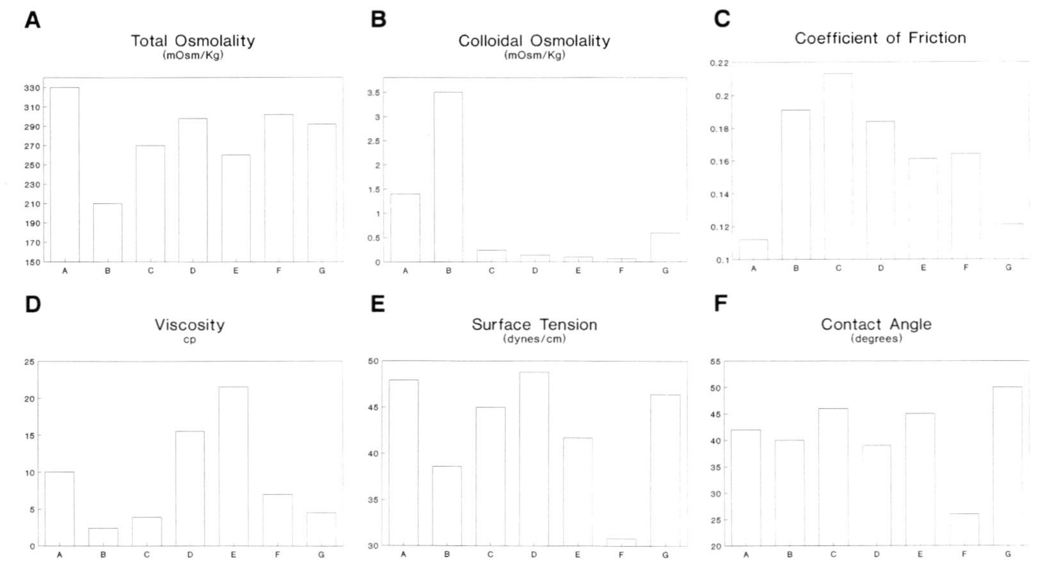


**FIG 13–5.**
Physical characteristics of tear substitutes. *A,* Adsorbotear (Alcon); *B,* HypoTears (IOLAB); *C,* Liquifilm Tears (Allergan); *D,* Neo-Tears (Barnes-Hind); *E,* TearGard (Bio Products Ophthalmic); *F,* Tears Naturale (Alcon); *G,* Tears Plus (Allergan). (Data from Holly FJ, Esquivel ED: *J Ocular Pharm* 1:327, 1985; and Kalachondra S, Shah DO: *Ann Ophthalmol* 17:708, 1985.)

the eye. Most of its buffering capacity to acids is due to the bicarbonate system, whereas buffering against alkalis occurs mainly via tear proteins (Fig. 13–4).[14]

## COEFFICIENT OF FRICTION

The lubrication value of an ophthalmic solution may be measured by the coefficient of friction as measured between a polymethylmethacrylate (PMMA) or nylon stylus rotating in a tract of a rotating PMMA plate. The frictional drag seems to be an independent property that depends on the confirmation of the polymers of the solutions. It was not found to correlate with viscosity, surface tension, or contact angle (Fig. 13–5).[15]

## OPTICAL EFFICACY

Patients wearing contact lenses who complained of blurred vision used various marketed wetting solutions to clear their view. Stopwatch timing indicated that the optical benefit of such solutions lasted for only 1 to 2 minutes.[15]

## METHYLCELLULOSE

Methylcellulose is a viscous, transparent, nonirritating, water-soluble compound used in ophthalmology as a lubricant and as a vehicle that substantially prolongs the contact time of topically applied drugs. Methylcellulose is nearly inert chemically and is entirely compatible with the drugs commonly used in ophthalmology. It is stable and may be sterilized by boiling. Growth of microorganisms is not supported by methylcellulose.[16]

Methylcellulose is nonirritating to ocular tissue and may be used without fear of eye damage. Topical instillation of 1% solutions can be continued indefinitely without altering the appearance of the normal eye. The healing of experimental corneal epithelial wounds is not slowed by a 2% methylcellulose solution.[17] Subconjunctival injection (in rabbits) of 0.1 ml of a 1% methylcellulose solution causes no irritation.[16]

### Intraocular Use

The tolerance of the rabbit eye to 1.4% polyvinyl alcohol in isotonic saline solution and to 0.5% methylcellulose in isotonic saline solution was studied by introducing 0.2 ml of each solution into the anterior chamber.[18] Mild to moderate conjunctival hyperemia was the result in five of 24 polyvinyl alcohol–treated eyes and in 28 of 36 methylcellulose eyes. Corneal edema occurred in eight of the methylcellulose-treated eyes but in none of the polyvinyl alcohol–treated eyes.[18] This reaction has subsequently been shown to be caused by a 0.9% sodium chloride solution. When 0.1 ml of 0.5% methylcellulose in balanced salt solution (a mixture of electrolytes designed to approximate the composition of tissue fluids[19]) was injected into the anterior chamber, no irritation resulted other than would be expected from the trauma of the needle. After such injection, traces of methylcellulose are detectable in the aqueous humor for 3 days.[20]

Before the demonstration that 0.9% saline solution was responsible for the mild iridocyclitis, ophthalmologists were advised not to use methylcellulose solutions during intraocular surgery. However, there now appears to be no reason to fear that clinically useful concentrations of highly purified methylcellulose will affect the intraocular structures adversely. Under no circumstances should solutions containing preservatives be introduced into the eye.

Experimentally, glaucoma may be produced by filling the anterior chamber with 2.5% methylcellulose. This solution is too viscous to escape through the trabecular spaces and produces an acute rise in pressure.[21]

## Preparation

The 4,000-cp viscosity of methylcellulose is preferable for ophthalmic use. It is not readily dissolved in water; hence, the following procedure is recommended. The methylcellulose fibers should be boiled for 20 to 30 minutes in half the desired volume of water. The suspension is then cooled to 5° to 10° C, and the remaining water is added. Methylcellulose is more soluble in cold water than in hot, but the resistance of the dry fibers to wetting is decreased by boiling. Concentrations of 0.5% to 2% are used in ophthalmology.

## Clinical Use

Methylcellulose, 0.5%, in a 0.9% sodium chloride solution makes excellent artificial tears. Lubrication with such a solution is helpful to patients with keratoconjunctivitis sicca, neuroparalytic keratopathy, or exposure keratopathy.

At least in theory, lacrimal substitutes (artificial tears) should correspond in chemical composition to the precorneal film. This precorneal film seems to be a most complex fluid sheet that resists evaporation, has excellent wetting characteristics, and is optically perfect. The film has both water and fat solubility characteristics. A hypothesis of the structure of the precorneal tear film suggests it is a thin sheet of water (and dissolved elements) lined both anteriorly and posteriorly by a monomolecular lipid layer.[22] One is led to speculate whether the ideal artificial tear might be some type of emulsion formulated to duplicate the lipid- and water-soluble, wetting, protective, and lubricating properties of the normal precorneal film. Clearly, such a simple substitute as normal saline solution is not an adequate tear replacement solution for therapeutic use.

Contact lenses may be moistened with methylcellulose solution. More viscous solutions (1%) are desirable for application of gonioscopic lenses, the three-mirror prism, and similar optical devices. The thick solution achieves a good contact with the cornea and is not readily lost during application.

In higher concentrations, methylcellulose becomes sufficiently viscous to be classified as an ointment. A 2.5% methylcellulose ointment may be used for gonioscopy and has the advantage of ensuring an optically tight fit with no tendency to leakage of coupling solution. A recommended formula is:

| | |
|---|---|
| Methylcellulose powder, 4,000 cp | 2.5 g |
| Methylparaben | 0.023 g |
| Propylparaben | 0.001 g |
| Sodium chloride | 1.2 g |
| Distilled water as needed | 100 ml |

If care is taken to prepare this ointment free of bubbles, it is optically perfectly clear. The preservatives maintain sterility and yet are nonirritating to the cornea.[23]

Currently available solutions for contact lens biomicroscopy include viscous solutions made from carboxymethylcellulose and also hydroxypropyl methylcellulose (Gonioscopic and Goniosol, respectively). These two solutions marketed for this purpose were compared against balanced saline solution and carboxymethylcellulose (Celluvisc). The comparison of the solutions was based on the ability to take fundus photographs after contact lens examination of the retina. None of the solutions prevented fundus photography after their use. The clarity with the fundus camera was somewhat worse after treatment 20% to 24% of the time, but in none of these cases was this of clinical importance.[24] Clinically it is somewhat easier to prolong contact lens-cornea contact without bubble formation with the more viscous solution. More viscous solutions, however, may affect subsequent visual acuity and visual field measurements. This fact should be kept in mind in glaucoma patients who might undergo further testing after gonioscopy.

The abrasive effect of a tonometer on the cornea may be reduced by instillation of a 1% methylcellulose solution immediately before tonometry.[25] The methylcellulose may be incorporated in the anesthetic vehicle; however, this prolongs the anesthetic duration somewhat, which itself causes minor corneal damage. The viscosity of a 1% methylcellulose solution does not alter tonometer readings, but stronger solutions may slow plunger movement because of capillary attraction.

The incorporation of methylcellulose in ophthalmic solutions causes the medication to remain in contact with the cornea for a longer time and thereby enhances its effect. The effect of a methylcellulose vehicle for a 2% pilocarpine concentration was compared with a 2% aqueous solution of pilocarpine in 17 patients with chronic simple glaucoma.[26] After 1 week without medication, these patients received 1 drop of aqueous pilocarpine in the right eye and 1 drop of methylcellulose pilocarpine in the left eye. The following week the solutions were placed in the opposite eyes. Pupil size was measured by photography before and 6 hours after medication. Average intraocular pressure was 22.2 mm Hg after aqueous pilocarpine and 20.5 mm Hg after methylcellulose pilocarpine.

In an experimental study in which *Pseudomonas* organisms were injected into a rabbit cornea and followed by hourly instillations of neomycin in different vehicles, 76% of the infections were prevented by 1% neomycin in a methylcellulose vehicle compared with 44% in a polyvinyl alcohol vehicle and 38% in a polyvinylpyrrolidone vehicle. Presumably the results were caused by enhanced contact time with the methylcellulose vehicle.[27]

Actually, the contact time of topical medications with the eye is far shorter than one would imagine. Computed microscintigraphy using technetium-99m will show the rate of loss of the labeled vehicle from a human eye. After 90 seconds, only 2.9% of radioactivity remains when a saline vehicle is used. Only 4.3% remains with polyvinyl alcohol 1.4%. Only 8.8% remains with hydroxypropyl methylcellulose 0.5%.[28] Of course, 90 seconds later, a comparable percentage drop of the remaining material will again occur. Obviously, medication contact time is not very long.

Electroretinographic eye contact electrodes are coupled to the cornea by various types of wetting solutions. The higher the electrical conductivity of the solution, the stronger will be the electrical signal. An 80% increase in the amplitude of the electroretinogram was obtained with a 0.2% hydroxyethylcellulose solution compared with a 1.6% solution.[29]

## POLYVINYL ALCOHOL

Polyvinyl alcohol, 1.4%, in water or isotonic saline solution, is another vehicle useful in prolonging the ocular contact of ophthalmic medications.[30] It is nontoxic, compatible with most ophthalmic medications and preservatives, and readily sterilized by autoclaving or filtering.

Studies of the regeneration of damaged corneal epithelium suggest that polyvinyl alcohol instillation only slightly retards regeneration of corneal epithelium. The variability of these experiments precluded a definite conclusion as to whether epithelial regeneration was more rapid with isotonic saline solution, methylcellulose, or polyvinyl alcohol. Actually all three types of drops were reported to slow healing of rabbit corneas slightly more than no treatment at all.

Polyvinyl alcohol is much less viscous than methylcellulose. A 1.4% solution has a viscosity of 4.4 cp in contrast to 50 cp for a 0.5% solution of methylcellulose.

Because it remains in the aqueous vehicle and does not penetrate the corneal epithelium, nickel chloride was selected as a test substance to determine ocular contact time after topical application in various solutions (0.5% methylcellulose, 1.4% polyvinyl alcohol, and isotonic saline solution). The time in minutes after application of a 0.5% nickel chloride solution was measured until nickel was no longer demonstrable on the conjunctiva by the dimethylglyoxime test. In saline solution the nickel disappeared in 9 to 12 minutes; in methylcellulose, 10 to 13 minutes; and in polyvinyl alcohol, 11 to 13 minutes. Although contact time is prolonged by both methylcellulose and polyvinyl alcohol, their effect obviously lasts for only a few minutes and is not comparable with the effect of a long-lasting ointment vehicle.

Fluorescein concentrations in cornea and aqueous humor were measured after application of 2% fluorescein in water, 1.4% polyvinyl alcohol, or 0.5% hydroxypropyl methylcellulose. At 1 hour, the corneal concentrations were $3.2 \times 10^{-4}$, 2.6, and 4.6 mg/ml for these vehicles, respectively. The 1-hour aqueous concentrations were $3.2 \times 10^{-5}$, 2.5, and 4.8 mg/ml, respectively. To determine if drop size or multiple drops increased drug penetration, the cul-de-sac was flooded with fluorescein compared with the use of a single drop. No difference in fluorescein penetration resulted, indicating that excess amounts of medication are simply wasted. Only a tiny proportion of applied fluorescein penetrates the eye. The corneal concentration is only one hundred thousandth of the tear concentration; the aqueous concentration, only one millionth.[31]

## PRESERVATIVE TOXICITY

No tear replacement has been found that can actually substitute for normal tears. However, the presence of preservatives seems to exacerbate epithelial defects, particularly in the severely affected individual with keratoconjunctivitis sicca. These epithelial defects have been evaluated in vitro in a tissue culture model. Solutions containing edetate disodium (EDTA) and either benzalkonium chloride (BAK) or polyquaternium-1 (Poly-Quad) were compared with similar solutions that were unpreserved. Cell viability of this model decreased dramatically over the first 15 minutes of the solution preserved with BAK. The solution preserved with polyquaternium-1 was not as toxic as the BAK preserved solution but had decreased viability compared with the unpreserved solutions.[32]

The elimination of preservative entails a change in the container to a sterile unit dose form. This increases expense and also usually decreases convenience for the patient. Preserved tear substitutes are generally tolerated and appreciated by the mildly symptomatic dry eye, whereas unpreserved products are required for the severely affected patient with keratoconjunctivitis sicca requiring frequent use of tear substitutes greater than four to six times daily.[33, 34]

## POLYMER DERIVATIVES

Reasoning that the most important component of the normal tear film is the mucous layer and assuming that the mucus functions by adhering to the corneal epithelium and increasing its surface tension, researchers attempted to duplicate the characteristics of mucus with a mixture of ethylene glycol polymers and polyvinylpyrrolidone. This preparation also contains 0.5% hydroxyethyl cellulose, 0.004% thimerosal, and 0.1% EDTA. This "artificial mucus" was originally introduced as contact lens wetting solution but was found to be comparably effective in wetting the dry cornea.[34, 35] It binds persistently to solids and has a very high surface tension, thereby producing an easily wettable surface.[36]

Sodium hyaluronate had been found to be useful for the treatment of refractory dry eye symptoms. It is used as a 0.1% solution and can be made by mixing 0.5 ml of 1% sodium hyaluronate used for anterior segment surgery in 4.5 ml of nonpreserved balanced salt solution. The sodium hyaluronate must be sterilized by autoclave before mixture, and the solution must be refrigerated between uses. This solution is available in unit dose containers commercially in Canada under the trade name Hylorin. This solution was found to improve symptoms in 26 of 28 patients who were refractory to conventional therapy.[37] Sodium hyaluronate was found to improve keratitis and mucous strands better than a nonpreserved solution of polyvinyl alcohol (Refresh).[38]

Sodium hyaluronate (0.1%) was compared with 1% chondroitin sulfate and the commercially available tear substitute of 1% polyvinyl alcohol and polyethylene glycol containing BAK (HypoTears) in 20 patients with keratoconjunctivitis sicca. A fourth solution was prepared through mixing 0.38% chondroitin sulfate and 0.3% sodium hyaluronate. The 20 patients used the solutions every 2 hours while awake for 2 weeks for each solution. Of the 18 patients who had a preference, four preferred the chondroitin sulfate solution, four the chondroitin sulfate/sodium hyaluronate, seven the polyvinyl alcohol solution, and three the sodium hyaluronate solution. Those patients with the lowest Schirmer test results seemed to prefer the chondroitin sulfate solution most, and those with the highest Schirmer test results seemed to prefer the sodium hyaluronate solution most. The solution preserved with BAK was found to increase corneal staining during its use, another indication that frequent use of preserved tear solutions can cause corneal toxicity.[39]

## SOLID INSERTS

A small rod of hydroxypropylcellulose has been designed for insertion into the lower cul-de-sac (Lacrisert, Merck and Co., Inc., West Point, Pa.). Its gradual dissolution into the tears is supposed to stabilize the tear film and reduce symptoms. Use of this device will increase the mean tear breakup time from an original 4.7 seconds to a posttreatment 6.8 seconds[40] (normal 15 to 35 seconds; values less than 10 seconds indicate mucin deficiency). This increase of only 2 seconds does not sound very important; however, the average blink rate is once every 5 to 10 seconds. Renewal of the tear film more rapidly than it breaks should theoretically eliminate damage to the corneal surface. Half of patients experience improvement in foreign body sensation and irritation with use of this insert compared with 10% relieved by artificial tears.

A soluble succinylated collagen wafer was designed for gradual dissolution in the cul-de-sac. Its contact angle was 74 degrees and surface tension 44 dynes/cm, values comparable with those of other artificial tears. This wafer prolonged the tear breakup time by 5 to 10 seconds when measured 1 hour after wafer insertion. The total duration of effect lasted up to 7 hours.[41]

## ALTERNATIVE DRY EYE THERAPY

If the quantity and quality of tears are severely deficient, no replacement therapy is of benefit. Even the most refractory cases of dry eye syndrome can be treated by an alternate method that eliminates evaporation. By means of an airtight goggle treated with an antifogging agent and containing a moist cotton ball reservoir, the air in contact with the cornea may be kept totally saturated with water vapor. Ordinary swimmer's goggles may be used, or a dental alginate form may be cast on regular spectacle frames to fit exactly the facial contours. This method has cosmetic disadvantages, and periodic sterilization by washing in detergent is advisable to prevent infection; nevertheless, it is helpful in protecting the dry cornea against further damage and permitting healing.[42, 43]

Occlusion of the nasal lacrimal system through punctal plugs or cautery can improve the retention of natural tears and tear substitutes, improving symptoms. Evaluation of 18 dry eye patients given punctal plugs after failure on maximum conventional therapy showed that 11 of these had subjective improvement, allowing them to decrease the frequency of their tear substitutes. Punctal plug extrusion occurred in 22% (4 of 18) of patients within 2 weeks of placement. Interestingly, the metaplasia found with impression cytology persisted long after improvement in symptoms.[44]

Punctal plug extrusion can be avoided by cauterizing the puncta. This is most comfortably performed by injecting a small amount of lidocaine subcutaneously next to the puncta and then using a hand-held cautery with a crimped tip, placing the crimped tip into the puncta for a few seconds until the area 1 mm around the puncta has whitened. This will provide permanent closure of the puncta; however, spontaneous openings have rarely been reported. Because of the difficulty in reversing this closure, it is important to first ascertain whether epiphora will occur with punctal closure by first using either silicon punctal plugs or the dissolvable collagen plugs. Silicon plugs will protrude from the puncta and can cause irritation and extrude. The collagen plugs will occasionally migrate from the punctal and canalicular area into the common canaliculus, effectively occluding both the inferior and superior systems, confusing the test results.

Tear stimulation is the ultimate approach to keratoconjunctivitis sicca. Bromhexine, an oral secretory stimulant, has been used in Europe in the treatment of keratoconjunctivitis sicca. It is currently under clinical investigation in the United States.[45]

To avoid the side effects of the systemic bromhexine, investigations have evaluated the role of topical stimulators of tear secretion. Agents that increased either cyclic adenosine monophosphate or cyclic guanosine monophosphate levels increased tear volume or decreased tear osmolarity in a rabbit model of keratoconjunctivitis sicca. These agents included vasoactive intestinal peptide and related molecules, pro-opiomelanocortins, and forskolin. Interestingly, in this model, pilocarpine, a cholinergic antagonist, was not found to affect tear film osmolarity when applied to the previously anesthetized eye. These agents must act on the accessory lacrimal glands because this model of keratoconjunctivitis sicca involved cauterization of the external duct and orifice of the lacrimal gland.[46]

Sucralfate (Carafate) is an oral medication commonly used for mucosal protection in patients with duodenal ulcers. This was used topically as a 2% solution in a viscous vehicle containing oxypropyl methylcellulose. Twenty-two patients were treated for 1 to 19 months (mean 6 months) using this solution. Improvement in ocular surface changes as documented by rose bengal staining was found over the first 4 months. Extrapolating from the experience with duodenal ulcers, it may be that this solution clings to areas of focal dryness or epithelial erosion, allowing these to heal more quickly. Double-mask evaluations of this solution are necessary before any definite conclusions are made as to its efficacy.[47]

## SILICONE FLUIDS

Lubrication of artificial eyes with silicone fluids has increased the comfort of wearing such prostheses and has improved prosthesis appearance. In a series of 35 patients, 28 reported socket irritation to be reduced by silicone use.[48] In addition, the silicone prevented discharge from crusting on the lids and the prosthesis. The glistening silicone film on the prosthesis surface also imparted a more lifelike appearance to the artificial eye.

The silicone used was Medical Fluid 360. Viscosities of 100 and 350 centistokes were used, with almost equal patient acceptance (slight preference for the thinner fluid, 100 centistokes). Frequency of use was variable, depending on the patient's comfort, but was usually three or four times daily.

Silicone usage did not decrease the volume of discharge or otherwise benefit socket infection. Although silicones are inert and do not support bacterial growth, they have no antibacterial properties.

Silicone eye drops of 100 centistokes of viscosity are preferable to the use of methylcellulose drops for the lubrication of artificial eyes if the lids do not close during sleep. Dry crusts of methylcellulose and mucus form on the prosthesis if the lids do not close and may be irritating to the lids. However, silicone drops have the disadvantage of making the prosthesis water repellent. Once used, the silicone drop must be continued daily, because tears will not properly moisten and lubricate the prosthesis thereafter.[49]

Because wetting agents and preservative are almost universally present in commercial eye drop preparations, reference to the relevant federal regulations may be helpful.[50, 51]

## SUMMARY

In the future the treatment of dry eye syndrome and related problems will be based on the diagnosis of the underlying cause. This may include aqueous, lipid, or mucin deficiency of the tears. This may also include related abnormalities such as blepharitis, ectropion, or entropion. Diagnosis includes evaluation of factors such as topical and systemic medications, cosmetic makeup, contact lenses, and environmental and occupational factors. After this evaluation, along with clinical examination, specific therapy may be directed to the problem instead of the "shotgun" approach commonly used.

## REFERENCES


1. Holly FJ: Surface chemical evaluation of artificial tears and their ingredients: I. Interfacial activity at equilibrium, *Contact Lens* 4:14, 1978.
2. Lemp MA, Szymanski ES: Polymer adsorption at the ocular surface, *Arch Ophthalmol* 93:134, 1975.
3. Norn MS: Topical fluorescein penetration, *Am J Ophthalmol* 79:335, 1975.
4. Levenson JE: The effect of short-term drying on the surface ultrastructure of the rabbit, *Ann Ophthalmol* 5:865, 1973.
5. Gilbard JP, Farris RL, Santamaria J: Osmolarity of tear microvolumes in keratoconjunctivitis sicca, *Arch Ophthalmol* 96:677, 1978.
6. Holly FJ: Biophysical aspects of epithelial adhesion to stroma, *Invest Ophthalmol Vis Sci* 17:552, 1978.
7. Holly FJ: Surface chemical evaluation of artificial tears and their ingredients: II. Interaction with a superficial lipid layer, *Contact Lens* 4:52, 1978.
8. Lemp MA, Goldberg M, Roddy MR: The effects of tear substitutes on tear film breakup time, *Invest Ophthalmol* 14:255, 1975.
9. Doane MG: Interaction of eyelids and tears in corneal wetting and the dynamics of the normal human eyeblink, *Am J Ophthalmol* 89:507, 1980.
10. Holly FJ, Esquivel ED: Colloid osmotic pressure of artificial tears, *J Ocular Pharmacol* 4:327, 1985.
11. Motolko M, Breslin CW: The effect of pH and osmolarity on the ability to tolerate artificial tears, *Am J Ophthalmol* 91:781, 1981.
12. Gilbard JP, Kenyon KR: Tear diluents in the treatment of keratoconjunctivitis sicca, *Ophthalmology* 92:646, 1985.
13. Gonnering R, Edelhauser HF, Van Horn DL, and others: The pH tolerance of rabbit and human corneal endothelium, *Invest Ophthalmol Vis Sci* 18:373, 1979.
14. Carney LG, Mauger TF, Hill RM: Buffering in human tears: pH responses to acid and base challenge, *Invest Ophthalmol Vis Sci* 30:747, 1989.
15. Poster MG: Optical efficacy of rewetting and lubricating solutions, *Contact Lens Forum* 6:25, 1981.
16. Swan KW: Use of methylcellulose in ophthalmology, *Arch Ophthalmol* 33:378, 1945.
17. Alexander CM, Newell FW: The effect of various agents on corneal epithelization, *Am J Ophthalmol* 48:210, 1959.
18. Krishna N, Mitchell B: Polyvinyl alcohol as an ophthalmic vehicle, *Am J Ophthalmol* 59:860, 1965.
19. Merrill DL, Fleming TC, Girard LJ: The effects of physiologic balanced salt solutions and normal saline on intraocular and extraocular tissues, *Am J Ophthalmol* 49:895, 1960.
20. Fleming TC, Merrill DL, Girard LJ: Studies of the irritating action of methylcellulose, *Arch Ophthalmol* 61:865, 1959.
21. Virno M, Bucci MG, Pecori-Giraldi J, and others: Intravenous glycerol–vitamin C (sodium salt) as osmotic agents to reduce intraocular pressure, *Am J Ophthalmol* 62:824, 1966.
22. Ehlers N: The precorneal film, *Acta Ophthalmol* 81(suppl):1, 1965.

23. Miller D, Aquino MV, Fiore AS: Gonioscopy ointment, *Am J Ophthalmol* 67:419, 1969.
24. Pepsin SR, Olk RJ: A comparison of three contact-lens biomicroscopy coupling solutions, *Am J Ophthalmol* 112:732, 1991.
25. Jervey JW: Tonometry and the cornea, *Arch Ophthalmol* 56:109, 1956.
26. Haas JS, Merrill DL: The effect of methylcellulose on responses to solutions of pilocarpine, *Am J Ophthalmol* 54:21, 1962.
27. Bach FC, Riddel G, Miller C, and others: The influence of vehicles on neomycin sulfate prevention of experimental ocular infection in rabbits, *Am J Ophthalmol* 69:659, 1970.
28. Trueblood JH, Rossomondo RM, Carlton WH, and others: Corneal contact times of ophthalmic vehicles, *Arch Ophthalmol* 93:127, 1975.
29. Declercq SS: The coating agent on the corneal contact lens in electroretinography, *Am J Ophthalmol* 83:267, 1977.
30. Krishna M, Brow F: Polyvinyl alcohol as an ophthalmic vehicle, *Am J Ophthalmol* 57:99, 1964.
31. Waltman SR, Patrowicz TC: Effects of hydroxypropyl methylcellulose and polyvinyl alcohol on intraocular penetration of topical fluorescein in man, *Invest Ophthalmol* 9:966, 1970.
32. Adams J, Wilcox MJ, Trousdale MD, and others: Morphologic and physiologic effects of artificial tear formulations on corneal epithelial derived cells, *Cornea* 11:234, 1992.
33. Laflamme MY, Swieca R: A comparative study of two preservative-free tear substitutes in the management of severe dry eye, *Can J Ophthalmol* 23:174, 1988.
34. Flanary LM, Block JH: Mucus substitutes for the dry-eye contact lens wearer, *J Contact Lens Soc Am* 4:36, 1970.
35. Barsam PC, Sampson WG, Feldman GL: Treatment of the dry eye and related problems, *Ann Ophthalmol* 4:122, 1972.
36. Holly FJ, Lemp MA: Surface chemistry of the tearfilm: implications for dry eye syndromes, contact lenses, and ophthalmic polymers, *J Contact Lens Soc Am* 5:12, 1971.
37. Lemp MD: Recent developments in dry eye management, *Ophthalmology* 94:1299, 1987.
38. Deluise VP, Peterson WS: The use of topical Healon® tears in the management of refractory dry-eye syndrome, *Ann Ophthalmol* 16:823, 1984.
39. Limberg MB, McCaa C, Kissling GE, and others: Topical application of hyaluronic acid and chondroitin sulfate in the treatment of dry eyes, *Am J Ophthalmol* 103:194, 1987
40. Merck Sharp & Dohme, Division of Merck & Co, West Point, Pa., data.
41. Bloomfield SE, Dunn MW, Miyata T, and others: Soluble artificial tear inserts, *Arch Ophthalmol* 95:247, 1977.
42. Poirier RH, Ryburn FM, Israel CW: Swimmer's goggles for keratoconjunctivitis sicca, *Arch Ophthalmol* 95:1405, 1977.
43. Savar DE, Runacre P, Godfrey CM: Moisture chamber spectacles, *Arch Ophthalmol* 97:1347, 1979.
44. Willis RM, Folberg R, Krachmer JH, and others: The treatment of aqueous deficient dry eye with removable punctal plugs, *Ophthalmology* 94:514, 1988.
45. Avisar R, Savir H: Our further experience with bromohexine in keratoconjunctivitis sicca, *Ann Ophthalmol* 20:382, 1988.
46. Gilbard JP, Rossi SR, Heyda KG, and others: Simulation of tear secretion by topical agents that increase cyclic nucleotide levels, *Invest Ophthalmol Vis Sci* 31:1381, 1990.
47. Praus JV: Beneficial effect of sodium-sucrose-sulfate on the ocular surface of patients with severe KCS in primary Sjogren's syndrome, *Acta Ophthalmol (Copenh)* 69:417, 1991.
48. Morgan JF, Hill JC: Silicone fluid as a lubricant for artificial eyes, *Am J Ophthalmol* 58:767, 1964.
49. Spivey BE, Allen L, Burns CA: The Iowa enucleation implant, a 10-year evaluation of technique and results, *Am J Ophthalmol* 67:171, 1969.
50. FDA monograph on over-the-counter ophthalmic drug products, *Fed Register* 45(89):30002, 1980.
51. Mullen W, Shepherd W, Labovitz J: Ophthalmic preservatives and vehicles, *Surv Ophthalmol* 17:469, 1973.

CHAPTER **14**

# Vasodilators

Robert B. Chambers

The history of the use of vasodilators in the therapy of various ocular diseases has been one of excitement and disappointment as the regulation of ocular blood flow, and in particular retinal blood flow, has become better understood. Diseases that may be affected by ocular blood flow range from some external diseases such as allergic conjunctivitis to glaucoma to retinal and choroidal vascular diseases. Retinal vascular occlusive diseases have been of particular interest because medical and surgical treatment options have been of rather limited value in these frequently devastating problems.

The pharmacology of glaucoma medications is covered in Chapter 4, but recent developments in the use of vasodilators in lowering intraocular pressure (IOP) make a few comments on these advances appropriate here. The primary aim of this chapter is the discussion of the factors affecting the dual supply to the retina, namely, the choroidal and retinal circulations.

## VASODILATORS IN GLAUCOMA

A new class of ocular hypotensive agents has been extensively studied in light of recent evidence indicating that hormonal regulation of guanylate cyclase may play a role in the control of IOP.[1] In rabbits treated with topical preparations of nitroglycerin, isosorbide dinitrate, sodium nitrate, hydralazine, minoxidil, and sodium nitroprusside, IOP was rapidly lowered in a dose-related fashion. The duration of action and peak effect was relatively short, and there was some evidence of tolerance and local side effects. The mechanism of action was postulated as an increased facility of outflow through the trabecular meshwork. The actions appeared to be local rather than systemic.

Other experimental evidence for potential new IOP-lowering drugs comes from work on fenoldopam mesylate, an adenyl cyclase stimulator.[2] Fenoldopam stimulation of adenyl cyclase through direct activation of dopamine-1 receptors in the trabecular meshwork raises IOP. This suggests that dopamine-1 receptor blockade may be useful in lowering IOP. It is likely that given the highly vascular nature of the ciliary body and the multiplicity and diversity of receptor sites in the trabecular meshwork, pharmacologic manipulation of IOP will offer new strategies in the management of glaucoma.

## REGULATION OF CHOROIDAL BLOOD FLOW

The outer one third of the retina, the ciliary body, some portions of the optic nerve, and other parts of the globe are supplied by the choroidal circulation. The flow of the blood to the choroid is through the long and short posterior arteries, which are branches of the ophthalmic artery off the internal carotid. Venous drainage is through a series of collector venous channels leading to four or more large vortex veins exiting the sclera posterior to the equator. These lead to the superior and inferior orbital veins and then to the cavernous sinus. A small contribution to this drainage is made by the ciliary body and anterior ciliary veins.

The choroidal circulation has a higher blood volume per unit area than any other tissue in the body, including the brain.[3] Important in understanding the pharmacology of blood flow in the choroid is the fact that choroidal blood flow is under autonomic control from the sympathetic nervous system.[4] This is in contradistinction to the retinal circulation, which is essentially autoregulatory and independent from autonomic control.

This fact seems to suggest that choroidal blood flow should be affected by systemically administered vasodilators. However, early experiments with radioactively tagged red blood cells showed no increase in radioactivity in the eye when systemic vasodilators such as papaverine, niacin, tolazoline, or phentolamine[5] were administered. More recent data confirm the relative stability of the choroidal circulation despite a pharmacologic lowering of peripheral vascular resistance and choroidal perfusion pressure.[6]

Carbon dioxide, a powerful local retinal vasodilator, had been shown in early experiments to dramatically affect choroidal circulation. However, more recent work indicates that even this potent vasodilator has little or no effect on normal choroidal blood volume.[5, 7, 8]

If one attempts to increase choroidal blood flow through local administration of such drugs as papaverine, tolazoline, or sodium nitrate, there is no significant effect.[9, 10] Paradoxically, systemic vasoconstrictors such as epinephrine and angiotensin can cause increased systemic peripheral resistance but actually lead to an increase in choroidal blood flow.[11]

Manipulation of the sympathetic chain by sympathectomy will decrease choroidal blood volume, whereas stimulation of the sympathetics will increase blood flow.[4, 10, 12, 13] Loss of sympathetic control is seen clinically in patients with such diseases as hypertension and diabetes and can be manifested in the onset of macular and choroidal edema or a worsening of preexisting edema. Numerous theories have been proposed to explain the role of the choroid in macular edema, all of which depend on maintenance of homeostatic conditions in choroidal blood flow preventing excessive outflow of plasma and plasma proteins into the extravascular space. Despite these data suggesting autonomic circulatory control is more significant than local autoregulatory mechanisms, pharmacologic manipulation of the sympathetic nervous system has little role in clinical practice in control of blood flow to the choroid directly. Control of systemic hypertension and hyperglycemia has been shown to be effective in stabilization and reversal of macular edema, and the mechanism may be through restoring normal autonomic control over the choroidal blood flow.

## REGULATION OF RETINAL BLOOD FLOW

The inner two thirds of the retina is supplied by the retinal circulation. The central retinal artery is a branch of the ophthalmic artery off the internal carotid. It pierces the sheathes of the optic nerve before entering the globe where it branches to supply the nasal and temporal retina. The larger branches lie just beneath the internal limiting membrane penetrating no deeper than the inner plexiform layer. Precapillary arterioles lead to a complex of capillaries and then to postcapillary venules in the inner nuclear layer and throughout the retina except in the capillary free zone in the macula and in a small border zone surrounding the major arterioles. Venules lead to branches of the central retinal vein that exits the eye.

The retinal circulation is somewhat unique in the body in that its flow is not regulated by the autonomic nervous system. This is particularly striking given its juxtaposition to the sympathetically regulated choroidal circulation. Rather, regulation of the retinal circulation depends on local servo-feedback systems. Within a limited range, deficiencies in choroidal blood flow can be compensated for by autoregulatory changes in the retinal circulation.[14]

The primary drive of the autoregulation

of retinal blood flow is tissue oxygen concentration.[15–18] Perfusion pressure also plays a role in the autoregulation of retinal circulation. Acute increases in retinal oxygen pressure ($Po_2$) levels lead to vasoconstriction of the retinal arteriolar tree. This was demonstrated by Deutsch[19] in experiments with oxygen breathing where retinal vascular vasoconstriction was observed after normal subjects breathed high concentrations of oxygen. Breathing $CO_2$ did not seem to have much effect on vascular dilatation. These data are in conflict with earlier work suggesting a more significant role for retinal $Po_2$ levels in regulation of retinal blood flow. In light of this, the often proposed treatment for acute embolic retinal arteriolar occlusion (i.e., $CO_2$ rebreathing or breathing 5% concentrations of $CO_2$) would appear to be of questionable value. The theoretic value of mixing oxygen and carbon dioxide in treatment of arteriolar occlusion is attractive in that the increase in $Po_2$ level might better oxygenate the tissues and $CO_2$ might dilate the vessels.

Sublingual nitroglycerin does increase the caliber of retinal arterioles, but the corresponding decrease in retinal venous blood oxygen saturation makes measurements of retinal blood flow based on observed retinal arteriole caliber changes suspect. Blood flow to the retina may actually decrease in these situations.

Studies of the relation of arterial perfusion pressure to retinal circulation have documented the importance of maintenance of normal IOP for proper retinal circulatory homeostasis. Acute rises in IOP led to vasodilation in experiments by Ffyche[20] and Russell.[21] The mechanism of this is questionable, but it appears that an initial vision loss as a result of raised IOP less than that required to occlude the central retinal artery is not sustained longer than 1 minute with return to normal levels. This may be another example of autoregulation where increased IOP leads to tissue anoxia, which, in turn, leads to autoregulatory feedback mechanisms and restoration of visual thresholds through improved tissue oxygenation.

Attempts of pharmacologic treatment of various retinal diseases caused by ischemic conditions in the retina with vasodilating agents have been largely ineffective. There are, however, studies to suggest that systemically administered drugs may have an effect on retinal circulation. Experimentally induced arterial vasospasm can be relieved by intravenously and topically administered papaverine, tolazoline, and caffeine sodium benzoate.[22] Vision loss caused by acute vasospasm may be helped by prompt administration of the drugs, but clinically these conditions are rarely seen, and medical treatment with these powerful vasodilators is seldom indicated. Venous caliber does not seem to be affected, and there does not seem to be a role for vasodilators in the treatment of venous occlusive diseases.

In a trial of nifedipine in patients with sickle cell disease and related genetic variants, ocular ischemic effects of the disease were reversed in the retina and conjunctiva. Color vision also improved.[23] Buflomedil has been reported to improve microcirculation through vasodilation. Diabetic patients were evaluated by vitreous fluorophotometry while being treated with buflomedil. The drug may act by improving blood flow, as evidenced by pH measurements on capillary blood that increased in patients on treatment.[24] Calcitonin gene–related peptide can dilate retinal arterioles.[25]

## REFERENCES

1. Nathanson JA: Nitrovasodilators as a new class of ocular hypotensive agents, *J Pharmacol Exp Ther* 260:956, 1992.
2. Elliot WJ, Karnezis TA, Silverman RA, and others: Intraocular pressure increases with fenoldopam, but not nitroprusside, in hypertensive humans, *Clin Pharmacol Ther* 49:285, 1991.
3. Alm A, Bill A: Ocular and optic nerve blood flow at normal and increased intraocular pressures in monkeys (macac irus): a study with radioactively labelled microspheres including flow determinations in brain and some other tissues, *Exp Eye Res* 15:15, 1973.
4. Bill A: Autonomic nervous control of uveal blood flow, *Acta Physiol Scand* 56:70, 1962.
5. Bettman JW, Fellows V: Effects of peripheral vasodilator and vasoconstrictor drugs on the intraocular (choroidal) blood vol-

ume, *Trans Am Acad Ophthalmol* 66:480, 1962.
6. Ernest JT, Goldstick TK: The effect of perfusion pressure on uveal blood flow, *Invest Ophthalmology Vis Sci* 19:83, 1980.
7. Friedman E, Chandra SR: Choroidal blood flow: III. Effects of oxygen and carbon dioxide, *Arch Ophthalmol* 87:70, 1972.
8. Wilson TM, Strang R, MacKenzie ET: The response of the choroidal and cerebral circulations to changing arterial $P_{CO_2}$ and acetazolamide in the baboon, *Invest Ophthalmol Vis Sci* 16:576, 1977.
9. Paul SD, Leopold IH: The effect of vasodilating drugs on choroidal circulation, *Am J Ophthalmol* 42:899, 1956.
10. Potts AM: An hypothesis on macular disease, *Trans Am Acad Ophthalmol Otolaryngol* 70:1058, 1966.
11. Dollery CT, Hill DW, Hodge JV: The response of normal retinal blood vessels to angiotensin and nonadrenaline, *J Physiol* 165:500, 1963.
12. Varma SD, Kinoshita JH: Sorbitol pathway in diabetic and galactosemic rat lens, *Biochem Biophys Acta* 338:632, 1974.
13. Weiter JJ, Schacher RA, and Ernest JT: Control of intraocular blood flow: II. Effects of sympathetic tone, *Invest Ophthalmol* 12:332, 1973.
14. Demant E, Kunihiko N, Gunter N: Effects of changes in systemic blood pressure on the electroretinogram of the cat: evidence for retinal autoregulation, *Invest Ophthalmol Vis Sci* 23:683, 1982.
15. Deutsch RA, Read JS, Ernest JT, and others: Effects of oxygen and carbon dioxide on the retinal circulation in man, *Invest Ophthalmol Vis Sci* 22(suppl):195, 1982 (abstract).
16. Frayser R, Hickam JB: Retinal vascular response to breathing increased carbon dioxide and oxygen concentrations, *Invest Ophthalmol Vis Sci* 3:427, 1964.
17. Petrig BL, Riva CE, Sinclair SH, and others: Quantification of changes in leukocyte velocity in retinal macular capillaries during oxygen breathing, *Invest Ophthalmol Vis Sci* 22(suppl):194, 1982 (abstract).
18. Riva CE, Grunwald JE, Petrig BI, and others: Effect of breathing pure oxygen on human retinal blood flow measured by Doppler velocimetry, *Invest Ophthalmol Vis Sci* 22(suppl):194, 1982 (abstract).
19. Deutsch TA, Read JS, Ernest JT, and others: Effect of oxygen and carbon dioxide on the retinal vasculature in humans, *Arch Ophthalmol* 101:1278, 1983.
20. Ffyche TJ, Bulpitt CJ, Kohner EM, and others: Effect of changes in intraocular pressure on the retinal microcirculation, *Br J Ophthalmol* 58:514, 1974.
21. Russel RW: Evidence for autoregulation in human retinal circulation, *Lancet* 2:1048, 1973.
22. Ellis PP, Lende RA: Induced spasm in the retinal arterioles of cats: II. Influences of physical factors and drugs, *Arch Ophthalmol* 71:706, 1964.
23. Rodgers GP, Roy MS, Noguchi CT, and others: Use of selective vasodilation in treatment of sickle cell disease, *Am J Pediatr Hematol Oncol* 10:351, 1988.
24. Kjaergaard JJ, Ditzel J: The effect of buflomedil in diabetic retinopathy estimated by ocular fluorophotometry, *Int J Microcirc Clin Exp* 6:257, 1987.
25. Prieto D, Benedito S, Nielsen PJ, and others: Calcitonin gene-related peptide is a potent vasodilator of bovine retinal arteries in vitro, *Exp Eye Res* 53:339, 1991.

CHAPTER **15**

# Vitamins

**Robert B. Chambers**

Vitamins are chemical compounds that the human body needs in small amounts. Vitamins regulate chemical reactions by which the body converts food to energy in living tissues. There are 13 vitamins. Five are produced by the body itself. Of these, only biotin, pantothenic acid, and vitamin K are produced in sufficient quantity that supplementation by diet is not necessary. The rest must be supplied in the diet. Vitamins are essential to proper ocular structure and function, and specific vitamin deficiencies can cause eye disease. In addition, excessive dosages of vitamins A, D, and K can cause ocular toxicity. The recommended daily dosage for vitamins with specific ocular activity are listed in Table 15-1. In spite of a growing trend toward use of vitamin supplementation and use of "megadose" vitamin supplementations, there is no evidence that in otherwise healthy individuals the use of these megadoses is useful in enhancing ocular function. In fact, in some instances the use of these megadoses of vitamins may actually cause toxicity.

## VITAMIN A

Vitamin A, also called retinol, is a fat-soluble vitamin that has been shown to be important to maintaining structure and function of the cornea and retina. The primary dietary source for vitamin A is carotenoids. Carotenoids are found in milk, fish liver oils, eggs, butter, and green and yellow vegetables. The most active carotenoid is β-carotene. It is absorbed readily from the small intestine and stored in the liver. There is evidence that vitamin A may be stored in the retinal pigment epithelium as well.[1] There are a number of storage forms of vitamin A in the retina and retinal pigment epithelium. A combination of the aldehyde derivative of vitamin A with a visual protein (opsin) results in an important visual pigment, rhodopsin. This is the visual pigment of the rod system. The visual process involves the conversion of an active 11-*cis* isomer of vitamin A into the *trans* form when stimulated by light striking the retina. Enzyme systems within the retinal pigment epithelium then reconvert the *trans* form to the *cis* form for reuse in the visual process.[2] Vitamin A can cause disease through both deficiency states and toxicity. Deficiency states may exist at plasma levels of 0.6 IU/ml. Nyctalopia is an early symptom of vitamin A deficiency. Even as the patient with severe vitamin A deficiency complains of night blindness, the abnormal electrophysiologic testing during dark adaptometry and electroretinography can be demonstrated. Eventually permanent structural changes occur within the retina and retinal pigment epithelium. Some of these are visualized ophthalmoscopically. The peripheral retina is the most common site for these yellow-white opacities in the retina caused by vitamin A deficiency. Fluorescein angiography shows retinal pigment epithelial window defects in these areas, and these correspond with constriction of the peripheral visual field.[3] Animal models show that vitamin A deficiency decreases the rate of rod

**TABLE 15–1.**
Recommended Daily Vitamin Doses

| Vitamin | Dose | |
|---|---|---|
| Vitamin A | 1,200 IU (men) | 1,000 IU (women) |
| Vitamin $B_1$ | 0.3–0.5 mg (infants) | 1.0–1.5 mg (adults) |
| Vitamin $B_6$ | 2 mg | |
| Vitamin $B_{12}$ | 3 μg (adults) | 0.3 μg (infants) |
| Vitamin C | 45–80 mg | |
| Vitamin D | 400 IU | |
| Vitamin E | 15 IU | |
| Vitamin K | Unknown | |

outer segment production.[4] These structural changes appear to be irreversible even with treatment. Individuals in industrialized nations with well-balanced diets seem to be protected against vitamin A deficiency by the liver's ability to store quantities of vitamin A against short-term dietary deficiencies. Vitamin A metabolism is altered with age and may be related to vision changes during senescence.[5] Vitamin A deficiency has also been shown to occur during the third trimester of pregnancy.[6] Vitamin A deficiency is a major cause of pediatric ocular morbidity, with more than 5 million children developing xerophthalmia annually worldwide. About one fourth of these will become blind. It is a major pathway for measles-associated blindness, particularly in Africa. Recommended treatment is 200,000 IU of oral vitamin A on 2 successive days with a maintenance dose of 2,000,000 IU every 3 to 6 months.[7] In a study in southern India, children with persistent diarrhea appeared to be at high risk of having vitamin A deficiency develop. Of the children with documented vitamin A deficiency, 68% had abnormal corneal epithelial cell shape and absent goblet cells, leading to xerophthalmia. The prevalence of hypovitaminosis A in preschool children of Senegal was estimated at 11.4%, with 19.4% at risk of the deficiency. Thirty-seven percent also had protein and caloric malnutrition, and only 0.2% had Bitot spots. Vitamin A–deficient children tended to grow more slowly and become more anemic. They also tended to have more infections. Vitamin A supplementation decreased the death rate by 30% to 60%.[8] Vitamin A deficiency can also occur in fat malabsorption syndromes such as chronic alcoholic pancreatitis. It can also occur in cystic fibrosis because of the lack of sufficient pancreatic enzymes for intestinal absorption of vitamin A. One study of cystic fibrosis patients observed that 10% had frank conjunctival xerosis and 19% had abnormal dark adaptation even when given vitamin A and pancreatic enzyme replacement.[9, 10]

Bitot's spots have been long known to be external signs of vitamin A deficiency. One study cautioned against using the appearance and disappearance of Bitot's spots in monitoring therapy of children with vitamin A deficiency, because severe deficiency may exist in the absence of Bitot's spots.[11]

Sommer[12] summarized the effects of vitamin A deficiency on the ocular surface. Early ocular surface changes include keratinization of the conjunctiva with corneal staining in a pattern consistent with superficial punctate keratopathy. As the vitamin A deficiency becomes more severe, keratinization extends from the conjunctiva onto the cornea, ultimately leading to ulceration necrosis and possible perforation. Vitamin A is necessary for normal developing and differentiation of nonsquamous epithelium, and its absence leads to abnormal keratinization. Vitamin A is also necessary for proper production and maintenance of goblet cells in the conjunctiva, making xerophthalmia a contributing factor to this keratinization and ulceration. These changes rapidly respond to systemic supplementation.

Vitamin A ointment has been used as a treatment for keratoconjunctivitis sicca. A study by Gilbard et al.[13] showed little efficacy compared with placebo in patients without demonstrable vitamin A deficiency. In 1987, Kastl et al.[14] reported that topical vitamin A ointment increased healing of cataract incisions. The study was based on evidence from previous workers that topical vitamin A preparations increased wound healing by causing an increase in the epithelial mitotic index of wound tissue. Vitamin A also stimulated epithelial migration and granulation tissue formation, and reversal of cortisone retarded healing of wounds.[15]

Anorexia nervosa is an eating disorder characterized by severe malnutrition. In a study of patients with anorexia nervosa, absence of nyctalopia, Bitot's spots, and xerosis with normal conjunctival goblet cell counts indicated that vitamin A deficiency was not a common complication of patients with anorexia.[16]

Ubels et al.[17] suggested that topically applied retinoids may be effective in treatment of persistent and recurring corneal epithelial defects. In a study by Ohashi et al.,[18] topical vitamin A eye drops were used to treat superior limbic keratoconjunctivitis in 12 patients; 83% of patients experienced some improvement without recurrences while using the topical medications. Topical retinoids continue to be prescribed for acne by many dermatologists. A case report warned against the development of acute myopia as an idiosyncratic reaction to the use of isotretinoin.[19] The question as to whether prophylactic treatment with vitamin A is useful in a patient population at risk of development of oral vitamin A deficiency was addressed in a randomized trial by Djunaedi et al.[20] in 2,500 preschool children in northern Sumatra. Results indicate that there was a dramatic decline in the prevalence of xerophthalmia.

The effect of topically applied retinoids and butyrate on fibroblast growth and contracture of collagen matrix was studied by Kim and Stern.[21] Both retinoic acid and butyrate have been shown to modulate growth in differentiation of normal and neoplastic cells. These investigators demonstrated that dermofibroblast proliferation was unaffected by vitamin A and stimulated by retinoic acid but inhibited by butyrate. Scleral fibroblast proliferation in contrast was stimulated by both vitamin A and retinoic acid. All three agents tested had negative effects on fibroblast contraction of collagen matrices. Their conclusions suggested that fibroblast mediation in ocular wound healing may, in fact, be modulated by these compounds.

### Toxicity

Excessive dosages of vitamin A can also produce toxicity. Vitamin A poisoning usually affects children receiving excessive dosages and rarely affects adults. The effects do not appear until after many months of treatment. Large single dosages, for example, 350,000 units for an infant, may cause an acute rise in cerebrospinal fluid pressure. Toxic manifestations include increased intracranial pressure with papilledema, very mild exophthalmos, alopecia, rash, and exfoliation of the skin. Widespread migratory arthritic pains, hypoprothrombinemia, hepatomegaly and splenomegaly with menstrual changes, and generalized malaise may also occur. Retinal damage can occur as a result of chronic vitamin A toxicity. The retinal pigment epithelial cells are particularly at risk. The neurosensory retina can also be damaged.[22] The increased intracranial pressure probably results from hypersecretion of cerebrospinal fluid. Typical ophthalmoscopic manifestations include papilledema with headaches and extraocular muscle paresis and resulting diplopia. Drugs that affect the processing of vitamin A in the retina or the pigment epithelium can cause ocular toxicity. In one study topical retinoic acid used for treatment of skin disorders was found to cause night blindness. It was shown to inhibit the ocular retinolol dehydrogenases, leading to a decrease in the formation of visual 11-*cis*-retinol, leading to night blindness.[23] Topical isotretinoin therapy is becoming increasingly common in the treatment of numerous skin diseases. Both systemic use of isotretinoin and topical use for cystic acne can lead to ocular toxic side effects, including anterior segment inflammation, keratitis sicca, contact lens intolerance, altered refraction, photosensitivity, and nyctalopia.[24]

## VITAMIN $B_1$

Vitamin $B_1$ (thiamine) is a water-soluble vitamin. It is found in yeast, meat, whole grain enriched breads, cereals, nuts, peas, potatoes, and most vegetables. Information on nutritional amblyopia comes primarily from examination of prisoners of war and concentration camp victims, as well as individuals malnourished because of chronic alcohol or drug abuse. These individuals frequently complain of decreased central vision based on central and cecocentral sco-

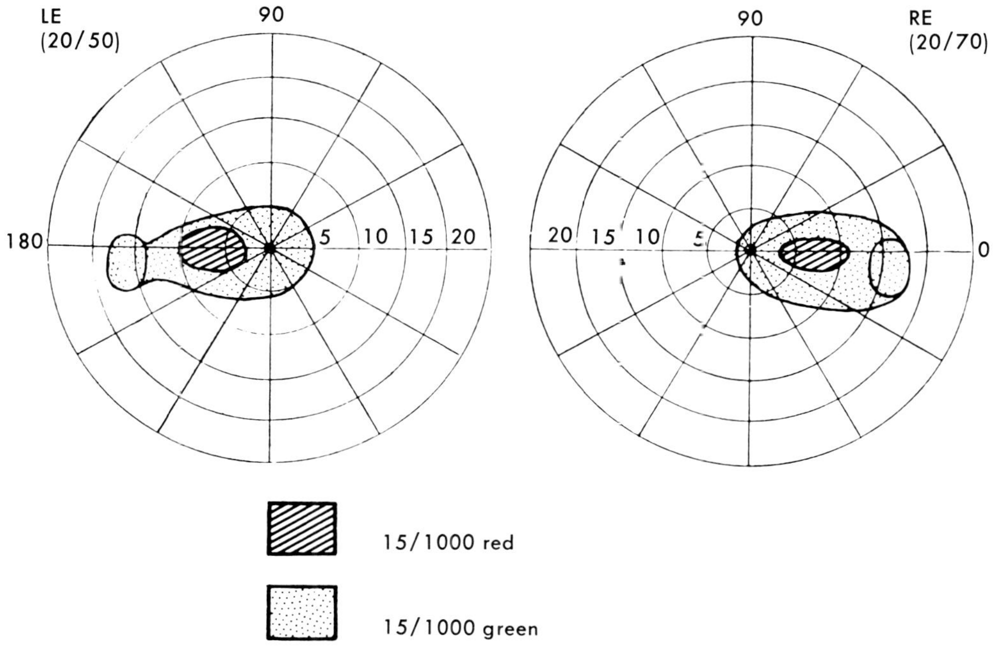


**FIG 15–1.**
Typical cecocentral scotoma of thiamine deficiency in chronic alcoholic. (From Victor M, Mancall EL, Dreyfus PM: *Arch Ophthalmol* 64:1, 1960. Used by permission.)

tomas. These dense central, paracentral, and cecocentral scotomas are characteristic of thiamine deficiency amblyopia (Fig. 15-1). Therapeutic dosage of thiamine for documented cases of dietary deficiency is 5 to 50 mg/day. The involvement of the optic nerves in vitamin $B_1$ deficiency was usually bilateral and often irreversible without ophthalmoscopically visible signs of optic atrophy. Although the precise role of thiamine in the development of tobacco-alcohol amblyopia and nutritional amblyopia is not clear, Dreyfus[25] was able to demonstrate a reduction in the amount of transketolase in patients with nutritional amblyopia. It is known that this enzyme is thiamine dependent. Wernicke's encephalopathy includes ophthalmoplegia and nystagmus and is known to be associated with vitamin $B_1$ deficiency. It is also associated with chronic alcoholism malnutrition and may be seen in patients on intravenous hyperalimentation when supplemental vitamins are not provided.[26] An additional patient developed Wernicke's encephalopathy after long-term intravenous treatment after surgery, and it is recommended that malnourished patients receive 100 mg of parenteral thiamine when glucose infusions are introduced long term postoperatively.[27] Toxicities from thiamine are not known.

## VITAMIN $B_6$

Vitamin $B_6$, also called pyridoxine, is necessary for proper metabolism of amino acids. It is necessary for maintenance of healthy teeth, gums, vasculature, nervous system, and hemopoietic system. It is found in yeast, whole grain cereals, meat, poultry, fish, and most vegetables. Deficiencies in pyridoxine cause vascular congestion, hyperkeratosis, and hair loss of the eyelid margins. Corneal neovascularization has also been seen in patients with this deficiency. The enzyme ornithine amino transferase in the presence of vitamin $B_6$ converts ornithine to glutamic acid. Gyrate atrophy of the retina is a progressive disease of the retina, eventually leading to severe vision loss, and is associated with hyperornithinemia. After an initial report by Gunby,[28] and after Weleber et al.[29] treated four patients with gyrate atrophy by using vitamin $B_6$

supplementation, it was seen that serum ornithine levels could be lowered. The electroretinogram and electrooculogram also improved. It is unclear whether the overall prognosis for maintenance of visual acuity can be directly associated with lowering systemic hyperornithinemia, however. Electromicroscopic examination of the histopathologic specimen with vitamin $B_6$–responsive gyrate atrophy showed abnormalities of the mitochondria of the corneal endothelium and of the nonpigmented ciliary epithelium. There were similar but less severe mitochondrial abnormalities present in the photoreceptors.[30]

## VITAMIN $B_{12}$

Vitamin $B_{12}$, also called cyanocobalamin, is essential for proper development of red blood cells and development and function of the central nervous system, including myelination of nerve fibers. It is found in eggs, meat, milk, and milk products. Retrobulbar neuritis with typical central scotomata may be caused by pernicious anemia seen in vitamin $B_{12}$ deficiency. This may be associated with general symptoms of pernicious anemia or with a numbness and tingling of the extremities typical of subacute combined sclerosis. Although folic acid stimulates hematopoiesis and can eliminate the megaloblastic anemia associated with pernicious anemia, it does not prevent the neurologic complications of pernicious anemia. Adequate treatment with vitamin $B_{12}$ can cure the retrobulbar neuritis of pernicious anemia. Several months of treatment are required before disappearance of the scotoma.

Although cyanocobalamin is the commonly used form of vitamin $B_{12}$, hydroxocobalamin has been reported to be considerably more effective. As little as 10 mg of hydroxocobalamin may maintain elevated vitamin $B_{12}$ levels for as long as 1 year. In contrast, comparable cyanocobalamin treatment may be effective for only 1 month. Subnormal levels of vitamin $B_{12}$ were found in patients with tobacco amblyopia. The theory was advanced that tobacco amblyopia is a result of the failure to detoxify cyanide derived from tobacco smoke. Apparently vitamin $B_{12}$ is necessary for this detoxification. Vitamin $B_{12}$ deficiency appears to be an independent factor unrelated to tobacco smoking.

A very similar neurologic syndrome is produced by a deficiency of thiamine, nicotinic acid, and riboflavin and by tobacco amblyopia. Amblyopia caused by drinking of Jamaican ginger and Nigerian tropical amblyopia are also related conditions. Apparently the common mechanism for the latter three conditions is cyanide inhibition of cytochrome oxidase. In the Nigerian patients a cassava diet contains a glycoside metabolized to hydrocyanic acid. Diffuse neurologic malfunction characterizes this tropical amblyopia, with impaired vision being present in 80% of cases. These patients were deficient in hydroxycobalamine, which detoxifies cyanide. Vitamin $B_{12}$ deficiency also occurs in severe alcoholic liver disease and in severe parasitic infestations. A deficiency can occur despite an adequate dietary intake if a certain glycoprotein called intrinsic factor is not present in the gastric mucosa. Malabsorption of this vitamin in the small intestine is the result of absent intrinsic factor. Vitamin $B_{12}$ deficiency results in inadequate myelin synthesis affecting the optic, peripheral, and cranial nerves.

## VITAMIN C

Vitamin C is a water-soluble vitamin also called ascorbic acid. It is essential for normal tissue metabolism and wound healing, as well as sound bones and teeth. It is found in citrus fruits, tomatoes, raw cabbage, potatoes, strawberries, and canteloupe. Ascorbic acid enhances proline hydroxylation and is thereby an important cofactor for collagen synthesis and wound healing. In experimental tissue cultures, 50 to 100 μg of ascorbic acid/ml are required to achieve maximal collagen synthesis.

Vitamin C has been shown to lower intraocular pressure. The mechanism is a lowering of the serum osmolarity. The effect of this elevated serum osmolarity is short lived, because vitamin C rapidly penetrates the blood-eye barrier, reducing the ocular hypotensive effect. A maximum hypotensive effect in humans from an intravenous sodium ascorbate dosage of 1 g/kg obtained a maximum hypotensive effect within 60 to 90 minutes. The hypotensive effect lasted 6 to 8 hours. There is some evidence that ascorbate receptors may exist and participate in the hypotensive effect.[31]

Severe acid and alkali burns or mechanical injury to the eye will lower the aqueous concentration of ascorbic acid. These levels can be lowered to as little as two thirds normal.[32] Topical administration of ascorbic drops (10%) given frequently for 6 weeks significantly reduces the instance of corneal ulcers after alkali burns. Subcutaneous injections of the vitamin may also help reduce the incidence of corneal ulceration and perforation. Topical citrate (10%) has also been found to reduce the incidence of corneal ulceration (possibly more effectively than ascorbate) by reducing polymorphonuclear infiltration. Both ascorbate and citrate therapy must be initiated early in the course of a chemical burn because they have little effect once ulceration begins. The majority of the data on ascorbate and citrate treatment of chemical burns is animal data. Large-scale human studies have not been performed to date. It is interesting to note, however, that thermal burns have a poorer outcome if ascorbic acid is given.[34]

Ascorbic acid is actively metabolized by the corneal endothelium.[35] It is thought that ascorbic acid can be concentrated in various compartments within the eye theoretically to protect animal species against the damaging effects of ultraviolet radiation. Radiolabeled ascorbic acid was seen to be actively taken up by endothelial cells. Interestingly, the oxidated product dehydro-L-ascorbic acid was taken up much more rapidly than the ascorbic acid itself. The uptake was inhibited by cyanide and iodoacetamide but is unaffected by ouabain. This suggests that total ascorbic acid of the aqueous humor is in the reduced state.

Premature infants possess a 35% to 50% higher level of retinal vitamin C than that found in the mature retina. The significance of this is not known at the present time.[36]

Vitamin C can be measured in significant levels in human tears.[37] The basal level of ascorbic acid in human tears ranged from 3.9 to 23 mg/dl. Reflex tears induced by noxious stimulants, however, showed that there was a decreased level of ascorbic acid in these artificially induced tears, but even in these reflex tears the ascorbic acid content was higher than that in the blood plasma.

## VITAMIN D

Vitamin D is another vitamin produced by the body. It is essential for calcium and phosphorus metabolism. It is found in fish liver oils, fortified milk, eggs, tuna, salmon, and sunlight. Excessive dosages of vitamin D may cause pathologic calcification in many areas of the body. Conjunctival and corneal opacities (typically a band-shaped keratopathy) appear in such patients.[38] Scleral calcification has also occurred in patients with rheumatoid arthritis predisposed to scleral disease. Excessive vitamin D administration during infancy has been recognized as the cause for idiopathic hypercalcemia. Severe cases can include osteosclerosis and may result in narrowed optic foramina. Optic atrophy may be the result. Systemic abnormalities include anorexia and vomiting, mental retardation, dwarfism, craniostenosis, and renal damage with hypertension.

Vitamin D deficiency affects eye growth, resulting in refractive error. Therapeutic blood levels of calcitonin to treat vitamin D intoxication may be reached by ocular administration rather than intravenous administration.

## VITAMIN E

Vitamin E, also called tocopherol, helps prevent oxidation of polyunsaturated fatty acids in cell membranes and other body structures. It is found in whole grain cereals, lettuce, and vegetable oils. It is a fat-soluble vitamin, and the most active is α-tocopherol. Normal vitamin E levels probably protect photoreceptor membranes from oxidative damage and retard the accumulation of cellular debris within the retinal pigment epithelium. Rats on vitamin E–deficient diets show marked outer segment disruption and increase in pigment cell lipofuscin granules.[39] The question as to the use of vitamin E supplementation in premature or low birth weight infants stems from the discovery that neonates with birth weights of less than 1,500 g have serum and retinal vitamin E levels from 5% to 12% of those found in mature newborns.[40] Initial trials suggested there may be some therapeutic value in administering oral and parenteral dosages of vitamin E to newborn infants of low birth weight or prematurity. However, the weight of evidence since these early studies suggests that there is little or no benefit to administration of vitamin E in these infants. Finer et al.,[41] Puklin et al.,[42] Schaffer et al.,[43] and Phelps et al.[44] in large trials of vitamin E therapy failed to show treatment benefit.

Vitamin E deficiencies can be produced by malabsorption syndromes. The ocular signs and symptoms associated with these malabsorption syndromes include extraocular muscle palsies, hemorrhagic retinopathy, and nystagmus, which respond to vitamin E therapy. Vitamin E theoretically prevents auto-oxidative reaction induced by light within the eye, reducing the amount of oxygen free radicals produced and thus limiting retinal damage. Therefore, there are clinical trials with vitamin E in an attempt to reduce the damage to the retina produced by age-related macular degeneration. Varma[45] suggests a scientific basis for therapy of cataracts by antioxidants such as vitamin E. The theoretic value of reduction of oxygen free radicals in the prophylactic treatment of cataracts by use of vitamin E was postulated. However, its use remains controversial. Katz and Robinson[46] investigated the effect on vitamin E in the retina of light and aging. The state of light adaptation had no influence on the α-tocopherol levels in the neural retina at any of the ages examined. However, in the retinal pigment epithelium, choroid, and sclera, the α-tocopherol levels were substantially higher in light adapted than in dark adapted at all three age levels studied. The effect of light adaptation on α-tocopherol levels in retinal pigment epithelium, choroid, and sclera was most pronounced in the oldest age group.

## VITAMIN K

Vitamin K is essential for normal clot formation. It is found in leafy green vegetables such as cabbage, cauliflower, kale, and spinach. Pork liver is also a source. Vitamin K is manufactured in the human small intestine by bacteria. Deficiency states of vitamin K are relatively rare. Excessive amounts of vitamin K or its analogs will cause a prothrombin deficiency. Indiscriminate and excessive use of vitamin K in the management of bleeding problems unrelated to prothrombin deficiency is a common therapeutic error. Hemorrhage glaucoma, postoperative hyphema, and spontaneous vitreous hemorrhage rarely result from defective coagulation mechanisms, and treatment with vitamin K is not beneficial.[47] Several investigations of administration of vitamin K have been initiated to assess retinal hemorrhages in newborn infants after labor and delivery.[48, 49] Vitamin K was administered to women before delivery, and there appeared to be a decreased incidence of retinal hemorrhages in the infants after delivery.

More recently, Kleis et al.[50] published a case report of a 72-year-old woman who had been taking warfarin in whom uncontrolled bleeding from a subconjunctival hemorrhage developed. Although doses of vitamin K reduced the prothrombin time, the bleeding was not controlled until administration of fresh, frozen plasma.

## TRACE ELEMENTS

### Zinc

Recent reports in the literature of the use of oral zinc in treatment of patients with macular degeneration have generated interest in the medical and general press. A report by Newsome et al.[51] suggested a treatment benefit for patients with macular degeneration based on zinc's role in the metabolic function of enzyme systems in the chorioretinal complex. This paper and others have spurred research interest into the use of trace elements and particularly antioxidants such as vitamin E in treatment and prevention of age-related macular degeneration. Newsome et al.[52] also reported that zinc was taken up directly by the retinal pigment epithelium and choroid in primate eyes. Zinc may also play a role in the maintenance of normal tear function. A finding of low serum zinc levels in 12 of 16 patients with Leber's congenital amaurosis adds further to the body of evidence that zinc is necessary for proper maintenance of the retinal pigment epithelial photoreceptor cell complex.[53] The Long-Evans rat was used in a study to test the significance of maternal zinc deficiency on the development of the eye.[54] Fetuses from these zinc-deficient rats showed abnormalities in the development of the optic nerve and choroidal fissure with resulting colobomas and retinal folds. Some of the fetuses were anophthalmic at birth. Caution should be exercised before expensive vitamin supplementations are recommended to elderly individuals often on fixed incomes. Although there is a suggestion that the use of vitamins and trace metals that act as antioxidants may provide some treatment benefit in patients with age-related macular degeneration, there is no evidence that special combinations have any more benefit than the usual vitamin supplements, which can usually be obtained at significant savings to the patient.

## REFERENCES


1. Robison Jr WG, Kuwabarat T: Vitamin A storage and peroxomes in retinal pigment epithelium and liver, *Invest Ophthalmol Vis Sci* 16:10, 1977.
2. Hollyfield JG, Fliesler SJ, Rayborn ME, and others: Synthesis and secretion of interstitial retinol-binding protein by the human retina, *Invest Ophthalmol* VisSci 26:58, 1985.
3. Borsf F: Reversal of the complications of self-induced vitamin A deficiency, *Br J Ophthalmol* 55:210, 1971.
4. Herron Jr WL, Reigel BW: Production rate and removal of outer segment material in vitamin A deficiency, *Invest Ophthalmol* 13:36, 1974.
5. Carlier C, Mourey MS, Luzeau R, and others: Assessment of vitamin A status in an elderly French population using impression cytology with transfer, *Int J Vitam Nutr Res* 59:1337, 1989.
6. Sommer A: New imperatives for an old vitamin A, *J Nutr* 119:96, 1989.
7. Sommer A: Xerophthalmia, keratomalacia and nutritional blindness, *Int Ophthalmol* 14:195, 1990.
8. Carlier C, Moulina-Pelat JP, Ceccon JF, and others: Prevalence of malnutrition and vitamin A deficiency in the Diourbel Fatic and Kaolack regions of Senegal: an epidemiologic study, *Am J Clin Nutr* 53:70, 1991.
9. Neugebauer MA, Vernon SA, Brimlow G, and others: Nyctalopia and conjunctival xerosis indicating vitamin A deficiency in cystic fibrosi, *Eye* 3:360, 1989.
10. Lindenmuth KA, Del-monte M, Marino LR: Advanced xerophthalmia as a presenting sign in cystic fibrosis, *Ann Ophthalmol* 21:189, 1989.
11. Semba R, Wirasasmita S, Natadisastra G, and others: Response of Bitot's spots in pre-school children to vitamin A treatment, *Am J Ophthalmol*, 110:416, 1990.
12. Sommer A: Effects of vitamin A deficiency on the ocular surface, *Ophthalmology* 90:592, 1983.
13. Gilbard J, Huang A, Belldegrund R, and others: Open labeled crossover study of vitamin A ointment as a keratoconjunctivitis sicca, *Ophthalmology* 96:224, 1989.
14. Kastl P, Rosenthal W, Batlle I, and others: Topical vitamin A ointment increases healing of cataract incisions, *Ann Ophthalmol* 19:175, 1987.
15. Prutkin L: Wound healing and vitamin A acid, *Acta Dermatol* 52:489, 1972.
16. Gilbert JM, Weiss JS, Sattler AL, and others: Ocular manifestations and impression cytology of anorexia nervosa, *Ophthalmology* 97:1001, 1990.
17. Ubels JL, Edelhauser H, Austin K: Healing of experimental corneal wounds treated with topically applied retinoids, *Am J Ophthalmol* 95:353, 1983.
18. Ohashi Y, Hitoshi W, Kinoshita S, and others: Vitamin A eye drops for superior limbic keratoconjunctivitis, *Am J Ophthalmol* 105:523, 1988.
19. Palestine H: Transient acute myopia resulting from isotretinoin (accutane) therapy, *Ann Ophthalmol* 16:660, 1984.
20. Djunaedi E, Sommer A, Pandji A, and others: Impact of vitamin A supplementation on xerophthalmia: a randomized control community trial, *Arch Ophthalmol* 106:218, 1988.

21. Kim RY, Stern WH: Retinoids and butyrate modulate fibroblast growth factor and contraction of collagen matrixes, *Invest Ophthalmol Vis Sci* 31:1183, 1990.
22. Amemiyat: Vitamin A and the retina, *Eye Ear Nose Throat Mon* 50:341, 1971.
23. Law WC, Randoe RR: The molecular basis of retinoic acid induced night blindness, *Biochem Biophys Res Comun* 161:825, 1989.
24. Caffery BE, Joseph JE: Ocular side effects of Isotretonin therapy, *J Am Optom Assoc* 59:221, 1988.
25. Dreyfus DM: Blood transketolase levels in tobacco-alcohol amblyopia, *Arch Ophthalmol* 74:617, 1965.
26. Cramer J, Goodwin JA: Wernicke's encephalopathy complication of intravenous hyperalimentation, *JAMA* 238:2176, 1977.
27. Ferrari V, Baratelli E, Colombo C, and others: Wernicke's Korsakoff syndrome caused by prolonged infusion therapy during the postoperative, *Recent Prog Med* 82:672, 1991.
28. Gunby P: Vitamin $B_6$ appears to be useful in treating choroid disorder, *JAMA* 243:1792, 1980.
29. Weleber RG, Kennaway NG, Buist NR: Vitamin B and management of gyrate atrophy of choroid and retina, *Lancet* 2:1213, 1978.
30. Wilson DJ, Weleber RG, Green WR: Ocular clinicopathologic study of gyrate atrophy, *Am J Ophthalmol* 111:24, 1991.
31. Lamb KW, Lee P, Fox R: Aqueous ascorbic concentrations in hereditary buphthalmic rabbits, *Arch Ophthalmol* 94:1565, 1976.
32. Phister RR, Patterson CA, Hayes SA: Topical ascorbate decreases the instance of corneal ulceration after experimental alkali burns, *Invest Ophthalmol Vis Sci* 17:1019, 1978.
33. Pfister RR, Nicolaro ML, Paterson CR: Sodium citrate reduces the incidence of corneal ulcerations and perforations in extreme alkali burned eyes—acetylcysteine and ascorbate have no favorable effect, *Invest Ophthalmol Vis Sci* 21:486, 1981.
34. Phan TM, Zelt RP, Kenyon KR, and others: Ascorbic acid therapy in a thermal burn model of corneal ulceration in rabbits, *Am J Ophthalmol* 99:74, 1985.
35. Bode AM, Vanderpool SS, Carlson EC, and others: Ascorbic acid uptake and metabolism by the corneal endothelium, *Invest Ophthalmol Vis Sci* 32:2266, 1991.
36. Nielsen JC, Nash M, Anderson RE: Regional distribution of vitamin E and C in mature and premature human retinas, *Invest Ophthalmol Vis Sci* 29:22, 1988.
37. Patterson CA, O'Rourke MC: Vitamin C levels in human tears, *Arch Ophthalmol* 105:376, 1987.
38. Harley RD, DiGeorge AM, Mabry CC, and others: Idiopathic hypercalcemia of infancy: optic atrophy and other ocular changes, *Trans Am J Ophthalmol Otolaryngol* 69:977, 1965.
39. Robison WG, Kuwabara T, Bieri JG: Vitamin E deficiency and the retina: photoreceptor and pigment epithelial changes, *Invest Ophthalmol Vis Sci* 18:683, 1979.
40. Neal PR, Erikson D, Baenziger JC, and others: Serum vitamin E levels vary in the very low birth weight infant during oral supplementation, *Pediatrics* 77:636, 1986.
41. Finer NN, Schindler RF, Peters KL, and others: Vitamin E and retrolental fibroplasia improved visual outcome with early vitamin E, *Ophthalmology* 90:4328, 1983.
42. Puklin JE, Simon RM, Ehrenkranz RA: Influence on retrolental fibroplasia of intramuscular vitamin E administration during respiratory syndrome, *Ophthalmology* 89:96, 1982.
43. Schaffer DB, Johnson L, Quinn GE, and others: Vitamin E and retinopathy of prematurity, *Ophthalmology* 92:1005, 1985.
44. Phelps DL, Rosenbaum AL, Eisenberg SJ, and others: Tocopherol efficacy and safety in preventing retinopathy of prematurity: a randomized control double masked trial, *Pediatrics* 79:489, 1987.
45. Varma SD: Scientific basis for medical therapy of cataracts by anti-oxidants, *Am J Clin Nutr* 53:3358, 1991.
46. Katz ML, Robinson Jr WG: Light and aging effects on vitamin E in the retina and retinal pigment epithelium, *Vision Res* 27:1875, 1987.
47. Smith Jr AM, Custer RP: Toxicity of vitamin K, *JAMA* 23:173, 1960.
48. Hellman LM, Shettles LB: Factors influencing plasma prothrombin in the newborn infant, *Bull Johns Hopkins Hosp* 65:138, 1939.
49. Maumenee AE, Hellman LM, Shettles LB: Factors influencing plasma prothrombin in the newborn infant: IV. The effect of antenatal administration of vitamin K on the incidence of retinal hemorrhage in the newborn, *Bull Johns Hopkins Hosp* 68:158, 1941.
50. Kleis W, Hernandez-Denton G, Hernandez-Morales F: An unusual complication of an-

ticoagulant therapy: bloody tears, *Bol Asoc Med PR* 81:275, 1989.
51. Newsome DA, Swartz M, Leone NC, and others: Oral zinc in macular degeneration, *Arch Ophthalmol* 106:192, 1988.
52. Newsome DA, Oliver PD, Deupree DM, and others: Zinc uptake by primate retinal pigment epithelium and choroid, *Curr Eye Res* 11:213, 1992.
53. Zen GLH: Clinical findings and trace metals (zinc and copper) in Leber's congenital amaurosis, *Chung Hua Yen Ko Tsa Chih* 26:26, 1990.
54. Rogers JM, Hurley LS: Effects of zinc deficiency on morphogenesis of the fetal rat eye, *Development* 99:231, 1987.

CHAPTER **16**

# Drugs That Affect Clotting:
## Coagulants, Anticoagulants, and Thrombolytics

Thomas F. Mauger

### HEMOSTASIS

Maintenance of vascular integrity is achieved through the complex interaction of a myriad of coagulation processes (Fig. 16–1). Key elements of this system include the vascular endothelium, blood rheology, platelets, and a vast array of chemical mediators. Each element is individually important, and their effects may either be to inhibit, amplify, or curtail this explosive, cascading coagulation process. Understanding the use of various drugs to control both intravascular and perivascular clotting events can be extremely important in surgical procedures and medical treatment.

#### Vascular Endothelium

The healthy vascular endothelium is nonthrombogenic through several mechanisms. Prostaglandin $I_2$ ($PGI_2$) and lipoxygenase products, inhibitors of platelet aggregation and adhesion, respectively, are produced by the vascular endothelium. The endothelium can bind and assist in the inactivation of thrombin. Thrombin is inhibited by the endothelium through the release of two factors, thrombomodulin and heparin. Thrombomodulin is a protein surface receptor that binds thrombin, decreasing its ability to activate coagulation factors. Thrombin bound to thrombomodulin promotes the anticoagulant activity of protein C, which inhibits factors $V_a$ and $VIII_a$ and stimulates the release of plasminogen activator. Protein C, a vitamin K–dependent protein, is such an important factor that congenital absence is associated with disseminated clotting and death.[1] Heparin sulfate on the endothelial surface potentiates thrombin inactivation by circulating antithrombin III (ATIII). In addition to thrombomodulin and heparin sulfate, the vascular endothelium elaborates plasminogen activators that promote fibrinolysis.

Vascular endothelial damage may occur by direct physical injury, immune complexes, infectious agents, proteolytic enzymes released during inflammation, hemodynamic stress, and atherosclerosis. This damage leads to platelet adherence. Contact activation of the coagulation system occurs when blood elements come in contact with the vascular endothelium. Proenzyme factor XII is converted to enzyme factor $XII_a$ through this contact mechanism. This intrinsic pathway is largely calcium dependent, with the exception of the interaction of thrombin and fibrinogen.

#### Platelets

Platelet adherence to normal uninjured vascular endothelium is physically inhibited because both are negatively charged. $PGI_2$ produced by stimulated endothelial cells will also prevent platelet

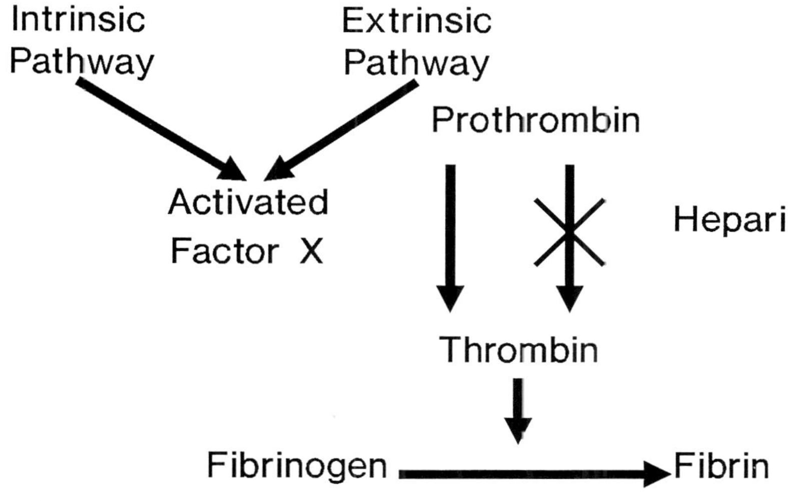


**FIG 16–1.**
Overview of coagulation.

aggregation. Platelets eagerly adhere to specific amino acid sequences in the collagenase components of the subendothelial matrix exposed by endothelial loss or injury. Turbulent flow, such as produced in an ulcerated carotid artery plaque, promotes platelet adherence. Plasma proteins such as von Willebrand's factor may be a necessary connection between the platelets and the subendothelium. Platelet aggregation will rapidly occur unless inhibited by other factors ($PGI_2$). Thrombin, adenosine diphosphate (ADP), epinephrine, collagen, and arachidonic acid potentiate platelet aggregation. Many of these processes are calcium dependent and operate via receptors on the platelet surface. Fibrinogen bound to platelet surface receptors is also necessary for platelet aggregation.

Platelets accelerate the generation of thrombin by catalyzing the interactions of coagulation factors. A number of coagulation reactions occur directly on the platelet surface at specific receptor and binding sites through calcium-dependent processes.

### Fibrinolytic System

The fibrinolytic system consists of a plasma and a cellular component. The plasma component involves the conversion of a β-globulin plasminogen to the active enzyme plasmin mediated by plasminogen activators. Plasmin hydrolyzes fibrin and fibrinogen. Inhibitors modulate the fibrinolytic system by affecting the activation of plasminogen and plasmin. Plasminogen is bound to fibrin in the developing thrombus. Tissue plasminogen activator (tPA) binds to fibrin and is activated thereafter, being produced from adjacent vascular endothelium. Plasmin is inactivated by $\alpha_2$-antiplasmin and other inhibitors, including $\alpha_2$-macroglobulin. It is necessary to overwhelm these inhibitors to achieve adequate thrombolytic therapy (Fig. 16–2).

The cellular component is composed of proteolytic enzymes with fibrinolytic activity produced by leukocytes attracted by the chemotactic products of platelets.

Intraplatelet granules, containing ADP among other mediators, may be released as a result of this stimulation and lead to further platelet activation. Surface receptors for plasma clotting factors occur during platelet activation. Cyclic adenosine monophosphate (cAMP) is increased in the presence of $PGD_2$ in platelets and $PGI_2$ in endothelial cells. cAMP inhibits platelet aggregation, secretion, and surface adhesion and is the most important regulator of platelet function.

The reader will recognize that platelet function is as important as platelet numbers. This explains the clinical improvement in idiopathic thrombocytopenia with systemic corticosteroids before an increase in the platelet count.

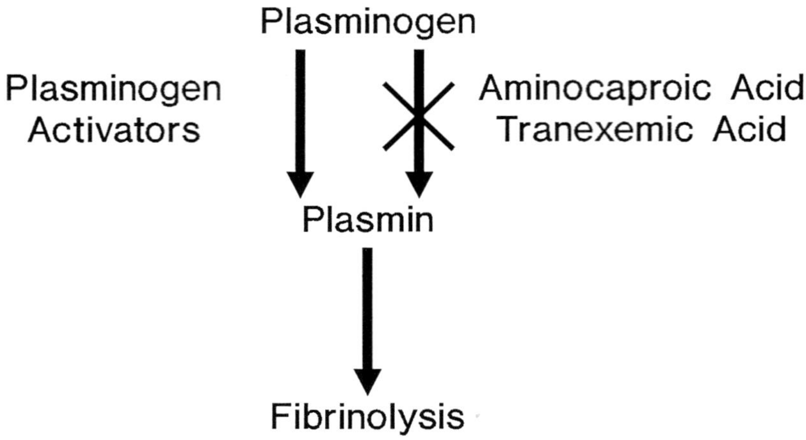


**FIG 16–2.**
Overview of fibrinolysis.

## GOAL OF THERAPY

Prevention of uncontrolled intravascular clotting is obviously the single best therapy. Controlling diet, tobacco use, and hypertension will decrease endothelial damage. Early mobilization of patients after surgery and pneumatic stockings to physically pump venous blood in the lower extremities of bedridden patients have been shown to reduce stasis of blood and prevent clotting.

Anticoagulant therapy (heparin, warfarin, aspirin) will prevent the formation of thrombi and the extension of previously formed thrombi. Thrombolytic therapy involves the acceleration of thrombolysis. Thrombolytic agents include urokinase, streptokinase, and tPAs. Systemic thrombolytic therapy is more dangerous and expensive than anticoagulant therapy and is thus reserved for life-threatening situations such as acute coronary artery thrombosis.

## HEPARIN

Heparin acts through binding to ATIII (heparin cofactor), changing the structure of the molecule. Heparin catalyzes the irreversible complexing of ATIII with thrombin and factor $X_a$, greatly accelerating their neutralization.[2, 3] Heparin has also been found to accelerate the in vitro inactivation of antithrombin by neutrophil elastase, which could equate to localized thrombogenesis on the vascular endothelium.[4] Coagulation factors IX, XI, and XII and plasmin are also neutralized by ATIII in the presence of heparin. Low doses of heparin catalyze the neutralization of mainly factor $X_a$ but not thrombin. Full-dose heparin therapy neutralizes thrombin and inhibits activation of fibrin-stabilizing factor. Anticoagulant activity is immediate on intravenous administration of heparin. There is a 20- to 60-minute delay in action after subcutaneous injection. Heparin is a heterogeneous anionic sulfated glycosaminoglycan, which is an integral component of the vascular endothelial cell wall and is present in most cells. It is prepared from porcine intestinal mucosa or bovine lung tissue. Intravenous heparin is the initial treatment of choice for most cases of deep venous thrombosis and pulmonary embolus. In deep venous thrombosis, heparin may be given as continuous intravenous, intermittent intravenous, or subcutaneous at the dose of approximately 30,000 units daily. Intramuscular injection is not recommended because of the high incidence of hematomas. It is not absorbed through the gastrointestinal tract. Subcutaneous heparin may be used as prophylaxis (5,000 units every 8–12 hours) against deep venous thrombosis in predisposed patients. A bolus dose of 10,000 to 20,000 units may be used with pulmonary embolus to prevent further platelet aggregation to the embolus. After full-dose therapy is achieved, follow-up anticoagulation is usually continued with a coumarin derivative.

The clotting times, activated coagulation time, and partial thromboplastin time all have been recommended to monitor heparin's effect. These values should be maintained between 1.5 to 2.5 times normal baseline. A considerable range of heparin's sensitivity exists in the population, making laboratory monitoring critical to prevent gross underdosing or overdosing.[5]

Of 2,656 heparin-treated patients, 9.1% had a bleeding episode during the first week of full-dose treatment. Of these 238 hemorrhages, 35 were severe. The risk of bleeding is, of course, cumulative with the duration of therapy and reached 12.8% at 10 days of treatment and 19.5% after 20 days. Heavy drinkers of alcohol had a sevenfold increased risk of bleeding. Simultaneous use of aspirin increased the risk of bleeding by 2½ times. Patients more than 60 years old bled three times more often than those less than age 40 years. Heparin is a major cause of drug-attributable death in otherwise reasonably healthy patients.

Hemorrhage occurred in 12% of 134 patients monitored with activated clotting times during heparin therapy. Hemorrhages occurred in half of the 10.5% of patients whose activated clotting times rose above the targeted range. All episodes of major bleeding, requiring either transfusion or cessation of heparin, occurred in this group. Hemorrhage occurs less frequently with low-dose heparin therapy.

### Intraocular Heparin

Heparin has been found to reduce postoperative intraocular fibrin response in rabbits. Heparin added to the vitrectomy infusion (5–10 IU/ml), as well as intravenous and anterior chamber heparin, caused fibrin clearing in 20% to 40% of the time necessary in control eyes. Subcutaneous heparin started at the time of surgery did not alter fibrin clearing. The addition of subcutaneous heparin did not cause significant change in the bleeding time after cutting a retinal vessel.[8–10]

Heparin has other important biologic effects. Among these are the inhibition of cellular contractility and proliferation, as well as collagen polymerization. The combined actions on the coagulation and wound healing pathways serve to minimize fibrin clot formation when heparin is infused during vitrectomy.[11]

### Antidotes

The neutralization of heparin is accomplished by the administration of protamine sulfate. It is a simple, low molecular weight, cationic protein prepared from the sperm of some fish. Vasectomized men have been reported to have IgG antibodies to protamine, putting them at risk for hypersensitivity reactions. Negatively charged heparin combines with positively charged protamine in a 1:1 ratio. The resulting complex has no activity. An in vitro protamine titration will determine the proper amount of protamine to be administered. Protamine sulfate is injected in a 1% solution over a period of a few minutes. It has a rapid onset of action, usually within 5 minutes. The dose should not exceed 50 mg every 2 to 4 hours because protamine itself is a thromboplastin antagonist preventing the conversion of prothrombin to thrombin. Hexaclimethrine is an alternative intravenous preparation. Hypotension, dizziness, and generalized discomfort occur if it is given too rapidly. Tolonium chloride is an oral antiheparin medication. It has a slower onset of action; therefore, it has limited clinical usefulness.

## COUMARIN AND INDANEDIONE DERIVATIVES

Coumarin anticoagulants act by depressing synthesis in the liver of factors II, IV, V, IX, and X by interfacing with the actions of vitamin K. Coumarin derivatives include warfarin and dicumarol. Anisindione is an indanedione derivative. Coumarin, like heparin, acts to prevent new thrombosis and limit extension of existing thrombosis. Coumarin will not lyse established thrombi.

The action of coumarin and indanedione derivatives is dose dependent. Many drugs or disease states may potentiate or inhibit the effects of warfarin. Aspirin and acetaminophen are two common drugs that can potentiate the action of warfarin, leading to unwanted bleeding.[12] Coumarin and indanedione derivatives' resistance may occur with familial deficiency of ATIII, inadvertent ingestion of vitamin K, or drug interaction, such as with alcohol ingestion. Minor hemorrhagic episodes occur in 2% to 10% of patients receiving these drugs. These usually involve the gastrointestinal or genitourinary tract. Spontaneous subconjunctival hemorrhage and hyphema may occur secondary to coumarin and indanedione derivative treatment.[13] These drugs may complicate age-related macular degeneration, causing massive subretinal or vitreous hemorrhage. A total of 19% to 27% of hemorrhages occurring in patients with age-related macular degeneration are associated with the use of anticoagulants. Patients with known disciform scars or subretinal neovascular membranes who are concurrently on anticoagulant therapy should consider discontinuing anticoagulant use if it is not medically contraindicated, or the subretinal lesion should be treated to prevent further hemorrhage.[14]

Coumarin and indanedione derivatives are sufficiently similar chemically to vitamin K to compete with it in the enzyme structure responsible for prothrombin synthesis. Dysfunctional factors II, VII, IX, and X are formed. This effect is reversible and can be overcome by providing an excess of vitamin K. Coumarin and indanedione derivatives have no anticoagulant effects in vitro.

Because of the time required for disappearance of existing prothrombin supplies or for synthesis of new prothrombin, the response to these drugs or to their antidotes is much slower than the heparin anticoagulant effect. One to 3 days must elapse before effective anticoagulant levels are reached. The dosage is governed by prothrombin time determinations with the intent of maintaining prothrombin activity at about 30% to 50% of normal. Considerable individual variation exists as to drug response; therefore, close laboratory control is essential. Coumarin and indanedione derivatives affect factors involved in both the intrinsic and extrinsic coagulation systems, therefore affecting both the prothrombin time (extrinsic system) and the activated partial thromboplastin time (intrinsic system). Patients with liver and kidney disease are particularly likely to be sensitive to these anticoagulants. The vitamin K antagonist embryopathy syndrome affects 15% to 25% of infants exposed to anticoagulants during gestation. This syndrome includes optic atrophy, mental retardation, faulty epiphyseal development affecting facial and extremity growth, hemorrhage, and death. Anticoagulant therapy is hazardous to the infant at any time during pregnancy.[15]

Ocular surgery on patients taking coumarin and indanedione derivatives is an area of great concern to the ophthalmic surgeon. Bleeding complications may involve orbital, eyelid, incisional areas, anterior chamber, iris, vitreous, retina, and choroid. Most of these bleeding episodes are minor and clear spontaneously with no effect on final visual acuity. Bleeding complications occur even when anticoagulants are discontinued before surgery and the prothrombin time is found to be normal. This is because of the relatively short half-life of factor VII (6 hours) compared with the much longer half-life of factor II (60 hours). Prothrombin time is much more sensitive to factor VII and can, therefore, be normal while factor II levels may still be low. Factor II measurement would be a more accurate way of evaluating the patient on warfarin, dicumarol, or anisindione therapy before surgery, but this measurement is not widely available. Life-threatening thrombotic complications may occur when anticoagulants are discontinued even for a short time. Communication with the physician managing the anticoagulation therapy is necessary to determine whether discontinuation is possible. Meticulous attention to incision hemostasis and size, as well as minimizing the manipulation of vascular tissue, is helpful in preventing unwanted bleeding during ophthalmic surgery on patients who are taking anticoagulants.[16, 17]

If serious hemorrhage should occur, any vitamin K antagonist should be discontinued immediately. Vitamin K (phytonadione) should be given orally in a dosage of 5 to 25 mg. In emergencies, this may be given as an intravenous infusion, diluted in normal saline solution or 5% dextrose, at a rate not to exceed 1 mg/min. Acute vascular collapse or anaphylactic reactions may occur in response to intravenous dosage, which must be given slowly and cautiously. Phytonadione does not reverse the anticoagulant effect of heparin, which should be inhibited with protamine. Because formation of sufficient prothrombin to arrest bleeding may take 6 hours or more, plasma or blood transfusion is necessary to stop severe bleeding promptly.

Excessive dosage of vitamin K will restore prothrombin time to normal and will make the patient temporarily refractory to antiprothrombin drugs. If the thrombotic condition under treatment still persists, large doses of vitamin K will again create the hazard of intravascular clotting that existed before anticoagulant therapy. Hence, if the patient has an unduly low prothrombin time but is not bleeding, only small doses (5–15 mg) of vitamin K should be given.[5]

## ASPIRIN

Aspirin is unique among salicylates in its ability to inhibit platelet aggregation induced by epinephrine or low concentrations of collagen. It does not inhibit platelet aggregation induced by thrombin or high concentrations of collagen. Aspirin prevents the release of ADP and platelet factor IV from platelets. Aspirin inactivates cyclooxygenase in circulating platelets and megakaryocytes. Cyclooxygenase is not regenerated in circulating platelets; therefore, the platelet dysfunction persisted for their total life span (4–7 days). Usually hemostasis returns to normal when 20% of the platelets have been replaced (1½ days). Other nonsteroidal antiinflammatory agents (e.g., ibuprofen, indomethacin, and naproxen) can inhibit platelet aggregation through their effects on prostaglandin synthesis.

Frequent use of nonsteroidal antiinflammatory agents (NSAIDs), particularly aspirin, may lead to unwanted bleeding during and after ocular surgery. Platelets have a turnover rate of 10% per day; therefore, low-dose aspirin should be discontinued 2 to 3 days before surgery, if possible. High doses of aspirin and other NSAIDs should be stopped 2 weeks before surgery, if possible. Macular hemorrhage associated with age-related macular degeneration and aspirin use has been reported anecdotally. The macular photocoagulation study showed no significant increase in hemorrhage or recurrence after laser treatment of age-related macular degeneration with subretinal neovascular membranes in patients using aspirin.[5, 18–21]

## THROMBOLYTIC AGENTS

Thrombolytic agents are a group of compounds that convert plasminogen into plasmin (see Fig. 16-2). Plasmin, in turn, degrades fibrin, fibrinogen, and factors V, VIII, and XII. This occurs through the hydrolysis of the arginine$^{560}$-valine$^{561}$ peptide bond in plasminogen. Plasminogen activators of interest to ophthalmologists are streptokinase (sPA), urokinase (uPA), and tPA. Fibrinolysis using plasminogen activators has been an area of active investigation in both cardiovascular and ophthalmic medicine. Plasminogen activators have been used systemically to treat coronary artery occlusion, arterial thrombosis, and pulmonary embolus.[22] Toxicity caused by solution impurities hindered the initial intraocular use of plasminogen activators. Improved purification, including human recombinant techniques, have allowed these powerful compounds to play a major role in postsurgical intraocular fibrinolysis.

## STREPTOKINASE

sPA is a natural product of the group C β-hemolytic streptococci. It is a nonenzymatic protein that complexes with plasminogen, subsequently converting free plasminogen to plasmin. Unlike tPA, it is independent of fibrin. When used systemically, this increases the risk of unwanted bleeding because of the uncontrolled degradation of fibrinogen. Circulating anti-streptococcal antibodies are often found because of the ubiquitous presence of group C β-hemolytic streptococci. sPA is strongly antigenic, and repeat dosing will elicit antibodies to the drug. These antibodies will partially inactivate sPA and must be saturated before achieving therapeutic effect. Systemic immunologic responses, including fever and rarely anaphylaxis, may occur after administration of sPA. Treatment of coronary artery thrombus with sPA should be instituted within 1 hour of onset of symptoms with an intravenous dose of 1.5 million IU over 60 minutes. Intracoronary sPA is given as a bolus at 10,000 to 30,000 IU.[23–25]

Ocular bleeding associated with systemic sPA has been reported and includes hyphema, subconjunctival, and choroidal hemorrhages. Severe intraocular hemorrhage was usually associated with a preexisting ocular condition such as retinal telangiectasia or recent surgery.[26]

Initial investigation on the use of sPA to clear anterior chamber and subconjunctival hemorrhage showed significant toxicity, including corneal endothelial damage and localized inflammation. These toxic reactions were the result of impurities and contaminants. Highly purified streptokinase has recently been used successfully to clear intraocular fibrin associated with vitrectomy. A single intraocular injection of 1,000 IU of sPA in 0.1 ml of solution clears fibrin clinically in 4 hours. Higher doses may be associated with ocular toxicity, including cataract formation, increased intraocular pressure, inflammation, corneal abnormalities, vitreous haze, and retinal degeneration. sPA may be particularly valuable intraocularly because the depletion of fibrinogen associated with its use may actually prevent the formation of fibrin. Increased systemic bleeding does not appear to be a factor when sPA is used intraocularly.

Urokinase is isolated from human kidney tissue cultures and is therefore much less antigenic than sPA both systemically and intraocularly and at much greater exposure levels. Fourteen patients with acute central retinal artery occlusion were treated with uPA (11 patients) or tPA (3 patients) through a microcatheter directly in the ophthalmic artery. A dose of 500,000 to 1 million IU of uPA or 30 mg of tPA was given over 90 minutes. Three patients given uPA had dramatic improvement in vision to 20/40 or better. Five other patients receiving uPA or tPA experienced significant visual improvement. No significant morbidity was found. Prognosis was poor with visual loss longer than 6 hours or if macular arterioles were still occluded after uPA or tPA administration. Initial vision of worse than hand motions at 1 m and massive retinal edema were also found to be signs of a poor prognosis with treatment.[27]

### Tissue Plasminogen Activators

A serine protease, tPA enzymatically converts the zymogen plasminogen to the fibrinolytic enzyme plasmin on the surface of the clot. Unlike sPA, this process is optimized by the binding of tPA to fibrin. This clot-specific process provides a negative feedback loop diminishing the possibility of unwanted bleeding through uncontrolled fibrinogenolysis. In high doses tPA may consume the plasmin inactivator $\alpha_2$-antiplasmin, leading to a severe fibrinolytic state. Intravascular tPA has been used successfully to treat coronary and pulmonary artery occlusions. Human recombinant technology allows the creation of highly purified tPA of low antigenicity in either single stranded (altepase) or double stranded (duteplase) form. Intravenous altepase may lyse acute retinal artery occlusion.

A study of 41,299 patients was conducted in the United Kingdom comparing the effects of sPA, tPA, and anisoylated plasminogen streptokinase activator complex (APSAC) in the treatment of acute myocardial infarction. tPA (a human protein) produced less fever and allergic symptoms than sPA or APSAC. APSAC and tPA lysed coronary artery clots more rapidly than sPA. All agents had similar mortality and reinfarction rates.[28]

Arterial thrombi were created in the retina of spontaneously hypertensive, stroke-prone rats by direct photocoagulation. The thrombus was lysed in four of six animals given 1 mg of intravenous recombinant tPA/kg while in the control eyes the arteries were still occluded 1 hour after intravenous injection with saline solution.[29] Intravenous recombinant tPA infusion may be considered for the rare patient who has a fresh retinal artery occlusion before irreversible retinal damage occurs.

Plasminogen activator is found naturally in human aqueous humor. This is an important factor in the resolution and recurrence of hyphema.[30] The plasminogen activator/plasminogen activator inhibitor/plasmin system is locally disrupted in the tears and at the corneal surface during various diseases and after surgeries. A corneal alkali burn is associated with the conversion of plasminogen activator from a latent to an active form in cultured corneal epithelial cells. These changes stimulate secretion of latent collagenase from cultured fibroblasts. Latent collagenase may be activated by plasmin. Alkali corneal ulceration and melting result from activation of these proteolytic enzymes.[31]

Recombinant human tPAs (altepase) are used in the treatment of anterior chamber or vitreous fibrin and in hyphema and subretinal hemorrhage. Intraocular fibrin deposition is a serious complication of complex anterior and posterior segment surgery or trauma. It can lead to the failure of glaucoma-filtering surgery, synechiae, increased intraocular pressure, cyclitic membranes, and proliferative vitreoretinopathy. Intracameral injection of tPA after penetrating keratoplasty, anterior segment reconstruction, or glaucoma-filtering surgery may result in rapid clearing of the fibrin. Minimal ocular toxicity is found after a single 25 μg dose.[32–36]

Subconjunctival hemorrhage may occur after glaucoma-filtering surgery, particularly with concomitant use of subconjunctival 5-fluorouracil. Plasminogen activator may be given subconjunctivally in a dose of 25 mg to lyse the clot and restore filtration in selective cases. Similarly, intracameral recombinant tPA may be used to lyse clots obstructing the internal filtration site.[37]

Vitrectomized diabetic eyes are particularly susceptible to fibrin formation because of the associated hypercoagulable state and dysfunctional fibrinolytic system.[38] Proliferative vitreoretinopathy and endophthalmitis also represent situations in which recombinant tPA may be used in reducing postvitrectomy fibrin. Intravitreal injection of 2.5 to 25 μg of tPA in rabbit eyes with experimentally induced fibrin formation through injection of citrated plasma showed rapid clearing (< 6 hours) of fibrin with no evidence of ocular toxicity in the electroretinogram, histopathology, or slit-lamp examination.[39] Fibrin reaction produced through vitrectomy and cyclocryotherapy showed no evidence of fibrin clearing compared with controls 3 to 4 hours after injection of 25,000 to 100,000 IU (50–200 μg) of tPA intravitreally. Significant clearing occurred in all treatment groups 24 hours after injection. No evidence of toxicity was found histologically with these larger doses.[40]

Intraocular injection of 25 μg of recombinant tPA has been reported to alleviate fibrin-induced pupillary block after vitrectomy in aphakic eyes. Lysis of the fibrin pupillary membrane occurred within 4 hours after anterior chamber or intravitreal injection of recombinant tPA. Intraocular pressure was 8 to 39 mm Hg less than it was 3 days after injection. Repeat injection was necessary in one of the seven treated patients because of recurrence of the fibrin pupillary block. No short-term complications were found.[36]

Intracameral and intravitreal tPA is extremely effective in lysing postvitrectomy fibrin formation in humans. Fibrin clears rapidly within 6 hours after injection of 25 μg of tPA. Anterior chamber hemorrhage complicated tPA injection in two of 23 eyes in one study. All of these eyes had preexisting severe rubeosis, which predisposed them to bleeding.

Although tPA is effective in lysing the massive fibrin deposition found in some diabetic eyes after vitrectomy, it does not prevent recurrent fibrin accumulation. The use of 25 μg of recombinant tPA cleared pupillary and vitreous membranes in seven diabetic eyes after vitrectomy. Five of six traction retinal detachments resolved; however, all but one redetached. Most eyes in this study had severe ischemic diabetic retinopathy with rubeosis. The vascular endothelium and blood-eye barrier were undoubtedly damaged, leading to ongoing fibrin deposition after initial clearing by recombinant tPA.[40–42]

Hyphemas created by injection of whole blood clear rapidly with only 1,800 IU (2.5 μg) of intraocular tPA. Total hyphemas showed 80% clearing within 24 hours and complete clearance in 6 days. Control eyes did not completely clear until 2 weeks after injection. Experimentally created traumatic hyphemas (disruption of iris vessels with the neodymium-YAG laser) cleared much more slowly than those created by injection of blood. A modest increase in clearing rate was found with traumatic hyphemas treated with 1,800 IU of recombinant tPA. Higher doses of recombinant tPA (5,000 and 10,000 IU) resulted in recurrent bleeding (20 and 83.3% respectively).[43, 44]

Intravitreal recombinant tPA (50,000 IU) only modestly cleared passively created vitreous hemorrhage in rabbits. The effect on visibility of retinal detail by single or sequential recombinant tPA injection was insignificant clinically. An increased incidence of traction retinal detachment was found with recombinant tPA used to clear this vitreous hemorrhage. More than half (52%) of tPA-treated eyes experienced retinal detachments compared with only 21% of the control eyes. The authors postulate that the release of free fibrin produced by the recombinant tPA causes morphologic changes in the retinal pigment epithelial cells, leading to traction retinal detachment.[39]

Subretinal hemorrhage secondary to chorioretinal disease or surgery can lead to overlying retinal degeneration within 1 day. Autologous blood was injected subretinally in the rabbit eyes to evaluate the role of tPA. Subretinal injection of either 2.5 or 25 μg of recombinant tPA accelerated clearing of the subretinal hemorrhage.[45, 46] Overlying retinal degeneration was not prevented by the recombinant tPA alone, however. Dilution of the subretinal blood with either 0.1 ml of recombinant tPA (25 μg) or balanced salt solution decreased the secondary retinal degeneration. Clot lysis, combined with dilution or drainage, may be necessary to prevent or reduce retinal degeneration associated with subretinal hemorrhage.

## THROMBIN

Intravitreal thrombin may be used to control intraocular hemorrhage during vitrectomy. The addition of thrombin (100 units/ml) to the vitrectomy infusate will significantly shorten intraocular bleeding time.[47] A significant inflammatory response occurred in 20% of the patients given intravitreal thrombin. This may be caused by impurities in the thrombin solution, which could be minimized using solution produced by DNA recombinant techniques. Minimizing the amount of thrombin instilled will decrease the postoperative inflammation. This may be accomplished by infusing thrombin through an intraocular instrument at the site of bleeding only when the bleeding is encountered and limited to the time necessary to control the bleeding with cautery. Irrigation of all thrombin from the eye is also essential.[48] Thrombin causes significant ultrastructural corneal endothelial changes when human corneas are profused with 1,000 units of thrombin/ml. Delays in deswelling times occurred with profusion of 100 units of thrombin/ml in human corneas. These effects may result from the secondary hyperosmolarity, impurities, or preservatives found in the thrombin solution. Sheep corneal endothelium exposed to thrombin of 100 and 1,000 units/ml were more resistant than human corneas, showing no morphologic changes with specular microscopy after 6 hours.[49–51]

Thrombin is a useful adjunct to maintain hemostasis during complicated intraocular surgery. However, significant corneal endothelial toxicity and intraocular inflammation is possible with long periods of perfusion. This may, in part, be minimized with the use of purified formulations that are isotonically balanced for intraocular use. Intraocular thrombin use does not preclude the postoperative use of fibrinolytic agents; however, the chance of unwanted hemorrhage may be high if there is a history of active bleeding during surgery.

## ANTIFIBRINOLYTIC AGENTS

Antifibrinolytic agents, such as ϵ-aminocaproic acid and tranexamic acid, inhibit the activation of plasminogen by plasminogen activators. The action of plasmin is also inhibited. They may be used systemically in cases of hemorrhage secondary to excessive fibrinolysis.

Antifibrinolytic agents are used systemically in ophthalmic practice to prevent recurrent hyphema.[52, 53] Tranexamic acid and ϵ-aminocaproic acid are examples of this group of drugs. Both of these agents affect fibrinolysis through inhibition of plasminogen activators. They are contraindicated in the presence of active intravascular clotting. Unwanted thrombosis are among its side effects. Retinal artery occlusion has been associated with systemic tranexamic acid use.[54] Tranexamic acid is ten times more potent in vitro than ϵ-aminocaproic acid. ϵ-Aminocaproic acid has a higher rate of gastrointestinal side effects than tranexamic acid.

### Hyphema

Traumatic hyphema is a common ophthalmic problem occurring in 0.017% of children per year. Recurrent hemorrhage occurs in 0.4% to 38.9%. Recurrent hyphema most commonly occurs 2 to 6 days after the original hemorrhage. The recurrent hyphema may be of greater severity than the original hyphema. Secondary hemorrhage is associated with a poorer visual prognosis than after a single bleed.[55] Rebleeds occur more frequently after large initial hyphemas but may occur even after a microhyphema. Recurrent hyphema has been associated with aspirin use.[56, 57] Cycloplegia and ocular patching do not diminish the frequency of recurrent hyphema. Oral ϵ-aminocaproic acid and prednisone have been shown to decrease the rate of rebleeding after traumatic hyphema in several randomized studies. One study found identical rebleed rates with either ϵ-aminocaproic acid or prednisone use. ϵ-Aminocaproic acid is used in a dosage of 50 to 100 mg/kg every 4 hours up to 30 g daily. Adverse reactions to ϵ-aminocaproic acid include nausea, vomiting, muscle cramps, conjunctival suffusion, nasal stuffiness, headache, rash, pruritus, dyspnea, tonic toxic confusional states, cardiac arrhythmias, and systemic hypotension. Gastrointestinal side effects are similar with either 50 or 100 mg/kg dosing.[58] Dizziness and hypotension were less common when the lower dosage was used. Therapeutic blood levels of ϵ-aminocaproic acid were achieved with either the 50 or 100 mg/kg regimens. ϵ-Aminocaproic acid inhibits the conversion of plasminogen to plasmin, delaying clot resolution. After discontinuation of ϵ-aminocaproic acid, clots may then dissolve rapidly. Intraocular pressure elevations have been found after discontinuation of systemic antifibrinolytic medications (e.g., ϵ-aminocaproic acid) used for traumatic hyphema.[59] This is most likely the result of obstruction of a trabecular meshwork by free red blood cells and fibrin during the rapid clot lysis found after discontinuation of the drug. The drugs should be continued for a full 5 to 6 days to achieve maximal clinical effectiveness. ϵ-Aminocaproic acid reduces the rebleed rate from 0 to 7%.

Therapeutic aqueous levels are found in animals after the topical application of ϵ-aminocaproic acid.[60] Topical solutions (600–735 g of ϵ-aminocaproic acid/L) prepared with polyvinyl alcohol and carboxypolymethylene produce aqueous levels comparable with that found after intravenous injection. Plasma levels were only 5% to 33% that of intravenous injection. Topical aminocaproic acid may be an attractive alternative to systemic delivery in the treatment of traumatic hyphema. Optimal topical concentration to maximize aqueous levels and minimize corneal epithelial toxicity is 30% ϵ-aminocaproic acid in 2% carboxypolymethylene.[61]

Tranexamic acid is another antifibrinolytic agent that reduces the incidence of rebleeding after traumatic hyphema. A retrospective analysis of 340 children with traumatic hyphema shows an improvement in rebleeding rate from 9.6% to 0.8% with the use of 25 mg of tranexamic acid/kg three times daily for 3 to 5 days. No incidents of gastrointestinal side effects were reported.[62]

Oral prednisone has been found to reduce the rebleed rate after traumatic hyphema to 7% to 13%. Fifty-six patients receiving oral prednisone for 5 days were compared with an equal number of those receiving oral ϵ-aminocaproic acid. There were no statistically significant differences in the groups when intraocular pressure

**TABLE 16–1.**
Uses and Dose of Drugs That Affect Coagulation

| Medications | Potential Ocular Uses | Dose |
|---|---|---|
| Heparin | Prevention of postoperative fibrin | 5–10 IU/ml vitreous infusion |
| Streptokinase | Dissolution of intraocular fibrin | 1,000 IU intraocular injection |
| Tissue plasminogen activator | Dissolution of intraocular fibrin, hyphema, vitreous hemorrhage, Subretinal hemorrhage | 2.5–100 μg intraocular injection |
| Thrombin | Control of intraocular bleeding | 100 units/ml vitreous infusion |
| ϵ-Aminocaproic acid | Prevent rebleeding after traumatic hyphema | 50–100 mg/kg orally q4h |
| Tranexamic acid | Prevent rebleeding after traumatic hyphema | 25 mg/kg orally 3 times daily |

and rebleed rates (7.1%) were compared. The prednisone group showed quicker clearance of hyphema (3.5 vs. 4.5 days), but this was not statistically significant.[63] Topical corticosteroids and ϵ-aminocaproic acid have not been compared prospectively with oral prednisone or ϵ-aminocaproic acid to determine if they may either singly or in combination reduce the rate of rebleeds comparable with that found with systemic delivery.

Hyphema associated with sickle cell anemia, trait, sickle-thal, or sickle-C is a special case deserving particular attention. Delay in clearing is common because of poor passage of the sickle cells through the trabecular meshwork. Control of intraocular pressure is important because of concurrent poor optic nerve perfusion. Drugs that may decrease aqueous or plasma pH (carbonic anhydrase inhibitors) or decrease aqueous oxygen pressure (epinephrine) should be avoided because of the possibility of increased sickling. Consideration should be given to early hemorrhage evacuation if intraocular pressure is elevated.

## CHONDROITIN SULFATE

Viscoelastic agents such as sodium hyaluronate and sodium chondroitin sulfate have been widely used during intraocular surgery to protect tissue and create and maintain spaces. They may be used to mechanically stop bleeding. Chondroitin sulfate has been found to inhibit clotting via heparin-like antithrombin action. Use of this viscoelastic to mechanically block hemorrhage may have an unintentional antithrombin effect on local hemostasis. Hyaluronate did not manifest an increase in clotting time and may, therefore, be the best choice of viscoelastic if significant intraocular hemorrhage is expected.[64]

## SUMMARY

The pharmacologic modification of the clotting system is one of the most rapidly developing areas in ophthalmology. Intraocular anticoagulants and thrombolyic agents are used to prevent or clear induced fibrin formation when its presence threatens the integrity of ocular tissues or the success of clotting is of benefit such as the use of intraoperative infusion of thrombin during vitreous surgery to control unwanted retinal hemorrhage. Plasminogen activators can be used to clear intraocular or subretinal hemorrhages or clots. Oral or topical antifibrinolytic therapy with or without systemic corticosteroids may be important in preventing recurrent hemorrhaging in patients with hyphemas. It is clear that the appropriate use of these agents to manipulate and control the coagulation process can improve the success rate in virtually all areas of ophthalmic therapy (Table 16–1).

## REFERENCES

1. Rick ME: Protein C and protein S: Vitamin K-dependent inhibitors of blood coagulation, *JAMA* 263:701, 1990.
2. Fareed J, Walenga JM, Williamson K, and others: Studies on the antithrombotic effects and pharmacokinetics of heparin frac-

tions and fragments, *Semin Thromb Hemost* 11:56, 1985.

3. Fareed J: Heparin: its fractions, fragments, and derivatives, *Semin Thromb Hemost* 11:1, 1985.
4. Jordan RE, Kilpatrick J, Nelson RM: Heparin promotes the inactivation of antithrombin by neutrophil elastase, *Science* 237:777, 1977.
5. Coagulants and anticoagulants. In McEvoy EK, editor: *American Hospital Formulary Service drug information 92,* Bethesda, MD, 1992, ASMP.
6. Walker AM, Jick M: Predictors of bleeding during heparin therapy, *JAMA* 244:1209, 1980.
7. Mattersley PG, Mitsuoka C, King JM: Heparin therapy for thromboembolic disorders, *JAMA* 250:1413, 1983.
8. Johnson RN, Balyeat E, Stern WM: Heparin prophylaxis for intraocular fibrin, *Ophthalmology* 94:597, 1987.
9. Johnson RN, Blankenship G: A prospective, randomized, clinical trial of heparin therapy for postoperative intraocular fibrin, *Ophthalmology* 95:312, 1988.
10. Iverson DA, Katsura M, Hartzer MK, and others: Inhibition of intraocular fibrin formation following infusion of low-molecular-weight heparin during vitrectomy, *Arch Ophthalmol* 109:405, 1991.
11. Blumenkranz MS, Hartzer MK: The mechanism of action of drugs for the treatment of vitreoretinal scarring. In Ryan SJ, editor-in chief: *The retina: surgical retina,* vol 3, St Louis, 1989, Mosby, p 408.
12. Bartle WR, Blakely JA: Potent action of warfarin anticoagulation by acetaminophen, *JAMA* 265:1260, 1991 (letter).
13. Koehler MP, Sholiton DB: Spontaneous hyphema resulting from warfarin, *Ann Ophthalmol* 15:858, 1983.
14. Baba FE, Jarrett WH, Harbin TS, and others: Massive hemorrhage complicating age-related macular degeneration, *Ophthalmology* 93:1581, 1986.
15. Stevenson RE, Burton M, Ferlauto EJ, and others: Hazards of oral anticoagulants during pregnancy, *JAMA* 243:1546, 1980.
16. Gainey SP, Robertson DM, Fay W, and others: Ocular surgery on patients receiving long-term warfarin therapy, *Am J Ophthalmol* 108:142, 1989.
17. Havener WH: Thrombophlebitis, anticoagulant therapy, and cataract extraction: questions and answers, *JAMA* 251:3010, 1984.
18. Klein ML: Macular degeneration: Is aspirin a risk for progressive disease? Questions and answers, *JAMA* 266:2279, 1991.
19. Macular Photocoagulation Study Group: Recurrent choroidal neovascularization after argon laser photocoagulation for recurrent maculopathy, *Arch Ophthalmol* 104:503, 1986
20. Macular Photocoagulation Study Group: Persistent and recurrent neovascularization after krypton laser photocoagulation for neovascular lesions of age-related macular degeneration, *Arch Ophthalmol* 108:825, 1990.
21. Werblin TP, Peiffer RL: Persistent hemorrhage after extracapsular surgery associated with excessive aspirin ingestion, *Am J Ophthalmol* 104:426, 1987.
22. Topol ES, Bell WR, Weisfeldt ML: Coronary thrombolysis with recombinant tissue-type plasminogen activator, *Ann Intern Med* 103:837, 1985.
23. Friedman MW: Streptokinase in ophthalmology, *Am J Ophthalmol* 35:1184, 1952.
24. O'Rourke JF: Evaluation of intraocular streptokinase, *Am J Ophthalmol* 39:119, 1952.
25. Cherfen GM, Maghraby AE, Tabbara KF, and others: Dissolution of intraocular fibrous exudate by streptokinase, *Ophthalmology* 98:870, 1991.
26. Sunderraj P: Intraocular hemorrhage associated with intravenous administered streptokinase, *Am J Ophthalmol* 112:734, 1991.
27. Schmidt D, Schumacher MD, Wakhloo AK: Microcatheter urokinase infusion in central retinal artery occlusion, *Am J Ophthalmol* 113:429, 1992.
28. ISIS-3: a randomised comparison of streptokinase vs tissue plasminogen activator vs anistreplise and of aspirin plus heparin vs aspirin alone among 41299 cases of suspected acute myocardial infarction, *Lancet* 339:753, 1992.
29. Vine AK, Maguire PT, Martonyi C, and others: Recombinant tissue plasminogen activator to lyse experimentally induced retinal arterial thrombi, *Am J Ophthalmol* 105:266, 1988.
30. Tripathi RC Park JK, Tripathi BJ, and others: Tissue plasminogen activators in human aqueous humor and its possible therapeutic significance, *Am J Ophthalmol* 106:719, 1988.
31. Wang M, Berman M, Law M: Latent and active plasminogen activator in corneal ulceration, *Invest Ophthalmol Vis Sci* 26:511, 1985.
32. Lambrou FM, Snyder RW, Williams GA, and

others: Treatment of experimental intravitreal fibrin with tissue plasminogen activator, *Am J Ophthalmol* 104:619, 1987.
33. Snyder RW, Sherman MD, Allinson RW: Intracameral tissue plasminogen activator for treatment of excessive fibrin response after penetrating keratoplasty, *Am J Ophthalmol* 109:483, 1990.
34. Johnson RN, Olsen K, Hernandez E: Tissue plasminogen activator treatment of postoperative intraocular fibrin, *Ophthalmology* 95:592, 1988.
35. Snyder RW, Lambrou FM, Williams GA: Intraocular fibrinolysis with recombinant human tissue plasminogen activator, *Arch Ophthalmol* 105:1277, 1987.
36. Jaffe GJ, Lewis M, Man DP, and others: Treatment of post-vitrectomy fibrin pupillary block with tissue plasminogen activator, *Am J Ophthalmol* 108:170, 1989.
37. Ortiz JR, Walker SD, McManus PE, and others: Filtering bleb thrombolysis with tissue plasminogen activator, *Am J Ophthalmol* 106:624, 1988.
38. Jones RL, Peterson CM: Reduced fibrinogen survival in diabetes mellitus, *Clin Invest* 63:485, 1979.
39. Johnson RN, Olsen KR, Hernandez E: Intravitreal tissue plasminogen activator treatment of experimental vitreous hemorrhage, *Arch Ophthalmol* 107:891, 1989.
40. Jaffe GJ, Abrams GW, Williams GA, and others: Tissue plasminogen activator for postvitrectomy fibrin formation, *Ophthalmology* 97:184, 1990.
41. Dabbs CK, Aaberg TM, Aguiter ME, and others: Complications of tissue plasminogen activator therapy after vitrectomy for diabetes, *Am J Ophthalmol* 110:354, 1990.
42. Williams GA, Lombrou FM, Jaffe GJ, and others: Treatment of postvitrectomy fibrin formation with intraocular tissue plasminogen activator, *Arch Ophthalmol Surg* 106:1055, 1988.
43. Howard GR, Vukica J, Fiscella RE, and others: Intraocular tissue plasminogen activator in a rabbit model of traumatic hyphema, *Arch Ophthalmol* 109:272, 1991.
44. Lambrou FM, Snyder RW, Williams GA: Use of tissue plasminogen activator in experimental hyphema, *Arch Ophthalmol* 105:995, 1987.
45. Johnson MW, Olsen KR, Hernandez E: Tissue plasminogen activator treatment of experimental subretinal hemorrhage, *Retina* 11:250, 1991.
46. Lewis M, Resnick SC, Flennery JG, and others: Tissue plasminogen activator treatment of experimental subretinal hemorrhage, *Am J Ophthalmol* 111:197, 1991.
47. Thompson JT, Glaser BM, Michiels RG, and others: The use of intravitreal thrombin to control hemorrhage during vitrectomy, *Ophthalmology* 93:279, 1986.
48. Cowan GM: Microinfusion of thrombin solution in vitreous surgery, *Am J Ophthalmol* 105:685, 1988.
49. Mannis MJ, Sweet E, Landers MB, and others: Uses of thrombin in ocular surgery effects on the corneal endothelium, *Arch Ophthalmol* 106:251, 1988.
50. McDermott ML, Edelhausen MF, Mannis MJ: Intracorneal thrombin and the corneal endothelium, *Am J Ophthalmol* 106:414, 1988.
51. Aaberg TM: Balancing the benefits and risks of intracorneal thrombin, *Am J Ophthalmol* 106:485, 1988.
52. McGetrick JJ, Jampol LM, Goldberg MF, and others: Aminocaproic acid decreases secondary hemorrhage after traumatic hyphema, *Arch Ophthalmol* 101:1031, 1983.
53. Kraft SP, Christianson MD, Crawford JS, and others: Traumatic hyphema in children. Treatment with epsilon-aminocaproic acid, *Ophthalmology* 94:1232, 1987.
54. Parsons MR, Merritt DR, Ramsay RC: Retinal artery occlusion associated with tranexamia acid therapy, *Am J Ophthalmol* 105:688, 1988.
55. Agapitos PJ, Noel L, Clarke WN: Traumatic hyphema in children, *Ophthalmology* 94:1238, 1987.
56. Crawford JS, Lewandoski RL, Chan W: The effect of aspirin on rebleeding in traumatic hyphema, *Am J Ophthalmol* 80:543, 1978.
57. Gorn RA: The detrimental effect of aspirin on hyphema rebleed, *Ann Ophthalmol* 11:351, 1979.
58. Palmer DJ, Goldberg MF, Frenkel M, and others: A comparison of two dose regimens of epsilon aminocaproic acid in the prevention and management of secondary traumatic hyphemas, *Ophthalmology* 93:102, 1986.
59. Dieste MC, Hersh PS, Kylstra JA, and others: Intraocular pressure increase associated with epsilon-aminocaproic acid therapy for traumatic hyphema, *Am J Ophthalmol* 106:383, 1988.
60. Allingham RR, Williams PB, Crouch ER, and others: Topically applied aminocaproic acid concentrates in the aqueous humor of the rabbit in therapeutic levels, *Arch Ophthalmol* 105:1421, 1987.
61. Ehlers WH, Crouch ER, Williams PB, and

others: Factors affecting therapeutic concentrations of topical aminocaproic acid in traumatic hyphema, *Invest Ophthalmol Vis Sci* 31:2389, 1990.

62. Vusitalo RJ, Ranta-Kemppainen L, Tarkkanen A: Management of traumatic hyphema in children: an analysis of 340 cases, *Arch Ophthalmol* 106:1207, 1988.
63. Farber MD, Fiscella R, Goldberg MF: Aminocaproic acid versus prednisone for the treatment of traumatic hyphema: a randomized clinical trial, *Ophthalmology* 98:279, 1991.
64. Medner MP: The effect of sodium hyaluronate and sodium chondroitin sulfate on the coagulation system in vitro, *Ophthalmology* 91:864, 1984.

CHAPTER 17

# Surgical Pharmacology

Thomas F. Mauger

SECTION ONE

## α-Chymotrypsin

α-Chymotrypsin is a proteolytic enzyme useful in ophthalmology because of its relatively selective action on zonular fibers. α-Chymotrypsin is an excellent example of the rapid change in medicine and ophthalmology in general and ocular surgery specifically. Ten years ago when the last edition of this book was prepared, α-chymotrypsin was a very important surgical agent, and 20 pages with 63 references were appropriately included. Now it is virtually a footnote among other more important pharmaceutical agents used in the treatment of surgical problems. In fact, it has been used only one time in more than 2 years.

### PHARMACOLOGY

#### Enzymatic Action

The main proteolytic effect of α-chymotrypsin is to split peptide bonds only at the location of certain amino acids. The most susceptible bonds are those of L-tyrosine, L-phenylalanine, and L-tryptophan; L-methionine and L-leucine may also be affected. α-Chymotrypsin may also hydrolyze some other types of chemical linkage. These amino acids occur widely throughout ocular tissues and not only in the zonular fibers; therefore, it would be expected that α-chymotrypsin would damage other protein structures within the eye besides the zonular fibers.

#### Potency

The potency of commercial preparations of α-chymotrypsin is measured in Armour proteolytic activity (APA) units. One unit releases 1 μg of tyrosine from a hemoglobin substrate. Assay of α-chymotrypsin powders shows their potency to vary between 750 and 1,300 APA units/mg. Because of this variability, concentrations are expressed as units rather than by weight. For instance, crystalline Alpha-Chymar assays at 1,150 APA units/mg, whereas Quimotrase assays at 750 APA units/mg. Optimum zonulysis is obtained with 150 APA units/ml, which is the strength of a 1:5,000 dilution of Quimotrase. The comparable 1:5,000 concentrations of the other brands also contain 150 APA units/ml, but the actual weight of drug dispensed in the commercial vial varies, depending on its potency. Hence, the 150 APA units/ml, or 1:5,000 dilution, of the various preparations will by definition provide equal proteolytic activity for all, regardless of the potency per milligram of drug.[1]

#### Stability

Solutions of α-chymotrypsin are relatively unstable. After 9 days at room temperature, solutions have lost half of their enzymatic activity.[2] Refrigeration at 2° C maintains full activity of the solution for at least 1 month. From the practical standpoint these findings indicate that the surgeon need not fear decomposition of α-chymotrypsin during the course of an operation even if a solution is not prepared immediately before use. Because α-chymotrypsin is relatively inexpensive, it is usually no more practical to save it from one operation to another than it is to save other solutions. The commercial preparations are sterilized by filtration, do not contain preservative chemicals, and therefore may easily become contaminated if saved for multiple use. To ensure sterility, one should prepare solutions immediately before use.

### Preparation

The enzymatic effect of the α-chymotrypsin is readily inactivated by many chemicals present in operating rooms, and inactivation has been reported to cause instances of complete failure of zonulysis. Inactivating chemicals include soaps, detergents, alkalies, acids, and antiseptics (e.g., alcohol). If a detergent is used to cleanse containers and syringes, it should be rinsed off before sterilization. If chemical sterilization is employed, naturally the equipment used in preparation of the enzyme must be thoroughly rinsed before use.

## EFFECTS ON EYE

Although the clinical use of α-chymotrypsin with appropriate precautions is surprisingly free of undesirable side effects, it must not be assumed that the enzyme is nontoxic. Extensive experimental studies of the ocular response to α-chymotrypsin indicate that it is a highly potent and destructive drug that must be used with caution and respect.

### Cornea

Fortunately, the corneal epithelium and endothelium are resistant to the effect of 1:5,000 concentrations of α-chymotrypsin, and when they are intact, they protect the corneal stroma against the enzymatic effect. When the epithelium and endothelium have been damaged, or if the enzyme is injected directly into the corneal stroma, considerable destruction and swelling of the cornea ensue.

Irrigation of a human eye with 1:500 α-chymotrypsin resulted in full dilatation of the pupil within a few minutes. Subsequently, the iris atrophied, leaving the appearance of aniridia. The cornea and vitreous were undamaged.[3]

Because most cataracts are removed through limbal incisions, evaluation of limbal rather than corneal wound strength would seem most logical in a study of the effect of α-chymotrypsin on wound healing. This was done in a series of 10 white rabbits.[4] An 8-mm limbal incision was irrigated with 0.2 ml of a 1:25,000 solution of α-chymotrypsin at 2-minute intervals for 4 doses. The control incisions in the fellow eyes were irrigated with the saline-heparin diluent. Wound disruption was induced 6 days after suture removal by means of oxygen introduced intraocularly under gradually increasing pressure. Pounds per square inch required to burst the α-chymotrypsin incisions averaged 10.9 compared with 11.1 for the controls—an insignificant difference.

### Iris

The iris is relatively resistant to clinically used concentrations of α-chymotrypsin injected into the anterior chamber. Iritis frequently accompanies the posterior ocular inflammation caused by intravitreal enzyme injection.

### Zonular Membrane

Zonulysis with α-chymotrypsin is a diffusely occurring fragmentation of the entire length of the zonular fiber.[5] These fibers are broken into relatively uniform fragments approximately 1,000 Å in length. This uniformity suggests the presence of a regularly located amino acid linkage that is selectively destroyed by the enzyme.

The fragmentation does not become visible until 10 to 15 minutes after enzyme application in contrast to destruction of the equatorial pericapsular membrane of the lens within 5 minutes. Up to 30 minutes is required for complete lysis of the entire zonular membrane.

The effective site of the action of α-chymotrypsin in cataract surgery is the zonular attachment to the lens. In these patients only 0.3 ml of a 1:5,000 solution of α-chymotrypsin was used, and it was thoroughly irrigated out after 2 to 4 minutes of action.

### Ciliary Body

Electron microscopy of the nonpigmented ciliary epithelium of monkey eyes after zonulysis by 1:5,000 solution of α-chymotrypsin shows no change in this membrane.[5] When the centripetal pull of the zonules is destroyed, the ring of ciliary processes increases in diameter.

### Lens

Electron microscopy of the lens capsule shows that there is a pericapsular membrane near the equator identical in structure to the zonular fibers. This membrane is not demonstrable in the central portions of the capsule. After zonulysis with α-chymotrypsin, the equatorial pericapsular membrane fragments and disappears, but the lens capsule proper shows no recognizable changes.[5]

### Lens-Vitreous Attachments

The lens-vitreous attachments of the young monkey and also of the young humans after autopsy are very resistant to α-chymotrypsin. These attachments are not lysed even when the enzyme exposure time is prolonged far beyond the time required to disintegrate the zonules completely.[5]

### Vitreous Face

The effect of α-chymotrypsin on the anterior hyaloid face has been studied in human eyes enucleated within 2 hours postmortem.[6] The cornea, iris, and lens were removed, and the vitreous was caused to protrude by equatorial pressure on the eye. α-Chymotrypsin in the higher concentration of 1:1,000 was then continuously applied to the exposed vitreous face for 40 minutes. Even 1 hour later there was still no noticeable decrease in the strength of the vitreous face or any increased tendency to protrusion of the vitreous. Such findings suggest that use of α-chymotrypsin could not predispose the eye to vitreous loss resulting from rupture of its face.

The resistance of the vitreous structure to dissolution by α-chymotrypsin is caused by its collagen content (collagen is not readily susceptible to the action of α-chymotrypsin).[7]

### Retina

Although relatively innocuous in the anterior chamber, α-chymotrypsin in even small quantities is quite toxic when injected intravitreally. As little as 0.002 mg in the rabbit vitreous causes infiltration of inflammatory cells into the retina and irregular partial destruction of the ganglion cell layer.[8] Increased dosage causes greater damage, until at the level of 2 mg the entire retina is destroyed, leaving only Müller's fibers, and the optic nerve itself is necrotic. Intermediate doses cause varying amounts of retinal hemorrhage, inflammation, and permanent destruction. By contrast, 0.2 mg injected into the rabbit anterior chamber causes no recognizable retinal damage. Presumably this results because the outflow of aqueous carries the enzyme anteriorly, and it does not readily diffuse into the intact vitreous body.

When these milligram values are compared with clinically used concentrations, somewhat less than 1 mg of α-chymotrypsin is contained in 5 ml of the comparable 1:5,000 solution used clinically. Only 0.01 ml of this clinically used concentration is required to contain 0.002 mg of enzyme—the amount that causes recognizable damage to the rabbit retina when injected intravitreally.

The intraocular damage resulting from injection of 0.4 ml of a 1:5,000 solution of α-chymotrypsin into the anterior axial rabbit vitreous is outlined in Table 17–1. The most serious of the enzyme-induced changes was retinal degeneration. During the 14 days of this experiment, 70% of

**TABLE 17–1.**
Incidence of Intraocular Changes After Intravitreal Injection of Normal Saline Solution and of α-Chymotrypsin in Saline Solution

| | Control (%) | α-Chymotrypsin (%) |
|---|---|---|
| Iritis | 15 | 40 |
| Cyclitis | 15 | 45 |
| Zonulysis | 0 | 77 |
| Hyalitis | 61 | 95 |
| Retinal holes | 7 | 18 |
| Retinolysis | 0 | 70 |

Modified from O'Malley C, Moskovitz M, Straatsma B: *Arch Ophthalmol* 66:539, 1961. Used by permission.

the α-chymotrypsin-treated eyes developed definite retinal damage.[9]

The enzyme-inhibiting property of human aqueous humor was evaluated after a 15-minute incubation period of equal volumes of 1:5,000 α-chymotrypsin and of human secondary aqueous. The resulting inhibitory activity destroyed from 5% to 67% of the α-chymotrypsin potency in the aqueous samples studied from 10 eyes. No enzyme activity could be detected in secondary aqueous obtained from five eyes in which α-chymotrypsin had been used for cataract extraction (0.4 ml of a 1:5,000 solution allowed to stand for 2 minutes). On the basis of these findings, there seems to be no need to irrigate or neutralize the enzyme when it is used for cataract extraction.[10] Primary human aqueous has also been shown to inactivate α-chymotrypsin.[11]

## Clinical Use

Relatively specific dissolution of the zonular attachments to the lens may be achieved without causing the intraocular toxic effects resulting from experimental use.[12]

Either a 1:5,000 or 1:10,000 concentration of enzyme may be used. Different authors advocate amounts ranging from 0.3 to 4.0 ml of solution. The good results reported with such different amounts indicate that the enzymatic action results from a relatively small amount of solution and that large excesses of fluid run harmlessly out of the incision.

Because the site of zonulysis is at the equatorial insertion of the fibers, the solution is introduced by various types of irrigating tips that are inserted behind the iris and are manipulated so as to direct the solution about the anterior lens equator. This distribution of the enzyme behind the iris is important; it should not simply be placed into the anterior chamber.

Immediately after enzyme injection, the conjunctiva and the incision edges may be irrigated with saline solution. Despite the previously noted animal experiments indicating that α-chymotrypsin does not interfere with corneoscleral wound healing, there is a clinical suspicion that wound complications are more frequent after zonulysis. For this reason, multiple sutures and a conjunctival flap are advised.

Zonulysis is usually achieved within 1 to 2 minutes and is recognized by either anterior displacement of the lens, a more rounded lens contour, or the ease with which it may be removed. At the end of 2 minutes, or sooner if zonulysis is recognized, gentle saline irrigation may be used to remove debris from the anterior chamber. If the zonule is unusually resistant, a second application of enzyme may be helpful in rare cases.

## Glaucoma

Use of α-chymotrypsin predisposes transient glaucoma to develop during the postoperative period. In a series of 343 cataract extractions (178 with α-chymotrypsin and 165 without), this glaucoma (defined as a pressure of at least 24.4 mm Hg Schiøtz and detected by daily tonometry) was found in 72.5% of enzyme-treated eyes in contrast to 23.6% of control eyes.[13] Carefully controlled analysis included the possibility that other factors might have caused the increased pressure (including type of iridectomy, instruments used, preexisting glaucoma, age of patient, number of sutures, technique of extraction, etc.). That the diluent vehicle or the irrigating cannula did not cause the glaucoma was proved by irrigation with diluent alone in 17 eyes, only 17.6% of which developed glaucoma.

α-Chymotrypsin-induced glaucoma is dose related in that its frequency and severity increase with use of a larger volume

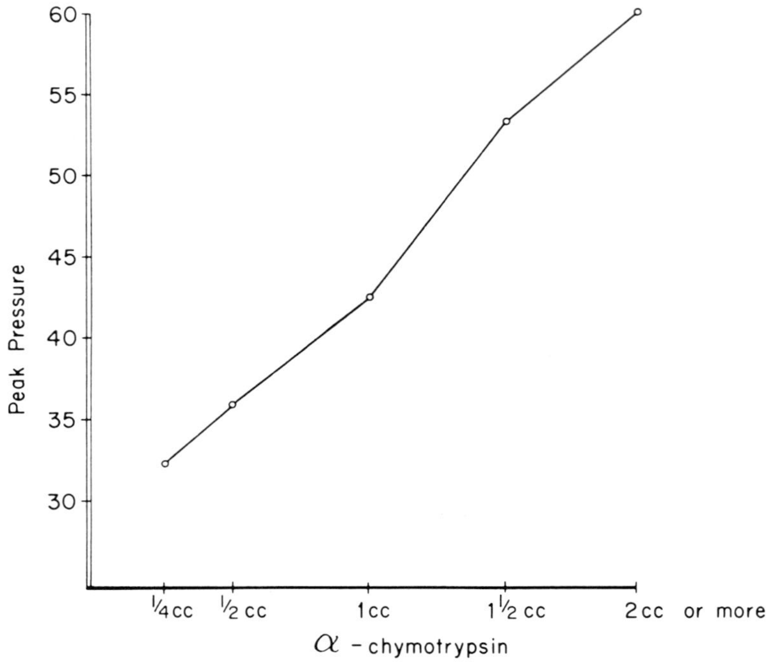


**FIG 17–1.**
Highest intraocular pressure occurring in each dosage group of α-chymotrypsin-treated patients undergoing cataract extraction. (Modified from Kirsch RE: *Arch Ophthalmol* 75:774, 1966. Used by permission.)

of enzyme solution. Fig. 17–1 charts the highest (not average) pressure encountered in groups of 20 cataract extractions performed with a given volume of 1:5,000 α-chymotrypsin. Obviously the use of a greater volumes causes substantial pressure increases. Even the smallest volume used (0.25 ml) caused postoperative pressures of 24 mm Hg or higher in 55% of cases. Use of 1.5 ml increased this to 70%. The cataract surgeon is advised to use the smallest dose of α-chymotrypsin necessary to produce satisfactory zonulysis. The reader is reminded that 2 to 4 ml of 1:5,000 α-chymotrypsin was routinely used when Kirsch[14] discovered this form of postoperative glaucoma.

Posterior chamber introduction of sufficient enzyme causes tissue breakdown. This tissue debris then flows forward and becomes trapped in the trabecular structure. Glaucoma ensues and lasts until this debris is absorbed. Corticosteroids are not beneficial because the mechanism is noninflammatory.

Confirmation of this hypothesis was achieved through scanning electron microscopy. Both in monkeys[15] and in human eyes,[16] scanning electron microscopy shows that the zonular fibers, especially those near the lens, swell up into a very loose, spongelike mass (Fig. 17–2). Fragments of these partially digested zonular fibers become trapped in the trabecular meshwork (Fig. 17–3).

Further evidence supporting the hypothesis of trabecular blockage by zonular debris was obtained by injections of the enzyme into the anterior chamber of monkey eyes.[17] Dissected specimens of the lens, zonular membrane, and ciliary body were discarded. Injection of the residual solution into the anterior chamber of a monkey eye resulted in typical enzyme-induced glaucoma. When this solution was cleared of particulate debris by microfiltration (Millipore filter), it did not cause glaucoma when injected.

If a monkey eye is already aphakic (zonular membrane already digested and removed), injection of α-chymotrypsin will not cause any pressure elevation. Aqueous from a monkey with enzyme-induced glaucoma will not cause pressure elevation when injected into another eye.

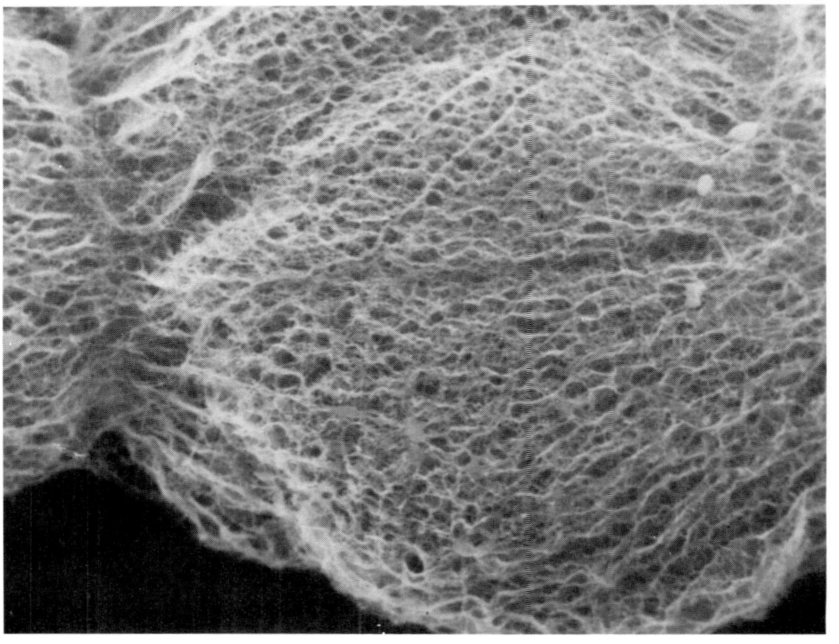

**FIG 17–2.**
Swollen human zonular fiber after α-chymotrypsin digestion. (Scanning electron microphotograph, ×2,000.) (From Worthen DM: *Am J Ophthalmol* 73:637, 1972. Used by permission.)

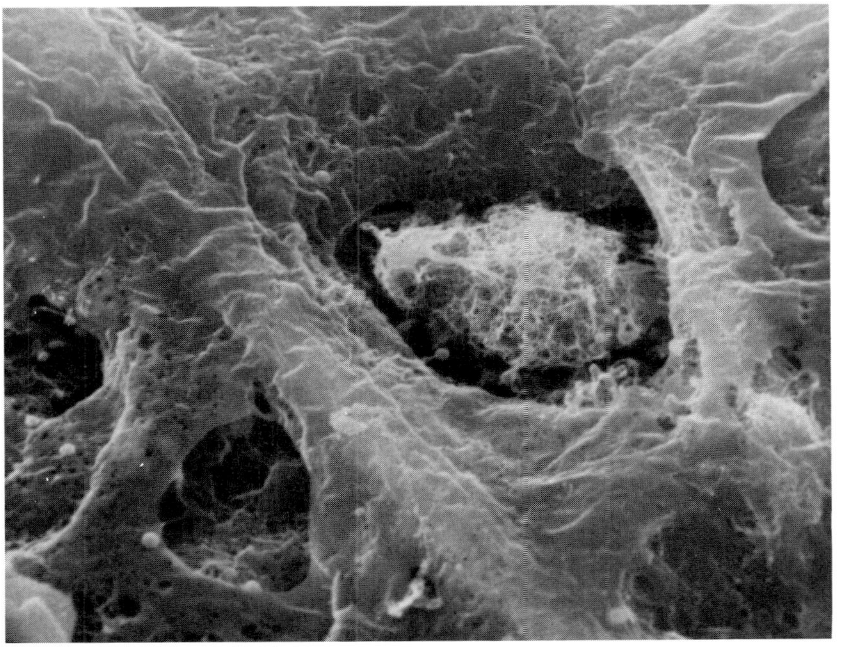

**FIG 17–3.**
Fluffy mass of α-chymotrypsin digested zonular fiber trapped in interstices of trabecular meshwork. (Scanning electron microphotograph, ×2,000.) (From Worthen DM: *Am J Ophthalmol* 73:637, 1972. Used by permission.)

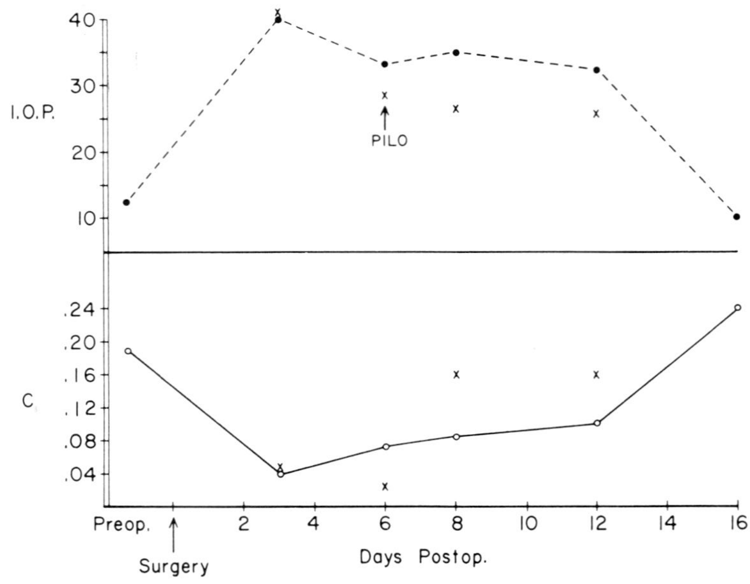


**FIG 17–4.**
Representative case of enzyme glaucoma. (Modified from Kirsch RE: *Trans Am Acad Ophthalmol Otolaryngol* 69:1011, 1965. Used by permission.)

Enzyme-induced glaucoma is accompanied by a decrease in facility of outflow (Fig. 17–4).[18] A deep anterior chamber and an open angle differentiate enzyme glaucoma from pupil-block glaucoma.

## SUMMARY

α-Chymotrypsin use in ophthalmic surgery is becoming negligible. Its main use in my hands is in the partially subluxated crystalline lens that still has some strong zonular attachments such as found after blunt injury. Even in these eyes extracapsular techniques such as endocapsular phacoemulsification are preferable if they can be performed. Unless a novel use of α-chymotrypsin is found, it will soon be only of limited clinical interest.

SECTION TWO

# Viscoelastic Substances

The development of viscoelastic substances for ophthalmic surgery ranks with the operating microscope, intraocular irrigating solutions, and fine suture materials as major breakthroughs. Viscoelastic substances are used in surgery to maintain spaces, move tissue, and protect surfaces. The physical properties responsible for these beneficial functions are related to the molecular structure and intramolecular and intermolecular interactions (Table 17–2).[1, 2]

The physical characteristics of importance in viscoelastic substances are viscosity, shear flow, elasticity, cohesiveness, and coatability.[3] The viscosity of the substance determines its resistance to flow. A simple way to measure viscosity is by measuring the time it takes for the solution to flow through a tube under the force of gravity compared with a controlled substance. This has the disadvantage that it does not take into account surface tension and shear flow issues that are related to the diameter of the tube. More accurate measures of viscosity can be made in the laboratory that allow control of these important variables. Higher viscosity may be obtained by having larger molecular weight molecules and a higher concentration of these in solutions. Because of the limitations of osmolarity on an intraocular substance, the only practical way to obtain higher viscosity is to increase molecular weight while maintaining osmolarity at a physiologic level. Viscosity is measured in centipoises. High viscosity is desirable to maintain spaces such as the anterior chamber with incisions or perforations present that would allow less viscous material such as saline solution to drain out immediately, collapsing the space.

The shear flow is the measure of the friction as two plates are moved over one another with the substance in question between. A meaningful example of shearing is the injection of viscoelastic material through a small cannula into the anterior chamber. The faster the material moves through the cannula, the higher the shear forces. For a nonnewtonian substance, for example, hyaluronate, viscosity decreases as the shear force is increased. This allows injection of the higher viscous material through a small cannula. Chondroitin sulfate is a newtonian fluid in which viscosity is independent of shear rate. The viscosity changes that occur with sodium hyaluronate in relation to shear rate are termed pseudoplasticity.

Viscosity prevents the easy leakage of the material from the eye. Elasticity is the property that allows the shape of the space such as the anterior chamber to be maintained despite manipulations of the eye. The property of elasticity is due to the ability of long-chain molecules to be deformed and then recover their original conformation. Elasticity has several important clinical implications. It may dampen high-frequency vibrational forces associated with phacoemulsification and, along with pseudoplasticity aid in the ability of injection of a substance through a small cannula.[3]

The cohesiveness of a viscoelastic substance is determined by the molecular weight of the substance, with larger molecules having greater attachments to one another and the entire volume of the substance tending to remain as one large mass. This can be observed in anterior segment surgery when a high molecular weight substance (e.g., sodium hyaluronate) is irrigated from the anterior chamber and comes out as a large mass, whereas a substance with much lower molecular weight (e.g., 2% hydroxypropyl methylcellulose [HPMC; Occucoat]) will come out slowly. Cohesiveness will, like viscosity, prevent the substance from leaving the eye, but it can also lead to the blockage of the trabecular meshwork and elevated intraocular pressure.[3]

Finally, the last physical property of importance is the ability of the viscoelastic to coat surfaces. In cataract surgery this is important in the protection of the endothelium during phacoemulsification. Coating is determined by surface tension and contact angle. As with contact lens solutions, a lower surface tension and lower wetting angle will allow better coating. Chondroitin sulfate has a better coating action than sodium hyaluronate. When a lens implant is inserted, it is desirable to have the viscoelastic coat the implant. Hyaluronate with greater cohesive-

**TABLE 17–2.**
Viscoelastics

| Name | Manufacturer | Preparation | pH | Osmolarity (mOsm) | Viscosity (cps)* |
|---|---|---|---|---|---|
| Vitrax | Allergan Medical Optics | 30 mg/ml Hyaluronate | 7–7.5 | 310 | 40,000 |
| Healon | Kabi Pharmacia Ophthalmic, Inc. | 10 mg/ml Hyaluronate | 7–7.5 | 302 | 40,000–64,000 |
| Healon GV | Kabi Pharmacia Ophthalmic, Inc. | 14 mg/ml Hyaluronate | 7–7.5 | — | 80,000 |
| Amvisc | IOLAB | 12 mg/ml | 6.5–7.2 | 318 | 40,000–42,000 |
| Amvisc Plus | IOLAB | 16 mg/ml Hyaluronate | 7.2 | 340 | 55,000 |
| Viscoat | Alcon | Chondroitin sulfate, 40 mg/ml Hyaluronate, 30 mg/ml | 7.2 | 325 | 40,000 |
| Occucoat | Storz | 2% Hydroxypropylmethylcellulose | 7.2 | 285 | 4,000 |

*Viscosity measured at a shear rate of 2/sec, 25° C.

ness and high wetting angle tends to slide off the implant during insertion, whereas chondroitin sulfate or HPMC may cling to the implant better and, because it has less cohesiveness, not be entirely stripped off during insertion.

The perfect viscoelastic for all purposes has not yet been created. Sodium hyaluronate with high viscosity, elasticity, and cohesiveness is excellent for maintaining the anterior chamber, whereas chondroitin sulfate and HPMC have superior coating ability and less cohesiveness and may be advantageous in coating of the endothelium during phacoemulsification and coating of the lens implant during insertion. These issues are controversial and are dependent primarily on surgical technique and the individual preferences of the surgeon.

## SODIUM HYALURONATE

Sodium hyaluronate was introduced to ophthalmic surgery in the late 1970s.[4–6] Sodium hyaluronate is found in the body as an extracellular substance in connective tissues. It is a natural shock absorber and is found in both the aqueous and vitreous humor of the eye. As previously described, it has a high molecular weight and high viscosity. Practically, the material can be obtained from rooster comb and with bacterial fermentation. It is currently used in a concentration of 10 mg/ml (Healon, Amvisc), 14 mg/ml (Healon GV), and as 16 mg/ml solution (Amvisc Plus). The higher concentration is associated with higher viscosity and also higher osmolarity. The solution can be obtained with a yellow tint caused by the addition of fluorescein in a concentration of 0.005 mg/ml (Healon Yellow). The yellow tint improves visualization of the sodium hyaluronate during procedures and helps to confirm total removal after irrigation.

Sodium hyaluronate (Healon) was compared with a balanced salt solution in a perspective study of intracapsular cataract surgery.[7] Healon was used to fill the anterior chamber after the incision was made and then to refill the anterior chamber at the end of surgery. The Healon was not removed at the conclusion of surgery. There was no difference in intraocular pressure measured at any point postoperatively compared with the balanced salt solution eyes. Corneas were thinner when Healon was used. A 9% corneal edema was found 1 day after surgery with Healon as opposed to 23% when balanced salt solution was used. The incision was corneoscleral. This difference was not found if a corneal incision was used. Both groups had approximately 15% edema 1 day after surgery with the corneal incision. The endothelial density was slightly better in eyes with corneoscleral incision that received Healon compared with balanced salt solution. Endothelial density was significantly lower with the corneal incision compared with the corneoscleral incision. This study documents not only the beneficial effects of sodium hyaluronate with intracapsular surgery but also the benefits of corneoscleral incision as opposed to corneal incision in protecting the endothelium from surgical damage.

Of more importance in the 1990s is the use of sodium hyaluronate in extracapsular surgery, particularly phacoemulsification. Phacoemulsification done entirely in the anterior chamber was evaluated in the early 1980s.[8] This type of procedure should have a large impact on the endothelium and corneal thickness and would be most likely to show any beneficial effects of a viscoelastic substance. Again, Healon was not irrigated out of the eye at the end of the procedure. A 39% corneal thickness was found only when balanced salt solution (BSS) was used compared with a 21% increase with Healon. This decreased to 8% by 10 days compared with 16% with BSS. Average intraocular pressure did not rise with Healon; however, three patients had pressures greater than 30 mm Hg, and one had pressure greater than 50 mm Hg on the first postoperative day. No similar pressure rises occurred with balanced salt solution. Endothelial cell loss was found using both solutions, but there was a significant difference in patients greater than 55 years old, Healon having a 23% cell loss and BSS a 54.6% loss in these older patients. These early studies of viscoelastic use demonstrated their practical value and stimulated increased clinical use and investigation.

Sodium hyaluronate was compared with BSS in nuclear expression extracapsular cataract surgery in rabbits.[9] Eighteen rabbit eyes were followed for 4 weeks after nuclear expression extracapsular cataract surgery in which corneal thickness, endothelial cell count, and intraocular pressure were measured. A 20% to 33% increase in the intraocular pressure occurred during the first 4 days postoperatively, but there was no difference between the two groups. There was also no difference in endothelial cell count or corneal thickness. The authors did find that the procedure was simpler with the sodium hyaluronate because the anterior chamber depth was maintained.

## Endothelial Protection

In addition to the studies already recorded, there are other investigations indicating the protective effects of sodium hyaluronate on the corneal endothelium. A prospective, randomized trial evaluated the use of sodium hyaluronate to fill the anterior chamber before the anterior capsulotomy in nuclear expression extracapsular cataract surgery. In both the control and experimental groups sodium hyaluronate was used after cortex removal to expand the capsular bag. A total of 200 patients were enrolled in the study. Two months after surgery endothelial loss was 6.1% in the group receiving sodium hyaluronate before capsulotomy and 7.6% in which sodium hyaluronate was not used before capsulotomy. Intraocular pressure rise was similar between the two groups despite removal of the sodium hyaluronate after lens insertion. A mean increase of almost 4 mm Hg was found with both groups 1 day after surgery. Corneal thickness was not different from preoperative corneal thickness 2 months after surgery in either group.[10]

Different techniques of nuclear evacuation were evaluated along with the role of sodium hyaluronate and extracapsular cataract extractions.[11, 12] Despite variations in technique, cell loss using sodium hyaluronate was approximately half that of cell loss if only BSS was used. This was consistent whether human or cat eyes were evaluated. Similar findings in corneal thickness change were also noted. These measurements were made 6 weeks postoperatively.

A report indicated that acute corneal decompensation might be caused by instillation of denatured sodium hyaluronate in cataract surgery.[13] Denaturization can occur with autoclaving. Denatured sodium hyaluronate was evaluated in the cat model and found to be nontoxic. Sudden onset of corneal decompensation after uneventful cataract surgery with normal preexisting endothelium may be caused by accidental instillation of detergents or germicides.[14]

## Epithelial Protection

Preservation of the epithelium is crucial in ocular surface disease and after penetrating keratoplasty. The intraoperative use of sodium hyaluronate to coat the corneal surface during penetrating keratoplasty was evaluated perspectively in 38 consecutive corneal transplant patients. The control group was given BSS drops during the suturing of the graft, and the experimental group had thin coatings of Healon placed on the cornea on three separate occasions during the surgery. Punctate epithelial keratitis was much less severe in the group that was given sodium hyaluronate topically compared with that found in the control eyes. The epithelium is crucial in the success of corneal transplantation, and the application of Healon would seem to be a wise choice. Unfortunately, this study did not evaluate a sterile bland ocular emollient to determine whether this effect resulted from the special properties of sodium hyaluronate or just from prolonged lubrication under the bright microscope light that could not be afforded by the balanced salt solution. Obviously a huge difference in cost would be found if an ocular emollient could be used instead of sodium hyaluronate. If, however, residual Healon remains at the end of penetrating keratoplasty and it would otherwise be thrown away, you could consider this treatment virtually free.[15]

Sodium hyaluronate was found to provide more protection to chicken embryo corneal epithelium than hydroxymethylcellulose or a phosphate buffered solution. It also reduced the toxicity of benzalkonium chloride.[16] Sodium hyaluronate has been diluted in a 1:10 ratio with artificial tears and given in cases of ocular surface disease. This solution seems to have both subjective and objective beneficial effects, particularly in patients unresponsive to conventional therapy.[17, 18] Sodium hyaluronate is used as a goniogel during vitreoretinal procedures to maintain good contact with the cornea preventing air bubbles from intruding. One paper suggests using the residual viscoelastic from other ocular procedures, maintaining sterility by removing the injection cannula.[19] Our institute conducted an uncontrolled trial of sterile bland methylcellulose solution as a substitute for the use of sodium hyaluronate for this purpose. It was found to be much inferior to sodium hyaluronate, leading to significant bubble formation and loss of contact from the contact lens to the cornea. Sodium hyaluronate's cohesiveness is probably responsible for this excellent coupling ability.

### Other Surgical Uses

In addition to cataract surgery, sodium hyaluronate has been used to good effect in both anterior segment and posterior segment procedures.[20–21] Its use in corneal transplantation surgery will limit endothelial cell loss, and it is associated with thinner corneas than those treated with air bubble or balanced salt solution.[20] It is very useful in breaking peripheral anterior synechiae during corneal transplantation, especially in patients undergoing removal of anterior chamber intraocular lenses. The viscoelastic can be used to hydraulically separate, break, and maintain the anterior chamber after breakage of synechiae. Its use in penetrating keratoplasty is associated with a small rise in intraocular pressures during the first 24 to 48 hours because it is often difficult to entirely irrigate the viscoelastic from the anterior chamber.[21] Care must be taken in the aphakic eye not to overinflate the eye, delivering a large load of viscoelastic into the vitreous.

Sodium hyaluronate is very useful in the traumatized eye. Eyes sustaining blunt trauma with subluxation of the crystalline lens can be treated through injection of the viscoelastic beneath the crystalline lens, elevating it and maintaining it in the pupillary area, where it can then safely be removed.[22] In cases of penetrating injuries viscoelastics can be used to maintain the anterior chamber during repair, as well as break synechiae and reposition the iris.[23, 24] Because of its ability to move tissue, sodium hyaluronate has been used to reposition a striped Descemet's membrane occurring with cataract surgery.[25] I have managed similar cases through the combined use of viscoelastics to reposition the striped Descemet's membrane along with an air bubble that will help maintain the position of the Descemet's membrane with a superior detachment. Interestingly, a case of detachment of Descemet's membrane associated with injection of sodium hyaluronate has been reported. Care must be taken with viscoelastics to not create real spaces where unwanted potential ones exist.[26]

Sodium hyaluronate has been used in conjunction with vitrectomy techniques to position the retina during repair of rhegmatogenous retinal detachments. It may be used to flatten a folded retina associated with giant retinal tear.[27] In diabetic eyes undergoing membranectomies, sodium hyaluronate may be used to mechanically tamponade the vessels, possibly decreasing the risk of vitreous hemorrhage.[28, 29] It may be used to clear hyphema from the visual axis to allow vitrectomy.[30]

Sodium hyaluronate has been used in extraocular ophthalmic surgery. Its use in ocular adnexal surgery includes identification of the lacrimal sac during dacryocystorhinostomy and also the severed canaliculus with a nasolacrimal duct laceration.[31] Sodium hyaluronate may also serve to reduce adhesions that sometimes accompany strabismus surgery.[32]

## CHONDROITIN SULFATE

Chondroitin sulfate is a polysaccharide found in cartilage and other hard connective tissues in the body. It is harvested from the cartilage of shark fins. In the eye it is found chiefly in the cornea. It is a much smaller molecule than sodium hyaluronate; its molecular weight is only 20,000 daltons and chain link is 50 nm compared with 10,000 nm with sodium hyaluronate. To achieve high enough viscosity to maintain spaces, one would have to use concentrations high enough to make the solution hyperosmotic. Therefore, chondroitin sulfate is not available as an isolated product for intraocular use. Viscoat is a combination of 40 mg of chondroitin sulfate/ml and 30 mg of sodium hyaluronate/ml mixed in a 1:3 ratio. The sodium hyaluronate used in Viscoat is produced by bacterial fermentation, whereas the chondroitin sulfate is obtained from the cartilage in shark fins. Theoretically, Viscoat would combine the viscosity, pseudoelasticity, and cohesiveness of sodium hyaluronate with the coating properties of chondroitin sulfate.[3]

A prospective evaluation of sodium hyaluronate (Healon) and Viscoat was performed in 60 randomly assigned patients who were having extracapsular cataract extraction and lens implantation by either the nuclear expression technique or phacoemulsification. Healon was used in 20 patients, and Viscoat was used in 40 patients. Viscoat was removed at the end of surgery in 20 of the eyes and left in the anterior chamber of the remaining 20 eyes. Healon was removed in all of the eyes. Intraocular pressures 4 to 6 hours after surgery were significantly higher in patients in which Viscoat was left in the eye. The average intraocular pressure in this group was 26.5 mm Hg compared with 21.2 in eyes in which Viscoat was aspirated and 13.3 in which Healon was used and aspirated. The intraocular pressure peaked in the Healon group at 24 hours postoperatively with a pressure of 20.8 mm Hg, whereas the group with Viscoat left in the eye had dropped to 22.9 mm Hg and with Viscoat aspirated was 17.0 mm Hg. Thirty percent of eyes in which Healon was used had pressures greater than 25 mm Hg, whereas only 15% of eyes in which Viscoat was aspirated had pressures of this magnitude. Fifty-five percent of eyes in which Viscoat was left in the anterior chamber had pressures greater than 25 mm Hg. Endothelial cell counts and corneal thickness were similar 2 months after surgery in all three groups. The surgeon[33] believed the Healon was better at maintaining the anterior chamber, dilating the pupil, and opening the capsular bag, whereas Viscoat coated the lens and endothelium better. Another study of intraocular pressure effects of Viscoat and Healon found no significant difference in the pressure rises associated with both when the substances were removed at the end of surgery. The peak intraocular pressure rise for both was found at 6 hours postoperatively and was 28.4 mm Hg with Viscoat and 28.8 mm Hg for Healon. Five of the 11 eyes in the Viscoat group had intraocular pressures greater than 29 mm Hg during the initial 24-hour postoperative period, whereas six of 13 eyes in the Healon treated group had intraocular pressures greater than 39 mm Hg during the initial 24-hour period.[34]

The endothelial protective effects of Viscoat were compared with Healon in the rabbit model. In 14 rabbits Viscoat was used in one eye and BSS Plus (see later discussion) was used in the second eye; in another group of 14 rabbits Viscoat was used in one eye and Healon in the fellow eye. Phacoemulsification and cortical aspiration were then performed in all eyes. In half of the eyes a polymethylmethacrylate (PMMA) implant was then inserted. The endothelium was evaluated with the light microscope using trypan blue and alizarin red stain by masked observers. The percentage of damaged endothelial cells in this model after phacoemulsification and cortical aspiration alone was 9.3% and 13.7% using Viscoat, 12.7% with BSS Plus, and 21.3% with Healon. Viscoat was not different from the fellow eye in either of these paired groups. In the eyes in which the lens implant was placed, the implant and the corneal endothelium were pressed together with 25 g of pressure, and then the endothelium was examined with staining and light microscopy. In this group of unusual endothelial trauma the percent of damaged cells with Viscoat was 17.4% and 21.1%, whereas that with BSS Plus was 76.2% and with Healon was 41.4%. The authors[35] postulate that the Viscoat remains in the anterior chamber, protecting the endothelium because of its better coating abilities, less cohesiveness, and newtonian characteristics, whereas the Healon was largely irrigated out during phacoemulsification and cortical aspiration.[35]

It was obvious from these data that each substance has its own particular characteristics that would make it advantageous in different situations. Unfortunately, we are unable to predict which eye will have a situation in which one or the other viscoelastic would be the most appropriate. An example would be the instance of a flat anterior chamber right after lens implantation in which Viscoat would have been a better choice. Another example would be the case of intraoperative miosis, which might be better managed with sodium hyaluronate than with a chondroitin sulfate/sodium hyaluronate combination. As with the selection of ophthalmic surgical instruments and suture material, viscoelastic use will continue to be an individual choice tailored to the surgeon's needs.

Chondroitin sulfate has been found to have an in vitro anticoagulant effect that is not found with 1% sodium hyaluronate; therefore, Viscoat would not be an appropriate substitute for sodium hyaluronate for the mechanical tamponade of vitreous hemorrhage.[36]

Sterile endophthalmitis has been reported in the use of Viscoat intraocularly.[3] A calcific band keratopathy occurred in some patients who received Viscoat during surgery. This occurred within days of surgery and appeared as a diffuse subepithelial deposit. The precipitate was more likely to occur if BSS Plus was used and when the Viscoat was not irrigated from the anterior chamber. Reformulation of the product seemed to clear up this problem. This does, however, emphasize the importance of irrigation of any viscoelastic from the anterior chamber at the end of surgery.[37, 38]

Chondroitin sulfate has been used in corneal preservation to maintain endothelial cells longer. Corneas preserved with chondroitin sulfate will swell significantly after surgery because of increased osmolarity. This can be counteracted through the addition of dextran.[39–43]

## HYDROXYPROPYL METHYLCELLULOSE

HPMC is marketed as a 2% solution (Occucoat) and has physical properties markedly different from sodium hyaluronate. It has few viscoelastic properties but has a low contact angle and surface tension that make it very adherent to lens implants and the endothelium. Sodium hyaluronate is much better at maintaining the anterior chamber. A study comparing 2% HPMC with 1% sodium hyaluronate with nuclear expression extracapsular cataract extraction and posterior chamber lens implants in 70 patients showed similar intraocular pressure responses and endothelial damage. The highest intraocular pressure in the sodium hyaluronate group was 41 mm Hg and in the HPMC was 30 mm Hg 1 day after surgery. The average intraocular pressures 1 day after surgery were 18 mm Hg in the sodium hyaluronate group and 16.91 mm Hg in the HPMC group. These were not significantly different. Some surgeons may find HPMC an inexpensive substitute for other viscoelastics in routine cataract surgery. It does not have the theoretical advantages of sodium hyaluronate in complicated anterior segment surgery and trauma because of its low cohesiveness, viscosity, and elasticity.[43, 44]

## DRUG BINDING

An important consideration for any intraocular substance is its ability to bind other drugs and chemicals that may adversely affect the eye. Viscoelastic agents are particularly important because a small amount of the substance remains in the eye at the conclusion of surgery. Drug binding to Amvisc, Healon, and Viscoat was evaluated using chloramphenicol, dexamethasone, epinephrine, and pilocarpine in an in vitro model. The drug binding was extremely low in this in vitro model, with the highest percent bound chemical being for epinephrine at 1.48% in Viscoat. Drug binding for the rest of the viscoelastic agents ranged from 0% to 0.57%.[45] Care should be exercised to prevent contamination of viscoelastic agents with drugs or detergents that might be toxic to the eye.

## SUMMARY

Other viscoelastic agents are currently being developed to somehow combine the desirable characteristics of high viscosity, elasticity, and cohesiveness with good adherence and coatability. As these are being developed, they must be evaluated for purity, availability, and expense, as well as their intraocular characteristics and protective functions.[1]

SECTION THREE

# Ophthalmic Irrigants

Before the advent of extracapsular cataract extraction, phacoemulsification, and vitrectomy, the significance of intraocular irrigants was minimal because their volume and time of irrigation was minimal. Today it is not unusual for several hundred milliliters of fluid to be irrigated through the anterior chamber during the course of a phacoemulsification. It has been found that normal saline solution causes significant toxicity to the corneal endothelium during irrigation. In rabbit eyes a 45-minute irrigation with either normal saline or BSS was associated with a twofold to fivefold delay in corneal clearing.[1–3] Dikstein and Maurice[4] developed glutathione bicarbonate Ringer's (GBR) solution by the addition of glutathione and adenosine to a bicarbonate Ringer's solution. This solution is associated with a lower corneal swelling rate than any previously developed solution (Fig. 17–5).[4–6] The GBR solution is in the reduced form and therefore unstable. Adenosine is also a labile compound. BSS Plus was developed by Alcon to avoid these stability problems. It contains stable oxidized glutathione and no adenosine. This solution is delivered as a two-part system mixed just before use, a stable pH being maintained for 24 hours using a bicarbonate buffer system.

Comparing BSS Plus with BSS in 100 extracapsular cataract extractions with posterior chamber intraocular lens implantation found a 15.4% endothelial cell loss with BSS Plus compared with a 22.7% cell loss with BSS. These differences were signifi-

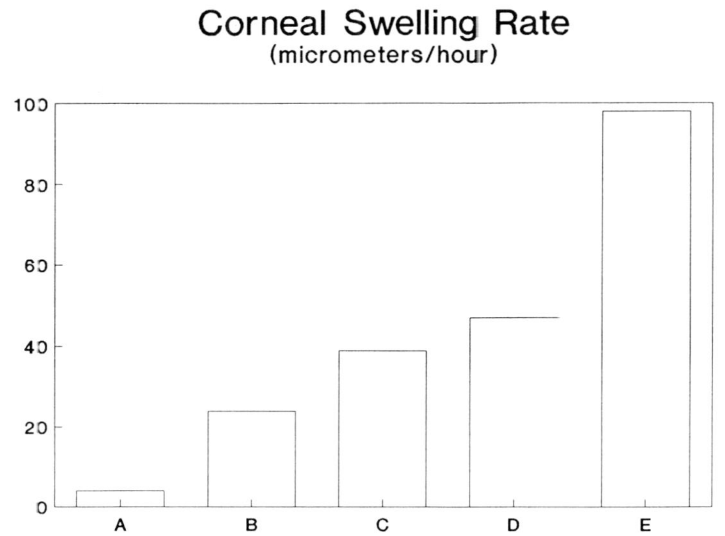


**FIG 17–5.**
Swelling rates of rabbit corneas perfused for 3 hours with *(A)* glutathione bicarbonate Ringer's, *(B)* BSS, *(C)* lactated Ringer's, *(D)* plasma-lyte 148, and *(E)* 0.9% NaCl. (Modified from Edelhauser HF, Van Horn DL, Schultz RO, and others: *Am J Ophthalmol* 81:473, 1976. Used by permission.)

**TABLE 17–3.**
Composition of Irrigating Solutions (mM/L)

| | Normal Saline | Lactated Ringer's | GBR | BSS | BSS Plus |
|---|---|---|---|---|---|
| Sodium chloride | 154 | 102 | 111.6 | 110 | 122.2 |
| Potassium chloride | | 4 | 4.8 | 10 | 5.08 |
| Magnesium chloride | | | 0.78 | 1.5 | 0.98 |
| Calcium chloride | | 3 | 1.1 | 0.3 | 1.05 |
| Sodium lactate | | 28 | | | |
| Sodium acetate | | | | 29 | |
| Sodium citrate | | | | 6 | |
| Sodium acid phosphate | | | 0.86 | | |
| Disodium phosphate | | | | | 3.0 |
| Sodium bicarbonate | | | 29.2 | | 25.0 |
| Dextrose | | | 5.01 | | 5.11 |
| Glutathione (reduced) | | | 0.30 | | |
| Glutathione (oxidized) | | | | | 0.30 |
| Adenosine | | | 0.50 | | |
| pH | 4.5–7.2 | 6.0–7.2 | 7.4 | 7.4 | 7.4 |
| Osmolality (mOsm) | 290 | 277 | 274 | 305 | 305 |

Modified from McDermott ML, Edelhauser HF, Hack HM, and others: *Ophthalmol Surg* 19:724, 1988. Used by permission.

cant. These endothelial counts were performed 6 months after surgery. Viscoelastic substances were not used in these surgeries.[7]

The barrier function of the corneal endothelium is an important measure of endothelial integrity. Both GBR solution and BSS Plus were found to cause less change in the endothelial barrier function than a citrate–acetate bicarbonate solution without glutathione (Table 17–3).[8]

A dextrose bicarbonate lactated Ringer's solution was compared with BSS Plus in eyes undergoing extracapsular cataract extraction with manual aspiration of the cortex. The corneal endothelial cells sizes were measured preoperatively and postoperatively no sooner than 2 months after surgery. There were no significant differences in the average endothelial cell sizes between the BSS Plus group and the dextrose bicarbonate lactated Ringer's group. There were, however, three patients in the dextrose bicarbonate lactated Ringer's group who had large increases in endothelial cell size. Although not specifically stated in the paper, one would predict a fairly low volume of irrigation considering that manual cortical removal was used and that greater volumes and longer irrigations (found with automated techniques) may be necessary to obtain the statistical differences noted in the animal models.[9]

To evaluate the effect of ocular irrigants on a fresh cornea transplant, stored corneas were perfused in irrigation solutions with measurement of corneal thickness during a 3-hour period. BSS was compared with BSS Plus. The corneas perfused in BSS Plus had a corneal swelling rate of 4 μm/hr, whereas the corneas perfused in BSS swelled at a rate of 26 μm/hr. This study indicates that corneas will be thinner if BSS Plus is left in the anterior chamber after cornea transplantation than if BSS were used. It does not take into account the effects of residual viscoelastics in the anterior chamber or the long-term significance of the intraocular irrigant.[10]

Intraocular irrigating solutions have been evaluated for use in pars plana vitrectomy. In aphakic eyes the irrigant solution is critical to the maintenance of corneal endothelium. Because of the large volumes of irrigation that occur during vitrectomy, BSS Plus should be used. In phakic eyes little difference can be found in the corneal endothelium after vitrectomy.[11, 12]

SECTION FOUR

## Vitreous Substitutes

Vitreous substitutes are used primarily in the reattachment of complicated proliferative vitreoretinopathy and traction retinal detachments associated with diabetic retinopathy. The ophthalmologist's enthusiasm for their use greatly exceeds the Food and Drug Administration's ability to evaluate these substances for approval; therefore, their use occurs investigationally. These agents, whether they be liquid or gaseous, are useful in tamponading the retina into position after membrane peeling as described by Machemer[1] in 1976.

## SILICONE OIL

Silicone oil has been used extensively in Europe and investigationally in the United States for the long-term reattachment of complicated retinal detachments. The oil may be used as a permanent vitreous replacement or temporarily in hopes of avoiding the long-term complications.[2] Animal studies and clinical experience have shown that vitreous substitutes, as well as other surgical maneuvers, are of little success if performed during the active phase of proliferative vitreoretinopathy.[3] If used in the proper clinical circumstance, silicone oil can greatly improve success rates in eyes that have failed standard treatment for retinal detachment and advanced proliferative vitreoretinopathy. An evaluation of 44 consecutive patients who had failed treatment of retinal detachment and proliferative vitreoretinopathy with standard therapy of vitrectomy, membrane peeling, and scleral buckling had successful anatomic retinal reattachment in 64% of the eyes. Forty-four percent of aphakic eyes and 30% of pseudophakic eyes developed corneal decompensation in this series of patients. The oil was removed in 69% of the successfully treated eyes without development of recurrent retinal detachment.[4] In another study, 51 consecutive patients with retinal detachment and advanced proliferative vitreoretinopathy who had failed standard treatment were treated with silicone oil. Sixty-five percent achieved anatomic reattachment of the retina.[5]

Giant retinal tears with proliferative vitreoretinopathy are one of the most difficult problems for the retinal surgeon to manage. Silicone oil was used to successfully reattach 18 of 19 eyes with giant retinal tears and proliferative vitreoretinopathy. Periretinal membranes recurred in all 18 eyes, and four had recurrent tractional retinal detachments develop.[6]

Silicone oil was used in the treatment of 10 patients with either rhegmatogenous retinal detachments with proliferative vitreoretinopathy or proliferative diabetic retinopathy. Three of these ten patients had retinal reattachment, with two patients regaining usable vision.[7] Many other studies demonstrated both the short- and long-term results of silicone oil in otherwise untreatable retinal detachments.[8–13] Silicone oil used during vitrectomy for patients with iris neovascularization have poor results related to the severe ischemic status of the eye.[14]

The density of silicone oil is less than that of vitreous, and therefore it is more useful in the treatment of superior retinal detachments than inferior ones. A higher-density fluorinated silicone oil was evaluated in a rabbit model and showed edema of the inner and outer retinal layers but was well tolerated clinically. These fluorosilicone oils have high viscosity and because they are newtonian liquids will be very difficult to pass through a small-gauge needle compared with sodium hyaluronate, which has nonnewtonian characteristics with lower viscosity at higher shear flow rates. Because of this characteristic, silicone and fluorosilicone oil are usually pumped into the vitreous rather than injected with a syringe.[15] Emulsification of silicone and fluorosilicone oil has been related to some of the ocular complications that have been seen. During emulsification, silicone and fluorosilicone droplets will develop between the body of the oil and the surrounding intraocular fluids or at the surfaces of intraocular tissues. These droplets may then migrate, entering into the anterior chamber, causing keratopathy and glaucoma. Low molecular weight components of silicone and fluorosilicone oils have also been linked to toxicity. These elements may be eliminated through solvent extraction.[16, 17] These factors, along with oil contamination, were found to have little long-term effect on in vitro human retinal pigment epithelial cells.

Proliferation of retinal pigment epithelial cells occurred despite different formulations of the silicone oil.[18, 19] Another evaluation of the effects of silicone oil emulsification was performed using in vivo rabbit eyes. The emulsified silicone oil was found to penetrate the inner retinal layer, causing epiretinal membrane formation after several weeks, whereas the nonemulsified oil produced no retinal toxicity during the 12 weeks in which the eyes were followed after intraocular injection.[20]

## Toxicity

Silicone oil has been found to adversely effect many intraocular tissues. It will cause cataract formation and corneal decompensation. It may fill the trabecular meshwork, causing glaucoma, or may lead to pupillary block. It has also been found in the retina being engulfed by Müller's cells. Epiretinal membranes may form at the surface of the silicone oil.[21] The electroretinogram (ERG) is masked by the presence of a large amount of silicone oil in the vitreous, but the ERG response will return after the silicone oil is removed. This result does not mean that the retina is not functional.[22, 23]

An eye that had silicone oil injection 12 years previously for a complicated retinal detachment was removed after perforation of the globe and migration of the encircling band. The eye was evaluated histopathologically, and silicone droplets were found throughout the eye, including the anterior chamber angle, iris, ciliary body, retina, and optic nerve.[24]

These toxic effects may occur from extraction of retinal and retinal-like substances, along with cholesterol from the intraocular tissues, as well as from the silicone and fluorosilicone oils. Cholesterol has been found in silicone oil removed from the vitreous of a human eye.[25] Ocular complications of silicone oil injection in 150 consecutive eyes included recurrent retinal detachments in 22% of eyes, pupillary block glaucoma in 3%, epiretinal and subretinal proliferations in 15%, and subconjunctival deposits of oil in 3%.[26] Cataracts developed in 100% of the phakic eyes after silicone oil injection. The cataracts were posterior subcapsular, occurring 3 to 6 months after surgery. Diabetic patients had cataract formation earlier than did nondiabetics. The aphakic patients with silicone oil to corneal endothelial touch had band keratopathy develop in every case. Similar to cataract formation, these changes were quicker to develop in the diabetic eye (3 months) than in the nondiabetic eye (5 months). An inferior iridectomy is recommended because the silicone oil is lighter than vitreous and would quickly plug a superior iridectomy. Fifteen of 105 inferior iridectomies (14.3%) closed, causing forward displacement of the oil. This was treated with removal of oil in 10 of 15 cases. Chronic uveitis developed in 6.7%, which might be related to the underlying ocular disease. Chronic increased intraocular pressure developed in 10% of the eyes, and 3.3% had pupillary block. The authors[27] of this report recommend removing the oil within 3 months of the initial procedure to limit the complications. The late complications of silicone oil are similar to those occurring early in the course and include cataract, glaucoma, keratopathy, and recurrent retinal detachment.[27] The optic nerve seems to tolerate intravitreal silicone oil well, as evaluated by electrophysiologic methods.[28]

A significant rise in intraocular pressure (>10 mm Hg) was found in 56% of 48 eyes receiving intravitreal silicone. Mechanisms for intraocular pressure rise include neovascular glaucoma, pupillary block, inflammation, phacolyses, corticosteroid responder, and hemorrhage or silicone oil.[29] Both Goldmann applanation tonometer and the Oculab Tono-Pen were found to be reliable measures of the intraocular pressure in silicone-filled eyes.[30] Patients developing glaucoma because of blocked inferior iridectomy may be treated by positioning the patient in a face-down position. These authors also recommend small iridectomies that are peripheral as a preventive measure.[31]

Two of 30 patients receiving silicone oil for complicated retinal detachment were found to have a marked postoperative hypopyon and anterior chamber fibrin. It is difficult to separate the underlying ocular disease, surgical treatment, and the possibil-

**TABLE 17–4.**
Vitreous Substitutes

| | Silicone[90] | Fluorosilicone[90] | Perfluorocarbons[114] | Sodium Hyaluronate |
|---|---|---|---|---|
| Viscosity (cp) | 1,000–12,500 | 1,000–10,000 | 0.8–2.7 | 40,000–64,000* |
| Specific gravity | 0.97 | 1.28–1.30 | 1.76–1.94 | 1.0084[45] |

*Sodium hyaluronate is a nonnewtonian fluid and has lower viscosity at higher shear rates.[21]

ity of impurities in the silicone oil as causes of this phenomenon. The condition resolved with aggressive topical corticosteroids; therefore, it was believed to be sterile inflammation.[32] A case of bacterial endophthalmitis has been reported in an eye filled with silicone oil for repair of a giant retinal tear. The organism was *Pseudomonas aeruginosa,* and despite removal of the silicone oil and instillation of gentamicin and cefazolin, the eye became blind. The infection was compartmentalized because of the silicone oil, and the authors postulate this may have resulted in a more severe necrosis of the retina than would ordinarily be expected in a postoperative endophthalmitis.[33]

Silicone oil keratopathy occurs eventually in every patient with silicone oil to endothelial touch. This has been evaluated in rabbit eyes, and in addition to endothelial thinning, the oil also causes increased permeability of the endothelium.[34] Ten patients evaluated with silicone oil keratopathy had corneal edema, corneal hypesthesia, endothelial opacification, band keratopathy, and peripheral corneal vascularization. Retrocorneal membrane formation also occurs.[35] Corneal transplantation was performed in 14 patients for silicone oil keratopathy. Silicone oil was removed at the time of corneal transplantation in eight of 14 eyes but left in the remaining six eyes. Graft rejections occurred in four patients. Graft failure was more frequent when the silicone oil was left in the eye (67%) than when it was removed (25%).[36]

If cataract extraction is to be performed in an eye with silicone oil replacing the vitreous, the intraocular lens calculation should be altered appropriately. Silicone oil, having a higher index of refraction than aqueous or vitreous, will decrease the effective power of the posterior surface of an intraocular lens, resulting in a hyperopic refraction if this is not accounted for.[37]

Many medical and nonmedical grades of silicone oil are available. It is a polymer of dimethylsiloxane. Obviously, a highly purified and sterile form of this substance is desirable. Viscosity may range from 1,000 to 12,500 cp (Table 17–4). Recommendations concerning specific silicone oil products are unclear and beyond the scope of this chapter.

## INTRAOCULAR GAS

Intravitreal gas may be used to temporarily tamponade the retina while subretinal fluid is reabsorbed and retinal-retinal pigment epithelial adhesions occur. Expansible gases persist longer in the vitreous than air and are usually preferred. Sulfur hexafluoride and perfluorocarbons (perfluoroethane; perfluoropropane) are the expansible gases in current use (Table 17–5). Complications may include elevated intraocular pressure and cataract. These may be more common with the higher expansible and longer duration gases. The gases are helpful in small superior breaks and in locations where the bubble can be located by head positioning in cooperative patients with or sometimes without vitrectomy.[38–41]

**TABLE 17–5.**
Expansile Gases

| Gas | Expansion | Duration (Days) |
|---|---|---|
| Air | 0 | 5–7 |
| Sulfur hexafluoride | 1.9–2.0 | 10–14 |
| Perfluoroethane | 3.3 | 30–35 |
| Perfluoropropane | 4.0 | 55–65 |

Modified from Chang S: Intraocular gases. In Ryan SJ, editor: *Retina,* 1989, Chicago, Mosby, p 247. Used by permission.

## PERFLUOROCARBON LIQUID

Another investigational substance for vitreous replacement is perfluorocarbon liquid. This class of compounds is characterized by a low viscosity and high specific gravity that allow injection into the vitreous and the settling of the substance inferiorly, flattening the retina (see Table 17–4). Once the retina is flattened, endolaser, epiretinal membrane stripping, and other retinal manipulations can be performed before removal of the liquid. Three examples of perfluorocarbon liquids include perfluorotributylamine, perfluoroctane, and perfluorodecalin with molecular weights of 671, 438, and 462 daltons, respectively. Specific gravities range from 1.76 to 1.94. Viscosities are remarkably low, ranging from 0.8 to 2.7 cp. Because these liquids are heavier than the vitreous, they can be used to elevate dislocated crystalline lenses, nuclei, and intraocular lens implants. Although small amounts of perfluorocarbon liquid have remained in human eyes after removal without severe side effects, animal models indicate retinal changes with long-term perfluorocarbon of the vitreous.[42, 43]

SECTION FIVE

# Tissue Adhesives

The primary tissue adhesive of ophthalmic interest is butyl-2-cyanoacrylate (Embucrilate). It has been found to be very useful in the closing of small corneal perforations. In an evaluation of 80 patients with either pending or full-thickness corneal perforations that were treated with either *N*-butyl-cyanoacrylate or isobutyl cyanoacrylate, 44% healed without surgery. The glue remained in place an average of 50 days. Complications that occurred included elevated intraocular pressure in two patients and bacterial corneal infiltrates in seven.[1] Even in patients with perforations deemed too extensive to allow long-term closure with cyanoacrylate, it can be used along with sodium hyaluronate to obtain a normotensive eye that can ease trephination before penetrating keratoplasty. This technique allows protection of the lens-iris diaphragm during trephination and would allow a more controlled trephination. By first deepening the anterior chamber with sodium hyaluronate or other viscoelastics, one can then apply the glue without adhering the cornea to the iris or the lens.[2]

In addition to its ability to seal small perforations, it has been found to have a modest bacteriostatic activity. This was most prominent against gram-positive organisms without any real effect against gram-negative organisms.[3]

Butyl-2-cyanoacrylate (Histoacryl) has been used to secure orbital implants in the repair of fractures of the orbital walls. It has been used successfully to adhere orbital implants without the use of wires.[4]

Complications of tissue adhesive use in perforated corneas include production of anterior synechiae because of gluing the cornea to the lens-iris diaphragm with a flat anterior chamber. Infectious corneal ulcers may occur as a result of the persistent foreign body and also the underlying corneal disease. Both bacterial and fungal keratitis have been reported after gluing. Close follow-up is necessary because the clinical signs and symptoms may be masked by the presence of the glue.[5] If possible, the tissue adhesive should be covered with a bandage soft contact lens; otherwise a superior tarsal conjunctivitis will form. This may take the appearance of a giant papillary conjunctivitis.[6]

A series of papers have been published describing the use of *N*-butyl-2-cyanoacrylate transvitreally in repair of rhegmatogenous retinal detachments. It has been used successfully in both animal models and human eyes.[7–10] Twenty-five eyes with complicated retinal detachments that failed traditional retinal surgery, including vitrectomy, membrane peeling, scleral buckling, and intraocular tamponade with gas or silicone oil, were treated with transvitreal cyanoacrylate. In these patients with advanced proliferative vitreoretinopathy, all but one had inferior retinal breaks that made them difficult to repair. As with corneal and conjunctival adhesion, it is important to have a dry surface with retinal adhesion, and this was accomplished through fluid aspiration during the procedure. A special microinjector was used to deliver small amounts of a combination cyanoacrylate and iophendylate to the site. Iophendylate was used to delay polymerization so that it occurred over 2 to 3 seconds, which was deemed to be manageable in this situation. The results of this technique showed retinal reattachment in 72% of eyes, with 40% of the eyes achieving usable vision. A localized inflammatory response was seen at the cyanoacrylate site in the animal models; however, no other ocular side effects were found, and the glue appeared to be tolerated well in the human.[10]

Cyanoacrylate may be used to anchor buckling elements into place over a thin sclera or to apply donor sclera or silicone in areas of staphylomas. This avoids the use of sutures in an area where perforation or suture "cheese wiring" may occur.[11]

Fibrin tissue adhesive has been used in Europe for many purposes, including treatment of corneal perforations.[12,13] Fibrin glue may be prepared from homologous blood. Fibrin glue was used to secure a fascia eye graft over an orbital fistula in a patient with previous blowout fracture. The fibrin adhesive is produced through the conversion of fibrinogen to fibrin polymer via thrombin in the presence of factor XIII. A double-barrel syringe is used with one barrel containing fibrinogen and factor XIII and the other containing thrombin and calcium chloride. Bonding occurs slowly within 2 minutes, and maximum strength occurs between 30 and 90 minutes. Similar to cyanoacrylate, the surface needs to be dry. Because of its slow bonding, this formulation would be difficult to use in corneal perforations, conjunctival bleb leaks, or repair of retinal detachments. It eventually resorbs, which makes it a good selection for orbital work.[12]

SECTION SIX

# Chelating Agents

## BRITISH ANTILEWISITE

British antilewisite (BAL, 2,3-dimercapto-1-propanol) is an effective antiarsenic agent that is of definite value in the treatment of various types of arsenic poisoning encountered in civilian practice, as well as in treatment of war gas casualties.[1] When used within 5 minutes after doses of lewisite sufficient to cause corneal perforation in 11 days, BAL treatment reduces corneal damage to only slight residual scarring. The longer the interval between lewisite burn and BAL application, the less effective is the therapeutic effect. Some benefit results from treatment as late as 30 minutes after the burn, but treatment after 1 hour is useless.[2]

Two drops of a 5% solution or 0.1 ml of 5% ointment provides a large excess of BAL over that required to react with whatever arsenic is likely to be in the eye. Three percent concentration is as effective as 5%. Ten percent preparations and prolonged irrigations have no demonstrable additional therapeutic effect. A second BAL instillation is desirable, however, to be certain that an adequate amount of medication actually enters the eye.

BAL is itself most irritating to the eye. A 5% solution or ointment will produce severe lacrimation and blepharospasm lasting from 2 to 5 minutes. Marked conjunctival injection lasts for 1 hour after the use of 5% solution of BAL. Ten percent preparations are more irritating but cause no permanent rabbit corneal damage. Concentrations of 20% or higher cause irreparable corneal scarring.

BAL is unstable in aqueous solution but is quite stable (no loss of therapeutic efficiency at room temperature for 6 weeks) in ethylene glycol solution or in ointment bases. Ointment and liquid preparations are equally effective therapeutically; however, from the practical standpoint, a gassed soldier can rub ointment into the eye much easier than instilling drops (e.g., ointment can even be rubbed into an eye while lying face down).[3] BAL is rapidly oxidized by iron or copper; hence, it cannot be dispensed in ordinary metal tubes.

Aqueous chamber concentrations of BAL as high as 0.1% may be attained within 5 minutes after the repeated application of a 5% BAL solution to the surface of rabbit eyes.[4] Aqueous solutions penetrate two to four times more effectively than do ointment preparations. Unfortunately, aqueous solutions are too unstable to be of practical value.

The arsenical war gas lewisite rapidly penetrates the cornea and can be demonstrated in the aqueous within 2 minutes. Ten minutes after exposure, irreversible corneal changes can already be detected. A single instillation of a 5% BAL solution or ointment within 2 to 5 minutes after exposure to lewisite will prevent this corneal destruction.[5]

Two percent sodium bicarbonate solution (1 teaspoon in a glass of water) is said to be helpful as an immediate first-aid treatment for eye burns by war gases such as lewisite or phosgene.[6] This is, of course, not nearly as effective as a specific antidote such as BAL but has the advantage of availability.

Hydrogen peroxide and potassium permanganate have also been recommended for lewisite poisoning but are definitely less effective than BAL.

## DESFERRIOXAMINE

Desferrioxamine mesylate (Desferal) is a potent and specific iron-chelating agent capable of forming a highly stable bond with ferric ions. Because it is a relatively nontoxic chemical, it may be used clinically for selective removal of pathologic iron deposits from the tissues of the body.

### Mechanism of Action

Apparently intraocular iron is toxic by liberation of iron ions that diffuse to the cells, combine with vital enzymes, and thereby destroy the more sensitive cells (e.g., of the retina). More resistant cells (e.g., uveal cells) may detoxify and store the iron. Ultimately the iron becomes firmly bound in the form of nontoxic siderin pigments.

Desferrioxamine acts by chelating free iron ions or those that may be loosely attached to the acid mucopolysaccharides of the vitreous. Such chelation of free (toxic) iron will prevent inactivation of vital intracellular enzymes. Desferrioxamine cannot liberate iron from the secure binding of hemosiderin, hemoglobin, or siderin pigments (nontoxic). Cells already dead from enzyme destruction will not be revived by desferrioxamine.

### Ocular Toxicity

No toxic effects result from topical ocular application of 10% desferrioxamine in 0.5% methylcellulose. Solutions of 20% or greater strength are irritating and cause conjunctival chemosis.[7]

Subconjunctival injection of as much as 100 mg does not damage the rabbit eye, but a dose of 200 mg causes uveal congestion and exudative detachment of the retina. Daily subconjunctival injection of 50 mg to a total of 2,000 mg did not cause intraocular damage.[8]

As much as 6 mg may safely be injected into the anterior chamber; however, as little as 3 mg injected intravitreally causes retinal necrosis and hemorrhagic destruction of the uveal tract.

### Ocular Penetration

The transcorneal penetration of desferrioxamine B is poor, producing an aqueous concentration of less than 30 ppm after topical instillation of 25% solution. Although higher levels are reached by subconjunctival injection, this route of administration is difficult for a drug requiring frequent dosage. Actually, because the prognosis of ocular siderosis is dependent primarily on the toxic effect of iron on the retina, and because intramuscular injection is the only practical method of obtaining therapeutically effective retinal drug concentrations, intraocular siderosis probably cannot be treated by topical application of desferrioxamine. In contrast, an effective drug concentration can easily be achieved on the cornea surface, as would be needed to remove rust staining from superficial foreign bodies.

### Clinical Use

Nonsurgical chemical removal of iron stains is applicable to the treatment of small corneal rust stains.[7] Experimental corneal rust stains were produced binocularly in 50 rabbits by embedding a 500-mg iron filing for 10 hours in each cornea. Ten percent desferrioxamine was instilled in the right eye of each animal four times daily. In all but one rabbit, visible rust staining was eliminated within 2 weeks. The rust stains of 95% of the control eyes persisted unchanged for periods up to 40 days.

Another obvious application of this drug would seem to be in the treatment of corneal bloodstaining. However, unpublished data indicate that experimental iron staining of the rabbit cornea does not clear more rapidly with desferrioxamine treatment.[9]

### Therapeutic Results

Experimental vitreous hemorrhage was not benefited by subconjunctival injection of 25 mg of desferrioxamine every 3 days for 10 weeks. There was no difference in rate of clearing of the vitreous or in the incidence of retinal detachment in treated or untreated eyes.[9] The problem of a ferrous intraocular foreign body was studied by introduction of a 2-mm iron wire into the rabbit vitreous, with subsequent treatment by subconjunctival injection of 25 mg of desferrioxamine every 3 days for 6 months. Desferrioxamine treatment prevented the development of siderosis, as evidenced by normal clinical appearance, absence of rust, normal ERG findings, and minimal histologic evidence of stainable iron.

A case report outlines the course of a patient with ocular siderosis treated with systemic desferrioxamine for almost 1 year.[10] The foreign body was deeply embedded and could not be removed surgically. The average daily dosage of desferrioxamine B was 500 mg given intramuscularly. The effectiveness of the drug was demonstrated by measuring urinary iron excretion, which was 366 μg daily without treatment but increased to 2,266 μg daily with treatment. Topical application only of 5% desferrioxamine ointment four times daily increased iron excretion to 1,100 μg daily. Both systemic and topical routes of administration were used. Visual acuity remained approximately 20/50 during the period of treatment, and the already subnormal ERG findings did not indicate further deterioration. The dark brown siderotic iris became normal in color and the dilated pupil returned to normal size.

If the cause of a discolored and possibly siderotic iris is uncertain, a diagnostic "Desferal test" may be of value. Apparently, intramuscular injection of 500 mg of desferrioxamine greatly increases urinary iron excretion if pathologic amounts of iron exist anywhere in the body. Normally the daily urinary excretion of iron after such an injection will not exceed 1 mg. Higher values would indicate the iris discoloration was siderotic, providing no other iron abnormality was present in the patient.

Perhaps a period of desferrioxamine B treatment should be considered after surgical removal of a foreign body if recognizable siderosis is present. Such therapy might prevent further retinal damage from the action of ferric salts remaining within the eye. Although of considerable theoretical interest, desferrioxamine seems of limited value in ocular therapy. The removal of a magnetic intraocular foreign body is more practicable than long-term repeated injections.

Solutions of desferrioxamine B lose their chelating properties rapidly; however, ointments are stable for at least 6 months.

Deferoxamine is relatively nontoxic and may be given in doses as high as 5 $g/m^2$. In cases of iron overload from transfusion, this will mobilize up to 90 mg of iron daily.[11]

## ETHYLENEDIAMINETETRAACETIC ACID

Ethylenediaminetetraacetic acid (EDTA, edathamil) is a chelating agent with a high affinity for many metals. This affinity may be clinically useful in the removal of toxic alkalies from the cornea.[12]

Irrigation of the human cornea for periods of 15 to 20 minutes with a 0.01M solution of sodium EDTA at pH 8.0 does not cause recognizable ocular damage. As much as 100 ml or more may be used during this period of irrigation. The corneal epithelium should be mechanically scraped off before irrigation with EDTA. Concentrations as strong as 0.1M, pH 7.5, are definitely irritating, causing stromal edema, which lasts for several days. Experimentally, this treatment demonstrably reduces the toxic effect of beryllium, yttrium, lanthanum, thorium, nickel, copper, silver, and mercury. Evidence that metal has actually been removed from the cornea by EDTA treatment has been obtained by assay. For instance, EDTA-bathed corneas retained only one fourth as much yttrium as corneas bathed in the same manner with physiologic saline solution.[12]

The disodium salt of EDTA may also be used to dissolve calcific deposits within Bowman's membrane (e.g., band keratopathy). Because EDTA does not penetrate the intact corneal epithelium, it must be mechanically scraped off before application of the chelating agent. Prolonged irrigation (20 minutes) with 0.37% solution will visibly dissolve these calcific changes. Because no delayed benefit accrues, the desired amount of clearing must be achieved at the time of treatment.[13–16]

Although some reports imply that chelation will rapidly dissolve the calcific plaque, the actual removal of a band may be much more difficult than this. In one case, 400 ml of EDTA was irrigated on the cornea for an entire hour, accompanied by massage with an applicator stick and scraping with a knife.[17]

Zinc chloride, the flux used in soldering, causes severe corneal damage by rapid tissue fixation. Chelation with EDTA will bind zinc ions and minimize tissue damage but only if applied within 2 minutes. Beyond this time, chelation is no more effective than washing with normal saline solution.[18]

A study of corneal toxicity showed a diffuse ground-glass stromal opacity resulting from four times daily instillation of a 0.2M solution of calcium disodium EDTA on corneas denuded of epithelium. This drug, as well as acetylcysteine, may be used to inhibit continuing destruction of an ulcerated cornea by collagenase. Under these circumstances, corneal scarring is expected as a sequel to the disease but could also be attributable to the treatment. Topical 20% acetylcysteine also caused stromal haze but to a lesser extent than resulted from the EDTA.[19]

Intramuscular injection of EDTA into pregnant rats causes gross malformations of the offspring. Because this embryopathy can be prevented by dietary zinc supplementation, zinc chelation with resultant deficiency is presumed to be the cause of the teratogenic effect.[20]

## PENICILLAMINE

Penicillamine is a chelating agent for copper, mercury, zinc, and lead that may be used to treat toxicity from these metals. Penicillamine can give excellent results in Wilson's hepatolenticular degeneration, not only preventing its ravages but actually resulting in clinical improvement.

Another possible use for this drug stems from its ability to prevent cross-linking of collagen fibers. Such cross-linkage is the basis for the tensile strength of collagen. Experimental intravitreal injection of 2 mg of penicillamine in the treatment of rabbit eyes with a double-perforating injury resulted in less dense vitreal scarring and band formation.[21]

## REFERENCES

### SECTION ONE


1. Thorpe HE: Enzymatic zonulolysis, *Am J Ophthalmol* 49:531, 1960.
2. Watts Jr LR, Margin CJ: Stability of alpha chymotrypsin, *Trans Am Acad Ophthalmol* 64:17, 1960.
3. Barraquer J, Troutman RC, Rutlan J: *Surgery of the anterior segment of the eye,* vol 1, New York, 1964, McGraw-Hill.
4. Bedrossian RH, Lalli RA: Clinical application of new laboratory data on alpha-chymotrypsin, *Arch Ophthalmol* 67:616, 1962.
5. Ley AP, Holmberg AS, Yamashita T: Histology of zonulolysis with alpha-chymotrypsin employing light and electron microscopy, *Am J Ophthalmol* 49:67, 1960.
6. Geeraets WJ, Chan G, Gueery D: The effect of alpha-chymotrypsin on zonular fibers and anterior hyaloid membrane, *Guildcraft,* September 1960, p 35.

7. Hogan MJ, Zimmerman LE: *Ophthalmic pathology*, ed 2, Philadelphia, 1962, WB Saunders.
8. Sekiguchi J: Histological studies on the ocular toxicity of alpha-chymotrypsin, *Jpn J Ophthalmol* 4:104, 1960.
9. O'Malley C, Moskovitz M, Straatsman B: Experimentally induced adverse effects of alpha-chymotrypsin, *Arch Ophthalmol* 66:539, 1961.
10. Bedrossian RH, Weimar V: Inhibitory effect of aqueous humor on alpha-chymotrypsin, *Trans Am Acad Ophthalmol* 67:822, 1963.
11. Scheie HG, Yanoff M, Tsou KC: Inhibition of alpha-chymotrypsin by aqueous humor, *Arch Ophthalmol* 73:399, 1965.
12. Barraquer J: Enzymatic zonulolysis in lens extraction, *Arch Ophthalmol* 66:32, 1961.
13. Kirsch RE: Glaucoma following cataract extraction associated with use of alpha-chymotrypsin, *Arch Ophthalmol* 72:612, 1964.
14. Kirsch RE: Dose relationship of alpha-chymotrypsin in production of glaucoma after cataract extraction, *Arch Ophthalmol* 75:774, 1966.
15. Anderson DR: Scanning electron microscopy of zonulolysis by alpha-chymotrypsin, *Am J Ophthalmol* 71:619, 1971.
16. Worthen DM: Scanning electron microscopy after alpha-chymotrypsin perfusion in man, *Am J Ophthalmol* 73:637, 1972.
17. Chee P, Hamasaki DI: The basis for chymotrypsin-induced glaucoma, *Arch Ophthalmol* 85:103, 1971.
18. Kirsch RE: Further studies on glaucoma following cataract extraction associated with the use of alpha-chymotrypsin, *Trans Am Acad Ophthalmol* 69:1011, 1965.


## SECTION TWO


1. Arshinoff SA: Comparative physical properties of ophthalmic viscoelastic materials, *Curr Can Ophthalmic Pract* 7:1, 1989.
2. *PDR for ophthalmology 1992. Medical economics data*, Montvale, NJ, 1992.
3. Liesegang TJ: Viscoelastic substances in ophthalmology, *Surv Ophthalmol* 34:268, 1990.
4. Miller D, O'Connor P, Williams J: Use of Na-hyaluronate during intraocular lens implantation in rabbits, *Ophthalmic Surg* 8:58, 1977.
5. Balazs EA: Ultrapure hyaluronic acid and the use thereof, US patent no 4. 141.973, 1973. Oct 17, 1979.
6. Miller D, Stegmann R: Use of Na-hyaluronate in anterior segment eye surgery, *Am Int Implant Soc* 66:13, 1980.
7. Holmberg AS, Philipson BT: Sodium hyaluronate in cataract surgery: I. Report on the use of Healon in two different types of intracapsular cataract surgery, *Ophthalmology* 91:45, 1984.
8. Holmberg AS, Philipson BT: Sodium hyaluronate in cataract surgery: II. Report on the use of Healon in extracapsular cataract surgery using phacoemulsifications, *Ophthalmology* 91:53, 1984.
9. Rappazzo JA, Ho KF, Waltman SR: Sodium hyaluronate use during lens expression in extracapsular cataract surgery in rabbits, *Ophthalmic Surg* 15:123, 1984.
10. Bourne WM, Liesgang TJ, Waller RR, and others: The effect of sodium hyaluronate on endothelial cell damage during extracapsular cataract extraction and posterior chamber lens implantation, *Am J Ophthalmol* 98:759, 1984.
11. Alpar JJ: Endothelial cell loss in different non-automated extracapsular nuclear evacuation techniques and the role of sodium hyaluronate, *Ophthalmic Surg* 17:719, 1986.
12. Alpar JJ: Use of Healon in different cataract surgery techniques: endothelial cell count study, *Ophthalmic Surg* 18:529, 1987.
13. Kim HJ: Intraocular inflammation of denatured viscoelastic substance in cases of cataract extraction and lens implantation, *J Cataract Refract Surg* 13:537, 1987.
14. Ohguro N, Matsuda M, Kinoshita S: The effects of denatured sodium hyaluronate on the corneal endothelium in cats, *Am J Ophthalmol* 112:424, 1991.
15. Reed DB, Mills JF, Mannis MJ, and others: Corneal epithelial healing after penetrating keratoplasty using topical Healon versus balanced salt solution, *Ophthalmic Surg* 18:525, 1987.
16. Wysenbeek YS, Loya N, Sira IB, and others: The effect of sodium hyaluronate on the corneal epithelium, *Invest Ophthalmol Vis Sci* 29:194, 1988.
17. Stuart JC, Lin JG: Dilute sodium hyaluronate (Healon) in the treatment of ocular surface disorders, *Ann Ophthalmol* 17:190, 1985.
18. Nelson JD, Farris RL: Sodium hyaluronate and polyvinyl alcohol artificial tear preparation. A comparison in patients with

keratoconjunctivitis sicca, *Arch Ophthalmol* 106:484, 1988.
19. Rosen E, Wright G: Use of sodium hyaluronate as a goniogel, *Cataract* 1:7, 1984.
20. Alpar JJ: The use of Healon in corneal transplant surgery with and without intraocular lenses, *Ophthalmic Surg* 15:758, 1984.
21. Guss RB, Koenig SB, Berkowitz RA, and others: Use of sodium hyaluronate (Healon), *J Ocular Ther Surg* 2:224, 1983.
22. Toczolowski JR: The use of sodium hyaluronate (Healon) for the removal of severely subluxated lenses, *Ophthalmic Surg* 18:214, 1987.
23. Stegmann R, Miller D: Use of sodium hyaluronate in severe penetrating ocular trauma, *Ann Ophthalmol* 18:9, 1986.
24. Drews RL: Sodium hyaluronate (Healon) in the repair of perforating injuries of the eye, *Ophthalmic Surg* 17:23, 1986.
25. Donzis PB, Karioglu ZA, Insler MS: Sodium hyaluronate (Healon) in the surgical repair of Descemet's membrane detachment, *Ophthalmic Surg* 17:735, 1986.
26. Graether JM: Detachment of Descemet's membrane by injection of sodium hyaluronate (Healon), *J Ocular Ther Surg* 3:178, 1984.
27. Brown GC, Benson WE: Use of sodium hyaluronate for the repair of giant retinal tears, *Arch Ophthalmol* 107:1246, 1989.
28. Folk JC, Weingeist TA, Packer AJ, and others: Sodium hyaluronate (Healon) in closed vitrectomy, *Ophthalmic Surg* 17:299, 1986.
29. Packer AJ, McCuen BW, Hutton WL, and others: Procoagulant effects of intraocular sodium hyaluronate (Healon) after phakic diabetic vitrectomy, *Ophthalmology* 96:1491, 1989.
30. Portis JM, Verne A, Milton GF: Sodium hyaluronate, *Am J Ophthalmol* 101:788, 1986.
31. Lerner HA, Boynton JR: Sodium hyaluronate (Healon) as an adjunct to lacrimal surgery, *Am J Ophthalmol* 99:365, 1985.
32. Searl SS, Metz JS, Lindahl KJ: The use of sodium hyaluronate as a biologic-sleeve in strabismus surgery, *Ann Ophthalmol* 19:259, 1987.
33. Alpar JJ, Alpar AJ, Baca J, and others: Comparison of Healon and viscoat in cataract extraction and intraocular lens implantation, *Ophthalmic Surg* 19:636, 1988.
34. Barron BA, Busin M, Page C, and others: Comparison of the effects of viscoat and Healon on postoperative intraocular pressure, *Am J Ophthalmol* 100:377, 1985.
35. Glasser DB, Katz HR, Boyd JE, and others: Protective effects of viscous solutions in phacoemulsification and traumatic lens implantation, *Arch Ophthalmol* 107:1047, 1989.
36. Hedner MP: The effect of sodium hyaluronate and sodium chondroitin sulfate on the coagulation system in vitro, *Ophthalmology* 91:864, 1984.
37. Coffmar MR, Mann PM: Corneal subepithelial deposits after use of sodium chondroitin, *Am J Ophthalmol* 102:279, 1986.
38. Binder PS, Deg JK, Kohl S: Elastic bond keratopathy after intraocular chondroitin sulfate, *Arch Ophthalmol* 105:1243, 1987.
39. Bourne WM, Lindstrom RL, Doughman DJ: Endothelial cell survival on transplanted human corneas preserved by organ culture with 13.5% chondroitin sulfate, *Am J Ophthalmol* 100:789, 1985.
40. Stein RM, Bourne WM, Campbell J: Chondroitin sulfate for corneal preservation at 4° C, *Arch Ophthalmol* 104:1358, 1986.
41. Keates RH, Robin B: Extending corneal storage with 2.5% chondroitin sulfate (K-sol), *Ophthalmic Surg* 19:817, 1988.
42. Lass JH, Reinhart WJ, Skelnik DL, and others: An in vitro and clinical comparison of corneal storage with chondroitin sulfate corneal storage medium with and without dextran, *Ophthalmology* 97:96, 1990.
43. Wlakenbach RJ, Corwin JG, Ye G: Corneal functions after storage in commercial eye bank medium, *Invest Ophthalmol Vis Sci* 32:1551, 1991.
44. Liesegang TJ, Bourne WM, Ilstrap DM: The use of hydroxypropyl methylcellulose in extracapsular lens implantation, *Am J Ophthalmol* 102:723, 1986.
45. McDermott ML, Edelhauser HF: Drug binding of ophthalmic viscoelastic agents, *Arch Ophthalmol* 107:261, 1989.

## SECTION THREE

1. McDermott ML, Edelhauser HF, Hack HM, and others: Ophthalmic irrigants: a current review and update, *Ophthalmic Surg* 19:724, 1988.
2. Harper JY, Pomerat CM: In vitro observations on the behavior of conjunctival and

corneal cells in relation to electrolytes, *Am J Ophthalmol* 96:269, 1958.

3. Merrill JK, Flemming TC, Gerard LJ: The effects of physiologic balanced salt solution and normal saline on intraocular and extraocular tissues, *Am J Ophthalmol* 49:895, 1960.
4. Dikstein S, Maurice DM: The metabolic basis to the fluid pump in the cornea, *J Physiol* 221:29, 1972.
5. McCarey BE, Edelhauser HF, Van Horn DL: Functional and structural changes in the corneal endothelium during in vitro perfusion, *Invest Ophthalmol* 12:410, 1973.
6. Edelhauser HF, Van Horn DL, Schultz RO, and others: Comparative toxicity of intraocular irrigating solutions on the corneal endothelium, *Am J Ophthalmol* 81:473, 1976.
7. Kline OR, Symes DJ, Lorenzetti OJ, and others: Effect of BSS Plus on the corneal endothelium with intraocular lens implantation, *J Toxical Cutan Ocular Toxicol* 2:243, 1983.
8. Araie M: Barrier function of corneal endothelium and the intraocular irrigating solutions, *Arch Ophthalmol* 104:435, 1986.
9. Kramer KK, Thomassen R, Evaul J: Intraocular irrigating solutions: a chemical study of BSS Plus and dextrose bicarbonate lactated Ringer's solution, *Ann Ophthalmol* 23:101, 1991.
10. McDermott HM, Snyder R, Slack J, and others: Effects of intraocular irrigants on the preserved human corneal endothelium, *Cornea* 10:402, 1991.
11. Rosenfeld SI, Waltman SR, Olk J, and others: Comparisons of intraocular irrigating solutions in pars plana vitrectomy, *Ophthalmology* 93:109, 1986.
12. Matsuda M, Tano Y, Edelhauser HF: Comparison of intraocular irrigating solutions used for pars plana vitrectomy and prevention of endothelial cell loss, *Jpn J Ophthalmol* 28:230, 1984.

## SECTION FOUR

1. Machemer R: Massive periretinal proliferation: a logical approach to therapy, *Trans Am Ophthalmol Soc* 75:556, 1977.
2. Gonovers M: Temporary silicone oil tamponade in the management of retinal detachment with proliferative vitreoretinopathy, *Am J Ophthalmol* 100:239, 1985.
3. Fastenberg DM, Diddie KR, Delmage JM, and others: Intraocular injection of silicone oil for experimental proliferative vitreoretinopathy, *Am J Ophthalmol* 95:663, 1983.
4. McCuen BW, Linders MB, Machemer R: The use of silicone oil following failed vitrectomy for retinal detachment with advanced proliferative vitreoretinopathy, *Ophthalmology* 92:1029, 1985.
5. Cox MS, Trese MT, Murphy PL: Silicone oil for advanced proliferative vitreoretinopathy, *Ophthalmology* 93:646, 1986.
6. Glaser BM: Treatment of giant retinal tears combined with proliferative vitreoretinopathy, *Ophthalmology* 93:1193, 1986.
7. Rinkoff JS, deJuan E, McCuen BW: Silicone oil for retinal detachment with advanced proliferative vitreoretinopathy following failed vitrectomy for proliferative diabetic retinopathy, *Am J Ophthalmol* 101:181, 1986.
8. Laqua H, Lucke K, Foerster M: Results of silicone oil surgery, *Jpn J Ophthalmol* 31:124, 1987.
9. Yeo JH, Glaser BM, Michels RG: Silicone oil in the treatment of complicated retinal detachments, *Ophthalmology* 94:1109, 1987.
10. Sell CH, McCuen BW, Linders MB, and others: Long-term results of successful vitrectomy with silicon oil for advanced proliferative vitreoretinopathy, *Am J Ophthalmol* 103:24, 1987.
11. Lucke KH, Foester MH, Laqua H: Long-term results of vitrectomy and silicone oil in 500 cases of complicated retinal detachments, *Am J Ophthalmol* 104:624, 1982.
12. Antoszyk AN, McCuen BW, deJuan E, and others: Silicone oil injection after failed primary vitreous surgery in severe ocular trauma, *Am J Ophthalmol* 107:537, 1989.
13. Zilis JD, McCuen BW, deJuan E, and others: Effects of silicone oil removal in advanced proliferative vitreoretinopathy, *Am J Ophthalmol* 108:15, 1989.
14. McCuen BW, Rinkoff JS: Silicone oil for progressive anterior ocular neovascularization after failed diabetic vitrectomy, *Arch Ophthalmol* 107:677, 1989.
15. Miyamoto K, Refajo MF, Tolentine FI, and others: Fluorinated oils as experimental vitreous substitutes, *Arch Ophthalmol* 104:1053, 1986.
16. Nakamura K, Refajo MF, Crabtree DV: Fac-

tors contributing to the emulsification of intraocular silicone and fluorosilicone, *Invest Ophthalmol Vis Sci* 31:647, 1990.

17. Nakamura K, Refajo MF, Crabtree DV, and others: Analysis and fractionation of silicone and fluorosilicone oils for intraocular use, *Invest Ophthalmol Vis Sci* 31:2059, 1990.
18. Lembrov FM, Burke JM, Aaberg TM: Effect of silicone oil on experimental traction retinal detachment, *Arch Ophthalmol* 105:1269, 1987.
19. Friberg TR, Verstraeten TC, Wilcox DK: Effects of emulsification, purity, and fluorination of silicone oil on human retinal pigment epithelial cells, *Invest Ophthalmol Vis Sci* 32:2030, 1991.
20. Ohira A, Wilson GA, deJuan E, and others: Experimental retinal tolerance to emulsified silicone oil, *Retina* 11:259, 1991.
21. Suzuki M, Okada T, Takevchi S, and others: Effect of silicone oil on ocular tissue, *Jpn J Ophthalmol* 35:282, 1991.
22. Foerster MH, Esser J, Laqua H: Silicone oil and its influence on electrophysiologic findings, *Am J Ophthalmol* 99:201, 1985.
23. Doslak MJ: A theoretical study of the effect of silicone oil on the electroretinogram, *Invest Ophthalmol Vis Sci* 29:1881, 1988.
24. Ni C, Want W, Albert DM, and others: Intravitreous silicone injection histopathologic findings in a human eye after 12 years, *Arch Ophthalmol* 101:1399, 1983.
25. Refago MF, Leong F, Chung H, and others: Extraction of retinal and cholesterol by intraocular silicone oil, *Ophthalmology* 95:614, 1988.
26. Federman JL, Schubert HD: complications associated with the use of silicone oil in 150 eyes with retina-vitreous surgery, *Ophthalmology* 95:870, 1988.
27. Chan C, Okun E: The question of ocular tolerance to intravitreal liquid silicone. A long-term analysis, *Ophthalmology* 93:651, 1986.
28. Kellner V, Lucke K, Foerster MH: Effect of intravitreal liquid silicone on optic nerve function, *Am J Ophthalmol* 106:293, 1988.
29. de Correl LR, Cohen SB, Peyman GA: Effect of intravitreal silicone oil on intraocular pressure, *Ophthalmic Surg* 18:446, 1987.
30. Alfaro DV, Tran VT: A clinical comparison of oculab Tono-Pen with the Goldmann applanation tonometer in eyes filled with silicone oil, *Retina* 11:219, 1991.
31. Bartov E, Huna R, Ashkenazi I, and others: Identification, prevention, and treatment of silicone oil pupillary block after an inferior iridectomy, *Am J Ophthalmol* 111:501, 1991.
32. Johnson RN, Flynn HW, Parel J, and others: Transient hypopyon with marked anterior chamber fibrin following pars plana vitrectomy and silicone oil injection, *Arch Ophthalmol* 107:683, 1989.
33. Chong LP, deJuan E, McCuen BW, and others: Endophthalmitis in a silicone oil filled eye, *Am J Ophthalmol* 102:660, 1986.
34. Norman BC, Oliver J, Cheeks L, and others: Corneal endothelial permeability after anterior chamber silicone oil, *Ophthalmology* 97:1671, 1990.
35. Foulks GN, Hatchell DL, Proia AD, and others: Histopathology of silicone oil keratopathy in humans, *Cornea* 10:29, 1991.
36. Noorily SW, Foulks GN, McCuen BW: Results of penetrating keratoplasty associated with silicone oil retinal tamponade, *Ophthalmology* 98:1186, 1991.
37. McCartney DL, Miller KM, Stark WJ, and others: Intraocular lens style and refraction in eyes treated with silicone oil, *Arch Ophthalmol* 105:1385, 1987.
38. Lincoff HA, Mardirossian J, Lincoff A, and others: Intravitreal longevity of three perfluorocarbon gases, *Arch Ophthalmol* 98:1610, 1980.
39. Chang S, Lincoff HA, Coleman DJ, and others: Perfluorocarbon gases in vitreous surgery, *Ophthalmology* 92:651, 1985.
40. Chang S: Intraocular gases. In Ryan SJ, editor: *Retina,* St Louis, 1989, Mosby, pp 245–259.
41. Bochow TW, Olk RJ, Hershey JM: Pneumatic retinopathy perfluoroethane ($C_2F_6$) in the treatment of rhegmatogenous retinal detachment, *Arch Ophthalmol* 110:1723, 1992.
42. Shapira MJ, Resnick KI, Kim SH, and others: Management of the dislocated crystalline lens with perfluorocarbon liquid, *Am J Ophthalmol* 112:401, 1991.
43. Chang S, Ozmert E, Zimmerman NJ: Intraoperative perfluorocarbon liquids in the management of proliferative vitreoretinopathy, *Am J Ophthalmol* 106:668, 1988.

## SECTION FIVE

1. Weiss JL, Williams P, Lindstrom RL, and others: The use of tissue adhesion in cor-

neal perforations, *Ophthalmology* 90:610, 1983.

2. Maguen E, Nesburn AB, Macy JI: Combined use of sodium hyaluronate and tissue adhesive in penetrating keratoplasty of corneal perforations, *Ophthalmic Surg* 15:55, 1984.
3. Eiferman RA, Snyder JW: Antibacterial effect of cyanoacrylate glue, *Arch Ophthalmol* 10:958, 1983.
4. Tse DT: Cyanoacrylate tissue adhesion in securing orbital implants, *Ophthalmic Surg* 17:577, 1986.
5. Cavanaugh TB, Gottsch JD: Infectious keratitis and cyanoacrylate adhesive, *Am J Ophthalmol* 111:466, 1991.
6. Carlson AN, Wilhelmis KR: Giant papillary conjunctivitis associated with cyanoacrylate glue, *Am J Ophthalmol* 104:437, 1982.
7. McCuen BW, Hida T, Sheta SM, and others: Experimental transvitreal cyanoacrylate retinopexy, *Am J Ophthalmol* 102:195, 1986.
8. Sheta SM, Hida T, McCuen BW: Experimental transvitreal cyanoacrylate retinopexy through silicone oil, *Am J Ophthalmol* 102:717, 1986.
9. Hida T, Sheta SM, Proia AD, and others: Experimental transvitreal cyanoacrylate retinopexy in a primate model, *Am J Ophthalmol* 103:1987.
10. McCuen BW, Hida T, Sheta SM: Transvitreal cyanoacrylate retinopexy in the management of complicated retinal detachment, *Am J Ophthalmol* 104:127, 1987.
11. Folk JC, Dreyer RF: Cyanoacrylate adhesive in retinal detachment surgery, *Am J Ophthalmol* 101:486, 1986.
12. Bartley GB, McCaftrey TV: Cryoprecipitated fibrinogen (fibrin glue) in orbital surgery, *Am J Ophthalmol* 109:227, 1990.
13. Lagoutte FM, Gauthier L, Comte PRM: A fibrin sealant for perforated and preperforated corneal ulcers, *Br J Ophthalmol* 73:757, 1989.

## SECTION SIX

1. Leopold IH, Adler FH: Specific treatment of ocular burns due to lewisite (β-chlorovinyldichloroarsine), *Arch Ophthalmol* 38:174, 1947.
2. Adler FH, Fry WE, Leopold IH: Pathologic study of ocular lesions due to lewisite (β-chlorovinyldichloroarsine), *Arch Ophthalmol* 38:89, 1947.
3. Mann I, Pirie A, Pullinger BD: The treatment of lewisite and other arsenical vesicant lesions of the eyes of rabbits with British anti-Lewisite (BAL), *Am J Ophthalmol* 30:421, 1947.
4. Leopold IH, Steele WH: Penetration of locally applied BAL into the anterior chamber of the rabbit eye, *Arch Ophthalmol* 38:192, 1947.
5. Hughes WF: Treatment of lewisite burns of the eye with dimercaprol (BAL), *Arch Ophthalmol* 37:25, 1947.
6. Cordes FC: Nonsurgical aspects of ocular war injuries, *Am J Ophthalmol* 26:1062, 1943.
7. Galin MA, Harris LS, Papariello GJ: Nonsurgical removal of corneal rust stains, *Arch Ophthalmol* 74:674, 1965.
8. Wise JB: Treatment of experimental siderosis bulbi, vitreous hemorrhage and corneal bloodstaining with deferoxamine, *Arch Ophthalmol* 75:698, 1966.
9. Bollheimer D: Personal communication, 1965.
10. Valvo A: Desferrioxamine B in ophthalmology, *Am J Ophthalmol* 63:98, 1967.
11. Blume KG, Beutler E, Chillar RK, and others: Continuous intravenous deferoxamine infusion, *JAMA* 239:2149, 1978.
12. Grant WM, Kern HL: Cations and the cornea, *Am J Ophthalmol* 42:167, 1956.
13. Grant WM: A new treatment for calcific corneal opacities, *Arch Ophthalmol* 48:681, 1952.
14. Grant WM, Kern HL: Action of alkalies on the corneal stroma, *Arch Ophthalmol* 54:931, 1955.
15. Breinin GM: Correction, *Arch Ophthalmol* 53:618, 1955.
16. Breinin GM, DeVoe AG: Chelation of calcium with edathamil calcium-disodium in band keratopathy and corneal calcium affection, *Arch Ophthalmol* 52:846, 1954.
17. Bloomfield SE, David DS, Rubin AL: Acute corneal calcification, *Ann Ophthalmol* 10:355, 1978
18. Johnstone MA, Sullivan WR, Grant WM: Experimental zinc chloride ocular injury and treatment with disodium edetate, *Am J Ophthalmol* 76:137, July 1973.
19. Sugar A, Waltman SR: Corneal toxicity of collagenase inhibitors, *Invest Ophthalmol* 12:779, 1973.
20. Gasset AR, Akaboshi T: Embryopathic effect of ophthalmic EDTA, *Invest Ophthalmol* 16:652, July 1977.
21. Weiss JF, Belkin M: The effect of penicillamine on posttraumatic vitreous proliferation, *Am J Ophthalmol* 92:625, 1981.

CHAPTER 18

# Prescribing Information (Label With the Name of Drug)

Elson L. Craig

Modern medicine continues to produce a number of new therapeutic agents and procedures, which places a significant responsibility on the treating physician to be aware of their pharmacologic characteristics and therapeutic applications. Labeling of medications is an important requirement of manufacturers and distributors and indicates that a drug has been approved for a specific use and has been adequately tested for efficacy and safety. Additional information concerning the drug such as chemical content, method of administration, recommended dosage, and adverse reactions and contraindication to its use may also be part of the label or insert. Lee and Yang[1] point out that the Food, Drug, and Cosmetic Act of 1938 prohibits the marketing of drugs unless they have been adequately tested for safety in the uses indicated on their labels and forbids false and misleading labeling. Requiring that labels accurately reflect the approved use of a drug provides important information to the prescribing physician and a necessary safeguard to the patient. The label further assures the physician that a given drug has gone through the scientific method required to develop a drug and that the drug has then gone through clinical evaluation under the guidelines of the Food and Drug Administration (FDA, phases 1–4) and has been approved for use. This long and costly process for the development of new drugs in ophthalmology has been carefully reviewed by Novack.[2] He reported that the interval and cost involved from chemical synthesis to marketing approval average 12 years and $114 million (1987 dollars). Clearly, such a costly and arduous process further protects the physician and patient from ineffective and unsafe drugs, and, indeed, approximately 99.9% of compounds synthesized do not become marketable products because of inadequate efficacy, unacceptable toxicity, or for other reasons.

Lee and Yang[1] also point out that once a drug had been approved for any use by the FDA, that drug may be prescribed by individual physicians for any indication without violating federal law, such prescribing being considered by the FDA as the "practice of medicine." Physicians must be aware that the nonapproved use of an approved drug or the use of unlabeled drugs may violate applicable standards of care. However, these authors suggested that when a standard of care exists to support such use and consent is obtained, the possibility of liability should be minimal.[1]

For the patient, family, and other physicians and medical personnel involved in the care of the patient, the label on the drug implies a number of certain necessary events have occurred. First and foremost, it should indicate that the physician has gone through the process of thoroughly evaluating the patient's past history and presenting symptoms and signs, has completed a physical examination, has obtained appropriate studies, and has developed a working diagnosis and plan of treatment. Medical history includes a detailed history of prescription and over-the-counter medications the patient is taking and any history of drug reactions or intolerances. This may be particularly difficult to ascertain in elderly patients because they may not have been made aware of the details of their medication usage or may not remember. In ophthalmology most patients are elderly, and approximately 80% of patients greater than age 65 years have at least one chronic disease (46% have heart disease), and 30% of all drugs are prescribed for this group. The average number of drugs being used daily in persons greater than age 65 years is five to 12, and two thirds take at least one or more drugs regularly. Cadieux[3] suggested that because of changes in metabolism, some drugs stay in the body of an elderly person longer; this, added to the increased incidence of chronic disease and multiple drug use, makes the possibility of drug interaction greater.[3] A careful history of medications being taken is therefore essential. Prescribing medications for any patient without the benefit of a history and physical examination is potentially dangerous for the patient and the physician and should be avoided.

The label on the medication should indicate that the prescribing physician has communicated with the patient about the need for the drug, the expected results, and the possible side effects and adverse reactions. Communicating with patients about their medications has become increasingly important in our complex medical system. Most patients are being treated by more than one physician, usually in more than one facility and, as previously discussed, are taking multiple drugs. Patients may remember their pills only by color or their drops by the color of the bottle. Mismedication or overmedication because of lack of patient education about their medications is increasing significantly. According to the National Council on Patient Information and Education, 40% to 50% of patients mishandle their medication, and approximately 10% of hospital admissions are a consequence of this problem. Kulig[4] reported that in one urban hospital, overdoses and other drug-related emergencies were responsible for 38% of visits to the emergency department. The misuse of drugs and the medical complications related to it are known to contribute greatly to the costs of health care in this country. The literature on adverse drug reactions, which has increased rapidly over the past few years, has been reviewed and can be found in the fourth edition of *Textbook of Adverse Drug Reactions* edited by Davis.[5]

Communicating with the patient about his or her medications and educating the patient and family about their appropriate use involves the prescribing physician primarily but often includes other medical personnel as well. Kessler,[6] in his article about communicating with patients about their medication, seems to suggest that the physician and the pharmacist are the most likely people to carry this out and that patient education about their medications is best accomplished by counseling reinforced by written material. Federal law passed as part of the Omnibus Budget Reconciliation Act of 1990, which went into effect January 1, 1993, places considerable emphasis on the role of the pharmacist and requires all pharmacists who fill prescriptions for Medicaid patients to counsel the patient about the use, storage, and dosage of the prescribed drug. Some states (e.g., Ohio) have passed laws that would extend this mandate to cover all persons filling or refilling a prescription and further requires pharmacists to not only counsel the patient but to also maintain detailed patient records and review patient histories for possible abuse or misuse of drugs.

## SUMMARY

Labeling with the name of the drug provides an essential identification marker for the patient, other physicians caring for the patient, the family, and all other involved persons. It is also an identification guide making it easier to determine the pharmacologic characteristics of the drug. The label is an essential means by which the patient can distinguish one drug from another, determine the method and amount of administration, and possibly avoid mismedication and abuse. Labeling the medication has minimal benefit if the prescribing physician does not communicate with the patient or family adequately to reasonably assure adherence to the prescribed therapy. Other medical personnel can and should have input and assist the patient in understanding how to use the medication, but the ultimate responsibility rests with the prescribing physician who directs-label with the name of the drug.

## REFERENCES

1. Lee PP, Yang JC: The nonapproved use of medications, *Ophthalmology* 98:1071, 1991.
2. Novack GD: The development of new drugs for ophthalmology, *Am J Ophthalmol* 114:357, 1992 (perspectives).
3. Cadieux RJ: Drug interaction in the elderly. How multiple drug use increases risk exponentially, *Postgrad Med* 86:179, 1989.
4. Kulig K: Initial management of ingestions of toxic substances, *N Engl J Med* 326:1677, 1992.
5. Davis DM, editor: *Textbook of adverse drug reactions,* ed 4, New York, 1991, Oxford University Press.
6. Kessler DA: Communicating with patients about their medications, *N Engl J Med* 325:1650, 1991.

# Index

## O